TEXTBOOK OF
Pediatric Rheumatology

TEXTBOOK OF
Pediatric Rheumatology

Sixth Edition

James T. Cassidy, MD, FAAP, MACR

Professor Emeritus of Child Health and Internal
  Medicine
University of Missouri School of Medicine
Columbia, Missouri;
Professor Emeritus of Pediatrics and Internal
  Medicine
University of Michigan Medical School
Ann Arbor, Michigan

Ronald M. Laxer, MDCM, FRCPC

Professor of Pediatrics and Medicine
University of Toronto;
Staff Rheumatologist, Division of Rheumatology
Department of Pediatrics
The Hospital for Sick Children
Toronto, Ontario, Canada

Ross E. Petty CM, MD, PhD, FAAP, FRCPC

Professor, Division of Rheumatology
Department of Pediatrics
University of British Columbia
British Columbia Children's Hospital
Vancouver, British Columbia, Canada

Carol B. Lindsley, MD

Professor of Pediatrics
Chief, Pediatric Rheumatology
Department of Pediatrics
University of Kansas Medical Center
Kansas City, Kansas

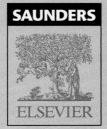

SAUNDERS

ELSEVIER

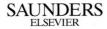

1600 John F. Kennedy Blvd.
Ste 1800
Philadelphia, PA 19103-2899

TEXTBOOK OF PEDIATRIC RHEUMATOLOGY   ISBN: 978-1-4160-6581-4
Copyright © 2011, 2005 by Saunders, an imprint of Elsevier Inc.

Library of Congress Cataloging-in-Publication Data

Textbook of pediatric rheumatology / [edited by] James T. Cassidy ... [et al.]. — 6th ed.
    p. ; cm.
  ISBN 978-1-4160-6581-4
  1. Pediatric rheumatology. 2. Rheumatism in children. I. Cassidy, James T.
  [DNLM: 1. Rheumatic Diseases. 2. Arthritis. 3. Child. 4. Connective Tissue Diseases. 5. Vasculitis.
WE 544 T355 2010]
  RJ482.R48.C37 2010
  618.92'723—dc22
                                                                        2010002720

Acquisitions Editor: Pamela Hetherington
Publishing Services Manager: Deborah Vogel
Team Manager: Radhika Pallamparthy
Project Manager: Joanna Dhanabalan/Bryan Hayward
Design Direction: Ellen Zanolle

Printed in Canada

Last digit is the print number: 9 8 7 6 5 4 3 2 1

To
Nan, Beryl, Edda and Bart

PREFACE

The first edition of the *Textbook of Pediatric Rheumatology* was completed in 1982. Progress in understanding the rheumatic diseases during the intervening decades occupies an important part of this sixth edition, to be published concurrent with the 2010 annual meeting of the American College of Rheumatology. These years have encompassed an enormous increase in our understanding of the pathophysiologic mechanisms operative in the pediatric rheumatic diseases. The recent developments in investigations specific to the younger age groups have afforded opportunities for better diagnosis and treatment. Yet much remains to be accomplished.

The journey from aspirin and gold compounds to targeted biologics, and silver emulsion to digitalized tomography, has been one that the editors have lived through and endured. Antinuclear antibodies and rheumatoid factors to genomic studies of polygenic mechanisms of inflammation have all been part of this landscape. Recent acceleration of developments in scientific studies specific to the younger age group have afforded opportunities for more timely diagnosis and treatment of children with rheumatic disorders. Diagnosis remains, however, primarily the province of observation and examination by an expert clinician.

This edition was reorganized in order to provide comprehensive information regarding the rheumatic diseases of childhood for specialists concerned with their care and for those in primary fields of medicine. Significant advances in practice and knowledge have been incorporated including exhaustive reviews of the major clinical syndromes, now numbering more than 100, and efforts toward validation of their classifications.

The present edition continues the tradition of reassessment of authorship with the enlistment of 29 new contributors, and represents a complete revision of the original text with the addition of 11 new chapters. Chapter divisions, tables and charts are now in color in order to facilitate understanding, and many photographs are in color in their place in the text.

We trust this edition will reflect the clinical science of pediatric rheumatology, its codification as a distinct specialty, and the gratifying maturity that it has achieved.

It is our belief that the advances in this field described herein are increasingly recognized as an integral and essential element of the clinical, investigative, and educational programs of academic institutions of medical training and research. The specialty is essential to the complete education of a pediatrician. Many new members are entering this specialty although serious geographic and institutional deficits in coverage still exist. Much of what is known is central to the developed nations, and insufficient effort so far has been expended on understanding these disorders in other areas of the world.

References have been extensively updated, retaining those regarded as "classics" or having historic importance. In fact, publications in this field are now so extensive that one can only suggest the depth of the investigations. To give due credit to all would require substantial additional text; therefore references in excess of 60 per chapter, not essential to understanding, have been placed on the Elsevier web page at www.expertconsult.com.

In addition to our colleagues, we are deeply indebted to our families and spousal support throughout this process of revision spanning more than three years. We trust that this sixth edition of the *Textbook of Pediatric Rheumatology* will aid physicians caring for these children to interpret the complex web of symptoms, signs, and laboratory abnormalities that are characteristic of these disorders, and their often inherent ambiguity; will inspire students of medicine to recognize the challenges and excitement of this pediatric discipline; and ultimately will ensure the provision of prompt and optimal care to the hundreds of thousands of children and their families around the world who endure the pain and limitations imposed by these disorders. It is not too much to expect that their adaptations to a normal life, and happiness, will be much enlarged in the ensuing years for them and their families.

James T. Cassidy
Ross E. Petty
Ronald M. Laxer
Carol B. Lindsley

CONTRIBUTORS

Salvatore Albani, MD, PhD
Professor and Director of Translational Research
    Inflammatory and Infectious Diseases Center
Sanford-Burnham Medical Research Institute
La Jolla, California

Khaled Alsaeid, MD
Professor of Pediatrics and Rheumatology
Kuwait University and Mubarak Hospital
Jabriya, Kuwait

Balu H. Athreya
Teaching Consultant, AI Dupont Hospital for Children
Wilmington, Delaware;
Professor Emeritus, Department of Pediatrics
University of Pennsylvania School of Medicine
Thomas Jefferson University
Philadelphia, Pennsylvania

Tadej Avčin, MD, PhD
Associate Professor of Pediatrics
Department of Pediatrics
University of Ljubljana, Faculty of Medicine
Head
Department of Allergology, Rheumatology and Clinical
    Immunology
Children's Hospital, University Medical Center
Ljubljana, Slovenia

Paul Babyn, MD, FRCPP
Radiologist-in-Chief
Hospital for Sick Children;
Associate Professor
Department of Medical Imaging
University of Toronto
Toronto, Ontario, Canada

Arvind Bagga, MD, FAMS
Professor
Division of Nephrology, Department of Pediatrics
All India Institute of Medical Sciences
New Delhi, India

Karyl S. Barron, MD
Deputy Director, Division of Intramural Research
National Institute of Allergy and Infectious Diseases
National Institutes of Health
Bethesda, Maryland

Susanne Benseler, MD
Associate Professor of Pediatrics
Research Director, Division of Rheumatology
Associate Scientist, Research Institute
Faculty, Health Policy, Management and Evaluation
University of Toronto
The Hospital for Sick Children
Toronto, Ontario, Canada

Paul Brogan, BsC Hon, MBChBHon, MCRCPCH, MSc, PhD
Senior Lecturer
Honorary Consultant
Department of Pediatric Rheumatology
Great Ormond Street Hospital for Children;
Department of Rheumatology
University College London Institute of Child Health
London, United Kingdom

Hermine I. Brunner, MD, MSc, MBA
Associate Professor of Pediatrics
Division of Rheumatology
Cincinnati Children's Hospital Medical Center;
University of Cincinnati
Cincinnati, Ohio

Prof. Rubén Burgos-Vargas, MD
Senior Investigator
Department of Rheumatology, Hospital General de
    México
Professor of Medicine
Faculty of Medicine, Universidad Nacional Autónoma
    de México
Mexico City, Mexico

Jill P. Buyon, MD
Professor
Associate Director
Division of Rheumatology
New York University School of Medicine;
Vice-Chairman,
Department of Rheumatic Diseases
Hospital for Joint Diseases
New York, New York

David A. Cabral, MBBS
Associate Professor and Head
Division of Rheumatology, Department of Pediatrics
British Columbia Children's Hospital and University of
    British Columbia
Vancouver, British Columbia, Canada

James T. Cassidy, MD
Professor Emeritus of Child Health and Internal
  Medicine
University of Missouri School of Medicine
Columbia, Missouri;
Professor Emeritus of Pediatrics and Internal Medicine
University of Michigan Medical School
Ann Arbor, Michigan

Prof. Rolando Cimaz
A. Meyers Children's Hospital;
University of Florence
Florence Italy

Robert A. Colbert, MD, PhD
Chief, Pediatric Translational Research Branch
National Institute of Arthritis and Musculoskeletal and
  Skin Diseases
National Institutes of Health
Bethesda, Maryland

Iris L. Davidson, BSR
Physical Therapist
Department of Pediatric Rheumatology
Mary Pack Arthritis Program and British Columbia
  Children's Hospital
Vancouver, British Columbia, Canada

Fabrizio De Benedetti, MD, PhD
Ospedale Pediatrico Bambino Gesù
Rome, Italy

Michael J. Dillon, MB, BS, FRCP, FRCPCH, DCH
Emeritus Professor of Paediatric Nephrology
Nephro-Urology Unit
UCL Institute of Child Health;
Great Ormond Street Hospital for Children
London, United Kingdom

Andrea Schwarz Doria, MD, PhD, MSc
Associate Professor
Department of Medical Imaging
University of Toronto;
Radiologist, Scientist
Department of Diagnostic Imaging
Hospital for Sick Children
Toronto, Ontario, Canada

Frank Dressler, MD
Department of Pediatrics
Hannover Medical School
Kinderklinik der Medizinischen Hochschule Hannover
Hannover, Germany

Ciarán M. Duffy, MB, BCh, MSc, FRCPC, FRCPI
Director, Division of Rheumatology and Associate
  Physician in Chief
Montreal Children's Hospital;
Professor and Associate Chair
Department of Pediatrics
McGill University
Montreal, Quebec, Canada

Allison A. Eddy, MD
The Robert O. Hickman Endowed Chair in Pediatric
  Nephrology
Professor of Pediatrics
University of Washington;
Head, Division of Pediatric Nephrology
Director, Tissue and Cell Sciences Center
Seattle Children's Hospital and Research Institute
Seattle, Washington

Fernanda Falcini, MD
Associate Professor
Pediatric Consultant
Department of Biomedicine, Division of Rheumatology
University of Florence
Florence, Italy

Brian M. Feldman MD, MSc, FRCPC
Professor
Pediatrics, Medicine, Health Policy Management
  & Evaluation
The Dalla Lana School of Public Health
University of Toronto;
Senior Scientist and Head
Department of Pediatric Rheumatology
The Hospital for Sick Children
Toronto, Ontario, Canada

Polly J. Ferguson, MD
Director, Pediatric Rheumatology
Department of Pediatrics
Roy J. and Lucille A. Carver College of Medicine
University of Iowa
Iowa City, Iowa

Robert C. Fuhlbrigge, MD, PhD
Associate Professor of Pediatrics and Dermatology
Harvard Medical School;
Attending Rheumatologist
Division of Immunology
Children's Hospital Boston;
Director of Research
Department of Dermatology
Brigham and Women's Hospital;
Boston, Massachusetts

Marco Gattorno, MD
Department of Pediatrics
University of Genoa;
Pediatria II Reumatologia
Istituto G. Gaslini
Genoa, Italy

Edward H. Giannini, MSc, DrPH
Professor, Division of Rheumatology
Cincinnati Childrens Hospital Medical Center;
Department of Pediatrics
University of Cincinnati College of Medicine
Cincinnati, Ohio

David N. Glass, MB, ChB
Professor of Pediatrics
University of Cincinnati;
Associate Director
Cincinnati Children's Research Foundation
Cincinnati Children's Hospital Medical Center
Cincinnati, Ohio

Alexei A. Grom, MD
Associate Professor of Pediatrics
University of Cincinnati, College of Medicine;
Associate Professor of Pediatrics and Attending
   Physician
Division of Rheumatology
Cincinnati Children's Hospital Medical Center
Cincinnati, Ohio

Kristin Houghton, MD, MSc, FRCPC, FAAP, Dip Sports Med
Clinical Assistant Professor
Division of Rheumatology, British Columbia Children's
   Hospital;
Department of Pediatrics, University of British Columbia
Vancouver, British Columbia, Canada

Hans-Iko Huppertz, MD
Professor of Pediatrics
Head and Director
Children's Hospital (Prof.-Hess-Kinderklinik);
Bremen, Germany
Children's Hospital
Georg-August-University
Göttingen, Germany

Norman T. Ilowite, MD
Chief, Division of Rheumatology
Children's Hospital at Montefiore
Professor of Pediatrics
Albert Einstein College of Medicine
Bronx, New York

Daniel L. Kastner, MD, PhD
NIH Distinguished Investigator
Clinical Director and Chief, Laboratory of Clinical
   Investigation, NIAMS
Deputy Director for Intramural Clinical
   Research, National Institutes of Health
Bethesda, Maryland

Gay Kuchta, OT
Occupational Therapist
Department of Pediatric Rheumatology
Mary Pack Arthritis Program and British Columbia
   Children's Hospital
Vancouver, British Columbia, Canada

Wietse Kuis, MD, PhD
Faculty of Medicine
Utrecht University;
Professor
Wilhelmina Children's Hospital;
University Medical Center Utrecht;
Utrecht, The Netherlands

Ronald M. Laxer, MDCM, FRCPC
Professor of Pediatrics and Medicine
University of Toronto;
Staff Rheumatologist, Division of Rheumatology
Department of Pediatrics
The Hospital for Sick Children
Toronto, Ontario, Canada

Claire LeBlanc, MD, FRCPC, Dip Sports Med
Department of Pediatrics
Division of Rheumatology
University of Alberta, Canada
Edmonton, Alberta, Canada

Carol B. Lindsley, MD
Professor of Pediatrics
Chief, Pediatric Rheumatology
University of Kansas Medical Center
Kansas City, Kansas

Alberto Martini, MD
Professor of Pediatrics
University of Genoa;
Head Pediatria II Reumatologia
Istituto G, Gaslini
Genoa, Italy

Peter A. Nigrovic, MD
Assistant Professor of Medicine
Harvard Medical School;
Attending Rheumatologist
Division of Immunology, Program in Rheumatology
Children's Hospital Boston;
Director, Center for Adults with Pediatric Rheumatic
   Illness
Division of Rheumatology, Immunology and Allergy
Brigham and Women's Hospital
Boston, Massachusetts

Kathleen M. O'Neil, MD
Associate Professor of Pediatrics
University of Oklahoma Health Sciences Center;
The Children's Hospital at Oklahoma University
   Medical Center
Oklahoma City, Oklahoma

Kiem G. Oen, MD
Professor
Pediatrics and Child Health
University of Manitoba;
Head, Section of Pediatric Rheumatology
Pediatrics and Child Health
Children's Hospital, Health Sciences Centre
Winnipeg, Manitoba, Canada

Seza Özen, MD
Professor of Pediatrics
Hacettepe University
Ankara, Turkey

Peri Hickman Pepmueller, MD
Associate Professor of Internal Medicine and Pediatrics
Internal Medicine and Pediatrics
Saint Louis University Hospital;
Department of Internal Medicine, Division of
Rheumatology
Cardinal Glennon Children's Medical Center
Division of Rheumatology
Saint Louis University
Saint Louis, Missouri

Berent J. Prakken, MD, PhD
Department of Pediatric Immunology
University Medical Centre Utrecht;
Wilhelmina Children's Hospital
Utrecht, The Netherlands

Michael A. Rapoff, PhD
Department of Pediatrics
Ralph L. Smith Professor of Pediatrics
University of Kansas Medical Center
Kansas City, Kansas

Lisa G. Rider, MD
Deputy Chief
Environmental Autoimmunity Group
Program of Clinical Research
National Institute of Environmental Health Science,
National Institutes of Health
Bethesda, Maryland

Carlos D. Rosé, MD, CIP, FAAP
Professor, Pediatrics
Thomas Jefferson University;
Division Chief, Rheumatology
AI DuPont for Children Hospital
Wilmington, Delaware

James T. Rosenbaum, MD
Edward E. Rosenbaum Professor of Inflammation
Research
Professor of Ophthalmology, Medicine,
and Cell Biology
Chair, Division of Arthritis and Rheumatic Diseases
Oregon Health & Science University
Portland, Oregon

Alan M. Rosenberg, MD
Section of Rheumatology
Department of Pediatrics
University of Saskatchewan
Saskatoon, Saskatchewan, Canada

Rayfel Schneider, MBBCh, FRCPC
Associate Professor
Department of Paediatrics
University of Toronto;
Associate Chair (Education) and Staff, Division
of Rheumatology
Department of Paediatrics
The Hospital for Sick Children
Toronto, Ontario, Canada

David D. Sherry, MD
Director, Clinical Rheumatology
Professor of Pediatrics
Children's Hospital of Philadelphia;
University of Pennsylvania
Philadelphia, Pennsylvania

Earl D. Silverman, MD, FRCPC
Professor of Pediatrics and Immunology
Ho Family Chair on Pediatric Autoimmunity
Hospital for Sick Children
Toronto, Ontario, Canada

Robert P. Sundel, MD
Associate Professor of Pediatrics
Harvard Medical School;
Director of Rheumatology
Department of Medicine, Division of Immunology
Children's Hospital Boston
Boston, Massachusetts

Susan D. Thompson, PhD
Associate Professor
Department of Pediatrics
University of Cincinnati College of Medicine;
Associate Director
Division of Rheumatology
Cincinnati Children's Hospital Medical Center
Cincinnati, Ohio

Lori B. Tucker, MD
Clinical Associate Professor of Pediatrics
University of British Columbia;
Pediatric Rheumatologist
British Columbia's Children's Hospital
Vancouver, British Columbia, Canada

Joris van Montfrans, MD, PhD
Department of Pediatric Immunology
Wilhelmina Children's Hospital;
University Medical Centre Utrecht
Utrecht, The Netherlands

Janitzia Vázquez-Mellado, PhD
Senior Investigator
Department of Rheumatology, Hospital General de México;
Professor of Medicine
Faculty of Medicine, Universidad Nacional Autónoma
de México
Mexico City, Mexico

Deborah Wenkert, MD
Associate Director
Center for Metabolic Bone Disease and Molecular
Research, Shriners Hospital for Children;
Associate Adjunct Clinical Professor of Pediatrics
Assistant Adjunct Clinical Professor of Internal Medicine
Saint Louis University School of Medicine
St. Louis, Missouri

Carine H. Wouters, MD, PhD
Professor of Pediatrics
University of Leuven
Consultant Pediatric Rheumatology
Leuven University Hospital
Leuven, Belgium

Nico Wulffraat
Associate Professor, Pediatric Rheumatology
Department of Pediatric Immunology
Wilhelmina Children's Hospital
University Medical Center Utrecht
Utrecht, The Netherlands

Francesco Zulian, MD
Professor, Chief
Division of Pediatric Rheumatology
Universita di Padova
Padua, Italy

CONTENTS

INTRODUCTION TO THE STUDY OF RHEUMATIC DISEASES IN CHILDREN

James T. Cassidy and Ross E. Petty

Pediatric rheumatology, the study of rheumatic diseases in children, had its origins in the first half of the 20th century, principally as a study of chronic arthritis; however, children with these disorders were occasionally recognized prior to then,[1-7] and archeological evidence supports the existence of chronic arthritis in children as long ago as 900 AD.[8,9]

The eminent British rheumatologist, Dr. Eric Bywaters, in referring to the origins of the specialty, said, "Pediatric rheumatology is one of the latest arrivals and one of the smallest, although I would not say premature. I think I can say I saw it arrive, although I cannot specify its birthday or place and I am damned if I can read the father's signature on the birth certificate."[10] Dr. Bywaters and his colleague Dr. Barbara Ansell, at the Canadian Red Cross Memorial Hospital in Taplow, England, were among the earliest workers in the field (1940s, 1950s). Dr. Elizabeth Stoeber, at Garmisch-Partenkirchen, Germany, also pioneered the field. The second generation of pediatric rheumatologists emerged in the 1950s and 1960s in the United States, Canada, and many countries in Europe, and in 1976 the first pediatric rheumatology meeting, Park City I, set the groundwork for the development of the discipline.[11] Reminiscences of seven of the pioneers of pediatric rheumatology are recommended to the interested reader.[12-18]

Contemporary pediatric rheumatology is rooted in pediatrics, adult rheumatology, immunology, and orthopaedics; however, as experience with rheumatic diseases in children accumulated, it became apparent that many aspects of these disorders demand a uniquely pediatric approach. Many of the diseases or their complications are confined to the childhood and adolescent population but have lasting effects on health and socioeconomic well-being throughout life.

RHEUMATIC DISEASES OF CHILDHOOD: HISTORICAL ASPECTS

Although chronic arthritis has always been the core of pediatric rheumatology, the broader scope of the discipline gradually emerged with the recognition in children of systemic lupus erythematosus (SLE),[19] dermatomyositis,[20-23] vasculitis,[24-26] infection-related disorders, such as Lyme disease,[27] and, most recently, the autoinflammatory disorders.[28,29]

A summary of the history of arthritis in children has been published by Hayem.[30] The first English-language reference to rheumatism in children is the 1545 text by Thomas Phaire, *The Regiment of Life Whereunto Is Added a Treatise of the Pestilence, with The Boke of Chyldren*.[31] In this work, the author refers to the "stifnes or starckenes of the limmes" resulting from exposure of a child to cold, a complaint that may not represent any specific rheumatic disease. In 1864, Cornil described a woman in whom polyarthritis had developed when she was 12 years old.[1] The disease pursued a chronic relapsing course and resulted in her death in a uremic coma at 28 years of age. Necropsy documented myocardial degeneration, nephrotic syndrome, and ankylosis of some joints and synovial proliferation with marked destruction of cartilage in others. This girl may have had amyloidosis complicating chronic polyarticular arthritis. In 1870, Moncorvo[3] described childhood arthritis in one of his own patients in Brazil and in eight children from the literature; in 1873, Bouchut described chronic rheumatism in six children.[2] West's *Lectures on the Diseases of Infancy and Childhood* in 1881 noted that "chronic rheumatic arthritis in children is a rare occurrence."[4]

In 1883 Barlow, a mentor to George Frederic Still at the Hospital for Sick Children, Great Ormond Street,

London, chaired a discussion on rheumatism in childhood at the meeting of the British Medical Association, Section of Diseases of Children.[32] In the report of this meeting, the term *rheumatism* was used to describe poststreptococcal disease, including acute rheumatic fever. Barlow recognized the extent and complexity of these disorders in childhood: "For there are in children many affections of joints, and of structures around joints, which do not suppurate, and yet are not rheumatic; and there is much rheumatism in children which does not affect joints." Disorders known today as toxic synovitis of the hip, acute pyogenic arthritis, syphilitic arthritis, hemophiliac arthropathy, Henoch-Schönlein purpura, poststreptococcal arthritis, and acute rheumatic fever, including carditis, arthritis, nodules, erythema marginatum, and chorea, are all identifiable in this paper. Barlow excluded rickets and scurvy, because he considered that the joint itself was not primarily involved in these conditions.

In 1891, Diamant-Berger published the first detailed account of chronic arthritis in 38 children whom he had seen or whose cases had been documented in the literature.[5] He noted the heterogeneity of onset of the disease and its predominance in girls, the involvement of the cervical spine and temporomandibular joints, and the occurrence of ocular inflammation. He also stated that the prognosis of arthritis in children was generally better than the prognosis of chronic arthritis in adults.

In 1896, Still described 22 cases of acute and chronic arthritis in children, almost all of whom were observed at the Hospital for Sick Children, London.[6] This treatise, written under the mentorship of Barlow,[33] documented the clinical characteristics and the differing modes of onset of disease in these children. Still was the first English physician to confine his practice to diseases of children and the first Professor of Paediatrics at King's College Hospital Medical School, London. After his classic study, he rarely returned to the field of pediatric rheumatology, although his scholarly work was comprised of 108 papers and five books, including the *History of Paediatrics* in 1931 and *Common Diseases in Children* (1909). In the same year, Koplick[7] described the first American child with chronic arthritis.

Although these publications describing arthritis in childhood rank as the most important milestones in the early development of pediatric rheumatology, other rheumatic diseases began to be identified in children in the 19th century. The clinical characteristics of leukocytoclastic vasculitis were described by Schönlein[24] and Henoch[25] in the early to mid-1800s. Juvenile dermatomyositis was first identified by Unverricht[23] and others in 1887, although it was not until the mid-1960s that significant experience with this disease in childhood was reported. SLE has been recognized in children at least since 1904.[34] The original description of scleroderma was in a 17-year-old girl,[35] but the disease was rarely diagnosed in a child until the early 1960s. Ankylosing spondylitis was perhaps first identified in a child;[36] it was certainly known to occur in childhood in the 1950s,[37] but specific studies of the disorder in children did not emerge until the late 1960s.[38,39]

More recent additions to the family of rheumatic diseases in children include Kawasaki disease, which was described in detail in 1967,[26] although its clinical characteristics in infants dying of "polyarteritis nodosa" were described by Munro-Faure in 1959.[40] Other rheumatic diseases, such as chronic infantile neurological, cutaneous, and articular (CINCA) syndrome, and the other autoinflammatory disorders, and neonatal lupus, have more recently been identified. Noninflammatory musculoskeletal pain syndromes are more recent additions to the expanding list of disorders that cause musculoskeletal pain and dysfunction in children and adolescents.

Little further information about these rheumatic diseases was published until the last half of the 20th century. This development coincided with the availability of penicillin and the retreat of acute rheumatic fever in Europe and North America. Until the mid-1940s, this disease was the major rheumatic disease, and it still is in many areas of the developing world. With its control in Europe and North America, attention shifted to the chronic nonstreptococcal rheumatic diseases, principally chronic arthritis. Today the specialty of pediatric rheumatology is concerned with a diverse group of disorders described in this book, most of which are systemic disorders that require great expertise for prompt diagnosis and optimal management. Of all of the specialties, rheumatology, one of the most stimulating and challenging areas in all of medicine, may deal with the broadest spectrum of disease, both organ-specific and systemic. It is sometimes considered a "gray area" of medicine, because there are few useful diagnostic tests, sparse pathognomonic clinical signs, and therapy that often lacks specificity. This specialty requires a diagnostic and therapeutic approach to the "whole" child and family unit, patience, careful observation over long periods, and a heightened ability to tolerate ambiguity and uncertainty. Sometimes only the passage of time makes a diagnosis possible.

THE BURDEN OF DISEASE

It has been difficult to accurately establish the extent of childhood rheumatic disease in defined populations.[41] In many of the most densely populated areas of the world, incidence and prevalence data for such diseases do not exist. In the developed world, inconsistencies of definition and classification, the rarity of occurrence for many of these disorders, and the brevity of follow-up have prevented accumulation of any substantial body of epidemiological data.

Fundamental to estimating the burden of pediatric rheumatic diseases in a society is the question: "How many children and adolescents have each of the identifiable rheumatic diseases?" Three national registries from 1996 provided some comparative insights concerning the relative prevalence of the rheumatic diseases of childhood in the United States,[42] Canada,[43] and the United Kingdom[44] in pediatric rheumatology clinics (Table 1–1). Conspicuously underrepresented are children with acute rheumatic fever, which is the major rheumatic disease of childhood in much of the world. Also, many children with noninflammatory disorders, such as pain amplification syndromes, are cared for in the pediatric rheumatology clinic setting[45] (Table 1–2). Community-based studies

Table 1–1

Relative frequencies of rheumatic diseases in pediatric rheumatology clinics in North America and the United Kingdom

	U.S.A. [51]	CANADA [52]	U.K. [53]
Juvenile rheumatoid arthritis/juvenile chronic arthritis	33.1	50.0	61.7
Mechanical/orthopaedic	34.9	40.6	32.6
Vasculitis	10.2	3.0	1.9
Systemic lupus erythematosus	7.1	3.9	1.3
Juvenile dermatomyositis	5.2	1.6	2.3
Systemic scleroderma	0.9	0.2	0.2
Rheumatic fever/ poststreptococcal arthritis	8.6	0.7	0
Total	100.0	100.0	100.0

Table 1–2

Classification of patients seen in a pediatric rheumatology ambulatory clinic

Category	%
Juvenile idiopathic arthritis	36
Orthopaedic/mechanical	12
Connective tissue diseases	11
Vasculitis	10
Nonrheumatic	8
Unclear diagnosis	8
Uveitis	6
Pain syndromes	5
Autoinflammatory diseases	3
Other	1

Data from Pediatric Rheumatology Clinic, British Columbia's Children's Hospital, Vancouver 2008-2009.

provide insight into disease prevalence that is more representative than those originating from tertiary care centers. A study by Manners and Diepeveen[46] in Western Australia documented that many cases of chronic arthritis in children went undiagnosed and untreated. If this is the case in a developed area of the world with readily available expert medical care, the proportion of such children in geographical areas where medical care is less accessible may be even higher. In Finland, Kunnamo and colleagues[47] surveyed all children under 16 years of age who had swelling or limitation of joint motion, walked with a limp, or had hip pain, as determined by a primary care physician, pediatrician, or orthopaedic surgeon. All of these patients were subsequently examined by a single group of pediatric rheumatologists. Overall, the incidence of arthritis was estimated at 109 per 100,000 children per year. Transient synovitis of the hip accounted for 48%, other acute transient arthritis for 24% (Henoch-Schönlein purpura, serum sickness), chronic arthritis for 17%, septic arthritis for 6%, and reactive arthritis for 5%. Connective tissue diseases such as SLE were not identified in this survey.

Determination of the lifelong burden of a pediatric rheumatic disease requires more precise and comprehensive data than those currently available. The effect of childhood rheumatic diseases on life expectancy, their contribution to morbidity and costs of medical care, and the effect on quality of life are all important outcome parameters for which little information exists, even in North America and Europe; there is no information whatsoever on the global scene. There can be little doubt, however, that a child with, for example, arthritis beginning at 2 or 3 years old, will carry a lifelong burden in one or more of these areas. The expense and inconvenience for other members of the family are also significant.

A number of studies have estimated the cost of caring for a child with juvenile idiopathic arthritis.[48-51] It is likely that children with connective tissue diseases, such as systemic lupus, dermatomyositis, and vasculitis will incur even higher costs to the family and to society as a whole. Although newer therapies such as the biological

response modifiers are expensive, the added cost of the therapy is at least partially offset by the reduced morbidity and improved quality of life.[52]

ADVANCES AND CHALLENGES IN PEDIATRIC RHEUMATOLOGY

Dramatic advances in understanding the nature of inflammation and the possibility of specifically regulating the aberrant immune inflammatory response are revolutionizing the treatment of rheumatic diseases of childhood. Better understanding of the genetics of rheumatic diseases, including polymorphisms of inflammatory mediators, are pointing the way to therapeutic targeting at an even more fundamental level: the gene. Cloning of the human genome opens the way to a myriad of approaches to understanding pathophysiology and developing new therapeutic approaches.

Mortality from diseases, such as chronic arthritis complicated by amyloidosis, dermatomyositis, and SLE, has been dramatically reduced since the 1970s. Disability associated with many rheumatic diseases has been minimized, and the quality of life has been enhanced. Nonetheless, major challenges remain. Although diminished, morbidity and mortality remain serious threats to the child with SLE, vasculitis, scleroderma, or other diseases. Although there have been major improvements in the short- and medium-term outcomes of these and other rheumatic diseases, there remains the challenge of the often disappointing long-term outcome. For example, one half of children with chronic arthritis have active disease 10 years after onset,[52] and children with SLE accumulate visceral damage with the passage of time, which affects the quality of life, in spite of much better control of acute life-threatening events.

The reasons for these improvements in outcomes are multiple; chief among them are the establishment of a body of knowledge and expertise and involvement of a multidisciplinary team of health professionals in diagnosis and care. Improved applications of old techniques and the development of new approaches have been important contributors to an improved prognosis. Therapeutic landmarks of importance to the child with a rheumatic disease must include the introduction of cortisone for treatment of rheumatoid arthritis: its influence on pediatric rheumatology has been profound. Intraarticular corticosteroid therapy has improved management of children with oligoarthritis, and methotrexate has radically improved the course and outcome of children with polyarthritis. More judicious use of glucocorticoids and cytotoxic drugs has minimized toxicity and maximized effectiveness in diseases such as SLE and dermatomyositis. Now the biological agents acting against effector molecules such as TNF-α, IL-1, and IL-6 mark a new dawn in antirheumatic therapy in the present decade. Pharmacogenetics promises the possibility of fine-tuning therapy, both with respect to dose of drug used, and with the selection of a drug which is likely to be most effective and least likely to produce side-effects.

The identification of the cause of Lyme disease, the pathogenesis of neonatal lupus, and the aggressive treatment of Kawasaki disease with intravenous immunoglobulin represent landmarks of progress. Recognition of the autoinflammatory diseases and their genetic basis illuminates a heretofore obscure and confusing group of childhood disorders.

The recognition of the appropriateness of patient and family involvement at all stages of decision-making and care has enabled individualized treatment options and improved compliance. Family support organizations, such as the American Juvenile Arthritis Organization in the United States and similar groups in many other countries, help promote education and research and provide psychosocial support for patients and families.

Increasing communication and collaboration in research worldwide is leading to a better understanding of the childhood rheumatic diseases. It is recognized that for the patient to receive the best available medical care, early recognition and diagnosis are critical. Limited exposure of medical students and trainees in pediatrics to learning clinical examination skills and the fundamentals of pediatric rheumatology must therefore be addressed.[54] The enhanced effectiveness of collaborative research is increasingly recognized through participation in clinical trials led by the Pediatric Rheumatology Collaborative Study Group (PRCSG), the Pediatric Rheumatology International Trials Organization (PRINTO), the Childhood Arthritis and Rheumatology Research Alliance (CAARA), and the Canadian Association of Pediatric Rheumatology Investigators (CAPRI). Such organizations enable the study of therapeutic interventions in chronic arthritis and rarer connective tissue diseases.

REFERENCES

1. M.V. Cornil, Mémoir sur des coincidences pathologiques du rhumatisme articulaire chronique, C.R. Soc. Biol. (Paris) 4 (3) (1864) 3–25.
2. E. Bouchut: Traite pratique des Malades des Enfants, sixth edition, JB Baillière et fils, Paris, 1875.
3. C.A. Moncorvo: Du Rhumatisme Chronique Noueux Des Enfants, O Doin et fils, Paris, 1875.
4. C. West, Lectures on the diseases of infancy and childhood, seventh ed. Blanchard and Lea, Philadelphia, 1881.
5. M.S. Diamant-Berger: Du Rhumatisme Noueux (Polyarthrite Déformante), Chez Les Enfants, Paris, 1891, Lecrosnier et Babe (Reprinted by Editions Louis Parente, Paris, 1988).
6. G.F. Still, On a form of chronic joint disease in children, Med Chir Trans 80 (1897) 47, Reprinted in Am. J. Dis. Child 132(12) (1978) 195–200.
7. H. Koplick, Arthritis deformans in a child seven years old, Arch. Pediatr. 13 (1896) 161.
8. J.F. Buikstra, A. Poznanski, A. Cerna, et al., A case of juvenile rheumatoid arthritis from pre-Columbian Peru, in: J.F. Buikstra (Ed.), A life in science: papers in honor of J Lawrence Angel, Center for American Archeology, Kampsville, Ill, 1990, 99–137.
9. B.A. Lewis, Prehistoric juvenile rheumatoid arthritis in a precontact Louisiana native population reconsidered, Amer. J. Physical Anthropol. 106 (1998) 229–248.
10. E.G. Bywaters, The history of pediatric rheumatology, Arthritis Rheum 20 (Suppl.) (1977) 145–152.
11. Schaller JG, Hanson V (Eds.), Proceedings of the first ARA Conference on the Rheumatic Diseases of Childhood, Arthritis Rheum. 20 (Suppl.) (1977) 145–638.
12. J.S. Stillman, The history of Pediatric Rheumatology in the United States, Rheum. Dis. Clin. North Am. 13 (1987) 143–147.
13. V. Hanson, Pediatric rheumatology: a personal perspective, Rheum. Dis. Clin. North Am. 13 (1987) 155–159.
14. J.E. Levinson, Reflections of a pediatric rheumatologist, Rheum. Dis. Clin. North Am. 13 (1987) 149–154.
15. B.M. Ansell, Taplow reminiscences, J. Rheumatol. 19 (Suppl. 33) (1992) 105–107.
16. E.J. Brewer Jr., The last thirty and the next ten years, J. Rheumatol. 19 (Suppl. 33) (1992) 108.
17. E. Stoeber, Zur Geschichte Der Kinderklinik und Rheumakinderklinik in Garmisch-Partenkirchen 1932-1986, Umschloggestaltung Christa J. Burges, Garmisch-Partenkirchen, 1986.
18. E.J. Brewer Jr., A peripatetic pediatrician's journey into pediatric rheumatology, Parts I – III, Pediatr. Rheumatol. Online. J. 5 (2007) 11. 5:14; 5:17.
19. J.H. Sequeira, H. Balean, Lupus erythematosus: a clinical study of seventy-one cases, Br J Dermatol 14 (1902) 367–379.
20. P. Hepp, Uber einen Fall von acuter parenchymatoser myositis, welche Geschwulste bildete und Fluctuation vortauschte, Klin Wochenschr 24 (1887) 89.
21. H. Jackson, Myositis universalis acuta infectiosa, with a case, Boston Med. Surg. J. 116 (1887) 498.
22. E. Wagner, Ein Fall von acuter Polymyositis, Dtsch. Arch. Klin. Med. 40 (1987) 241.
23. H. Unverricht, Uber eine eigentumliche Fomr von acuter Muskelentzundung mit einem der Trichinose ahnelnden Kranheitsbilde, Munch. Med. Wochenschr 34 (1887) 488.
24. J.L. Schönlein, Allgemeine und specielle Pathologie und Therapie, Literatur-Comptois, Herisau, Germany, 1837.
25. Henoch E Über eine eigenthümliche Form von Purpura, Berliner Klin Wochenschr 11 (1874) 641, Reprinted in Am. J. Dis. Child. 128 (1974) 78-79.
26. T. Kawasaki, Acute febrile mucocutaneous syndrome with lymphoid involvement with specific desquamation of the fingers and toes in children, Arerugi 16 (1967) 178–222.
27. A.C. Steere, S.E. Malawista, D.R. Snydman, et al., Lyme arthritis. An epidemic of oligoarticular arthritis in children and adults in three Connecticut communities, Arthritis Rheum. 20 (1977) 7–17.
28. A.M. Prieur, C. Griscelli, Arthropathy with rash, chronic meningitis, eye lesions, and mental retardation, J. Pediatr. 99 (1981) 79–83.
29. J.P. Drenth, C.J. Haagsma, J.W. van der Meer, Hyperimmunoglobulinemia D and periodic fever syndrome, The clinical spectrum in a series of 50 patients, International Hyper-IgD Study Group, Medicine (Baltimore) 73 (1994) 133–144.
30. F. Hayem, The history of chronic joint diseases in children, Rev. Rhum. Engl. Ed. 66 (1999) 499–504.
31. T. Phaire, The Regiment of Life. Whereunto is Added a Treatise of the Pestilence, with the Boke of Children, Newly Corrected and Enlarged, London, 1545, Edw Whitechurch Reprinted by E&S Livingstone, London, 1955.
32. T. Barlow, 51st Annual Meeting of the British Medical Association. Section of Diseases of Children, Br. Med. J. 2 (1883) 509–519.
33. J.H. Keen, George Frederic Still– registrar, Great Ormond Street Children's Hospital, Br. J. Rheumatol. 37 (1998) 1247.
34. W. Osler, On the visceral manifestations of the erythema group of skin diseases, Am. J. Med. Sci. 127 (1904) 1.

35. Watson R: An account of an extraordinary disease of the skin, and its cure, extracted from the Italian of Carlo Crusio, accompanied by a letter of the Abbe Nollet, FRS to Mr William Watson FRS. Philos. Trans. R. Soc. Lond. 48, 1754 (Cited by Rodnan GP, Benedek TG: A historical account of the study of progressive systemic sclerosis [diffuse scleroderma], Ann. Intern. Med. 57:305-319, 1962).

36. Travers B: Curious case of anchylosis of a great part of the vertebral column probably produced by an ossification of the intervertebral substance, Lancet 5:254, 1814 (Cited by Bywaters EGL, In Moll JMH: Ankylosing spondylitis, Edinburgh, 1980, Churchill Livingstone).

37. F.D. Hart, N.F. Maclagan, Ankylosing spondylitis: a review of 184 cases, Ann. Rheum. Dis. 14 (1955) 77–83.

38. J. Schaller, S. Bitnum, R.J. Wedgwood, Ankylosing spondylitis with childhood onset, J. Pediatr. 74 (1969) 505–516.

39. J.R. Ladd, J.T. Cassidy, W. Martel, Juvenile ankylosing spondylitis, Arthritis Rheum. 14 (1971) 579–590.

40. H. Munro-Faure, Necrotizing arteritis of the coronary vessels in infancy: case report and review of the literature, Pediatrics 23 (1959) 914–926.

41. R.C. Lawrence, C.G. Helmick, F.C. Arnett, et al., Estimates of the prevalence of arthritis and selected musculoskeletal conditions in the United States, Arthritis Rheum. 41 (1998) 778–799.

42. S. Bowyer, P. Boettcher, Pediatric rheumatology clinic populations in the United States: Results of a three year survey, Pediatric Rheumatology Database Research Group, J. Rheumatol. 23 (1996) 1968–1974.

43. P.N. Malleson, M. Fung, A.M. Rosenberg, The incidence of pediatric rheumatic diseases: Results from the Canadian Pediatric Rheumatology Association Disease Registry, J. Rheumatol. 23 (1996) 1981–1987.

44. D.P.M. Symmons, M. Jones, J. Osborne, et al., Pediatric Rheumatology in the United Kingdom: data from the Pediatric Rheumatology Group National Diagnostic Register, J. Rheumatol. 23 (1996) 1975–1980.

45. A.M. Rosenberg, Longitudinal analysis of a pediatric rheumatology clinic population, J. Rheumatol. 32 (2005) 1992–2001.

46. P.J. Manners, D.A. Diepeveen, Prevalence of juvenile chronic arthritis in a population of 12-year old children in urban Australia, Pediatrics 98 (1996) 84–90.

47. I. Kunnamo, P. Kallio, P. Pelkonen, Incidence of arthritis in urban Finnish children. A prospective study, Arthritis Rheum. 29 (1986) 1232–1238.

48. J. Thornton, M. Lunt, D.M. Ashcroft, et al., Costing juvenile idiopathic arthritis: examining patient-based costs during the first year after diagnosis, Rheumatology (Oxford) 47 (2008) 985–990.

49. K. Minden, M. Niewerth, J. Listing, et al., Burden and cost of illness in patients with juvenile idiopathic arthritis, Ann. Rheum. Dis. 63 (2004) 836–842.

50. K. Minden, What are the costs of childhood-onset rheumatic disease? Best Prac. Res. Clin. Rheumatol. 20 (2006) 223–240.

51. S. Bernatsky, C. Duffy, P. Malleson, et al., Economic impact of juvenile idiopathic arthritis, Arthritis. Rheum. 57 (2007) 44–48.

52. J. Haapasarri, H.J. Kautiainen, H.A. Isomäki, M. Hakala, Etanercept does not essentially increase the total costs of the treatment of refractory juvenile idiopathic arthritis, J. Rheumatol. 33 (2004) 2286–2289.

53. K. Oen, P. Malleson, D. Cabral, et al., Disease course and outcome of juvenile rheumatoid arthritis in a multicenter cohort, J. Rheumatol. 299 (2002) 1989–1999.

54. S. Jandial, A. Myers, E. Wise, et al., Doctors likely to encounter children with musculoskeletal complaints have low confidence in their clinical skills, J. Pediatr. 154 (2009) 267–271.

Chapter 2

STRUCTURE AND FUNCTION

Ross E. Petty and James T. Cassidy

Connective tissues provide the supporting structures of the body (bone, periosteum, cartilage); permit the action of muscles through tendons, ligaments, and fasciae; support internal organs (dermis, capsules, serosal membranes, basement membranes); and provide support for blood vessels and the bronchopulmonary tree. Inflammation of the structures of the musculoskeletal system, particularly joints, connective tissues, and muscles, is common to almost all rheumatic diseases; inflammatory processes affecting blood vessels characterize many of the systemic connective tissue disorders and vasculitides. An appreciation of some fundamental aspects of the development, structure, and biology of the connective tissues and the components of the musculoskeletal system is important to the study of pediatric rheumatology. This chapter is intended as a brief overview of selected aspects of the anatomy and biology of tissues important to the basic understanding of rheumatic diseases of childhood and as a stimulus for further study.

BONES

Bones are the structural components of the skeleton. Through articulations and attachments of muscles, tendons, and fascia, they permit movement and provide stability.

Classification of Bones

Bones can be classified as *membranous* or *endochondral*, depending on the manner of their ossification. Bones of the skull, face, and the clavicle are membranous bones, and ossification takes place within mesenchymal tissue condensations. Bones of the remainder of the skeleton ossify within a cartilaginous matrix (endochondral ossification). The cortex of tubular bones is also influenced by membranous (subperiosteal) bone formation.

Structure of Bones

Bones consist of cortical bone, which forms the external surface, and trabecular bone, which lies beneath the cortex. Trabecular bone predominates in the vertebral bodies and the flat bones of the pelvis and skull, whereas tubular bones of the appendicular skeleton have prominent cortical bone, which provides strength.

Long bones of the appendicular skeleton have four parts: the epiphysis that is separated from the metaphysis by the physis, and the diaphysis that joins the two metaphyses and provides length. Apophyses, such as the tibial tuberosity, are like epiphyses in that they are the site of new bone formation, but they do not contribute to bone length; instead, they lay down new bone in response to traction. The microscopic structure of bone is discussed in Chapter 50.

Growth of Bones

Linear growth of bone occurs at the physis or growth plate. Circumferential growth is accounted for by periosteal deposition of new bone, and, to some extent, by the physis through the zone of Ranvier. Hyaline cartilage cells are arranged in columns in the metaphysis subjacent to the physis. Proliferation of these cells results in elongation of the long bone (Fig. 2–1). The relative contributions to growth at the major physes of the limbs are shown in Table 2–1. Growth of the appendicular skeleton ceases at the time of completion of ossification of the iliac apophyses, although height of the vertebral bodies may continue to increase and contribute to overall height until the third decade of life. Skeletal bone age can be determined by radiographic identification of the onset of secondary ossification in the long bones and by physeal closure. In general, ossification centers appear earlier, and physes fuse earlier in girls than in boys.

Factors that influence growth at the physis include thyroxine, growth hormone, and testosterone. Growth hormone and insulin-like growth factor (IGF-1) act together to facilitate the achievement of peak bone mass during puberty. Testosterone stimulates the physis to undergo rapid cell division, with resultant physeal widening during the growth spurt (the anabolic effect). Estrogens suppress the growth rate by increasing calcification of the matrix, a prerequisite to epiphyseal closure. For a discussion of bone mineral metabolism, see Chapter 49.

Vascular Supply

The arterial supply to the diaphysis and metaphysis of a long bone arises from a nutrient artery that penetrates the diaphysis and terminates in the child in end-arteries

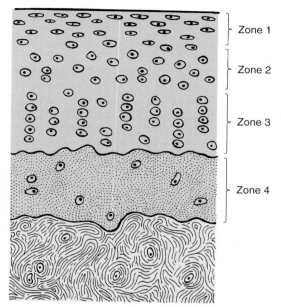

FIGURE 2–1 Organization of articular cartilage. In zone 1, adjacent to the joint space, the chondrocytes are flattened. In zone 2, the chondrocytes are more rounded, and in zone 3 they are arranged in perpendicular columns. The tide mark separates zone 3 from zone 4, which is impregnated with calcium salts. Bone is beneath zone 4. (Courtesy of J.R. Petty.)

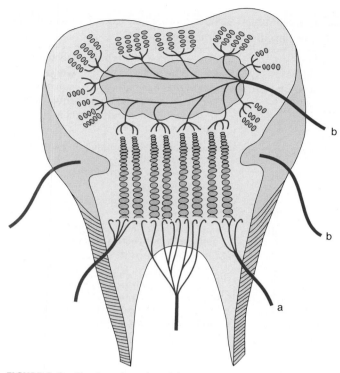

FIGURE 2–2 Blood supply to the epiphysis and metaphysis. End-arteries (a) at the epiphyseal plate arise from the medullary arteries. Juxtaarticular arteries (b) supply epiphysis and synovium. (Courtesy of J.R. Petty.)

Table 2–1			
Relative contributions of individual physes to the length of the bone and limb			
Contribution to Total Growth (%)			
Growth Area		Of Bone	Of Limb
Humerus	Proximal	80	40
	Distal	20	10
Radius/Ulna	Proximal	20	10
	Distal	80	40
Femur	Proximal	30	15
	Distal	70	40
Tibia/Fibula	Proximal	55	27
	Distal	45	18

Data from Ogden JA: *Skeletal injury in the child*, Philadelphia, 1982, Lea & Febiger.

at the epiphyseal plate.[1,2] The epiphyseal blood supply arises from juxtaarticular arteries, which also supply the synovium via a complex network of arterial and arteriovenous anastomoses and capillary beds, which William Harvey called the *circulus articularis vasculosus*. (Fig. 2–2) Not until growth has ceased, and the epiphyseal plate has ossified, does arterial communication begin between the metaphyseal and epiphyseal-synovial circulations, an important phenomenon that explains the predisposition of the immature diaphysis to infection and aseptic necrosis after trauma.

JOINTS

Classification of Joints

Joints may be classified as *fibrous, cartilaginous,* or *synovial* (Table 2–2). Fibrous joints (synarthroses) are those in which little or no motion occurs, and the bones are separated by fibrous connective tissue. Cartilaginous joints (amphiarthroses) are those in which little or no motion occurs, but the bones are separated by cartilage. Diarthrodial joints are those in which considerable motion occurs, and a joint space lined with a synovial membrane is present between the bones. The synovial joint is the site of inflammation in most of the chronic arthritides of childhood. Diarthrodial joints may be further classified according to their shape (Table 2–3).

Development of Diarthrodial Joints

Within the mesenchyme of the limb buds, cells destined to become chondrocytes are surrounded by the perichondrium (the source of new chondrocytes). Between the developing bones, the perichondrium is called the "interzone." Subsequently, cavitation occurs in this location, resulting in the formation of a joint "space."[3] Whether this results from enzymatic action or apoptosis is not certain. It is suggested that differential growth rates result in slight negative pressure in the more slowly growing interzone, thereby facilitating separation of the interzone from the underlying cartilage and, together with a high concentration of hyaluronan at the site, the attraction

Table 2–2

Joints classified by structure

Fibrous	Bones separated by fibrous connection
Suture	Bones of the skull
Syndesmosis	Bones united by interosseous ligament
	Sacroiliac interosseous ligament
	Distal tibiofibular and radioulnar interosseous membranes
Cartilaginous	Bones separated by cartilage and allowing minimal movement
Symphysis	Bones separated by cartilaginous disc
	Symphysis pubis
	Sternomanubrial joint
	Intervertebral disk
Synchondrosis	Temporary joints in fetal life; bones separated by hyaline cartilage
	Growth plate (physis)
Synovial	Bones covered by hyaline cartilage are separated by joint "space" lined with synovial membrane producing synovial fluid (SF), surrounded by a joint capsule, and allowing free movement

Table 2–3

Synovial (diarthrodial) joints classified by shape

Plane joints	Intercarpal, intertarsal
Spheroidal	Hip, shoulder
Cotylic	Metacarpophalangeal
Hinge	Interphalangeal
Condylar	Knee, temporomandibular joint
Trochoid or pivot	Radioulnar, atlanto-odontoid
Sellar	Carpometacarpal joint

of water into the newly forming joint space.[4] The most important signals for joint morphogenesis are provided by the cartilage-derived morphogenetic protein 1 (CDMP1) and the bone morphogenetic proteins (BMPs).[5-7] The joint "cavity" is occupied at first by hyaluronic acid–rich joint fluid secreted by fibroblast-like cells lining the synovial membrane. Continued development of the diarthrodial joint depends on fetal movement,[8] which induces formation of cartilage and synovial membrane and without which the "cavity" regresses and becomes filled with fibrous tissue.[9] The synovial lining forms from the interzone subsequent to cavitation, and the development of other structures, such as bursae, intraarticular fat, tendons, muscle, and capsule, quickly ensues. The whole process takes place between the fourth and seventh weeks of gestation, except for the temporomandibular joint[10] and the sacroiliac joint,[11] which develop several weeks later.

Anatomy of Synovial Joints

The bones of the articular surfaces of diarthrodial (synovial) joints are usually covered by hyaline cartilage. The synovial membrane attaches at the cartilage–bone junction so that the entire joint "space" is surrounded by either hyaline cartilage or synovium. The temporomandibular joint is unusual in that the surface of the condyle is covered by fibrocartilage (fibroblasts and type I collagen).[12] In the sacroiliac joint, the sacral side is covered by thicker hyaline cartilage, whereas the iliac side of the joint is covered by fibrocartilage.[13] In some synovial joints, intraarticular fibrocartilaginous structures are present. A disk (or meniscus) separates the temporomandibular joint into two spaces; the knee joint contains two menisci that separate the articular surfaces of the tibia and femur; and the triangular fibrocartilage of the wrist joins the distal radioulnar surfaces. Other intraarticular structures include the anterior and posterior cruciate ligaments of the knee, the interosseous ligaments of the talocalcaneal joint, and the triangular ligament of the femoral head. These structures are actually extrasynovial, although they cross through the joint space.

ARTICULAR CARTILAGE

The hyaline cartilage, which covers subchondral bone, facilitates relatively frictionless motion and absorbs the compressive forces generated by weight-bearing.[14-20] The cartilage is firmly fixed to subchondral bone in adults by collagen fibrils, although there is little collagen at the osteochondral interface in the growing child.[14] Its margins blend with the synovial membrane and the periosteum of the metaphysis of the bone. In children hyaline cartilage is white or slightly blue and is somewhat compressible. It is composed of chondrocytes within an extracellular matrix (ECM) and becomes progressively less cellular throughout the period of growth; the cell volume in adult articular cartilage is less than 2%.[20] The matrix consists of collagen fibers, which contribute to tensile strength, and ground substance composed of water and proteoglycan, which contributes resistance to compression.[21-24]

Cartilage Zones

Articular hyaline cartilage is organized into four zones (Fig. 2–1). Zones 1, 2, and 3 represent a continuum from the most superficial area of zone 1, in which the long axes of the chondrocytes and collagen fibers are parallel to the surface; through zone 2, in which the chondrocytes become rounder and the collagen fibers are oblique; to zone 3, in which the chondrocytes tend to be arranged in columns perpendicular to the surface. The *tidemark*, a line that stains blue with hematoxylin and eosin, separates zone 3 from zone 4 and represents the level at which calcification of the matrix begins. Chondrocytes in each of the cartilage zones differ not only in appearance but also in metabolic activity, gene expression, and response to stimuli.[25] In the child end-capillaries proliferate in zone 4, eventually leading to replacement of this area by bone. This is probably the manner in which the chondrocytes are nourished, although, in the adult, constituent replacement (through the exchange of synovial fluid [SF] with cartilage matrix) may play the predominant role.

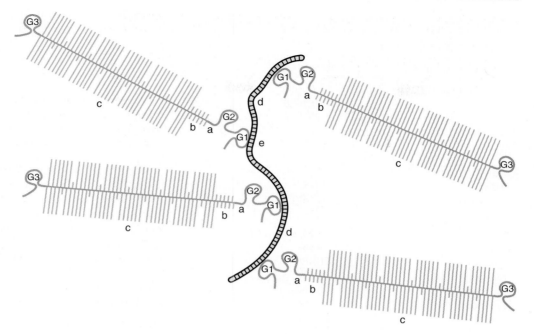

FIGURE 2–3 The structure of the proteoglycan aggregate of cartilage. The proteoglycan monomer consists of a core protein (a) of variable length that contains three globular domains: G1 (located at the aminoterminus and containing the haluronate binding region) G2, and G3. Link protein (e) stabilizes the aggregate by binding simultaneously to the hyaluronate chain (d) and G1. Glycosaminoglycan molecules are attached to the core protein in specific regions: keratan sulfate (b) and chondroitin sulfate (c).

Chondrocytes

Chondrocytes are primarily mesodermal in origin and are the sole cellular constituents of normal cartilage. Their terminal differentiation determines the character of the cartilage (hyaline, fibrous, or elastic). This complex process has been recently reviewed.[26] Chondrocytes in articular cartilage persist and do not ordinarily divide after skeletal maturity is attained.[27] Those in the epiphyseal growth plate differentiate to facilitate endochondral ossification, after which they may undergo apoptosis or become osteoblasts.[27] Chondrocytes are responsible for the synthesis of the two major constituents of the matrix, collagen and proteoglycan, and enzymes that degrade matrix components (collagenase, neutral proteinases, and cathepsins).[27] This dual function places the chondrocyte in the role of regulating cartilage synthesis and degradation. Immediately surrounding the chondrocyte is the pericellular region, which contains type VI collagen and the proteoglycans decorin and aggrecan.[20] Chondrocytes in zone 1 produce superficial zone protein (lubricin), which is important in maintaining relatively frictionless joint motion. Synthesis of this protein is defective in the camptodactyly-arthropathy-coxa vara-pericarditis syndrome.[28]

Extracellular Matrix (ECM)

The ECM of hyaline cartilage consists of collagen fibers, which contribute tensile strength, water, diverse structural and regulatory proteins, and proteoglycans (mainly aggrecan). The ECM is heterogeneous and can be subdivided into three compartments. A thin inner rim of aggrecan-rich matrix surrounds the chondrocytes and lacks cross-linked collagen. An outer rim contains fine collagen fibrils. The remainder of the ECM consists primarily of aggrecan, which binds via the link protein to hyaluronan (Fig. 2–3).[25] The endoskeleton of hyaline cartilage consists of a network of collagen fibrils, 90% of which are type II collagen, with minor components of collagen types IX and X.[20]

Proteoglycans

Proteoglycans are macromolecules consisting of a protein core to which 50 to 100 unbranched *glycosaminoglycans* (chondroitin sulfate [CS] and O-linked keratan sulfate [KS]) are attached.[29-31] At least five different protein cores have been defined. The principal proteoglycan of hyaline cartilage is called aggrecan. Its attachment to hyaluronan is stabilized by link protein to form large proteoglycan aggregates with molecular weights of several million (Fig. 2–3).[20,21,23] With increasing age, the size of the proteoglycan aggregate increases, the protein and KS content increase, and the CS content decreases.[31,32] CS chains also become shorter with increasing age, and the position of the sulfated moiety changes, from a combination of 4-sulfated and 6-sulfated N-acetylgalactosamine at birth to mainly 6-sulfated N-acetylgalactosamine in the adult.[32-34] Dermatan sulfate and chondroitin-4-sulfate are the principal mucopolysaccharides in skin, tendon, and aorta; heparan sulfate is present in basal lamina. The significance to inflammatory joint disease, if any, of these and other age-related changes, is unknown.

Collagens

Collagens, the most abundant structural proteins of connective tissues, are glycoproteins with high proline and hydroxyproline content.[35-37] Many are tough, fibrous proteins that provide structural strength to the tissues of the body.[38] There are at least 29 different collagen α chain trimers grouped into three major classes: fibril forming, fibril-associated collagens with interrupted triple helices (FACIT), and non-fibril forming (Table 2–4).[39-41] Types I, II, and III are among the most common proteins in

Table 2–4

Some Types of collagen

Subclass and Type	Composition	Tissue Distribution
Fibril-Forming Collagens		
Type I	α1(I), α2(I)	Most connective tissues; abundant in bone, skin, and tendons
Type II	α1(II)	Cartilage, intervertebral disk, vitreous humor
Type III	α1(III)	Most connective tissues, particularly skin, lung, and blood vessels
Type V	α1(V), α2(V), α3(V)	Tissues containing type I collagen, quantitatively minor component
Type XI	α1(XI), α2(XI), α3(XI)	Cartilage, intervertebral disk, vitreous humor
Type XXIV	α1(XXIV)	Fetal skeleton
Type XXVII	α1(XXVII)	Fetal skeleton
FACIT collagens		
Type IX	α1(IX), α2(IX), α3(IX)	Cartilage, intervertebral disk, vitreous humor
Type XII	α1(XII)	Tissues containing type I collagen
Type XIV	α1(XIV)	Tissues containing type I collagen
Type XVI	α1(XVI)	Several tissues
Type XIX	α1(XIX)	Rhabdomyosarcoma cells
Type XX	α1(XX)	Corneal epithelium
Type XXI	α1(XXI)	Fetal blood vessel walls
Non-Fibril Forming Collagens		
Type IV	α1(IV), α2(IV), α3(IV), α4(IV), α5(IV), α6(IV)	Basement membranes
Type VIII	α1(VIII), α2(VIII)	Several tissues, especially endothelium
Type X	α1(X)	Hypertrophic cartilage
Type VI	α1(VI), α2(VI), α3(VI)	Most connective tissues
Type VII	α1(VII)	Skin, oral mucosa, cervix, cornea
Type XIII	α1(XIII)	Endomysium, perichondrium, placenta, mucosa of the intestine, meninges
Type XVII	α1(XVII)	Skin, cornea
Type XXIII		Prostate
Type XXV		Neurons
Type XV	α1(XV)	Many tissues, especially skeletal and heart muscle, placenta
Type XVIII	α1(XVIII)	Many tissues, especially kidney, liver, and lung
Type XXVI	"Not a FACIT Collagen"	Testes and ovaries

humans. Type II collagen, the principal constituent that accounts for more than one half the dry weight of cartilage, is a trimer of three identical α-helical chains. Collagen types III, VI, IX through XII, and XIV are all present in minute quantities in the mature cartilage matrix.[33] The content of types IX and XI collagen is greater in young animals (20%) than in mature animals (3%).[35]

Collagen synthesis is minimal in the mature animal. The degree of stable crosslinking of collagen fibers increases with advancing age up to the fourth decade of life.[42] This results in increased resistance to pepsin degradation and may contribute to the increased rigidity and decreased tensile strength of old cartilage.[43]

Collagen undergoes extensive changes in primary and tertiary structure after it is secreted from the fibroblast into the extracellular space as a triple-helical procollagen.[44] Specific peptidases cleave the amino and carboxyl extension peptides, yielding collagen molecules that form crosslinks and fibrils via lysyl and hydroxylysyl residues in some types. Glycosylation also occurs at this posttranslational stage (Fig. 2-4).

Collagen genes are named for the type of collagen (e.g., COLI) and the fibril (e.g., A1), and they encode the large triple-helical domain common to human collagens. Mutations in the collagen genes account for human diseases, such as Ehlers-Danlos syndrome and osteogenesis imperfecta[41] (see Chapter 50).

Other Connective Tissue Constituents

In addition to collagens, a number of specialized tissues derived from embryonic mesoderm contribute to connective tissue structures other than cartilage. *Elastin* occurs in association with collagen in many tissues, especially in the walls of blood vessels and in certain ligaments.[45] Fibers of elastin lack the tensile strength of collagens but can stretch and then return to their original length. Elastin is produced by fibroblasts and by smooth muscle cells. *Fibronectin* is a dimeric glycoprotein with a molecular weight of 450,000 that acts as an attachment protein in the ECM.[46] It is produced by many different cell types, including macrophages, dedifferentiated chondrocytes, and fibroblasts, and has the ability to bind to collagens,

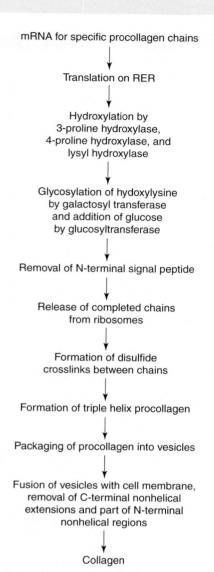

mRNA for specific procollagen chains

↓

Translation on RER

↓

Hydroxylation by
3-proline hydroxylase,
4-proline hydroxylase, and
lysyl hydroxylase

↓

Glycosylation of hydroxylysine
by galactosyl transferase
and addition of glucose
by glucosyltransferase

↓

Removal of N-terminal signal peptide

↓

Release of completed chains
from ribosomes

↓

Formation of disulfide
crosslinks between chains

↓

Formation of triple helix procollagen

↓

Packaging of procollagen into vesicles

↓

Fusion of vesicles with cell membrane,
removal of C-terminal nonhelical
extensions and part of N-terminal
nonhelical regions

↓

Collagen

FIGURE 2–4 Schematic representation of collagen biosynthesis. Triple-helical procollagen is secreted from the fibroblast. Specific procollagenases produce collagen by cleaving the ends of the molecules. The collagen molecules (except for type IV collagen) then form fibrils that undergo crosslinking to form collagen fibers. (Adapted from Nimni ME: Collagen: structure, function, and metabolism in normal and fibrotic tissues, *Semin Arthritis Rheum* 13:1, 1983.)

Table 2–5		
Proteinases and inhibitors for collagen and cartilage substrates		
Enzyme	**Substrate**	**Inhibitor**
Metalloproteinases		
Collagenase	Various collagens and GAGs	Tissue inhibitor of metalloproteinases (TIMP)
Gelatinase	Denatured collagens	TIMP
Stromelysin	Fibronectin, GAG, elastin, collagens	TIMP
Serine proteinases		
Plasmin	Metalloproteinases	α_2-Antiplasmin
Elastase	Various collagens and GAGs	α_1-Plasminogen inactivator
Cathepsin G	GAGs, type II collagen, elastin, TIMP	α_1-Plasminogen inactivator
Plasminogen activator	Proplasminogen	
Cysteine proteinases		
Cathepsin B	Type II collagen, GAGs, link protein	Cystatins
Cathepsin L	Type I collagen, GAGs, link protein, elastin	Cystatins
Aspartic proteinases		
Cathepsin D	GAGs, type II collagen	α_2-Macroglobulin

GAG: Glycosaminoglycan

proteoglycans, fibrinogen, actin, and to cell surfaces and bacteria. Fibronectin is present in plasma and as an insoluble matrix throughout loose connective tissues, especially between basement membranes and cells. *Laminin* is a major constituent of the basement membrane together with type IV collagen.[47] *Reticulin* may be an embryonic form of type III collagen. It is present as a fine branching network of fibers widespread in the spleen, liver, bone marrow, and lymph nodes.

Proteinases for Collagen and Cartilage

The proteinases (endopeptidases) are proteolytic enzymes active in homeostatic remodeling of the ECM during health and in its degradation during inflammation. These enzymes occur both intracellularly and extracellularly in tissue fluids and plasma and have been classified into four categories based on functional catalytic groups:[48]

the *metalloproteinases* and *serine proteinases*, which are active at neutral to slightly alkaline pH, and the *cysteine* and *aspartic proteinases*, which are most active at acid pH (Table 2–5).

The metalloproteinases, which are activated by calcium and stabilized by zinc ions, consist of at least ten well-characterized enzymes.[49] They are active in the degradation or remodeling of collagens and are known to be synthesized by rheumatoid synovium. Collagenases are inhibited naturally by α_2-macroglobulin and by the *tissue inhibitor of metalloproteinase (TIMP)*. *Stromelysin* is a neutral proteinase synthesized by cultured fibroblasts and synovium. Other members of this family, the *gelatinases*, are secreted by many cells in culture and are active in the remodeling of collagen-containing tissues.

The serine proteinases are a family of endopeptidases that participate in matrix degradation either directly or by activating precursors of the metalloproteinases. They include many of the enzymes of pathways involving coagulation, fibrinolysis, complement activation, and kinin generation: plasmin, plasminogen activator, kallikrein, and elastase. Serine proteinase inhibitors constitute 10% of the plasma proteins. The cysteine proteinases that degrade ECM include cathepsins B and L, which are lysosomal enzymes associated with inflammatory reactions. The aspartic proteinases are primarily lysosomal proteinases active at acid pH. Cathepsin D is the major representative of this family that degrades proteoglycans and is present in the lysosomes of most cells.

SYNOVIUM

Synovial Membrane

The synovial membrane is a vascular connective tissue structure that lines the capsules of all diarthrodial joints and has important intraarticular regulatory functions.[50,51] The synovium consists of specialized fibroblasts,[52] one to three cells in depth, overlying a loose meshwork of type I collagen fibers containing blood vessels, lymphatics, fat pads, unmyelinated nerves, and isolated cells such as mast cells.[53,54] (Fig. 2–5) There is no basement membrane separating the joint space from the subsynovial tissues. The synovial membrane is discontinuous, and within the joint space there are so-called *bare areas* between the edge of the cartilage and the attachment of the synovial membrane to the periosteum of the metaphysis.[55] These bare areas are especially vulnerable to damage (erosion) by inflamed synovium (pannus) in inflammatory joint diseases. Folds, or villi, of synovium provide for unrestricted motion of the joint and for augmented absorptive area.

The synoviocytes are of two predominant types, a subdivision that may reflect different functional states rather than different origins. Synovial A cells are capable of phagocytosis and pinocytosis, have numerous microfilopodia, a prominent Golgi apparatus, and synthesize hyaluronic acid. Synovial B cells are more fibroblast-like, have a prominent rough endoplasmic reticulum, and synthesize fibronectin, laminin, types I and III collagen, enzymes (collagenase, neutral proteinases), and catabolin.

Synovial Fluid (SF)

SF, present in very small quantities in normal synovial joints, has two functions: lubrication and nutrition.[56,57] Normal fluid is clear and pale yellow; SF is a combination of a filtrate of plasma, which enters the joint space from the subsynovial capillaries, and hyaluronic acid, which is secreted by the synoviocytes. Hyaluronic acid provides the high viscosity of SF and, with water, its lubricating properties.[58] Concentrations of small molecules (electrolytes, glucose) are similar to those in plasma, but larger molecules (e.g., complement components) are present in low concentrations relative to plasma unless an inflammatory state alters vasopermeability. Notably absent from SF are elements of the coagulation pathway (fibrinogen, prothrombin, factors V and VII, tissue thromboplastin, and antithrombin).[59] As a result, normal SF is resistant to clotting. There appears to be free exchange of small molecules between SF of the joint space and water bound to collagen and proteoglycan of cartilage. Characteristics of normal SF are listed in Table 2–6.

Synovial Structures

Synovium lines bursae, tendon sheaths, and joints.[14] Bursae facilitate frictionless movement between surfaces, such as subcutaneous tissue and bone, or between two tendons. Bursae located near synovial joints frequently communicate with the joint space. This is particularly evident at the shoulder, where the subscapular bursa or recess communicates with the glenohumeral joint; and around the knee, where the suprapatellar pouch, the posterior femoral recess, and occasionally other bursae communicate with the knee joint. Tendon sheaths lined with synovial cells are prominent around tendons as they pass under the extensor retinaculum at the wrist and at the ankle. Although they are closely associated with joints, tendon sheaths do not communicate with the synovial space.

Table 2–6		
Normal synovial fluid		
Characteristic	Mean or Representative Value*	Reference No.
Volume	0.13–3.5 mL (adult knee)	60
pH	7.3–7.4	64
Relative viscosity	235	60
Cl, HCO$_3$	Slightly higher than serum	60
Na, K, Ca, Mg	Slightly lower than serum	60
Glucose	Serum value ± 10%	61
Total protein	1.7–2.1 g/dL	67
Albumin	1.2 g/dL	68
α1 globulin	0.17 g/dL	
α2 globulin	0.15 g/dL	
β globulin	0.23 g/dL	
γ globulin	0.38 g/dL	
Immunoglobulin G	13% of serum value	65
Immunoglobulin M	5% of serum value	
Immunoglobulin E	22% of serum value	66
α$_2$-Macroglobulin	3% of serum value	65
Transferrin	24% of serum value	
Ceruloplasmin	16% of serum value	
CH$_{50}$	30–50% of plasma value	63
Hyaluronic acid	300 mg/dL	62
Cholesterol	7.1 mg/dL	68
Phospholipid	13.8 mg/dL	68

CONNECTIVE TISSUE STRUCTURES

Tendons

Tendons are specialized connective tissue structures that, via the enthesis, attach muscle to bone.[61] In addition to water, they contain type I collagen and small amounts of elastin and type III collagen, the latter forming the *epitenon* and *endotenon*. The type III collagen fibers are densely packed in a parallel configuration in a proteoglycan matrix containing elongated fibroblasts.

Ligaments and Fasciae

Ligaments and fasciae join bone to bone and, like tendons, are composed of type I collagen. So-called elastic ligaments, such as the ligamenta flava and ligamentum nuchae, predominantly contain elastin.

Entheses

An enthesis is the site of attachment of tendon, ligament, fascia, or capsule to bone. Unlike tendon or ligament, the enthesis is an active metabolic site, particularly in the child. It includes the peritenon, which is continuous with the *periosteum;* collagen fibers of the tendon or ligament, which insert into the bone *(Sharpey's fibers);* the adjoining cartilage; and bone not covered by periosteum.[62] In 1998, a highly informative commentary was published on the strongest tendon in the body, the Achilles tendon, and its enthesis.[63] Entheses have been the subject of a recent extensive review.[64]

SKELETAL MUSCLE

Anatomy

Skeletal muscle makes up approximately 40% of the adult body mass and consists of about 640 separate muscles that support the skeleton and permit movement and locomotion. Skeletal muscle forms during embryogenesis from mesodermal stem cells that differentiate into the various types of muscle, bone, and connective tissue.

A skeletal muscle is surrounded by the connective tissue *epimysium.* Within the muscle *fascicles* are covered by connective tissue *perimysium.* Each fascicle contains many individual muscle fibers, which are the basic structural units of skeletal muscle (Fig. 2–6). Muscle fibers are elongated, multinucleated cells surrounded by connective tissue *endomysium* (reticulin, collagen), which is richly supplied with capillaries. Within each fiber is a large number of *myofibrils,* consisting of highly organized interdigitated *myofilaments* of actin and myosin.[65] Each myofilament has approximately 180 myosin molecules with a molecular weight of 500,000, a long tail, and a double head. The myofilament is composed of the myosin tails; the myosin heads project in a spiral arrangement. Lying parallel to the myosin molecules are *actin filaments* (F-actin) composed of globular subunits of G-actin with a molecular weight of 42,000. Two actin filaments are coiled around each other as a helix, with a second protein, *tropomyosin B,* lying in the groove. A regulatory protein, *troponin,* is located at intervals along this structure. This complex structure is demonstrable by light or electron microscopy as striations. *Creatine kinase* is bound to the myosin filaments at regular intervals.[66]

Muscle Contraction

The functional ability of muscle to produce coordinated movements is governed by the conversion of chemical to mechanical energy by actomyosin.[67,68] Calcium diffusion in the myoplasm and binding to thin-filament regulatory proteins are stimulated by the action potential of the α-motor neuron. Variation in the properties of the types of motor fibers and motor units and recruitment of motor units result in the specific patterns of movement. The

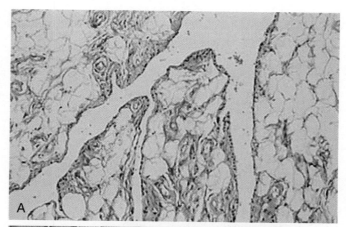
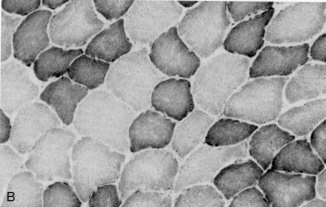

FIGURE 2–5 **A,** Normal synovial membrane histology. **B,** Normal muscle histologsy.

properties of the motor unit are influenced by the genetic makeup of the individual, muscular conditioning, and the presence of any disease that results in joint pain or immobilization, or metabolic, hormonal, or nutritional disturbances.[69,70]

Types of Muscle Fibers

Muscle fibers constitute 85% of muscle tissue. There are two major types of fibers, which differ in structure and biochemistry (Table 2–7).[69-71] Most muscles contain both types. Type I (slow) fibers are narrower, have poorly defined myofibrils, are irregular in size, have thick Z bands, and are rich in mitochondria and oxidative enzymes but poor in phosphorylases. Type II (fast) fibers have fewer mitochondria and are poor in oxidative enzymes but rich in phosphorylases and glycogen. Types I and II muscle fibers can be differentiated histochemically.[72] Muscles differ in the proportions of each fiber type. The diaphragm contains predominantly "slow" fibers, and small muscles contain predominantly "fast" fibers. Muscle conditioning leads to adaptations in the contractile and structural proteins and fiber species within the genetic potential of the individual. Strength training results in hypertrophy of type IIB fibers, and endurance training leads to metabolic alterations in type I and type IIA fibers.[73-76]

Table 2–7

Classification of muscle fiber types

Characteristic	Type I	Type IIA	Type IIB	Type IIC
Size	Moderate	Small	Large	Small
Color	Red	White	White	White
Myoglobin content	High	Medium	Low	High
Mitochondria	Many	Intermediate	Few	Intermediate
Blood supply	+++	+	+	+
ATPase (pH 4.4)	High	Low	Low	–
ATPase (pH 10.6)	Low	High	High	–
Lipid	High	Low	Low	–
Glycogen	Low	High	High	Variable
Metabolic characteristics				
Oxidative (aerobic)	High	Intermediate	Low	High
Glycolytic (anaerobic)	Moderate	High	High	High
Function				
Contraction time	Slow and sustained	Fast twitch	Fast twitch	Moderate twitch
Resistance to fatigue	High	Moderate	Low	Moderate

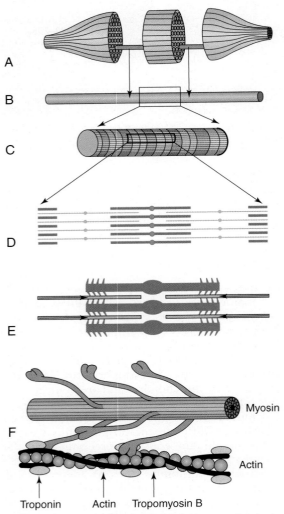

A, Fascicle; B, Fiber; C, Myofibrils; D, Actin and myosin; E and F, Enlargement of actin and myosin filaments.

Myosin

Actin

Troponin   Actin   Tropomyosin B

FIGURE 2–6 Schematic representation of the anatomy of skeletal muscle: **A**, Fascicle; **B**, Fiber; **C**, Myofibrils; **D**, Actin and myosin; **E** and **F**, Enlargement of actin and myosin filaments showing the actin filaments coiled around each other and associated with tropomyosin B lying in the groove. (Courtesy of J.R. Petty.)

REFERENCES

1. M. Liew, W.C. Dick, The anatomy and physiology of blood flow in a diarthrodial joint, Clin. Rheum. Dis. 7 (1981) 131–148.
2. J.C. Edwards, V. Morris, Joint physiology relevant to the rheumatologist? Br. J. Rheumatol. 37 (1998) 121–125.
3. C.W. Archer, G.P. Dowthwaite, P. Francis-West, Development of synovial joints, Birth Defects Res. Part C: Embryo Today 69 (2003) 144–155.
4. A.D. Knight, J.R. Levick, Pressure-volume relationships above and below atmospheric pressure in the synovial cavity of the rabbit knee, J. Physiol. Lond. 328 (1982) 403–420.
5. C.J. Edwards, P.H. Francis-West, Bone morphogenetic proteins in the development and healing of synovial joints, Semin. Arthritis Rheum. 31 (2001) 33–42.
6. A.H. Reddi, Cartilage morphogenetic proteins: role in joint development, homoeostasis, and regeneration, Ann. Rheum. Dis. 62 (Suppl. II) (2003) ii73–ii78.
7. R.J.U. Lories, F.P. Luyten, Bone morphogenetic proteins signalling in joint homeostasis and disease, Cytokine Growth Factor Rev. 16 (2005) 287–298.
8. D.B. Drachman, L. Sokoloff, The role of movement in embryonic joint development, Dev. Biol. 14 (1966) 401.
9. A.A. Pitsillides, Identifying and characterizing the joint cavity-forming cell, Cell Biochem. Funct. 21 (2003) 235–240.
13. V. Bowen, J.D. Cassidy, Macroscopic and microscopic anatomy of the sacroiliac joint from embryonic life until the eighth decade, Spine 6 (1981) 620–628.
17. H.E. Jasin, Structure and function of the articular cartilage surface, Scand. J. Rheumatol. 10 (Suppl.) (1995) 51–55.
18. L.C. Dijkgraaf, L.G. de Bont, G. Boering, et al., Normal cartilage structure, biochemistry, and metabolism: a review of the literature, J. Oral Maxillofac. Surg. 53 (1995) 924–929.
20. A.R. Poole, T. Kohima, T. Yasuda, et al., Composition and structure of articular cartilage, Clin. Orthop. 391S (2001) S26–S33.
21. D. Heinegard, A. Oldberg, Structure and biology of cartilage and bone matrix noncollagenous macromolecules, FASEB J. 3 (1989) 2042–2051.
23. N.P. Cohen, R.J. Foster, V.C. Mow, Composition and dynamics of articular cartilage: structure, function, and maintaining healthy state, J. Orthop. Sports Phys. Ther. 28 (1998) 203–215.
24. V.C. Mow, C.C. Wang, C.T. Hung, The extracellular matrix, interstitial fluid and ions as a mechanical signal transducer in articular cartilage, Osteoarthritis Cartilage 7 (1999) 41–58.
25. S. Chubinskaya, K.E. Kuettner, Regulation of osteogenic proteins by chondrocytes, Int. J. Biochem. Cell Biol. 35 (2003) 1323–1340.

26. L. Shum, G. Nuckolls, The life cycle of chondrocytes in the developing skeleton [review], Arthritis. Res 4 (2002) 94–106.

27. C.W. Archer, P. Francis-West, The chondrocyte, Int. J. Biochem. Cell Biol. 35 (2003) 401–404.

29. A.D. Lander, Proteoglycans: master regulators of molecular encounter? Matrix Biol. 17 (1998) 465–472.

30. P.J. Roughley, The structure and function of cartilage proteoglycans, Eur. Cells Mater. 12 (2006) 92–101.

31. J.T. Gallagher, The extended family of proteoglycans: social residents of the pericellular zone, Curr. Opin. Cell Biol. 1 (1989) 1201–1218.

32. R.V. Iozzo, Matrix proteoglycans: from molecular design to cellular function, Annu. Rev. Biochem. 67 (1998) 609–652.

33. M.T. Bayliss, S.Y. Ali, Age-related changes in the composition and structure of human articular-cartilage proteoglycans, Biochem. J. 176 (1978) 683–693.

34. P.J. Roughley, Age-associated changes in cartilage matrix, Clin. Orthop. 391S (2001) S153–S160.

35. D. Eyre, Articular cartilage and changes in arthritis: collagen of articular cartilage, Arthritis Res. 4 (2002) 30–35.

36. M.E. Nimni, Collagen: structure, function, and metabolism in normal and fibrotic tissues, Semin. Arthritis Rheum. 13 (1983) 1–86.

37. M. van der Rest, R. Garrone, Collagen family of proteins, FASEB J. 5 (1991) 2814–2823.

41. E.M. Carter, C.L. Raggio, Genetic and orthopedic aspects of collagen disorders, Curr. Opin. Pediatr. 21 (2009) 46–54.

43. H. Muir, P. Bullough, A. Maroudas, The distribution of collagen in human articular cartilage with some of its physiological implications, J. Bone Joint Surg. Br. 52 (1970) 554–563.

45. L.B. Sandberg, N.T. Soskel, J.G. Leslie, Elastin structure, biosynthesis, and relation to disease states, N. Engl. J. Med. 304 (1981) 566–579.

46. E. Ruoslahti, E. Engvall, E.G. Hayman, Fibronectin: current concepts of its structure and functions, Coll. Relat. Res. 1 (1981) 95–128.

47. K. Beck, I. Hunter, J. Engel, Structure and function of laminin: anatomy of a multidomain glycoprotein, FASEB J. 4 (1990) 148–160.

48. T.E. Cawston, Proteinases and inhibitors, Br. Med. Bull. 51 (1995) 385–401.

50. J. Edwards, Second international meeting on synovium: cell biology, physiology and pathology, Ann. Rheum. Dis. 54 (1995) 389–391.

51. O. FitzGerald, B. Bresnihan, Synovial membrane cellularity and vascularity, Ann. Rheum. Dis. 54 (1995) 511–515.

52. J.C. Edwards, Synovial intimal fibroblasts, Ann. Rheum. Dis. 54 (1995) 395–397.

54. N.A. Athanasou, Synovial macrophages, Ann. Rheum. Dis. 54 (1995) 392–394.

55. U. Muller-Ladner, R.E. Gay, S. Gay, Molecular biology of cartilage and bone destruction, Curr. Opin. Rheumatol. 10 (1998) 212–219.

56. C.W. McCutchen, Lubrication of joints, in: L. Sokoloff (Ed.), The joints and synovial fluid, Academic Press, New York, 1978.

57. P.A. Simkin, Synovial perfusion and synovial fluid solutes, Ann. Rheum. Dis. 54 (1995) 424–428.

58. J.R. Levick, J.N. McDonald, Fluid movement across synovium in healthy joints: role of synovial fluid macromolecules, Ann. Rheum. Dis. 54 (1995) 417–423.

60. M.W. Ropes, W. Bauer, Synovial fluid changes in joint disease, Harvard University Press, Cambridge, MA, 1953.

61. J.J. Canoso, Bursae, tendons and ligaments, Clin. Rheum. Dis. 7 (1961) 189–221.

62. G.A. Niepel, S. Sit'aj, Enthesopathy, Clin. Rheum. Dis. 5 (1979) 857–872.

63. J.J. Canoso, The premiere enthesis, J. Rheumatol. 25 (1998) 1254–1256.

64. M. Benjamin, T. Kumai, S. Milz, et al., The skeletal attachment of tendons: tendon "entheses," Compar. Biochem. Physiol. A 133 (2002) 931–945.

65. B.A. Gowitzke, M. Milner, Scientific basis of human movement, Williams & Wilkins, Baltimore, 1988.

67. J. Squire, The structural basis of muscular contraction, Plenum Press, New York, 1981.

68. A.M. Kelly, N.A. Rubinstein, Development of neuromuscular specialization, Med. Sci. Sports Exerc. 18 (1986) 292–298.

69. J.A. Faulkner, T.P. White, Adaptations of skeletal muscle to physical activity, in: C. Bouchard, R.J. Shephard, T. Stephens (Eds.), Exercise, Fitness, and Health, Human Kinetics, Champaign, IL, 1990.

70. R.R. Heffner Jr., (Ed.), Muscle pathology, Churchill Livingstone, New York, 1984.

71. F.E. Stockdale, Mechanisms of formation of muscle fiber types, Cell Struct. Funct. 22 (1997) 37–43.

72. R.S. Staron, Human skeletal muscle fiber types: delineation, development, and distribution, Can. J. Appl. Physiol. 22 (1997) 307–327.

74. F.W. Booth, B.S. Tseng, M. Fluck, et al., Molecular and cellular adaptation of muscle in response to physical training, Acta Physiol. Scand. 162 (1998) 343–350.

76. A.W. Taylor, L. Bachman, The effects of endurance training on muscle fibre types and enzyme activities, Can. J. Appl. Physiol. 24 (1999) 41–53.

Chapter 3

IMMUNOLOGY AND RHEUMATIC DISEASES

Marco Gattorno and Alberto Martini

The immune system, which protects against infections, comprises two branches: a more primitive one called *innate* (natural, native) immunity and a highly sophisticated one called *adaptive* (specific) immunity. Innate and adaptive immunity function as an integrated system of host defense, sharing bidirectional interactions fundamental to both the inductive phase and the effector phase of the immune response. The innate immune system constitutes the first line of host defense against infection and therefore plays a crucial role in the early recognition and subsequent triggering of the proinflammatory response to invading pathogens. The adaptive immune system is responsible for elimination of pathogens in the late phase of infection and in the generation of immunological memory.

The cells of the immune system originate from the pluripotent hematopoietic stem cells that give rise to stem cells of more limited potential (lymphoid and myeloid precursors) (Fig. 3–1) (online only). The immune system functions through a complex network of cellular interactions that involve cell surface proteins and soluble mediators, such as cytokines.

INNATE IMMUNITY

The innate immune system is the first line of defense against microorganisms and is conserved in plants and animals. It is phylogenetically ancient compared with the more evolved form of adaptive immunity, which exists only in vertebrates. The principal components of innate immunity are (1) physical and chemical barriers, such as epithelia and antimicrobial substances, produced at epithelial surfaces; (2) circulating effectors proteins, such as the complement components and cytokines; and (3) cells with innate phagocytic activity: neutrophils, macrophages, and natural killer (NK) cells.

Phagocyte surface receptors recognize highly conserved structures characteristic of microbial pathogens that are not present in mammalian cells. The binding of microbial structures to these receptors triggers the cell to engulf the bacterium and induces cytokines, chemokines, and costimulators that recruit and activate antigen-specific lymphocytes and initiate adaptive immune responses. Thus, innate immunity not only represents an early effective defense mechanism against infection but also provides the "warning" of the presence of an infection against which a subsequent adaptive immune response has to be mounted.[1]

Phagocytes

The cells of the phagocyte system originate from a common lineage in the bone marrow, circulate in the blood in inactive form, and are recruited and activated in the peripheral tissues in case of infection, tissue injury, or other proinflammatory stimuli. Monocytes (Mos) are characterized by a granular cytoplasm with many phagocytic vacuoles and lysosomes. Once they enter the tissues, Mos mature into macrophages. Macrophages are present in all tissues, where they act as "sentinels" to recognize and respond to microbes and to amplify the response against a potentially harmful stimulus. Depending on the tissues in which they are found, macrophages are known by a number of different names: Kupffer cells in the liver, microglial cells in the central nervous system, alveolar macrophages in the airways. These cells are the prototypes of the effector cells of innate immunity. Once activated, macrophages initiate a number of crucial events, which include phagocytosis and destruction of ingested microbes, and production of proinflammatory cytokines and other mediators of inflammation that lead to further recruitment of cells of innate immunity (Mos, neutrophils) and provide signals to cells (T and B cells) of adaptive immunity.[2]

Neutrophils (polymorphonuclear leukocytes) are the other major group of phagocytes and are the most abundant type of circulating leukocytes. The cytoplasm is characterized by the presence of two types of granules. The so-called specific granules contain a number of enzymes, such as lysozyme, elastase, and collagenase. The azurophilic granules are lysosomes containing enzymes and microbicidal substances. Neutrophils are the first cells to enter the site of infection and represent the prevalent cell type in the early phases of the inflammatory response. Within one or two days, neutrophils are almost completely replaced by newly recruited Mos-macrophages, which are the dominant effector cells in the later stages of inflammation.[2]

Pattern Recognition Receptors

The innate immune response relies on recognition of evolutionarily conserved structures on pathogens, termed *pathogen-associated molecular patterns (PAMPs)*, through a limited number of germ line–encoded *pattern recognition receptors (PRRs)* present on the surfaces of macrophages, dendritic cells (DCs), and B lymphocytes, where they act as "tissue sentinels" (Table 3–1).[3] PAMPs are invariant among entire classes of pathogens and distinguishable from "self." This characteristic allows a limited number of germ-line encoded PRRs to detect the presence of different microbial infections. Because PAMPs are essential for microbial survival, mutations or deletions are lethal, which greatly reduces the possibility that microbes undergo PAMP mutations in order to escape recognition by the innate system.[6]

Among the PRRs, the family of *Toll-like receptors (TLRs)* has been studied most extensively.[4,5] The TLRs are a large class of PRRs characterized by an extracellular leucine-rich repeat (LRR) domain and an intracellular Toll/IL-1 receptor (TIR) domain (Fig. 3–2). To date, ten TLRs have been identified in humans, and they each recognize distinct PAMPs derived from various microbial pathogens, including viruses, bacteria, fungi, and protozoa (Table 3–2).[3,7]

PAMP-TLR interaction induces receptor oligomerization, which triggers intracellular signal transduction, ultimately resulting in the generation of an antimicrobial proinflammatory response that is also able to involve and orientate the adaptive branch of the immune system (see later discussion).

In addition to transmembrane receptors on the cell surface and in endosomal compartments, there are intracellular (cytosolic) receptors that function in the pattern recognition of bacterial and viral pathogens. These include nucleotide-binding oligomerization domain (NOD)-like receptors (NLRs)[8,9] and the intracellular sensors of viral nucleic acids, such as retinoic-acid-inducible gene I (RIG-I) or melanoma differentiation-associated gene 5, which are grouped under the term RIG-I-like receptors[10] (see Fig. 3–2).

NLRs include at least 23 intracellular proteins with a common protein-domain organization, but with diverse functions[10] (Table 3–3). NLRs are multi-domain proteins composed of a variable N-terminal effector region, consisting of caspase recruitment domain (CARD), pyrin domain, acidic domain, a centrally located NOD (or NACHT (Domain conserved in NAIP, CIITA, HET-E and TP1)) domain that is critical for activation, and C-terminal LRRs that sense PAMPs (see Fig. 3–2). NOD and NALP subfamilies are the best characterized NLRs.

The proteins of the NOD subfamily, NOD1 and NOD2, are both involved in sensing bacterial molecules derived from the synthesis and degradation of peptidoglycan.[11]

The NLRP (Nucleotide-Binding Oligomerization Domain, Leucine Rich Repeat and Pyrin Domain Containing) or NALP subfamily of NLRs has 14 members, some involved in the induction of the inflammatory response mediated by the interleukin (IL)-1 and IL-18.[12] These cytokines are synthesized as inactive precursors that need to be cleaved by the proinflammatory caspases, such as caspases 1, 4, and 5. These caspases are activated in a multisubunit complex called the inflammasome (see later discussion).

Most of the PRRs "sense" not only pathogens but also misfolded/glycated proteins or exposed hydrophobic portions of molecules released at high levels by injured cells, which are known as *damage-associated molecular patterns (DAMPs)*.[13] DAMP molecules, including high mobility group box 1 protein (HMGB-1), heat-shock proteins (HSPs), uric acid, altered matrix proteins, and S100 proteins, represent important danger signals that mediate inflammatory responses through TLRs or NLRP, or other specific receptors for advanced glycation end-products (RAGE), after release from activated or necrotic cells. The terms "alarmins" have also been proposed for DAMP molecules.[13]

Table 3–1

Examples of pathogen-associated molecular patterns (PAMPs) and pattern recognition receptors (PRRs)

Molecular Pattern	Origin	Receptor	Main Effector Function
LPS	Gram-negative bacteria	TLR4, CD14	Macrophage activation
Unmethylated CpG nucleotides	Bacterial DNA	TLR9	Macrophage, B cell, and plasmacytoid cell activation
Terminal mannose residues	Microbial glycoprotein and glycolipids	1. Macrophage mannose receptor	Phagocytosis
		2. Plasma mannose-binding lectin	Complement activation osponization
LPS, dsRNA	Bacteria, viruses	Macrophage scavenger receptor	Phagocytosis
Zymosan	Fungi	TLR2, Dectin-1	Macrophage activation
dsRNA	Viral	TLR3, RIG-I*	IFN type I production
ssRNA	Viral	TLR7/8, MDA5*	IFN type I production
N-formylmethionine residues	Bacteria	Chemokine receptors	Neutrophil and macrophage activation and migration
MDP	Gram-positive and-negative bacteria	NOD2*, NLRP1*	Macrophage activation

dsRNA, double-stranded RNA; IFN, interferon; LPS, lipopolysaccharide; MDP, muramyl dipeptide; ssRNA, single-stranded RNA; TLR, Toll-like receptor.
*Cytoplasmatic

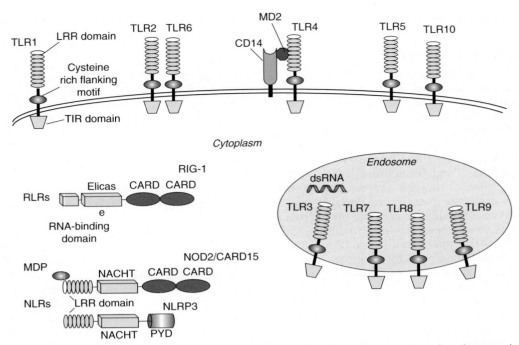

FIGURE 3–2 Localization and structure of cellular pattern recognition receptors. Toll-like receptors (TLRs) are membrane-bound receptors localized at the cellular or endosomal membranes. In addition, there are intracellular (cytosolic) receptors that function in the pattern recognition of bacterial and viral pathogens. Nucleotide-binding oligomerization domain (NOD)2/caspase recruitment domain (CARD)15 and NALP3 belong to the NOD-like receptors (NLRs) family. Most NLRs contain a leucine-rich repeat domain for pathogen-associated molecular patterns recognition, such as muramyl dipeptide for NOD2/CARD15. Retinoic-acid-inducible gene I (RIG-I) represents an example of a class of intracellular sensors of viral nucleic acids grouped under the term of RIG-I-like receptors. Thanks to its C-terminal helicase domain RIG-I bind viral RNA and become activated to transduce CARD-dependent signaling, ultimately resulting in an antiviral response mediated by type I interferon production.

Table 3–2

Toll-like receptors

TLR	Cellular Localization	Ligand(s)	Microbial Source
TLR1	Cell surface	Lipopeptides	Bacteria, mycobacteria
TLR2	Cell surface	Zymosan	Fungi
		Peptidoglycans	Gram-positive bacteria
		Lipoteichoic acids	Gram-positive bacteria
		Lipoarabinomannan	Mycobacteria
		Porins	Naisseria
		Envelope glycoproteins	Viruses (e.g., measles, HSV, CMV)
TLR3	Cell surface/endosomes	dsRNA	Viruses
TLR4	Cell surface	LPS	Gram-negative bacteria
		Lipoprotein	Many pathogens
		HSP60	Chlamydia pneumoniae
		Fusion protein	RSV
TLR5	Cell surface	Flagellin	Bacteria
TLR6	Cell surface	Diacyl lipoptides	Mycoplasma
		Lipoteichoic acid	Gram-positive bacteria
TLR7	Endosome	ssRNA	Viruses
TLR8	Endosome	ssRNA	Viruses
TLR9	Endosome	Unmethylated CpG DNA	Bacteria, protozoa, viruses
TLR10	Cell surface	Unknown	-

Downstream Effects of the Stimulation of PRRs

The activation of cells of innate immunity by different PAMPs and DAMPs leads to the induction of the pro-inflammatory response through the synthesis and secretion of inflammatory mediators, including chemokines, cytokines, vasoactive amines, eicosanoids, and products of proteolytic cascades.

On engagement of TLRs by individual PAMPs, signal transduction is mediated initially by a family of adaptor molecules, which in part determines the specificity of the response.[14] Recruitment of one or several adaptor

Table 3–3

The human NLR family classification

Name*	Other Names	Microbial Motifs Recognized	NLR family
CIITA	NLRA, C2TA		NLRA
NAIP	NLRB1, BIRC1		NLRB
NOD1	NLRC1, CARD4,	GM-tripeptide	NLRC
NOD2	NLRC2, CARD15, BLAU	MDP	
NLRC3	NOD3	Flagellin from Salmonella, Shigella, Listeria, Pseudomonas	
NLRC4	CARD12, IPAF		
NLRC5	NOD27		
NLRP1	NALP1, CARD7	MDP	NLRP
NLRP2	NALP2, PYPAF2	Bacterial RNA, viral RNA, uric acid crystals, LPS, MDP	
NLRP3	NALP3, CIAS1, Cryopyrin, PYPAF3		
NLRP4	NALP4, PYPAF4		
NLRP5	NALP5, PYPAF8		
NLRP6	NALP6, PYPAF5		
NLRP7	NALP7, PYPAF3		
NLRP8	NALP8, NOD16		
NLRP9	NALP9, NOD6		
NLRP10	NALP10, NOD8		
NLRP11	NALP11, PYPAF6, NOD17		
NLRP12	NALP12, PYPAF2, Monarch1		
NLRP13	NALP13, NOD14		
NLRP14	NALP14, NOD5		
NLRXI	NOD9		NLRX

*According to the Human Genome Organization Gene Nomenclature Committee (HGNC)
CIITA = MHC Class II Transactivator Gene
NALP = NLR Family, Apoptosis Inhibitory Protein
NOD = Nucleotide Binding and Oligomerization Domain
NLRC = NLR Family, Card Domain containing Nucleotide-Binding Domain and Leucine-rich Repeat

molecules to a given TLR is followed by activation of downstream signal transduction pathways via phosphorylation, ubiquitination, or protein-protein interactions, ultimately culminating in activation of transcription factors that regulate the expression of genes involved in inflammation and antimicrobial host defense[6] (Fig. 3–3). TLR-induced signaling pathways can be broadly classified because of their use of different adaptor molecules, e.g., dependent on or independent of the adaptor MyD88 or TIR domain-containing adaptor inducing interferon (IFN)-γ, and, additionally, their respective activation of individual kinases and transcription factors.[14] The three major signaling pathways responsible for mediating TLR-induced responses are (1) nuclear fact or kB (NF-kB), (2) mitogen-activated protein kinases (MAPKs), and (3) IFN regulatory factors (IRFs).[15] Whereas NF-kB and MAPKs play central roles in induction of a proinflammatory response, IRFs are essential for stimulation of IFN production[6] (see Fig. 3–3).

NF-kB exists in an inactive form in the cytoplasm physically associated with its inhibitory protein called inhibitor of NF-kB (IkB). After an inflammatory stimulus occurs, IkB is phosphorylated and degraded, and it releases NF-kB dimers, which translocate to the nucleus. Phosphorylation of IkB is performed by a kinase complex called IkB kinase. NF-kB binds to promoters or enhancers of target genes in the nucleus, which leads to increased transcription and expression.[7,16]

MAPKs are involved in rapid downstream inflammatory signal transduction, resulting in activation of several nuclear proteins and transcription factors.[17]

Unlike most cytokines, IL-1β (together with IL-18 and IL-33) lacks a secretory signal peptide and is externalized by monocytic cells through a nonclassical pathway, arranged in two steps.[18,19] First, TLR ligands, such as lipopolysaccharide (LPS), induce gene expression and synthesis of the inactive IL 1b precursor (pro-IL-1b). The activation of caspase-1 later catalyzes the cleavage of the IL-1 precursor pro-IL-1b in the 17kd active form.[12,20] A protein complex responsible for this catalytic activity has been termed the *inflammasome*.[21] The inflammasome is composed of the adaptor ASC (apoptosis-associated specklike protein containing a CARD), pro-caspase-1, and an NLR family member (such as NLRP1, NLRP3 or ice protease-activating factor [Ipaf]).[21] Oligomerization of these proteins through CARD/CARD interactions results in activation of caspase-1, which subsequently cleaves the accumulated IL-1 precursor, eventually resulting in secretion of biologically active IL-1.[12]

Several families of inflammasomes have been identified, each recognizing different danger signals or PAMPs through their respective NLRPs.[21]

Both NLRP3 and NLRP1 have been demonstrated to mediate caspase-1 activation in response to bacterial MDP.[22] The binding of microbes to phagocytes through PRRs also initiates the process of phagocytosis of the invading microorganism and its subsequent killing in phagolysosomes. Activation of phagocytes through PRRs also induces effector molecules, such as inducible nitric oxide synthase and other antimicrobial peptides that can directly destroy microbial pathogens, especially polymorphonuclear leukocytes, the major contributors to the immediate innate immune response.

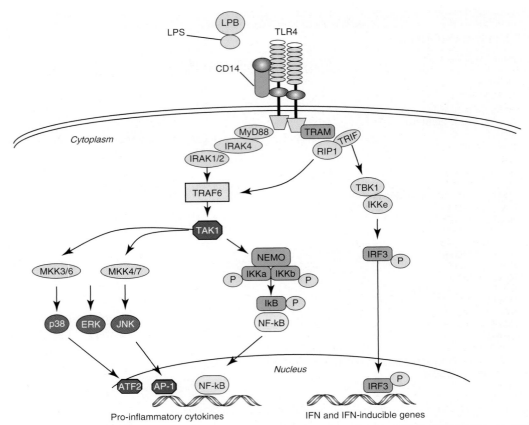

FIGURE 3–3   Toll-like receptors (TRLs) signaling pathways: MyD88-dependent and -independent activation of TLR4. Lipopolysaccharide (LPS) bind to the CD14 molecule present on phagocyte surface. Then the LPS-CD14 complex associates to TLR4 for the subsequent intracellular signaling. The lipopolysaccharide binding protein is a circulating protein that binds to LPS in the blood or extracellular fluid, which forms a complex that facilitates LPS binding to CD14. The MyD88-dependent signaling pathway is responsible for the early-phase NF-κB and mitogen-activated protein kinases (MAPKs) activation, which controls the induction of proinflammatory cytokines (see text). The MyD88-independent pathway ultimately activates interferon (IFN) regulatory factor 3 (IRF3), which is required for the induction of IFN-β and IFN-inducible genes. This latter pathway also mediates the late-phase NF-κB and MAPK activation through the activation of TRAF-6 and TAK1.

Peptides generated from microbial proteins are presented by *dendritic cells (DC)* to T cells to initiate the adaptive immune response. During this process, phagocytosis, upregulation of costimulatory molecules (including CD80, CD86, CD40, and antigen-presenting MHC molecules), switches in chemokine receptor expression, and cytokine secretion are all events regulated through the recognition of pathogens by PRRs expressed on DCs (Fig. 3–4).

This section focuses on the pathways of activation of phagocytes during the early response after pathogen recognition. However, cells of innate immunity also play a crucial role as the effector arm of the later immune response driven by the adaptive immunity. Macrophages can also be activated by TH1-oriented lymphocytes through the production of IFN-γ (see later discussion), and both macrophages and neutrophils are also activated by immune complexes and complement fragments through the binding with immunoglobulin (Ig) and complement receptors expressed on their surface (Fig. 3–5).

Dendritic Cells

DCs are specialized antigen-presenting cells that originate from the bone marrow and play a critical role in the processing and presentation of antigen to T cells during the

adaptive immune response.[23,24] DCs should be considered as a bridge between innate and adaptive immunity.

At their immature stage of development, DCs act as sentinels in the epithelia of the skin (Langerhans cells), gastrointestinal, and respiratory systems, continuously sampling the antigenic environment. These cells are morphologically identified by their extensive membrane projections. Recognition of microbial or viral products through the same PRRs present on the surface of phagocytes initiates the migration of DCs to lymph nodes where they mature (express costimulatory molecules) to present antigen to T cells.[23] Under the control of DCs, T helper (TH) cells acquire the capacity to produce IFN-γ to activate macrophages to resist infection by facultative and obligate intracellular microbes (TH1 cells); or IL-4, -5, and -13 to mobilize white cells that resist helminths (TH2 cells); or IL-17 to mobilize phagocytes at body surfaces to resist extracellular bacilli (TH17 cells). Alternatively, DCs can guide T cells to become suppressive by making IL-10 (T regulatory cells [Tregs]) or by differentiating into FOXP3 positive T-Cells (Tregs).[25] The role of DCs in antigen presentation and in the regulation of the immune response is described in more detail in the discussion of the adaptive immune response.

Plasmacytoid DCs (PDCs), also called plasmacytoid IFN producing cells,[26] are a distinct subtype of DCs that

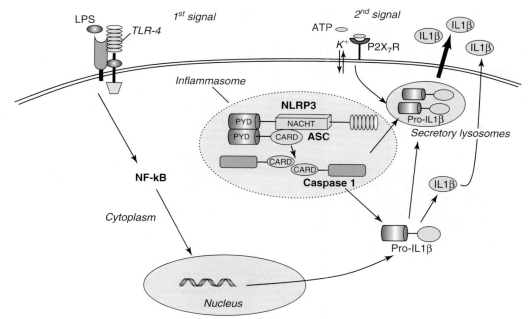

FIGURE 3–4   Role of Cryopyrin NLRP3 in the activation of inflammasome and induction of interleukin (IL)-1β secretion. TLR ligands, such as lipopolysaccharide, are the first signal for gene expression and synthesis of the inactive IL 1β precursor (pro-IL-1β). After stimulation, NLRP3 oligomerizes and becomes available for the binding of the adaptor protein ASC (Apoptosis associated Speck-like protein containing a CARD). This association activates two molecules of Caspase-1 directly, which then converts pro-IL-1β to the mature and active 17 kDa form. A second stimulus, such as exogenous ATP, strongly enhances proteolytic maturation and secretion of IL-1β.

display the unique capacity to secrete large amounts of type I IFN (α/β) in response to viral nucleic acids and self nucleoproteins internalized in the form of immune complexes. The triggering of TLR7 and TLR9 expressed by PDCs, lead to type I IFN production.[27]

Natural Killer Cells

Natural killer (NK) cells are large lymphocytes characterized by the presence of numerous cytoplasmic granules containing many proteins (perforin, granzymes) with proteolytic activities. They lack antigen-specific receptors, such as Ig or T cell receptors, and are able to kill abnormal cells, such as some tumor cells and virus-infected cells[28] without a need for activation by other cell types or soluble molecules (as is the case for CD8+ cytolytic T lymphocytes). Activation of NK cells is regulated through activating and inhibitory cell surface receptors.[29] The inhibitory receptors bind to self class I MHC molecules, which are normally expressed on the surface of the majority of cell types (Fig. 3–6A) [online only]. The ligands for activating receptors are only partially known. The engagement of both inhibitory and activating receptors results in a dominant effect of the inhibitory receptors. The infection of the host cells, especially by some viruses, leads to the loss of class I MHC from their surface and exposes these cells to the exclusive activity of activating receptors (see Fig. 3–6A,B [online only]).[28] Once activated, NK cells release the contents of their granules. Perforin creates pores in target cell membranes, permitting granzymes to enter and inducing the death of target cells by apoptosis. Other important activities of NK cells include their ability to recognize (via Fc receptors) and destroy antibody-coated cells through a process called antibody-dependent cell-mediated cytotoxicity or ADCC, and to

produce high amounts of IFN-γ, a potent stimulator of macrophage activity. In turn, activated macrophages produce IL-12, a potent inducer of NK cell IFN-γ production and cytolytic activity (see Fig. 3–6C,D [online only]).

Fibroblasts

Fibroblasts are specialized in secreting collagenous extracellular matrix (ECM), providing a supporting framework for the ECM, and functioning in repair mechanisms. Tissue fibroblasts play an active role in the effector arm of the inflammatory response. During inflammation, the proinflammatory cytokines produced by tissue macrophages activate mature tissue fibroblasts to produce cytokines, chemokines, prostaglandins (PGs), and proteolytic enzymes (i.e., metalloproteinases) with the final goal to promote tissue rearrangement and subsequent repair. The failure to switch off activated tissue fibroblasts has been proposed as a possible mechanism leading to chronic inflammation, through the persistent overexpression of chemokines and proinflammatory cytokines and consequent continuous recruitment of leukocytes within tissues.[30]

Mature fibroblasts have a lesser capacity of transformation, but immature fibroblasts, also called *mesenchymal* fibroblasts, are capable of differentiating into several different cell lineages. Moreover, fibroblast precursors with a multipotent character also circulate in blood and, due to their similarity with stromal cells of bone marrow, are called *mesenchymal stem cells.*

Mesenchymal stem cells may exert an important role in the modulation of the immune response. The molecular basis related to this phenomenon and the possible clinical implications for the autoimmune disorders has been recently reviewed.[31]

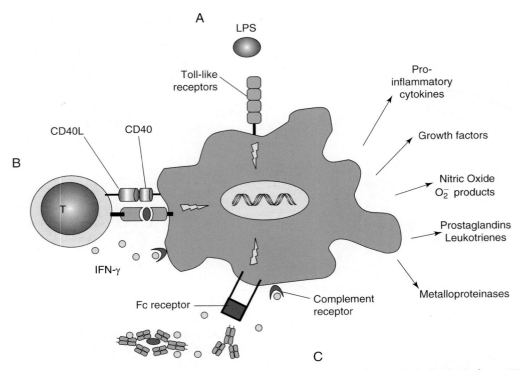

FIGURE 3–5 Different modalities of macrophage activation. **A,** Recognition of conserved molecular constituents of microbes (in the figure: LPS, lipopolysaccharide) by specific receptors (i.e., TLRs, mannose-receptor, scavenger-receptor); **B,** T-cell mediated activation via IFN-γ and CD40-CD40-ligand (L) interaction; **C,** Recognition of antibodies, immune complexes, and complement by the membrane receptors for the Fc fragment of immunoglobulins and complement receptors. The main effector soluble mediators produced after macrophage activation are also shown.

Molecules of Innate Immunity

The Complement System

The complement system consists of several normally inactive plasma proteins that, after activation, generate a number of products that mediate important effector functions, including promotion of phagocytosis and lysis of microbes, and stimulation of inflammation. Activation of complement involves sequential proteolytic steps that generate an enzymatic cascade similar to that of the coagulation system.[32]

There are three major pathways of complement activation (Fig. 3–7). The *alternative pathway* is related to the direct binding of one of the complement proteins, C3b to microbial cells. The *classic pathway* involves a more sophisticated mode of activation, in which a plasma protein C1 binds to the CH2 domains of IgG or to the CH3 domains of IgM that have bound antigen (see later discussion). The same proteins involved in the classic pathway can be activated in the absence of antibodies by a plasma protein called mannose-binding lectin, which binds to mannose residues on microbial glycoproteins and glycolipids (*lectin pathway*). The three pathways of complement activation converge in a central protein C3, which is cleaved into two fragments. The larger fragment C3b becomes covalently attached to microbes, where it acts as opsonin to stimulate phagocytosis and activates C5 with a subsequent generation of C5b, which is the initiator of the formation of a complex of the complement proteins C6, C7, C8 and C9, which are assembled on the membrane of microbes forming the membrane attack complex (MAC).

The MAC forms a pore that causes lysis of the target cell. During complement activation, smaller complement fragments, C3a, C4a, and C5a, are generated and released into the circulation. Also known as anaphylatoxins, they exert several proinflammatory effects, including activation of mast cells and neutrophils and an increase in vascular permeability.[32,33] Another function of complement is to bind to antigen-antibody complexes, promoting their solubilization and their clearance by phagocytes. Complement has a pivotal role in the clearance of apoptotic blebs by the phagocytic system,[34] and the possible implications of this mechanism in the pathogenesis of systemic lupus erythematosus (SLE) have been recently pointed out.[32,35]

The biological activities of complement are mediated by the binding of complement fragments to membrane receptors. Receptors for the fragments of C3 are best characterized in Table 3–4. Type 1 complement receptor, CR1, CD35, is expressed by almost all blood cells and promotes phagocytosis of C3b-coated microbes. CR1 expressed on erythrocytes binds to circulating immune-complexes with attached C3b. In this way, circulating erythrocytes are able to transport immune-complexes to the liver and spleen, where they are removed from erythrocyte surface and cleared. Type 2 complement receptor, CR2, CD21, is present on B lymphocytes and follicular DCs of lymph node germinal centers (GCs). Its main function is to act as coreceptor for B cell activation by antigen (see later discussion) and to stimulate the trapping of antigen-antibody complexes in GCs. Type 3 and type 4 complement receptors are members of the integrin family and are expressed by the cells of innate

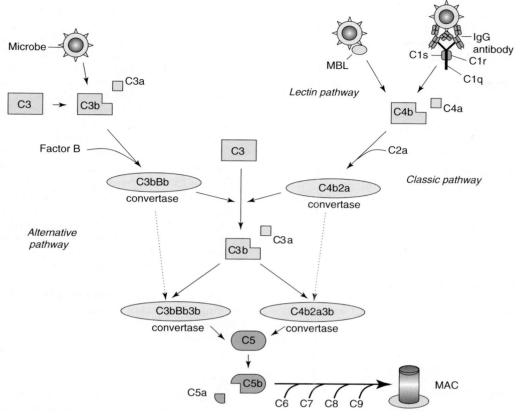

FIGURE 3–7   The complement cascade. The *alternative pathway* is activated by C3b binding to microbial cell wall, after spontaneous cleavage of free circulating C3. Thereafter, C3b binds to factor B forming a C3bBb convertase. The *classic pathway* is initiated by the binding of the trimolecular complex C1 (C1q, C1r, C1s) to antigen-antibody complexes. The same proteins involved in the classic pathway can be activated in absence of antibodies by a plasma protein called mannose-binding lectin (MBL), which binds to mannose residues on microbial glycoproteins and glycolipids (*lectin pathway*). The following binding with the C4b and C2a subunits leads to the formation of the C4b2a convertase. The three pathways of complement activation converge into a central protein, C3, which is cleaved into two fragments. The larger fragment (C3b) activates C5 with subsequent generation of C5b, which is the initiator of the formation of a complex of the complement proteins C6, C7, C8 and C9, which is assembled on the membrane of microbes (membrane attack complex, MAC).

Table 3–4			
Complement receptors			
Receptor	**Cell Types**	**Ligands**	**Function**
CR1 (CD35)	B and T cells Erythrocytes Monocytes, macrophages Eosinophils FDC, neutrophils	C3b, C4b, iC3b	C3b and C4b decay Clearance of immune complexes Phagocytosis
CR2 (CD21)	B cells FDCs Upper airway epithelium	C3d, C3dg, iC3b	Activation of B cell (coreceptor) Antigen presentation in germinal centers Receptor for EBV
CR3 (CD11b/CD18)	Macrophages Neutrophils, NK cells Dendritic cells, FDC	iC3b, ICAM	Phagocytosis Adhesion to endothelium (via ICAM)
CR4 (CD11c/CD18)	Macrophages Neutrophils, NK cells Dendritic cells	iC3b	Phagocytosis

EBV, Epstein-Barr virus; FDC, follicular dendritic cell; ICAM, intracellular adhesion molecule. NK, natural killer;

immunity (neutrophils, NK cells, mononuclear phago-cytes). The binding of CR3 or CR4 promotes the activation of these cells and the phagocytosis of microbes opsonized with C3b.

Genetic deficiencies of classic pathway components, C1q, C1r, C2 and C4, may cause a disease that resembles systemic lupus erythematosus.[36] This may be related to the role of the early complement components in the clearance of apoptotic cells and circulating immune-complexes. Deficiency of C3 is associated with serious pyogenic infections. Defects of the terminal complement components, C5-C9, are associated with an increased risk of disseminated *Neisseria* infections, including *Neisseria meningitides*.

Activation of the complement cascade is regulated by a number of circulating and cell membrane proteins that prevent activation on normal host cells and limit the duration of complement activation on microbial cells and antigen-antibody complexes. The C1 esterase inhibitor, C1 INH, regulates the proteolytic activity of C1, the initiator of the classic pathway of complement activation. Deficiency of this protein causes an autosomal dominant inherited disease called *hereditary angioneurotic edema*, characterized by intermittent acute edema in the skin and mucosae, which causes gastrointestinal symptoms and potentially life-threatening airway obstruction. A number of membrane proteins, membrane cofactor protein (MCP), type 1 complement receptor (CR1), decay-accelerating factor (DAF), and the plasma protein Factor H prevent the activation of C3b if it is deposited on the surfaces of normal mammalian cells. The deficiency of an enzyme required for the linkage of DAF with the cell membrane causes a disease called *paroxysmal nocturnal hemoglobinuria*, characterized by recurrent attacks of intravascular hemolysis due to unregulated complement activation on the surface of erythrocytes. Similarly, the rare deficiency of Factor H is characterized by an excess alternative pathway activation leading to C3 consumption and glomerulonephritis.

Other Circulating Proteins

A number of circulating proteins behave as secreted PRRs (see earlier discussion), which recognize microbial PAMPs and promote innate immunity. *Mannose binding ligand* (MBL) belongs to the collectin family of proteins with a collagen-like domain separated by a neck region from a calcium-dependent (C-type) lectin.[37] MBL is structurally similar to the C1q component of the complement system, binds the C1q receptor present on phagocytes, and may activate complement. Thus, MBL is able to opsonize microbes and induce phagocyte activation via the C1q receptor.

C-reactive protein (CRP) and *serum amyloid protein (SAP)* are plasma proteins belonging to the family of *pentraxins*.[38] They are abundantly produced during the acute phase of inflammation by the liver. They bind to phosphorylcholine present on microbial membranes. Moreover, they are also able to activate the classic complement pathway and to act as opsonins for neutrophils.

The lipopolysaccharide binding protein (LPB) is a circulating protein that binds to LPS in the blood or extracellular fluid forming a complex that facilitates LPS binding to CD14 (see earlier discussion).

Other circulating proteins that participate in innate immunity include *defensins*, which are diverse members of a large family of antimicrobial peptides, contributing to the antimicrobial action of granulocytes, mucosal host defense in the small intestine, and epithelial host defense in the skin and elsewhere.[39,40]

ADAPTIVE IMMUNITY

The main characteristics of adaptive immunity are the capacity to recognize microbes with a high level of molecular specificity and to remember and respond more promptly and vigorously to subsequent exposure to the same microbe (immunological memory). Any substance capable of being recognized by the adaptive immune system is called an antigen. Lymphocytes, the cells responsible for adaptive immunity, consist of various cell subsets that are morphologically similar but different in their functions. They are the only cells capable of recognizing different soluble or membrane-bound antigenic determinants by specific antigen receptors.

The adaptive immune response can be divided into three phases. The *recognition phase* consists of the binding of antigens to specific lymphocyte receptors. The *activation phase* is the sequence of events induced in lymphocytes after specific antigen recognition. Lymphocytes first proliferate and then differentiate into either effector cells, which are aimed at eliminating the antigen, or memory cells, which survive and are ready to respond promptly to antigen reexposure. In the *effector phase*, activated lymphocytes perform their function of eliminating the antigen. Many effector functions require the participation of molecules or cells that belong to the innate immune system. For instance, some antibodies activate complement, whereas T lymphocytes release cytokines that stimulate the function of phagocytes and the inflammatory response. The immune system is able to recognize and eliminate a foreign antigen but does not normally react harmfully to self molecules (*self-tolerance*).

Lymphocytes display common morphological features but differ in their origin, in how they recognize antigens, and in their functions. Immature lymphocytes that have not encountered antigen are called *naïve*. These cells are small lymphocytes of 8 to 10 µL in diameter, with a large nucleus and a small amount of cytoplasm containing mitochondria and ribosomes but no specialized organelles. After antigenic stimulation, naïve lymphocytes enter into the cell cycle, become larger (10 to 12 µL), and have more cytoplasm and organelles (lymphoblasts).

There are two main types of lymphocytes: B lymphocytes, which mature in the bone marrow, and T lymphocytes, which mature in the thymus. B lymphocytes produce antibodies and are responsible for humoral immunity. Their antigen receptors are membrane-bound antibodies that can recognize soluble antigens. Cell activation leads to a sequence of events that culminates in the generation of plasma cells that secrete antibodies. T lymphocytes are responsible for cell-mediated immunity. The T-cell receptor (TCR) recognizes cell surface–associated, but not soluble antigens. The TCR recognizes peptide antigens that are generated inside *antigen-presenting cells (APCs)* and brought to the cell surface in association with specialized molecules of the major histocompatibility complex (MHC). This allows the immune system to detect intracellular pathogens. There are two functionally distinct populations of circulating T lymphocytes: TH lymphocytes and cytotoxic T lymphocytes. TH lymphocytes play the pivotal role in adaptive immunity and activate other cells, such as B lymphocytes, macrophages, and cytotoxic T cells, to perform their effector functions. Cytotoxic T lymphocytes lyse cells that are infected by virus or other intracellular microorganisms. More recently, a distinctive subpopulation of circulating T lymphocytes with a suppressor activity (defined as *naturally occurring Tregs*) has also been characterized (see later discussion).

Some antigen-stimulated B and T lymphocytes differentiate into *memory cells*, which mediate a rapid and enhanced response to a subsequent exposure to the specific antigen. These cells survive in a quiescent state for many years, not requiring antigen recognition for their prolonged survival *in vivo*.

Naïve lymphocytes (so-called because they have not yet encountered antigens) migrate through specialized tissues, called peripheral (or secondary) lymphoid organs, which are able to concentrate antigens that are introduced through the skin or the gastrointestinal and respiratory tracts. In the peripheral lymphoid organs, naïve lymphocytes recognize antigens and are activated; the generated effector and memory lymphocytes circulate in the blood and localize in the peripheral site of antigen entry, where they exert their effector functions.

Different subsets of lymphocytes express different membrane proteins that identify their particular stage of differentiation and function. The membrane proteins are defined by specific monoclonal antibodies and are designed by the abbreviation of CD *(cluster of differentiation)*.

B Lymphocytes

B lymphocytes develop in the bone marrow and are found mainly in secondary lymphoid organs and, in low number, in the circulation. B lymphocytes express cell surface Igs that act as antigen receptors.[41]

B Cell Development and Maturation

B cell development takes place in the bone marrow and spleen and can be subdivided into various stages based on the expression of different cell-surface and intracellular markers and the rearrangement status of the cell's Ig-heavy (IgH) and Ig-light (IgL) chains.

The earliest B-lineage cell type found in the bone marrow is the pro/pre-BI cell. This cell type is characterized by the expression of CD19 and CD117 (c-kit) and the IgH chain loci are in a rearranged D–J configuration. Pro/pre-BI cells are the direct precursors of large pre-B cells, which have lost CD117 expression and have gained the expression of CD25.

At this stage of differentiation, the IgH chain loci are V to D–J rearranged and those that have done this successfully (synthesized an m-heavy [mH] chain) are positively selected within this compartment. Upon down-modulation of surface pre-BCR (B-cell receptor) expression, cells stop proliferating and enter the small pre-B compartment. At this developmental stage, rearrangement of the IgL chain loci takes place. Those cells that have made a productive light chain rearrangement will enter the IgM positive immature B-cell pool.[41,42]

Immature B cells exiting the marrow acquire cell surface IgD, CD21, and CD22. The daily output of new B cells from the bone marrow accounts for about 5% to 10% of total B cells in the peripheral blood. Most of them die in their short-lived immature status. The failure of the most newly formed B cells to survive is due to the competition for the access to the follicles in the peripheral lymphoid tissues. In fact, the follicle provide signals necessary for B-cell survival, particularly BAFF (B cell activating factor belonging to the TNF family) that interacts with its receptor BAFF-R, which is expressed by B cells.[43]

Antigen activation of mature B cells initially leads to GC development, the transient generation of plasmablasts that secrete antibody while still dividing and short-lived extrafollicular plasma cells that secrete antigen-specific germ line–encoded antibodies (Fig. 3–8). GC-derived memory B cells generated during the second week of primary antibody responses express mutated BCRs with enhanced affinities, the product of somatic hypermutation. Memory B cells persist after antigen challenge, rapidly expand during secondary responses, and can terminally differentiate into antibody-secreting plasma cells.[44]

Marginal zone B cells reside in the marginal sinus of the white pulp in the spleen. They express a high level

Table 3–5				
Fc receptors				
Receptor	**Structure**	**Cell Type**	**Ig Binding (Affinity)**	**Function**
FcγRI (CD64)	2 subunits: α chain (72 kDa, CD64) γ chain (9 kDa)	Macrophages Neutrophils Eosinophils Dendritic cells	IgG1, IgG3 (Kd: 10^{-9})	Activation of phagocytes and phagocytosis
FcγRIIA (CD32)	α chain (40 kDa) with a γ–like domain	Macrophages Neutrophils Eosinophils Platelets	IgG1 (Kd: 10^{-7})	Phagocytosis
FcγRIIB (CD32)	α chain (40 kDa) with an ITIM domain	B cells Mast cells	IgG1, IgG3 (Kd: 10^{-7})	Inhibition of activation
FcγRIIIA (CD16)	2 subunits: α chain (50 kDa) γ chain	NK cells	IgG1, IgG3 (Kd: 10^{-6})	Antibody-dependent cell mediated cytotoxicity
FcεRI	3 subunits: α chain (CD64) β chain (33 kDa) γ chain (9 kDa)	Mast cells Basophils Eosinophils	IgE (Kd: 10^{-10})	Cell activation (degranulation)
FcαR (CD89)	2 subunits α chain (55 kDa, CD89) γ chain (9 kDa)	Macrophages Neutrophils Eosinophils	IgA1, IgA2 (Kd: 10^{-7})	Cell activation

of the MHC class I-like molecule CD1 and two receptors for the C3 fragment of complements CR1 and CR2. They have restricted antigen specificities, mainly toward common environmental and self-antigens, and provide a quick response if such an antigen enters in the bloodstream in a T-independent manner (see Fig. 3–8).[45]

The B-1 cells are another subset of circulating B cells (almost 5%) that express the cell-surface protein CD5 (also called CD5+ B cells), high levels of IgM but little IgD, and are found primarily in the peritoneal and pleural cavity fluid (see Fig. 3–8).[46]

The functions of marginal zone B cells and CD5+ B cells are being clarified. Their location suggests a role for B-1 cells in the body cavities and, for marginal zone B cells, in defense against pathogens that penetrate the bloodstream. Their restricted repertoire of receptors seems to give them a function in the recognition of common bacterial antigens, which allows them to contribute in the very early phase of the adaptive immunity response, especially against carbohydrate antigens.[44]

Immunoglobulins

Antibodies, or Igs, are the antigen-specific products of B cells. Igs (1) serve as membrane-bound B cell antigen receptors (see later discussion), (2) are produced and released by antigen-activated B cells, (3) bind their specific antigen, and (4) recruit other molecules or cells to destroy the target to which they have bound. The Ig variable region (Fab) binds to the antigen; the constant region (Fc) binds to a limited number of effector molecules and cells.

The Ig structure is substantially the same for all five main Ig classes or isotypes (IgM, IgD, IgG, IgA, and IgE). Antibodies are Y-shaped molecules composed of two identical heavy (H) chains (each 50 or 70 kD) and two identical light (L) chains (each about 25 kD). In all antibodies, there are only two types of functionally equivalent L chains, which are called lambda (l) and kappa (k) chains. The aminoterminal sequence of both L and H chains (variable, or V, region), which vary greatly among different antibodies, form pairs to generate two identical antigen-binding sites that lie at the ends of the arms of the Y. The carboxyterminal sequences are constant (constant, or C, region) among Ig chains of the same heavy-chain isotype (Fig. 3–9A) (online only). Within the variable regions, there are hypervariable (HV) regions. These HV regions, also called the complementarity-determining regions or CDRs (CDR1, CDR2, CDR3), are localized to a particular part of the surface of the molecule, so that when the VH and the VL regions pair in the antibody molecule, the hypervariable regions are brought together, creating a single hypervariable site that forms the binding site for antigens. Thus, final antigen specificity is particularly determined by the juxtaposition of the CDRs. The molecular region that is recognized specifically by an antibody is called the *antigenic determinant*, or *epitope*.

B Lymphocytes Activation

In addition to the binding of surface Ig (the antigen receptor) to its specific epitope, a second signal is required to activate B cells. The second signal is usually delivered by an already-primed CD4 cell (for thymus-dependent, or TD,

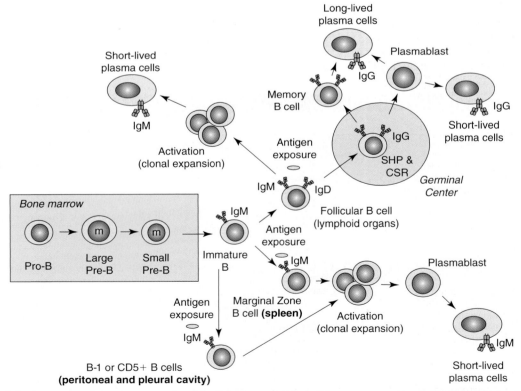

FIGURE 3–8 B cell development. The figure shows an outline of B cell developmental stages in bone marrow and lymphoid organs in humans (see text). CSR, class switch recombination; SHM, somatic hypermutation.

antigens). In other cases the second signal is provided by the pathogen itself (thymus-independent, or TI, antigens).

THYMUS-INDEPENDENT ACTIVATION

The so-called TI antigens[47] are nonprotein antigens that stimulate antibody production in athymic persons. The most important TI antigens are polymeric polysaccharides or glycolipids present in the bacterial cell wall. These antigens induce maximal crosslinking of membrane Igs, leading to activation of B cells without the requirement of T-cell help. Moreover, many polysaccharides activate the alternative pathway of the complement system, generating C3d, which binds to the antigen and provides the second signal to the B cell receptor complex (Fig. 3–10 A).

Three tyrosine kinases (Fyn, Blk, and Lyn) are associated with the receptor complex. The antigen activates the signaling cascade by crosslinking the surface Ig molecules and therefore bringing receptor-associated tyrosine kinases together with the ITAMs (Immunoreceptor Tyrosine-Based Activation Motif) they phosphorylate. When phosphorylated on tyrosine, the ITAMs are recognized by cytoplasmic molecules that activate a cascade of events resulting in cell activation. Surface Ig function is also modulated by a particular coreceptor complex, present on cell membrane, which contains at least three cell surface molecules, known as the CR2-CD19-CD81 complex (see Fig. 3–10A). Coligation of the surface Igs with this coreceptor complex greatly increases the efficiency of cell activation. CR2 is a receptor for the complement protein C3d, generated by the proteolysis of C3, and many microbes activate complement by the alternative pathway in the absence of antibody.[48] Therefore, as for T cell activation, the innate immune response to microbes provides signals that are essential also for B cell activation. In most instances, however, the activation of B cells requires the presence of other additional signals, the most important of which is delivered by TH cells that recognize antigen on the surface of B cells. The antibody response to TI antigens occurs mainly in the marginal zones of lymphoid follicles of the spleen. In these sites, macrophages are particularly efficient at trapping polysaccharides. Antibodies produced in the absence of T cell help are generally of low affinity and consist mainly in IgM because of a lack of T-mediated isotype switching processes.

THYMUS-DEPENDENT ACTIVATION

Antibody responses to protein antigens require antigen-specific T-cell help.[41] Antigen-specific TH cells must therefore be primed earlier during the course of the immune response. B cells internalize the antigen bound to their surface Ig, degrade it, and present peptides on the cell surface in association with MHC class II molecules for recognition by specific TH cells (see Fig. 3–10B).

The functional interaction between T and B cells takes place in peripheral lymphoid organs (lymph nodes, spleen, mucosal immune system). In lymphoid organs, naïve B and T cells are anatomically segregated but are induced to migrate toward one another after activation with antigen. Recognition of the specific peptide–MHC complex on the surface of B cells activates TH cells to express the cell surface molecule CD40L and secrete cytokines. The interaction between CD40L expressed on activated TH cells and CD40 constitutively expressed on B cells lead to further activation of B cells. This mechanism, common also to other interactions between T cells and APC, is particularly important for the activation and differentiation of B cells in a TD response (see Fig. 3–10B).

The interaction with CD40L leads to the oligomerization of CD40 molecules. This induces the association of cytoplasmic proteins (TRAFs [TNF receptor-associated factors]) with the cytoplasmic domains of CD40, initiating the enzymatic cascade that leads to the activation of transcription factors, such as NF-kB and AP-1. These intracellular events also play an important role in the induction of isotype switching. The isotype switching is a DNA recombination process during which the same variable region of the clonally expanded B cell is associated with different constant regions.[49] B cells initially express IgM and IgD; later in the immune response, the same variable region may be associated with other constant portions, giving

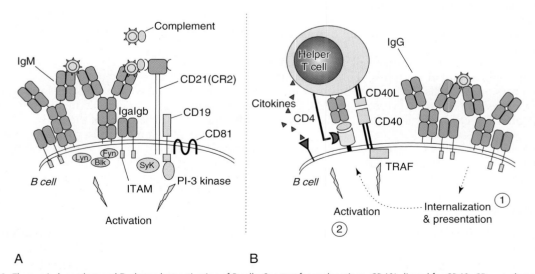

A   B

FIGURE 3–10 **A,** Thymus-independent and **B,** dependent activation of B cells. See text for explanations. CD40L, ligand for CD40; CR, complement receptor; ITAM, immunoreceptor tyrosine activation motif; TRAF, TNF receptor-associated factor.

rise to IgG, IgA, or IgE. The second TH-dependent mechanism of B cell activation and differentiation is related to the production of cytokines by activated T cells. Cytokines play two principal functions in antibody response: they increase the proliferation of B cells and promote the switch of Ig classes. Three different T-derived cytokines (IL-2, IL-4 and IL-5) are known to enhance B cell proliferation; moreover, IL-6 produced by activated T cells and macrophages acts as an important growth factor on already differentiated and antibody-secreting B cells. IL-4 preferentially induces switching to IgE. TGF-β induces switching to IgA, whereas IL-5 augments IgA production by cells that have already undergone switching. Although TH1 cells are poor inducers of antibody production, the release of IFN-γ induces switching to IgG3 subclass, which binds to high-affinity Fcγ receptors and complement.

Effector Functions of Antibody-Mediated Immunity

The first humoral response is characterized by the production of low-affinity IgM. IgM is also produced in the secondary immune response and after somatic hypermutation, but other isotypes dominate the later phases of the response. An important function of antibodies is related to their capacity to neutralize microbes and circulating microbial toxins blocking their binding to the host cellular receptors.

IgG is the principal Ig in the blood and extracellular fluid, whereas IgA is the principal immunoglobulin in mucosal secretions. The different Ig isotypes have distinct properties that enable them to induce different effector mechanisms. Antibodies can activate a variety of effector cells that bear a receptor for their Fc portion. *Fc receptors* make up a family of related molecules with different affinities for different isotypes; the isotype, therefore, determines which effector cell is preferentially activated (Table 3–5)[50]. Only Fc portions of Igs that have interacted with their antigens can activate Fc receptors. This occurs because of aggregation of Ig on the pathogen surface or because of conformational changes in the Fc portion occurring after antigen binding, or because of both.

Antibodies coat (opsonize) the surface of microbes. The recognition of antibodies by Fc receptors on phagocytes triggers phagocytosis and killing of the opsonized microbes by phagocytes (see Fig. 3–5).

Fc receptor may also activate other cell types, such as mast cells, basophils, and eosinophils. Through their action, Fc receptors on NK cells and eosinophils may initiate *antibody dependent cellular cytotoxicity (ADCC)* of antibody-coated infected cells and destroy them (see Fig. 3–6C).

Binding of antibodies to the C1 part of complement is an important modality of activation of the complement cascade (classic pathway) (see Fig. 3–7).

T Lymphocytes

Igs bind antigens in the blood and the extracellular space. However, some bacteria and parasites and all viruses replicate inside cells, where they cannot be recognized by antibodies. These pathogens are destroyed by T cells, which are responsible for cell-mediated immunity and recognize

Table 3–6

Immunological disease continuum

Rare Monogenic Diseases	FMF, Hyper IgD syndrome, TRAPS, CAPS, Blau syndrome, DIRA, PAPA syndrome, NLRP12-mediated periodic fever
Polygenic Autoinflammatory Diseases	Crohn disease, ulcerative colitis Gout and other crystal arthropathies Storage/congenital diseases associated with tissue inflammation Nonantibody associated vasculitis (giant cell and Takayasu arteritis) Idiopathic uveitis Recurrent pericarditis Acne and acneiform-associated diseases Erythema nodosum-associated diseases, including sarcoidosis Recurrent pericarditis Systemic onset juvenile idiopathic arthritis Adult Still's disease Schnitzeler syndrome
*Mixed Pattern Diseases**	Ankylosing spondylitis Reactive/psoriatic arthritis Behçet syndrome HLA-B27 associated uveitis
Classic Polygenic Autoimmune Diseases (Organ-Specific and Nonspecific)	Rheumatoid arthritis Autoimmune uveitis (sympathetic ophthalmia) Coelic disease Primary biliary cirrhosis Autoimmune gastritis/pernicious anemia Autoimmune thyroid disease Addison disease Pemphigus, vitiligo Myasthenia gravis Goodpasture syndrome ANCA associated vasculitis Type 1 diabetes Sjogren syndrome Systemic lupus erythematosus
Rare Monogenic Autoimmune Diseases	ALPS, IPEX, APECED

Adapted by Mc Gonagle and Mc Dermott, ref n. 168
*With evidence of acquired component (MHC class I association and autoinflammatory features)

only antigens displayed on the cell surface, to which they are presented by specialized, highly polymorphic molecules encoded by the genes of the MHC. Moreover, T cells are essential in helping B cells; therefore, both cellular and humoral immune responses to protein antigens depend on antigen recognition by T lymphocytes.[51,52]

Infectious agents may replicate inside the cell either in the cytosol or in the vesicular system (endosomes and lysosomes). Cells infected with viruses or bacteria that live in the cytosol are killed by cytotoxic T cells, which are distinguished by the presence of the cell surface molecule CD8.[53] Pathogens or their products internalized by the cell in the vesicular system are detected by T cells that express the cell surface molecule CD4. CD4 T cells, also called TH cells, do not directly kill the infected cells but activate other types of effector cells. TH cells are comprised of different cell types, the best characterized being TH1 cells, which activate macrophages to kill intravesicular bacteria; TH2 cells, which activate B cells to make antibodies and activate the response against helminths; and TH17 cells, which activate neutrophils and macrophages against extracellular bacteria and fungi.[52]

The antigen receptor of T cells (TCR), is a heterodimer composed of two different transmembrane glycoprotein chains (α and β) bound in a structure that is very similar to the Fab fragment of the Ig molecules (see Fig. 3–9b).[54] The organization of the gene segments encoding the TCR is very similar to that of Igs.[55] Each TCR locus consists of variable (V), joining (J), and constant (C) region genes; the b locus also contains the diversity (D) gene segments. As for Igs, the different gene segments coding for the variable regions of the TCR are present in multiple copies and undergo a process of gene rearrangement that, if successful, leads to the production of a functional TCR. The TCR recognizes the complex formed by the peptide and the presenting HLA molecule. Moreover, T cells recognize and respond to antigens presented by an APC only if that APC expresses MHC molecules that the T cell recognize as self; in other words, they are self-MHC restricted.[56]

Although the vast majority of T cells have the earlier-described a:b TCR, some lymphocytes have another type of TCR consisting of a heterodimer formed by g and d polypeptide chains (g:d TCR).[57] Both are associated with a CD3 complex on the cell membrane. The true function of g:d T cells is still unknown, but it appears that these cells represent a link between innate and adaptive immunity. They account for less than 5% of blood T cells; are present in epithelia of the gut, lungs, and skin; and appear to be able to recognize pathogens as well as stress-associated antigens expressed on cell surfaces. Growing evidence supports the possible relevant role of g:d T cells in the regulation of immune response at the tissue level.[58]

The TCR specifically recognizes the peptide–MHC complex but is independently incapable of activating the T cell. This function is carried out by a complex of proteins, the CD3 complex, which is associated with the TCR on the cell surface. Like the Iga and Igb chains associated with membrane Ig, the cytoplasmic domains of the CD3 proteins contain sequences called ITAM that allow them, after receptor stimulation, to associate with tyrosine kinases and signal to the interior of the cell that antigen binding has occurred (see Fig. 3–10B).[59]

TH cells and cytotoxic T cells are characterized by the presence of the cell surface coreceptor proteins CD4 and CD8, respectively. CD4 binds to invariant parts of MHC class II molecules, and CD8 binds to invariant parts of MHC class I molecules. During antigen recognition, they associate on the cell membrane with components of the TCR, participate in signal transduction, and bring about a 100-fold increase in the sensitivity of the T cell to the antigen presented by MHC molecules (see Fig. 3–10B).[60]

MHC class I and class II molecules have different functions and are differently expressed on cells. MHC class I molecules present peptides to cytotoxic T cells. Unlike antibodies that can recognize both conformational and continuous epitopes on a protein surface, T cells respond only to continuous short amino acid sequences that bind to the cleft of the outer surface of the MHC molecule. Because the composition of the MHC peptide-binding cleft is highly polymorphic, different allelic variants of MHC molecules bind preferentially to different peptides of suitable length that share common anchor residues. MHC molecules bind peptides as an integral part of their structure and are unstable in the absence of peptides. This phenomenon prevents peptide exchange at cell surfaces that would impair the efficiency of intracellular antigen recognition.[61]

T Cell Development and Selection

T cells originate in the bone marrow and migrate at a very early stage to the thymus, where they undergo TCR gene rearrangement. In the thymus, thymocytes proliferate and mature into T cells through a series of events characterized by rearrangement of the TCR genes and expression on the cell membrane of the TCR, coreceptors CD4 and CD8, and other surface molecules that reflect the functional maturation of the cell.[62]

Thymocytes enter the thymic cortex and, during maturation, migrate from the cortex toward the medulla, encountering epithelial cells, macrophages, and DCs. Thus, the medulla contains mostly mature T cells, and only mature CD4-positive or CD8-positive T cells exit the thymus and enter the blood.

A fundamental step in thymocyte maturation (after expression of the TCR, CD4, and CD8 molecules) is the selection of cells that will make up the repertoire of mature T cells in the periphery. Mature T cells recognize only peptides bound to MHC molecules. As previously discussed, T cells are self-restricted, which means that only those T cells that recognize the body's own MHC molecules will be able to contribute to the adaptive immune response. On the other hand, the random generation of TCR can give rise not only to lymphocytes that do not recognize self-MHC molecules (and are therefore useless) but also to lymphocytes that recognize complexes of self-peptides/self-MHC molecules with high affinity (and are therefore potentially harmful). The dual need of selecting only cells that recognize self-MHC molecules and eliminating autoreactive cells is accomplished through processes of positive and negative selection (Fig. 3–11) that occur once thymocytes have rearranged their α:β TCR genes.[63]

Evidence from fetal thymic organ cultures suggests that these processes, which shape the future immunological repertoire, are driven by the differential avidity for self-peptide/self-MHC complexes.[64] Thymocytes that express a TCR with low but measurable avidity for a self-peptide/self-MHC complex are allowed to differentiate into mature T cells, whereas immature lymphocytes that express TCRs that have no or no strong avidity for self-peptide/self-MHC complexes die by apoptosis. More than 95% of developing thymocytes are thought to die in the thymus by apoptosis because they do not recognize self-MHC molecules or undergo negative selection. Cells that survive this dual selection process leave the thymus as mature naïve T cells.

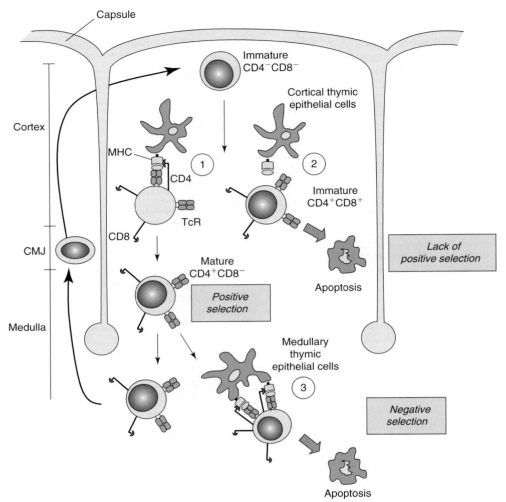

FIGURE 3–11 Processes of thymocyte maturation and selection in the thymus. Precursors of T cells (CD4⁻CD8⁻TcR⁻) coming from the bone marrow arrive into the thymic cortex, where they mature into pre-T thymocytes (bearing a pre-T cell receptor formed by a β chain and a pre-T α chain). In the following maturation, thymocytes express a complete T cell receptor together with CD4 and CD8 (double positive thymocytes). During their migration from the cortex to the medulla CD4+CD8+, thymocytes go into the process of thymic selection. (1) The engagement of thymocyte TcR in a low-affinity interaction with a self-MHC molecules expressed on a thymic epithelial cell rescue it from programmed cell death and allows the progression of thymocyte maturation as naïve CD4+ (or CD8+) mature T cell (*positive selection*); (2) if the thymocyte TcR does not engage any interaction with peptide-MHC molecule complexes, it will die by apoptosis (*lack of positive selection*); (3) the high affinity or avidity binding between the thymocyte TcR and the peptide-MHC complex expressed by thymic antigen-presenting cell induces the death of thymocyte for apoptosis (*negative selection*).

T Lymphocyte Activation and Effector Functions

TWO SIGNALS

The TCR's recognition of the specific peptide presented in the context of MHC molecules is necessary but not sufficient to activate T cells. To induce cell activation, TCR recognition must be simultaneously accompanied by the delivery of a second, costimulatory signal. This may occur when T cells interact with APCs. Although DCs appear to function exclusively as APCs, macrophages and B cells are also targets of activated T cells. The activation of T cells upon the initial encounter with the specific peptide on the surface of an APC (priming) occurs in peripheral lymphoid organs

The initial interaction between naïve T cells and APCs is mediated by adhesion molecules. If the naïve T cell recognizes its specific peptide–MHC complex on the surface of an APC, signaling through the TCR induces conformational changes in the adhesion molecules that enhance the adhesiveness between the two cells. However, if no recognition takes place, the T cell dissociates from that APC and samples other APCs. The binding of the TCR and of the coreceptors (CD4 or CD8) transmits a first signal to the cell indicating that the specific antigen has been recognized. The second signal is delivered through specialized molecules called *costimulatory molecules*,[65,66] the best known of which are two structurally related molecules B7.1 (CD80) and B7.2 (CD86). The receptors for B7 molecules on T cells are two similar molecules called CD28, which is constitutively expressed on most T cells, and CTLA-4. Once the first signal has been provided, ligation of CD28 by B7 molecules induces lymphocyte activation. T-cell activation also induces the expression on cell surface of CTLA-4, which has a

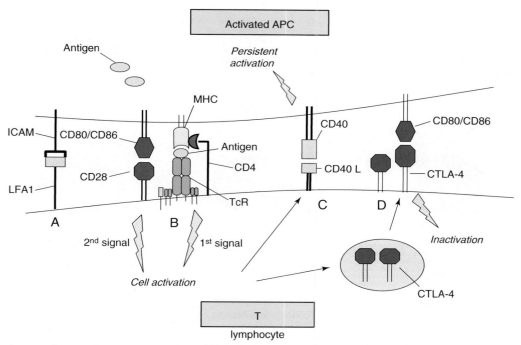

FIGURE 3–12 Mechanisms of T-cell activation and regulatory role of CTLA-4. **A,** Adhesion molecules are involved in the interactions between T cell and antigen presenting cell (APC); ICAM, intracellular adhesion molecule 1; LFA, leukocyte function-associate antigen. **B,** Crosslinking of CD28 delivers the costimulatory signal for T cell activation and induces the expression of CD40 ligand (C) and CTLA-4 (D). See text for explanations.

higher affinity for B7 molecules than CD28 and delivers a negative signal to the cell, thereby limiting the proliferative response of activated T cells. The CD28/CTLA-4 and B7-1/B7-2 interactions, therefore, provide a regulation system that ensures that immune responses are turned on when needed and turned off when not needed (Fig. 3–12).[67] A number of additional molecules with costimulatory function have been identified on the membrane of T lymphocytes. One of them, *inducible costimulator (ICOS)*, presents many homologies with CD28, and its ligand is highly homologous to B7.1 and B7.2. ICOS plays a role in the regulation of T-dependent antibody responses and germinal-center reactions.[68] In the same way, molecules other than CTLA-4 have been found to mediate a negative signal for T cell activation. An example is programmed death-1(PD-1), that exerts its negative regulatory function mainly in peripheral tissues.[69]

Approximately 100 specific peptide–MHC complexes are required on a target cell to trigger a T cell. Then TCR aggregation initiates the events that lead to T-cell activation. One of these events involves a cytoplasmic phosphatase called *calcineurin,* which activates nuclear activation factor of T cells (NAFT), which binds to the promoter region of the IL-2 gene and is necessary to activate transcription. Because NAFT is a T-cell–specific factor, blockade of the signaling pathway leading to NAFT is a way specifically to inhibit the T-cell response. Both cyclosporin and FK506 inhibit calcineurin and therefore prevent the activation of NAFT.

T-cell activation leads to a 100-fold increase in IL-2 production, to the expression of anti-apoptotic proteins of the Bcl family, and to the synthesis of the α chain of the IL-2 receptor. Resting T cells express a low-affinity IL-2 receptor composed of αβ and αγ chain. The association

of the α chain with the β and γ chains generates a receptor with a much higher affinity. Interaction of IL-2 with its receptor activates cell proliferation, which leads to the production of many T cells, all bearing an identical TCR (clonal expansion). Activation also induces the expression of CD40 ligand (CD40L) on T lymphocytes. CD40L specifically binds to the CD40 molecule constitutively expressed on APC. This interaction induces and sustains the further activation of APC. This latter mechanism plays a pivotal role in the activation and differentiation of B cells during the response to protein antigens (see later discussion).[70]

Once activated, CD4 T lymphocytes can differentiate into TH1, TH2. or TH17 cells (see later discussion). Due to their highly destructive effects, naïve CD8 T cells are kept under strict control and require high levels of costimulatory activity to be activated by APCs.[71]

The delivery to the naïve T cell of signal 1 alone not only fails to activate the cell but also induces a state of unresponsiveness (anergy) in which the T cell is refractory to activation. The most important change induced in anergic T cells is their inability to produce IL-2. The need of the second c-stimulatory signal for T-cell activation and the fact that this signal is provided only by APCs is important in preventing autoimmune diseases, because not all potentially self-reactive T cells are deleted in the thymus. On the other hand, the inhibition of the positive T cell costimulation represents an important strategy for the treatment of autoimmune diseases.[72,73]

FUNCTIONAL DEVELOPMENT OF T HELPER CELLS

Historically, the two best characterized subsets of TH cells were called TH1 and TH2 and were distinguished by the cytokines they produce: IL-2, IFN-γ, and TNF-α

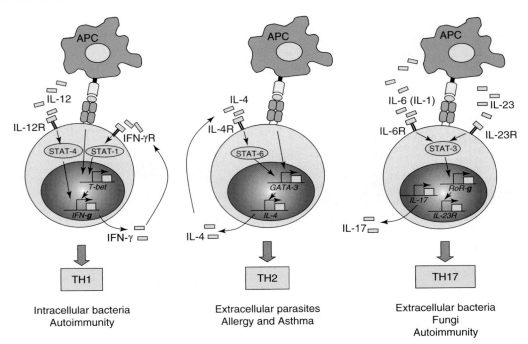

FIGURE 3–13 Development of TH1, TH2, and TH17 effector T cells. Cytokines produced in the innate immune response to microbes or early in adaptive immune response influence the differentiation of naive CD4+ T cells into TH1, TH2, and TH17 cells. IL-12 produced by antigen presenting cells induces the transcription of interferon (IFN)-γ (TH1 development) through a STAT-4 dependent pathway. The transcription factor T-bet produced in response to IFN-γ amplifies TH1 response. The stimulation of naive T cells in presence of IL-4 favors the differentiation of TH2 cells through a STAT-6 dependent pathway. The transcription factor GATA-3 is critical for TH2 differentiation. In humans, IL-1, IL-6, and IL-23 induce the transcription of IL-17 (TH17 development) through a STAT-3 dependent pathway. The transcription factor RoR-γt is critical for IL-17 and expression of IL-23 receptor that is essential for the stabilization and amplification of TH17 response. For sake of simplicity, other cytokines produced by TH1 (IL-2, tumor necrosis factor-α, lymphotoxin), TH2 (IL-5, IL-10, IL-13), and TH17 (IL-21, IL-22) are not reported in the present figure.

for TH1 cells and IL-4, IL-5, IL-10, and IL-13 for TH2 cells.[74-76]

IL-12, a heterodimeric cytokine composed of p35 and p40 subunits, is the most important cytokine that stimulates the development of TH1 cells and is produced by macrophages and DCs. IFN-γ, which is produced by macrophages, NK cells, and TH1 cells themselves, enhances IL-12 secretion by macrophages, probably has a direct TH1-inducing effect, and inhibits the development of TH2 cells.

IL-4, produced by TH2 cells, stimulates TH2 development; both IL-4 and IL-10 inhibit the generation of TH1 cells. It has been hypothesized that activated CD4 cells produce small amounts of IL-4, leading to TH2 differentiation unless they are counteracted by the presence of TH1-inducing cytokines. The differing capacity of pathogens to interact with macrophages and NK cells may therefore influence the overall balance of cytokines produced early during the immune response and thus determine the preferential development of TH1 or TH2 cells.[75,76]

The intracellular signals that regulate TH1 or TH2 commitment of CD4+ T cells have been the subject of intense investigations. During antigen presentation in secondary lymphoid organs, the regulatory cytokines IL-12 and IL-4 play a critical role in the orientation of the functional phenotype through the activation of signal transducer and activator of transcription 4 (STAT-4) or STAT-6 signaling pathways, respectively (see Fig. 3–12)[52,77] (Fig. 3–13).

NEW T CELL SUBSET: TH17

Until 2003, the action of TH1 cells was assumed responsible for many autoimmune diseases, including multiple sclerosis, rheumatoid arthritis (RA), and their experimental models, due to their ability to induce IFN-γ production and subsequent macrophage activation. However, the identification of the functional role of a cytokine homologue to IL-12, called IL-23, partially changed the view on the pathogenesis of autoimmune disorders and on some crucial aspects of the immune response.[78,79]

IL-23 is in fact constituted by a IL-12p40 chain (in common with IL-12) paired with a distinctive (p19) chain.[78] The discovery of IL-23 helped the understanding of some paradoxical findings observed in some studies related to the induction of experimental autoimmune encephalomyelitis (EAE), a mouse model for multiple sclerosis. In these experiments, neutralizing or knocking out IL-12 and IFNg had different effects on the induction EAE.[79] In fact, IL-12 p40 knockout mice were resistant to EAE induction, whereas IFNg knockout mice were more sensitive. The discovery of IL-23 led to a reassessment of the relative contributions of IL-12 and IL-23 in EAE induction, with a major role of this latter cytokine.[79]

As described later, IL-23 is mainly produced by DCs at the moment of antigen presentation, and, in collaboration with other cytokines, it plays a pivotal role in the induction of a subpopulation of CD4+ T cells characterized by the prevalent production of IL-17. This observation lead to the identification of a new Th lineage, named TH17.[80,81]

TH17 cells are different from classic TH1/TH2 cells based on the following evidence: TH17 cells do not produce the "classic" TH1/TH2 cytokines; TH17 cells express low levels of T-bet and GATA-3; and the TH1/TH2 signature cytokines, IL-4, and IFNg suppress TH17 cell differentiation.[82]

TH17 cells can be induced in vitro from naïve mouse CD4 T cells by stimulation through their TCR in the presence of IL-6 and TGF-β.[83,84] RORgt was identified as the master regulator gene for TH17 cells[82] and activator of transcription 3 (STAT3) required for signal transduction in TH17 development[82] (see Fig. 3–13).

For TH1 and TH2 T cells, the differentiation of naïve T cells into proinflammatory TH17 cells is closely dependent to the extracellular environment now of their activation. IL-6 and TGF-β are critical for the induction of TH17 in mice.[83,84] In contrast, IL-1, together with IL-23 and IL-6, is essential for the differentiation of IL-17 producing cells in humans.[85-87]

T HELPER EFFECTOR FUNCTIONS

The principal TH1 effector cytokine is IFN-γ, which activates macrophages to destroy microbes and stimulates the production of IgG antibody subclasses that bind to complement and high-affinity Fcγ receptors and are the principal antibodies involved in microbe opsonization and phagocytosis. An additional mechanism of macrophage activation is represented by the expression on TH1 cells of CD40 ligand, which activates the CD40 molecule on the surface of macrophages. Activated macrophages undergo several changes that augment their antimicrobial capacity and potentiate the immune response (e.g., upregulation of B7 molecules, further IL-12 secretion).[52,76] TH1 cells also are fundamental in recruiting macrophages to the site of infection. This occurs through the secretion by TH1 cells of several additional different cytokines, which include (1) IL-3 and granulocyte/macrophage colony-stimulating factor (GM-CSF), which stimulate the production of new phagocytic cells in the bone marrow; (2) TNF-α which induce the expression of adhesion molecules on endothelial cells; and (3) macrophage chemotactic factor (MCF) and other chemokines that direct the migration of macrophages from the endothelium to the site of infection. Many autoimmune disorders (rheumatoid arthritis (RA), Crohn disease) are characterized by infiltration and activation of TH1 lymphocytes in the inflamed tissues, leading to tissue damage.

TH2 cells induce the production of IgM and non-complement-fixing IgG subclasses. IL-4 is the main inducer of B-cell switch to IgE production, and IL-5 is the principal cytokine that activates eosinophils. TH2 cells typically mediate the immune response to helminths, stimulating the production of specific IgE antibodies that opsonize the parasites. Eosinophils activated by IL-5 bind to IgE-coated helminths through Fc receptors specific for ε heavy chain, and release their granule contents. The same mechanism of activation via IgE is also the cause of mast cell degranulation in the immediate hypersensitivity immune response in allergic diseases.[52,76]

TH17 cells are characterized by secretion of IL-17 and IL-22.[81] IL-17 and IL-22 can induce expression of several proinflammatory cytokines and chemokines by a broad range of cellular targets, including epithelial cells, endothelial cells, and macrophages, but the most potent effects of both IL-17 and IL-22 are mobilization, recruitment, and activation of neutrophils.[82] The role of TH17 cells in the pathogenesis of autoimmunity has been emphasized, primarily because the apparent limitations of the TH1/TH2 paradigm forced a reconsideration of the mechanisms of these disorders and thereby led to the understanding of the role of this new subset. However, it should be obvious that the evolutionary pressure for this specialized subset likely came from its role in host defense. As discussed, the receptor for IL-17 is widely expressed on many cell types, where it induces the expression of chemokines, proinflammatory cytokines, and colony-stimulating factors. These cytokines and chemokines in turn induce the recruitment of neutrophils and other myeloid cells, which is a critical feature of many infectious diseases.[88]

Accordingly, it has been established that IL-17 is critical for protection against gram-negative bacteria, including *Klebsiella pneumoniae*.[88] If fact, IL-17R, IL-12/IL-23, p40, IL-23, and p19 knockout mice are more susceptible to the *Klebsiella pneumoniae* infection. Moreover, TH17 cells are also involved in antifungal defense in both the mouse and human.[52,89] Zymosan, a cell wall polysaccharide of yeast, and w-1,3-glucan from C. *albicans*, preferentially induce IL-23 production.[90]

It would appear that in contrast to TH1 and TH2 cells, which protect against intracellular bacteria and helminths, a major function of TH17 cells is to protect against extracellular bacteria and fungi.

The recent description of the selective deficit in development of TH17 cells in patients with hyper-IgE syndrome (HIES or Job syndrome) strikingly validates this concept.[89] HIES patients have a genetically determined inability to signal through Stat3, due to dominant negative mutations in the SH2 domain or the DNA-binding domain of this molecule.[89] As already stated, in both humans and mice, the three major inducers and/or sustainers of TH17 differentiation, IL-6, IL-21 and IL-23, each use Stat3 for signal transduction. The principal difficulties HIES patients face, recurrent staphylococcal and fungal infections, are precisely those observed in mice that cannot develop TH17 cells, strikingly validating the importance of the CD4 T-cell differentiation concept.

EFFECTOR FUNCTIONS OF CYTOTOXIC T CELLS

CD8+ cytolytic T lymphocytes (CTL) function to eradicate intracellular microbes. Because such microbes cannot be eliminated by T cell-mediated activation of phagocytes, killing infected cells is the only way to eliminate the infection. After recognition of a specific class I MHC-associated antigen and subsequent activation, CTLs deliver their cytoplasmic cytotoxic granule proteins (*perforin* and *granzymes*) to the target cell (Fig. 3–14 (online only)).[91] Perforin is a pore-forming protein, also present in NK cells, that has the capacity to polymerize in the lipid bilayer of the target cell membrane, thus forming an aqueous channel. Granzymes are serine proteases that enter the target cell through the perforin-induced channels and activate intracellular enzymes, called caspases, which play an important role in the induction of apoptosis. Activated CTLs may also induce apoptosis through cell surface expression of the Fas ligand (FasL), which binds to and activates Fas on the cellular surface of target cell (see later discussion).

Regulation of Lymphocytes Activation (Immune Homeostasis)

During the course of a normal immune response, after the eliciting foreign antigen has been eliminated, the immune system must terminate its activation and return to a state of rest. Moreover, because lymphocytes bearing receptors capable of recognizing self-antigens are generated constantly, the immune system must be able to prevent or abort potentially self-reactive responses. Several mechanisms, only partly understood, fulfill these control functions (Fig. 3–15).[92] The disruption of these mechanisms may lead to autoimmune phenomena.

1. Negative Costimulators

A number of the possible control mechanisms have already been described for T cells. CTLA-4 appears three or four days after T cell activation and has a much higher affinity for B7.1 and B7.2, the same ligands on APCs of the T cell proactivating CD28 molecule (see Fig. 3–15).[66] Thus, CTLA-4 represents an important mechanism for the physiological termination of T-cell activation; disruption of the CTLA-4 gene in mice results in massive accumulation of activated lymphocytes in lymph nodes and the spleen and infiltration of tissues by activated lymphocytes.[93]

2. Counterregulatory Cytokines

Another important mechanism of T lymphocytes homeostasis is cytokine counterregulation. As previously noted, cytokines (IL-4, IL-13) released by TH2 cells inhibit macrophage activation and therefore control TH1-mediated immunity. Conversely, IFN-γ, released by TH1 cells, inhibits IL-4–stimulated B-cell switching to IgE. Therefore, cytokines released by different T-cell populations are able to suppress different types of immune responses. The TH1/TH2 signature cytokines, IL-4 and IFNg, suppress TH17 cell differentiation.[52]

3. Regulatory T Cells

This class of cells was discovered by Sakaguchi and colleagues (1995), who observed that depletion of the minor population of CD4+ T cells that coexpress CD25 from a population of normal adult CD4+ T cells generated a population of cells that induced a spectrum of autoimmune diseases when transferred to an immunocompromised recipient. Cotransfer of the CD25+ cells prevented the development of autoimmunity.[80] In 2001, the autoimmune Scurfy mice and a human immune dysregulation, polyendocrinopathy, enteropathy, X-linked (IPEX) patient were found to have mutations in Foxp3.[94] In 2003, Foxp3 was reported as the master transcriptional regulator for Treg cells.[95]

Numerous studies have proposed and demonstrated that Tregs are generated in the thymus (natural Tregs) through MHC class II dependent TCR interactions, resulting in high avidity selection.[96] In recent years it became evident that Foxp3+ Tregs could also be generated outside the thymus (adaptive Tregs) under a variety

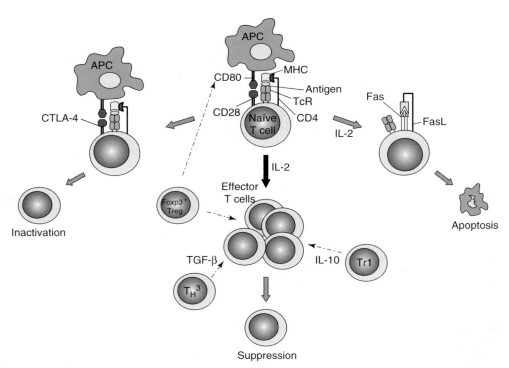

FIGURE 3–15   Different strategies for the regulation of lymphocytes activation (immune homeostasis). See text for explanations. APC, antigen-presenting cell; FasL, ligand for Fas; IL, interleukin; MHC, major histocompatibility complex; TCR, T cell receptor; TGF: transforming growth factor.

of conditions. It is now clear that activated naïve CD4 T cells stimulated by TGF-β in the absence of proinflammatory cytokines develop into adaptive Tregs (Fig. 3–16).

Several mechanisms can explain the capacity of Tregs to suppress directly responder Foxp3- T cells. Tregs may secrete suppressor cytokines (i.e., IL-10, TGF-β, IL35) that can directly inhibit the function of responder T cells and myeloid cells (see Fig. 3–16). Tregs express high CD25, the IL-2 receptor a chain, and have the capacity to compete with effector T cells for IL-2, resulting in cytokine-mediated deprivation of the effector cells and thus inducing apoptosis. Most studies have demonstrated that Tregs mediate suppression by inhibiting the induction of IL-2 mRNA (and mRNA for other effector cytokines) in the responder Foxp3- T cells. Tregs may also compete with Foxp3-T cells for IL-2, consume it, and inhibit the proliferation of Foxp3- T cells, resulting in a form of apoptosis dependent on the proapoptotic factor Bim.[97]

Activated Foxp3+ Tregs may function as cytotoxic cells and may directly kill effector cells in a manner similar to CD8+ cytotoxic cells. Human CD4+CD25+Foxp3+ Tregs can be activated by a combination of antibodies to CD3 and CD46 to express granzyme A and kill activated CD4+ and CD8+ T cells and other cell types in a perforin-dependent, Fas-FasL-independent manner.[98] Activated Tregs may express known (e.g., galectin-1) or unknown molecules on their cell surface that can interact with receptors on effector T cells, resulting in cell cycle arrest[99] (see Fig. 3–16). All of these mechanisms may also

be used by Tregs to inhibit the function of APCs or other cells of the innate immune system (i.e., DCs, B cells, macrophages, NK cells).

4. Apoptosis

Upon exposure to antigen, clonal expansion of specific T and B lymphocytes increases their frequency by more than 1000-fold within a week. After one to three months, the number of specific lymphocytes returns to baseline levels, leaving long-lived, functionally quiescent memory cells. This rapid decline in antigen-specific lymphocyte numbers is due to their elimination by apoptosis, a further important mechanism for immune homeostasis.

Apoptosis occurs by two main pathways (Fig. 3–17). Lymphocytes that are deprived of survival stimuli, such as costimulators and cytokines, lose expression of specialized antiapoptotic proteins, mainly belonging to the Bcl family[100] and die "by neglect." This mechanism leading to apoptosis is called passive cell death and is probably the most important mechanism that downregulates the immune response once the eliciting antigen has been eliminated and the innate immune response subsides. The stimuli that maintain quiescent and viable naïve and memory cells are probably sufficient to maintain the expression of antiapoptotic proteins and therefore to prevent cell death. Passive cell death has to be distinguished from the other mechanism, activation-induced cell death, in which apoptosis is actively induced. Although these two mechanisms are distinct in their

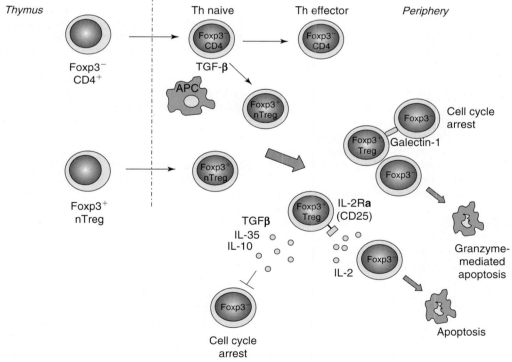

FIGURE 3–16 Thymic and peripheral generation of Foxp3+ Tregs and schematic representation of the mechanisms by which Treg can directly suppress responder Foxp3- T cells. Natural Treg (nTreg) cells differentiate in the thymus and migrate to peripheral tissues. Adaptive Foxp3+ Treg (aTreg) cells differentiate in secondary lymphoid organs and tissues under the influence of TGFβ, now of antigen presentation (see text). Tregs may secrete suppressor cytokines that can directly inhibit the function of responder T cells. Tregs express high CD25, express the IL-2 receptor a chain, and have the capacity to compete with effector T cells for IL-2, resulting in cytokine-mediated deprivation of the effector cells. Activated Foxp3+ Tregs may function as cytotoxic cells and directly kill effector cells in a manner similar to CD8+ cytotoxic cells. Finally, activated Tregs may express galectin-1 on their cell surface that can interact with receptors on effector T cells, resulting in cell cycle arrest.

induction and function, they share the same terminal biochemical pathway.

Activation-induced cell death is important in preventing uncontrolled T-cell activation and as an effector mechanism of CD8 cytotoxic T cells and NK cells.[101] It is usually the result of the interaction of two molecules that are co-expressed on activated cells: the surface receptor Fas (CD95) and its ligand (Fas ligand or CD95L). Fas belongs to a family of proteins that includes TNF receptors (TNFR) I and II and the B cell-activating molecule CD40. This family of proteins dictates signals that can induce cell survival and proliferation or apoptotic death.[101]

Fas is expressed on different cell types, and in lymphocytes its levels increase after antigen stimulation. Fas ligand is expressed on activated T lymphocytes; therefore, activated, mature T cells express both Fas and Fas ligand. The interaction of Fas ligand with Fas induces a series of intracellular events that lead to apoptosis. These events are initiated by the cytoplasmic region of Fas, which contains a sequence called the death domain and involves a proteolytic system, the central component of which is represented by a family of proteases called caspases (see Fig. 3–17 [online only]).

In mice, mutations in the Fas receptor (lymphoproliferation phenotype [lpr]) or its ligand (generalized lymphoproliferative disease [gld]) are associated with massive lymphadenopathy and lupuslike autoimmunity.[102] In humans, Fas mutations cause the so-called autoimmune lymphoproliferative syndrome (ALPS) 122, characterized by lymphadenopathy and autoimmunity.

PATHOGENESIS OF CHRONIC INFLAMMATORY DISEASES

Multifactorial Origin of the Rheumatic Diseases

Inflammatory rheumatic diseases are thought to be secondary to the loss of the mechanisms of immunological tolerance by adaptive immunity, leading to the induction, activation, and proliferation of autoreactive T and B cells and production of autoantibodies. The recent identification of some monogenic inflammatory diseases caused by mutations of genes involved in the regulation of the innate response (autoinflammatory diseases) has also raised a great interest in the central role of this latter branch of the immune response as primary inducer of a number of immune-mediated diseases.

Autoimmunity: Breaking the Immunological Tolerance

Immunological tolerance is the antigen-induced functional inactivation or death of specific lymphocytes that results both in the inability to respond to that antigen and in the inhibition of lymphocyte activation during subsequent administration of the same antigen in an immunogenic form.[103] Antigens that induce an immune response are called immunogens, whereas antigens that induce tolerance are called tolerogens. Self-antigens are normally

tolerogens; many foreign antigens, depending on their physicochemical form, dose, and route of administration, may act as immunogens, tolerogens, or both. For instance, protein antigens administered subcutaneously or intradermally are usually immunogenic, whereas large amounts of protein antigens administered intravenously or orally often induce unresponsiveness.

The random generation of antigen receptors during lymphocyte maturation can give rise to lymphocytes that are specific for self-antigens. Lymphocytes with high avidity for abundant self-antigens constitutively expressed in all cells (and therefore present in high concentration in the thymus and the bone marrow) are deleted during their development in central lymphoid organs (central tolerance). Although this is an efficient process, not all self-antigens are expressed in central lymphoid organs or gain access to it. Lymphocytes that are specific for these antigens, therefore, survive and must be eliminated or held in check by other mechanisms. These mechanisms, only partly understood, are responsible for peripheral tolerance and include not only clonal deletion but also clonal anergy, active suppression, and ignorance.

Central Tolerance

The process of central tolerance seeks to eliminate or impair T cells that express a high affinity receptor for self-antigens, because these cells hold the potential to mediate autoimmunity. The hallmarks of central tolerance are the clonal deletion of autoreactive T cells and the selection of Tregs, which control self-reactive T cells.

During their maturation in the primary lymphoid organs, lymphocytes encounter a number of antigens to which they respond by developing tolerance rather than activation. Lymphocytes that recognize with high affinity, self-antigen presented in association with MHC molecules by medullary thymic epithelial cells (mTECs) die by apoptosis (negative selection). This fundamental process avoids the possibility that lymphocytes with high affinity receptors for ubiquitous self-antigens may reach maturation (see Fig. 3–11). The process affects both class I and class II MHC-restricted T cells and is therefore important for tolerance in CD8 and CD4 lymphocytes subpopulations.[104]

Medullary TECs acts as DCs, as they express costimulatory molecules (CD40, CD80, CD86) and MHC class II molecules.[105] mTECS selectively express the so-called transcriptor factor *autoimmune regulator (AIRE)* that is responsible for the ectopic expression of many tissue-restricted self-antigens (TRAs), that represent as many self-antigens expressed outside of the thymus as necessary to establish and maintain self-tolerance. During negative selection, these encoded TRAs are presented by mTECs to differentiating thymocytes as self-antigens, leading to the induction of tolerance by clonal deletion, functional inactivation, or clonal deviation of self-reactive T cells.

Mutations in the human AIRE gene *cause autoimmune polyendocrinopathy candidiasis ectodermal dystrophy (APECED)*, a syndrome that is characterized by the presence of autoantibodies specific for multiple self-antigens; this leads to lymphocytic infiltration of endocrine glands and autoimmune disorders localized at these organs.[104,106,107]

Mice with mutations in the AIRE gene have pathological autoimmune features similar to those of patients with APECED, including multiorgan lymphocytic infiltration and autoantibody production.[108] In recent years, many studies have shown that AIRE is a crucial factor for the promiscuous expression of TRAs in the thymus, and that mutations in this gene lead to the escape of self-reactive T cells from the thymus, which results in autoimmunity.[104]

Negative thymic selection is not entirely efficient and inadvertently permits the emigration of some autoreactive T cells with a low affinity TCR for self-antigens. One additional mechanism that occurs in the thymus is the generation of Tregs, which control self-reactive T cells and thereby maintain immune system homeostasis and tolerance to self-antigens (see earlier discussion).

The expression of Foxp3 (the master gene for Treg development) during T lymphopoiesis is first noted in a very small fraction of late double positive thymocytes and then detected in approximately 5% of CD4 single positive cells within the thymus, displaying a TCR repertoire that is highly enriched for receptors with a high affinity for self-antigens.[109] Given the stringent selection processes during thymocyte differentiation, Treg may arise by positive selection of highly self-reactive T cells and/or by resistance of differentiated Foxp3+ single positive thymocytes to negative selection.[110]

Peripheral Tolerance

The mature lymphocyte repertoire still contains cells capable of recognizing self-antigens that are exclusively expressed in the peripheral tissues. Thus, other mechanisms of tolerance are required to avoid the response of these mature self-reacting lymphocytes. Most of the mechanisms involved in the peripheral tolerance are related to the strategy of control of lymphocyte homeostasis.

As previously noted, activation of CD4+ T cells after recognition of antigens presented by APCs requires the simultaneous presence of a second signal given by the costimulatory molecules, which are expressed only by activated APCs and not by resting APCs. In the absence of such costimulatory signal, T cells are able to survive, but are rendered incapable of responding to the same antigen in a future encounter (clonal anergy). The continuous presentation to mature T cells of self-antigens by resting APCs makes many self-reacting T cells anergic.[103]

Many self-proteins are presented too poorly to T cells to be recognized. These self-antigens are called cryptic epitopes and are collectively referred to as cryptic self. T cells that are specific for these epitopes are not tolerant because they can respond if the antigen is presented appropriately. They are considered ignorant because they are not aware of the existence of the self-antigen they are able to recognize. Strictly speaking, ignorance is not a mechanism of tolerance because it represents a lack of response rather than an actively induced immunological unresponsiveness. Ignorance may also be related to the difficulty of T cells to gain access to some tissues, such as brain, gonads, and eye ("immunologically privileged sites") because of the existence of blood–tissue barriers.[111]

A further important mechanism of peripheral tolerance is related to Tregs.[95,112] The major population of Tregs is represented by natural or adaptive FoxP3-positive CD4+CD25+ T cells. The generation and functional properties of these cells are described earlier and in Figure 3–16.

Other T cell subpopulations may presumably play a similar regulatory function using different mechanisms (see Fig. 3–15). Antigen-specific T cells selectively producing high level of the antiinflammatory cytokine IL-10 (also called Tr1) are able to inhibit the development of experimental autoimmune colitis.[113] The same cytokine-mediated regulatory mechanism was also observed for cells displaying high production of TGF-β and was defined as TH3.[114]

Another mechanism of peripheral tolerance is represented by the deletion of self-reactive T cells by *activation-induced cell death*. As previously described in the mechanisms of immune homeostasis, repeated stimulation of T cells by persistent antigens induces the death of the activated cells by a process of apoptosis. It is believed that Fas-mediated activation induced death is responsible for the elimination of T cells specific for abundant peripheral self-antigens most likely responsible for the repeated activation of T cells (see Fig. 3–15). As previously mentioned, mutations in the Fas receptor are associated with massive lymphoproliferative disorder associated with a lupuslike autoimmunity.[102,115]

B Cell and Immunological Tolerance

The process of tolerance for B cells is essentially defined as the elimination, editing, or silencing of self-reactive cells to prevent ultimately the excessive production of pathogenic autoantibodies. At least in animal models, B cell tolerance is established through multiple mechanisms, either during B cell development in the bone marrow and in the peripheral lymphoid organs,[41,115a] including: (1) arrest of maturation leading to premature death and clonal deletion[116]; (2) elimination of the antibody autoreactivity by rearrangement of a new light chain (receptor editing)[117]; and (3) induction of anergy in chronically stimulated autoreactive cells.[118]

During the immature B cell development, the strength of the BCR signal determines whether the BCR-triggered cells progress in development (positive selection) or undergo receptor editing to be rescued. Immature B cells that express a nonautoreactive receptor with an efficient combination of IgH and IgL chains receive the right amount of BCR signaling, which allows them to progress in development and be positively selected. These cells can switch off RAG expression controlling Ig rearrangement and then be allowed to migrate to the spleen.[119]

Conversely in immature B cells expressing an autoreactive BCR, an encounter with their self-antigen generates a stronger BCR signal, which induces receptor editing. The strong BCR signaling prevents these autoreactive cells from progressing in their development and switches off RAG expression. The latter phenomenon allows them to undergo secondary IgL chain rearrangements that can lead to the generation of a new IgL chain. If the resulting new BCR is nonautoreactive, and the new IgL chain pairs well their IgH chain, these cells will be positively selected. This mechanism rescues immature B cells that express an autoreactive BCR from apoptosis and clonal deletion. Alteration of this important checkpoint is associated with the development of autoimmunity.[120]

Autoreactivity at the mature stage can also be enforced by additional mechanisms during antigen-induced T cell-dependent GC reactions.

This peripheral tolerance is related to different possible mechanisms that may have a combinatory effect in the induction of tolerance: (1) induction of apoptosis of autoreactive B cells by FasL on activated T cells or by self-antigen-induced BCR signaling; (2) prevention of autoreactive plasma cell differentiation by BCR signaling; (3) lack of interaction with follicular TH cells; and (4) attenuation of autoreactivity by BCR modification, either through somatic hypermutation or receptor revision.[121]

Role of Dendritic Cells

In the absence of inflammatory signals, resident tissue specific DCs remain in an immature or resting state characterized by low expression of costimulatory molecules and cytokines.[121] Immature DCs show weak migratory activities and T-cell priming properties, and more importantly, are able to induce antigen-specific T-cell tolerance. Tolerance induction by immature DCs includes several mechanisms: silencing of differentiated antigen-specific T cells,[121] transfer of regulatory properties to effector T cells,[122] activation and expansion of naturally occurring CD25+ Tregs,[123] and the differentiation of naïve CD4+ T cells into Tregs[124] (see Fig. 3–16).

The local micromilieu controls the functional differentiation of DCs, ranging from immunostimulatory to tolerogenic.[25]

Development of Autoimmune Diseases

The development of an autoimmune disease is presumably initiated by an aberrant, genetically regulated, immune response to environmental antigens. The importance of environmental factors in eliciting disease is indicated by the relatively low disease concordance in monozygotic twins and by the fact that migrant populations tend to acquire the disease prevalence of the geographical area to which they move. The importance of the genetic component varies among diseases. The frequency of a given disease in relatives of an index case (the recurrent risk) is about 4 for RA and approaches 50 to 100 for SLE and spondyloarthropathies; similarly, the concordance in twins is between 25% and 50% for SLE and nearly 10-fold lower for RA.[29] The combination of environmental and genetic factors determines the development and expression of an autoimmune disorder.

Only a few autoimmune syndromes have been shown to be caused by single gene mutations. These mutations usually affect genes that regulate pivotal mechanisms involved in central and/or peripheral tolerance. As previously mentioned, mutations of the autoimmune regulator AIRE gene lead to an autosomal recessive disease APECED,[108] whereas mutations of FoxP3 gene (which causes the complete loss of the regulatory functions of CD4+CD25+ Tregs) provokes IPEX syndrome,[125] and mutations of the Fas gene cause the ALPS.[115a] However, most of the known autoimmune diseases are not inherited in a simple mendelian way.

The human and animal genomes contain a pool of allelic variants or DNA mutations that affect the control of the immune response. Although the complex genetic mechanisms that predispose to autoimmune diseases have not yet been elucidated, it appears that some of these genetic variants, in combination with other genes, confer increased susceptibility to autoimmunity and affect the wide variability of disease manifestations and outcome.

The mechanisms that normally prevent autoimmunity may be considered as a succession of checkpoints. Each checkpoint plays a partial role in preventing antiself-response, but all of them together act synergistically to provide efficient protection against autoimmunity. During the last decades, a number of genes that predispose to autoimmunity in human and animal autoimmune diseases have been localized.

There appear to be genes that both cause general defects in immune regulation and are shared between different diseases, and genes that are unique to a given disease and may confer susceptibility of the target organ to the autoimmune process. Some conclusions have been drawn from the analysis of murine autoimmune disease models: (1) no single allele but rather a combination of genes causes the disease, and more than one combination may exist; (2) the risk of the disease depends on the number of susceptibility alleles at unlinked loci; (3) some alleles have a greater effect than others; and (4) several predisposing alleles have a weak effect and are therefore difficult to map.[125a]

Role of Environmental Factors

Infection appears to be the most important exogenous factor in the induction of autoimmunity. However, how infections trigger the activation of autoaggressive T cells and cause tissue destruction is unknown. Different mechanisms have been hypothesized.

According to the bystander activation hypothesis, the local inflammatory response induced by an infection may lead to the activation of preexisting self-reactive bystander lymphocytes. Proinflammatory mediators secreted from APCs at the site of local inflammation, and the increased expression of costimulatory molecules may lead to the activation of self-reactive lymphocytes that are not specific for the antigens of the pathogens. Moreover, cell death associated with tissue destruction secondary to the infection may also provoke a release of self-antigens, potentiating antigen presentation and activation of self-reactive lymphocytes. Thus, products of microorganisms, such as bacterial and virus DNA or LPS, acting as adjuvants, might play a role in eliciting autoimmunity. Notably, coadministration of a microbial adjuvant together with the relevant antigen or peptide is necessary for inducing experimental autoimmune disease.[126]

Some pathogens associated with autoimmune diseases express protein or carbohydrate antigens that share structural similarities with self-antigens and could elicit a pathogenic immune response that crossreacts with self-antigens (*molecular mimicry*).[127]

Many experimental autoimmune animal models are generated by hyperimmunization of genetically susceptible strains with foreign proteins that are homologous to tissue-specific self-proteins. Although in this case the triggering antigen is a homologous nonmicrobial antigen, the mechanism is equivalent to that which may occur after infection with a pathogen whose antigens, although nonhomologous, share structurally related epitopes with self-antigens.[128]

Molecular mimicry is involved in triggering disease in many animal models of autoimmune disease. These models include Thelieur's murine encephalomyelitis virus (TMEV)-induced demyelinating disease[129]; some models of type I diabetes[130]; and autoimmune myocarditis associated with coxsackievirus.[131] Bacterial peptides have also been implicated in human autoimmune diseases by molecular mimicry, such as streptococcus in rheumatic carditis.[132]

Superantigens are a distinct class of bacterial-derived antigens that stimulate a primary T-cell response similar to a response to allogenic MHC molecules. However, unlike other protein antigens they can be recognized by T cells without being processed into peptides that are captured by MHC molecules. Bacterial superantigens primarily bind to the Vb CDR2 loop of MHC molecules, and each superantigen is specific for one or a few of the different Vb gene products. The binding with MHC leads to the activation of T cells, bearing the specific Vb chain with a massive production of cytokines by CD4+ T cells. Among bacterial superantigens are the staphylococcal enterotoxin, which causes food poisoning, and the toxic shock syndrome toxin-1 that is the etiological principle in toxic shock syndrome.[133] Superantigens may also induce a potent polyclonal immune response and could trigger autoimmune diseases either by driving anergic autoreactive T cells out of their nonresponsive state or by facilitating activation of ignorant T cells that are specific for cryptic epitopes. Superantigen-induced immune activation could also be a cause of disease exacerbation in already established autoimmune diseases.[134,135]

Mechanisms of Perpetuation and Amplification of Autoimmune Response at the Site of Tissue Inflammation (Epitope Spreading)

During the course of an autoimmune disease, a T-cell response may develop not only to the original immunizing peptide but also to novel antigens processed and presented by B cells. At the site of the autoimmune-mediated inflammation, activated B lymphocytes can take up their specific autoantigens by endocytosis, process, and present them to T cells. During this process, a number of new autoantigens (also named cryptic epitopes) can be revealed. Autoreactive T cells responding to theses epitopes can provide help to any B cells presenting this peptide and recruit additional B cells for the production of a greater variety of autoantibodies (Fig. 3–18). This mechanism is thought to play a crucial role in spreading autoantibody specificity during the course of systemic lupus erythematosus and therefore in the perpetuation of the autoimmune response.[136]

How Environmental Factors May Contribute to the Breakdown of Tolerance. The Example of Plasmocytoid Dendritic Cells (PDC) in the Pathogenesis of SLE

PDC, or natural type I IFN-producing cells (IPC), are a distinct small subset of circulating leukocytes, characterized by their typical (plasma cell-like) morphology[137,138] and by their capacity to produce large amounts of type I IFNs

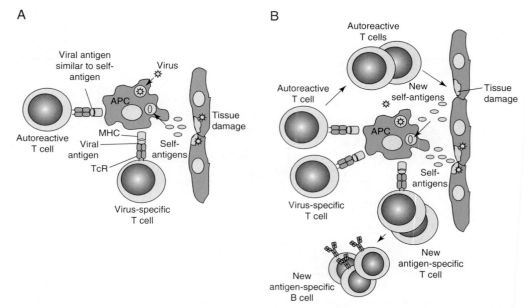

FIGURE 3–18 Mechanisms of infection-induced autoimmunity. **A,** Autoreactive T cells can be activated through a mechanism of molecular mimicry that involves crossreactive recognition of a viral antigen that has similarity to self-antigen. **B,** Self-antigen that is released from damaged tissue can be taken up by activated APCs, processed and presented to autoreactive T cells (concomitant with presentation of virus antigen to virus-specific T cells) in a process known as bystander activation. Further tissue destruction by activated T cells and inflammatory mediators causes the release of more self-antigen from tissues. The T-cell response can then spread to involve T cells specific for other self-antigens in a process known as epitope spreading. Autoreactive T cells responding to theses epitopes can provide help to any B cells presenting this peptide, recruiting additional B cells for the production of new autoantibodies. TCR, T cell receptor.

(α and β) in response to viral infections[139,140] or bacterial DNA containing unmethylated CG dinucleotide (CpG motifs).[26,141,142] IPCs are found in secondary lymphoid organs, express MHC class II molecules, and, upon stimulation, mature to antigen presenting cells and are therefore included in the DC family[23] (see earlier discussion).

As major type I IFN producers, PDCs play an important role in regulation of immune responses by influencing T-cell activation and functional orientation,[26,143,144] DC maturation,[27] B-cell activation, and plasma-cell differentiation.[145]

Through their direct effect on B cells, type I IFNs enhance primary antibody responses to soluble proteins and upregulate CD38, a GC B cell and plasma cell marker, on B lymphocytes and BAFF on Mos and mDCs. BAFF in turn contributes to the survival of autoreactive B lymphocytes. IFN-α also promotes the differentiation of activated B lymphocytes into plasmablasts and antibody-secreting plasma cells.[146]

If dysregulated, IFN-α might lead to autoimmune diseases.[147,148] It was shown that serum levels of type I IFN correlate with disease activity and severity,[149] and genomic studies on blood cells of patients with SLE indicate that many patients overexpress IFN-induced genes.[150] In addition, polymorphisms of IFN-related genes were found

to be associated with an increased susceptibility for the development of SLE.[151] In mice, a null mutation of type I IFN bred with lupus-prone mice, exhibited decreased morbidity and prolonged survival.[152] IFN accelerates the development of autoimmune symptoms in lupus-prone NZB/NZW mice.[152]

According to a recent hypothesis, viral infections induce type I IFN production by pDC and the release of auto-antigens. In susceptible individuals this can lead to the breakdown of tolerance with the subsequent production of autoantibodies against DNA and/or RNA (Fig. 3–19). These autoantigens, together with autoantibodies, form immune complexes that can act as endogenous IFN inducers, leading to persistent IFN-α production. Type I IFN will induce maturation of Mos into DCs, and activate B cells and both CD4 and CD8 T cells. This could amplify the production of type I IFN and the differentiation of autoreactive plasma cells with further production of autoantibodies, which perpetuates this pathogenic loop[146] (see Fig. 3–19).

New Role for Innate Immunity: Autoinflammation versus Autoimmunity

The study of a number of inherited inflammatory diseases caused by mutations of genes of importance in the regulation of the innate immune response (autoinflammatory

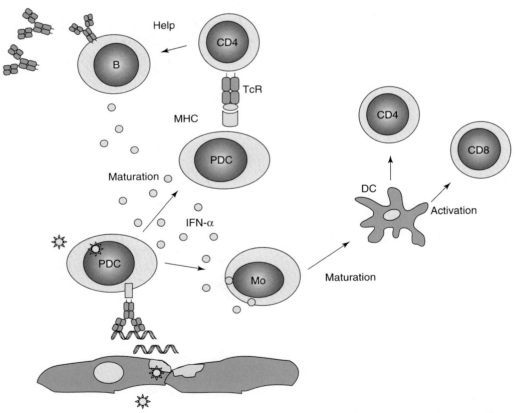

FIGURE 3–19 Possible pathogenic role of viral infections and plasmocytoid dendritic cells activation in the induction and maintenance of autoimmunity. Viral infections induce the release of autoantigens from tissue (including DNA or RNA) and activation of plasmocytoid dendritic cells (PDC) with production of type I interferon (IFN-α and β). In susceptible individuals, tolerance can break and cause production of autoantibodies against DNA and/or RNA containing autoantigens. These immune complexes are bound by the Fc receptors on PDC and represent a further source of activation of these cells via Toll-like receptor-7 and -9, representing endogenous IFN inducers and leading to persistent IFN-α production. Type I IFN will induce maturation of PDCs and differentiation of monocytes (Mo) into dendritic cells (DC). These latter cells can activate both CD8 and CD4 T cells with subsequent help for a further activation of autoreactive B cells. IFN also directly stimulate B cell activation and differentiation (modified, by Ronnblom and Pascual ref n. 146).

diseases, see Chapter 43) has modified some paradigms concerning the origin and maintenance of many chronic inflammatory diseases.[153]

The prototype of these diseases are the so-called cryopyrin-associated periodic syndromes (CAPS) that are all caused by activating, gain-of-function mutations in NLRP3 (originally denoted CIAS1 for cold-induced auto-inflammatory syndrome 1 and also known as cryopyrin, NALP3, or PYPAF1).[154,155] As described earlier, a crucial role in IL-1β processing is played by the inflammasome, a multi-protein complex responsible for activation of the IL-1 converting enzyme (ICE) (or Caspase-1), which in turn converts pro-IL-1β to the mature, active 17 kDa form.[18,19]

Experimental mouse models revealed that Mos from knockout mice deficient in cryopyrin cannot activate caspase-1 upon LPS and ATP stimulation, which results in lack of IL-1β secretion.[20] On the contrary, mutations in the cryopyrin gene in humans are associated with its gain of function that lead to an excessive production of IL-1β,[156] even in absence of a second signal, such as extracellular ATP.[15] Specific inhibition of IL-1 is able to dampen dramatically the severe systemic inflammatory picture of CAPS patients.[158]

The discovery of disease-associated mutations in NLRP3 sheds new light in the understanding of the role in the induction of acute and chronic inflammation of the downstream events following the activation of PRRs of the innate immunity.[159]

Of note, proteins mutated in other autoinflammatory diseases may directly or indirectly interact with the NLRP3 inflammasome complex, influencing its function. Pyrin (mutated in familial Mediterranean fever) modulates the inflammasome by interacting with both ASC and Caspase-1,[160,161] whereas PSTPIP1 (mutated in the PAPA syndrome) binds to pyrin, forming a trimolecular complex with ASC[162] (Fig. 3–20).

On the other hand, mutations of the NACHT domain of another cytoplasmatic PRR, NOD2/CARD15, result in overexpression of the proinflammatory pathway, leading to NF-kB activation and are associated with a chronic granulomatous condition known as Blau syndrome (see Fig. 3–20).[163] Notably, mutations of the LRR domain of the same gene are associated with Crohn disease, another chronic granulomatous disease.[164]

As shown earlier, PRRs are not only able to sense various microbial products but also a number of endogenous "danger signals" (DAMPs). The NLRP3 protein is activated by endogenous molecules, such as ATP or monosodium urate (MSU) and calcium pyrophosphate dihydrate (CPPD), which shows that innate immunity is also able to react towards the self.

Martinon and colleagues[165] elegantly showed that NLRP3 is important in gout. Both MSU and CPPD crystals increase caspase-1 activation and IL-1β secretion from macrophages stimulated with LPS, but this does not occur in ASC- or Nlrp3- deficient macrophages.[165]

This and other observations raised interest in the role of the inflammasome in the regulation of the inflammatory response, not only in gout but also in autoinflammatory diseases, Crohn disease,[164] systemic onset juvenile arthritis,[166] recurrent pericarditis,[167] and other inflammatory diseases that do not present the classic hallmarks of adaptive immunity.[168]

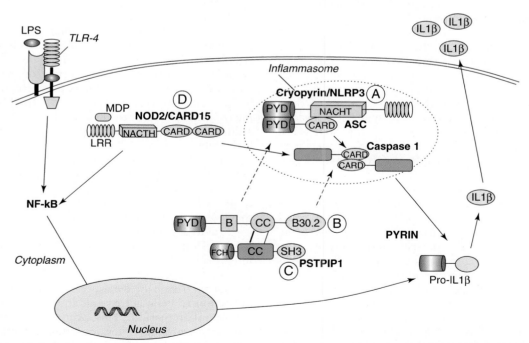

FIGURE 3–20 Schematic representation of the functional role of genes involved in autoinflammatory diseases in the control of NF-kB activation and IL-1β secretion. **A,** Cryopyrin (NLRP3) play a pivotal role in the activation of inflammasome and induction of IL-1β secretion (see Fig. 3–4). **B,** Pyrin modulates the inflammasome by interacting with both ASC and Caspase-1 with the pyrin and SPRY domains, respectively (see text). **C,** PSTPIP1 binds to pyrin. Disease-associated mutations in PSTPIP1 enhance pyrin binding, forming a trimolecular complex with ASC. **D,** CARD15/NOD2 is an intracellular sensor for pathogen-associated molecular patterns, such as muramyl dipeptide (MDP). After stimulation, NOD2/CARD15 is able to induce both NF-kB activation and the release of bioactive IL-1β in a Caspase 1 dependent-manner.

Based on these observations, a new schema for the classification of immune-mediated inflammatory diseases has been proposed[168] (Table 3–6). The spectrum of self-reactive immunological diseases represents a continuum between autoimmune disorders based primarily on lesions of the adaptive immune system and autoinflammatory conditions rooted primarily in the innate immune system.

MECHANISMS OF TISSUE INJURY IN IMMUNE-MEDIATED DISEASES

The clinical and pathological manifestations of a given autoimmune or autoinflammatory disease are determined by several factors, including the nature and location of the trigger stimulus and the type of effector mechanisms that the immune system uses to eliminate the aberrant stimulus.

Inflammatory Response

The acute inflammatory response triggered by infection or tissue injury involves the coordinated delivery of plasma and leukocytes through postcapillary venules to the site of infection or injury. The activated endothelium of the blood vessels allows selective extravasation of neutrophils and, later, other leukocytes.

During bacterial infections, this response is triggered by PRRs of the innate immune system, such as TLRs and membrane or intracellular sensors. This initial recognition of infection is mediated by tissue resident macrophages and mast cells, leading to the production of a variety of inflammatory mediators (vasoactive amines, cytokines, chemokines, eicosanoids, products of proteolytic cascades).[169]

After their recruitment to the site of infection, neutrophils become activated, either by direct contact with pathogens or through the actions of cytokines secreted by tissue-resident cells. The neutrophils attempt to kill the invading agents by releasing the toxic contents of their granules, which include reactive oxygen species, reactive nitrogen species, and proteolytic enzymes (proteinase 3, cathepsin G and elastase 5). Due to the lack of specificity of these highly potent effectors, host tissue may be damaged as a collateral effect.[169]

A successful acute inflammatory response results in the elimination of the infectious agents, followed by a resolution and repair phase. Conversely, if the acute inflammatory response fails to eliminate the pathogen, the inflammatory process persists and acquires new characteristics. In this case, the neutrophil infiltration is gradually replaced by recently-immigrated Mos differentiating into macrophages, and T cells (see the type IV delayed type hypersensitivity in later). The characteristics of this inflammatory state can differ depending on the effector class of the T cells (TH1, TH2, TH17) that are present according to the pathogens involved (see earlier discussion).

If the combined effect of these cells is still insufficient, a chronic inflammatory state ensues, involving the formation of tertiary lymphoid tissues and granulomas.[170] Unsuccessful attempts by macrophages to engulf and destroy pathogens or foreign bodies can lead to the formation of granulomas, in which the intruders are walled off by layers of macrophages, in a final attempt to protect the host.

As already described, chronic inflammation can result not only from the persistence of pathogens, but also from other causes of tissue damage such as autoimmune or autoinflammatory responses, owing to the persistence of self-antigens or DAMPs.

Recruitment of Leukocytes into Inflamed Tissue

The migration of leukocytes from the circulation to the site of inflammation is a multistep process leading to the attachment of circulating cells to endothelial cells and migration through the endothelium (Fig. 3–21).[171] The capture and rolling of circulating cells by activated endothelium is followed by the activation of cells and their firm adhesion to endothelium, and finally the migration of cells across the endothelium (diapedesis).[171]

A proinflammatory stimulus leads to the production of proinflammatory cytokines (TNF-α, IL-1β) by the resident cells of innate immunity. These cytokines induce the expression of glycoproteins (selectins) that act as adhesion molecules for circulating leukocytes[172] (Table 3–7). In particular, endothelial (E)-selectin and platelet (P)-derived selectin are selectively expressed on the surface of cytokine-activated endothelial cells. Circulating leukocytes flowing in the bloodstream first loosely adhere to the endothelium through constitutively expressed surface glycoproteins (sialyl Lewis-X for E-selectin, P-selectin glycoprotein ligand 1 [PSGL-1] for P-selectin.) The second step of leukocyte migration needs their firm adherence to endothelial cells. This is ensured by other surface molecules, constitutively expressed on circulating leukocytes, called integrins.[173,174] Integrins are a large family of heterodimeric proteins composed of two noncovalently linked polypeptide chains β (see Table 3–7). Proinflammatory cytokines (IL-1β, TNF-α) mediate the overexpression of the ligands that are specific for high affinity integrins. In this way, a firm adhesion between leukocytes and endothelium occurs. During inflammation, the very late antigen (VLA)-4 (or α4β1) is selectively expressed on leukocytes and mediates their adhesion to activated endothelial cells expressing its ligand, vascular cell adhesion molecule (VCAM)-1.[174] Similarly, the leukocyte function-associated antigen-1 (LFA-1 or CD11aCD18) binds to its specific ligand, the intracellular adhesion molecule (ICAM). The specific inhibition of integrins involved in leukocyte recruitment is a therapeutic target in autoimmune diseases.[174]

The final step in leukocyte recruitment is the transmigration of cells across the endothelial lining into the site of inflammation. This process is facilitated by the interaction among other integrins expressed on leukocytes and their specific ligands present at the level of the adherence junction between the endothelial cells (platelet-endothelial cell adhesion molecule [PECAM-1]; junctional adhesion molecule [JAM–family]), or in the subendothelial ECM (fibronectin, osteopontin, collagen) (see Table 3–7).[175]

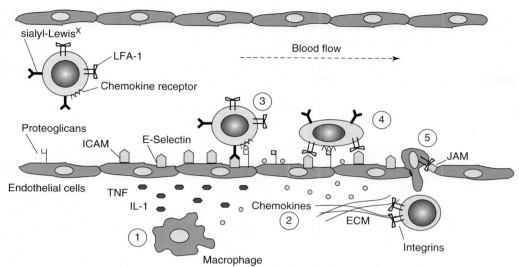

FIGURE 3–21   Recruitment of leukocytes into the inflammatory site. **(1)** Proinflammatory cytokines produced by macrophages stimulate the expression of adhesion molecules (selectins and integrin ligands) on the endothelial cells. (2) Chemokines produced by stromal cells, inflammatory cells, and endothelial cells specifically attract leukocytes bearing specific chemokine receptors. (3) Leukocytes bearing selectin ligands (i.e., Sialyl Lewis^X) weakly adhere to endothelium (*rolling*). (4) Leukocytes display a process of integrin affinity maturation stimulated by chemokines. In this way, a firm adhesion between leukocytes and endothelium occurs (*adhesion*). (5) Transmigration of cells across the endothelial lining into the site of inflammation. The progression of cells through the endothelial cells is allowed by the interaction between other integrins expressed on leukocytes and their specific ligands present at the level of the adherence junction between the endothelial cells (i.e., junctional adhesion molecule [JAM]-family) or in the subendothelial extracellular matrix. ECM, extracellular matrix; ICAM, intracellular adhesion molecule; IL, interleukin; LFA-1, leukocyte function-associated antigen-1; TNF, tumor necrosis factor.

Table 3–7

Adhesion molecules

Family	Name	Cell Distribution	Ligands	Main Functions
1. Selectins	P-selectin (CD62P) E-selectin (CD62E) L-selectin (CD62L)	Endothelium,* PLT Endothelium* Leukocytes	Sialyl Lewis^X PSGL-1 GlyCAM-1, CD34, MadCAM-1	Initiate leukocyte-endothelium interactions

2. Integrins
β_1 α_{1-2-3}
    α_{4-5}
    α_6
    α_v
	VLA-1/3
	VLA-4-5
	VLA-6
	CD51CD29
		Leukocytes	Laminin, collagens
			JAM-B
			Fibronectin, laminin
			Vitronectin, fibronectin
				Cell matrix-adhesion
				Homing to inflamed tissues

β_2 α_L α_M	LFA-1 MAC-1	Leukocytes	ICAM-1/3, JAM-A	Leukocyte adhesion to endothelium Interaction T cell-APC
β_3 α_V	Vitronectin receptor	Leukocytes, endothelium, osteoclasts	Fibronectin, fibrinogen, osteopontin, vitronectin, thrombospondin	Cell matrix-adhesion Leukocyte activation Osteoclast activation Angiogenesis
β_4 α_6	CD49CD104	Leukocytes	Laminin	Cell matrix-adhesion
β_5 α_V		Leukocytes, endothelium	Vitronectin	Cell matrix-adhesion Angiogenesis
β_6 α_V		Leukocytes	Fibronectin	Cell matrix-adhesion
β_7 α_4	LPAM-1	Leukocytes	VCAM-1, fibronectin	Homing to lymphoid tissues
3. Immunoglobulin Superfamily	ICAM-1 (CD54) ICAM-2 (CD102) VCAM-1 (CD106) PECAM-1 (CD31)	Endothelium* Dendritic cells Endothelium** Leukocytes, endothelium	LFA-1, MAC-1 LFA-1 VLA-4 PECAM-1, $\alpha_V\beta_3$	Cell adhesion Ligands for integrins
4. Cadherins	VE-cadherin	Endothelium lateral junctions	VE-cadherin	Cell to cell adhesion

*Activated endothelial cells
**Resting endothelial cells
APC, Antigen presenting cells; ICAM, intracellular adhesion molecule; JAM, junctional adhesion molecule; LFA, leukocyte function-associated antigen; LPAM1, Lymphocyte peyer's patch adhesion molecule 1; MAC-1, membrane attack complex; MadCAM-1, mucosal addressin cell-adhesion molecule-1; PECAM-1, platelet-endothelial cell adhesion molecule; PLTs, platelets; PSGLs, P-selectin glycoprotein ligands 1; VLA, very late antigen; VE-cadherin, vascular endothelial cadherin.

Table 3–8

Immunopathogenic mechanisms of immune-mediated diseases

Type of Hypersensitivity	Immune-Pathological Mechanisms	Mechanism of Tissue Damage	Human or Animal Model of Autoimmune Diseases
Type I Immediate hypersensitivity	IgE antibody	Activation of mast cells and release of vasoactive mediators	Allergic manifestations (bronchial asthma, anaphylactic shock, urticaria)
Type II Antibody-mediated hypersensitivity	IgM or IgG against cellular or extracellular antigens	1. Recruitment and activation of leukocytes by complement and Fc receptors 2. Opsonization of target cells and complement activation 3. Alteration of normal tissue function	Autoimmune hemolytic anemia Autoimmune thrombocytopenic purpura Goodpasture syndrome Pemphigus vulgaris Acute rheumatic fever Antiphospholipid syndrome Neonatal lupus Myasthenia gravis Graves' disease
Type III Immune-complex mediated hypersensitivity	Tissue deposition of circulating immune-complexes	Recruitment and activation of leukocytes by complement and Fc receptors	Systemic lupus erythematosus Mixed cryoglublinemia Rheumatoid arthritis (rheumatoid factor)
Type IV T cell mediated hypersensitivity	1. Delayed hypersensitivity (CD4 T cells) 2. T-cell mediated cytolysis (CD8 T cells)	Activation of tissue macrophage Direct lysis of target cells	Insulin-dependent diabetes Rheumatoid arthritis Multiple sclerosis Autoimmune myocarditis

During acute inflammation, mast cells and platelets degranulate and secrete histamine and serotonin that increase vascular permeability and vasodilation. Other vasoactive peptides that are stored in sensory neurons, such as substance P, can be released after their activation or generated by proteolytic processing of inactive precursors in the extracellular fluid (e.g., kinins, fibrinopeptide A, fibrinopeptide B, fibrin degradation products). Finally, C5a (and, to a lesser extent, C3a and C4a) promote granulocyte and Mo recruitment and induce mast cell degranulation.[169]

Immune Hypersensitivity

The effector mechanisms in autoimmunity are the same observed during a normal immune response against microbes or other foreign antigens (Table 3–8). The majority of autoimmune diseases are the result of a complex combination of humoral and cellular-mediated immune responses in which multiple effector mechanisms operate.

Type I Hypersensitivity

Immediate (or type I) hypersensitivity is the mode of tissue damage during IgE-mediated allergic diseases. Mast cells involved in this type of response also play a role in non-IgE-mediated autoimmune diseases.[176] However, in the vast majority of autoimmune diseases, the other three types of hypersensitivity predominate.

Type II Hypersensitivity

In humans, transplacental transfer of pathogenic maternal autoantibodies to the fetus causes *neonatal lupus*,[177] "autoimmune" thyroiditis,[178] and "autoimmune" thrombocytopenia.[179]

Antibodies cause tissue damage by different mechanisms (Fig. 3–22). In *type II hypersensitivity*, antibodies opsonize the target cells and activate the complement cascade. Phagocytes of the reticuloendothelial system of secondary lymphoid organs, especially the spleen, are activated by the binding of their Fc or C3 receptors. Antibodies may also activate the complement cascade that ultimately leads to cell lysis. These mechanisms are responsible for cellular destruction in *autoimmune hemolytic anemia* or *autoimmune thrombocytopenic purpura*. Tissue damage is mediated by release of proteolytic agents from phagocytes. This occurs in *acute rheumatic fever,* in which antibodies directed to streptococcal cell wall antigen crossreact with myocardial antigens; *Goodpasture syndrome,* in which the tissue target for autoantibodies is a noncollagenous protein in the basement membranes of kidney glomeruli and lung alveoli; and *pemphigus vulgaris,* in which antibodies are directed against epidermal cadherin. In other circumstances, autoantibodies do not cause inflammation but interfere with the cell receptors' function and cause disease without eliciting tissue damage. This is the case with *Graves' disease,* which is caused by antibody-mediated stimulation of TSH receptors, and with *myasthenia gravis,* in which antibodies inhibit acetylcholine binding and downmodulate receptors.[180]

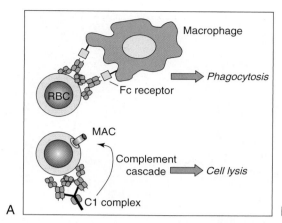
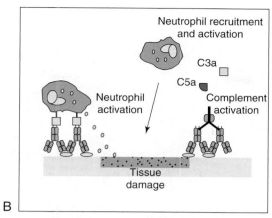

FIGURE 3–22 Examples of antibody-mediated mechanisms of tissue or cellular damage. **A,** Two different modalities of destruction of red blood cells (RBCs) during the course of autoimmune hemolytic anemia are shown. RBC coated by specific antibodies are recognized and are destroyed by macrophages of the reticular endothelial system of secondary lymphoid organs (prevalently the spleen). Antibodies activate the complement cascade that ultimately leads to cellular lyses in the circulation. **B,** Antibodies recruit leukocytes and activate them directly through their Fc receptors and/or indirectly through the complement cascade.

Type III Hypersensitivity

This mechanism of tissue damage is similar to that described for antibodies directly bound to tissue antigens but is mediated by organ deposition of circulating immune complexes. The preferential deposition of immune complexes in small arteries, with particular tropism to those structures in which the blood is ultrafiltered, such as kidney glomeruli and synovia, cause immune complex-mediated diseases, including vasculitis, arthritis, systemic lupus erythematosus, and mixed cryoglobulinemia.[180,181] In both type II and type III hypersensitivity, antigen-specific TH cells are important in the activation and maturation of B cells for the subsequent production of high-affinity autoantibodies.

Type IV Hypersensitivity

In type IV delayed type hypersensitivity (DTH), T cells are responsible for tissue damage. In most instances, damage is induced by the secretion (by TH1 and TH17 subsets of CD4+ T cells, and CD8+ T cells) of cytokines, which activates tissue macrophages (IFN-γ), induces inflammation (TNFα), and recruits and activates neutrophils (IL-17). Occasionally, self-reactive CD8+ cytolytic (CTL) T cells directly kill target cells (see Fig. 3–16).

The findings of T lymphocytes and macrophages in close anatomical proximity in tissue infiltrates and the predominant TH1 orientation of T cells isolated from tissue lesions are evidence of the major involvement of a DTH in many autoimmune disorders. Diseases in which DTH is believed to play a major role are *multiple sclerosis,*[182] *insulin-dependent diabetes mellitus,*[202] *RA*[183] and *juvenile idiopathic arthritis*[184,185] *(JIA)*. However, the recent identification of the role of IL-17 producing cells (TH17) in the generation of autoimmunity has raised the possibility of a role of this T cell subpopulation in DHT. Both IFN-γ and IL-17 producing cells are highly represented in the inflammatory tissue infiltrate in different autoimmune diseases.[186]

A typical example of a DHT-like reaction is represented by the synovitis of JIA. The dramatic hyperplasia of synovial tissue is also due to infiltration of the lining layer

with Mo-derived macrophages recruited from the circulation. These cells, together with the resident fibroblastlike cells, are activated by IFN-producing CD4+ T cells and play the major role in the determining cartilage and bone destruction (Fig. 3–23). However, TH17 T cells are able to play a direct role in the pathogenesis of bone and cartilage damage. IL-17 also promotes bone erosion through the upregulation of RANKL,[186] a key regulator of osteoclast neogenesis. Among the downstream effects of IL-17 is the production of metalloproteinases and proteoglycan breakdown, which leads to cartilage destruction.[187]

A significant infiltration of B cells and plasma cells can also be found in inflamed synovial tissue, with the possible formation of GC-like structures.[188] Figure. 3–23 is a schematic representation of the complex network of various cell interactions in determining tissue damage in chronic synovitis.

Soluble Mediators of Inflammation and the Immune Response

A large number of soluble mediators are involved in the initiation and maintenance of the inflammatory and immune responses.

CYTOKINES

Cytokines and chemokines are proteins secreted by the cells of the innate and adaptive immune systems in response to a possible harmful exogenous stimulus, and they mediate the immune and inflammatory responses. Cytokines usually act locally in autocrine or paracrine fashion. Their functions are mediated via cellular receptors. All cytokine receptors consist of one or more transmembrane protein, whose extracellular portions are responsible for cytokine binding, whereas the cytoplasmatic portions mediate the triggering of the intracellular signaling pathway. According to their functional activity and to the cells producing them, cytokines may be classified into four main categories: (1) cytokines of innate immunity, produced mainly by mononuclear phagocytes in response to infectious agent (Table 3–9); (2) cytokines of adaptive immunity, produced by T lymphocytes after

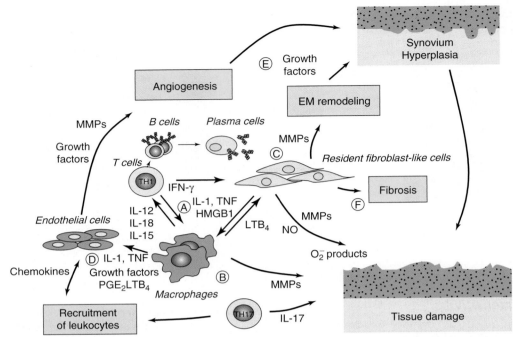

FIGURE 3–23 Schematic representation of the complex network of cells, proinflammatory molecules, and pathogenic events leading to tissue damage during chronic synovitis. Different cell types are involved in the disease process at the level of synovial membranes. **A,** Effector T cells (TH1 and TH17) express a number of cytokines that activate macrophages (IFN-γ) for the production of proinflammatory cytokines, growth factors, and other soluble products or directly contribute to tissue damage (IL-17). **B,** Resident fibroblastlike cells proliferate and become activated. **C,** B cells may cluster in a follicularlike structure with maturation of a large number of antibody-secreting plasma cells. **D,** Proinflammatory cytokines produced by inflammatory cells activate endothelial cells for the continuous recruitment of leukocytes from peripheral blood. **E,** Growth factors and proteolytic enzymes, such as matrix metalloproteinases (MMPs), sustain the continuous remodeling of extracellular matrix (ECM) and formation of new blood vessels from preexisting microvascular (angiogenesis). These are the two key mechanisms for the continuous growth of synovial tissue (hyperplasia), leading to the progressive invasion and destruction of joint cartilage and bones. **F,** Mechanisms involved in the control of tissue inflammation ultimately leads to synovial fibrosis. HMGB-1, High-mobility group box chromosomal protein 1; IFN, interferon; IL, interleukin; LTB$_4$, leukotriene B$_4$; NO, nitric oxide; PGE$_2$, prostaglandin E$_2$; TNF; tumor necrosis factor.

specific recognition of foreign antigens (Table 3–10); (3) chemokines, produced by various cell types that stimulate and regulate leukocyte migration (Table 3–11); and (4) growth factors, produced by bone marrow stromal cells and leukocytes that stimulate the differentiation and proliferation of immature leukocytes and sustain angiogenesis.

Tumor necrosis factor (TNF), is a proinflammatory cytokine produced by activated phagocytes.[189] TNF-α was originally identified in the sera of animals treated with LPS, which displayed the ability to cause tumor necrosis *in vivo*.[190] TNF-α is synthesized as a membrane protein that is expressed as a homodimer. It is cleaved by membrane-associated metalloproteinases and is released as a 17-kD polypeptide, three of which polymerize to form a 51-kD TNF protein. The various biological actions of TNF are mediated by two distinct receptors: the 55 kD TNF receptor I (TNFRI or p55 receptor) and the 75 kD TNFRII (or p75 receptor).[191] The binding of circulating TNF-α to TNFRs leads to the recruitment of cytoplasmic proteins, called TNF receptor-associated factors (TRAFs) that initiate the intracellular signaling leading to the activation of transcription factors, such as NF-kB and activation protein 1 (AP-1), that ultimately cause the production of inflammatory mediators and anti-apoptotic proteins[191] (Fig. 3–24A). Notably, in the case of TNFRI, the binding with TNF-α may lead to

either inflammation or apoptosis. In the latter case, different signaling proteins (TNF receptor-associated death domain [TRADD]) are involved. The activation of this particular intracellular pathway leads to the activation of caspases that eventually result in cell apoptosis (see Fig. 3–24A). This latter mechanism is similar to Fas-mediated apoptosis involved in activation-induced cell death (see Fig. 3–17) and represents an important strategy for self-limitation of cell activation.

The principal function of TNF-α during inflammation is to stimulate the recruitment of phagocytes into the site of tissue damage (Table 3–12). TNF also induces the expression of adhesion molecules and chemokines by endothelial cells and enhances the affinity of leukocyte integrins for their ligands. It can activate recently recruited Mos and stimulate the proinflammatory activity of resident fibroblasts (see Fig. 3–23). When produced in large amounts, TNF-α enters the bloodstream and acts at distant sites as an endocrine hormone. TNF-α is then able to stimulate the hypothalamus to induce fever, to act on hepatocytes for the production of acute phase reactants, and to promote metabolic changes leading to the wasting of muscle and of fat cells (cachexia). Very high levels of circulating TNF-α (> 10-7 M) play a major role in the pathogenesis of septic shock induced by LPS.

The potentially lethal effects of TNF-α are balanced by a strategy for the downregulation of TNF-α activity that

Table 3–9

Main cytokines of innate immunity

Cytokine	Size and Form	Receptors	Main Cell Source	Main Biological Effects
IL-1α IL-1β	17kD, monomer 33kD (precursors)	CD121a, b (IL-1RI and II)	Macrophages, endothelial cells, epithelial cells	Fever Activation of endothelial cells and macrophage Acute phase reactants
TNF-α	17kD homotrimer	p55, p75 (TNFRI, TNFRII)	Macrophages, T cells, NK cells	Fever Activation of endothelial cells, macrophage, and neutrophils Acute phase reactants Apoptosis Cachexia
TNF-β (LT-α)	Homotrimer	p55, p75 (TNFRI, TNFRII)	T cells, B cells	Killing, endothelial activation
Type I IFNs	IFNα: 15-21 kD IFNβ: 20-25 kD monomers	CD118 (IFNAR2)	Leukocytes Fibroblasts	Antiviral response Activation of NK cells
IL-6	19-26 kD, monomer	IL-6R, gp130	T cells, macrophages, endothelial cells	Fever Activation of endothelial cells Acute phase reactants B cell proliferation
IL-7	monomer	CD127, CD132	Non-T cells	Growth of pre-B cells and pre-T cells
IL-10	34-40 kD homodimer	IL-10 Rα CRF2-4	Macrophages T cells (TH2, Treg)	Suppression of macrophage function
IL-12	Heterodimer of 35 and 40 kD*	IL-12 Rβ1 IL-12 Rβ2	DC, B cells Macrophages	Differentiation of TH1 cells Synthesis of IFN-γ by T cells and NK cells
IL-15	13 kd monomer	IL-15 R (CD122)	Macrophages and other non-T cells	NK cells and T cell proliferation
IL-18	17 kD, monomer	IL-1Rrp (α chain) AcPL (β chain)	Macrophage	Synthesis of IFN-γ by T cells and NK cells
IL-23	Heterodimer of 19 and 40 kD*	IL-12 Rβ1 IL-23R	DC	Differentiation TH17 cells
IL-27	P28 and EBI3 heterodimer	WSX-1 + CD130c	Monocytes, macrophages, DC	Induces IL12R on T cells

*IL-12 and IL-23 share the same p40 subunit.
DC, dendritic cells; IFN, interferon; IL, interleukin; NK, natural killer; R, receptor; TNF, tumor necrosis factor; Treg, regulatory T cell.

Table 3–10

Cytokines of adaptive immunity

Cytokine	Size and Form	Receptors	Main Cell Source	Main Biological Effects
IL-2	14-17 kD, monomer	CD25 (α chain) CD122 (β chain) CD132 (γ chain)	T cells	Proliferation and activation of T cells, NK cells Proliferation of B cells and antibody synthesis Fas-mediated apoptosis
IL-4	18 kD, monomer	CD124	T cells (TH2)	Isotype switching to IgE TH2 differentiation Inhibition of IFN-γ- mediated macrophage activation TH1 suppression
IL-5	45 kD homodimer	CD125	T cells (TH2)	Activation and proliferation of eosinophils B cell proliferation and IgA production
IL-13	15 kD, monomer	IL-13 R	T cells (TH2)	B cell proliferation Isotype switching to IgE Inhibition of macrophage activation
IL-17	150 kD monomer	IL-17AR	TH17 T cells, NK cells, CD8 T cells	Neutrophil migration Activation of endothelial cells, macrophage and neutrophils
IL-22	146 homodimer	IL-22Rαc IL10Rβc	TH17 T cells, NK	Acute phase proteins Proinflammatory
IL-25	145 monodimer	IL17BR	TH2 cells, mast cells	Promote TH2 cytokine production

Continued

Table 3–10

Cytokines of adaptive immunity—cont'd

Cytokine	Size and Form	Receptors	Main Cell Source	Main Biological Effects
IFN-γ	50 kD homodimer	CD119 (IFNGR2)	T cells, NK cells	Macrophage activation Ig class switching to opsonizing and complement fixing IgG antibodies TH1 differentiation TH2 suppression
LT-β	Trimerizes with LT-α	LTβR	T cells, B cells	Lymph node development
TGF-β	25 kD homodimer	TGF-βR	T cells (Treg), macrophages	Inhibition of proliferation and effector function of T cells Inhibition of B cell proliferation

IL, interleukin; LT, lymphotoxin; NK, natural killer; TGF, transforming growth factor; Treg, regulatory T cells.

Table 3–11

Main chemokines and chemokine receptors

Class	Name (Previous)	Major Sources	Receptor	Cells Attracted	Main Functions
1. CXC	CXCL1 (Gro-α)	M, F, EC	CXCR2	N, M, Tc, NK	Leukocyte recruitment
	CXCL2 (Gro-β)	M, F, EC	CXCR2	N, M, Tc, NK	Leukocyte recruitment
	CXCL3 (Gro-γ)	M, F, EC	CXCR2	N, M, Tc, NK	Leukocyte recruitment
	CXCL5 (ENA78)	M, F, EC	CXCR2	N	Leukocyte recruitment
	CXCL6 (GCP-2)	M, F, EC	CXCR1	N, M, Tc, NK	Leukocyte recruitment
	CXCL7 (NAP-2)	M, F, EC	CXCR2	N	Neutrophils activation, angiogenesis
	CXCL8 (IL-8)	M, Mo, F, EC	CXCR1/2	N, M, Tc, NK	Neutrophils recruitment and activation
	CXCL9 (MIG)	M, Tc, F, EC	CXCR3	Tc, NK, M	Leukocyte recruitment
	CXCL10 (IP-10)	M, Tc, F, EC	CXCR3	Tc, NK, M	Leukocyte recruitment, TH1 response
	CXCL11 (I-TAC)	M, Tc, F, EC	CXCR3	Tc, NK, M	Leukocyte recruitment
	CXCL12 (SDF-1)	Sc	CXCR4	Naive Tc, Bc	Lymphocyte recruitment
	CXCL13 (BCA-1)	Sc	CXCR5	B cells	Lymphocyte homing to lymphoid organs
2. CC	CCL1 (I-309)	M, Tc, EC	CCR8	M, Tc	Leukocyte recruitment
	CCL2 (MCP-1)	M, F	CCR2	M, NK, Tc, F	Activate macrophage and basophils, TH2 response
	CCL3 (MIP1α)	M, Tc, Mc, F	CCR1/5	M, NK, B, Dc	Leukocyte recruitment, TH1 response
	CCL4 (MIP1β)	M, Mo, N, EC	CCR5	M, NK, Tc, Dc	Leukocyte recruitment, HIV coreceptor
	CCL5 (RANTES)	Tc, EC, P	CCR1/5/3	M, NK, Tc, B, E, Dc	Activation of basophils and Tc Chronic inflammation
	CCL7 (MCP-3)	M, F, P, EC	CCR1/2	E, B, NK	Leukocyte recruitment
	CCL8 (MCP-2)	M, F, EC	CCR2	E, B	Leukocyte recruitment
	CCL11 (Eotaxin)	EC, M, Ep, Tc	CCR3	E, M, Tc (TH2)	Allergy, TH2 response
	CCL13 (MCP-4)	EC, M, Ep	CCR2/4	E, B, Tc	Leukocyte recruitment
	CCL17 (TARC)	EC, M, Ep	CCR4/8	E, B, Tc	T cell and basophil recruitment
	CCL19 (ELC)	SC, EC	CCR7	Tc, Dc	Lymphocyte and Dc recruitment in lymphoid organs
	CCL20 (MIP-3α)	M, Tc, DC, E, Mc	CCR6	Tc, Dc	Lymphocyte and Dc recruitment
	CCL21 (SLC)	SC, EC	CCR7	Tc, Dc	Lymphocyte and Dc recruitment in lymphoid organs
	CCL22 (MDC)	EC, M, Ep	CCR4	E, B	T cell and basophil recruitment
	CCL25 (TECK)	Ep	CCR9/11	Tc	T cell migration
	CCL27 (CTACK)	K, EC	CCR10	Tc	T cell migration to skin
	CCL28 (MEC)	Ep	CCR3/10	Tc	T cell migration to skin
3. C	XCL1 (lymphotactin)	Tc	XCR1	Dc, NK, Tm	Lymphocyte trafficking and development
4. CX₃C	CX₃CL1 (fractalkine)	M, Ec, Mig	CX₃CR1	M, Tc	Leukocyte-endothelium adhesion Brain inflammation

B, basophils; Bc, B cells; DC, dendritic cells; E, eosinophils; Ec, endothelial cells; Ep, epithelial cells; F, fibroblasts; K, keratinocytes; M, monocytes/macrophages; Mc, mast cells; Mig, microglial cells; Mo, macrophages; NK, natural killer cells; P, platelets; Sc, stromal cells; Tc, T cells; Tm, thymocytes.

A

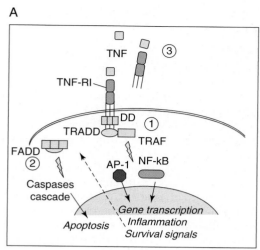

B

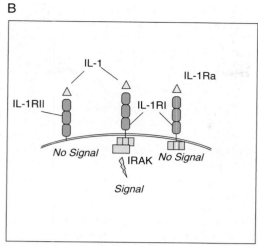

FIGURE 3–24 Mechanisms of cell activation induced by proinflammatory cytokines and strategies for their downregulation. **A,** (1) The binding of circulating TNF-α to TNF receptors (TNFR) leads to the recruitment of cytoplasmatic proteins, called TNF receptor associated factors (TRAFs) that initiate the intracellular signalling; DD, death domain. (2) In the case of TNFRI, the binding with TNF-α may lead to either inflammation or apoptosis. In the latter case, different signalling proteins (Fas-associated death domain [FADD]) are involved. The activation of this particular intracellular pathway, due to the loss of survival signals, leads to the activation of caspases cascade that eventually results in cell apoptosis, representing an important strategy for self-limitation of cell activation. (3) Shedding of TNF receptors from the surface of activated cells and prevention of free TNF-α binding to cellular receptors. **B,** Type I receptor is constitutively expressed on many cell types and mediates the intracellular transmission of the signal after binding with soluble IL-1 through the activation of the IL-1 receptor-associated kinase (IRAK) that eventually leads to cell activation. Type II receptor (decoy receptor) is expressed only after cell activation and lacks a cytoplasmatic tail. Thus, the binding with IL-1 does not result in intracellular signal transmission. Activated macrophages also secrete a protein with a close structural homology to IL-1 that bind to the same surface receptors but is biologically inactive; IL-Ra, IL-1 receptor antagonist.

is related to the shedding of TNFRs from the surface of activated cells, thus generating circulating soluble receptors that prevent the binding of free TNF-α to cell-bound receptors (see Fig. 3–24A). This strategy has been successfully adopted for the therapeutic blockade of TNF activities.[189]

IL-1 shares many biological functions with TNF.[176,192] Like TNF, its major source is activated macrophages, although neutrophils, epithelial cells, and endothelial

cells can also produce IL-1. There are two different 33-kD isoforms of circulating IL-1 (IL-1α and IL-1β). Biologically active IL-1β is a 17-kD protein released from the cell after cleavage by caspase-1 after activation of the inflammasome (see Fig. 3–4).

There are two different membrane receptors for IL-1. Type I receptor is constitutively expressed on many cell types and mediates the intracellular transmission of the signal after binding with soluble IL-1 through the activation of the IL-1 receptor-associated kinase (IRAK), which eventually leads to activation of NF-kB and AP-1 transcription factors (Fig. 3–24B).[193] Type II receptor is expressed only after cell activation and lacks a cytoplasmic tail; consequently, binding with IL-1 does not result in intracellular signal transmission. Thus, its major function is to downmodulate the biological action of IL-1, acting as a "decoy" receptor in competition with type I receptor (see Fig. 3–24B).[194]

A second strategy also downmodulates IL-1 activities. Activated macrophages secrete a protein with a close structural homology to IL-1, which binds to the same surface receptors but is biologically inactive (IL-1 receptor antagonist [IL-Ra]) (see Fig. 3–24B).[195]

This natural pathway of regulation of IL-1 biological activity has been adopted with the use of recombinant IL-1Ra in the treatment of many inflammatory conditions.[166,196,197] A genetic defect in the expression of IL-1Ra has been recently associated to a severe neonatal autoinflammatory disease, called deficiency of IL-1 receptor antagonist (DIRA).[198]

The biological functions of IL-1 largely overlap, both locally and systemically, with those described for TNF (see Table 3–12).

Table 3–12

Main systemic biological effects of IL-1, TNF-α, and IL-6 during inflammation

	IL-1	TNF-α	IL-6
CNS			
Fever	++	+	+++
Production CRH	+	+	++
Liver			
Acute phase reactants	+	+	++
Endothelium			
Chemokine expression	++	++	+
Adhesion molecules	+++	+++	+
Neoangiogenesis	++	+++	-
Bone Marrow			
Myelopoiesis	++	-	++
Thrombocytopoiesis	-	-	+++
Inhibition of erythropoiesis	++	++	++

CNS, central nervous system; CRH, corticotrophin-releasing hormone; IL, Interleukin; TNF, tumor necrosis factor.

IL-6 is produced by macrophages, endothelial cells, and tissue fibroblasts during acute and chronic inflammation.[182, 199] Its biological actions are mediated by binding with an IL-6 receptor present on cell membranes or in soluble form; this complex then binds to a signal transducing subunit called gp130, which is also involved in signal transduction for other cytokines.[200]

IL-6 has many proinflammatory functions (see Table 3–12). It stimulates the synthesis of acute phase reactants by the liver and the production of neutrophils from bone marrow. It induces endothelial cell activation, fibroblast proliferation, and osteoclast activation. A large body of evidence has stressed the central role of this cytokine in systemic JIA. Many of the clinical features peculiar to this disease (chronic anemia, severe growth retardation, osteoporosis, thrombocytosis, amyloidosis) have been related to the biological actions of IL-6.[201-203] Recently, the use of anti-IL-6 receptor monoclonal antibodies has been shown to be a promising therapeutic option for systemic JIA.[204]

Cells of innate immunity isolated from inflamed tissues characterized by a prevalent DHT response also produce other cytokines, which facilitate the crosstalk between cells of innate and adaptive immune response. IL-12, IL-18, and IL-23 (together with IL-1 and Il-6) are key inducers of cell-mediated immunity that may contribute to the differentiation of recently recruited CD4+ TH cells into IFN-γ producing TH1 cells or IL-17 producing TH17 cells.

CHEMOKINES

Chemokines (chemotactic cytokines) are small cytokines (8-15 kDa) that control the trafficking of leukocytes.[205] According to the motif displayed by the first two cysteine residues near the amino terminus, chemokines are classified into four families: CC, CXC, C, and CX3C (see Table 3–11). Chemokines are produced by leukocytes and by endothelial cells, fibroblasts, and epithelial cells. Chemokines can be broadly classified in two main classes: inflammatory and lymphoid (or homing).[162] The inflammatory chemokines are produced by leukocytes in response to a proinflammatory stimulus. Homing chemokines are constitutively expressed in the microenvironment of lymphoid tissues, skin, and mucosa and are involved in the continuous leukocyte trafficking between circulation and lymphoid structures. Examples include CCL19, CCL21, and CXC13, together with their specific cellular receptors CCR7 and CXCR5 in secondary lymphoid organs.[206]

The chemokines induce cytoskeletal rearrangements by stimulating alternating polymerization and depolymerization of actin filaments that eventually lead to cell mobilization. Expression of different chemokine receptors on the surface of circulating leukocytes is closely related to their specific function, state of differentiation, and degree of activation (see Table 3–11).

Many inflammatory chemokines and leukocytes displaying their specific surface receptors have been identified in inflamed tissues. In particular, some receptors for inflammatory chemokines CCR1, CCR2, CCR5, and CXCR3 are regularly detected in tissues where inflammation is characterized by chronic infiltration of macrophages and predominantly T lymphocytes (i.e., RA and Crohn disease).[207] The selective blockade of inflammatory chemokines and their cellular receptors is

a promising possible strategy for the treatment of many autoimmune disorders.[208]

GROWTH FACTORS

During chronic inflammation, growth factors are secreted by inflammatory cells. Platelet-derived growth factor (PDGF), basic fibroblast growth factor (bFGF), transforming growth factor β (TGF-β), epidermal growth factor (EGF), and vascular endothelial growth factor (VEGF) play a role in the induction of angiogenesis,[209] whereby new blood vessels develop from preexisting microvascular bed. During chronic inflammation, this process provides oxygen and nutrients to meet the high metabolic requirement of resident cells and permits the migration and progressive infiltration of newly recruited inflammatory cells. Angiogenesis supports the extensive vascularization occurring during the proliferation of rheumatoid pannus (see Fig. 3–23).[210]

Prostaglandins and Leukotrienes

Prostaglandins (PGs) and *leukotrienes (LTs)* are acid lipids derived from enzymatic cleavage of the membrane lipid arachidonic acid and are produced by most mammalian cells in response to mechanical, chemical, and immunological stimuli. The activation of the enzyme phospholipase A2 releases arachidonic acid that is further metabolized by two main enzymatic pathways leading to the final production of a class of mediators belonging to the family of bioactive eicosanoids (Fig. 3–25 (online only)).

Cyclooxygenases (COX) are responsible for the production of PGs both in physiological and pathological conditions. Two different isoforms of COX are currently known. COX-1 is constitutively expressed at a constant level in most tissues. Indeed, PGs are physiologically produced in many tissues and regulate many functions, including platelet-dependent homeostasis, renal blood flow, and gastric mucosal integrity. Conversely, COX-2 is normally undetectable in normal tissues, but it can be rapidly induced by fibroblasts, Mos, and endothelial cells upon proinflammatory stimulation. Thus, activation of COX-2 is thought to play a major role in the inflammatory reactions.[211] Together with the mast cell-derived PGD2, the most abundant separately COX-2 product is PGE2. It can sensitize nerve endings to painful chemical and mechanical stimuli and acts as a potent vasodilator. Furthermore, PGE2 has a crucial role in the induction of fever after stimulation of specialized endothelial cells in hypothalamic tissue by endogenous pyrogens (such as TNF and IL-6).

LTs are derived from the combined actions of 5-lipoxygenases (5-LOX) and 5-LOX–activating protein (FLAP) with initial formation of 5-hydroperoxyeicosatetraenoic acid (5-HPETE), followed by LTA4 and LTA4B. LTB4 is rapidly synthesized by neutrophils and macrophages upon challenge with stimuli, such as microbial pathogens, toxins, aggregated Igs, and proinflammatory cytokines. LTB4 is one of the most powerful chemoattractants, and it induces neutrophil aggregation, degranulation, and macrophage production of proinflammatory cytokines 02- and PGE2.[212]

Lipoxins (LXs) are efficient endogenous mediators of inflammation resolution.[213] LXs are produced after activation of two distinct intracellular pathways depending on the cell involved and the mode of activation. Activation of adherent platelets leads to the activation of 12-LOX that ultimately results in the production of lipoxin A4 and B4.[213] A second pathway of LX production occurs in Mos and macrophages exposed to IL-4 and IL-13. In this case, LX production is initiated by a 15-LO that leads to the generation and release of 15S-hydroxy eicosatetraenoic acid (HETE), which is rapidly taken up and converted by polymorphonucleates to LXs.[213] Therefore, in peripheral blood neutrophils, a switch in ecoisanoid biosynthesis from predominantly proinflammatory molecules (PGE2 and LTB4) to antiinflammatory LX production occurs. Notably, PGE5 itself promotes both 5-LOX and 12-LOX gene expression, thus initiating a mechanism of self limitation of inflammation. LXs display a number of antiinflammatory activities in many animal models of inflammatory diseases, mainly to the inhibition of recruitment of inflammatory cells.[169]

Nitric Oxide and Reactive Oxygen Products

Nitric oxide (NO) is produced by mammalian cells by the action of NO synthetase (NOS).[214] During inflammation, inducible NOS is activated by proinflammatory cytokines (IFN-γ, IL17, TNF, IL-1). This enzyme catalyzes the production of NO and L-citrulline from L-arginine and molecular oxygen. The induction of NO under conditions of immune activation can be both beneficial, in the eradication of micro-organisms, and harmful by causing tissue damage.[214]

Generation of reactive oxygen products is essential for the microbicidial activity of phagocytes and directly mediated tissue damage in acute and chronic inflammatory conditions. Their generation is mediated by the activation of NADPH oxidase, an enzyme located in the plasma membrane of phagocytes. The activation of NADPH oxidase leads to the formation of superoxide (O_2^-). O_2^- spontaneously dismutases into hydrogen peroxide (H_2O_2), which may react with chloride ions to form the toxic hypochlorous acid (HOCl) in a reaction catalyzed by myeloperoxidase. This latter enzyme is abundantly present in the preformed granules of phagocytes, and it is rapidly released after cell activation.[215]

Proteolytic Enzymes

Myeloperoxidase and a number of other proteolytic enzymes are abundantly present in the granules of professional phagocytes, such as neutrophils.[216] Among them are serine proteinases (elastases, cathepsin G), acid hydrolases (β-glucuronidase, α-mannosidoses), and other peptides with bactericidal activity (lysozyme, defensins, lactoferrin, azurocidin).

Matrix metalloproteinases (MMPs) are proteolytic enzymes produced by fibroblasts, macrophages, neutrophils, and chondrocytes upon stimulation with proinflammatory cytokines and growth factors.[217] Their main function is the remodeling of ECM during tissue resorption. Thus, the proteolytic activity of MMPs is a crucial component of both physiological (embryonic development, organ morphogenesis, angiogenesis) and pathological (chronic inflammatory diseases, tumors) conditions. MMPs are one of the most important classes of final mediators of tissue damage in many chronic inflammatory conditions, including RA.[218]

REFERENCES

1. R. Medzhitov, C. Janeway Jr., Innate immunity, N. Engl. J. Med. 343 (2000) 338–344.
2. C. Nathan, Neutrophils and immunity: challenges and opportunities, Nat. Rev. Immunol. 6 (2006) 173–182.
3. R. Medzhitov, Recognition of microorganisms and activation of the immune response, Nature 449 (2007) 819–826.
4. R. Medzhitov, Toll-like receptors and innate immunity, Nat. Rev. Immunol. 1 (2001) 135–145.
5. K. Takeda, S. Akira, Toll-like receptors in innate immunity, Int. Immunol. 17 (2005) 1–14.
6. S. Akira, S. Uematsu, O. Takeuchi, Pathogen recognition and innate immunity, Cell 124 (2006) 783–801.
7. T.H. Mogensen, Pathogen recognition and inflammatory signaling in innate immune defenses, Clin. Microbiol. Rev. 22 (2009) 240–273.
8. J.M. Wilmanski, T. Petnicki-Ocwieja, K.S. Kobayashi, NLR proteins: integral members of innate immunity and mediators of inflammatory diseases, J. Leukoc. Biol. 83 (2008) 13–30.
9. L. Franchi, N. Warner, K. Viani, et al., Function of Nod-like receptors in microbial recognition and host defense, Immunol. Rev. 227 (2009) 106–128.
10. M. Yoneyama, M. Kikuchi, T. Natsukawa, et al., The RNA helicase RIG-I has an essential function in double-stranded RNA-induced innate antiviral responses, Nat. Immunol. 5 (2004) 730–737.
11. T.D. Kanneganti, M. Lamkanfi, G. Nunez, Intracellular NOD-like receptors in host defense and disease, Immunity 27 (2007) 549–559.
12. L. Agostini, F. Martinon, K. Burns, et al., NALP3 forms an IL-1beta-processing inflammasome with increased activity in Muckle-Wells autoinflammatory disorder, Immunity 20 (2004) 319–325.
13. M.E. Bianchi, DAMPs, PAMPs and alarmins: all we need to know about danger, J. Leukoc. Biol. 81 (2007) 1–5.
14. L.A. O'Neill, A.G. Bowie, The family of five: TIR-domain-containing adaptors in Toll-like receptor signalling, Nat. Rev. Immunol. 7 (2007) 353–364.
15. T. Kawai, O. Takeuchi, T. Fujita, et al., Lipopolysaccharide stimulates the MyD88-independent pathway and results in activation of IFN-regulatory factor 3 and the expression of a subset of lipopolysaccharide-inducible genes, J. Immunol. 167 (2001) 5887–5894.
16. C. Wang, L. Deng, M. Hong, et al., TAK1 is a ubiquitin-dependent kinase of MKK and IKK, Nature 412 (2001) 346–351.
17. L. Chang, M. Karin, Mammalian MAP kinase signalling cascades, Nature 410 (2001) 37–40.
18. A. Rubartelli, F. Cozzolino, M. Talio, et al., A novel secretory pathway for interleukin-1 beta, a protein lacking a signal sequence, EMBO J. 9 (1990) 1503–1510.
19. C. Andrei, C. Dazzi, L. Lotti, et al., The secretory route of the leaderless protein interleukin 1beta involves exocytosis of endolysosome-related vesicles, Mol. Biol. Cell 10 (1999) 1463–1475.
20. S. Mariathasan, D.S. Weiss, K. Newton, et al., Cryopyrin activates the inflammasome in response to toxins and ATP, Nature 440 (2006) 228–232.
21. F. Martinon, K. Burns, J. Tschopp, The inflammasome: a molecular platform triggering activation of inflammatory caspases and processing of proIL-beta, Mol. Cell 10 (2) (2002) 417–426.
22. F. Martinon, L. Agostini, E. Meylan, et al., Identification of bacterial muramyl dipeptide as activator of the NALP3/cryopyrin inflammasome, Curr. Biol. 14 (2004) 1929–1934.
23. J. Banchereau, R.M. Steinman, Dendritic cells and the control of immunity, Nature 392 (1998) 245–252.
24. F. Sallusto, A. Lanzavecchia, Understanding dendritic cell and T-lymphocyte traffic through the analysis of chemokine receptor expression, Immunol. Rev. 177 (2000) 134–140.
25. R.M. Steinman, J. Banchereau, Taking dendritic cells into medicine, Nature 449 (2007) 419–426.
26. N. Kadowaki, S. Ho, S. Antonenko, et al., Subsets of human dendritic cell precursors express different toll-like receptors and respond to different microbial antigens, J. Exp. Med. 194 (2001) 863–869.
27. P. Blanco, A.K. Palucka, M. Gill, et al., Induction of dendritic cell differentiation by IFN-alpha in systemic lupus erythematosus, Science 294 (2001) 1540–1543.

28. A. Moretta, E. Marcenaro, S. Parolini, et al., NK cells at the interface between innate and adaptive immunity, Cell Death Differ. 15 (2008) 226–233.
29. L. Moretta, C. Bottino, D. Pende, et al., Human natural killer cells: their origin, receptors and function, Eur. J. Immunol. 32 (2002) 1205–1211.
30. C.D. Buckley, D. Pilling, J.M. Lord, et al., Fibroblasts regulate the switch from acute resolving to chronic persistent inflammation, Trends Immunol. 22 (2001) 199–204.
31. A. Uccelli, L. Moretta, V. Pistoia, Mesenchymal stem cells in health and disease, Nat. Rev. Immunol. 8 (2008) 726–736.
32. H. Molina, Complement and immunity, Rheum. Dis. Clin. North Am. 30 (2004) 1–18.
33. R.F. Guo, P.A. Ward, Role of C5a in inflammatory responses, Annu. Rev. Immunol. 23 (2005) 821–852.
34. P.R. Taylor, A. Carugati, V.A. Fadok, et al., A hierarchical role for classical pathway complement proteins in the clearance of apoptotic cells in vivo, J. Exp. Med. 192 (2000) 359–366.
35. H.T. Cook, M. Botto, Mechanisms of disease: the complement system and the pathogenesis of systemic lupus erythematosus, Nat. Clin. Pract. Rheumatol. 2 (2006) 330–337.
36. M. Botto, M. Kirschfink, P. Macor, et al., Complement in human diseases: lessons from complement deficiencies, Mol. Immunol. 46 (2009) 2774–2783.
37 D.C. Kilpatrick, T.E. Delahooke, C. Koch, et al., Mannan-binding lectin and hepatitis C infection, Clin. Exp. Immunol. 132 (2003) 92–95.
38. B. Bottazzi, C. Garlanda, A. Cotena, et al., The long pentraxin PTX3 as a prototypic humoral pattern recognition receptor: interplay with cellular innate immunity, Immunol. Rev. 227 (2009) 9–18.
39. T. Ganz, Defensins: antimicrobial peptides of innate immunity, Nat. Rev. Immunol. 3 (2003) 710–720.
40. J. Wehkamp, M. Schmid, E.F. Stange, Defensins and other antimicrobial peptides in inflammatory bowel disease, Curr. Opin. Gastroenterol. 23 (2007) 370–378.
41. T.W. LeBien, T.F. Tedder, B lymphocytes: how they develop and function, Blood 112 (2008) 1570–1580.
42. R.R. Hardy, Y.S. Li, D. Allman, et al., B-cell commitment, development and selection, Immunol. Rev. 175 (2000) 23–32.
43. B. Schiemann, J.L. Gommerman, K. Vora, et al., An essential role for BAFF in the normal development of B cells through a BCMA-independent pathway, Science 293 (2001) 2111–2114.
44. L.J. Heyzer-Williams, M.G. Heyzer-Williams, Antigen-specific memory B cell development, Annu. Rev. Immunol. 23 (2005) 487–513.
45. T. Lopes-Carvalho, J. Foote, J.F. Kearney, Marginal zone B cells in lymphocyte activation and regulation, Curr. Opin. Immunol. 17 (2005) 244–250.
46. K. Hayakawa, S.A. Shinton, M. Asano, et al., B-1 cell definition, Curr. Top. Microbiol. Immunol. 252 (2000) 15–22.
47. S. Fagarasan, T. Honjo, T-Independent immune response: new aspects of B cell biology, Science 290 (2000) 89–92.
48. D.T. Fearon, M.C. Carroll, Regulation of B lymphocyte responses to foreign and self-antigens by the CD19/CD21 complex, Annu. Rev. Immunol. 18 (2000) 393–422.
49. J. Stavnezer, J.E. Guikema, C.E. Schrader, Mechanism and regulation of class switch recombination, Annu. Rev. Immunol. 26 (2008) 261–292.
50. M. Raghavan, P.J. Bjorkman, Fc receptors and their interactions with immunoglobulins, Annu. Rev. Cell Dev. Biol. 12 (1996) 181–220.
51. W.E. Paul, R.A. Seder, Lymphocyte responses and cytokines, Cell 76 (1994) 241–251.
52. L. Zhou, M.M. Chong, D.R. Littman, Plasticity of CD4+ T cell lineage differentiation, Immunity 30 (2009) 646–655.
53. P. Wong, E.G. Pamer, CD8 T cell responses to infectious pathogens, Annu. Rev. Immunol. 21 (2003) 29–70.
54. J.D. Ashwell, Antigen-driven T cell expansion: affinity rules, Immunity 21 (2004) 603–604.
55. S.A. Muljo, M.S. Schlissel, Pre-B and pre-T-cell receptors: conservation of strategies in regulating early lymphocyte development, Immunol. Rev. 175 (2000) 80–93.
56. R.M. Zinkernagel, P.C. Doherty, The discovery of MHC restriction, Immunol Today 18 (1997) 14–17.
57. H. Li, M.I. Lebedeva, A.S. Llera, et al., Structure of the delta domain of a human gammadelta T-cell antigen receptor, Nature 391 (1998) 502–506.
58. A.C. Hayday, [gamma][delta] cells: a right time and a right place for a conserved third way of protection, Annu. Rev. Immunol. 18 (2000) 975–1026.
59. E.J. Peterson, G.A. Koretzky, Signal transduction in T lymphocytes, Clin. Exp. Rheumatol. 17 (1999) 107–114.
60. M.A. Basson, R. Zamoyska, The CD4/CD8 lineage decision: integration of signalling pathways, Immunol. Today 21 (2000) 509–514.

Entire reference list is available online at www.expertconsult.com.

Chapter 4

INFLAMMATION

Berent J. Prakken and Salvatore Albani

INTRODUCTION

The previous chapter described the elements of the immune system in great detail. This chapter highlights immunity and inflammation in relation to chronic inflammatory arthritis. The delicate balance between inflammation and immune tolerance is normally tightly controlled but the balance is broken in autoimmune diseases such as Juvenile Idiopathic Arthritis (JIA) and Rheumatoid Arthritis (RA). New insights into how the immune system normally handles inflammation have greatly added to our understanding of the pathogenesis of these and other autoimmune diseases.

WHAT INITIATES CHRONIC INFLAMMATION?

In normal circumstances, the inflammatory immune response is self-limiting. This is not the case in diseases such as JIA and RA, however, as the normal self-limiting immune response is turned into a nonremitting process, which leads to damage. This damage by itself attracts more proinflammatory mediators that continue to promote the ongoing inflammatory reflex. Thus, it leads to self-sustaining loops of inflammation, which are resistant to the normal feedback mechanisms.[1] What initiates this chronic inflammatory immune response becomes, at this point, less relevant, unless the causing agent is still present and is provoking the inflammatory response. Lyme arthritis could be an example of chronic arthritis maintained by persistence of a microorganism fueling the immune response.[2,3] However, in most instances, this is not the case. By the time the patient comes to see the physician with complaints of chronic arthritis, the supposed originally initiating micro-organism already has disappeared. Thus, although a potential causal agent sets off the inflammatory reflex, it does not actively contribute to the chronicity of the disease. This is called a "hit and run" scenario,[4] which includes the premise that not one but various, possibly very different, environmental factors can be involved in the development of a chronic inflammatory response. Despite various very extensive studies, no definite proof of any single microorganism causing human autoimmune diseases exists.[2,5,6]

THE PATHOLOGICAL IMMUNE RESPONSE

As discussed earlier, it appears that multiple triggers can cause a chronic inflammatory response in genetically susceptible individuals. The resulting inflammatory responses, however, are remarkably similar and nonspecific. In JIA, the synovial tissue (ST) becomes hyperplastic and is infiltrated by a large variety of cells of both the innate and adaptive immune systems.[7,8] Innate immunity cells involved in the inflammatory process are neutrophils, macrophages, and fibroblasts. There is also an infiltration of cells of the adaptive immune system, such as CD4+ and CD8+ T cells, dendritic cells (DCs) and B cells.[9,10] The following discussion will focus on the major players in the regulation of inflammation in JIA: innate immunity, focusing on damage- or pathogen- associated molecular patterns (DAMP or PAMP); adaptive immunity, focusing on the role of T cells in both promoting and down-regulating inflammation; and cytokines, the soluble mediators that drive both innate and adaptive immunity.

INNATE IMMUNITY AND INFLAMMATION

As discussed in Chapter 3, the innate immune system forms the first line of defense against a pathogen and initiates the inflammatory response. Though not specific for a particular antigen, most innate immune cells harbor pattern recognition receptors (PRRs), including toll-like receptors (TLRs) that can respond to identifiable damage- or pathogen-associated molecular patterns (DAMPs or PAMPs). The activation of TLRs sets off an inflammatory cascade that leads to the activation of the cells of the innate immune system and the production of cytokines and other soluble mediators. Normally, activation of cells of innate immunity through PRRs will further increase the inflammatory response. To minimize risks to the host, mechanisms are in place to limit the innate immune activation through PRRs. First of all, almost simultaneously with immune activation there is also activation of down-regulatory mechanisms. These mechanisms include the production of IL-10 by innate cells and a temporary unresponsiveness to subsequent signaling through PRRs, as in so-called endotoxin tolerance.[11,12] These counter-regulatory loops help limit the inflammatory response. A second mechanism has more recently been described. Consistent with the danger concept, it has been demonstrated that signaling through PRRs is fundamentally different between sterile and nonsterile organs. In sterile organs, activation of PRRs by PAMPs always leads to immune activation, which makes sense because sterile organ pathogens should not be present. However, recently it was shown that in nonsterile organs such as the gut, the continuous interaction between PAMPS and innate immune receptors does not normally lead to full activation.[13,14] This organ-specific innate immune response is part of the symbiotic relationship with the abundantly present micro-organisms.[15-17] The innate immune system can judge danger and, depending on specific organ physiology, act differently as a result.

Understanding the molecular pathways that underlie the physiological organ-specificity of innate immunity could pave the way for new therapeutic approaches based on these physiological mechanisms.

S100 Proteins Leading the Way

PRRs and the molecules that can activate them are crucial for the first phase of the inflammatory response. They are also pivotal contributors to the pathological process of chronic inflammation, as in JIA. For this reason, DAMP molecules are suggested as biomarkers of inflammation. This concept has been strongly advanced by studies on a group of DAMP molecules known as calcium binding proteins or myeloid-related proteins (MRPs), which are also called S100 proteins.[18-20] S100 proteins are expressed intracellularly in granulocytes, monocytes, and macrophages during early differentiation stages and are released when cells are activated or damaged. They act as mediators of the inflammatory reflex; they have strong proinflammatory effects on other cells by acting as endogenous activators of PRRs, including TLRs.[4] Most information about arthritis and inflammation comes from various studies performed with MRP-8 (S100A8) and MRP-14 (S100A9). S100A8 and S100A9 form a heterodimeric complex and are secreted after cell activation. These proteins are present in elevated concentration in the blood and synovial fluid (SF) from patients with varying forms of chronic arthritis.[21-25] The high levels in SF suggest that they are released locally by phagocytes that infiltrate the synovium. Notably, serum levels of S100A8/9 correlate better with joint inflammation and destruction than CRP and erythrocyte sedimentation rate. This is even more striking in systemic JIA. In these patients, elevated levels of S100A8/A9 can help to differentiate systemic JIA not only from healthy controls but also from patients with infections and even leukemia. Recent data showed that elevated levels of these proteins in patients with polyarticular JIA, who are in long-term remission while on MTX therapy, predict a higher risk for relapse after discontinuing MTX therapy. This is an important finding, because no clinical or other laboratory data show evidence of residual diseases activity in these patients. Elevated levels of S100A8/A9 reveal subclinical inflammation in patients who otherwise appear to be completely in remission. This unnoticed inflammation could be important in guiding therapy in patients with JIA. Also, as S100A8/A9 proteins clearly correlate with disease activity, they may be targets for immune therapy.

Another calcium-binding molecule, S100A12 (EN-RAGE), is markedly elevated in serum of patients with Kawasaki disease and is a more reliable predictor of the disease than conventional parameters of inflammation such as CRP and ESR.[25a]

Levels of calcium-binding proteins reflect local and systemic inflammation in JIA, Kawasaki disease, and various other autoimmune diseases, which makes them both potential biomarkers and targets for immune therapy.

Cytokines in Inflammatory Arthritis

Inflammation in JIA and RA is characterized by a chronic activation of both adaptive and innate immunity. The result is an ongoing and nonremitting inflammation, in which it is extremely difficult to dissect the contribution of various individual immune cells. All immune cells that play a role in the synovial inflammation rely on the production of soluble mediators: cytokines, chemokines, and other mediators, such as S100 proteins, for their proinflammatory effect. Cytokines are an important driving force in this ongoing inflammatory reflex.[26,27] This is underlined by the fact that cytokines can both activate and regulate cells from both adaptive and innate immunity. Therefore, they form a crucial link among the different cells that contribute to synovial inflammation. The importance of cytokines in the pathogenesis of JIA and RA has been highlighted by the success of therapeutic approaches directed against cytokines and cytokine receptors. Apart from being targets of therapy, measurement of cytokines during an inflammatory response provides insight into the ongoing inflammation and serves as a biomarker for an immune mechanism.

Cytokines themselves are nonspecific, as very different cells and cell types can produce them. They are characterized by their redundancy and pleiotropy: multiple cytokines can target the same receptor, whereas a single cytokine can have multiple, even contradictory, immunological effects. Therefore, measurement of single cytokines has very limited value. However, cytokine signatures that include multiple cytokines in plasma can reveal different clustering of cytokines among patients with different inflammatory diseases.[28,29] Cytokine concentrations in plasma of patients with JIA increase significantly during active disease.[30-34] This is more clearly seen in SF than in plasma, with a remarkable increase of many chemokines with both Th1 (IL-6, IL-15, CCL2, CCL3, CCL5, CXCL8, CXCL9 and CXCL10) and Th2 signatures (CCL11 and CCL22)[7] (see Chapter 3). These chemokines may have a dual function in JIA. On the one hand, they can attract more inflammatory cells, while they also can have a role in counterbalancing the dominant inflammatory milieu by attracting regulatory T cells.

Furthermore, there is a clear difference in the cytokine pattern between systemic JIA and oligoarticular or polyarticular JIA, indicating that inflammation in systemic JIA probably has a different immune pathogenesis. In systemic JIA the inflammatory profile is strongly biased toward cytokines from the IL-1 family, such as IL-1 and IL-18, similar to the profile of autoinflammatory diseases.[35-38] In JIA, even during apparent clinical remission, levels of several inflammatory proteins are increased in plasma, which is consistent with the earlier-mentioned observation that a significant proportion of JIA patients in full clinical remission on MTX therapy still have markedly elevated levels of the calcium-binding proteins S100A8/A9. This subclinical inflammation may determine the risk of disease reactivation after stopping therapy. It is conceivable that in the future biomarker profiles that include S100 proteins, cytokines, and yet to be determined soluble markers of inflammation may allow the physician to make a more evidence-based and individualized decision about discontinuing, continuing, or even intensifying treatment of patients with similar clinical features.

THE ADAPTIVE IMMUNE RESPONSE AND INFLAMMATION

The innate immune system is crucial both for the rapid induction of an immune response and for sustaining a pathological response, but its mode of action is nonspecific. The adaptive immune response is highly specific and is needed to mount an inflammatory response tailor-made for the inflammatory insult whether the danger signal involves an external antigen (pathogen) or a self-antigen. This again may involve various cell types, most importantly B cells, dendritic cells, and T cells.

B Cells and Pathological Inflammation

That B cells play a role in autoimmune inflammation has been suggested ever since the first description of autoantibodies in human autoimmune diseases. The relationship between rheumatoid factor (RF), cyclic citrullinated peptide (CCP) antibodies, and RA has underscored this relationship. The realization that CCP antibodies in otherwise healthy individuals increases the risk for the subsequent development of RA also clearly points to a direct association between B cells and the development of an autoimmune disease. The mechanisms by which anti-CCP and RF contribute to the pathological inflammatory response in RA are still largely unknown. However, the remarkable success of anti-B cell therapy with rituximab in RA has confirmed the importance of B cell-mediated immunity in chronic arthritis. The pathological immune response in RF-positive JIA is probably similar to RA. It is far less clear what role B cells play in RF-negative JIA.[39,40] Antinuclear antibodies are present, especially in oligoarticular JIA, and their presence relates to subtype, prognosis, and additional risk factors.[41] However, there is no indication

that those antibodies are directly related to the immune pathogenesis of inflammation in those patients. It is more likely that their presence reflects the type of inflammation but is not directly involved in the pathological process.

Dendritic Cells Direct the Adaptive Inflammatory Response

Dendritic cells are central regulators of the adaptive inflammatory response and are crucial for mounting an appropriate immune response in the periphery. There are several subtypes of DCs, and their precise role is dependent on their lineage and maturation stage. One DC subtype, human plasmacytoid DCs, can induce T cells to differentiate into suppressor or regulatory T cells (Tregs) that can contribute to down-regulation of inflammation. These "tolerogenic DCs" act through various mechanisms, which are not yet fully understood but include the production of cytokines, such as IL10 and TGFβ, and the expression of tolerogenic costimulatory molecules (PD1/PDL-l, BT7.2, ICOS). This process of regulation of inflammation steered by DCs is not a one-way route as Tregs can down regulate the expression of costimulatory molecules on DCs.[42-46] This can inhibit effective antigen presentation to other neighboring effector T cells and thus may lead to spreading or "infectious tolerance."

Given the central role of DCs in regulating the inflammatory response, it is highly attractive to think of therapeutic application of this characteristic with the purpose of specifically down regulating a pathogenic inflammatory response. Indeed several approaches are now being explored in both experimental models and proof of concept studies in humans to specifically target DCs. This is achieved by pharmacological approaches with immunosuppressive drugs or by manipulation of DC's *ex vivo*.[45,48]

T Cells and Inflammation

In concert with DCs, T cells are central in the regulation of inflammatory processes. In JIA, there is ample evidence for a role of T cells in directing the autoimmune inflammation.

First of all, JIA is associated with multiple HLA class II genes, suggesting that susceptibility for JIA is based, at least in part, on the shaping of the T cell repertoire.[49-53] Moreover, inflamed synovial tissue (ST) from JIA patients is characterised by an infiltrate that contains activated T cells, clustered around antigen-presenting (dendritic) cells.[7-10,54-56] These T cells are clonally expanded in the synovial fluid (SF) compared with peripheral blood, and have an activated, memory phenotype that implies selective recruitment into the synovial infiltrate.

It is assumed that T cells initiate the first autoimmune inflammatory insult by triggering a pathological immune response toward self-antigens. However, with the exception of Borrelia, no single autoimmunity triggering self-antigen has been identified in chronic childhood arthritis. Given the heterogeneous genetic background of JIA, it is more likely that multiple different environmental triggers can set off autoimmune inflammation in a genetically predisposed subject. This presumption makes the search for disease triggering autoantigens in JIA both difficult and of less interest. Even if an individual patient's disease triggering self-antigens can be identified, they will be of little use in patient management, because, by the time the diagnosis is made, the inflammatory process is no longer T cell dependent, as many other cell types are now involved.[57-59] As described earlier, most of the ultimate effector responses determining the severity of inflammation are nonspecific and involve various innate immune activating mechanisms. At this point in time, the inflammatory response has become T cell independent, which may explain the failed therapeutic approaches to directly target CD4 T cells in RA.

That does not mean that in these later stages T cells are not important in regulating the response and does not even exclude the possibility to target T cells for therapeutic approaches. On the contrary, there is growing evidence for a very active role of T cells in both sustaining and regulating pathological inflammation in JIA. Two T cell subtypes that are crucial for JIA inflammation are Th17 cells and T regulatory cells. Deciphering the roles of these two T cell lineages in JIA may lead to novel therapeutic strategies to specifically regulate inflammation.

TH17 CELLS: CULPRITS IN SYNOVIAL INFLAMMATION?

IL-17A (often referred to as IL-17) is part of the family of IL-17 cytokines, which include IL-17E (IL-25), a cytokine involved in allergic inflammation. Th17 cells are responsible for its production.[60] In various experimental models of autoimmunity, Th17 cells (and Th1 cells to a lesser extent) were found to be responsible for the onset and maintenance of pathological inflammation.[61,62] Data on human Th17 cells are rapidly expanding, but are inconclusive. Seemingly conflicting data have emerged on how Th17 cells are induced. Th17 cells are associated with a number of human autoimmune diseases, most notably psoriasis.

In recent years the evidence for a pathological role of Th17 cells in human arthritis has also grown substantially, although many questions remain. Surprisingly the Th17 cells are not increased in number in the SF of RA patients.[63-66] In JIA Th17 cells are enriched in the SF of patients with a bad prognosis, namely there with extended oligoarticular JIA.[9,67] This enrichment may be the consequence of factors that promote selective recruitment of these cells in the synovial infiltrate. In this respect there is evidence for a role of a chemokine gradient. Th17 cells can express the chemokine receptor CCR6, while its ligand, CCL20, is elevated in the SF of JIA patients.

There are some remarkable and still poorly explained similarities between Th17 cells and Tregs that are involved in controlling inflammation. Tregs and Th17 cells both can express similar chemokine receptors (CCR4 and CCR6), suggesting that they can be recruited simultaneously under certain circumstances.

Biological agents that specifically target Th17 cells are now under development,[63-68] but they will have to be applied in young children with caution. Th17 cells play an important role in protection against various bacteria, mycobacteria, and fungi. Targeting them could lead to a selected immune deficiency and increase the risk of opportunistic infections. Studies are now underway in inflammatory bowel disease. Similar studies need to dissect the role of Th17 cells and their relationship to the other crucial cell lineage in JIA, namely Tregs.

T CELL TOLERANCE TO PREVENT AUTOIMMUNE INFLAMMATION

As discussed earlier, the maintenance of T cell tolerance to self-antigens to prevent autoimmune inflammation involves both central and peripheral mechanisms. Deletion of self-reactive T cell clones during thymocyte differentiation is the predominant means of eradicating cells expressing potentially pathogenic T cell receptors. However, this process is imperfect; self-reactive clones do escape but are prevented from initiating potentially disastrous autoimmune reactions by a variety of mechanisms generally termed peripheral tolerance. T cells that are able to suppress immune responses were described first in the early 1970s. However, only recently has a specific population of CD4$^+$CD25$^+$CD127 low Tregs been shown to inhibit CD4$^+$ effector T cell function and to protect against the onset of autoimmunity.[69] These so-called Tregs have various phenotypical characteristics, such as the high ("bright") expression of gamma chain of the IL-2 receptor (CD25), which are typical but not unique to these T cells. The expression of the transcription factor FOXP3 is crucial for their *in vitro* and *in vivo* functions and constitutes their most important marker.[70] The importance of FOXP3$^+$ Tregs was underscored by the discovery that IPEX (immune dysregulation, polyendocrinopathy, enteropathy, X-linked), a disease characterized by very serious chronic inflammation and autoimmunity, is caused by a single mutation in the FOXP3 gene. The discovery of Tregs and their amazing capacity in experimental models to specifically suppress other cells and regulate autoimmunity has raised high hopes for new and more targeted approaches. However, questions still remain with regard to their specific function in humans *in vivo*.

REGULATORY T CELLS AND THE CONTROL OF INFLAMMATION

The role of Tregs is now well described in animal models of autoimmunity, but their potential therapeutic role in human autoimmune diseases is far less defined. The increased levels of FOXP3$^+$ cells at sites of inflammation in human autoimmune diseases raises the question, are these cells activated effector cells that temporarily express FOXP3 rather than true suppressor cells.

Most evidence for a true regulatory role of Tregs in human autoimmune diseases comes from self-remitting oligoarticular JIA. In this disease, the presence and function of both natural and adaptive (induced) CD4+FOXP3+ Tregs is associated with disease remission.

In oligoarticular JIA, two types of Tregs are associated with disease remission. First, natural FOXP3+Tregs can be found in increased numbers both in peripheral blood and the SF of patients, and the suppressive capacity of such FOXP3+ Tregs at the site of inflammation correlates with a benign course.[71-73] Second, adaptive Tregs induced by heat shock protein 60 (HSP60) are present in the peripheral blood and SF of patients with oligoarticular JIA.[74,75] Heat shock proteins are highly conserved cellular proteins that are immune dominant and are up-regulated during cellular stress.[59,76] A large body of evidence points to a role for HSP60 in the regulation of the immune response in autoimmunity, especially for arthritis and diabetes mellitus type I. These HSP60-induced T cells in patients with oligoarticular JIA have characteristics of adaptive (induced) Tregs, as they are capable of producing IL-10 and TGF-beta, and of expressing CD30 and the Th2 gatekeeper transcription factor GATA-3. Not only whole HSP60 but also HSP60-derived peptides can induce CD4+T cells with a similar regulatory phenotype, excluding the possibility that even a low LPS contamination in recombinant HSP60 may be responsible for the observed effects.[74,77,78] Very recent data, obtained in healthy donors, show that these HSP60-induced Tregs can also express FOXP3. Thus, beside natural FOXP3+CD4+ Tregs, a second population of HSP- induced FOXP3+ T cells can be detected in the peripheral blood and SF of patients with JIA. Both types of FOXP3+ T cells are correlated with a favorable disease outcome in remitting oligoarticular JIA.

At the molecular level little is known about the role and function of these FOXP3+ cells, either at the periphery or at the sites of inflammation. Even less is known of the presence, role, and function of FOXP3+ T cells in nonremitting autoimmunity, such as polyarticular JIA.

RESTORING THE BALANCE

The inflammatory process in JIA is caused by a close and complex interaction between various innate and adaptive immune mechanisms. Innate immunity accounts for the most important effector mechanisms in JIA inflammation and involves many soluble factors, including cytokines and S100 proteins. Although nonspecific by nature, these soluble factors are both valuable targets for therapy and are potential biomarkers for the inflammatory process. In contrast, the adaptive immune system, especially DCs and T cells, holds the key to specifically regulating the inflammatory response. In naturally remitting oligoarticular JIA, Tregs play a central role in both amplifying and subsequently down-regulating inflammation. This regulatory function may be impaired in nonremitting JIA and other forms of autoimmunity. Restoring this naturally regulatory principle may be the key to develop future therapeutic strategies that are directed at not just temporary suppressing inflammation, but at permanently restoring the immune balance.

REFERENCES

1. G. Trinchieri, Regulatory role of T cells producing both interferon gamma and interleukin 10 in persistent infection, J. Exp. Med. 194, (2001) F53-F37.
2. C. Benoist, D. Mathis, Autoimmunity provoked by infection: how good is the case for T cell epitope mimicry? Nat. Immunol. 2 (2001) 797–801.
3. D.D. Bolz, J.J. Weis, Molecular mimicry to Borrelia burgdorferi: pathway to autoimmunity? Autoimmunity. 37 (2004) 387–392.
4. C. Munz, J.D. Lunemann, M.T. Getts, et al., Antiviral immune responses: triggers of or triggered by autoimmunity? Nat. Rev. Immunol. 9 (2009) 246–258.
5. C. Benoist, D. Mathis, Autoimmunity. The pathogen connection, Nature 394 (1998) 227–228.
6. B.J. Prakken, D.A. Carson, S. Albani, T cell repertoire formation and molecular mimicry in rheumatoid arthritis, Curr. Dir. Autoimmun. 3 (2001) 51–63.
7. D.S. Pharoah, H. Varsani, R.W. Tatham, et al., Expression of the inflammatory chemokines CCL5, CCL3 and CXCL10 in juvenile idiopathic arthritis, and demonstration of CCL5 production by an atypical subset of CD8+ T cells, Arthritis Res. Ther. 8 (2006) R50.
8. L.R. Wedderburn, P. Woo, Type 1 and type 2 immune responses in children: their relevance in juvenile arthritis, Springer. Semin. Immunopathol. 21 (1999) 361–374.
9. K. Nistala, L.R. Wedderburn, Th17 and regulatory T cells: rebalancing pro- and anti-inflammatory forces in autoimmune arthritis, Rheumatology (Oxford) 48 (2009) 602–606.
10. L.R. Wedderburn, A. Patel, H. Varsani, et al., Divergence in the degree of clonal expansions in inflammatory T cell subpopulations mirrors HLA-associated risk alleles in genetically and clinically distinct subtypes of childhood arthritis, Int. Immunol. 13 (2001) 1541–1550.
11. N. Koch, M. Jung, R. Sabat, et al., IL-10 protects monocytes and macrophages from complement-mediated lysis, J. Leukoc. Biol. 86 (2009) 155–166.
12. G. Grutz, New insights into the molecular mechanism of interleukin-10-mediated immunosuppression, J. Leukoc. Biol. 77 (2005) 3–15.
13. J. Lee, J.H. Mo, K. Katakura, et al., Maintenance of colonic homeostasis by distinctive apical TLR9 signalling in intestinal epithelial cells, Nat. Cell. Biol. 8 (2006) 1327–1336.
14. K. Takabayshi, M. Corr, T. Hayashi, et al., Induction of a homeostatic circuit in lung tissue by microbial compounds, Immunity 24 (2006) 475–487.
15. E. Raz, Mucosal immunity: aliment and ailments, Mucosal. Immunol. 3 (2010) 4–7.
16. J. Lee, J.M. Gonzales-Navajas, E. Raz, The "polarizing-tolerizing" mechanism of intestinal epithelium: its relevance to colonic homeostasis, Semin. Immunopathol. 30 (2008) 3–9.
17. P.J. Sansonetti, War and peace at the intestinal epithelial surface: an integrated view of bacterial commensalism versus bacterial pathogenicity, J. Pediatr. Gastroenterol. Nutr. 46 (Suppl. 1) (2008) E6–7.
18. T. Vogl, K. Tenbrock, S. Ludwig, et al., Mrp8 and Mrp14 are endogenous activators of Toll-like receptor 4, promoting lethal, endotoxin-induced shock, Nat. Med. 13 (2007) 1042–1049.
19. D. Foell, H. Wittkowski, J. Roth, Mechanisms of disease: a 'DAMP' view of inflammatory arthritis, Nat. Clin. Pract. Rheumatol. 3 (2007) 382–390.
20. D. Foell, H. Wittkowski, T. Vogl, et al., S100 proteins expressed in phagocytes: a novel group of damage-associated molecular pattern molecules, J. Leukoc. Biol. 81 (2007) 28–37.
21. H. Wittkowski, M. Frosch, N. Wulffraat, et al., S100A12 is a novel molecular marker differentiating systemic-onset juvenile idiopathic arthritis from other causes of fever of unknown origin, Arthritis Rheum. 58 (2008) 3924–3931.
22. D. Foell, H. Wittkowski, I. Hammerschmidt, et al., Monitoring neutrophil activation in juvenile rheumatoid arthritis by S100A12 serum concentrations, Arthritis Rheum. 50 (2004) 1286–1295.
23. F. Ye, D. Foell, K.I. Hirono, et al., Neutrophil-derived S100A12 is profoundly upregulated in the early stage of acute Kawasaki disease, Am. J. Cardiol. 94 (2004) 840–844.
24. M. Frosch, T. Vogl, S. Seeliger, et al., Expression of myeloid-related proteins 8 and 14 in systemic-onset juvenile rheumatoid arthritis, Arthritis Rheum. 48 (2003) 2622–2626.

25. N.M. Wulffraat, P.J. Haas, M. Frosch, et al., Myeloid related protein 8 and 14 secretion reflects phagocyte activation and correlates with disease activity in juvenile idiopathic arthritis treated with autologous stem cell transplantation, Ann. Rheum. Dis. 62 (2003) 236–241.

25a. H. Wittkowski, K. Hirono, F. Ichida, et al., Acute Kawasaki disease is associated with reverse regulation of soluble receptor for advance glycation end products and its proinflammatory ligand S100A12, Arthritis Rheum. 56 (2007) 4174–4181.

26. F.M. Brennan, I.B. McInnes, Evidence that cytokines play a role in rheumatoid arthritis, J. Clin. Invest. 118 (2008) 3537–3545.

27. I.B. McInnes, G. Schett, Cytokines in the pathogenesis of rheumatoid arthritis, Nat. Rev. Immunol. 7 (2007) 429–442.

28. H.J. van den Ham, W. de Jager, J.W. Bijlsma, et al., Differential cytokine profiles in juvenile idiopathic arthritis subtypes revealed by cluster analysis, Rheumatology (Oxford) 48 (2009) 899–905.

29. W. de Jager, B. Prakken, G.T. Rijkers, Cytokine multiplex immunoassay: methodology and (clinical) applications, Methods Mol. Biol. 514 (2009) 119–133.

30. F. De Benedetti, P. Pignatti, M. Massa, et al., Circulating levels of interleukin 1 beta and of interleukin 1 receptor antagonist in systemic juvenile chronic arthritis, Clin. Exp. Rheumatol. 13 (1995) 779–784.

31. F. De Benedetti, M. Massa, P. Pignatti, et al., Serum soluble interleukin 6 (IL-6) receptor and IL-6/soluble IL-6 receptor complex in systemic juvenile rheumatoid arthritis, J. Clin. Invest. 93 (1994) 2114–2119.

32. W. de Jager, E.P. Hoppenreijs, N.M. Wulffraat, et al., Blood and synovial fluid cytokine signatures in patients with juvenile idiopathic arthritis: a cross-sectional study, Ann. Rheum. Dis. 66 (2007) 589–598.

33. S. Chiesa, I. Prigione, F. Morandi, et al., Cytokine flexibility of early and differentiated memory T helper cells in juvenile idiopathic arthritis, J. Rheumatol. 31 (2004) 2048–2054.

34. M. Gattorno, L. Chicha, A. Gregorio, et al., Distinct expression pattern of IFN-alpha and TNF-alpha in juvenile idiopathic arthritis synovial tissue, Rheumatology (Oxford) 46 (2007) 657–665.

35. F. Allantaz, D. Chaussabel, J. Banchereau, et al., Microarray-based identification of novel biomarkers in IL-1-mediated diseases, Curr. Opin. Immunol. 19 (2007) 623–632.

36. F. Allantaz, D. Chaussabel, D. Stichweh, et al., Blood leukocyte microarrays to diagnose systemic onset juvenile idiopathic arthritis and follow the response to IL-1 blockade, J. Exp. Med. 204 (2007) 2131–2144.

37. V. Pascual, F. Allantaz, E. Arce, et al., Role of interleukin-1 (IL-1) in the pathogenesis of systemic onset juvenile idiopathic arthritis and clinical response to IL-1 blockade, J. Exp. Med. 201 (2005) 1479–1486.

38. V. Pascual, F. Allantaz, P. Patel, et al., How the study of children with rheumatic diseases identified interferon-alpha and interleukin-1 as novel therapeutic targets, Immunol. Rev. 223 (2008) 39–59.

39. H. Valleala, M. Korpela, T. Mottonen, et al., Rituximab therapy in patients with rheumatoid arthritis refractory or with contraindication to anti-tumour necrosis factor drugs: real-life experience in Finnish patients, Scand. J. Rheumatol. (2009) 1–5.

40. P. Roll, T. Dorner, H.P. Tony, Anti-CD20 therapy in patients with rheumatoid arthritis: predictors of response and B cell subset regeneration after repeated treatment, Arthritis Rheum. 58 (2008) 1566–1575.

41. A. Ravelli, A. Martini, Juvenile idiopathic arthritis, Lancet 369 (2007) 767–778.

42. C. Koble, B. Kyewski, The thymic medulla: a unique microenvironment for intercellular self-antigen transfer, J. Exp. Med. 206 (2009) 1505–1513.

43. M.N. Meriggioli, J.R. Sheng, L. Li, et al., Strategies for treating autoimmunity: novel insights from experimental myasthenia gravis, Ann. N. Y. Acad. Sci. 1132 (2008) 276–282.

44. S. Rutella, S. Danese, G. Leone, Tolerogenic dendritic cells: cytokine modulation comes of age, Blood 108 (2006) 1435–1440.

45. L. Adorini, Intervention in autoimmunity: the potential of vitamin D receptor agonists, Cell. Immunol. 233 (2005) 115–124.

46. R.M. Steinman, D. Hawiger, M.C. Nussenzweig, Tolerogenic dendritic cells, Annu. Rev. Immunol. 21 (2003) 685–711.

48. E. Gonzalez-Rey, A. Chorny, A. Fernandez-Martin, et al., Vasoactive intestinal peptide generates human tolerogenic dendritic cells that induce CD4 and CD8 regulatory T cells, Blood 107 (2006) 3632–3638.

49. A. Hinks, A. Barton, N. Shephard, et al., Identification of a novel susceptibility locus for juvenile idiopathic arthritis by genome-wide association analysis, Arthritis Rheum. 60 (2009) 258–263.

50. B. Pazar, P. Gergely Jr., Z.B. Nagy, et al., Role of HLA-DRB1 and PTPN22 genes in susceptibility to juvenile idiopathic arthritis in Hungarian patients, Clin. Exp. Rheumatol. 26 (2008) 1146–1152.

51. E. Zeggini, J. Packham, R. Donn, et al., Association of HLA-DRB1*13 with susceptibility to uveitis in juvenile idiopathic arthritis in two independent data sets, Rheumatology (Oxford) 45 (2006) 972–974.

52. W. Thomson, J.H. Barrett, R. Donn, et al., Juvenile idiopathic arthritis classified by the ILAR criteria: HLA associations in UK patients, Rheumatology (Oxford) 41 (2002) 1183–1189.

53. A. Smerdel, R. Ploski, B. Flato, et al., Juvenile idiopathic arthritis (JIA) is primarily associated with HLA-DR8 but not DQ4 on the DR8-DQ4 haplotype, Ann. Rheum. Dis. 61 (2002) 354–357.

54. L.R. Wedderburn, N. Robinson, A. Patel, et al., Selective recruitment of polarized T cells expressing CCR5 and CXCR3 to the inflamed joints of children with juvenile idiopathic arthritis, Arthritis Rheum. 43 (2000) 765–774.

55. L.R. Wedderburn, M.K. Maini, A. Patel, et al., Molecular fingerprinting reveals non-overlapping T cell oligoclonality between an inflamed site and peripheral blood, Int. Immunol. 11 (1999) 535–543.

56. M. Gattorno, I. Prigione, F. Morandi, et al., Phenotypic and functional characterisation of CCR7+ and CCR7- CD4+ memory T cells homing to the joints in juvenile idiopathic arthritis, Arthritis Res. Ther. 7 (2005) R256–R267.

57. B.J. Prakken, S. Albani, Using biology of disease to understand and guide therapy of JIA, Best. Pract. Res. Clin. Rheumatol. 23 (2009) 599–608.

58. B. Prakken, S. Albani, Exploiting T cell crosstalk as a vaccination strategy for rheumatoid arthritis, Arthritis Rheum. 56 (2007) 389–392.

59. B. Prakken, S. Albani, W.V. Eden, Translating immunological tolerance into therapy, Eur. J. Immunol. 37 (2007) 2360–2363.

60. M.L. Toh, P. Miossec, The role of T cells in rheumatoid arthritis: new subsets and new targets, Curr. Opin. Rheumatol. 19 (2007) 284–288.

61. L. Geboes, L. Dumoutier, H. Kelchtermans, et al., Proinflammatory role of the Th17 cytokine interleukin-22 in collagen-induced arthritis in C57BL/6 mice, Arthritis Rheum. 60 (2009) 390–395.

62. M. Fujimoto, S. Serada, M. Mihara, et al., Interleukin-6 blockade suppresses autoimmune arthritis in mice by the inhibition of inflammatory Th17 responses, Arthritis Rheum. 58 (2008) 3710–3719.

63. W.B. van den Berg, P. Miossec, IL-17 as a future therapeutic target for rheumatoid arthritis, Nat. Rev. Rheumatol. 5 (2009) 549–553.

64. S.L. Gaffen, The role of interleukin-17 in the pathogenesis of rheumatoid arthritis, Curr. Rheumatol. Rep. 11 (2009) 365–370.

65. F. Annunziato, L. Cosmi, F. Liotta, et al., Type 17 T helper cells-origins, features and possible roles in rheumatic disease, Nat. Rev. Rheumatol. 5 (2009) 325–331.

66. H.G. Evans, N.J. Gullick, S. Kelly, et al., In vivo activated monocytes from the site of inflammation in humans specifically promote Th17 responses, Proc. Natl. Acad. Sci. U. S. A. 106 (2009) 6232–6237.

67. K. Nistala, H. Moncrieffe, K.R. Newton, et al., Interleukin-17-producing T cells are enriched in the joints of children with arthritis, but have a reciprocal relationship to regulatory T cell numbers, Arthritis Rheum. 58 (2008) 875–887.

68. P. Miossec, Diseases that may benefit from manipulating the Th17 pathway, Eur. J. Immunol. 39 (2009) 667–669.

69. S. Sakaguchi, K. Wing, M. Miyara, Regulatory T cells - a brief history and perspective, Eur. J. Immunol. 37 (Suppl. 1) (2007) S116–S123.

70. S. Hori, T. Nomura, S. Sakaguchi, Control of regulatory T cell development by the transcription factor Foxp3, Science 299 (2003) 1057–1061.

71. I. de Kleer, B. Vastert, M. Klein, et al., Autologous stem cell transplantation for autoimmunity induces immunologic self-tolerance by reprogramming autoreactive T cells and restoring the CD4+CD25+ immune regulatory network, Blood 107 (2006) 1696–1702.

72. C.R. Ruprecht, M. Gattorno, F. Ferlito, et al., Coexpression of CD25 and CD27 identifies FoxP3+ regulatory T cells in inflamed synovia, J. Exp. Med. 201 (2005) 1793–1803.

73. I.M. de Kleer, L.R. Wedderburn, L.S. Taams, et al., CD4+CD25bright regulatory T cells actively regulate inflammation in the joints of patients with the remitting form of juvenile idiopathic arthritis, J. Immunol. 172 (2004) 6435–6443.

74. S. Kamphuis, W. Kuis, W. de Jager, et al., Tolerogenic immune responses to novel T-cell epitopes from heat-shock protein 60 in juvenile idiopathic arthritis, Lancet 366 (2005) 50–56.

75. I.M. de Kleer, S.M. Kamphuis, G.T. Rijkers, et al., The spontaneous remission of juvenile idiopathic arthritis is characterized by CD30+ T cells directed to human heat-shock protein 60 capable of producing the regulatory cytokine interleukin-10, Arthritis Rheum. 48 (2003) 2001–2010.

76. W. van Eden, R. van der Zee, B. Prakken, Heat-shock proteins induce T-cell regulation of chronic inflammation, Nat. Rev. Immunol. 5 (2005) 318–330.

77. M. Massa, M. Passalia, S.M. Manzoni, et al., Differential recognition of heat-shock protein dnaJ-derived epitopes by effector and Treg cells leads to modulation of inflammation in juvenile idiopathic arthritis, Arthritis Rheum. 56 (2007) 1648–1657.

78. H. de Jong, F.F. Lafeber, W. de Jager, et al., Pan-DR-binding Hsp60 self epitopes induce an interleukin-10-mediated immune response in rheumatoid arthritis, Arthritis Rheum. 60 (2009) 1966–1976.

Chapter 5

INTEGRATIVE GENOMICS

Robert A. Colbert, Susan D. Thompson and David N. Glass

When viewed from the perspective of the pediatric rheumatology clinic, few patients with arthritis appear to have genetically determined diseases. Family histories are rarely positive for the more common diseases, including juvenile idiopathic arthritis (JIA), and diseases with a Mendelian pattern of inheritance are especially uncommon. Few extended families with chronic pediatric rheumatological illnesses suitable for traditional linkage studies have been reported. Pediatric rheumatic diseases share this scenario with autoimmune diseases in which the absence of a family history of the specific disease is common, whereas a family history of autoimmunity in its various forms is frequent. One notable exception is ankylosing spondylitis (AS), where in some families the phenotype follows an autosomal dominant inheritance pattern linked to human leukocyte antigen (HLA)-B27 with penetrance as high as 20%. The paradoxical view that diseases without a family history are genetically based is considered in this context. In addition, it is commonly hypothesized that this genetic effect extends not only to a primary predisposition but also to variation in the phenotype including the extent and severity of disease and applies to JIA in its various forms,[1] systemic lupus erythematosus (SLE), scleroderma, and dermatomyositis.

The presence of HLA associations in most of these diseases provides some indication of their genetic nature, although for many years HLA or HLA-linked genes were not necessarily perceived to be central to pathogenesis. It is argued that they are a necessary part of genetic predisposition (although only a component) and that other non-major histocompatibility complex (MHC) genes predispose to the disease in a given individual with potential for an environmental contribution to pathogenesis.[2]

Current high-throughput molecular technology not only allows screening of deoxyribonucleic acid (DNA) polymorphisms but can also track newly identified genes; thus, the traditional approach starting from a disease phenotype and then identifying the gene can be reversed.[3] Also microarray gene expression technology allows investigation of the entire expressed genome as ribonucleic acid (RNA) and eventually as the proteome. The so-called functional genomics can be combined with data representing DNA polymorphisms to yield a comprehensive integrative genomic and systems biology approach to better understanding human diseases. We review knowledge of the genome with respect to genes and polymorphic variability before discussing the genetic components of pediatric rheumatic diseases and the manner of their inheritance.

THE GENOME

The *genome* can be defined as the individual's (or cell's) total genetic information. The related science of mapping, sequencing, and analyzing genomes is known as *genomics*. The Human Genome Project provides a strong basis for understanding gene function and its pathophysiology. A complete description of this project can be found at *www.nhgri.nih.gov/HGP/*.

Gene Structure and Polymorphisms

At the DNA level, genetic information consists of approximately 3.1×10^9 base pairs organized into three components: 22 paired autosomal chromosomes, two sex chromosomes, and mitochondrial DNA. A large part of this genetic material is aggregated into repetitive sequences that contribute, as either long or short interspersed sequences, to the familiar banding pattern that characterizes the morphology of chromosomes. The remainder (about 10% of the whole) is single copy DNA, which is primarily organized into genes of which only about 2% are protein coding genes and an additional 4% contain conserved sequence elements, which include promoter and other regulatory regions.[4] The number of genes encoding proteins, originally estimated to be in the range of 60,000 to 70,000, appears to be closer to 20,000 to 30,000. The number of genes expressed varies qualitatively and quantitatively in different organs: A metabolically complex organ, such as the liver, may have 20,000 genes expressed that are important for hepatic function; the synovium may well have fewer, varying with stage of development and appropriateness for the function of the tissue. Genes are divided into coding and noncoding compartments, exons and introns, respectively, with additional promoter and flanking sequences that are less well understood. The latter are a major part of the regulatory process, which determines when and where specific genes are expressed. Thus, the gene is a complex unit in both its structure and its regulation.

Polymorphic Elements

It is fundamental to the understanding of human diversity and of disease to recognize that, although the genome and gene structures are broadly the same for all persons (99.9% identity) and great similarity exists among species, variability is nevertheless substantial among individuals and this can be related to disease, the focus of this chapter. This variability may be local (gene specific) or part of a class of genome wide polymorphic elements.

Local Variability

Local variability in a given gene or segment of DNA containing several genes can range from a change or mutation in a single nucleotide to larger deletions, translocations, or to gene conversion. The resulting change in even a single expressed gene product can range from deleterious (including fatal), to neutral, or even to a gain in function. Clearly, the nature and site of the change (e.g., coding regions, regulatory regions) are critical in this regard and can be reflected in changed phenotypes and disease. It is true that although variability is local, the impact may be devastating for the patient. These types of structural changes affect relatively few patients but may also provide mechanistic insights. The complement deficiencies are examples of individual gene variability of relevance to autoimmunity; the chromosome 22 deletion associated with JIA[5] is another such example and, like trisomy 21 (Down's syndrome), may also have a considerable effect on gene expression in a given individual.[6] As a whole, the single nucleotide polymorphisms (SNPs) are a formidable tool as markers to evaluate the whole genome (see later discussion) or in local variability related to gene function.

Genome Wide Polymorphisms

A key aspect of research in the genetics of disease is associating sequence variations with heritable phenotypes. There are two major classes of variation that can be measured across the genome-variable number tandem repeats (VNTRs) and SNPs, with copy number variation and deletions contributing to additional polymorphism.

VARIABLE NUMBER TANDEM REPEATS

There are in excess of 10,000 VNTRs distributed randomly throughout the genome as microsatellites. Polymorphisms in these small, repetitive sequences of DNA can be distinguished by polymerase chain reaction (PCR)-based methods. Their utility is enhanced by the availability of genome-wide maps and by knowledge of their polymorphic information content, allowing the selection of an optimal set of markers. Their purpose is diminishing as the use of SNPs as markers accelerates, driven by cost and ease of high-throughput technologies.

SINGLE-NUCLEOTIDE POLYMORPHISMS

SNPs are much more common than VNTRs.[7] Resequencing efforts of the human genome have produced a collection, as of the summer 2009, of 15 million validated SNPs or about one in every 100 to 300 bases. The SNP datasets are changing rapidly as a major effort is being vested in their identification and in establishing their map position, in part for the so called HapMap project, which will describe the common patterns of human genetic variability (*http://hapmap.ncbi.nlm.nih.gov/*). Their frequency and widespread presence make them of considerable value as markers in genome-wide association studies (GWAS), a powerful tool for genomic studies that adds greater analytic power than is available through linkage analysis in affected sib pairs (ASPs). Although the very great number of SNPs, hundreds or more per gene, adds to the analysis,[8] their added use in the dissection of complex genetic traits can be illustrated by two SNPs that have been associated with components of a disease phenotype. These SNPs result in a coding amino acid change leading to a gain of function in the interleukin-4 receptor, which is associated with severe asthma, whereas the second SNP results in a functional change in a β_2-adrenergic receptor gene associated with greater resistance to adrenergic drugs.[9,10] For rheumatoid arthritis (RA), an SNP resulting in the amino acid coding change R620W in the PTPN22 gene marks predisposition and has important functional consequences, particularly increasing susceptibility for RA along with the shared epitope and other non-MHC gene polymorphisms in smokers.[2] The PTPN22 gene codes for a tyrosine phosphatase, with a potential function in the regulation of T cell and B cell activation.

Structure variations in DNA sequences can also be assessed using SNPs. Inheritable copy number alterations have been recently identified for numerous diseases, including a reported association of the beta-defensin gene region with psoriasis.[11] Investigations of copy number variants (CNV) have gained great popularity with the availability of SNP chips that can be used to interrogate CNV.

Whole Genome Sequencing. New methodologies permit a broader investigation of individual variation beyond the markers identified in the HapMap project, which focus on genetic variants that are present at a frequency of 5% or greater in the population. The 1000 Genomes Project, launched in January 2008, is an international research effort to establish a more detailed catalogue of human genetic variation (*www.1000genomes.org/*).

The genomes of at least 1000 anonymous participants from a number of different ethnic groups will be sequenced and will identify genetic variants that are present at a frequency of 1% across most of the genome and 0.5% or lower within genes. This will permit documentation of differences between individuals in the era of personalized medicine.

Maps

Genome-wide maps are being generated from different sources of information. Cytochemical approaches have been widely used to generate the familiar chromosome maps with banding patterns. The addition of fluorescent in situ hybridization combines cytochemical and molecular approaches. Although only broad localization is possible with these techniques, several thousand genes have been mapped by this process to specific chromosomes, albeit with low resolution. Now microarray technologies offer radically enhanced specificity and employ about one million probes. Creating a genetic map is a more detailed process in which the relationship of individual genes to each other and their eventual assignments to a chromosome region and linkage groups becomes possible. Sufficient genes or polymorphic markers are mapped to cover effectively the whole genome except mitochondria. Genes that cosegregate are a component of a linkage group. This sometimes involves genes of like function, the linkage group having arisen by gene duplication, but a cluster of genes do not necessarily have similar or related functions.

Examples of functional clusters are the HLA and T cell receptor genes, which each form close linkage groups. Linkage refers to the close association of two genes on the same chromosome that are inherited together. The statistical analyses used in such situations are logarithm of the odds (LOD) scores in which a score of 3.0 or more is the standard for establishing linkage between two genes. A particular linkage group may be inferred from findings in other species, a concept known as *synteny*. Although clustering of a particular set of genes may be shared across species, it may be that the same linkage group is found on a different chromosome in humans. The MHC linkage group is located on chromosome 6 in humans and on chromosome 17 in mice.

The recombination rate detected in families is a measure of the closeness of linkage. Recombination may be current or ancestral and translates into map distance, or centimorgans (cM). There are approximately 3500 cM in the human genome. This genetic distance that depends on recombination frequency may be different from the physical distance between linkage groups on the same chromosome.

Of particular relevance are approaches to linkage analysis, which include affected sibpair methods and transmission disequilibrium testing (TDT). These approaches do not depend on large kindreds and instead avoid confounding issues of population substructure because they use family-based controls.[12-15] Linkage studies that in the past relied on higher information content of VNTRs now can be SNP-based, because large-scale SNP typing is now affordable.

Physical Map and Linkage Disequilibrium

The advent of DNA sequencing allows definition of individual genes and their relationship to each other in terms of intervening DNA structure *(www.ncbi.nlm.nih.gov and www.nhgri.nih.gov)*. This process allows physical mapping of individual stretches of DNA; interim physical maps were based on VNTRs in the past but are more recently based on SNPs,[16,17] for which the MHC region, located on the short arm of chromosome 6 (6p21.3), is an example. The classical MHC (3.6 Mb or 0.1% of the genome) is densely packed with immunologically important genes.[18] As knowledge for the physical map became available, the MHC boundaries were revised to include 7.6 Mb. This new knowledge showed that the surrounding sequences, especially in the telomeric part, demonstrated synteny to the mouse MHC, contained MHC-similar genes, and displayed linkage disequilbrium that extended past the original MHC boundaries.[19] The entire extended MHC region should be considered in the study of genetic associations of autoimmune disease.

Across the genome, groups of alleles from closely linked genes inherited together are called *haplotypes*. It has long been recognized that alleles of closely linked genes may not occur at random, i.e., they show linkage disequilibrium. The most comprehensively documented haplotypes span the MHC region. The generation of SNP maps of the genome will allow definition of linkage disequilibrium throughout the genome, including the MHC region. So-called tag SNPs define haplotype blocks[20] and may effectively mark a particular haplotype. These specific tag SNPs can then be used as markers in genome-wide screens as a surrogate for large stretches of DNA. This allows a cost effective approach for genome-wide testing by a limiting the number of SNPs necessary to obtain maximum coverage.

Functional Map

The physical map identifies the genes and their location within the total genome but does not determine whether they are functional. Pseudogenes cannot be expressed because of a specific mutation. Pseudogenes need to be differentiated from a gene that, because of mutation, will not function. The nonfunctioning gene is known as a *null gene* and is allelic with functioning variants.

A functional map is based on the analysis of function of individual genes and gene networks.[21] Through the identification of expressed genes, assisted by technological advances such as arrays that measure RNA expression[22] and gene knockouts and knockdowns, it is possible to not only identify all expressed genes in a given tissue but also to consider their function. Comparisons between developing and developed tissues and disease and normal states will eventually result in a complete functional map.

Biotechnology and Bioinformatics

The Human Genome Project and the potential to establish the genetic basis of disease would not have been possible without parallel technological advances. The PCR is a method that allows the expansion of specific segments of DNA to make enough of them available for quantitative analysis, including sequencing. With respect to genomics, the widespread availability of polymorphic markers detectable by PCR for every part of the genome and the commercial availability of the appropriate PCR primers have created great opportunities for scientific advances in understanding the contributions of genetics to disease. These primer pairs are organized into sets that allow a genome-wide approach.[23]

MONOGENIC DISEASE IN PEDIATRIC RHEUMATOLOGY

The diseases referred to as Mendelian are controlled primarily by a single genetic locus and are typically inherited in an autosomal dominant or recessive fashion or are sex-linked. Although more than 10,000 Mendelian diseases are now recognized, only the fraction with musculoskeletal features present directly to a pediatric rheumatology clinic, which can include arthritis and periodic fever syndromes. With the increasing capacity to identify particular genes and their mutations as causative factors and the functional consequences that lead to particular phenotypes, molecular analysis becomes more practical and necessary, as is awareness of the phenotypes of these disorders.

The familial categories of inherited disease (dominant, recessive, X-linked) provide patterns of inheritance discernible if typically penetrant. A dominant disease should be evident in every generation, showing vertical transmission; a recessive disease occurs in approximately one in four children in an affected sibship and is more likely to occur in offspring of consanguineous marriages. X-linked recessive diseases become evident in male children whose mothers are the carriers, although female carriers may show some features of the disease consistent with the Lyon hypothesis of X chromosome inactivation. Not all of these disorders present in the classic or traditional Mendelian manner due to incomplete penetrance.

Athreya and colleagues categorized monogenic disease that affects the musculoskeletal system into three groups: arthritic (e.g., Lesch-Nyhan), those with contractures or stiff joints (e.g., Gaucher disease), and those with hypermobility (e.g., Ehlers-Danlos syndrome).[25] A total of 75 disorders were identified, probably representing only a portion of the whole.[26] In the late 1990s, the discovery of genes responsible for certain inherited periodic fever syndromes (familial Mediterranean fever [FMF], TNF receptor-associated periodic syndrome [TRAPS])[27,28] led to the concept of "autoinflammatory" disease (see Chapter 43). A classification system that incorporates other diseases whose genetic basis is now recognized but may not have all the features of classic autoinflammation has been proposed.[29]

COMPLEX GENETIC TRAITS

A complex genetic trait is dependent on multiple genes and has non-Mendelian inheritance patterns. It is likely that the chronic rheumatic diseases and other autoimmune diseases[30,31] are complex genetic traits. Examples of complex genetic traits include RA, AS, multiple sclerosis, psoriasis and psoriatic arthritis, scleroderma, SLE, and insulin dependent diabetes mellitus.[32]

Genomic screens are time-consuming and expensive ventures; some quantitation of familial risk for a given disease has helped to determine the probability that a given disease is or is not likely to be a complex genetic trait. The standard measure of risk of affected sibs is λs, calculated as the prevalence of the disease in sibs of the patient with the illness in question divided by the prevalence of disease in the general population.[12,33] For JIA one early estimate of λs is 15, similar to that of IDDM. AS, with greater penetrance, may have a λs of around 80.

JIA and its various subtypes display features that suggest a complex genetic trait,[34] including a definite but limited family history but with few or no extended affected kindreds, an increased presence of other autoimmune diseases in the family,[35] and HLA disease associations. Of these features, HLA associations have been extensively documented, and family history has been reported for JIA, e.g., when the disease affects the proband, but more commonly for autoimmune disease in general.

Individual components of the phenotype are likely to be regulated separately such that each component could be called a *Quantitative Trait Locus (QTL)*, with its own genetic basis. Vasculitis complicating SLE or uveitis complicating early-onset oligoarticular JIA may be viewed as individual QTLs. Some patients have these features in their disease phenotype; others do not. Studies of animal models support this QTL concept in rheumatological disease.[36] What has also been missing and important to predict is information regarding the likelihood that non-HLA genes in the MHC region are involved. It is likely that responses (or failures) to therapy are also QTLs and will prove to be genetically mediated as part of pharmacogenetics.

While some genetic associations are strong (e.g., HLA shared epitope alleles provide 11% of genetic risk in RA), these remain the minority.[79] The emerging picture is that the risk alleles identified in genomic screens are common in the general population, have a modest effect on risk, and together explain only a small part of the variance in disease risk. Whereas the actual causal mutation and causal gene for most loci remain to be determined, studies are beginning to reveal general themes: many risk loci are associated with more than one autoimmune disease, and many genes are associated with discrete biological pathways.[37] It has been estimated that for adult arthritis together all risk alleles identified thus far explain less than 5% of the variance in disease risk.[38] Identifying the numerous weak risk factors for pediatric rheumatic disease requires the study of multiple large cohorts, involving national and international collaboration.

Disease-Specific Susceptibility Genes versus General Autoimmunity Genes

Polymorphisms in genes with an immunological function may relate to a variety of autoimmune diseases in both patients and animal models. One such example is *fas* gene defects that affect apoptotic cell death.[39,40] This gives rise to the concept that both general autoimmune-predisposing genes and disease-specific susceptibility genes confer risk of autoimmunity. Striking examples of general autoimmune predisposing genes include *PTPN22*, which is associated with RA, JIA, SLE, type 1 diabetes, and autoimmune thyroid disease; and *TNFAIP3*, which predisposes to RA, SLE, and Crohn's Disease.[37] The number of genes involved in a particular complex trait may be as high as 20 to 30; confirmation of this concept is forthcoming as genome screens are completed in many autoimmune diseases. It is possible that phenotypic specificity will rest with susceptibility genes that do not overlap substantially between diseases, such as the various HLA associations on the short arm of chromosome 6. In this context, both general and disease specific polymorphisms may be found within the MHC.

Table 5–1 illustrates examples of common findings for associated genes for a variety of autoimmune diseases identified using SNP markers in GWAS. Equally important and not shown in this table are the genes unique to individual diseases. The recent identification of

Table 5-1

Common findings for associated genes in autoimmune disease.

		JIA	RA	AS	SLE	Ps	ATD	CD	CeD	MS	T1D
T cell differentiation	IL23R			•		•		•			
	IL2-IL21	•	•		•				•		•
	IL2RA	•	•						•	•	•
	STAT4	•	•		•						
Immune cell activation & signalling	CTLA4		•				•				•
	PTPN22	•	•			•		•			•
Innate Immunity & TNF signalling	PTPN2		•								•
	TRAF1-C5	•	•		•						•

Disease Abbreviations: JIA-Juvenile Idiopathic Arthritis, RA-Rheumatoid Arthritis, AS-Ankylosing Spondylitis, SLE-Systemic Lupus Erythematosus, Ps-Psoriasis, ATD-Autoimmune Thyroid Disease, CD-Crohn's Disease, CeD-Celiac Dis, MS-Multiple Sclerosis, and T1D-Type 1 Diabetes.

genes associated with more than one autoimmune disease could help explain a genetic basis of the shared pathogenesis of immune disorders. It is remarkable that most of the shared genes involve a few key pathways.[41] At the current stage of discovery, these pathways include T cell differentiation, immune-cell signaling, and the innate immune response. A catalogue of published GWAS is available (www.genome.gov/gwastudies).

Disease Phenotype as a Potential Complex Genetic Trait

Two strategies are commonly used in evaluating a disease as a complex trait. One is a candidate gene approach, including selected specific genes or chromosome regions that are tested for disease susceptibility; the other is a comprehensive genome screen. As the growing number of comprehensive or global screens in other autoimmune diseases identify chromosomal loci that confer disease susceptibility, a candidate gene approach for any potential autoimmune complex genetic trait becomes more feasible. Using candidate genes has the potential to reduce the overall workload, but they may miss loci or decrease the resolution, whereas the genome wide screen systematically examines every genetic region, albeit often at low resolution. However, a conservative approach allows both methods of ascertaining linkage or association to be tried in parallel. As the technology is enhanced, global approaches to association are being rapidly expanded. The importance of replication in independent populations is evident.

Candidate Genes

With most autoimmune diseases, evidence supports the involvement of individual genes or polymorphisms in susceptibility. For JIA, a recent review[34] identified 30 such potential genes or chromosome regions outside the MHC. Although the data supporting the candidacy of such entities are conflicting at best, the probability that several will be shown to be involved in disease susceptibility is high, especially for those chromosome regions in which selection is based on a metaanalysis of prior genome screens.[42] HLA-B27 is nearly uniformly and strongly associated with spondylarthritis.[43]

Genome-wide association studies have become the norm with certain provisos. The studies need to be large with extensive phenotype documentation, and the statistical ability to monitor population stratification. It is important to distinguish significant odds ratios from false positives resulting from multiple testing errors. In genome wide studies P values must be in the range of 10^{-7} to 10^{-9} to be considered as significant. Even studies with large numbers of DNA samples (e.g., 1000) are limited in their ability to detect associations. To combat these issues, SNPs are often chosen based on less stringent statistics for testing in replication cohorts. Building large cohorts and employing strategies that maximize power for discovery have been challenges in pediatric rheumatic disease genetic studies.

Replication and Extension of Findings

Initial findings suggestive of linkage or association in any genome-wide study require replication. Hence, a second set of DNA on a new population is a necessity to establish a gene or region for further evaluation. The method of approach, earlier through sib pairs or through case-control studies (see later discussion), need not be identical in design to the first study and could be focused on areas of potential interest (chromosome loci or genes) established in the initial study. For the next step to identify causal variation, different design strategies could be used, e.g., exon sequencing, sequencing complete gene regions, or studying samples with extreme phenotypes or the entire phenotypic distribution, but there is so far no consensus on the best approach.

PEDIATRIC RHEUMATIC ILLNESSES AS COMPLEX GENETIC TRAITS

To what extent are the common chronic pediatric rheumatic illnesses complex genetic traits? The subtypes of JIA, juvenile dermatomyositis, SLE, and scleroderma are undoubtedly all in this category. Supportive evidence is available for some diseases but not for others

For oligoarticular JIA with onset in young children, the relatively frequent occurrence of this illness has ensured that enough ASPs are available to demonstrate substantial

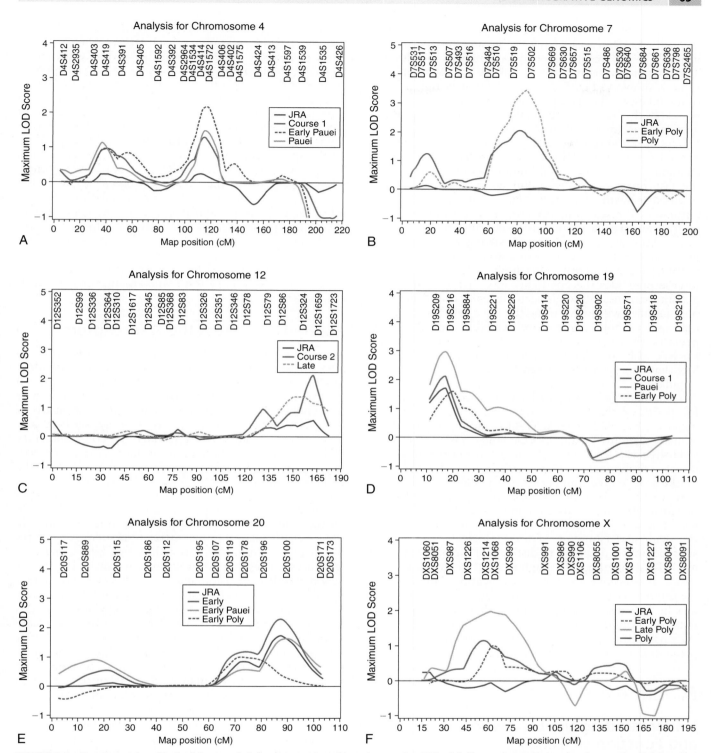

FIGURE 5-1 Nonparametric multipoint linkage analysis for chromosomes with peaks exceeding LOD= 2.0. The results are displayed as the negative 10th logarithm of the probability (p) value for indicated subphenotypes. The x-axis indicates the chromosome distance in centimorgans (cM), and the microsatellite markers are shown across the top. For each chromosome, all subphenotypes that have coincident peaks are shown.

concordance for disease.[44] HLA associations are well documented, although extended multiplex families are not available for linkage studies. HLA and JIA have been shown to be linked through two approaches by the TDT in 103 HLA-typed simplex families[45] and through allele

sharing in 53 ASPs.[46] Both of these studies used fewer numbers of families than has generally been the case in genomic studies in adults, suggesting that a genome-wide screen will be successful in identifying at least the major susceptibility, if not all of the minor susceptibility, loci.

An initial genome wide screen with eight regions identified with LOD scores of two or greater has been published.[47] These results depend on analyses of subsets. The nonparametric multipoint linkage for each chromosome is shown in Fig. 5–1. Simplex families and association studies will be required to resolve additional genetic issues. Both the candidate gene approach and genome-wide screens are feasible and in progress.

The selection of candidate genes can be based on evidence from studies of JIA, other arthropathies, and from candidate loci in other autoimmune diseases in general, the last being especially useful because such data are oriented toward non-HLA genes. The occurrence of autoimmune diseases in JIA families is documented,[35,48] as it is in juvenile dermatomyositis, in which, in addition to HLA associations, there is stronger evidence of an increased familial prevalence of autoimmune disease.[49] In juvenile dermatomyositis, the limited occurrence of the disease precludes the possibility of enough sib pairs for genome screens, although such sib pairs do occur. Simplex families will prove to be the most reliable resource, especially if both parents are available. For the other pediatric rheumatic disorders, studies in adults, especially for RA, SLE, and AS, will generate candidate genes and loci that can be readily tested for relevance in pediatric populations.[50-54]

Candidate genes studies have been completed in JIA for many of the findings described for adult arthritis including PTPN22, IL2RA, STAT4, and IL2-IL21.[55-57,57a] While a definitive genome-wide study has not yet been published for JIA, the best studied pediatric rheumatic disease, preliminary screens with a limited number of markers or limited number of patients have revealed the potential for novel genetic discovery in JIA and other pediatric rheumatic diseases including TRAF1-C5.[58,59] Genomic discovery in JIA may ultimately lead to a more thorough understanding of the biological basis for JIA subtypes and a potential to distinguish them at a subtype level. This will affect the diagnosis and treatment by providing an objective means for classification. Furthermore, identifying contributing genetic factors may provide insight into disease origins and pathogenesis, may promote development of more rationally conceived biologically based therapies, and may offer opportunities for the prevention of disease and disability.

FUNCTIONAL GENOMICS

Understanding the Expression and Function of Genes

For decades biologists have been interested in the temporal and spatial patterns of expression of genes and their protein products, interacting gene products, and the consequences for the individual when a gene product is altered or absent. Functional genomics refer broadly to the methods and techniques aimed at answering these questions systematically for all genes encoded in the genome and complement the global approaches to studying genome structure and its variability described in the preceding pages.

The exact number of genes encoded in the human genome is still unknown. Scientists at the National Human Genome Research Institute estimate the number of protein-coding genes (i.e., those where mRNAs encode functional proteins) to be in the range of 20,000 to 25,000. The number of genes expressed at a given time in a particular cell type depends on a variety of factors but is much smaller. Genes expressed in different cell types overlap but also differ considerably depending on the specialized function of the cell. Gene expression at the level of individual mRNA abundance is generally referred to as the "transcriptome," whereas the protein products that result from translation of these mRNAs (i.e., the protein products of the genome) are called the "proteome." Microarray (or "chip") technology has made assessing the transcriptome, both qualitatively and quantitatively, a routine laboratory practice. Although methods to detect and measure the proteome of a cell or tissue have improved significantly, difficulties remain.

Methods to Assess the Transcriptome

Microarray-based platforms are frequently used to assess comprehensively the abundance of individual mRNA transcripts. Oligonucleotide arrays use 25 to 60 nucleotide oligomers with perfect and single-base pair mismatched oligonucleotides to provide a measure of specificity. RNA samples are reverse transcribed, and then complementary RNA (cRNA) or complementary DNA (cDNA), containing fluorescent-labeled nucleotides, is synthesized. The product is hybridized to the chip, and the fluorescent signal intensity, which is proportional to the abundance of the particular mRNA species in the original sample, is measured at each location on the chip using a high-resolution scanner. Commonly used oligonucleotide microarrays include Affymetrix GeneChips®, Illumina Expression BeadChips®, and Agilent chips®. These vendors sell chips that provide virtually genome-wide expression analyses of known and characterized genes and ESTs (expressed sequence tags). Newer sequencing-based approaches to gene expression analysis are beginning to emerge (e.g., RNA-Seq) because of the availability of ultrahigh-throughput DNA sequencing or "deep sequencing." One advantage of this new technology is the potential for discovery of rare transcripts and alternative splicing events.[60,61] The Affymetrix Human Exon Array® also enables expression analysis at the exon level, and thus a view of alternative splicing events expected to translate into changes in the expression of a gene product.[62] cDNA arrays spotted onto glass slides can be used as an alternative to oligonucleotide arrays. Typically two mRNA samples for comparison are labeled with distinct fluorescent probes and then combined and hybridized to the chip. The signal intensity ratio for the two fluorescent probes provides a measure of the relative amount of the mRNA in the two samples. A detailed comparison of the strengths and weaknesses of these two methods is beyond the scope of this review. However, one advantage of the oligonucleotide-based microarrays is that with the one sample-one chip approach, multiple crosswise comparisons can be made. This is particularly important when comparing multiple clinical samples in large datasets.

Data Analysis

An in-depth discussion of data analysis for microarray-based gene expression studies is beyond the scope of this chapter. Nevertheless, a few important points should be considered. Issues of experimental design and quantity, quality, and efficient processing of samples are paramount to obtaining sufficient power to detect statistically significant and biologically meaningful differences. Delayed processing or exposure of cells to heat or cold stress can dramatically change gene expression patterns. Estimates of sample sizes depend on the questions being asked, the complexity of the sample (e.g., number of cell or tissue types represented), and variability between samples. For a relatively homogeneous disease state using peripheral blood, sample numbers can be expected to range from 20 to 40 or more, and with higher numbers enabling further heterogeneity to be discovered. Given the issues inherent in the analysis of data generated from 40,000 probe sets, conservative P value interpretation and/or multiple testing corrections are often necessary. Several software packages are available for identifying differentially expressed genes across multiple samples, recognizing clusters of genes with similar expression, identifying pathways with functional significance, and estimating overall similarity and differences between patterns of gene expression in complex samples. It is important to remember that the relative abundance of individual mRNA species does not always correlate with the abundance of the encoded protein. The turnover of many individual proteins is tightly regulated. Furthermore, in complex samples such as tissue, whole blood, or peripheral blood mononuclear cells (PBMCs), where several cell types are represented, increases or decreases in the expression of individual genes may represent differences in the abundance of cell populations.

Proteomics

Proteomics refers to the systematic study of the structure and function of all proteins encoded in the genome.[63] This may include identification and quantitation of all proteins expressed in a particular cell or tissue type, determining posttranslational modifications, subcellular locations, and interacting partners. Methods to assess the proteome have lagged significantly behind genomic techniques for a variety of reasons. Proteins are inherently more complex with 20 amino acid building blocks, rather than four nucleotides for DNA/RNA; they cannot be amplified *in vitro*; and there are considerable posttranslational modifications, such as glycosylation and phosphorylation that affect structure and conformation. Multiple translation products from differentially spliced mRNA and/or proteolytic processing further increase the complexity of the proteome. Thus, in many cases, a single gene locus may give rise to multiple molecular species because resolution of proteins based on migration in 2D gels depends primarily on two parameters, relative molecular mass (M_r), and isoelectric point (pI), there may be considerable overlap in a complex mixture containing thousands of cellular proteins. Methods such as mass spectroscopy (MS),

which provides precise mass measurements, are highly sensitive and provide greater resolution than 2D gel separations but are difficult to automate

Protein Identification by Mass Spectroscopy (MS) Peptide Fingerprinting

The identification of individual proteins separated from complex mixtures has become relatively routine. Single protein "spots" from 2D gel separations can be removed from the gel, be proteolytically digested into peptide fragments, and be subjected to MS analysis. Matrix assisted laser desorption ionization - time of flight provides highly precise fragment masses (fingerprints), which are matched against a database of calculated peptide fragment masses from "*in silico*" digested proteins based on the specificity of the protease

It is also possible to obtain peptide sequence information using tandem MS (MS/MS or MS^2), where peptide ion fragments in a complex mixture are isolated in the machine due to their mass (*m/z*), and then fragmented in the gas phase. Because peptides will fragment in a sequence-dependent fashion, in most cases, an unambiguous ordering of the amino acids can be obtained from the MS/MS spectrum. This technology has been instrumental in determining the sequences of complex mixtures of peptides derived from HLA class I and class II molecules.[64]

Methods for Studying the Proteome

Microarray-Based Methods

As indicated previously, the proteome is more difficult to study than the transcriptome. Two techniques are usually applied.

Protein or antigen arrays have been used successfully to assess autoantibody profiles from patients with various autoimmune diseases. Antibody to protein or peptide autoantigens attached to planar surfaces is visualized with anti-human secondary antibodies conjugated to fluoroprobes followed by scanning and quantitation. The arrays were more sensitive than conventional enzyme-linked immunosorbent assay (ELISAs) and offered parallel screening for multiple autoantibodies. Studies using MS or 2D gel methods have also revealed differences in proteins expressed in the synovial fluid or peripheral blood of RA patients compared with reactive or osteoarthritis controls.[65,66] An innovative approach is to tag monoclonal antibodies covalently with unique oligonucleotide sequences as a molecular "bar code."[67] After reacting with a sample of immobilized antigens or cells and removing unbound antibodies, the tags can be amplified enzymatically and be reacted with a DNA microarray to indirectly measure the analyte.

A second approach is to detect protein-protein interactions by genetic methods known as "yeast two-hybrid screens." Using molecular biological tools, a known or "bait" protein can be expressed as a fusion product with the DNA-binding domain of a transcriptional activator. A different protein ("prey") is expressed as a fusion product with the activation domain of the transcription factor. If the bait and prey interact when expressed in the yeast, the result is activation of transcription of a reporter gene that can easily be detected. This method can be used to study protein-protein interactions of known gene products or to screen entire libraries to discover interaction partners.

Functional Genomics in Pediatric Rheumatic Diseases

Functional and integrative genomics approaches have been applied to the study of pathogenesis of complex rheumatological diseases. Oligonucleotide microarrays were used to examine differential gene expression in PBMCs from patients with juvenile onset SLE,[68] and revealed prominent granulopoiesis and type I interferon (IFN)-response "signatures," with the latter correlating with disease activity scores (SLEDAI) and highlighting a role for IFN-α in SLE pathogenesis.[69] The granulopoiesis signature was more surprising, and further analysis of cell populations led to the identification of highly granular cells in the early stages of granulocyte development that purified with PBMC and were present in new-onset untreated patients. Similar evidence for upregulation of IFN-inducible genes in adult onset SLE[70,71] also correlated with disease severity, particularly with renal and hematological involvement. These studies supported the potential for targeting type I IFNs in SLE and have led to new ideas about pathogenesis. Furthermore, new biomarkers have been identified that may help investigators and eventually clinicians to follow disease activity and potentially even predict severity.

In early studies on juvenile arthritis, it became apparent that PBMC gene expression differences could distinguish patients with polyarticular juvenile RA (JRA, ACR criteria) from healthy controls.[71] This work also revealed possible differences between the polyarticular and pauciarticular subtypes and patients with juvenile onset AS. Interestingly, differentially expressed genes in the peripheral blood of polyarticular JIA patients tended to normalize when the patients responded to treatment.[72] Subsequent large studies have confirmed and significantly extended initial observations. First, it has been possible to distinguish the major subtypes of JIA, including oligoarticular, polyarticular, systemic, and enthesitis-related arthritis, based on PBMC gene expression differences at disease onset prior to any treatment with disease modifying antirheumatic drugs. In addition to distinguishing disease subgroups, there was evidence of upregulation of genes responsive to IL-10 in several subtypes (oligo- and polyarticular and systemic). Perhaps, not surprisingly, gene expression differences in active systemic JIA are quite profound and include evidence for IL-1 and IL-6 signaling, an erythropoiesis signature with overexpression of fetal hemoglobins, innate immune signaling, and downregulation of natural killer cell and T cell networks.[73-76]

Studies of large numbers of recent onset JIA patients have also revealed substantial heterogeneity within the polyarticular JIA subtype. In 59 subjects classified with polyarticular JIA, at least three subgroups were identified based on the relative strengths of three gene expression signatures.[77] One signature (I), most likely from monocytes, correlated with the presence of autoantibodies (RF and anti-CCP), and was present in two groups of polyarticular JIA subjects but not the third. Another signature (III) with low CD8 expression was associated with reduced numbers of CD8 T cells and increased plasmacytoid dendritic cells. Signature III was almost exclusively found in one group of polyarticular JIA subjects, and many of the gene expression differences were consistent with biological effects of TGFβ. Together with emerging genetic data, these results strongly support a molecular genetic and gene expression biomarker-based approach to JIA classification.

Although functional genomics studies in the pediatric rheumatic diseases are still emerging, these papers highlight several important points. First, it is striking that peripheral blood is such a rich source of information. Although this might have been expected in active SLE, it is perhaps more surprising in JIA and supports the concept that the joint inflammation might be an end result of immune dysregulation, rather than simply being a sight where joint antigens drive a crossreactive local inflammatory process. Second, analysis of complex cell mixtures, such as those present in peripheral blood and synovial fluid, can provide useful information, despite the complexity of the sample. It has been striking in these and other studies how powerful small changes in RNA abundance are for detecting differences in cell populations rather than simply up or downregulation of genes. Third, the comprehensive nature of microarrays affords several advantages, including the ability to measure simultaneously multiple gene products in a pathway, which can be more sensitive and more specific than analyzing individual genes or even levels of the cytokine responsible for the signature. Finally regardless of the actual identities of the differentially represented genes, consistent differences between the groups being compared can serve as gene expression biomarkers that help distinguish disease subtypes, and equally importantly, disease states.[78] It will be important to develop biological correlates of active and inactive disease states that will enrich our clinical definitions and will eventually provide a biological definition of remission. It may be possible to use information from these types of studies to predict outcome, e.g., identifying patients most likely to develop severe erosive arthritis involving multiple joints. There are currently few good predictors for these outcomes, but it is possible that genotyping for known susceptibility alleles combined with differential gene expression analyses will provide clues to some of these questions in the near future.

CONCLUSION

The immune-mediated inflammatory diseases most commonly encountered by pediatric rheumatologists are complex genetic traits that result from the interaction of multiple gene products in the context of environmental signals that generate immune responses. Eventually, diagnosis and prognosis will be based on such traits, and some combination of information derived from genetic polymorphisms and gene expression biomarkers will be used to predict responsiveness to therapy. Ultimately, therapy will be matched to an individual's genomic findings, a science known as *pharmacogenetics*. The methods now being developed to evaluate genomes will also allow gene therapy to be applied to chronic pediatric rheumatic illnesses.

REFERENCES

1. R.E. Petty, T.R. Southwood, P. Manners, et al., International League of Associations for Rheumatology classification of juvenile idiopathic arthritis: second revision, Edmonton, 2001, J. Rheumatol. 31 (2004) 390–392.

2. E. Lundstrom, H. Kallberg, M. Smolnikova, et al., Opposing effects of HLA-DRB1*13 alleles on the risk of developing anti-citrullinated protein antibody-positive and anti-citrullinated protein antibody-negative rheumatoid arthritis, Arthritis Rheum. 60 (2009) 924–930.

3. S.F. Grant, H. Hakonarson, Microarray technology and applications in the arena of genome-wide association, Clin. Chem. 54 (2008) 1116–1124.

4. E.T. Dermitzakis, A. Reymond, N. Scamuffa, et al., Evolutionary discrimination of mammalian conserved non-genic sequences (CNGs), Science 302 (2003) 1033–1035.

5. K.E. Sullivan, D.M. McDonald-McGinn, D.A. Driscoll, et al., Juvenile rheumatoid arthritis-like polyarthritis in chromosome 22q11.2 deletion syndrome (DiGeorge anomalad/velocardiofacial syndrome/conotruncal anomaly face syndrome), Arthritis Rheum. 40 (1997) 430–436.

6. X.S. Zhou, W. Cole, S. Hu, et al., Detection of DNA copy number abnormality by microarray expression analysis, Hum. Genet. 114 (2004) 464–467.

7. L. Kruglyak, The use of a genetic map of biallelic markers in linkage studies, Nat. Genet. 17 (1997) 21–24.

8. E. Pennisi, A closer look at SNPs suggests difficulties, Science 281 (1998) 1787–1789.

9. F.D. Martinez, P.E. Graves, M. Baldini, et al., Association between genetic polymorphisms of the beta2-adrenoceptor and response to albuterol in children with and without a history of wheezing, J. Clin. Vest. 100 (1997) 3184–3188.

10. G.K. Hershey, M.F. Friedrich, L.A. Esswein, et al., The association of atopy with a gain-of-function mutation in the alpha subunit of the interleukin-4 receptor, N. Engl. J. Med. 337 (1997) 1720–1725.

11. E.J. Hollox, U. Huffmeier, P.L. Zeeuwen, et al., Psoriasis is associated with increased beta-defensin genomic copy number, Nat. Genet. 40 (2008) 23–25.

12. N. Risch, Linkage strategies for genetically complex traits. II. The power of affected relative pairs, Am. J. Hum. Genet. 46 (1990) 229–241.

13. R.S. Spielman, R.E. McGinnis, W.J. Ewens, Transmission test for linkage disequilibrium: the insulin gene region and insulin-dependent diabetes mellitus (IDDM), Am. J. Hum. Genet. 52 (1993) 506–516.

14. R.S. Spielman, R.E. McGinnis, W.J. Ewens, The transmission/disequilibrium test detects cosegregation and linkage, Am. J. Hum. Genet. 54 (1994) 559–560. author reply 560-553.

15. R.S. Spielman, W.J. Ewens, A sibship test for linkage in the presence of association: the sib transmission/disequilibrium test, Am. J. Hum. Genet. 62 (1998) 450–458.

16. C. Dib, S. Faure, C. Fizames, et al., A comprehensive genetic map of the human genome based on 5,264 microsatellites, Nature 380 (1996) 152–154.

17. D. Cohen, I. Chumakov, J. Weissenbach, A first-generation physical map of the human genome, Nature 366 (1993) 698–701.

18. Complete sequence and gene map of a human major histocompatibility complex. The MHC sequencing consortium, Nature 401 (1999) 921–923.

19. R. Horton, L. Wilming, V. Rand, et al., Gene map of the extended human MHC, Nat. Rev. Genet. 5 (2004) 889–899.

20. The International HapMap Project, Nature 426 (2003) 789–796.

21. T. Strachan, M. Abitbol, D. Davidson, et al., A new dimension for the human genome project: towards comprehensive expression maps, Nat. Genet. 16 (1997) 126–132.

22. R.A. Heller, M. Schena, A. Chai, et al., Discovery and analysis of inflammatory disease-related genes using cDNA microarrays, Proc. Natl. Acad. Sci. U.S.A. 94 (1997) 2150–2155.

23. P.W. Reed, J.L. Davies, J.B. Copeman, et al., Chromosome-specific microsatellite sets for fluorescence-based, semi-automated genome mapping, Nat. Genet. 7 (1994) 390–395.

24. J.S. Ziegle, Y. Su, K.P. Corcoran, et al., Application of automated DNA sizing technology for genotyping microsatellite loci, Genomics. 14 (1992) 1026–1031.

25. E.C. Chalom, J. Ross, B.H. Athreya, Syndromes and arthritis, Rheum. Dis. Clin. North. Am. 23 (1997) 709–727.

26. S. Prahalad, R.A. Colbert, Genetic diseases with rheumatic manifestations in children, Curr. Opin. Rheumatol. 10 (1998) 488–493.

27. T.I.F. Consortium, Ancient missense mutations in a new member of the RoRet gene family are likely to cause familial Mediterranean fever, The International FMF Consortium, Cell 90 (1997) 797–807.

28. M.F. McDermott, I. Aksentijevich, J. Galon, et al., Germline mutations in the extracellular domains of the 55 kDa TNF receptor, TNFR1, define a family of dominantly inherited autoinflammatory syndromes, Cell 97 (1999) 133–144.

29. S.L. Masters, A. Simon, I. Aksentijevich, et al., Horror autoinflammaticus: the molecular pathophysiology of autoinflammatory disease*, Annu. Rev. Immunol. 27 (2009) 621–668.

30. E.S. Lander, N.J. Schork, Genetic dissection of complex traits, Science 265 (1994) 2037–2048.

31. N. Risch, K. Merikangas, The future of genetic studies of complex human diseases, Science 273 (1996) 1516–1517.

32. J.L. Davies, Y. Kawaguchi, S.T. Bennett, et al., A genome-wide search for human type 1 diabetes susceptibility genes, Nature 371 (1994) 130–136.

33. N. Risch, Linkage strategies for genetically complex traits. I. Multilocus models, Am. J. Hum. Genet. 46 (1990) 222–228.

34. P. Rosen, S. Thompson, D. Glass, Non-HLA gene polymorphisms in juvenile rheumatoid arthritis, Clin. Exp. Rheumatol. 21 (2003) 650–656.

35. S. Prahalad, E.S. Shear, S.D. Thompson, et al., Increased prevalence of familial autoimmunity in simplex and multiplex families with juvenile rheumatoid arthritis, Arthritis Rheum. 46 (2002) 1851–1856.

36. J.J. Weis, B.A. McCracken, Y. Ma, et al., Identification of quantitative trait loci governing arthritis severity and humoral responses in the murine model of Lyme disease, J. Immunol. 162 (1999) 948–956.

37. P.K. Gregersen, L.M. Olsson, Recent advances in the genetics of autoimmune disease, Annu. Rev. Immunol. 27 (2009) 363–391.

38. R.M. Plenge, Rheumatoid arthritis genetics: 2009 update, Curr. Rheumatol. Rep. 11 (2009) 351–356.

39. M. Adachi, R. Watanabe-Fukunaga, S. Nagata, Aberrant transcription caused by the insertion of an early transposable element in an intron of the Fas antigen gene of lpr mice, Proc. Natl. Acad. Sci. U.S.A. 90 (1993) 1756–1760.

40. G.H. Fisher, F.J. Rosenberg, S.E. Straus, et al., Dominant interfering Fas gene mutations impair apoptosis in a human autoimmune lymphoproliferative syndrome, Cell 81 (1995) 935–946.

41. A. Zhernakova, C.C. van Diemen, C. Wijmenga, Detecting shared pathogenesis from the shared genetics of immune-related diseases, Nat. Rev. Genet. 10 (2009) 43–55.

42. K.G. Becker, R.M. Simon, J.E. Bailey-Wilson, et al., Clustering of non-major histocompatibility complex susceptibility candidate loci in human autoimmune diseases, Proc. Natl. Acad. Sci. U.S.A. 95 (1998) 9979–9984.

43. S. Gonzalez-Roces, M.V. Alvarez, S. Gonzalez, et al., HLA-B27 polymorphism and worldwide susceptibility to ankylosing spondylitis, Tissue Antigens 49 (1997) 116–123.

44. M.B. Moroldo, M. Chaudhari, E. Shear, et al., Juvenile rheumatoid arthritis affected sibpairs: extent of clinical phenotype concordance, Arthritis Rheum. 50 (2004) 1928–1934.

45. M.B. Moroldo, P. Donnelly, J. Saunders, et al., Transmission disequilibrium as a test of linkage and association between HLA alleles and pauciarticular-onset juvenile rheumatoid arthritis, Arthritis Rheum. 41 (1998) 1620–1624.

46. S. Prahalad, M.H. Ryan, E.S. Shear, et al., Juvenile rheumatoid arthritis: linkage to HLA demonstrated by allele sharing in affected sibpairs, Arthritis Rheum. 43 (2000) 2335–2338.

47. S.D. Thompson, M.B. Moroldo, L. Guyer, et al., A genome-wide scan for juvenile rheumatoid arthritis in affected sibpair families provides evidence of linkage, Arthritis Rheum. 50 (2004) 2920–2930.

48. R.D. Rossen, E.J. Brewer, R.M. Sharp, et al., Familial rheumatoid arthritis: linkage of HLA to disease susceptibility locus in four families where proband presented with juvenile rheumatoid arthritis, J. Clin. Invest. 65 (1980) 629–642.

49. L.R. Ginn, J.P. Lin, P.H. Plotz, et al., Familial autoimmunity in pedigrees of idiopathic inflammatory myopathy patients suggests common genetic risk factors for many autoimmune diseases, Arthritis Rheum. 41 (1998) 400–405.

50. D. Jawaheer, M.F. Seldin, C.I. Amos, et al., Screening the genome for rheumatoid arthritis susceptibility genes: a replication study and combined analysis of 512 multicase families, Arthritis Rheum. 48 (2003) 906–916.

51. B.P. Tsao, R.M. Cantor, K.C. Kalunian, et al., Evidence for linkage of a candidate chromosome 1 region to human systemic lupus erythematosus, J. Clin. Invest. 99 (1997) 725–731.

52. J.J. Eskdale, P. McNicholl, B. Wordsworth, et al., Interleukin-10 microsatellite polymorphisms and IL-10 locus alleles in rheumatoid arthritis susceptibility, Lancet 352 (1998) 1282–1283.

53. K.L. Moser, B.R. Neas, J.E. Salmon, et al., Genome scan of human systemic lupus erythematosus: evidence for linkage on chromosome 1q in African-American pedigrees, Proc. Natl. Acad. Sci. U.S.A. 95 (1998) 14869–14874.

54. P.M. Gaffney, G.M. Kearns, K.B. Shark, et al., A genome-wide search for susceptibility genes in human systemic lupus erythematosus sib-pair families, Proc. Natl. Acad. Sci. U.S.A. 95 (1998) 14875–14879.

55. A. Hinks, A. Barton, X. Ke, et al., Association of juvenile idiopathic arthritiis (JIA) with the IL2RA gene, EULAR (2008).

56. A. Hinks, S. Eyre, X. Ke, et al., Overlap of disease susceptibility loci for rheumatoid arthritis (RA) and juvenile idiopathic arthritis (JIA), Ann. Rheum. Dis (2009).

57. S. Prahalad, S. Hansen, A. Whiting, et al., Variants in TNFAIP3, STAT4, and C12orf30 loci associated with multiple autoimmune diseases are also associated with juvenile idiopathic arthritis, Arthritis Rheum. 60 (2009) 2124–2130.

57a. A. Hinks, S. Eyre, X. Ke, et al., Association of the AFF3 gene and IL2/IL21 gene region with juvenile idiopathic arthritis, Genes Immun. 11 (2010) 194–198.

58. A. Hinks, A. Barton, N. Shephard, et al., Identification of a novel susceptibility locus for juvenile idiopathic arthritis by genome-wide association analysis, Arthritis Rheum. 60 (2009) 258–263.

59. E.M. Behrens, T.H. Finkel, J.P. Bradfield, et al., Association of the TRAF1-C5 locus on chromosome 9 with juvenile idiopathic arthritis, Arthritis Rheum. 58 (2008) 2206–2207.

60. Z. Wang, M. Gerstein, M. Snyder, RNA-Seq: a revolutionary tool for transcriptomics, Nat. Rev. Genet. 10 (2009) 57–63.

61. J.W. Bauer, H. Bilgic, E.C. Baechler, Gene-expression profiling in rheumatic disease: tools and therapeutic potential, Nat. Rev. Rheumatol. 5 (2009) 257–265.

62. T. Kwan, D. Benovoy, C. Dias, et al., Genome-wide analysis of transcript isoform variation in humans, Nat. Genet. 40 (2008) 225–231.

63. S.D. Patterson, R.H. Aebersold, Proteomics: the first decade and beyond, Nat. Genet. 33 (Suppl.) (2003) 311–323.

64. D.F. Hunt, R.A. Henderson, J. Shabanowitz, et al., Characterization of peptides bound to the class I MHC molecule HLA-A2.1 by mass spectrometry, Science 255 (1992) 1261–1263.

65. A. Sinz, M. Bantscheff, S. Mikkat, et al., Mass spectrometric proteome analyses of synovial fluids and plasmas from patients suffering from rheumatoid arthritis and comparison to reactive arthritis or osteoarthritis, Electrophoresis 23 (2002) 3445–3456.

66. H. Dotzlaw, M. Schulz, M. Eggert, et al., A pattern of protein expression in peripheral blood mononuclear cells distinguishes rheumatoid arthritis patients from healthy individuals, Biochim. Biophys. Acta. 1696 (2004) 121–129.

67. M.G. Kattah, J. Coller, R.K. Cheung, et al., HIT: a versatile proteomics platform for multianalyte phenotyping of cytokines, intracellular proteins and surface molecules, Nat. Med. 14 (2008) 1284–1289.

68. L. Bennett, A.K. Palucka, E. Arce, et al., Interferon and granulopoiesis signatures in systemic lupus erythematosus blood, J. Exp. Med. 197 (2003) 711–723.

69. P. Blanco, A.K. Palucka, M. Gill, et al., Induction of dendritic cell differentiation by IFN-alpha in systemic lupus erythematosus, Science 294 (2001) 1540–1543.

70. E.C. Baechler, F.M. Batliwalla, G. Karypis, et al., Interferon-inducible gene expression signature in peripheral blood cells of patients with severe lupus, Proc. Natl. Acad. Sci. U.S.A. 100 (2003) 2610–2615.

71. M.G. Barnes, B.J. Aronow, L.K. Luyrink, et al., Gene expression in juvenile arthritis and spondyloarthropathy: pro-angiogenic ELR+ chemokine genes relate to course of arthritis, Rheumatology (Oxford) 43 (2004) 973–979.

72. J.N. Jarvis, I. Dozmorov, K. Jiang, et al., Novel approaches to gene expression analysis of active polyarticular juvenile rheumatoid arthritis, Arth. Res. Ther. 6 (2004) R15–R32.

73. F. Allantaz, D. Chaussabel, D.L. Stichweh, et al., Blood leukocyte microarrays to diagnose systemic onset juvenile idiopathic arthritis and follow the response to IL-1 blockade, J. Exp. Med. 204 (2007) 2131–2144.

74. N. Fall, M. Barnes, S. Thornton, et al., Gene expression profiling of peripheral blood from patients with untreated new-onset systemic juvenile idiopathic arthritis reveals molecular heterogeneity that may predict macrophage activation syndrome, Arthritis Rheum. 56 (2007) 3793–3804.

75. M.G. Barnes, A.A. Grom, S.D. Thompson, et al., Subtype-specific peripheral blood gene expression profiles in recent-onset juvenile idiopathic arthritis, Arthritis Rheum. 60 (2009) 2102–2112.

76. E.M. Ogilvie, A. Khan, M. Hubank, et al., Specific gene expression profiles in systemic juvenile idiopathic arthritis, Arthritis Rheum. 56 (2007) 1954–1965.

77. T. Griffin, M.G. Barnes, N.T. Ilowite, et al., Gene expression signatures in polyarticular juvenile idiopathic arthritis demonstrate disease heterogeneity and offer a molecular classification of disease subsets, Arthritis Rheum. 60 (2009) 2113–2123.

78. N. Knowlton, K. Jiang, M.B. Frank, et al., The meaning of clinical remission in polyarticular juvenile idiopathic arthritis: gene expression profiling in peripheral blood mononuclear cells identifies distinct disease states, Arthritis Rheum. 60 (2009) 892–900.

79. D. van der Woude, J.J. Houwing-Duistermaat, R.E. Toes, et al., Quantitative heritability of anti-citrullinated protein antibody-positive and anti-citrullinated protein antibody-negative rheumatoid arthritis, Arthritis Rheum. 60 (2009) 916–923.

Chapter 6

PHARMACOLOGY AND DRUG THERAPY

Norman T. Ilowite and Ronald M. Laxer

The principal drugs used in pediatric rheumatology are drugs that suppress the inflammatory and immune responses. The targets of their therapeutic effects are predominantly the arachidonic acid metabolic pathways and the cells of the immune system and their products. This chapter outlines important general principles relating to use of these medications, particularly as they apply to children. The treatment of specific rheumatic disorders is discussed in detail in the relevant chapters.

CONCEPTS IN PHARMACOLOGY

Knowledge of the pharmacokinetics of drugs used to treat childhood rheumatic diseases contributes to understanding of their clinical applications. The following brief overview can be supplemented by referring to standard works in the field.[1,2]

Drug Absorption and Bioavailability

Drugs that are given by the oral route are absorbed mainly through the mucosa of the gastrointestinal (GI) tract, primarily in the small intestine. GI absorption may be influenced by numerous factors, including the presence or absence of food in the gastric lumen, luminal pH, gastric emptying time, and coadministration of other drugs. Drug bioavailability, the net result of these factors, is usually determined by sequential measurement of plasma drug concentrations. Three parameters are routinely considered: peak drug concentration, the time necessary to reach peak concentration, and the area under the time-concentration curve. The area under the curve after intravenous administration is considered equivalent to complete absorption after oral administration. Because the effects of many repeatedly administered drugs are cumulative except with drugs of extremely short half-life given at infrequent intervals, bioavailability is best determined at the mean steady-state concentration of the drug—that is, the point at which drug intake is equal to drug elimination.

Volume of Distribution

The volume of distribution is the volume of fluid into which a drug would need to be distributed to achieve a concentration equal to the concentration ultimately measured in plasma. If the drug stays in the plasma, its volume of distribution is smaller than if it is distributed widely in tissues.

Drugs in the body are either free or bound to plasma proteins or tissue lipids. The extent and nature of binding affect the volume of distribution of the drug, the rate of renal clearance (because only free drug is filtered by the glomerulus), the drug half-life, and the amount of free drug that reaches the target tissue or receptor.

Most acidic drugs are bound to plasma albumin, whereas the basic drugs are bound to lipoproteins, α_1-acid glycoproteins, and globulins. In inflammatory states, plasma albumin concentration decreases, and α_1-acid glycoproteins increase, although the extent of the decrease usually does not require any change in drug therapy. Drugs that are highly protein bound tend to stay within the vascular compartment and have a limited volume of distribution. Drugs that are widely bound to lipids in tissues have large volumes of distribution.

Half-life and Clearance

The half-life of a drug is the time necessary for the serum concentration to decrease by 50% during the elimination phase of a time-concentration curve. Clearance is a measure of the removal of a drug from the body as a whole or from a specific part of the body, such as liver or kidney. It is expressed as the volume of body fluid from which a drug is removed per unit of time.

The first-pass effect refers to the rapid breakdown of a drug when it passes through the intestinal mucosa or enters the liver for the first time. In this case, the drug reaches the systemic circulation predominantly in the form of metabolites that may be pharmacologically inactive. Avoidance of this effect requires intravenous administration.

When the rate of elimination of a drug is directly proportional to its concentration in the body, the drug is said to have first-order kinetics. Drugs that are eliminated at a constant rate, unrelated to the amount of the agent in the body, are said to follow zero-order kinetics. Some drugs obey capacity-limited kinetics: At low concentrations, first-order kinetics are observed; at higher concentrations, the enzymes used in metabolism of the drug are saturated, and zero-order kinetics is approached. Salicylate and its metabolites exhibit this phenomenon. Time-dependent kinetics may be altered by the effect of drug metabolites. For most drugs, a steady state is not reached until the passage of five half-lives. Blood levels measured before that time may be erroneous.

Drug Biotransformation

Drug biotransformation or metabolism principally occurs in the liver, kidney, skin, and GI tract. In the liver, biotransformation involves hydrolysis, oxidation, reduction, or demethylation and conjugation of the metabolite with glycine, glucuronide, sulfate, or hippurate with subsequent secretion into the bile. In the kidney, drugs may be filtered, filtered and secreted, filtered and passively reabsorbed (e.g., acetaminophen), or filtered or actively secreted and passively reabsorbed (e.g., salicylates).[3] Many drugs used to treat rheumatic diseases are active in the form in which they are administered; exceptions include sulindac, salsalate, prednisone, leflunomide, azathioprine, mycophenolate mofetil (MMF), and cyclophosphamide, which require biotransformation before they exert their principal effects.

Because the liver and kidney play such key roles in drug metabolism, dysfunction of these organs may require alteration in drug dose. Generally, additional toxicity caused by drugs that totally depend on the kidney for their elimination is not a danger, however, unless renal function is diminished by more than 50%.[2] In patients with significant renal or hepatic disease, monitoring of drug levels and attention to the potential of drug toxicity become more critical.

ANTIRHEUMATIC DRUGS

The pharmacological agents used to treat children with rheumatic disorders are grouped into five categories: nonsteroidal antiinflammatory drugs (NSAIDs); disease-modifying antirheumatic drugs (DMARDs) or slow-acting antirheumatic drugs; glucocorticoids; cytotoxic, immunosuppressive, and immunomodulatory agents; and biological response modifiers.

Nonsteroidal Antiinflammatory Drugs

Nonselective

NSAIDs provide symptomatic antiinflammatory relief; they are recommended for most patients with juvenile rheumatoid arthritis (JRA) and are used in many other rheumatic disorders. In the United States, acetylsalicylic acid (aspirin, ASA), tolmetin, naproxen, ibuprofen, etodolac, oxaprozin, meloxicam, and indomethacin are approved for pediatric use. NSAIDs that are commonly used in children are presented in Table 6–1.

Selective Cyclooxygenase-2 Inhibitors

Celecoxib is the only available cyclooxygenase-2 (COX-2) inhibitor that is approved by the U.S. Food and Drug Administration (FDA) for use in the treatment of chronic arthritis in children. Rofecoxib was also approved by the FDA for treatment of JRA signs and symptoms; however,

the manufacturer voluntarily withdrew it from the market in September 2004[4] after concerns regarding cardiovascular toxicity in adults surfaced.

Mechanism of Action

NSAIDs inhibit proinflammatory pathways that lead to chronic inflammation. The major antiinflammatory effect of NSAIDs is mediated by inhibition of the COX enzyme in the metabolism of arachidonic acid to prostaglandins, thromboxanes, and prostacyclins (Fig. 6–1) (see Chapter 3).[5] Currently available NSAIDs (except diclofenac and indomethacin) have little effect on the lipoxygenase pathway, the other major pathway of arachidonic acid metabolism.[6] Individual NSAIDs may have additional specific mechanisms of action. Indomethacin blocks the action of phosphodiesterase, increasing intracellular cyclic adenosine monophosphate.[7] This effect leads to a decrease in the generation of superoxide and hydroxyl radicals.[7-9] Indomethacin also inhibits the mobility of polymorphonuclear neutrophils in inflammatory sites. Similar to ASA and ibuprofen, indomethacin uncouples oxidative phosphorylation and decreases the synthesis of mucopolysaccharides.[10] Diclofenac and indomethacin also limit the availability of the substrate for prostaglandin and leukotriene synthesis by facilitating incorporation of arachidonic acid into triglycerides.[6,11] Piroxicam at high concentrations inhibits neutrophil migration, phagocytosis, lysosomal enzyme release,[12] and oxygen radical production by neutrophils.[13] Meclofenamate sodium may inhibit prostaglandin binding at its receptor and inhibits phospholipase A_2.[14] Meclofenamate also inhibits the lipoxygenase pathway of arachidonic acid metabolism.[15] Other differences in the mechanism of action of various NSAIDs have been reviewed elsewhere.[6,16]

There are two related but unique isoforms of the COX enzyme, COX-1 and COX-2, which are 60% identical in sequence, but are encoded by distinct genes and differ in their distribution and expression in tissues. COXs catalyze the conversion of arachidonic acid to prostaglandins G_2 and H_2 (see Fig. 6–1). COX-1, coded by the relatively stable gene *Ptgs-1*, is widely distributed and constitutively expressed in most tissues. *Ptgs-2* codes for COX-2 and is an immediate early gene activated by a wide variety of inflammatory and proliferative stimuli. It is suggested that COX-1 provides prostaglandins that are required for "housekeeping," or homeostatic function resulting in cytoprotection, platelet aggregation, vascular homeostasis, and maintenance of renal blood flow (see Fig. 6–1). In contrast, COX-2 is an inducible enzyme that is upregulated at sites of inflammation by various proinflammatory mediators, including interleukin-1 (IL-1), tumor necrosis factor-α (TNF-α), bacterial endotoxins, and various mitogenic and growth factors.

COX-2 plays the predominant role during disease states associated with inflammation and tumorigenesis. There is overlap, however, in that constitutive COX-2 expression is well recognized in brain, kidney, and the female reproductive tract, and evidence for COX-1 induction during lipopolysaccharide-mediated inflammation and cellular differentiation has been reported. COX-2 also seems to have a role in the central mediation of pain

Table 6–1

Nonsteroidal antiinflammatory drugs (NSAIDs) commonly used in children

Drug	Dose (mg/kg/day unless otherwise noted)	Maximal Dose (mg/day)	Doses per Day	Comments
Salicylates				
Acetylsalicylic acid (ASA)	Antiinflammatory dose: 80-100 (<25 kg); 2500 mg/m² (>25 kg)	4900	2-4	Kawasaki disease: high dose for initial and low dose for subsequent treatment
	Antiplatelet dose: 5			Therapeutic serum levels (for antiinflammatory therapy): 16-25 mg/dL (measure 5 days after initiation of therapy or alteration of dose)
				Nonlinear (zero-order) kinetics (see text)
				LFT abnormalities common (stop ASA if LFT >3 times normal)
				Association with Reye syndrome (see text)
				Watch for salicylism
Propionic Acid Group				
Naproxen*	10-20	1000	2	Most frequently used initial NSAID
				Overall favorable toxicity/efficacy profile
				Pseudoporphyria in fair-skinned children (see text)
				May have nonlinear pharmacokinetics at higher doses
Ibuprofen*	30-40	2400	3-4	Most favorable toxicity/efficacy profile
				Association with aseptic meningitis in patients with SLE
Ketoprofen	2-4	300	3-4	Least favorable toxicity/efficacy profile
Fenoprofen	35	3200	4	Significant risk of nephrotoxicity
Oxaprozin	10-20	1200	1	Available only in 600-mg tablets
Acetic Acid Derivatives				
Indomethacin*	1.5-3	200	3	Useful in spondyloarthropathies and treatment of fever or pericarditis in systemic-onset JRA
				Less favorable toxicity profile
				Headache common at initiation and may diminish with continuation of therapy
Tolmetin	20-30	1800	3-4	Least favorable toxicity/efficacy profile
				May cause false-positive result for urinary protein
Sulindac	4-6	400	2	Absorbed as a prodrug and converted to active metabolite
				Significant enterohepatic recirculation
				May be less nephrotoxic than other NSAIDs
Diclofenac	2-3	150	3	Similar potency to indomethacin
				Reports of significant hepatotoxicity
Etodolac	10-20	1000	1	Extended-release tablet available at 400-, 500-, 600-mg doses
Oxicams				
Meloxicam†	0.25	15	1	Once-daily dosing possible
				Relatively new agent
Piroxicam	0.2-0.3	20	1	Least favorable toxicity/efficacy profile
				Once-daily dosing possible—may be useful in older children or adolescents with poor medication compliance; little experience in young children
Nabumetone	30	2000	1	Once-daily dosing possible
				Tablets can be mixed in water to create a slurry
Pyrazole Derivative				
Celecoxib	>2 yr old, 10-25 kg: 100; >2 yr old, 25-50 kg: 200	200	2	Use lowest effective dose, shortest effective treatment
				Capsules can be opened and sprinkled on applesauce

*Available as a liquid

†Ruperto N, Nikishina I, Pachanov ED, et al. A randomized, double-blind clinical trial of two doses of meloxicam compared with naproxen in children with juvenile idiopathic arthritis: short- and long-term efficacy and safety results. Arthritis Rheum 2005;52:563-72.

LFT, liver function test; JRA, juvenile rheumatoid arthritis; SLE, systemic lupus erythematosus.

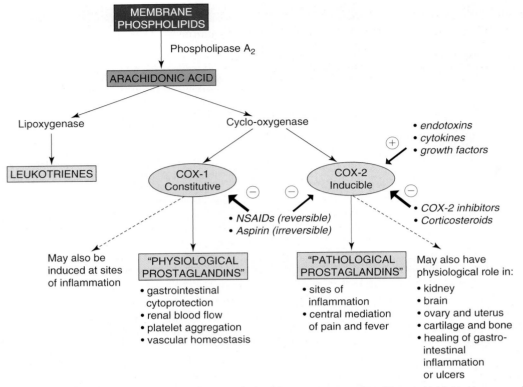

FIGURE 6–1   Synthesis of prostaglandins and leukotrienes. Sites of action of antiinflammatory agents and cytokines are highlighted by *arrows* (–, downregulation; +, upregulation). COX, cyclooxygenase; NSAIDs, nonsteroidal antiinflammatory drugs.

and fever. Absence of COX-2 results in severe disruption of postnatal kidney development, and female knockout mice are infertile because of failure of ovulation and embryo implantation. The cardiotoxic effects of COX-2 inhibition also support a constitutive role of COX-2 in maintaining cardiovascular health.

After the discovery of COX-2 in the early 1990s,[17] it was hypothesized that COX-1 mediated uniquely physiological prostaglandin production, whereas COX-2 mediated uniquely pathological prostaglandin production; consequently, the antiinflammatory effects of NSAIDs were considered to result from COX-2, and the adverse effects were considered to result from COX-1 inhibition. This hypothesis seems to have been an oversimplification, however.[18] COX-2 may also have a physiological function in certain tissues; it is expressed constitutively in structures such as the ovary, uterus, brain, kidney, cartilage, and bone.[19] COX-2 knockout mice have severe renal dystrophy, suggesting an important role for this isoenzyme in early renal development. Conversely, COX-1 may have nonphysiological functions and, similar to COX-2, may be upregulated at sites of inflammation. Each of the two isoforms of COX seems to have a role in physiological and pathological prostaglandin production and to have more broad and complex functions than originally thought.

Currently available NSAIDs inhibit both isoforms of COX, but most inhibit COX-1 preferentially, resulting in undesirable adverse effects such as GI toxicity while producing desirable antiinflammatory effects through concurrent inhibition of COX-2.[20] NSAIDs differ in the degree of inhibition of COX-2, compared with COX-1, that they produce. This difference has been found to correlate with their adverse-effect profiles: NSAIDs that are more selective for COX-2 seem to have more favorable adverse-effect profiles.[21]

In light of the differences between COX-1 and COX-2 isoenzymes and their binding sites for NSAIDs, there has been a profusion of research into a "safer" class of drugs that selectively bind to and inhibit COX-2 activity: the COX-2 inhibitors.[22] The degree of COX-2 suppression needed to produce antiinflammatory and analgesic effects in vivo is uncertain, however—a threshold degree of COX-2 inhibition that must be achieved with no associated COX-1 suppression cannot be clearly defined at this time.[23,24]

Many additional concerns remain about specific COX-2 inhibitors. Because COX-1 may also be induced at sites of inflammation, a specific COX-2 inhibitor may be less effective as an antiinflammatory or analgesic agent.[18,21,22]

The consequences of specific COX-2 inhibition in tissues wherein the COX-2 isoenzyme seems to have a physiological role, such as the renal medulla, ovary, and uterus, are also unknown.[21,22] Renal toxicity may occur with COX-2 inhibitors. The doses of existing NSAIDs that are required to reduce inflammation are generally higher than the doses needed to inhibit prostaglandin formation, suggesting the existence of other mechanisms by which their antiinflammatory effects are mediated. In addition to inhibiting prostaglandin production, current NSAIDs inhibit specific proteinases involved in degradation of proteoglycans and collagens of cartilage,[25] and inhibit the generation of oxygen radicals, particularly superoxide.[26-28] NSAIDs also have been shown to interfere with bradykinin release, response of lymphocytes to antigenic challenge, phagocytosis, and chemotaxis of granulocytes and monocytes.[29]

Pharmacology

The pharmacokinetic evaluation of NSAIDs in children with JRA has been variable, ranging from extensive for salicylates to minimal or none with newer agents; the interested reader is referred to reviews on the subject.[30,31] Studies in adults indicate that most NSAIDs share similar pharmacokinetic properties. They are weakly acidic drugs that are rapidly absorbed after oral administration, with most absorption occurring in the stomach and upper small intestine. Circadian rhythms in gastric pH and intestinal motility may lead to variability in NSAID absorption, with reduced absorption of a dose given at night compared with a dose given in the morning.[32]

Most NSAIDs are strongly protein bound, primarily to albumin, leading to a potential for drug-disease and drug-drug interactions. Hypoalbuminemia may occur as a manifestation of disease activity in JRA, especially in patients with systemic-onset disease, and may be one of the most important factors influencing the pharmacokinetics of NSAIDs in these children. Because clinical effects are determined by unbound or free drug levels, states of severe hypoalbuminemia may be associated with a corresponding increase in the unbound fraction and with a potential for increased toxicity. Most studies of NSAID pharmacokinetics in children do not report the level of disease activity, however.[33] Protein binding may also be reduced with renal or hepatic disease.

Although the strong plasma protein binding of NSAIDs also makes possible drug-drug interactions with other highly protein-bound drugs, significant clinical interactions are rare.[34,35] NSAIDs may potentially interact with methotrexate (MTX), however, through several mechanisms, including displacement from plasma protein-binding sites, competition for renal secretion, and impairment of renal function. Although the impact of NSAIDs on MTX clearance varies widely, and the potential for clinically significant interactions exists in some children,[36] MTX-NSAID interactions are rarely of clinical significance.

The kinetics of NSAIDs at their antiinflammatory sites of action (e.g., synovial fluid) may be more clinically relevant than their kinetics in plasma. The comparative kinetics of NSAIDs in plasma and synovial fluid are related to the half-life of the drug and to differences in protein binding at these sites. Studies in adults indicate that NSAIDs with short half-lives have less fluctuation in synovial fluid concentrations than in plasma concentrations over a given dosage interval.[35] This phenomenon may partially account for the fact that the dosage interval of these drugs is longer than their plasma half-life. In addition, because synovial fluid albumin concentrations are lower than plasma concentrations, the free fraction of NSAIDs in synovial fluid can be significantly higher than in plasma and has been shown to correlate with clinical effectiveness.[32] This higher free fraction of drug in synovial fluid

may account for clinical effects observed with relatively low plasma drug levels. Except for naproxen and ASA, plasma concentrations correlate poorly with antiinflammatory activity.[37]

NSAIDs are eliminated predominantly by hepatic metabolism; only small amounts are excreted unchanged in urine. Some NSAIDs, such as sulindac or indomethacin, are also secreted in significant amounts in bile and undergo enterohepatic recirculation.[35] Most NSAIDs are metabolized by first-order or linear kinetics, whereas salicylate is metabolized by zero-order or nonlinear kinetics. For this reason, dosage adjustments are frequently required with ASA therapy, and small changes in dose may lead to large fluctuations in serum levels of ASA at the higher end of the therapeutic range.[31] Naproxen may also show nonlinear pharmacokinetics at doses greater than 500 mg/day in adults because of the saturation of plasma protein-binding sites and associated increase in clearance.[31,32] Differences in the metabolic clearances of individual NSAIDs among patients may be marked, resulting in considerable variation in the extent of their accumulation at all sites throughout the body.[35] In children (especially younger children), NSAIDs may be eliminated more rapidly than in adults; children may require more frequent doses to maintain a clinical response.[33,38]

Differences in pharmacokinetics between short-term and long-term administration may be significant, but this has not been studied systematically.[39] Abnormalities of hepatic function are common in children with JRA, particularly children with systemic-onset disease. Because hepatic metabolism plays a major role in NSAID elimination, it is necessary to assess hepatic function before institution of NSAID therapy in these children. NSAIDs should not be started if there is significant elevation of transaminase levels (e.g., three times normal or higher).

General Principles of Nonsteroidal Antiinflammatory Drug Therapy

NSAIDs are generally good analgesic and antipyretic agents and weak antiinflammatory agents. They provide good symptomatic relief, but have traditionally not been considered to influence the underlying disease process or to affect long-term outcomes significantly. A more recent report suggested, however, that NSAIDs change the course of ankylosing spondylitis by preventing syndesmophyte formation.[40] The analgesic effect of NSAIDs is rapid, but the antiinflammatory effect takes longer and can require doses twice as large as those needed for analgesia.[41,42] NSAIDs are relatively safe for long-term use. Although toxicity, especially GI side effects, is frequent, it is seldom serious.[43-45] Given the wide variety of available NSAIDs, a few general principles can be applied in the selection of a particular NSAID for therapy in an individual patient.

First, according to empirical evidence from clinical experience and some studies in adults, response to NSAIDs seems to have some disease specificity. Indomethacin, a more potent NSAID, may be more useful in treating manifestations of systemic JRA, such as fever and pericarditis, and in managing spondyloarthropathies. Ibuprofen is also a very effective antipyretic agent in systemic-onset JRA. Sustained-release preparations of available NSAIDs given at night may be effective in reducing night pain or prolonged morning stiffness. Some NSAIDs, such as ASA or indomethacin, seem to be more toxic than others.[41]

Second, individual patient response to NSAIDs is variable and often unpredictable; a child may fail to respond to one drug and yet respond to another. Similarly, the frequency of toxicity may vary widely. A favorable initial response occurs in more than 50% of patients on the first NSAID chosen; of patients showing an inadequate response to the first NSAID, a further 50% improve when given another drug of the same class.[31] For a child whose condition has not responded to one NSAID or who is experiencing significant toxicity and still requires NSAID treatment, a subsequent trial with another agent is usually warranted. An adequate trial of any NSAID should be at least about 8 weeks;[46,47] although about 50% of children who respond favorably to NSAID therapy do so by 2 weeks, the mean time to therapeutic response can be 4 weeks, and 25% may not respond until after approximately 12 weeks of therapy.[48]

Third, additional factors, such as availability in liquid form, frequency of dosing, cost, and tolerability of any given NSAID, may influence patient preference. These factors can have a major impact on patient adherence to a particular treatment regimen and should be carefully evaluated when making therapeutic choices. A reasonable initial approach is to choose a drug that has a favorable toxicity and efficacy profile; can be taken on a convenient schedule (e.g., once or twice daily); is affordable; and, for young children, is available in a liquid formulation that is palatable. For these reasons, naproxen has become the initial drug of choice for most children with arthritis. It is generally well tolerated and safe, is administered twice daily, and is available in a palatable liquid form.[49] Nabumetone has advantages of being able to be administered at a dose of 30 mg/kg/day in a single dose and to be given as a liquid slurry.[50]

Generally, therapy should begin with the NSAID of choice at the lowest recommended dose, which can be titrated to the patient's clinical response. Use of multiple NSAIDs is not recommended because this approach has no documented benefit in terms of efficacy and can be associated with a greater potential for drug interactions and organ toxicity. The dose range and schedule of administration vary with the individual NSAID (see Table 6–1). Patients who are receiving long-term daily NSAID therapy should have a complete blood count and liver and renal function tests performed at baseline and every 6 to 12 months. Patients with active systemic disease should have more frequent monitoring of liver function, including serum albumin, particularly with any changes in dose. Although there are no good studies of NSAID discontinuation in children with juvenile idiopathic arthritis (JIA) to guide recommendations, the trend has been to use NSAIDs at the lowest dose and for the shortest duration possible. When used in conjunction with DMARDs or biological agents, NSAIDs may often be discontinued as the disease comes under control. Similarly, they may be stopped soon after joint injections if remission ensues. Adherence to NSAID regimens may be improved by various behavioral interventions.[51,52]

Toxicity

Serious toxicity associated with the use of NSAIDs seems to be rare in children.[42] Much of the available information regarding toxicity is derived from case reports, case series, or retrospective cohort studies, however, which makes it difficult to derive accurate figures for the incidence and prevalence of various toxicities. Generally, most toxicities are shared to a greater or lesser degree by all NSAIDs (Table 6–2), although individual patients may have fewer side effects with one drug than with another.[9,43,44,45,53,54]

CARDIOVASCULAR TOXICITY

Data from several clinical trials and observational studies in adults have suggested that there is an increased risk of cardiovascular toxicity (myocardial infarction, cerebrovascular ischemia, hypertension, and exacerbation of congestive heart failure) associated with several NSAIDs and COX-2 inhibitors. This cardiovascular toxicity not only led to the withdrawal of rofecoxib and valdecoxib from the market, but also resulted in more restricted, similar product labels in the United States for celecoxib and traditional NSAIDs.

In the Adenomatous Polyp Prevention on Vioxx (APPROVe) trial involving 2586 patients with a history

Table 6–2									
Relative toxicities of nonsteroidal antiinflammatory drugs									
Toxicity	**ASA**	**Ibuprofen**	**Naproxen**	**Indomethacin**	**Tolmetin**	**Etodolac**	**Oxaprozin**	**Meloxicam**	**Celecoxib**
GI irritation	+++	+	++	++++	++	+	+	+	+
Peptic ulcer	++	+	++	+++	++	+	+	+	+
CNS	+	+	+	++++	+	+	+	+	+
Tinnitus	+++	+	+	+	+	+	+	+	+
Hepatitis	++	+	+	+	+	+	+	+	+
Asthma	+	+	+	+	+	+	+	+	+
Renal function	+	+	+	++	++	+	+	+	+
Bone marrow	–	+	+	+	+	+	+	+	+
Cardiovascular	–	+	–	+	+	+	+	+	+
Skin	–	+	++	+	+	+	+	++	++

ASA, acetylsalicylic acid; CNS, central nervous system; GI, gastrointestinal.

of colorectal adenoma who were randomly assigned to either rofecoxib, 25 mg/day, or placebo, the incidence of cardiovascular events was significantly higher in the rofecoxib arm (3.6%) versus the placebo arm (2%).[55] The relative risk of a serious cardiovascular event on rofecoxib was 1.92 (95% confidence interval [CI] 1.19 to 3.11). Cardiovascular events that occurred more frequently in the subjects treated with rofecoxib were hypertension, congestive heart failure, and pulmonary edema, and events became apparent after about 5 months of continuous treatment. In the Adenoma Prevention with Celecoxib (APC) trial involving 2035 subjects, comparing two doses of celecoxib (200 mg and 400 mg given twice daily), there was a higher risk of death from cardiovascular causes that was dose related (hazard ratio 2.3 for the 200-mg dose group, CI 0.9 to 5.5; hazard ratio 3.4 for the 400-mg dose group, CI 1.4 to 7.8).[56]

The Prevention of Spontaneous Adenomatous Polyps (PreSAP) trial involving 1561 subjects did not show a significantly increased risk among patients on 400 mg/day of celecoxib compared with placebo.[57] In the Alzheimer Disease Anti-inflammatory Prevention Trial (ADAPT) involving 2400 subjects, analysis of preliminary data suggested increased cardiovascular events in the naproxen arm compared with placebo, but not in the celecoxib subjects.

These and other studies suggest that celecoxib seems to be safer than rofecoxib and valdecoxib, but that long-term use at high doses may also be associated with an increased risk of cardiovascular events. In a systematic review of 29 studies of NSAIDs and COX-2 inhibitors for primary prevention of colorectal cancer, cardiovascular harms (serious cardiovascular events, myocardial infarction, but not stroke or mortality) were found for non-naproxen, nonaspirin NSAIDs (ibuprofen, diclofenac) and COX-2 inhibitors.[58] In a similar review, hypertension was found to be associated with COX-2 inhibitor use.[59]

Meaningful data in children are scarce, so pediatric rheumatologists must to use adult data to help guide them in determining cardiovascular risk/benefit of long-term use of NSAIDs or COX-2 inhibitors in treatment of pediatric rheumatic diseases. Consideration of the underlying cardiovascular risk of the patient including the rheumatic disease being treated is likely to enter into the calculation (e.g., patients with systemic lupus erythematosus (SLE) and Behçet syndrome are known to be at higher risk for cardiovascular complications). A good general strategy seems to be to use the lowest dose for the shortest time possible.

The mechanisms by which some NSAIDs and COX-2 inhibitors are thought to lead to increased cardiovascular risk relate to the altered balance between reduced endothelial production of prostacyclin (which causes vasodilation, inhibits platelet aggregation, and inhibits vascular proliferation), whereas platelet production of thromboxane A_2 (which causes platelet aggregation, vasoconstriction, and smooth muscle proliferation) is unaffected.[60] Some NSAIDs and selective COX-2 inhibitors may predominantly inhibit prostacyclin production compared with nonselective NSAIDs and aspirin. Celecoxib was toxic to myocytes in the low micromolar concentration range. Additionally, interference of propionic acid derivatives (ibuprofen and naproxen) with

antiplatelet effects of concurrent aspirin may have led to the erroneous conclusion of naproxen-associated adverse cardiovascular outcomes in the ADAPT and APC trials. Appropriate timing of aspirin coadministration (2 hours before NSAIDs or COX-2 inhibitors) would minimize these effects.[60] It is believed that COX-2 inhibitors should be administered with low-dose aspirin in patients with cardiac risk factors.[61]

GASTROINTESTINAL TOXICITY

GI toxicity is common to all NSAIDs. The pathogenesis of gastroduodenal mucosal injury involves multiple mechanisms with local and systemic effects secondary to NSAIDs.[62] The systemic effects seem to have a predominant role and are largely the result of inhibition of prostaglandin synthesis, which leads to impairment of many cytoprotective actions, such as epithelial mucus production, secretion of bicarbonate, mucosal blood flow, epithelial proliferation, and mucosal resistance to injury.[62] The associated symptoms range from mild epigastric discomfort immediately after taking the medication to symptomatic or asymptomatic peptic ulceration.[63]

The average relative risk of developing a serious GI complication in adult patients exposed to NSAIDs as a group is fivefold to sixfold that of patients not taking NSAIDs.[64] Many of the studies on which these figures are based have limitations in ascertainment and attribution of adverse effects to NSAIDs, however, resulting in the potential for substantial underestimation or overestimation of NSAID adverse effects. Differences in patient populations, drugs used, dosages, and periods of exposure add to the variability in estimates of prevalence. Possible risk factors for GI complications during NSAID therapy include advanced age, past history of GI bleeding or peptic ulcer disease, and cardiovascular disease.[65] Most patients who have a serious GI complication requiring hospitalization have not had prior GI side effects, however.[62,63] Additional risk factors include longer disease duration, higher NSAID dose, use of more than one NSAID, longer duration of NSAID therapy, concomitant glucocorticoid or anticoagulant use, and serious underlying systemic disorders.[62,63] Many of the studies on which these conclusions are based do not account for the interaction of multiple factors or confounding by coexisting conditions.[62] Infection with *Helicobacter pylori* seems to increase the risk of gastroduodenal mucosal injury associated with NSAID use only minimally, if at all.[66]

The magnitude of this problem in children is poorly documented, but has traditionally been thought to be considerably less than in adults, partly because of the absence of the associated risk factors identified in adults. *H. pylori* has not been reported to be an important pathogen in children with JRA treated with NSAIDs.[67] Studies in children confirm that although mild GI disturbances are frequently associated with NSAID therapy, the number of children who develop clinically significant gastropathy seems to be low.[45] In many children who develop GI symptoms while receiving NSAIDs, alternative causes, such as the underlying disease process, psychosocial factors, and other concomitant medications, could account for their symptoms. The rigor with which these factors have been systematically evaluated and the definition of "clinically significant" gastropathy have varied considerably among studies, resulting in variability in reported rates for this complication.

A retrospective study of a cohort of 702 children receiving NSAID therapy for JRA who were monitored for at least 1 year found 5 children (0.7%) with clinically significant gastropathy defined as esophagitis, gastritis, or peptic ulcer disease.[68] The retrospective nature of this study may have resulted in a substantial underestimation of the prevalence of NSAID-associated gastropathy. A prospective study of a cohort of 203 children found that although 135 children (66.5%) had documented GI symptoms at some stage during NSAID therapy, only 9 (4.4%) had endoscopically detected ulcers or erosions; the most commonly reported GI symptoms were abdominal pain (49.7%) and appetite loss (32%).[69]

A prospective study reported on 45 children who underwent routine endoscopy (in association with general anesthesia for joint injections). Of these children, 19 (42%) had normal gastric and duodenal mucosa, and 20 had histologically mild gastritis. A clear association was seen between abdominal pain and gastroduodenal pathology, but the severity of gastric inflammation did not correlate with the duration of NSAID therapy.[70] Factors frequently associated with clinically significant gastropathy in children are abdominal pain at night, melanotic stools, and a previous history of gastropathy.[68] Endoscopic studies in very small numbers of highly selected groups of children with JRA receiving NSAIDs have reported a higher frequency of abnormalities.[71,72] These endoscopic lesions, which are usually mild, have not been found to correlate well with symptoms, and their clinical significance is unclear. Further prospective studies are needed.

Studies have shown differences in rates of serious GI complications associated with different NSAIDs. Systematic reviews have found ibuprofen to be associated with the lowest risk; indomethacin, naproxen, sulindac, and aspirin with moderate risk; and tolmetin, ketoprofen, and piroxicam with the highest risk.[73,74] In adults, endoscopic studies have shown that COX-2 inhibitors induce significantly fewer ulcers than traditional NSAIDs do.[75] Studies in children have found that tolmetin may be associated with higher risk.[68,69] GI symptoms can be minimized further by ensuring that NSAIDs are always given with food. Although some studies in healthy volunteers suggest that enteric coating may reduce acute gastric mucosal injury,[76] the use of enteric-coated preparations and parenteral or rectal administration of NSAIDs aimed at preventing topical mucosal injury have not been shown to prevent gastric ulceration.[62]

The development of "safer" NSAIDs offers considerable promise, but the clinical utility of these agents in children remains to be determined. These agents include COX-2 inhibitors, NSAIDs combined with proton pump inhibitors, phosphatidyl-conjugated NSAIDs, terminal prostaglandin synthase inhibitors, and new chemical agents obtained by the coupling of the gaseous mediators nitric oxide and hydrogen sulfide with NSAIDs to exploit the protective effect of these compounds in the gastric mucosa.[64,77]

The utility of antacids and histamine$_2$-receptor antagonists for prophylaxis against serious NSAID-induced GI complications is controversial. Although these medications suppress symptoms, they do not prevent significant GI events such as endoscopically documented gastric ulcers. Asymptomatic patients on acid-reduction therapies seem to be at greater risk for serious GI complications than patients not taking these medications, so their routine use in asymptomatic patients taking NSAIDs cannot be recommended.[62,63] Sucralfate also does not seem to offer any significant benefit in the prophylaxis of NSAID-induced gastric ulcers.[78]

Misoprostol, a synthetic prostaglandin E_1 analogue, has been shown in adults to be effective in prophylaxis[65,79] and treatment of NSAID-induced gastroduodenal damage, allowing continuation of NSAID therapy while achieving ulcer healing.[80,81] Studies of misoprostol cotherapy in children are limited, but also suggest that misoprostol may be effective in the treatment of GI toxicity symptoms in children receiving NSAIDs.[72,82] Misoprostol may also be associated with a protective effect on hemoglobin values in patients being treated with NSAIDs.[83,89] Omeprazole, a proton pump inhibitor, has been shown to be superior to ranitidine and misoprostol for the prevention and treatment of NSAID-related gastroduodenal ulcers in adults.[83,85] Prospective studies are needed to evaluate further the role of misoprostol, omeprazole, and other proton pump inhibitors such as lansoprazole cotherapy in children.

Recommendations for the treatment of established dyspeptic symptoms or active gastroduodenal ulceration, with or without continuation of NSAIDs, differ from recommendations for the prophylaxis of gastroduodenal injury. Symptoms of active gastroduodenal ulceration after discontinuation of NSAIDs can be treated empirically with a histamine$_2$-receptor antagonist or a proton pump inhibitor. If an ulcer develops, discontinuation of the NSAID is preferred, but if NSAID therapy needs to be continued, proton pump inhibitors are recommended.[62]

HEPATOTOXICITY

Hepatitis with elevation of transaminase levels can occur with any NSAID, but has most commonly been reported in children with JRA receiving ASA; 50% of these children may have some elevation of enzyme levels,[86] and 15% may require discontinuation of therapy for this reason.[43] In one retrospective study, transaminase levels were increased in 6% of children receiving naproxen.[43] A confounding factor is that transaminases can be elevated in untreated JRA, particularly in the systemic-onset subtype, and in SLE. Elevated transaminase levels are rarely of clinical significance and often resolve spontaneously, but they may necessitate reduction of the dose or temporary cessation of therapy. Rarely, hepatotoxicity is severe; NSAIDs have been associated with macrophage activation syndrome.[87,88] Liver function should be carefully monitored in children taking daily NSAIDs for extended periods, particularly children with systemic-onset JRA.

RENAL TOXICITY

Several types of renal complications have been associated with NSAID therapy, including reversible renal insufficiency and acute renal failure; acute interstitial nephritis; nephrotic syndrome; papillary necrosis; and sodium, potassium, and water retention.[89-93] Although these complications are reported more often in adults, with an estimated prevalence of 1% to 2%, numerous cases have been described in children.[92,94-97] The limited data on the prevalence of these complications in children suggest that they are considerably less prevalent than reported in adults.

A 4-year prospective study of 226 children with JRA treated with NSAIDs found the prevalence of renal and urinary abnormalities attributable to NSAID therapy to be only 0.4%;[98] an even lower prevalence of 0.2% was reported in another cohort of 433 children.[99] Several studies showed subclinical abnormalities of renal glomerular or tubular function in children with JRA, but the clinical relevance of these abnormalities as potential markers for the development of more serious renal complications is unclear.[100,101]

The various renal syndromes associated with NSAID therapy differ in their pathophysiologic basis, clinical presentation, frequency, and predisposing risk factors. The most commonly reported complication is reversible renal insufficiency, mediated through the effect of NSAIDs on prostaglandin synthesis. Inhibition of renal prostaglandin synthesis has little effect on renal function in healthy individuals. In states of hypovolemia or salt depletion, the adrenergic and renin-angiotensin system is activated, resulting in renal vasoconstriction. Prostaglandins are needed to maintain renal perfusion under such conditions by producing local vasodilation. Inhibition of prostaglandin synthesis with NSAID therapy may suppress this protective autoregulatory mechanism, resulting in unopposed vasoconstrictor activity and renal hypoperfusion.[89,91]

This type of renal insufficiency is usually reversible within 24 to 72 hours.[92] Risk factors include underlying renal disease (e.g., SLE) or, in healthy individuals, states of hypovolemia and salt depletion with high plasma renin activity (e.g., gastroenteritis, sepsis, congestive cardiac failure, cirrhosis, diuretic treatment).[102] Indomethacin is the NSAID most often implicated with this complication.[91,103] In addition to impairment of renal function, some children show signs of fluid retention, such as congestive heart failure, edema, or hypertension, when treated with NSAIDs. A modest decline in hematocrit value with ASA or other NSAIDs may result from mild degrees of sodium retention and hemodilution, rather than from anemia related to GI bleeding.[42]

Acute interstitial nephritis with nephrotic syndrome is far less commonly reported with NSAIDs. It occurs sporadically and is thought to represent a hypersensitivity-type reaction.[89] It typically has an abrupt onset with hematuria, heavy proteinuria, and flank pain. In contrast to classic drug-induced allergic nephritis, fever, rash, eosinophilia, and eosinophiluria usually are not present. Onset may be 2 weeks to 18 months after initiation of NSAID therapy, and resolution may take 1 month to almost 1 year after discontinuation of the NSAID.[89] Renal failure may be severe enough to require temporary dialysis support. Glucocorticoids have been used to treat this complication, but their efficacy is unproven. Interstitial nephritis with and without nephrotic syndrome has also been described in a few children.[42] This complication is more commonly reported with propionic acid (naproxen, fenoprofen) and acetic acid (tolmetin, indomethacin, sulindac) derivatives.[89,90]

Papillary necrosis is a chronic renal injury that has been most commonly associated with long-term analgesic abuse, particularly with phenacetin.[89,104] It has also been reported to occur with several NSAIDs, including ibuprofen, fenoprofen, phenylbutazone, and mefenamic acid. Medullary ischemia is thought to be the initiating factor in the production of papillary necrosis.[89] The syndrome is usually characterized by painless leukocyturia and hematuria, without impairment of renal function, and by demonstration of changes on intravenous pyelography.[89,95,105-110] Combination NSAID therapy seems to be a risk factor in adults and children.[42,106]

CENTRAL NERVOUS SYSTEM EFFECTS

Three general categories of central nervous system (CNS) side effects have been reported in association with NSAID therapy in adults: aseptic meningitis, psychosis, and cognitive dysfunction.[111] The NSAID most commonly reported to cause aseptic meningitis has been ibuprofen; susceptibility seems to be greater in patients with SLE. There does not seem to be any crossreactivity between NSAIDs for this complication. Indomethacin and sulindac have been reported to induce psychotic symptoms, including paranoid delusions, depersonalization, and hallucinations, in a few patients.[111] More subtle CNS effects, such as cognitive dysfunction and depression, can also occur and are probably underrecognized and underreported. Tinnitus may occur with any NSAID, but particularly with ASA.[42] A prospective study of 203 children with JRA found that CNS symptoms occurred in 55% of patients taking NSAIDs; the most common symptom was headache, which occurred in about one third of children.[69] Other reported symptoms included fatigue, sleep disturbance, and hyperactivity. Seizures were noted in two patients, both of whom were taking indomethacin.

CUTANEOUS TOXICITY

A diverse group of skin reactions, including pruritus, urticaria, morbilliform rashes, erythema multiforme, and phototoxic reactions, have been described.[42,112] Initially described in Australia,[113] the syndrome of pseudoporphyria occurring in association with naproxen therapy in children with JRA has now been reported in several case series.[113-118] Pseudoporphyria is a distinctive photodermatitis marked by erythema, vesiculation, and increased skin fragility characterized by easy scarring of sun-exposed skin (Fig. 6–2). Porphyrin metabolism is normal. All findings except scarring resolve with discontinuation of naproxen, but the vesiculation may persist for several months.[119]

Children with fair skin and blue eyes are particularly susceptible; one study reported a relative risk of 2.96 if the child had blue-gray eyes and was taking naproxen.[118] In one retrospective and parallel prospective study, young age, JIA itself, duration of therapy, evidence of systemic inflammation, and concurrent antimalarial therapy seemed to be additional risk factors for naproxen-induced pseudoporphyria.[120] Pseudoporphyria seems to be a common side effect even in geographic areas without high

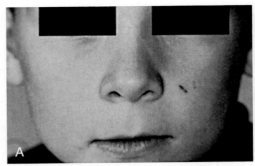 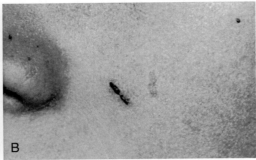

FIGURE 6–2 **A** and **B**, Distant and close-up views of the face of an 8-year-old boy with pseudoporphyria who was taking naproxen. Note a blistered lesion adjacent to a superficial scar. Superficial scars are also visible on the nose.

sun exposure; a 6-month prospective study of children seen in a rheumatology clinic in Halifax, Nova Scotia, reported a prevalence of 12% among children treated with naproxen;[116] similarly, there was a 10.9% incidence among NSAID-treated children with JIA in Edinburgh.[118] Although this complication has most often been reported with naproxen, many other NSAIDs have also been implicated.

EFFECTS ON COAGULATION

NSAIDs decrease platelet adhesiveness by interfering with platelet prostaglandin synthesis, such as that of thromboxane B_2, which promotes platelet aggregation. This inhibition is reversible in the case of all NSAIDs except ASA, which irreversibly acetylates and inactivates COX (see Fig. 6–1), an effect that persists for the life of the platelet; bleeding time returns to normal only as new platelets are released into the circulation.[42] NSAIDs also displace anticoagulants from protein-binding sites, potentiating their pharmacological effect. These effects of NSAIDs must be considered when any surgical procedure is planned.

REYE SYNDROME

Past editions of this textbook addressed Reye syndrome because of its epidemiologic association with salicylate treatment. That association has been called into question.[121] Reye syndrome seems to be related to salicylate treatment and the associated disease (chickenpox or flu) for which it was prescribed. Reye syndrome is rarely seen today, perhaps related to the decreased use of salicylates and perhaps related to other factors. The interested reader should see previous editions of this book for a more detailed discussion of the clinical features of Reye syndrome and its management.

HYPERSENSITIVITY AND MISCELLANEOUS EFFECTS

The precipitation of asthma or anaphylaxis with NSAIDs has been reported in adults as a unique syndrome associated with nasal polyps; 15% to 40% of patients with nasal polyps may experience bronchospasm when given aspirin.[20,122] Although this syndrome can theoretically be provoked by any NSAID, it has most commonly been reported with ASA or tolmetin; crossreactivity between NSAIDs may occur.[42] There seems to be a correlation, however, with the strength of COX inhibition: More potent NSAIDs such as indomethacin induce

bronchospasm at smaller doses than less potent NSAIDs such as ibuprofen.[123] Although "allergy" to ASA is often reported by patients or parents, true hypersensitivity to this drug is exceedingly rare in childhood. ASA hypersensitivity occurs in about 0.3% to 0.9% of the general population, in 20% of patients with chronic urticaria, and in 3% to 4% of patients with chronic asthma and nasal polyps.[124-126] Such patients are often hypersensitive to the other NSAIDs as well.[127]

Hematological toxicity, including aplastic anemia, agranulocytosis, leukopenia, and thrombocytopenia, has been reported but is uncommon.[42] Mild anemia occurs in about 2% to 14% of children[43] and may be due partly to hemodilution, hemolysis,[127] or occult GI blood loss secondary to NSAID therapy.[82]

Salicylates

The salicylates, a group of related drugs that differ by the nature of the substitutions on the carboxyl or hydroxyl groups of the molecule, include ASA, salsalate, choline salicylate, magnesium salicylate, and sodium salicylate. They are hydrolyzed in vivo to salicylic acid.

ASA is the oldest NSAID and has been used to treat the articular manifestations of rheumatic diseases for many years. Although newer NSAIDs have largely replaced ASA as the mainstay of antiinflammatory drug therapy in pediatric rheumatology, ASA continues to have a role in the management of Kawasaki disease (see Table 6–1) and in the treatment of patients who are predisposed to thromboses. The general principles of NSAID mechanism of action and pharmacology and the principles of therapy and the spectrum of known adverse effects have already been addressed with reference to salicylates where relevant. The salicylates differ from other NSAIDs, however, in many specific aspects; these are addressed in this section.

Mechanism of Action

ASA exerts its antiinflammatory, analgesic, and antipyretic effects in part by irreversibly acetylating and inactivating COX, inhibiting biosynthesis and release of the prostaglandins (see Fig. 6–1; see Chapter 3).[128,129] Other salicylates also inactivate this enzyme, but not irreversibly. A dose-dependent effect of ASA on the inhibition of prostacyclin (prostaglandin I_2) production by endothelial cells and of thromboxane A_2 production by platelets has also been noted and may be relevant in the management of Kawasaki disease or other types of vasculitis in children (see Chapter 33).[130,131] Large doses of ASA increase urinary excretion and decrease the serum concentration of urate; low doses have the opposite effect.[132] This phenomenon must not be confused with hyperuricemia or with gout, which is extremely rare in children.

Pharmacology

The plasma level of salicylate (ASA and salicylate ion) peaks 1 to 2 hours after a single dose, and the drug is virtually undetectable at 6 hours. ASA itself is bound very little to plasma protein, but salicylic acid binds extensively to albumin and erythrocytes. Salicylic acid is found in most body fluids (including cerebrospinal fluid, saliva, synovial fluid, and breast milk), and it crosses the placenta.

ASA is metabolized by hepatic microsomal enzymes by conjugation with glycine to form salicyluric acid and, to a lesser extent, by conjugation with the phenolic and acyl glucuronides, which are excreted by the kidneys. Renal clearance of these metabolites, which have longer half-lives than the parent drug, is augmented by alkalinization of the urine.

Administration

ASA is quickly absorbed from the stomach and proximal small intestine.[133,134] Some salicylates (methyl salicylate, salicylic acid) are well absorbed through the skin. The systemic antiinflammatory effects of ASA are maximal, and in most cases they are achieved only if serum steady-state levels are 15 to 25 mg/dL (1.09 to 1.81 mmol/L).[135,136] With levels less than 15 mg/dL, ASA does not function effectively as an antiinflammatory agent; at greater than 30 mg/dL (2.17 mmol/L), it is likely to be toxic. The dosage necessary to reach these concentrations is usually 75 to 90 mg/kg/day, divided into four doses given with food. Lower doses suffice in children weighing more than 25 kg. The plasma half-life of salicylate increases as the plasma concentration of the drug increases (capacity-limited kinetics). At a plasma concentration of 26 mg/dL, the half-life of ASA may be 16 hours, whereas at a plasma level of 4 mg/dL, it may be 2.5 hours.[31] Consequently, ASA need not be given as frequently when plasma concentrations are high, and toxic concentrations of the drug take much longer to decrease than would otherwise be anticipated.

Therapeutic levels are not reliably attained before 2 to 5 days of administration. Serum salicylate and serum liver enzyme levels should be checked 5 days after initiation of therapy or after any dose adjustment. Although it is the authors' practice to monitor salicylate concentrations in serum taken 2 hours after the morning dose, one study indicated that the timing of blood sampling was not crucial if the interval between doses was 8 hours or less, and a steady state had been achieved after 5 days of therapy.[137]

Toxicity: Salicylism

Salicylism (acute or chronic salicylate intoxication) can occur rapidly in a young child, and early signs such as drowsiness, irritability, or hyperpnea can easily be overlooked. In very young children, metabolic acidosis and ketosis occur, whereas older children may first experience respiratory alkalosis by direct action of ASA on the hypothalamus. Abdominal pain or vomiting may occur in some children. A child with fever and dehydration is prone to salicylism: In a child with intercurrent illness and nausea, vomiting, or diarrhea, the drug should be immediately discontinued.

Symptoms of salicylism include tinnitus, deafness, nausea, and vomiting. Early on, there is CNS stimulation (hyperkinetic agitation, excitement, maniacal behavior, slurred speech, disorientation, delirium, convulsions). Later, CNS depression (stupor and coma) supervenes. Because a young child, in whom there is a narrow margin between therapeutic and toxic levels,[138,139] may not effectively communicate symptoms of salicylism, the family must be thoroughly schooled in the signs of overdose.

Mild salicylate toxicity requires no treatment and often only a minor decrease in salicylate dose. If a child has persisting symptoms, evidence of CNS stimulation, or depression, the drug must be discontinued. The child should be monitored for evidence of acute salicylate toxicity—fever, acute renal failure, CNS depression, pulmonary edema, bleeding, and hypoglycemia. In situations of severe chronic salicylism or acute overdose, the stomach contents should be emptied, and activated charcoal (0.5 to 1 g/kg) should be administered. Urine output, body temperature, serum electrolytes, and glucose should be monitored, and glucose-containing intravenous fluids should be given as required. Alkaline diuresis induced with sodium bicarbonate and furosemide increases the rate of salicylate excretion in the urine, but must be carefully titrated in the presence of rapidly changing metabolic or respiratory function. Peritoneal dialysis or hemodialysis may be necessary. The reader is referred to the recommendations of Mofenson and Caraccio[140] for details of the management of severe salicylate poisoning.

Contraindications

ASA leads to hemolysis in children who have the enzyme defect glucose-6-phosphate dehydrogenase deficiency or pyruvate kinase deficiency. Use of ASA should be avoided in children who have bleeding disorders, such as hemophilia or von Willebrand disease, and in patients receiving thrombolytic agents or anticoagulants. ASA, or any NSAID for that matter, should not be given during the last trimester of pregnancy because of its effects on coagulation, platelet function, and ductus arteriosus closure.

Drug Interactions

ASA should be used with caution in children taking certain other drugs. Levels of MTX,[36] valproic acid,[141] phenytoin,[142] and other NSAIDs (tolmetin, diclofenac)[137,143] may be increased in children who are also receiving aspirin. ASA decreases the bioavailability of other NSAIDs by 20% to 50%,[140] and increases the digitalis concentration by 30%,[142] although the clinical significance of this interaction is uncertain. Glucocorticoids increase the rate of excretion of ASA,[144] and salicylism may occur if glucocorticoid drugs are abruptly discontinued in a child taking therapeutic amounts of ASA.

Disease-Modifying Antirheumatic Drugs

Numerous drugs used to treat JRA and certain other rheumatic diseases exert their beneficial effects weeks to months after initiation of therapy. These compounds—DMARDs or slow-acting antirheumatic drugs—currently include MTX, antimalarials, sulfasalazine, leflunomide, gold compounds, and penicillamine. As experience has increased with the use of these agents, there has been a tendency to start them earlier in the disease course than in the past based on an appreciation that irreversible damage occurs early; that active disease, leading to deleterious long-term effects, persists for many years;[145] and that MTX, the most frequently prescribed drug in this class, is safe and effective.[146-149] Gold, penicillamine, and antimalarials now are rarely used for JRA.

MTX is the most commonly used DMARD for JRA. Several DMARDs are also used to treat other rheumatic diseases (e.g., MTX in juvenile dermatomyositis [JDM], vasculitis, and uveitis; hydroxychloroquine in the management of SLE). In the treatment of arthritis, DMARDs are usually given in addition to an NSAID. The goal of treatment is to achieve disease control with drugs from this class and then to stop other treatments (e.g., NSAIDs, prednisone).

Methotrexate

Low-dose weekly MTX has emerged as one of the most useful agents in the treatment of rheumatic diseases in children, and it has become the first-choice second-line agent in childhood arthritis. Although MTX has been studied most extensively in adult rheumatoid arthritis and in children with JRA, it is used in many other chronic inflammatory disorders.[150]

MECHANISM OF ACTION

MTX (Fig. 6–3 [online only]) is a folic acid analogue and a potent competitive inhibitor of dihydrofolate reductase (DHFR) (Fig. 6–4). It may also inhibit thymidylate synthase and interfere with the metabolic transfer of single carbon units in methylation reactions, especially reactions involved in synthesis of thymidylate and purine deoxynucleosides, which are essential components of DNA.[151] It also interferes with de novo purine biosynthesis by inhibition of 5-aminoimidazole-4-carboxamide ribonucleotide (AICAR) transformylase, an enzyme in the purine biosynthetic pathway. MTX-induced inhibition of AICAR transformylase and secondary inhibition of adenosine deaminase leads to accumulation and enhanced release of adenosine, a potent inhibitor of neutrophil adherence.[152,153] It is believed that the effects of MTX are mediated primarily through the antiinflammatory action of adenosine acting through various receptors.[154] In one study, adenosine and MTX-polyglutamate concentrations in erythrocytes did not correlate significantly with serum adenosine concentrations, however, and serum adenosine concentrations did not differ in clinical responders compared with nonresponders. The authors postulate that local release of adenosine at inflamed tissues is responsible for its action.[155]

MTX acts at numerous intracellular levels. In addition to its action as an antimetabolite, it is an antiinflammatory and immunomodulatory agent. MTX modulates the

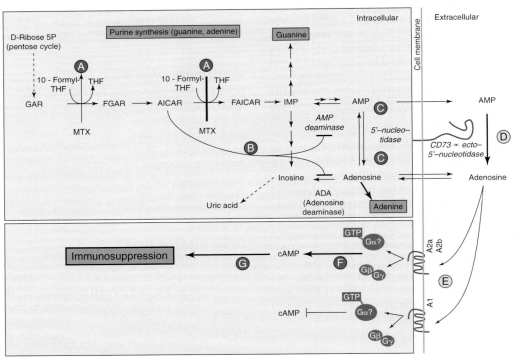

FIGURE 6–4   Steps in methotrexate (MTX) intracellular metabolism and possible sites of action. (F)AICAR, 5-aminoimidazole-4-carboxamide ribonucleotide; AMP, adenosine monophosphate; cAMP, cyclic adenosine monophosphate; (F)GAR, F1-glycinamide ribonucleotide GTP, guanosine triphosphate; THF, tetrahydrofolate; IMP, Inosinic acid (Redrawn from Cutolo M, Sulli A, Pizzorni C, et al: Anti-inflammatory mechanisms of methotrexate in rheumatoid arthritis, *Ann Rheum Dis* 60:729-735, 2001.)

function of many of the cells involved in inflammation and affects the production of various cytokines, including reducing the production of TNF-α, interferon-γ (IFN-γ), IL-1, IL-6, and IL-8, acting as a potent inhibitor of cell-mediated immunity.[151,154] By reducing the endothelial cell production of adhesion molecules, MTX may reduce the permeability of the vascular endothelium. In addition, adenosine inhibits adherence of stimulated neutrophils to endothelial cells, protecting the vascular endothelium from neutrophil-induced damage.[157,158] It may also have more direct effects in inflamed joints by inhibiting the proliferation of synovial cells and synovial collagenase gene expression.

Although the exact mechanism of action is the subject of intense study, it is not yet possible to distinguish clearly which of the many cellular and immune effects shown in vitro and in vivo are of particular relevance to the clinical effects of MTX. The reader is referred to reviews that explore this issue in greater detail.[151,156,157] The widespread biological effects of MTX may account for its observed efficacy in a wide variety of diseases with disparate pathogeneses, such as cancer, psoriasis, and various rheumatic and other chronic inflammatory diseases.

PHARMACOLOGY

There is significant intraindividual and interindividual variability in the absorption and pharmacokinetics of MTX after oral administration.[158] Although the average oral bioavailability is about 0.70 (compared with intravenous dosing), the range can be quite wide (0.25 to 1.49), with 25% of subjects in one study absorbing less than half their dose.[159] Factors such as age-related differences, the influence of food, and the effects of concurrently administered medications contribute to this variability. The effect of food on the oral bioavailability of MTX has been controversial.[160] A pharmacokinetic study showed that factors such as age, body weight, creatinine clearance, sex, dose, and fed versus fasted state significantly influenced the disposition of MTX in adults with rheumatoid arthritis.[161] The bioavailability of MTX has also been shown to be greater in the fasting state in children with JRA.[162]

The authors recommend that MTX be given on an empty stomach with water or clear beverages. Oral bioavailability generally is about 15% less than after intramuscular administration. Bioavailability of intramuscular and subcutaneous administration is similar,[163] with the latter being generally more acceptable for children who require parenteral MTX.

After a single dose of MTX, the drug is present in the circulation for a short period before it is redistributed to the tissues (Fig. 6–5). Peak serum levels are reached in approximately 1.5 hours (range 0.25 to 6 hours), with elimination half-life being approximately 7 hours in subjects with normal renal function.[164] Circulating levels diminish rapidly as the drug is distributed into tissue and eliminated. The predominant route of elimination is renal, with more than 80% of the drug eliminated unchanged via glomerular filtration and tubular secretion within 8 to 48 hours. A smaller but significant route of elimination is the biliary tract. The pharmacokinetics of MTX are triphasic. The initial rapid phase represents tissue distribution and renal clearance; the second phase is prolonged because of slow release from tissues, tubular

reabsorption, and enterohepatic recirculation; the third phase is flat between weekly doses, reflecting the gradual release of tissue MTX.[164]

Most MTX is delivered to cells as the parent compound and enters cells via active transport by reduced folate carriers. MTX competes with leucovorin for these carriers. Folic acid enters cells through a different set of receptors, the folate receptors. Their expression may be upregulated in inflamed synovium, allowing for more efficient transport of MTX into cells. These receptors are expressed variably, most likely under genetic control, and the interindividual variability may explain some of the differences in efficacy and toxicity. Similarly, removal of MTX from cells occurs via multidrug resistance-associated proteins, which may be enhanced in some patients and could again explain some interindividual variability in MTX response.

Of the parent drug, 3% to 11% is hydroxylated in the liver to 7-hydroxymethotrexate (7-OH-MTX). A portion of intracellular MTX and 7-OH-MTX is metabolized to MTX polyglutamates by the enzyme folyl-polyglutamyl synthetase. This enzyme also polyglutamates folic acid and folinic acid, which at high levels may overwhelm this enzyme system, preventing MTX polyglutamation and allowing it to efflux from cells.[151] MTX polyglutamates are long-lived derivatives that retain biochemical and biological activity within the cell.[164] These intracellular, polyglutamated MTX derivatives may be the active antiinflammatory agents,[154] and levels of polyglutamates in red blood cells have been shown to correlate with efficacy in patients with rheumatoid arthritis.[165]

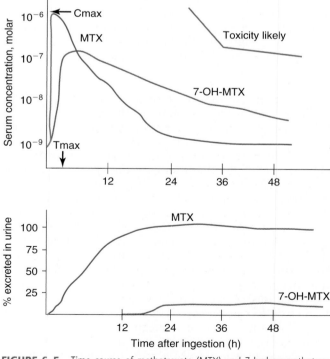

FIGURE 6–5 Time course of methotrexate (MTX) and 7-hydroxymethotrexate (7-OH-MTX) after an oral dose of 15 mg. (Redrawn from Hillson JL, Furst DE: Pharmacology and pharmacokinetics of methotrexate in rheumatic disease: practical issues in treatment and design, *Rheum Dis Clin North Am* 23:757-778, 1997.)

Plasma drug levels do not correlate well with clinical effects and are not useful in routine monitoring of MTX therapy.[157] Measurement of MTX levels in saliva also has not been helpful.[164,166] The pharmacokinetics of oral MTX in JRA seem to be age dependent, with more extensive metabolism of MTX in younger children.[167] This difference may account for the observation that children require higher doses of MTX than adults to obtain similar therapeutic effects.[168,169] Isocratic reversed phase chromatographic method with fluorescence detection quantifies the sum of all MTX polyglutamates in erythrocytes and was found to be suitable for monitoring JIA patients receiving MTX.[170]

At low doses, MTX is only moderately protein bound (11% to 57%), so the potential for interactions with other protein-bound drugs is small and usually is not clinically significant.[164] Studies in adults have not shown a consistent or clinically important interaction between MTX and NSAIDs. Several studies in children have shown an interaction between MTX and NSAIDs that may be clinically significant in individual patients, however, particularly patients with any renal dysfunction.[36,171] This interaction may be mediated through competition for protein-binding sites and through alteration of renal clearance.[150] The combination of MTX and trimethoprim-sulfamethoxazole should be avoided because it may lead to hematological toxicity through the synergistic effects of these drugs on dihydrofolate reductase.

Although the potential for interaction between MTX and various other drugs (e.g., sulfasalazine, hydroxychloroquine,[172,173] glucocorticoids, folate supplementation) exists, current clinical data do not support general avoidance of these combinations (see later discussion).[164] There seems to be an association of the methylene tetrahydrofolate reductase 677C/C polymorphism with a higher tolerability of MTX and of 1298A/A with lower clinical efficacy of MTX therapy in patients with JIA.[174]

EFFICACY

The short-term to medium-term efficacy of MTX in controlling the signs and symptoms of JRA is now well established. Benefits in initial retrospective and uncontrolled studies were subsequently confirmed in a combined U.S.-USSR placebo-controlled, randomized controlled clinical trial.[147] In this 6-month study of 127 children with resistant JRA (mean age 10.1 years; mean disease duration 5.1 years), 63% of the group treated with 10 mg/m² of MTX improved compared with only 32% of children treated with 5 mg/m² and 36% of the placebo group. The assessment of efficacy was based on a composite of clinical and laboratory parameters and subjective global assessment by physician and parent, but did not include any functional assessments or radiographic examinations. A Cochrane review, based on only two studies of 165 patients, concluded that MTX had minimal clinically significant effects (>20%) on patient-centered disability in patients with JIA.[175]

Various investigators have tried to determine whether MTX is more effective in some JRA subgroups than others. A randomized, controlled study from the United Kingdom concluded that MTX, at doses up to 20 mg/m², produced significant improvement in patients with extended oligoarticular JIA, but was much less effective in patients with systemic-onset JIA.[176] Ravelli and associates[177] studied the effects of MTX in patients with polyarticular, extended oligoarticular, and systemic-onset JIA (20, 23, and 37 subjects) and determined that the extended oligoarticular subtype was the best predictor of short-term clinical response. These patients also relapsed more quickly on discontinuation of MTX, supporting the conclusion that MTX may be most effective in patients with extended oligoarticular disease. Finally, a study from Saudi Arabia of 18 patients with systemic-onset JIA treated with MTX for a mean of 18 months found that systemic features resolved in all of the 10 patients who had such features at the start of treatment; the active joint count and functional class improved in 16 patients, and there was an overall reduction of the need for corticosteroid treatment.[178] Some children with systemic-onset JRA had worsening of their disease with MTX treatment, however.[179]

MTX may also slow the radiologic progression of disease in JRA, although the available data are inconclusive.[177,180] Some authors suggested that earlier treatment with MTX, possibly before the appearance of radiographic changes, may have a favorable influence on the outcome of MTX treatment in children with systemic-onset disease.[181] Similar results were found with early "aggressive" treatment in adults with recent-onset rheumatoid arthritis.[182] MTX results in improved health-related quality of life, particularly the physical domains. Determinants of poorer outcome include marked disability at baseline, initial levels of systemic inflammation, pain, and antinuclear antibody negative status.[183]

MTX is also used in many other rheumatic disorders, including SLE,[184] some vasculitides,[185,186] sarcoidosis,[187] systemic sclerosis,[188] localized scleroderma,[189] and uveitis.[190] The evidence for the efficacy of MTX in these conditions is less strong, however, and often is based on open, uncontrolled studies or extrapolated from the larger experience in adults, which is not always valid. The reader is referred to the specific chapters addressing these conditions for a fuller discussion of the role of MTX in their overall management.

DOSAGE, ROUTE OF ADMINISTRATION, AND DURATION OF METHOTREXATE THERAPY

Standard effective doses of MTX in children with JRA are 10 to 15 mg/m²/wk or 0.3 to 0.6 mg/kg/wk (Table 6–3). Improvement is generally seen by about 6 to 8 weeks on effective doses, but may take 6 months. Children seem to tolerate much higher doses than adults, and some series have described using 20 to 25 mg/m²/wk or 1.1 mg/kg/wk in children with resistant disease with relative safety in the short-term.[169] The efficacy of the use of doses greater than 15 mg/m² was not supported by a randomized controlled trial.[149]

Parenteral MTX administration should be considered in children who (1) have a poor clinical response to orally administered MTX (this may be due to poor compliance or to reduced oral bioavailability for various reasons); (2) need a dose greater than about 10 to 15 mg/m²/wk to achieve maximum clinical response (oral MTX absorption is a saturable process, whereas subcutaneous administration is not) (Fig. 6–6 [online only]);[191,192]

Table 6–3

Guidelines for use of methotrexate in treatment of juvenile idiopathic arthritis

Dose

Initially, 10 mg/m², once per week; give on an empty stomach with water, citrus, or carbonated beverage

Increase dose as tolerated or as needed to 15 mg/m²

Administer subcutaneously once per week if intolerance or nonadherence[193]

Administer with folic or folinic acid (see text)

Clinical Monitoring

Improvement should be seen by 6-12 wk

Monitor every 3-6 mo, depending on course

Reduce dose or discontinue if clinical or laboratory adverse events

Laboratory Monitoring

CBC with WBC count, differential, and platelet count; MCV; AST, ALT, albumin every 4-8 wk initially, then every 12-16 wk, unless risk factors are present (psoriasis, alcohol intake) (see also Table 6–5)

ALT, alanine aminotransferase; AST, aspartate aminotransferase; CBC, complete blood count; MCV, mean corpuscular volume; WBC, white blood cell.

Data from Ortiz-Alvarez O, Morishita K, Avery G, et al. Guidelines for blood test monitoring of methotrexate toxicity in juvenile idiopathic arthritis. J Rheumatol 2004;31:2501-6.

or (3) develop significant GI toxicity with orally administered MTX.[150,193] Studies in adult patients with rheumatoid arthritis suggest that oral absorption of MTX is considerably reduced at doses of 15 mg or more, and MTX should be administered parenterally.[194,195] Bypassing the enterohepatic circulation may also reduce hepatotoxicity. Some pediatric rheumatologists even advocate using parenteral MTX at initiation of treatment to ensure complete absorption and achievement of early disease remission.[150,196]

The issue of when, how, and by what criteria to attempt withdrawal of MTX therapy in JRA is currently undecided. There have been many studies in children treated with variable doses of MTX for variable periods in whom discontinuation of MTX was attempted after clinical "remission" of variable length was achieved.[168,177,198] The criteria for "remission" or "relapse" have usually not been well defined or standardized among various studies, and the assessment of outcomes has been nonblinded. Given these limitations, no firm conclusions can be drawn about the optimal time and mode of MTX discontinuation in children with JRA. MTX withdrawal may result in disease flare in more than 50% of patients; this rate may be even higher in younger children.[177,198]

A longer period on MTX treatment after remission may not prolong the duration of improvement after stopping treatment, but the duration of clinical remission may be predicted by the degree of subclinical synovial inflammation (using myeloid-basic protein 14) at the time of stopping MTX.[199] There are conflicting data about the ease with which remission can be reestablished when MTX is restarted after disease relapse, which may be related to the different doses of MTX used and the differing lengths of follow-up in the studies reported to date.

Prospective studies with more standardized assessments of outcome and durations of follow-up are needed to address these issues.

SAFETY

MTX is the second-line agent with the best toxicity/efficacy profile for treatment of various rheumatic diseases in children and adults. Although MTX is associated with many potential toxicities, the documented overall frequency and severity of adverse effects in children with arthritis have been low (Table 6–4).[148,150,200] Most side effects are mild and reversible and can be treated conservatively. The two areas of greatest concern and debate, especially in children, have been the potentially increased risk of hepatic cirrhosis in patients exposed to large cumulative doses of MTX and a possible increased risk of malignancies. Although the precise mechanism of all MTX-related toxicities is not clearly understood, at least some of its adverse effects are directly related to its folate antagonism and its cytostatic effects.[201] This relationship is especially evident in tissues with a high cell turnover rate, such as the GI tract and bone marrow, which have a high requirement for purines, thymidine, and methionine. Supplementation with folic or folinic acid may diminish these, but not other types of toxicities, which, along with MTX efficacy, may be mediated by different mechanisms (see later discussion).[201]

Gastrointestinal Toxicity. Abdominal discomfort and nausea, the most frequently reported symptoms, occur in about 12% of children with JRA who receive MTX. Stomatitis or oral ulcers are reported in about 3% of children.[150] Higher rates are reported in adults; 60% of patients taking low-dose MTX may develop GI adverse events in the form of stomatitis, anorexia, abdominal pain, indigestion, dyspepsia, nausea, vomiting, weight loss, or diarrhea.[202,203] MTX-related abdominal discomfort, anorexia, nausea, or oral ulcers usually occur within 24 to 36 hours after administration of the weekly dose and can be diminished by the addition of folic acid supplementation (see later discussion); by dose reduction; or, in some troublesome cases, by conversion to subcutaneous MTX administration, although the evidence for the effectiveness of this strategy is only anecdotal.

Liver Toxicity. The effect of MTX on liver function and the development of hepatic fibrosis has been extensively reviewed.[204] MTX is associated with the potential for acute and chronic hepatotoxicity. Mild acute toxicity, with elevations of transaminases, is common, occurring in about 9% of children with JRA treated with MTX.[150] These elevations are usually transient and resolve with either MTX discontinuation or lowered dose after a brief interval off treatment.[147,148,204] In some of these cases, concurrent administration of NSAIDs may contribute to the elevation in transaminases, and discontinuation of NSAID treatment may allow normalization of liver function.[171]

The issue of greatest concern with the long-term use of low-dose MTX in children has been the potential for significant liver fibrosis or cirrhosis. The risk of this complication in children with JRA may differ, however, from the risk in adults with rheumatoid arthritis or psoriasis

Table 6–4

Reported adverse effects in children treated with methotrexate*

	Study 1	Study 2	Study 3	Study 4	Study 5	Study 6	Study 7	Study 8	Totals
Patients (n)	19	23	12	19	30	62	86	27	277
Treatment duration (mo)									
Mean	10.5	19.2	6	18.5	—	27	6	—	—
Range	4-10	6-52	—	8-39	6-30	19-65	—	6-72	4-72
Methotrexate dose									
mg/m²/wk	4-17	—	8-25	6-15	—	6-20	5 or 10	10-15	—
mg/kg/wk	—	0.1-0.6	—	—	0.4-0.8	—	—	—	—
Adverse effects (no. patients)									
GI symptoms	2	0	1	2	6	14	8	0	33
Peptic ulcer	0	0	ND	0	0	4	0	1	5
Stomatitis	1	0	ND	1	0	0	2	1	5
Mouth ulcers	1	0	1	0	2	0	1	0	4
Rashes	0	0	ND	0	ND	0	1	0	1
Alopecia	ND	0	ND	0	ND	2	0	0	2
Jaundice	0	0	ND	0	ND	ND	0	1	1
Bacterial infections	0	0	ND	ND	ND	4	0	ND	4
Herpes zoster	1	0	0	0	1	1	0	ND	3
Mood changes	0	ND	1	ND	ND	ND	0	ND	1
LFT elevations	3	10	1	1	3	9	1	4	25
Hematuria	0	0	0	0	0	0	0	0	0
Leukopenia	0	0	0	0	1	0	0	0	1
Anemia	0	0	0	0	0	1	0	0	1
Proteinuria	3	0	0	0	0	0	0	0	3

GI, gastrointestinal; LFT, liver function tests; ND, no data.

treated with low-dose MTX. Long-term studies of MTX use in adults with rheumatoid arthritis have found a much lower incidence of liver fibrosis and cirrhosis than that initially reported in psoriatic patients; one retrospective study of 16,000 patients with rheumatoid arthritis reported a 5-year cumulative incidence of liver cirrhosis or failure of 1 in 1000 patients receiving MTX treatment.[205] A systematic review reported conflicting data on the risk of liver fibrosis or cirrhosis, but severe damage seems to be exceedingly rare.[206]

Another study suggested that the incidence may be higher, with a 5-year cumulative incidence of cirrhosis of 9.4 in 1000 patients with rheumatoid arthritis receiving MTX treatment.[207] A metaanalysis of patients with rheumatoid arthritis and psoriasis found that higher cumulative dose of MTX, heavy alcohol consumption, and presence of psoriasis were associated with higher risk of progressive liver histological abnormalities.[208] Other risk factors include preexisting liver disease, obesity, insulin-dependent diabetes mellitus, and renal insufficiency.[204,209,210]

The American College of Rheumatology (ACR) has suggested guidelines developed by consensus for laboratory monitoring of patients with rheumatoid arthritis (Tables 6–5 and 6–6).[211] Although a similar level of consensus does not exist for monitoring children with JRA receiving MTX treatment, most pediatric rheumatologists tend to follow these guidelines or a variation of them.[150] A study examining the relationship between hepatotoxic risk factors and liver histopathology in patients with JRA receiving MTX treatment found that serial biochemical abnormalities were significantly associated with Roenigk grade and the presence of liver fibrosis, suggesting that the guidelines for monitoring MTX hepatotoxicity in adults with rheumatoid arthritis may also be applicable to children with JRA.[212] Even close monitoring of liver function tests does not eliminate the possibility of progressive hepatic fibrosis, however. Erickson and colleagues[209] reported one patient in a series who developed cirrhosis despite normal results on liver function tests. These guidelines may not apply to patients receiving more than 25 mg/wk or a cumulative dose of greater than 10 g; surveillance liver biopsies may be indicated for these patients.[204]

In many small studies in children, liver biopsies were performed after cumulative doses of 3000 mg had been reached; none showed any cirrhosis.[148,213,214] A cross-sectional study[215] reported on results of liver histology in children exposed to even higher cumulative doses of MTX (>3000 mg or >4000 mg/1.73 m²), with the mean duration of treatment being about 6 years (with some children treated for up to 10 years); no significant fibrosis or cirrhosis was found. Thirteen (93%) of 14 biopsy specimens showed some histological abnormality, however, with only 1 graded as Roenigk grade II. In addition, higher weekly doses of MTX (≥20 mg/m²/wk) were not associated with significant hepatic fibrosis in 10 patients who underwent liver biopsy.[216]

Table 6–5

Recommendations for baseline evaluation for starting, resuming, or significant dose increase of a therapy in patients with rheumatoid arthritis receiving nonbiological and biological disease-modifying antirheumatic drugs*

Therapeutic Agents	CBC	Liver Transaminases	Creatinine	Hepatitis B and C Testing†	Ophthalmological Examination‡
Hydroxychloroquine	X	X	X		X
Leflunomide	X	X	X	X	
Methotrexate	X	X	X	X	
Minocycline	X	X	X		
Sulfasalazine	X	X	X		
All biological agents	X	X	X		

*Therapies are listed alphabetically. X = recommended test.
†If hepatitis risk factors are present (e.g., intravenous drug abuse, multiple sex partners in the previous 6 months, health care personnel). Evaluation might include tests for hepatitis B surface antigen, hepatitis B antibodies, hepatitis B core antibodies, or hepatitis C antibodies.
‡Ophthalmological examination is recommended within the first year of treatment. For patients in higher risk categories (e.g., liver disease, concomitant retinal disease, and ≥60 years old), the American Academy of Ophthalmology recommends an annual follow-up eye examination.[284]
CBC, complete blood count.
Data from Saag KG, Teng GG, Patkar NM, et al: American College of Rheumatology 2008 recommendations for the use of nonbiologic and biologic disease-modifying antirheumatic drugs in rheumatoid arthritis, *Arthritis Rheum* 59:762-784, 2008.

Table 6–6

Recommendations for optimal follow-up laboratory monitoring intervals for complete blood count, liver transaminase levels, and serum creatinine levels for rheumatoid arthritis patients receiving nonbiological disease-modifying antirheumatic drugs*

| Therapeutic Agents | Monitoring Interval Based on Duration of Therapy | | |
	<3 months	3-6 months	>6 months
Hydroxychloroquine	None after baseline	None	None
Leflunomide	2-4 wk	8-12 wk	12 wk
Methotrexate	2-4 wk	8-12 wk	12 wk
Minocycline	None after baseline	None	None
Sulfasalazine	2-4 wk	8-12 wk	12 wk

*More frequent monitoring is recommended within the first 3 months of therapy or after increasing the dose, and the outer bound of the monitoring interval is recommended beyond 6 months of therapy. Therapies are listed alphabetically.
Data from Saag KG, Teng GG, Patkar NM, et al: American College of Rheumatology 2008 recommendations for the use of nonbiologic and biologic disease-modifying antirheumatic drugs in rheumatoid arthritis, *Arthritis Rheum* 59:762-784, 2008.

Although these data are encouraging, their interpretation requires some caution: First, the number of children studied is small, so the statistical power for detection of infrequent events, such as cirrhosis, is low (type II error); second, only 58% of eligible patients receiving MTX treatment underwent biopsy, so selection bias may have occurred; and third, the clinical significance, if any, of the minor histological abnormalities detected in most of the biopsy specimens is unknown, and there were no control biopsy specimens to help distinguish the effects of disease (e.g., systemic-onset JRA) or concomitant medications (e.g., NSAIDs) on liver histology.

A follow-up study from Hashkes and associates[206] reported the results of 33 liver biopsies in 25 patients; 27 biopsy specimens (82%) were classified as Roenigk grade I; 4 (12%), as grade II; and 2 (6%), as grade IIIA; none showed significant fibrosis. The frequency of biochemical abnormalities and body mass index were the only risk factors found to relate significantly to the Roenigk grade.[215] The same limitations as with the earlier study apply, however, particularly with respect to the small number of patients studied (possibility of type II error) and the unknown significance of the minor histological abnormalities observed in most patients. Further long-term, prospective studies in larger numbers of children treated with MTX are needed to define more accurately the risk of MTX-related liver fibrosis or cirrhosis and to develop appropriate guidelines for monitoring therapy in JRA.

Infection. Although MTX potentially may increase the risk for common bacterial infections, herpes zoster, and opportunistic infections, these complications are infrequently reported in treated patients. One study of 62 children with JRA treated for a mean of 161 weeks reported only two cases of recurrent cellulitis, one of osteomyelitis, and one of an infected Hickman catheter site; there were eight viral infections, including one case of herpes zoster, one case of mononucleosis, and six cases of primary varicella. Many of the patients with varicella infection were also concurrently receiving glucocorticoids.[148] The randomized controlled clinical trial of

MTX treatment in JRA did not document an increased frequency of infection in children treated with MTX compared with placebo.[147]

Although the overall risk of infection seems to be low, it has not been precisely quantitated in adults or in children.[206] Infections in patients treated with MTX are usually common bacterial infections (e.g., lungs, skin) or herpes zoster. The development of hypogammaglobulinemia in patients treated with MTX may predispose to infection.[217] Opportunistic infections associated with MTX treatment are rare, unless there is concurrent treatment with high-dose glucocorticoids.[29,218] Immunization with inactivated vaccines is not contraindicated in children receiving MTX treatment, but immunization with live attenuated vaccines should be avoided.[219] There are currently no generally accepted guidelines regarding varicella immunization in these children. Active varicella immunization of susceptible children and family members may need to be considered before initiation of MTX therapy.[205] Family members of patients receiving MTX treatment who require polio immunization should receive inactivated vaccine. Administration of measles, mumps, rubella (MMR) or hepatitis B vaccine to patients with JIA, including patients taking MTX, did not result in flares of disease activity.[220,221]

Hematological Toxicity. Hematological toxicity includes macrocytic anemia, leukopenia, thrombocytopenia, and pancytopenia. In adults with rheumatoid arthritis, pancytopenia has been reported in about 1% to 2% of patients receiving MTX treatment.[222] Identified risk factors in this population include impaired renal function, advanced age, concurrent viral infection, alcohol ingestion, folate deficiency, hypoalbuminemia, and drug interactions (e.g., trimethoprim-sulfamethoxazole). MTX-associated pancytopenia has not been reported in children, and hematological toxicity is uncommon overall; a 1997 review of published studies, including 277 children treated with MTX, found only one case of leukopenia and one case of macrocytic anemia.[150] Although supplemental folate treatment results in lowering of the mean corpuscular volume in patients treated with MTX, whether this would prevent pancytopenia is not yet known. Spontaneous recovery is usual within 2 weeks after withdrawal of MTX in patients with mild bone marrow suppression. Patients with moderate to severe bone marrow suppression may require folinic acid rescue and supportive therapy (e.g., colony-stimulating factors).[202] MTX may have triggered the macrophage activation syndrome in one patient with systemic-onset JIA.[223] Reversible asymptomatic eosinophilia has also been described.[224]

Malignancy. The issue of whether MTX treatment is an independent risk factor for various malignancies is controversial and remains unresolved. Although in vitro studies have shown that MTX has mutagenic and carcinogenic potential, in vivo studies in animal models (mice, rats, hamsters) have failed to show any carcinogenicity. In humans, low-dose weekly MTX therapy has not been convincingly linked to malignancy.[224,225] There have been numerous case reports, however, of an association between MTX treatment and lymphoproliferative

diseases in adults with rheumatoid arthritis.[226,227] It has not been possible to determine whether these observations were merely coincidental or were causally linked to MTX or to the underlying disease process.[225] Rheumatoid arthritis is known to be associated with an increased risk of hematological malignancy.[228]

Several cases of Epstein-Barr virus (EBV)–associated lymphoma manifested during the course of MTX treatment for rheumatoid arthritis or dermatomyositis and regressed with discontinuation of MTX.[229] Some of the reported cases showed features typical of immunosuppression-induced lymphoproliferation, including extranodal location, large cell or polymorphous histology, geographic areas of necrosis, and the presence of EBV.[230] The association of MTX with reversible lymphoproliferation suggests a causative role. MTX has not been shown to increase the risk of lymphoproliferative disorders, however, when used in the treatment of other diseases such as psoriasis[231,232] or in bone marrow transplantation.[223] Several cases of Hodgkin lymphoma[233-236] and non-Hodgkin lymphoma[237,238] have been reported in children with JRA treated with MTX. In three of these cases, EBV was implicated.[236,238,239] Long-term prospective cohort studies, with appropriate controls, are needed to define the risk of hematological or other malignancies in MTX-treated patients.

Pulmonary Toxicity. Significant pulmonary toxicity occurring during the course of treatment with low-dose weekly MTX has been described in adults with rheumatoid arthritis; reported prevalence rates in published studies range from 0.3% to 18%, with a mean prevalence of 3.3%.[240] The actual frequency of this complication is difficult to estimate, however, because the literature has been unclear in defining toxicity related to the drug itself, rather than to secondary problems associated with MTX therapy (e.g., opportunistic lung infections). The issue is clouded further by the fact that rheumatoid arthritis itself is associated with interstitial lung disease. The mechanism of this toxicity and the risk factors for its development are poorly defined, although many studies implicate preexisting lung disease as an important predisposing factor in the development of MTX pneumonitis.[202,240,241] MTX-associated pneumonitis is rarely reported in psoriatic patients.

Prospective studies of lung function in children with various types of JRA have not shown any significant abnormalities in pulmonary function test results in children treated with MTX.[146,150,242-244] One case of possible MTX-induced pneumonitis was reported in an 11-year-old girl with rheumatoid factor (RF)–positive, polyarticular JRA,[245] but the clinical course of lung disease in this case was not typical of the course described in adults with MTX pneumonitis.

Accelerated Nodulosis. MTX has been associated with a syndrome of accelerated nodulosis, with an estimated prevalence of 8% in adults with rheumatoid arthritis.[203] The causal role of MTX has been called into question.[246] This association was described in two teenagers with RF-positive JRA and in one 3-year-old girl with systemic-onset JRA.[247] The nodules were similar in distribution and size to the nodules reported in adults and developed within 6 months after the initiation of MTX treatment in these children. Although discontinuation of MTX is associated with regression of nodulosis, some patients have been successfully treated with hydroxychloroquine[248] or colchicine,[249] allowing stabilization of nodulosis with continued MTX treatment of the underlying disease. MTX-associated nodulosis is thought to be mediated by MTX-enhanced adenosine production; therapies that inhibit adenosine production or interfere with adenosine A_1 receptor function may be effective in treating MTX-associated nodulosis.[203]

OTHER ADVERSE EFFECTS

Central Nervous System. Various CNS symptoms, including headaches, mood alterations, change in sleep patterns, irritability, fatigue, and impaired academic performance, have been reported to occur transiently in the 12 to 48 hours after the weekly dose of MTX.[150] These problems may be subtle and need to be differentiated from effects of underlying disease and from various psychosocial issues that may coexist. The anticipatory nausea and behavioral distress in anticipation of treatment that occurs in children taking MTX can be ameliorated in part by psychological intervention including behavioral therapy.[250]

Osteopathy. Animal studies have shown that prolonged administration of low-dose MTX is associated with suppression of osteoblast activity and stimulation of osteoblast recruitment, resulting in increased bone resorption and osteopenia.[251] Similar effects have been described in a few case reports in adults with rheumatoid arthritis or psoriasis treated with low-dose weekly MTX.[252,253] Although leg pain and spontaneous fractures attributed to MTX therapy in pediatric oncology have been recognized for some time, this phenomenon has been described in only one patient with polyarticular JRA and a disease duration of 25 years recently treated with low-dose MTX.[254]

Teratogenicity. MTX therapy is associated with spontaneous abortions.[255] A case of multiple congenital abnormalities in an infant whose mother was treated with low-dose MTX for JRA has been reported.[256] Although it is difficult to quantitate the risk of teratogenicity with low-dose weekly MTX treatment, women of childbearing age should be counseled to practice effective contraception during the course of treatment. Patients should be informed that past MTX use does not predispose to congenital abnormalities, and that, ideally, MTX should be discontinued before attempts at conception. There have not been any reports of azoospermia caused by low-dose MTX treatment of JRA.[150] MTX is excreted in breast milk in low concentrations, but it is unknown whether this affects the newborn. Women taking MTX should be advised not to breastfeed.[257-259]

FOLATE SUPPLEMENTATION

Numerous studies have examined the issue of minimizing MTX toxicities with the use of concurrent folic or folinic acid (leucovorin) supplementation in adults with rheumatoid arthritis.[260-263] These studies have evaluated the effect of folate supplementation on the efficacy and the toxicity of low-dose weekly MTX therapy. Although the doses and regimens of folic and folinic acid used in the various trials, the doses of concurrent MTX therapy, and the assessment of "toxicity" have not been standardized, there is evidence for overall effectiveness of folate supplementation.

A 1998 systematic review of all published clinical trials found that folic acid supplementation was associated with a significant reduction in mucosal and GI toxicity in adults with rheumatoid arthritis treated with MTX.[264] There was no adverse effect on efficacy except with high-dose folinic acid supplementation. In a post hoc analysis of two phase III randomized controlled trials of MTX and leflunomide in adults using propensity scores to adjust for differences in the baseline characteristics of folic acid users and nonusers, 9% to 21% fewer rheumatoid arthritis patients receiving MTX treatment and taking folic acid had ACR 20%, ACR 50%, or ACR 70% improvement at 52 weeks compared with patients who did not receive folic acid, suggesting folic acid may supplementation may have an adverse impact on efficacy.[265]

Data are insufficient to assess the effect of long-term folate supplementation on hepatic or hematological toxicities. It also is unclear whether folate supplementation should be started as prophylaxis with initiation of MTX therapy in all patients or as treatment if specific toxicities develop. No formal study has addressed this issue. Folic acid is cheaper and has a greater margin of safety in dosing compared with folinic acid. The two agents have not been directly compared, however, for their clinical effectiveness and cost.

Studies in children are limited. A short-term, randomized, double-blind, placebo-controlled, crossover trial of folic acid (1 mg/day) added to a stable dose of MTX (mean 9 to 9.7 mg/wk) in 19 children with JRA showed no effect on clinical efficacy.[266] There were no observable abnormalities of liver function, but no data about other toxicities are available from this small study. Folinic acid administered 24 hours after the weekly dose of MTX at doses of approximately one third of the MTX dose has been used effectively to treat manifestations of MTX toxicity in children with JIA,[204] but at high doses this treatment was associated with disease flares.[267]

At present, it is impossible to make firm recommendations about routine folate supplementation in children receiving MTX treatment. Based on the data from adult studies and the small trial in children with JRA, it seems that low-dose (1 mg/day) folic acid supplementation does not have any detrimental effect on disease control and confers a beneficial effect in terms of GI and mucosal toxicities associated with low-dose weekly MTX treatment. Folic acid supplementation should be considered at least in symptomatic patients. High-dose folinic acid rescue should be reserved for patients with severe, life-threatening toxicity (e.g., aplastic anemia).

Antimalarials

Hydroxychloroquine sulfate (Fig. 6–7 [online only]) is the first-line antimalarial to treat pediatric rheumatic diseases, although other antimalarial agents are occasionally used for recalcitrant skin disease in SLE or JDM.[268] Hydroxychloroquine is rapidly absorbed from the intestine. Equilibrium concentrations are reached after 2 to 6 months of a constant daily dose, and the half-life exceeds 40 days.[268,269] Tissue levels are much greater than plasma concentrations, and there is increased affinity of the drug for melanin and for the liver, pituitary, spleen, kidney, lung, and adrenals. Excretion is primarily via the kidney, although hepatic oxidative deamination accounts for part of the excretion.

Antimalarial drugs inhibit the synthesis of DNA, RNA, and protein by interacting with nucleic acid. These drugs alter lysosomal pH, interfering with ligand-receptor dissociation and antigen processing; stabilize lysosomal membranes;[270] inhibit antigen-antibody reactions;[271] suppress lymphocyte responses to mitogens; act as antioxidants;[270] inhibit phospholipase activity;[272] and inhibit neutrophil chemotaxis, nitric oxide production,[273] and phagocytosis.[274] They may also antagonize the action of some prostaglandins.[275] Antimalarials interfere with IL-1 release by monocytes;[271] interfere with production of TNF-α, IL-6, and IFN-γ;[276] inhibit natural killer activity;[268] and induce apoptosis.[277,278] They also have antiplatelet and antihyperlipidemic effects that are extremely important in patients with SLE.[279] There has been interest more recently in the toll-like receptor 7/9 antagonist effects of antimalarials.[280,281]

When used at recommended doses, antimalarials are considered extremely safe. At least four young children have died of respiratory failure after accidental ingestion of large doses (1 to 3 g) of chloroquine, however.[282] It is recommended that antimalarials be used with great caution in very young children because there is no antidote.

GI intolerance occurs in 10% of adults, but is probably less common in children. Antimalarials occasionally cause bleaching of the skin and hair. Skin hyperpigmentation has also been described.[283-286]

Rarely, neuropathy or myopathy occurs. CNS side effects are common, may be reversible with dose reduction, and may remit spontaneously. CNS effects include headache, lightheadedness, tinnitus, insomnia, and anxiety. Myasthenia and muscle weakness have been described.[287]

The major concerning side effect is retinal toxicity.[288-290] Antimalarials accumulate in the pigmented cells of the retina and persist for long periods after they have been discontinued; however, the binding to melanin may not be predictive of ocular damage. Retinal toxicity, although rare, can cause blindness, even after the medication has been stopped. Retinitis is sometimes, but not always, reversible.[290] Evidence in adults suggests that retinal toxicity does not occur if the dose of hydroxychloroquine is maintained at less than 6.5 mg/kg/day, even for as long as 7 years.[291] Early detection of premaculopathy prevents visual loss if the medication is discontinued and forms the basis for routine ophthalmological monitoring (every 6 months) with visual field testing, color vision testing, corneal examination, and visual acuity testing. A progressive loss of color vision may signify early retinopathy and is an indication for stopping the drug. Corneal deposits are not visually limiting, but are probably an indication to reduce the dose.

Debate continues regarding the necessity of an initial ocular examination or of biannual examinations. The authors' current policy is to continue to perform these examinations every 12 months, but not to perform a baseline examination. Recommendations differ in adults.[292] Each examination should include visual acuity, color vision testing, visual field corneal examination,[291,293] and retinoscopy. More recently, the use of a multifocal electroretinogram has been suggested to detect early changes of retinal dysfunction.[294] Retinal abnormalities or interference with vision, especially with foveal recognition of red,[295] is an absolute indication for discontinuing the medication. Use of hydroxychloroquine in children younger than 7 years may be limited by difficulty in obtaining satisfactory evaluation of color vision in this age group.

The dose of antimalarials is limited by retinal toxicity. For hydroxychloroquine, the recommended dose is less than or equal to 6.5 mg/kg/day to a maximum of 400 mg/day.[296] At this dose, there is no significant risk of toxicity until after 6 years of treatment.[297] The overall retinal toxicity seems to be related to daily dose rather than to cumulative dose. One study of children with JRA did correlate outcome with serum levels of hydroxychloroquine,[298] but levels are not measured in clinical practice.

Hydroxychloroquine crosses the placenta, but is considered safe to use during pregnancy.[299] Hydroxychloroquine does appear in breast milk, but the amount ingested per day by a breastfeeding infant would be very low.[300] It seems reasonable for a mother taking hydroxychloroquine to breastfeed if she had taken hydroxychloroquine during pregnancy.

Sulfasalazine

Sulfasalazine is an analogue of 5-aminosalicylic acids linked by an azo bond to sulfapyridine, a sulfonamide (Fig. 6–8 [online only]). Its development was based on the concept that rheumatoid arthritis might be an infectious disease and would respond to combination therapy with an antibacterial agent and an antiinflammatory drug.[301,302] Sulfasalazine has become a primary therapeutic choice in the treatment of mild to moderate inflammatory bowel disease, and it has been reported to be beneficial in the management of childhood arthritis,[303-311] particularly oligoarthritis,[312] psoriatic arthritis,[313] and reactive arthritis.[313] Its role in ankylosing spondylitis is controversial,[313-315] although it does seem to be effective for the peripheral arthritides.[316]

Sulfasalazine is poorly absorbed from the GI tract.[317-319] Peak serum concentrations are reached after 5 days of therapy. The half-life of the drug is 10 hours. Approximately one third of the dose is absorbed in the small intestine and excreted unchanged in the bile. The remaining 70% enters the colon intact, where the azo linkage is split by bacterial enzymes to sulfapyridine, which is absorbed and excreted in the urine, and 5-aminosalicylate, which reaches high concentrations in the feces. Approximately 90% of sulfapyridine is absorbed from the colon. Sulfapyridine is tightly protein bound and acetylated, hydroxylated, and conjugated with glucuronic acid in the liver. Sulfasalazine and sulfapyridine reach synovial fluid in concentrations comparable to those in serum. About one third of 5-aminosalicylic acid is absorbed, acetylated, and excreted in the urine. The rest is eliminated unchanged in the stool. The small amount of salicylate absorbed is insufficient to reach antiinflammatory levels in the plasma.

Several mechanisms of action may explain the antiinflammatory effect of sulfasalazine. Bacterial growth is reduced by sulfasalazine and sulfapyridine, and the bacterial antigenic load delivered to the gut-associated lymphoid tissue may be reduced. This mechanism may be important for patients with spondyloarthropathies, in whom bacteria may gain access through inflamed gut mucosa and stimulate the immune system. Sulfasalazine interferes with many enzymes that are important in inflammation, in the formation of leukotrienes and prostaglandins.[320] Sulfasalazine is a potent inhibitor of AICAR transformylase; as a result, there is an accumulation of extracellular adenosine with a consequent reduction in inflammation via occupancy of A_2 receptors on inflammatory cells.[321]

Levels of matrix metalloproteinase 3 (MMP-3) are decreased in patients with early rheumatoid arthritis responsive to sulfasalazine.[322] Sulfasalazine reduces the release of IL-1, IL-2, TNF-α, IL-6, and IFN-γ.[323,324] This effect is most likely mediated by inhibition of the degradation of Iκ-κB (inhibitor of nuclear factor-κB [NF-κB]), which results in an inhibition of NF-κB upregulation of gene transcription,[325] and by the induction of apoptosis through the activation of caspase 8.[326] Sulfasalazine decreases natural killer cell activity and induces neutrophil apoptosis in vitro.[327] In vitro effects on macrophages include suppression of production of IL-12, production of nitric oxide, and expression of major histocompatibility complex (MHC) class II molecules.[328] Sulfasalazine may also have antiangiogenic properties.[328,329]

Intolerance and toxic reactions occur in approximately 20% of sulfasalazine-treated adults with rheumatoid arthritis (range 5% to 55%).[322-353] In a placebo-controlled study of 35 children with JRA, 29% developed adverse effects that led to discontinuation of the drug.[354] Toxicity

---

Table 6–7

Guidelines for use of leflunomide in the treatment of juvenile idiopathic arthritis

Dose

<20 kg: loading dose of 100 mg for 1 day, followed by 10 mg every other day

20-40 kg: loading dose of 100 mg for 2 days, followed by 10 mg daily

>40 kg: loading dose of 100 mg for 3 days, followed by 20 mg daily

Clinical Monitoring

Improvement should be seen by 6-12 wk

Monitor every 3-6 mo depending on course

Reduce dose or discontinue and monitor for clinical or laboratory adverse events

Laboratory Monitoring

CBC with WBC count, differential, and platelet count; AST, ALT, albumin every 4-12 wk

ALT, alanine aminotransferase; AST, aspartate aminotransferase; CBC, complete blood count; WBC, white blood cell.

---

may be more common in patients with a slow acetylator phenotype, but there is no clinical indication to document a patient's acetylator status before starting sulfasalazine. Enteric-coated preparations probably cause fewer GI side effects (anorexia, nausea, vomiting, dyspepsia, diarrhea). Rashes occur in 1% to 5% of patients. A maculopapular rash occurring within 2 days after institution of therapy, especially on sun-exposed skin, is the most common dermatological complication.[336] In patients who develop hypersensitivity reactions (usually early), desensitization protocols can be carried out.

Oral ulcers[342] and Stevens-Johnson syndrome[330] are uncommon but important complications. Neutropenia can occur in 4.4% of patients treated with sulfasalazine.[343] Sulfasalazine-induced thrombocytopenia has also been reported,[351] and pancytopenia[345] and macrocytic anemia may occur[346]. Serious hematological toxicity can develop many months after starting treatment. Drug-induced SLE,[348] Raynaud Phenomenon,[333] interstitial pneumonitis, fibrosis, alveolitis, pulmonary syndromes,[340,353] and hepatitis (granulomatous hepatitis, elevated transaminases)[352] are rare complications of sulfasalazine therapy. Hypogammaglobulinemia and IgA deficiency have been reported,[354] and immunoglobulin levels should be monitored. Serious infections have not been reported, however. A reversible decrease in sperm count has been observed,[332] but there are no reports of increased fetal wastage or abnormalities.

The drug should not be used in infants or in patients with known hypersensitivity to sulfa drugs or salicylates, impaired renal or hepatic function, or specific disease contraindications (e.g., porphyria, glucose-6-phosphate dehydrogenase deficiency). Most authors also believe that sulfasalazine is contraindicated in patients with systemic-onset JRA because of an apparent increased risk of disseminated intravascular coagulation–like reactions[308,355] and in patients with adult-onset Still's Disease.[356]

The suggested dosage in children is 30 to 50 mg/kg/day in two to three divided doses, usually taken with food or milk.[303,357] Treatment is initiated at a lower dose (10 to 15 mg/kg/day) and increased weekly over 4 weeks to achieve maintenance levels. A satisfactory clinical response may occur within 4 to 8 weeks. Sulfasalazine should probably be continued for at least 1 year after disappearance of clinical disease before tapering is begun (Table 6–7). It has been reported that sulfasalazine can be used safely during pregnancy,[358] and that women can breastfeed while taking sulfasalazine.[359]

Leflunomide

Leflunomide (Fig. 6–9 [online only]) is an immunomodulatory agent that, through its active plasma metabolite, A77-1726, inhibits de novo pyrimidine synthesis by inhibiting the enzyme dihydroorotate dehydrogenase.[360] Activated lymphocytes require de novo pyrimidine synthesis for proliferation. As a result of the inhibition, p53 in the cytoplasm translocates to the nucleus and initiates cellular arrest in the G_1 phase of the cell cycle. It also inhibits tyrosine kinase,[361] inhibits leukocyte-endothelial adhesion,[362] and affects cytokine production leading to immunosuppression.[363]

In vitro, leflunomide inhibits the production of prostaglandin E_2, MMP-1, and IL-6, and modulates various tyrosine kinases and growth factor receptors.[364] Leflunomide treatment results in decreases in serum metalloproteinase activity similar to MTX.[365]

Leflunomide is rapidly converted to A77-1726, which is highly protein bound and has a prolonged half-life of up to 18 days.[366] As a result, loading doses have been recommended for the first 3 days of administration to achieve steady state rapidly, although this is unnecessary because it increases the frequency of GI toxicity.[367] Another result of this prolonged half-life is that the metabolite remains in the circulation for prolonged periods (Table 6–7).

Initial studies in adults with rheumatoid arthritis showed that after a 3-day loading dose of 100 mg/day, daily doses of 10 mg and 25 mg of leflunomide were more effective than placebo,[366,368] as effective as sulfasalazine over 24 weeks,[369] and as effective as MTX at 1 year[370] and at 2 years.[371] After a 3-day loading dose of 100 mg/day, daily doses of 10 mg, 20 mg, and 25 mg have shown benefit by 4 weeks and continuing improvement for 20 weeks, after which the clinical improvements are maintained. The major side effects from leflunomide have been related to the liver, with elevation of liver function tests occurring in approximately 5% of patients with rheumatoid arthritis. The risk of serious hepatic disease seems to be minimal, however, and, as with MTX, associated with preexisting liver disease, viral hepatitis, or heavy alcohol consumption. Side effects from leflunomide have been mild and dose related. These include GI side effects (abdominal pain, dyspepsia, anorexia, diarrhea, gastritis), allergic rash, reversible alopecia, mild weight loss, and elevation of liver function test results.[369,372] No increase in infection has been reported.

A randomized double-blind, placebo-controlled trial failed to show benefit of leflunomide in ankylosing spondylitis in a 24-week pilot study of 45 adults.[373] In a small randomized double-blind, placebo-controlled trial of 12 patients with SLE, reduction in the Systemic Lupus Erythematosus Disease Activity Index (SLEDAI) from baseline to 24 weeks was significantly greater in the leflunomide group than the placebo group.[374] In a randomized placebo-controlled trial of 100 patients, leflunomide was found to be safe and effective treatment for psoriatic arthritis and psoriasis.[375] Combination MTX and leflunomide was also shown to be safe and effective in the treatment of rheumatoid arthritis.[376]

Silverman and colleagues[367] compared the safety and efficacy of leflunomide with MTX in the treatment of patients with polyarticular course JRA in a multinational, randomized controlled trial. The dose of leflunomide depended on the weight of the child. A loading dose of 100 mg for 1, 2, or 3 days for weight less than 20 kg, 20 to 40 kg, or greater than 40 kg was followed by a dose of 10 mg every other day, 10 mg daily, or 20 mg daily for weight less than 20 kg, 20 to 40 kg, or greater than 40 kg. MTX was given at a dose of 0.5 mg/kg/wk (maximum 25 mg/wk). Pharmacokinetic studies were performed at week 16. At week 16, 68% of patients receiving leflunomide showed an ACR Pediatric 30 versus 89% of patients treated with MTX; the improvements achieved were maintained at a similar rate in a 32-week extension study. The median time to an ACR Pediatric 30

did not differ between the two groups (52 days in leflunomide, 56 days in MTX). Body weight was a significant determinant of response, and patients weighing less than 20 kg showed the greatest discrepancy between the two groups. The incidence of treatment-related adverse events was similar in both groups, although there was an increased frequency of liver transaminase elevations in the MTX group. The clinically active metabolite of leflunomide, M1, was lower in patients weighing less than 40 kg than associated with clinical responses in adult rheumatoid arthritis, which may have explained the discrepancy between responses in the patients weighing less than 40 kg. The authors do not use a loading dose of leflunomide.

Leflunomide is teratogenic.[377] Because of the very long half-life of this drug, it has been recommended that cholestyramine be administered, and that drug levels less than 0.02 mg/L be verified on two separate tests at least 2 weeks apart in men and women before attempting to conceive.[349] In addition, women of childbearing potential must have a negative pregnancy test before starting leflunomide and must practice contraception. Breastfeeding is contraindicated while patients are taking leflunomide.[258,259]

The place of leflunomide in the treatment of patients with JRA is not yet established. At present, it should be considered for patients who do not tolerate MTX.

Other Disease-Modifying Antirheumatic Drugs

The use of gold and penicillamine has declined dramatically since the introduction of MTX and the newer biological agents. The interested reader is referred to previous editions of this textbook or to a current textbook of adult rheumatology for updated information on the use of gold and penicillamine in arthritis, and to disease-specific chapters of this book.

Other Disease-Modifying Drugs

Colchicine

The primary use of colchicine (Fig. 6–10 [online only]) in pediatric patients is for treatment of familial Mediterranean fever (FMF), wherein it has been shown to reduce not only the frequency of attacks, but also the development of amyloidosis. Colchicine is also occasionally used for recurrent aphthous stomatitis, Behçet disease, and cutaneous vasculitis. Peak plasma levels are reached 1 to 3 hours after oral administration. Its bioavailability is less that 50%, and its half-life after oral administration is 9 ± 4 hours.[378] Colchicine is predominantly eliminated by biliary excretion through the stool. The multidrug transporter molecule ABCB1 mediates the extrusion of colchicine into the GI tract. Enteric and hepatic cytochrome P-450 3E4 is also important in colchicine metabolism.[379,380]

Polymorphisms in ABCB1 may explain some of the differences in treatment response in patients with FMF.[381] Its action is thought to depend on binding of two of its rings to cellular microtubules, inhibiting the movement of intracellular granules and preventing secretion of various components to the cell exterior.[382,383] Interaction with endothelial cells and neutrophils is inhibited by reducing the expression of adhesion molecules on the neutrophil membrane.[384] The drug is present in granulocytes to a much greater extent than in lymphocytes or monocytes, perhaps because of reduced activity of the P-glycoprotein efflux pump in these two cell types.[382] Drug interactions may occur either at the level of the intestine (reduced absorption)[385] or through the cytochrome P-450 system. Agents that inhibit this system may lead to colchicine toxicity; alternatively, drugs that are metabolized by this system may compete with colchicine, leading to a buildup of both agents.

The effect of colchicine on microtubules has raised concern about chromosomal and gonadal aberrations. In a group of patients with FMF receiving long-term treatment with colchicine, there were no differences between patients and controls in lymphocyte mitotic rate, percentage of tetraploidy, or chromosomal breakage.[386]

The amount of colchicine needed to reduce sperm motility is much greater than the amount used with standard therapy.[387] Azoospermia and oligospermia are more common in patients with Behçet's disease than in patients with FMF, which suggests that genetic makeup or the underlying disease may contribute to reduced sperm production.[388] Concerns regarding growth delay in children are unfounded.[389,390]

The therapeutic dose of colchicine ranges from 0.5 to 2 mg/day as needed to prevent or reduce significantly the frequency of FMF attacks. Toxicity is extremely rare with oral administration and is generally limited to the GI tract (nausea, vomiting, abdominal pain, diarrhea). In the case of serious overdose, treatment with colchicine-specific Fab could be considered.[391] Severe toxicity can result in dehydration, multiorgan failure, and a disseminated intravascular coagulation–like syndrome.[382] Colchicine treatment improves fertility in women with FMF by suppressing disease activity.[392] It is safe to take during pregnancy and breastfeeding.[392]

Thalidomide

Thalidomide (N-α-phthalimidoglutarimide), a major teratogen, has been shown to be effective in various immune-mediated disorders. Its immunosuppressive effects include inhibition of neutrophil chemotaxis,[393] decreased monocyte phagocytosis,[394] decrease in the ratio of T helper cells to T suppressor cells,[395] inhibition of expression of TNF-α and IL-6 messenger RNA (mRNA),[396] and inhibition of angiogenesis.[397,398] Its structure includes two ring systems (Fig. 6–11 [online only]). Mean peak plasma concentrations occur 4.39 ± 1.27 hours after a 200-mg dose.[399] It is metabolized primarily by spontaneous hydrolysis and has an elimination half-life of 3 to 7.3 hours. Once-daily or twice-daily administration is appropriate.[400]

Controlled trials have shown benefit of thalidomide compared with placebo in recurrent aphthous ulcers[401] and in recurrent oral ulceration in men with Behçet syndrome.[402] There is one report of response to thalidomide in an infant with Behçet disease.[403] In addition, several reviews[404,405] have described multiple case series reporting improvement in patients with various disorders, including cutaneous lupus[406-408] and graft-versus-host disease.[404] Single series or case reports have documented

improvement in patients with palmoplantar pustulosis, sarcoidosis, pyoderma gangrenosum, erythema multiforme, Weber-Christian disease, pemphigoid, Crohn Disease (including two children),[409,410] ulcerative colitis, rheumatoid arthritis,[411] spondyloarthropathies,[412] and adult-onset Still's Disease.[413] Numerous, more recent small series of children with systemic-onset JIA who have benefited from thalidomide treatment have been described.[414-416]

In addition to embryopathy (which can occur with 100 mg given between 34 and 50 days of gestation), the major side effects of thalidomide include peripheral neuropathy and drowsiness. Neuropathy is predominantly sensory and manifests as painful paresthesias in a glove-and-stocking distribution.[417] Neuropathy can progress despite discontinuation of thalidomide and may or may not be dose related; it has been reported in 1% to 70% of patients. Even after discontinuation of the drug, recovery may be delayed for several years. Baseline and routine follow-up electrophysiological testing should be performed, and the dose should be reduced or discontinued on detection of abnormalities.[418] Various other neurological effects, including carpal tunnel syndrome, muscle weakness and cramps, and signs of pyramidal tract involvement, may occur. Endocrine effects include hypothyroidism, hypoglycemia, and stimulation of adrenocorticotropic hormone (ACTH) and prolactin production or secretion.[419] A promising immunomodulatory analogue to thalidomide, lenalidomide, seems to have a better safety profile than thalidomide, with similar immunomodulatory effects.[420]

The dose of thalidomide ranges from 100 to 400 mg/day. Doses of 2.5 to 4 mg/kg/day have been suggested for children with SLE or systemic-onset JRA.[37,414,421] Birth control must be practiced. Excellent control is maintained in a postmarketing surveillance program and a restricted distribution program, the System for Thalidomide Education and Prescribing Safety program (STEPS), monitored by Boston University, Celgene Corporation, and the FDA.[422]

Glucocorticoid Drugs

Glucocorticoid drugs are the most potent antiinflammatory agents used the treatment of rheumatic diseases.[423] Reports of their use in children with rheumatic diseases, especially rheumatic fever, JRA, and SLE, began to appear in the 1950s and 1960s.[424-427] Specific aspects of therapy are discussed in the chapters on individual diseases and in reviews.[428-434] This section describes more general aspects, such as the pharmacology, physiology, and mechanism of action of glucocorticoids, and the indications and contraindications for systemic and local glucocorticoid therapy and their associated adverse effects.

PHARMACOLOGY

Glucocorticoid drugs are modeled on the principal naturally occurring glucocorticoid, hydrocortisone (cortisol). They are 21-carbon molecules that in active form have a hydroxyl group at C11. Synthetic preparations such as prednisone and cortisone must be metabolized to the active forms (prednisolone and hydrocortisone) (Fig. 6–12 [online only]). Glucocorticoids that are used topically (e.g., dexamethasone) or given by intraarticular injection (e.g., triamcinolone hexacetonide) have a hydroxyl group at C11 and are already in active form.[435] The different relative potencies and durations of biological action of the various synthetic analogues are outlined in Table 6–8.

Orally administered glucocorticoids (prednisone, prednisolone) are rapidly absorbed. Prednisone is converted to prednisolone in the liver and reaches a peak plasma concentration within 2 hours. Hydrocortisone and prednisolone bind to the serum proteins transcortin (high affinity) and albumin (low affinity). Methylprednisolone and dexamethasone are bound primarily to albumin.[435] Prednisolone has a large volume of distribution; about two thirds is taken up by muscle. After metabolism in the liver, excretion occurs principally via the bile.

PHYSIOLOGICAL AND PHARMACOLOGICAL EFFECTS

Glucocorticoids are unique among pharmacological agents used to treat rheumatic diseases because they are synthetic analogues of chemicals produced by the body and have a physiological and a pharmacological role. Glucocorticoids enter cells passively and bind to two distinct cytosolic receptors: mineralocorticoid (type I) and glucocorticoid (type II) receptors (GRs). Type I receptors have highest affinity for aldosterone and are found on epithelial cells of the kidney, colon, and salivary glands, and on nonepithelial cells in the brain and heart. Activation of mineralocorticoid receptors induces activity of epithelial sodium channels, leading to sodium retention and hypertension.

Type II receptors have highest affinity for dexamethasone and are present in virtually all cells, including cells of the immune system. The receptors are present in the cytoplasm and consist of a hormone-binding portion, a DNA-binding portion, and an immunogenic region. Binding of the hormone to the receptor causes translocation of the complex to the nucleus, where the DNA-binding portion binds to glucocorticoid-responsive elements of the DNA in the promoter or enhancer region of the responsive genes. This induces mRNA transcription of specific genes that encode for proteins important in inflammatory and immune responses, such as phospholipase A_2 inhibitory protein. The effect is reflected indirectly in decreased prostaglandin production.[436,437] Binding to negative glucocorticoid-responsive elements may repress gene transcription. This mechanism of glucocorticoid effect, mediated via binding to a cytosolic receptor, reflects traditional understanding of the therapeutic effects of glucocorticoids and can be categorized as "genomic" action. GRs may also interact via protein-protein interaction with other transcription factors (e.g., NF-κB), preventing activation of transcription.[438] Two forms of GR have been described, GRα and GRβ. GRβ does not bind glucocorticoids and may play a role in the glucocorticoid resistance of some diseases.[439]

The therapeutic effects of glucocorticoids occur in a modular fashion via genomic and nongenomic mechanisms (see Table 6–9).[440] This modular hypothesis postulates the following steps:

- *Module 1*: At very low dosages of glucocorticoids, genomic effects occur. These include the classic receptor-mediated actions that result in increased transcription of certain genes (e.g., genes coding for lipocortin) and decreased transcription of others (e.g., genes coding for various cytokines), resulting in net antiinflammatory and immunosuppressive effects. These genomic effects start at least 30 minutes after glucocorticoid administration and result from binding to cytosolic receptors.
- *Module 2*: As the dosage is increased to approximately 200 to 300 mg of prednisone equivalent per day, specific nongenomic effects occur owing to a greater occupation of receptors. It is postulated,

Table 6–8

Relative doses and equivalent potencies of glucocorticoids (compared with hydrocortisone)

Glucocorticoid[†]	Equivalent Dose‡ (mg)	Relative Antiinflammatory Potency	Relative Sodium-retaining Potency
Short-acting			
Hydrocortisone	20	1	1
Deflazacort	6	4	1
Intermediate-acting			
Prednisone	5	4	0.8
Prednisolone	5	4	0.8
Methylprednisolone	4	5	0.5
Long-acting			
Dexamethasone	0.75	25	0

†Biologic half-life, short acting, 8-12hr (deflazacort,~1.5hr); intermediate acting, 12-36hr; long acting, 36-72hr.
‡Oral or intravenous administration only.
Adapted from Goodman and Gilman's, eds: Goodman and Gilman's the pharmacological basis of therapeutics, 8th ed. New york; Pergamon Press, 1990. Reproduced with permission of the McGraw-Hill Companies.

Table 6–9

Dose-effect relationships of glucocorticoids

Level of Therapeutic Effect	Prednisone Equivalent (mol/L)	Mechanisms	Onset of Action
Module 1	$>10^{-12}$	Genomic actions	After at least 30 min
Module 2	$>10^{-9}$	Additional nongenomic, receptor-mediated actions	Seconds to 1-2 min
Module 3	$>10^{-4}$	Additional nongenomic, physicochemical actions	Within seconds

however, that a further increase in dosage may affect pharmacodynamics (e.g., receptor off-loading and reoccupancy), receptor synthesis, and receptor expression, and may bring additional therapeutic benefit via other mechanisms. In contrast to genomic actions, these receptor-mediated actions occur within minutes after glucocorticoid administration. The clinical correlates of these effects may include the negative feedback of ACTH production, behavioral changes, cardiovascular effects, and programmed cell death (apoptosis).

- *Module 3*: The assumed additional therapeutic effects of higher dosages could be obtained predominantly via nonspecific nongenomic mechanisms, mediated by membrane-bound receptors, initiated by even more rapid effects (within seconds) through physicochemical interactions with cellular membranes.[440] The antianaphylactic actions of glucocorticoids may be explained by this mechanism.

This hypothesis provides a modular system of increasing therapeutic effect with increasing dosage, occurring through recruitment of numerous nongenomic actions, with increasingly more rapid onset of effect than the classic genomic actions of glucocorticoids.

Glucocorticoids are essential for normal vascular integrity and responsiveness; they suppress leukocyte migration and immune reactions and stabilize cell membranes.[431,441-451] Glucocorticoids influence protein, carbohydrate, fat, and purine metabolism; electrolyte and water homeostasis; cardiovascular, nervous, and renal function; and bone and muscle integrity.

CARBOHYDRATE, PROTEIN, AND LIPID METABOLISM

Glucocorticoids stimulate the synthesis of glucose, diminish its peripheral use, and promote its storage as glycogen. They increase secretion of insulin by pancreatic islet cells. In the periphery, glucocorticoids mobilize amino acids from tissues, which are then diverted in the liver to the production of glucose and glycogen. This catabolic action results in lymphoid and muscular atrophy, osteoporosis, thinning of the skin, and negative nitrogen balance. Glucocorticoids stimulate fat cell differentiation and, in high doses, redistribution of fat in a typical cushingoid distribution. They increase the production of the peroxisome proliferator-activated receptor γ_2 (PPAR-γ_2), a nuclear hormone receptor important in adipogenesis. Various other effects on lipids have been reported, but most have not been conclusively shown to result from the direct actions of glucocorticoids themselves. There is no consistent alteration in plasma lipids in either hypercorticism or hypocorticism.[452]

ELECTROLYTE AND WATER BALANCE

Glucocorticoid analogues used in the treatment of rheumatic diseases have been modified to decrease their mineralocorticoid potency. In that manner, increased resorption of sodium ions from the distal renal tubules is moderated, as is increased urinary excretion of potassium and hydrogen ions. Patients on long-term therapy are nonetheless in positive sodium balance, have an increased extracellular fluid volume, and have a tendency toward hypokalemia and alkalosis. In practice, these changes are only moderate in severity, however, reflecting the relatively weak effect of glucocorticoids on electrolyte balance. Glucocorticoids also decrease the absorption of calcium from the intestine and increase its renal excretion, producing a negative calcium balance (discussed later).

ANTIINFLAMMATORY AND IMMUNOSUPPRESSIVE ACTIONS

Glucocorticoids have antiinflammatory and immunosuppressive effects.[428,430,431,441-449,453] These effects are largely mediated by the inhibition of specific functions of leukocytes, such as the elaboration or the action of various lymphokines.

Antiinflammatory Actions. Steroids inhibit the early stages of inflammation (e.g., edema, fibrin deposition, capillary dilation, migration of lymphocytes into inflamed areas, phagocytic activity) and the later manifestations (e.g., proliferation of capillaries and fibroblasts, deposition of collagen).[452] Many of these effects are mediated by inhibition of the elaboration of numerous chemokines and cytokines, including the following:

- Arachidonic acid and its metabolites (e.g., prostaglandins, leukotrienes). Glucocorticoids induce synthesis of lipocortins (also called annexins) by macrophages and other cells.[448,449,454] Lipocortins inhibit the binding of phospholipase A_2 to its substrate and reduce the generation of arachidonic acid, the substrate for the COX-mediated synthesis of prostaglandins and leukotrienes.
- Platelet-activating factor. This effect is also mediated by the induction of lipocortin.
- TNF.
- IL-1. Numerous inflammatory actions of IL-1 are inhibited, including stimulation of the production of prostaglandin E_2 and collagenase, activation of T lymphocytes, stimulation of fibroblast proliferation, and enhanced hepatic synthesis of acute-phase proteins.
- Mitogen-activated protein kinase (MAPK) phosphatase 1. Cytokines activate the MAPK cascade resulting ultimately in the transcription of inflammatory and immune genes. Glucocorticoid-induced MAPK phosphatase 1 dephosphorylates all members of the MAPK family of proteins.
- NF-κB. The cortisol-GR complex physically interacts with NF-κB to block its transcriptional activity.

In addition, glucocorticoids can inhibit the action of humoral regulators of inflammation, such as platelet-activating factor and macrophage migration inhibition factor.[455] Readers interested in the antiinflammatory effects of glucocorticoids are referred to the extensive review by Rhen and Cidlowski.[456]

Immunosuppressive Actions. Glucocorticoid effects on the immune system are mediated principally through T lymphocytes.[443] Acute administration of hydrocortisone produces a 70% decline in circulating lymphocytes. T lymphocytes are affected more than B lymphocytes, and T helper cells are affected more than T suppressor cells. Lymphocytopenia is probably a result of sequestration of cells in the bone marrow rather than cell lysis, although drug-induced apoptotic cell death may also be involved.[457] The most pronounced lymphopenia occurs 4 to 8 hours after a single dose of glucocorticoid and disappears by 24 hours. There is also a 90% decline in circulating monocytes within the initial 6 hours. Proliferative T cell responses to antigens (streptodornase-streptokinase), mitogens (concanavalin A), and cell surface antigens (as in the mixed leukocyte reaction) are reduced by glucocorticoids. IL-2 production by T cells in vitro is also reduced.[458]

Glucocorticoids cause an increase in the numbers of blood neutrophils by increasing the release of cells from the marginated neutrophil pool, prolonging their stay in the circulation, and reducing chemotaxis of neutrophils to sites of inflammation.[431] Another effect of the decreased action of phospholipase A_2 is reduction of neutrophil chemotaxis, which decreases accumulation of these cells at inflammatory sites.[446] No consistent effect of glucocorticoids on neutrophil phagocytosis or bacterial killing has been shown, however.[459]

Intravenous glucocorticoid causes a decrease in circulating IgG, but little discernible effect on the serum titer of specific antibodies. The protein catabolic effects of long-term administration may have consequences on the humoral immune system, however. Endothelial secretion of C3 and factor B of the complement cascade is inhibited by glucocorticoid.[460]

INDICATIONS FOR SYSTEMIC GLUCOCORTICOID THERAPY

When considering glucocorticoid use in children with rheumatic diseases, the risk/benefit ratio must be carefully weighed because these agents are associated with substantial toxicity when used systemically in the long-term (Table 6–10). Clinicians must review the specific indications for which glucocorticoids are to be used and the outcomes that would be monitored to measure response

and consequently determine the duration of therapy. The overall aim is to limit the dose and duration of steroid therapy to the lowest possible levels while achieving disease control. Administration of a single dose in the morning and use of alternate-day regimens, which have been shown to minimize the suppression of linear growth in children, should be used whenever possible.[461]

In JRA, the use of systemic glucocorticoids is mainly limited to treating the extraarticular features of systemic-onset disease. These include systemic "toxicity" and fevers unresponsive to NSAID therapy, severe anemia, myocarditis or pericarditis, and macrophage activation syndrome.[87,88] The presence of fever or arthritis alone in systemic-onset JRA is an insufficient indication for systemic glucocorticoid therapy. Low-dose, short-term systemic glucocorticoids may also be indicated in severe forms of polyarticular JRA with significant functional impairment and for chronic uveitis unresponsive to local therapy. High-dose systemic glucocorticoids are used in children with other inflammatory conditions such as SLE, JDM and vasculitis.

ADVERSE EFFECTS

Two broad categories of adverse effects are associated with the therapeutic use of systemic glucocorticoids: effects resulting from prolonged use of large doses and effects resulting from withdrawal of therapy. The major manifestation of the latter effects is acute adrenal insufficiency with too-rapid withdrawal after prolonged therapy (see later discussion). The adverse effects of glucocorticoid excess are many (see Table 6–10). The mechanisms involved in the development of these adverse events have been reviewed more recently.[438]

Cushing Syndrome. Cushing syndrome, a term used originally to identify the effects of idiopathic hypercortisism, may also be induced by prolonged glucocorticoid administration (Table 6–11). It is characterized biochemically by high plasma glucocorticoid levels and suppression of the hypothalamic-pituitary-adrenal axis. Cushing syndrome is characterized clinically by many features, including truncal obesity (Fig. 6–13), osteoporosis, thinning of the subcutaneous tissues, and hypertension.

Table 6–10

Adverse effects of glucocorticoid drugs

Cushing syndrome
Growth suppression
Effects on bone
  Osteoporosis
  Avascular necrosis of bone
Immunosuppression
Lymphopenia and neutrophilia
Central nervous system effects
  Psychosis
  Mood and behavioral disturbances
Cardiovascular system effects
  Hypertension
  Dyslipoproteinemia
Cataracts and glaucoma
Metabolic effects
  Impaired carbohydrate tolerance
  Protein wasting
  Metabolic alkalosis
Myopathy

Table 6–11

Comparison of idiopathic and iatrogenic Cushing syndromes

Prominent in Idiopathic Cushing Syndrome	Equal Frequency	Prominent in Iatrogenic Cushing Syndrome
Hypertension	Obesity	Avascular necrosis
Menstrual irregularities	Psychosis	Cataract, glaucoma
Impotence	Edema	Pseudotumor cerebri
Hirsutism	Growth restriction	Pancreatitis
Acne, striae		Panniculitis
Purpura, plethora		

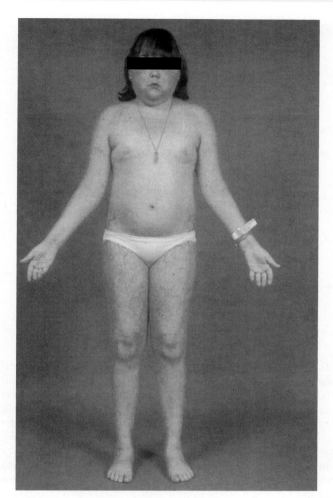

FIGURE 6–13 An 11-year-old girl with severe systemic-onset idiopathic arthritis requiring high-dose corticosteroid treatment. Cushingoid features shown include moon facies, truncal obesity, and cutaneous striae.

In Cushing syndrome, the distribution of fat is predominantly in the subcutaneous tissue of the abdomen and upper back (buffalo hump) and in the face (moon facies). Weight gain reflects fluid retention and increased caloric intake: Children taking prednisone are often ravenously hungry. Attempts to minimize weight gain by limiting caloric and sodium intake may be useful, but difficult. Skin changes, in addition to the characteristic purple striae on the lower abdomen, lower legs, upper arms, and chest, include hirsutism and acne. Hypertension is usually mild, but occasionally requires treatment or reduction of the glucocorticoid dose. Osteoporosis is one of the most troublesome consequences of long-term, high-dose glucocorticoid therapy and is discussed further later in this chapter.[462]

Few side effects occur at the start of therapy; the major manifestations of iatrogenic Cushing syndrome and other toxicities are related more directly to the total dose administered than to the length of time that the patient has been taking the drug. Cushingoid effects supervene when the long-term daily dose in a child (25 kg) exceeds approximately 5 mg of prednisone. Cushingoid appearance is an important source of distortion of body image and can

affect self-esteem and psychological well-being, particularly in adolescents and young adults. With the exception of skin striae, all of the physical features contributing to the cushingoid appearance are reversible, however, after cessation of glucocorticoid therapy.

Growth Suppression. Growth suppression is one of the most worrisome long-term adverse effects. It occurs in young children who are receiving prolonged therapy[463] in dosages equivalent to 3 mg/day of prednisone and increases with higher doses.[464,465] There may be substantial interindividual variability, however, in the severity of growth suppression and the minimal dose required to suppress growth.[466] The mechanism of glucocorticoid-associated growth suppression in children with arthritis is controversial. Glucocorticoids have been shown to inhibit production of insulinlike growth factor I (somatomedin C), resulting in decreased chondrocyte proliferation.[467,468] In addition, the general inhibitory effect of glucocorticoids on cell growth and cell division probably contributes to growth failure.[464] Although early studies showed that growth hormone did not always improve growth failure in children with glucocorticoid-induced inhibition of growth,[469] more recent reports have shown not only increased height velocity in many patients,[470,471] but also catch-up growth.[472]

Growth suppression may be a consequence of the underlying disease process, as in JRA.[424] Evidence suggests that when glucocorticoids are used, growth restriction is more severe in patients with JRA than in patients with SLE receiving equivalent doses.[473] Growth suppression seems to be worse in patients with systemic-onset disease compared with patients with polyarticular-onset or oligoarticular-onset disease.[473] Although alternate-day regimens have been shown to minimize this adverse effect,[424,474,475] the usefulness of such regimens for controlling the actual disease is unclear.

Effects on Bone: Osteoporosis and Avascular Necrosis. Osteoporosis is another serious consequence of long-term glucocorticoid therapy. There are multiple other contributing factors, including inadequate dietary intake of calcium and vitamin D, underlying disease activity (e.g., in children with polyarticular-onset or systemic-onset JRA),[478] reduced physical activity,[479] reduced exposure to sunlight (e.g., in children with JDM or SLE), and low body weight.[480]

Glucocorticoids are associated with a reduction in bone formation and an increase in bone resorption; the reduction in bone formation seems to be more important. Reduced bone formation is caused by a direct inhibitory effect on and apoptosis of osteoblasts. Glucocorticoids also directly inhibit gut absorption of calcium and cause increased urinary calcium excretion, potentially resulting in secondary hyperparathyroidism and increased bone resorption;[481,482] however, this mechanism seems to play a minor role, at least in adults.

The extent of bone loss seems to be related to the dose and the duration of glucocorticoid therapy, although these factors do not have a consistent relationship with fracture risk. Significant trabecular bone loss occurs with doses of 7.5 mg/day or greater in most adults.[483,484] Bone

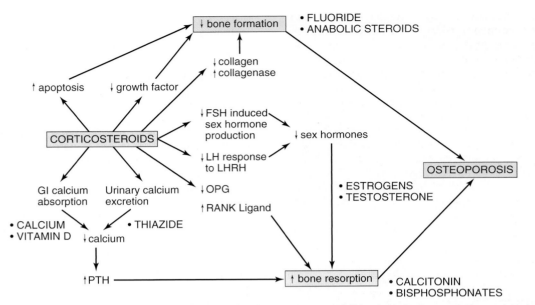

FIGURE 6–14 Approaches to the prevention and treatment of steroid-induced osteoporosis. FSH, follicle-stimulating hormone; GI, gastrointestinal; LH, luteinizing hormone; LHRH, luteinizing hormone–releasing hormone; OPG, osteoprotegerin; PTH, parathyroid hormone; RANK ligand, receptor-associated NF-κB ligand.

loss seems to occur rapidly within the first 6 to 12 months of therapy and then reaches a plateau.[484] Alternate-day glucocorticoid therapy may not be protective.[485] In adults, bone loss is predominantly trabecular (e.g., spine and ribs), rather than cortical, whereas in children the osteoporotic effect of glucocorticoids is more generalized. Not all patients exposed to long-term glucocorticoid therapy develop bone loss.[486] There are no reliable biochemical markers, however, that can be used to predict which children treated with glucocorticoids will experience significant bone loss.[487] Bone densitometry may be used to screen children who are at high risk for osteoporosis. Approaches to the prevention and treatment of glucocorticoid-associated osteoporosis are discussed later.

Some mechanisms by which glucocorticoids result in bone loss have been explored and are depicted in Figure 6–14. They include effects on the production of local growth factors, reduction of matrix proteins, increase in the production of enzymes that break down matrix, increase in apoptosis of osteoblasts and osteocytes, and increase in osteoclastogenesis secondary to decreased production of osteoprotegerin and increased production of receptor-associated NF-κB ligand (RANK ligand).[488-490]

High-dose glucocorticoids have also been associated with avascular necrosis of bone (AVN). Although the exact mechanism is unknown,[491] a variety of more recent observations may help explain this devastating complication. Intramedullary vascular compromise may result from the increased osteocyte apoptosis induced by glucocorticoids. Absence of clearance of these apoptotic osteocytes may result in reduced blood flow and bony ischemia.[492] Glucocorticoids induce adipocyte differentiation via the increased production of PPAR-γ_2, which may result in increased fat in the marrow.[492] Finally, glucocorticoids also increase the increased expression of endothelin-I, which may also lead to reduced intramedullary blood flow.[493] Many sites can be involved, but the most common

and clinically significant location for AVN is the femoral head. This complication is more frequently reported in patients with SLE (in which the underlying disease process can be a contributing factor) and possibly after high-dose intravenous methylprednisolone therapy, although the data to support the latter association are not strong.[304,499]

Infection and Immunity. Glucocorticoids interfere with the ability to resist infection through two main mechanisms: (1) They act as immunosuppressives and unpredictably decrease the patient's resistance to viral and bacterial infections. (2) They are also antiinflammatory agents and may mask the signs and symptoms of infection, including important signs such as fever or abdominal pain in peritonitis. Susceptibility to infections generally is related to the dose and duration of glucocorticoid administration. The minimal amount of systemic steroids and the duration of administration sufficient to cause immunosuppression in an otherwise healthy child are not well defined.[219] Additional factors that may affect the overall extent of immunosuppression in children with rheumatic diseases receiving steroid treatment include the effects of the underlying disease and concurrent immunosuppressive therapies.

The most profound effect of glucocorticoid administration is on cell-mediated immune reactions, including delayed hypersensitivity and allograft rejection. Patients receiving high doses of glucocorticoids for a prolonged period are prone to infections that are associated with defects of delayed hypersensitivity (e.g., tuberculosis). If possible, the Mantoux test (purified protein derivative [PPD], 5 tuberculin units) should be performed before glucocorticoids are started. The risk of complications of varicella infection must also be considered. A susceptible child being treated with glucocorticoids who is exposed to chickenpox should receive zoster immune globulin within 96 hours (for maximum effectiveness, as soon as possible after exposure) or acyclovir during the infectious illness itself.[219]

There is little information to guide decisions about the glucocorticoid regimen in varicella-infected children who have been on long-term steroid therapy; it would seem reasonable to try to minimize doses while maintaining disease control during the course of such an infection. If bacterial infection develops in a child treated with glucocorticoids, the dose may be maintained or increased, and the best available treatment for the infection should be vigorously administered. In patients with acquired immunodeficiency syndrome (AIDS) and moderate to severe *P. jiroveci* pneumonia, early adjunctive treatment with glucocorticoids has been shown to have a beneficial effect on the clinical course and outcome.[495] Although no controlled trials of glucocorticoids in young children have been performed, most experts recommend glucocorticoids as part of therapy for children with moderate to severe *P. jiroveci* pneumonia.[219] The impact of glucocorticoids in immunocompromised hosts without AIDS seems to be similar to that in patients with AIDS.[496]

Hematological System. Glucocorticoids decrease the number of circulating lymphocytes, monocytes, basophils, and eosinophils, but increase the number of circulating neutrophils.[497] Excess glucocorticoid may also cause polycythemia.

Central Nervous System. The effect of glucocorticoids on the CNS results from changes in the concentration of plasma glucose, circulatory dynamics, and electrolyte balance. These effects are reflected by changes in mood, behavior, and electroencephalographic studies.[498] Pseudotumor cerebri is rare, but may occur after rapid reduction of glucocorticoid dose.[499]

Most glucocorticoid-induced psychoses have an acute onset, are related to high doses, and occur within 96 hours after initiation of medication.[500,501] Psychosis is more common in idiopathic Cushing syndrome than in iatrogenic disease. Early on, there may be euphoria and mania; later in Cushing syndrome, depression tends to predominate. Other types of mood and behavioral disturbances, such as anxiety and insomnia, may occur.

A prospective cohort study of the adverse effects of high-dose intermittent intravenous glucocorticoids in 213 children with rheumatic diseases found behavioral changes in 21 (10%).[502] These abnormalities included altered mood in 14 children, hyperactivity in 4, sleep disturbance in 3, and psychosis in 2. In some cases, CNS effects may be related to the underlying disease (e.g., SLE). Behavioral abnormalities usually disappear after glucocorticoids are withdrawn.

Cardiovascular System. The major effect of glucocorticoids on the cardiovascular system is mediated by their influence on the regulation of renal sodium excretion, sometimes leading to hypertension. In addition, induction of angiotensin II receptors by glucocorticoids results in enhanced vasopressor responses. This complication is uncommon, however, in children with JRA who do not have underlying renal disease. The actual mechanism of glucocorticoid-induced hypertension is not fully explained. Sodium retention plays a role, and additional factors, such as increased plasma renin activity or antidiuretic hormone, may be involved.[452] Glucocorticoids also exert an important effect on capillaries, arterioles, and myocardium.[452] These influences are relevant in acute relative steroid deficiency when patients treated with long-term glucocorticoids are subject to physiological stress (see "Preventing Acute Adrenal Insufficiency [Addisonian Crisis]").

Other important possible long-term effects of long-term glucocorticoid administration include hyperlipemia and accelerated coronary atherosclerosis.[503] Patients with SLE, who often are treated with large doses of glucocorticoids for prolonged periods, are at increased risk for dyslipoproteinemia and coronary artery disease after about 10 years of disease. Although the pathogenesis of coronary artery disease in these patients is multifactorial, some studies have suggested that a long duration of glucocorticoid therapy may be an important risk factor.[504] A cross-sectional study of 40 children with SLE did not find steroids to be an independent risk factor for coronary artery disease.[505] These children had a median age of 15.9 years and median disease duration of 1.4 years at the time of study. In contrast to adults, children with abnormalities in coronary perfusion tended to have shorter median duration of prednisone use and lower cumulative dose of steroids and fewer intravenous pulsed doses of steroids. Although the study was small, and these were observed trends only and not statistically significant differences, they raise the possibility that coronary artery disease may be more a manifestation of the underlying disease process than of the glucocorticoid therapy used to treat it.

Cataracts and Glaucoma. Subcapsular cataracts[499,506,507] are more common with glucocorticoid therapy than in idiopathic Cushing syndrome. The risk of cataract development becomes significant when a dose of prednisone equal to or greater than 9 $mg/m^2/day$ has been maintained for longer than 1 year. Most children who have been treated with doses of glucocorticoid equivalent to 20 mg/day of prednisone for 4 years or longer develop cataracts.[499] These cataracts often do not progress, are functionally benign, and rarely affect vision. Children receiving long-term glucocorticoid therapy should also be monitored for glaucoma, especially if they have a history of uveitis.

Muscle Disease. Muscle wasting that results from high-dose glucocorticoid administration is associated with atrophy of muscle fibers, especially type IIB fibers. Steroid myopathy can complicate the clinical assessment of a patient with SLE or JDM (see Chapters 21 and 24). Myopathy induced by glucocorticoids usually affects proximal muscles, is seldom painful, and is usually associated with normal serum levels of muscle enzymes and an electromyogram suggestive of myopathy. A muscle biopsy may be needed to differentiate between steroid myopathy and active myositis. Glucocorticoid-induced hypokalemia may also lead to muscular weakness and fatigue. Recovery from steroid myopathy may be slow and incomplete.[508]

Other Side Effects. Glucose intolerance and glycosuria may occur after prolonged exposure to large doses of glucocorticoids, particularly if there is a genetic predisposition to diabetes.[509] Glucose intolerance can usually be managed with diet or insulin and should not preclude the use of glucocorticoid therapy in diabetic patients who need treatment.

The role of glucocorticoids in peptic ulceration is controversial. Although some authorities have suggested an increased risk, current evidence does not support a definitive association between peptic ulceration and glucocorticoid therapy independent of any other factors, such as NSAID therapy or concomitant illness.[510]

MINIMIZING TOXICITY

The deleterious effects of glucocorticoids can be minimized by choosing a drug with a short half-life (see Table 6–9).[511] Prednisone is the drug most often given for oral therapy. Its enhanced glucocorticoid and minimal mineralocorticoid actions give it the lowest risk/benefit ratio of any of the analogues in general use.[512] Adherence to the use of a single synthetic analogue simplifies communications with the patient, parents, and medical personnel and reduces the risk of an error in dose.

The GR-DNA interaction induces genes that code for antiinflammatory proteins (transactivation). Genes that code for proinflammatory proteins are regulated by transcription factors such as NF-κB (transrepression). In this situation, the GR operates via protein interactions, inhibits the activity of the transcription factors, and represses the expression of the proinflammatory proteins. Many glucocorticoid side effects seem to be mediated via binding to DNA elements, rather than protein elements. If synthetic glucocorticoids could be designed to operate via the latter rather than the former pathway, the result would be maintenance of antiinflammatory properties with reduction in toxicity. Work is in progress to develop such agents.[513]

Deflazacort, an oxazoline derivative of prednisone with antiinflammatory and immunosuppressive activity, may have a bone-sparing effect compared with prednisone.[514-516] There are at least two case reports, however, of children who developed symptomatic vertebral collapse while receiving deflazacort for vasculitis and a lupuslike syndrome.[478] Deflazacort is commonly used in patients with Duchenne muscular dystrophy, but not frequently in rheumatic diseases.

The antiinflammatory effect and the toxicity of glucocorticoids increase with larger doses and more frequent administration (Table 6–12). Four-times-daily administration is more effective than twice-daily administration of the same total dose. Daily administration is more effective than administration of the same total dose every other day.[424,515,517,518] Glucocorticoid administration should be as infrequent as is consistent with achieving disease control. Short-acting glucocorticoids given in the morning (on waking) do not suppress the pituitary as much as glucocorticoids given later in the day (which suppress the normal surge of ACTH that occurs during sleep).[452]

Reduction in glucocorticoid dose must be individualized for the child and the disease. At high doses (e.g., 60 mg/day), reductions of 10 mg are usually well tolerated; at lower doses (e.g., 10 mg/day), reductions of only 1 or 2 mg may be possible. An alternate-day regimen should be

Table 6–12

Systemic administration of glucocorticoid drugs

Schedule	Advantages	Disadvantages
Divided daily doses	Better disease control	More side effects
Single daily dose	Good disease control; fewer side effects	May not control severe disease
Alternate-day dose	Fewer side effects	Less disease control
IV pulse therapy	Less long-term toxicity	Acute toxicities

IV, intravenous.

the goal to minimize toxicity, although some patients do not tolerate this regimen. Glucocorticoid dose tapering is often fraught with difficulty because of the adaptation of the patient's metabolism to chronic steroid excess.[519,520] In some children, steroid pseudorheumatism may result from a rapid dose decrease.[521] Pseudotumor cerebri may occur under similar conditions.[499] These withdrawal effects gradually resolve over 1 or 2 weeks and are minimized if each decrement in daily prednisone is 1 mg or less per week (at the lower dose levels).

Many approaches for the prevention and treatment of corticosteroid-associated osteoporosis have been studied in adults (see Fig. 6–14), and several guidelines have addressed these issues.[522,523] Vitamin D and its analogues, calcitonin, and various bisphosphonates have been used. Calcitriol (vitamin D_3) or cholecalciferol (vitamin D), with or without calcitonin, was shown to prevent bone loss from the lumbar spine better than calcium alone in several randomized controlled clinical trials of adults starting long-term glucocorticoid therapy.[524,525] Treatment with calcium and vitamin D in adults receiving glucocorticoids effectively retards lumbar and forearm bone loss.[526] Reported adverse effects included mainly constipation (calcium) and hypercalcemia and hypercalciuria (calcitriol), although these may be less frequent with physiological doses.

The clinical significance of these findings needs interpretation in light of the fact that none of the studies was able to show any significant decrease in fracture incidence. This is probably a result of the lack of power for detection of infrequent events in these relatively small studies. Because none of the controlled studies included children with rheumatic diseases, the generalizability of results to this group of patients also requires caution. Treatment with calcium and vitamin D supplementation has now become the standard of practice in most centers for children with rheumatic disease receiving glucocorticoids.[477,527-529]

Bisphosphonates have also been studied as a potential treatment for glucocorticoid-induced osteoporosis. Etidronate, pamidronate, alendronate, and risedronate have been shown in randomized controlled trials to increase lumbar spine bone mineral density in adults receiving long-term glucocorticoids for various diseases.[481,530-533] These trials did not include children, however, and did not show any significant reduction in fracture incidence, which is the most clinically relevant outcome. Bisphosphonates have been studied in children with osteogenesis imperfecta and seem to be beneficial in reducing bone resorption, increasing bone density, and reducing the chronic bone pain associated with this condition.[534-542] In addition, although there are concerns regarding their effects on growth and remodeling, bisphosphonates have been found to be useful and safe in open-label studies of children with idiopathic juvenile osteoporosis[543] and osteoporosis associated with connective tissue diseases or induced by glucorticoids,[544-546] the latter accompanied by changes in markers reflecting bone turnover (resorption and formation).[547] The most frequently used regimen is alendronate, 5 mg/day for children weighing less than 20 kg and 10 mg for children weighing 20 kg or more, daily, after an overnight fast and remaining upright for 30 minutes after the dose to prevent esophagitis.

Although much is known about the mechanisms of glucocorticoid-induced osteoporosis, knowledge about how best to prevent and treat this complication, particularly in children, is limited. Standards of practice in this area are still evolving, and larger, prospective trials evaluating prevention and treatment of glucocorticoid-induced osteoporosis in children are also needed.

PREVENTING ACUTE ADRENAL INSUFFICIENCY (ADDISONIAN CRISIS)

The use of pharmacological doses of glucocorticoids for a 2-week period may result in transient suppression of endogenous cortisol production,[548] and prolonged therapy may lead to suppression of pituitary-adrenal function that can be slow in returning to normal. This is potentially the most serious and life-threatening adverse effect associated with glucocorticoid therapy. The magnitude of the effect on adrenal function of relatively low amounts of glucocorticoid, especially if given over prolonged periods, is often underestimated. The actual doses and duration of therapy that are associated with this suppression and the length of the recovery period after cessation of therapy are not well defined, however.[549,550] Some evidence suggests that a component of adrenal insufficiency may be a result of the underlying inflammatory process in some patients.[551]

If not recognized, suppression of the hypothalamic-pituitary-adrenal axis as a consequence of long-term glucocorticoid administration places a child at risk for vascular collapse, adrenal crisis, and death in situations that demand increased availability of cortisol.[552] Under conditions of stress (e.g., serious infection, trauma, surgery), all children who may be at risk for hypothalamic-pituitary-adrenal axis suppression require additional glucocorticoids.

Glucocorticoid supplementation should be prescribed before surgery in any patient who has received significant amounts of glucocorticoids at any time during the preceding 12 months (possibly as long as 36 months),[552] although the appropriate candidates and amount and duration of glucocorticoid taken are controversial.[553] For an elective procedure, "steroid preparation" consists of dexamethasone (0.05 to 0.15 mg/kg/24 hr) before the procedure in four divided intramuscular doses given 6 hours apart, and hydrocortisone (1.5 to 4 mg/kg/24 hr) as a continuous intravenous infusion beginning at the time of surgery and continuing for 24 hours postoperatively, or until the child has recovered or is able to take prednisone again by mouth.

This regimen is based on requirements for hydrocortisone during stress. Hydrocortisone (0.36 mg/kg/24 hr) is needed for physiological maintenance. During maximal stress, 1.5 to 4 mg/kg/24 hr is required. Dexamethasone sodium phosphate (0.75 mg has a mineralocorticoid effect approximately equivalent to 20 mg of hydrocortisone) is given preoperatively because of its long half-life; hydrocortisone is used during the procedure because of its immediate biological availability. These recommended doses should be modified according to the magnitude of the stress and the severity and duration of suppression of the hypothalamic-pituitary-adrenal axis by exogenous steroid administration.

The requirement of increased amounts of glucocorticoid during acute stress should be explained to the parents. In addition, the child should carry a card or wear a necklace or bracelet indicating that glucocorticoid medication is being taken. Such a warning can be of great value to emergency medical teams if the child is involved in an accident.

HIGH-DOSE INTRAVENOUS GLUCOCORTICOID THERAPY

Intravenous glucocorticoid "pulse" therapy is sometimes used to treat more severe, acute, systemic connective tissue diseases such as SLE, JDM, vasculitis, and macrophage activation syndrome.[554-557] It has also been used to treat the refractory systemic features of systemic-onset JRA.[558-561] The rationale of this approach is to achieve an immediate, profound antiinflammatory effect and to minimize toxicity related to long-term continuous therapy in moderate to high daily doses. The main benefit seems to be rapid clinical improvement. This rapid improvement may be useful in the context of concurrent treatment with a disease-modifying agent, which may take several weeks or months to begin to exert its effect.

Although oral pulse regimens have been reported,[562] most publications report studies in which intravenous pulse therapy has been used. Methylprednisolone has been the drug of choice, given in a dose of 10 to 30 mg/kg/pulse up to a maximum of 1 g, administered according to various protocols (Table 6–13): a single administration repeated as clinical circumstances warrant, a pulse each day for 3 to 5 days, or alternate-day pulses for three doses. Intravenous glucocorticoid pulse therapy, although possibly efficacious in selected circumstances (no controlled trials have been reported in children), may be associated with potentially serious complications (Table 6–14).

The most frequently reported short-term adverse effect in children is abnormal behavior in 10% of patients.[502] These behavioral changes included altered mood, hyperactivity, psychosis, disorientation, and sleep disturbances. Nonbehavioral adverse effects included headache, abdominal complaints, pruritus, vomiting, hives, hypertension, bone pain, dizziness, fatigue, lethargy, hypotension, tachycardia, and hyperglycemia.[502] Potential longer term effects, such as influences on bone metabolism and risk of AVN, have not been systematically studied. Although

Table 6–13

Suggested protocol for administration of intravenous methylprednisolone

Dose
Up to 30 mg/kg (maximum 1 g)

Preparation
Prepare drug with diluent provided with package
Calculated dose is added to 100 mL normal saline and infused over 1-3 hr

Monitoring
Temperature, pulse rate, respiratory rate, blood pressure before beginning infusion
Pulse and blood pressure every 15 min for first hour, every 30 min thereafter
Slow rate or discontinue infusion and increase frequency of monitoring if there are significant changes in blood pressure or pulse rate

Side Effects
Hypertension or hypotension, tachycardia, blurring of vision, flushing, sweating, metallic taste in mouth

Table 6–14

Potential acute toxicities of intravenous glucocorticoid pulse therapy

Cardiac arrhythmia secondary to potassium depletion
Hypertension secondary to sodium retention
Acute psychosis, convulsions
Hyperglycemia with or without ketosis
Anaphylaxis
Infection
Osteonecrosis

there have been many reports of AVN associated with intravenous pulse methylprednisolone,[563,564] a retrospective cohort study of patients with rheumatoid arthritis did not find an increased risk of AVN in patients treated with pulse methylprednisolone.[565]

INTRAARTICULAR STEROIDS

Injection of long-acting glucocorticoids directly into inflamed joints has emerged as a major advance in the management of various types of arthritis. Although intraarticular steroid (IAS) therapy has not been studied in randomized controlled clinical trials, multiple reports have documented its efficacy and safety in children (i.e., numerous uncontrolled, prospective cohort studies).[566-572] It is difficult to summarize the results of the available studies, however, because of the variability in the populations studied and in the type, dose, and frequency of steroids used; the lack of control groups; and the variability in the assessment of outcomes, which often were not blinded and did not use standard outcome measures or lengths of follow-up.

IAS therapy has been used most often in children with oligoarticular disease; indications for use have included lack of response to NSAIDs; significant NSAID

toxicity; and the presence of joint deformity, growth disturbance, or muscle wasting. These drugs may also have a role as an alternative to NSAIDs in children with oligoarticular disease. In polyarticular disease, multiple IAS injections at one time can be used as a temporizing measure while awaiting response to second-line agents given systemically. IAS may also be useful as an alternative to increasing systemic therapy in children with polyarticular disease who have significant inflammation in only a few joints.

Virtually all patients experience rapid resolution of symptoms and signs of joint inflammation within a few days after injection, resulting in improved physical function.[573] About two thirds achieve remission for at least 12 months after a single injection.[567,568] The duration of response seems to be longer in children with oligoarticular JRA than in children with polyarticular-onset or systemic-onset disease and in children with other forms of arthritis (e.g., spondyloarthropathies).[574,575] Younger patients and patients with shorter disease duration achieved longer remissions after IAS injection,[566] as did patients with higher mean erythrocyte sedimentation rates in another study.[576] Early use of IAS injections may result in less leg-length discrepancies in patients with asymmetrical pauciarticular JRA.[577] Neidel and associates[578] reported a 2-year remission rate of 58% after a single injection of 1 mg/kg (maximum 40 mg) of triamcinolone hexacetonide into inflamed hip joints; responses were better in children with pauciarticular or RF-negative polyarticular-onset disease (65%) compared with children with RF-positive polyarticular-onset or systemic-onset JRA. More recent data suggest efficacy of IAS injections into involved temporomandibular and subtalar joints.[579-581]

Type of Steroid, Dosage, and Frequency of Injection. Various preparations are available for IAS injection. The most frequently studied agents in children are the least soluble and longest acting forms of injectable steroid: triamcinolone hexacetonide (THA)[566-567,569] and triamcinolone acetonide.[568] These agents are completely absorbed from the site of injection over 2 to 3 weeks. Because of its lower solubility, THA is absorbed more slowly than triamcinolone acetonide, maintaining synovial levels for a longer period and creating lower systemic glucocorticoid levels.[582] THA is preferred by most pediatric rheumatologists. In comparative studies in patients with JIA, THA was found to be more effective than triamcinolone acetonide at equivalent doses.[583-585] Intraarticular THA is superior to betamethasone[586] and methylprednisolone.[587]

The dose of THA used in clinical studies has varied: Some data indicate that higher doses (about 1 mg/kg) may be associated with a better response.[566] Although there are no established rules regarding the choice of steroid, the dosage and frequency of injection have been outlined. Generally, children who weigh less than 20 kg receive 20 mg of THA in large joints. Children weighing more than 20 kg receive 30 to 40 mg THA in the hips, knees, and shoulders, and 10 to 20 mg in the ankles and elbows. In smaller joints such as the wrist, midtarsal, and subtalar joints, 10 mg is used. For injections into tendon sheaths and small joints of the hands and feet, 0.25 to 0.50 mL of a combination of methylprednisolone acetate mixed 1:1

with preservative-free 1% lidocaine (Xylocaine) is recommended. The shorter acting steroid is associated with less risk of damage to tendon sheaths or of local soft tissue atrophy caused by leakage of steroid from the smaller volume joints.

Repeated injections into the same joint are not performed more than three times per year, although there are few data on which to base this recommendation. There are also no controlled studies in children examining whether postinjection rest has a role. Although full immobilization of the injected joint is common practice in some clinics, the authors' recommendation is to limit ambulation for the first 24 hours for injections to the joints of the lower extremities and to avoid high-impact physical activity 24 to 72 hours after a joint injection.

Adverse Effects. Despite initial reservations about the safety of IAS therapy in children, clinical studies indicate an overall favorable adverse-effect profile. Iatrogenic septic arthritis is always a potential risk. It occurs very rarely in adults and can be avoided with appropriate aseptic precautions.[587] Transient crystal synovitis occurs in a few patients.[355] It is very similar to gouty arthritis and is self-limited, with resolution of symptoms within 3 to 5 days in most cases without any intervention.[571] The most frequent adverse effects are atrophic skin changes at the site of injection, particularly of smaller joints such as wrists, ankles, and interphalangeal joints in young children, and asymptomatic calcifications on radiographs in joints after multiple injections.[575] The frequency of these skin changes ranges from 5.6% of knees injected to 16% of ankles, 22% of wrists, and 50% of metatarsophalangeal joints.[588] The skin changes are attributed to leakage of long-acting steroids into subcutaneous tissues and can be minimized by clearing the needle track with injection of saline or local anesthetic as the needle is withdrawn from the joint. Most skin changes eventually resolve.[567,588] Radiographic reviews have shown joint calcifications in 6% to 50% of injected joints.[589,590] These are usually asymptomatic, but in one case surgical removal was required because of the size of the calcification.[591]

One of the main reservations about the use of IAS in young children was based on the theoretical potential for cartilage toxicity. Cartilage damage occurred after IAS injection in the rabbit model, but was not reproduced in higher species.[587] Clinical magnetic resonance imaging (MRI) studies in children to assess cartilage integrity up to 13 months after steroid injection of single joints showed no toxic effects on cartilage and no detrimental effects on statural growth.[592,593] Some children with multiple IAS injections (more than five per joint) who are monitored for longer periods (6 to 18 years) may have nonspecific abnormalities of cartilage on MRI.[594] The clinical significance of these findings is unclear.

Although most adverse effects associated with IAS injections are local, the injections are also associated with some systemic effects. Children develop transient suppression of endogenous cortisol production lasting 10 to 30 days after IAS injection.[595,596] Younger children may undergo a more prolonged period of suppression. The clinical significance of this finding in terms of effects on

linear growth or actual risk of adrenal crisis at times of stress is unknown. Although these complications have not been reported after single injections, whether there is any risk after multiple injections, particularly in younger children, needs further study. Systemic absorption of steroid may also be associated with altered salicylate kinetics, resulting in a transient decrease in serum salicylate levels. Diabetic children may require a temporary increase in insulin requirements.

Cytotoxic, Antimetabolic, and Immunomodulatory Agents

Cytotoxic drugs prevent cell division or cause cell death. They act primarily on rapidly dividing cells such as cells of the immune system, particularly T lymphocytes, and are immunosuppressive. Cytotoxic drugs have immediate antiinflammatory actions and delayed immunosuppressive effects. Pharmacological actions are usually considered to be either specific for the cell cycle phase or nonspecific. The cell cycle consists of the G_1 presynthetic phase, the S phase (synthesis of DNA), the G_2 resting (or postsynthetic) phase, and mitosis. Mercaptopurine and azathioprine inhibit biosynthesis of purine and nucleotide interconversions and act during the G_1 and S phases in proliferating cells. MMF reduces the pool of guanine nucleotide, interfering with purine biosynthesis; it also acts in the G_1 and S phases. Alkylating agents crosslink DNA and act during all phases of the cell cycle, whether or not a cell is replicating. These agents are maximally effective in inhibiting immunological responses when their administration coincides with the period of proliferation of the specific immunologically competent cells.

Although cytotoxic drugs have been used to treat children who are seriously ill with rheumatic diseases after other modes of therapy have proved ineffective, there have been no adequately controlled trials in children. In most instances, the effects of these drugs are delayed; they have proved to be more valuable in moderate-term to long-term therapy than in an acute crisis. The potential toxicity of these drugs is substantial. Although extensive experience has been accumulating with the use of these agents, each child's illness must be considered thoroughly before drugs from this class are recommended. As with most agents used in pediatric rheumatology, these agents are not approved for unrestricted use in children with rheumatic diseases and should be used only by physicians who are familiar with their administration, toxicity, and expected benefits. Occasionally, these agents are used for their steroid-sparing effect.

Azathioprine

Azathioprine (Fig. 6–15 [online only]), a purine analogue, is inactive until it is metabolized to mercaptopurine by the liver and erythrocytes.[597] Hypoxanthine phosphoribosyl transferase metabolizes mercaptopurine to thioinosinic acid, which suppresses the synthesis of adenine and guanine, interfering with DNA synthesis. Inosinic acid inhibits phosphoribosyl pyrophosphate conversion in purine nucleotide synthesis, conversion of inosinic acid to xanthylic acid by purine nucleoside phosphorylase, and incorporation of nucleotide triphosphates into DNA.

Azathioprine suppresses cell-mediated immune functions and inhibits monocyte functions.[598-601] These immunosuppressive effects are related primarily to inhibition of T cell growth during the S phase of cell division. A measurable decrease in antibody synthesis occurs with long-term administration; occasionally, a decrease in serum antibody concentration occurs.

Approximately 50% of the drug is absorbed after oral administration, of which one third is protein bound.[597] The plasma half-life is approximately 75 minutes. The kidneys are the major route of excretion. Azathioprine crosses the placenta. Because the fetal liver lacks the ability to convert azathioprine to its active metabolites, however, the fetus is generally protected from adverse effects, although rare cases of fetal bone marrow suppression have been reported.[602] It is best to avoid using azathioprine during pregnancy, although this is not always possible. Azathioprine appears in breast milk, and breast-feeding is not recommended.[603]

Toxicity to the GI tract (oral ulcers, nausea, vomiting, diarrhea, epigastric pain) is common.[604] Toxicity to the liver (mild elevation of serum concentrations of liver enzymes, cholestatic jaundice), lung (interstitial pneumonitis), pancreas (pancreatitis), or skin (maculopapular rash) is uncommonly associated with azathioprine therapy. Dose-related toxicity to the bone marrow results in leukopenia and, less commonly, thrombocytopenia and anemia.

An idiosyncratic arrest of granulocyte maturation that occurs shortly after initiation of therapy has been described and results from reduced activity of the enzyme thiopurine methyltransferase.[605,606] Thiopurine methyltransferase is responsible for inactivating mercaptopurine. Polymorphisms exist in the gene responsible for thiopurine methyltransferase, and at least eight alleles have been identified. Deficiency of the enzyme may result in severe toxicity, and high levels may require higher dosing of azathioprine. Most of the population has high enzymatic activity; approximately 0.03% of the population is deficient.[607] These latter patients may rapidly develop severe leukopenia on exposure to azathioprine. Lower levels of enzymatic activity have been observed in African Americans compared with whites.[608] Testing of thiopurine methyltransferase levels is now available and should be considered for patients who develop severe leukopenia while taking azathioprine.

The bone marrow effects of azathioprine may be increased by concomitant use of trimethoprim.[609] Although the risk of malignancy theoretically increases in patients treated with azathioprine, the long-term data are inconclusive. Data are insufficient with respect to childhood rheumatic diseases, but in adults with rheumatoid arthritis treated with azathioprine, the risk of malignancy did not seem to be greater than in similar patients who did not receive azathioprine.[610-612] The combination of azathioprine with infliximab is associated with increased hepatosplenic T cell lymphoma (see later discussion of TNF inhibitors).

The use of azathioprine has been reported anecdotally in many pediatric rheumatic diseases and in series of

Table 6–15

Guidelines for use of azathioprine

Dose
0.6-2.5 mg/kg/day, maximum 150 mg in a single dose (taken with food)

Clinical Monitoring
Clinical evaluation at 1-2 mo and then every 3 mo (or more often if disease uncontrolled)

Laboratory Monitoring
Consider testing thiopurine methyltransferase genotype or activity

CBC with WBC count, differential, and platelet count weekly until stable dose is achieved, then every 4-12 wk

Hepatic enzymes, BUN, serum creatinine initially and then monthly

Discontinue if WBC count <3500/mm³, platelet count <100,000/mm³, or elevated liver enzymes

BUN, blood urea nitrogen; CBC, complete blood count; WBC, white blood cell.

patients with JRA or SLE.[613,614] Starting doses should be 1 to 1.5 mg/kg/day, increasing as needed and as tolerated to 2 to 2.5 mg/kg/day, maximum 150 mg (Table 6–15).

Mycophenolate Mofetil

MMF has been found to be effective in various autoimmune diseases (Fig. 6–16 [online only]). Mycophenolic acid (MPA), a fermentation product of *Penicillium stoloniferum*, is the active immunosuppressant species, and MMF was developed to increase the oral bioavailability of MPA. Its major effect is on T and B lymphocytes, for which it is relatively selective. Action of MPA is mediated through noncompetitive binding to inosine monophosphate dehydrogenase, an enzyme crucial for de novo synthesis of guanine nucleotide, a pathway on which T and B lymphocytes are primarily dependent.

In vitro, MPA inhibits T and B cell mitogen proliferation,[615-617] antigen-specific antibody response of memory B cells,[616,618,619] suppression of the humoral immune response,[620] and attachment of monocytes to endothelial cells.[621] MPA enhances vascular cell adhesion molecules induced by TNF-α and E-selectin surface expression on endothelial cells.[622] Some of the improvement seen in renal disease in MRL/lpr mice may be associated with inhibition of renal nitric oxide production.[623,624] Because its effect seems to be at a late stage of T cell activation, MMF can be used safely with calcineurin inhibitors.

MMF is rapidly absorbed after oral administration and is hydrolyzed in the liver to biologically active MPA. MPA is 8% albumin bound, and the activity of the drug results from the unbound MPA. Peak plasma levels occur 1 to 3 hours after a single dose, with a second peak at 6 to 12 hours as a result of enterohepatic circulation. The oral bioavailability is approximately 94%. The elimination half-life is approximately 17 hours after oral administration.[625] Because of its extensive binding to albumin, MMF may interact with other albumin-bound drugs. Antacids containing aluminum and magnesium decrease absorption and should not be administered simultaneously.

There may be competition for renal tubular secretion with acyclovir (Table 6–16).

The effective adult dose in solid organ transplantation is 2 to 3 g/day in two divided doses. The dose used to prevent solid organ transplant rejection in children has been 46 mg/kg/day.[625,626] The recommended dose for children 13 months to 18 yrs is 600 mg/m² BID. Cyclosporine and, to a lesser extent, tacrolimus alter the kinetics of MMF so that higher doses are required in the transplantation setting.[627] In children with autoimmune diseases, mean doses reported have included 900 mg/m²/day[628] and 22 mg/kg/day.[629] Individual pharmacokinetic profiling is available and can be especially helpful in determining the lowest effective dose in patients experiencing side effects.[630,631] A high interindividual variability was shown for MPA area under the curve serum concentrations in patients treated with MMF for SLE, with concentration-effect relationship with immunological disease activity parameters suggesting that the dose should be individualized in patients with SLE.[632]

Adverse effects of MMF include GI toxicity, hematological effects (leukopenia, anemia, thrombocytopenia, pancytopenia), and opportunistic infections. GI side effects are usually improved by giving the dose three or four times a day instead of twice a day or by reducing it. Hematological toxicity usually responds to therapy cessation within 1 week. The incidence of lymphoma has been reported to be 0.6%, similar to the incidence associated with azathioprine.[633] Forty-one cases of pure red blood cell aplasia have been reported in patients treated with MMF; some cases were in patients treated in combination with other immunosuppressive agents (alemtuzumab, tacrolimus, and azathioprine).[634] In 16 of the reported cases, dose reduction or discontinuation led to resolution of the condition.

Although early reports of MMF use in patients with rheumatoid arthritis showed promise,[635] the availability of newer agents seems to have had an effect on further study in this area. MMF is being used increasingly, however, in patients with SLE,[629,636-641] systemic vasculitis[630,633,642] (although flares may be common[643]), or inflammatory eye disease.[644,645]

In a randomized, open-label noninferiority study of MMF in the treatment of class III, IV, or V lupus nephritis in adults, 3 g daily of MMF was at least as effective as cyclophosphamide as induction therapy. Fewer severe infections and hospitalizations, but more diarrhea occurred in patients receiving MMF.[646] Numerous uncontrolled or retrospective studies in children with SLE show similar efficacy and safety as induction therapy, maintenance therapy, or both.[647-650]

MMF crosses the placenta and is teratogenic in rats and rabbits. Several cases of structural malformations have been seen with MMF exposure during pregnancy in renal transplant recipients and others.[651,652] If immunosuppression is required, a switch to azathioprine is recommended. No human data are available regarding breastfeeding at this time.

Cyclophosphamide

Cyclophosphamide, an alkylating agent, is a nitrogen mustard derivative (Fig. 6–17 [online only]). It is well absorbed after oral administration and may be given intravenously (Tables 6–17 and 6–18). It is inactive until metabolized, principally in the liver, by the cytochrome P-450 mixed-function oxidase system to inactive intermediates and the active metabolite phosphoramide mustard. Phosphoramide mustard covalently binds to guanine in DNA, destroying the purine ring and preventing cell replication.[653,654] Cyclophosphamide potentially acts on all cells, including cells that are mitotically inactive (G_0 interphase) at the time of administration (e.g., memory T cells).[655,656] Excretion of the drug is primarily by the

---

Table 6–16

Guidelines for use of mycophenolate mofetil

Dose

Starting dose usually 250 mg bid, titrate up to 1.5 g bid as a maximum dose (see text for dosing guidelines)

At predicted optimal dose, consider measuring trough levels and area under the curve and adjusting dose accordingly

Clinical Monitoring

Clinical evaluation every 1-2 mo and then every 3 mo (or more often if disease uncontrolled)

Laboratory Monitoring

CBC with WBC count, differential, and platelet count every 4-12 wk

Discontinue if WBC count <3500/mm³, platelet count <100,000/mm³, or declining hemoglobin not related to disease activity

CBC, complete blood count; WBC, white blood cell.

Table 6–17

Suggested protocol for administration of intravenous cyclophosphamide

Dose

0.5-1 g/m² cyclophosphamide

Preparation

IV 0.9% sodium chloride 20 mL/kg (maximum 1 L) bolus

Cyclophosphamide is mixed with 5% dextrose and ½ normal saline to infuse over 6 hr

3 mesna doses equaling the total cyclophosphamide dose are administered intravenously in 5% dextrose in water: one third of the dose is given ½ hour before infusion, one third is given midway through infusion, and one third is given at end of infusion (alternatively, the last dose of mesna can be given orally, but at double the IV dose [i.e., two thirds of total cyclophosphamide dose])

Ondansetron (0.15 mg/kg/dose diluted in 0.9% sodium chloride) intravenously or orally, orally 30 min before cyclophosphamide and every 8 hr until infusion is complete. Ondansetron orally every 8 hours times 2 doses at home

Monitoring

Pulse, blood pressure, and respiratory rate every 30 min during infusion, then every 4 hr for next 24 hr

Urinalysis before and after infusion

Monitor urinary output: Empty bladder every 2-4 hr. If urinary output falls to <50% of IV input over any 4-hr period, give IV furosemide 1 mg/kg. Repeat at 2-4 mg/kg in 2 hr, if necessary

IV, intravenous.

kidney, and the dose must be reduced in patients with renal impairment (Table 6–19). Intravenous doses should be reduced by 20% to 30% in patients with severe renal insufficiency.[657] Because cyclophosphamide is dialyzable, it is important to delay hemodialysis until at least 12 hours after intravenous administration of the drug.[657] Acrolein, the other principal metabolite, is thought to be therapeutically inactive, but is responsible for bladder toxicity. The half-life of cyclophosphamide is approximately 7 hours.

Cyclophosphamide exerts antiinflammatory actions by its effects on mononuclear cells and cellular immunity. Alkylating agents cause B and T cell lymphopenia. B cells seem to be more sensitive than T cells to the effects of cyclophosphamide.[658] It has been suggested that the route of administration influences the nature of the effects of this drug; daily oral low-dose therapy may affect cell-mediated immunity more profoundly, whereas intermittent high-dose intravenous therapy predominantly affects B cell immunity.[659,660] In humans, IgG and IgM synthesis is depressed, and there is a measurable decrease of serum antibody concentration after long-term administration.[655,656]

Alkylating agents have prominent toxic effects.[661-669] Short-term side effects are common; although troublesome to the child, they are seldom serious. These include anorexia, nausea and vomiting, and alopecia. Alopecia seems to be related to dose and duration of treatment and is usually reversible. Pulmonary fibrosis has been reported in a few patients receiving daily cyclophosphamide therapy.[670,671]

Leukopenia and thrombocytopenia are the most common adverse reactions, although with careful monitoring they are seldom clinically significant. The cyclophosphamide dose should be adjusted to maintain the total granulocyte count at 1500/mm^3 (1.5 × 10^9/L) or higher. The nadir of granulocytopenia with intravenous therapy occurs between the first and the second weeks of therapy, and the dose should be adjusted accordingly based on the complete blood count and differential white blood cell count obtained on days 7, 10, and 14 after intravenous cyclophosphamide administration. Lymphocyte counts less than 500/mm^3 (0.5 × 10^9/L) are also an indication to reduce the dose. Glucocorticoids probably aid in protecting bone marrow from the neutropenia-inducing effects of cyclophosphamide.

Cyclophosphamide is administered in one of two ways: either orally each day or by intravenous bolus every 2 to 4 weeks (see Table 6–19). Intravenous pulse administration is less toxic and at least as efficacious for lupus nephritis;[672] in some systemic vasculitides, it is unclear whether the intravenous route is as effective as oral administration.[660,673] Bladder toxicity (cystitis, fibrosis, transitional cell carcinoma) is a major risk of cyclophosphamide therapy and results from prolonged contact of acrolein with the bladder mucosa.[664-666] In rats, toxicity seems to be mediated through nitric oxide produced by inducible nitric oxide synthase.[674] To prevent cystitis, adequate hydration and frequent voiding must be emphasized for children receiving daily cyclophosphamide. Persistent nonglomerular hematuria is an indication for cystoscopy; if cystitis is observed, the dose should be reduced or the drug stopped. Intravenous pulse therapy reduces the risk of toxicity, including hemorrhagic cystitis, and confines the risks to a short period each month instead of every day. Prophylactic mesna should be considered a part of any intravenous cyclophosphamide protocol to minimize contact of acrolein with the bladder mucosa.

The syndrome of inappropriate antidiuretic hormone secretion has been reported in patients receiving large doses of cyclophosphamide and is exacerbated by the large fluid load that must be administered.[675] With the large doses of cyclophosphamide administered by intravenous bolus, children must be encouraged to empty their bladders every 2 hours and must be awakened during the night to do so; if this is impossible, furosemide should be given, and catheterization should be considered to prevent significant contact of the bladder mucosa with acrolein. Nausea and vomiting can be a significant problem; prophylactic use of a potent antiemetic (e.g., ondansetron) is encouraged.

An important consideration with the use of alkylating agents is their effect on fertility for men and women.[676] The stage of sexual maturity is crucial in terms of inducing gonadal dysfunction; the further beyond puberty, the greater the chance of infertility with an equivalent dose of cyclophosphamide.[677] In female patients with lupus nephritis, amenorrhea and oligomenorrhea occur more

---

Table 6–18

Guidelines for use of daily cyclophosphamide

Dose
0.5-2 mg/kg/day in single oral dose
0.5-2 mg/kg/day as IV pulse (with ample IV fluids for 24 hr)
Encourage fluid intake to minimize risk to bladder
Encourage frequent emptying of bladder

Clinical Monitoring
Clinical evaluation every month

Laboratory Monitoring
CBC with WBC count, differential, and platelet count, and urinalysis every week until stable dose is achieved, then every month
Hepatic enzymes, BUN, serum creatinine initially and then every month
Discontinue drug if WBC count <1500/mm^3 (1.5 × 10^9/L), platelet count <100,000/mm^3 (100 × 10^9/L), or hematuria

BUN, blood urea nitrogen; CBC, complete blood count; IV, intravenous; WBC, white blood cell.

Table 6–19

Recommended reductions of cyclophosphamide dose in patients with impaired renal function

Serum Creatinine Concentration (μmol/L)	Oral Cyclophosphamide Dose (mg/kg/day)
<250	2
250-500	1.75
>500	1.5

frequently with higher total dose and with increased age at administration.[678-681] Use of intravenous bolus administration at currently recommended doses results in a much lower total cumulative dose than daily oral administration and should be the preferred route, presuming equivalent effectiveness. Ovarian destruction attributable to cyclophosphamide was reported in one child.[661] In children with SLE, amenorrhea more likely results from disease activity and damage than cyclophosphamide treatment.[682]

Luteinizing hormone–releasing hormone may protect the ovary against cyclophosphamide-induced damage and may be effective in patients treated with cyclophosphamide, as was shown in a study of women with lymphoma who received gonadotropin-releasing hormone agonist.[683,684] A systematic review concluded that gonadotropin-releasing hormone agonist seemed to improve ovarian function and the ability to achieve pregnancy after chemotherapy.[685] Oocyte or ovarian tissue cryopreservation holds potential promise for the future. In male patients, sperm cryopreservation may be considered before cyclophosphamide treatment is instituted. Additional approaches include the use of testosterone.[686]

Cyclophosphamide is associated with an increased risk of malignancy in adults with rheumatoid arthritis, a risk that is dose related and increases with duration of follow-up. One case-control study showed a fourfold elevation of myeloproliferative disorders,[667] and there are increased risks of bladder and skin cancer.[688] The incidence of bladder cancer in adults with Wegener granulomatosis treated with cyclophosphamide is 5% at 10 years and 16% at 15 years; the incidence is related to total dose and duration of treatment. Nonglomerular hematuria identified a subgroup of patients at high risk for bladder cancer.[689]

Monthly intravenous cyclophosphamide is used commonly in patients with severe lupus nephritis (World Health Organization class IV) and other life-threatening complications of SLE. Because of the well-known toxicity of cyclophosphamide and the effectiveness of agents such as MMF and azathioprine in maintaining remission, it has been recommended that the duration of intravenous treatment be shortened to 3 months in some patients with lupus nephritis.[690]

Cyclophosphamide crosses the placenta and is teratogenic. It is contraindicated during pregnancy and during breastfeeding.[603]

Chlorambucil

Chlorambucil (Fig. 6–18 [online only]), similar to cyclophosphamide, is an alkylating agent that preferentially reduces B cell numbers, with less effect on memory T cells and natural killer cells, and acts by crosslinking macromolecules, interfering with several cellular functions. It is usually prescribed for oral administration at a dose of 0.1 to 0.2 mg/kg/day, but can be given intravenously as well. Because of serious toxicity, use of chlorambucil is reserved for very narrow indications, including uveitis.[691] The very high risk of malignancy, 7.5% in some cases,[692] precludes its use in all but the most severe cases. In addition to the risk of malignancy, male infertility is very common when total doses of 25 mg/kg are reached.[693] Thrombocytopenia and infection are also common.[691,694]

Cyclosporine, Tacrolimus, and Sirolimus

Cyclosporine (Fig. 6–19 [online only]), a cyclic peptide of fungal origin, has been shown to have profound effects on the immune system.[695] The observation that cyclosporine could virtually eliminate mitogen-induced proliferation by T cells, but had little effect on other cell types,[696] indicated the potential of this drug in the treatment of immunologically mediated disease. It has had a major impact on the prevention of solid organ transplant rejection. Cyclosporine is inactive until complexed with its intracellular receptor, cyclophilin. Tacrolimus, a macrolide antibiotic (formerly FK-506), binds to a set of cytoplasmic proteins—the FK-506 binding proteins, which are different from proteins bound by cyclosporine, with similar downstream immunomodulatory effects, converging on the calcium-dependent and calmodulin-dependent serine threonine protein phosphatase calcineurin.[697]

In the process of T or B cell activation, cell receptor signaling leads to a release of intracellular calcium, which binds to calmodulin, activating the protein serine/threonine phosphatase calcineurin.[698] When activated, calcineurin stimulates the translocation of nuclear factor of activated T cells, a transcription factor that is an important stimulus for IL-2 gene transcription[699] and cell-mediated immune responses.[696,700-702] The cyclosporine-cyclophilin (or tacrolimus–FK-506 binding protein) complex binds to calcineurin, inhibiting the early phase of T cell activation and IL-2 production. A related drug, sirolimus, binds to the FK binding protein 12 to form a complex that has no effect on calcineurin, but inhibits a key regulatory protein (the mammalian target of rapamycin) suppressing cytokine-driven T cell proliferation.[703]

Cyclosporine inhibits the production of IL-3, IL-4, IFN-γ,[704,705] and IL-15,[706,707] and it enhances the production of transforming growth factor-β_1 protein.[708] It is also antiangiogenic, as shown by the inhibition of vascular endothelial growth factor expression in several systems.[709,710]

Cyclosporine and tacrolimus may also result in immunosuppression by inhibiting degradation of I-κB.[711] In addition, they may modulate antiinflammatory effects by inhibiting monocyte production of tissue factor, a potential stimulus of the coagulation cascade via inhibition of NF-κB.[712] They may also result in apoptosis of T and B cells.[713]

Whether cyclosporine affects antigen presentation is uncertain. Some studies have shown that the drug has no effect on macrophage function in antigen presentation,[714] whereas others have suggested that the drug interferes with antigen presentation by dendritic cells[715] and Langerhans cells.[716]

Cyclosporine is incompletely and variably absorbed from the GI tract, bound principally to serum albumin and erythrocytes, metabolized by the liver, and excreted in the bile. The absorption of cyclosporine, but not tacrolimus, depends on bile salts. Cyclosporine has a half-life of approximately 18 hours; tacrolimus has a half-life of 9 hours. Mean half-life of sirolimus ranged from 26 to 40 hours.[717] A microemulsion formulation of cyclosporine has been developed to improve absorption and bioavailability;[718] this preparation has more consistent interpatient and intrapatient pharmacokinetics.

Cyclosporine crosses the placenta and is present in breast milk. Several significant drug interactions are associated with cyclosporine,[37] and considerable toxicity is associated with the use of this drug, including impaired renal function,[719,720] hypertension, hepatic toxicity,[721] tremor, mucous membrane lesions, and nausea and vomiting. Hypertrichosis, paresthesias, and gingival hyperplasia have been observed. Renal toxicity may result in hypertension from interstitial fibrosis or tubular atrophy, even in adults treated with relatively low dosages (3 to 5 mg/kg/day orally). Concomitant use of NSAIDs may exacerbate this toxic effect of the drug. Sirolimus pharmacokinetics display large interpatient and intrapatient variability, which may change in specific patient populations because of disease states or concurrent immunosuppressants or other interacting drugs, and monitoring of levels is required.[722]

Cyclosporine is effective in the treatment of rheumatoid arthritis alone[723] and in combination with MTX.[724,725] Several open trials have shown improvement in children with JRA,[725-729] JDM,[730] and uveitis.[731,732] Tacrolimus was reported to be beneficial in two patients with systemic-onset JIA.[733] Sirolimus has been found to be effective in murine models of lupus[734] and in one patient with dermatomyositis.[735] The addition of cyclosporine to MTX was associated with significant clinical improvement in 8 of 17 patients with JIA.[736] Side effects are common, however, and often necessitate reduction or discontinuation of treatment, particularly as a result of reduced renal function or hypertension.[728] Cyclosporine has been reported to have dramatic beneficial effects in patients with macrophage activation syndrome.[87,88] Patients with membranous lupus nephritis and patients with World Health Organization class III or IV lupus nephritis and heavy proteinuria[737] may benefit from cyclosporine treatment. These agents may be especially helpful as steroid-sparing agents.[738] Cyclosporine may also be effective in cases of Behçet disease with ocular involvement.[739] Despite concern, a case-control series[740] did not show any increased risk of malignancy over a 5-year follow-up period in adults treated with cyclosporine compared with controls.

Current guidelines for cyclosporine use are outlined in Table 6–20; these apply to tacrolimus as well. Factors that most commonly limit clinical use of cyclosporine are hypertension and an increase in serum creatinine of greater than 30% from baseline. Long-term renal damage can occur despite normal serum creatinine levels during the course of therapy.[718] In the rheumatic diseases, the goal has been to achieve a whole-blood trough level between 125 μg/mL and 175 μg/mL. Grapefruit juice increases cyclosporine and cyclosporine metabolite levels significantly.[741]

Small Molecules

MAPKs are part of a larger class of serine/threonine protein kinases that permit transduction of extracellular stress to the cell nucleus. They seem to be expressed in multiple cell types in response to stress, extracellular stimuli, shock, proinflammatory cytokines, and other triggers. Increased expression of MAPK p38 leads to increased production of IL-1, IL-6, TNF, nitric oxide, prostaglandins/prostacyclins, COX-2, and MMPs; MAPK p38 represents a potential target for therapy. The α-isoform of the enzyme is believed to be the most appropriate target because it seems to be the most important in inflammation.[742]

Many inhibitors are in various stages of development. Because these inhibitors are small molecules, they can be taken by mouth. The small molecule pamapimod was not as effective as MTX in one short-term study of adults with rheumatoid arthritis, and more infections occurred in the group treated with pamapimod.[743] Other p38 MAPK inhibitors studied in rheumatoid arthritis, Crohn disease, and psoriasis were found to be ineffective or to have unacceptable toxicity.[742] Many of the studies reported initial reduction of C-reactive protein levels with return to baseline by the second week of therapy. Enthusiasm is waning for this previously promising strategy in the treatment of chronic arthritis.

Tyrosine kinases also have a role in mediating inflammation. Three main tyrosine kinase families—Src, Tec, and Syk—are intimately involved in toll-like receptor signaling, the crucial first step in cellular recognition of invading pathogens and tissue damage. Their activity results in signaling regulating expression of proinflammatory and antiinflammatory cytokines.[744] The Syk kinases are important modulators of immune signaling in B cells and other cells bearing Fcγ receptors. R788 is a relatively selective inhibitor of Syk kinase and was studied in an ascending-dose, double-blind, placebo-controlled phase II trial.[745] The trial randomly assigned 189 patients to active drug or placebo. Doses of 100 mg and 150 mg twice daily were significantly superior to placebo or 50 mg twice daily at week 12. Serum IL-6 and MMP-3 levels also decreased. Dose-related diarrhea (45% with 150-mg dose) and neutropenia (15% overall) were the major adverse events. Syk kinase is a viable new target for the treatment of rheumatoid arthritis. Longer term studies are needed.

Table 6–20

Guidelines for use of cyclosporine

Dose
3-5 mg/kg/day orally

Clinical Monitoring
Blood pressure every week for first month, then monthly

Laboratory Monitoring
Renal function studies (BUN, creatinine, urinalysis) at start of therapy and every month

Hepatic enzymes, CBC with WBC count, differential, and platelet count every month

Maintain 12-hr whole-blood trough drug levels 125-175 ng/mL (RIA method)

Reduce dose if serum creatinine increases by ≥30%

BUN, blood urea nitrogen; CBC, complete blood count; RIA, radioimmunoassay; WBC, white blood count.

Other promising targets include the Janus kinases 1 and 2.[746,747] Much progress is likely to be made in the area of small molecules in the near future.

Antibiotics

The concept that rheumatoid arthritis was caused by microbial pathogens led to early use of antimicrobial therapy. Gold was first introduced as a treatment for rheumatoid arthritis for that reason. Sulfasalazine was synthesized to take advantage of its antimicrobial properties. More recently, antibiotics have again been considered in the treatment of inflammatory rheumatic disease.

Penicillin plays a key prophylactic role in preventing the recurrence of acute rheumatic fever and perhaps in preventing poststreptococcal arthritis.[748] Cutaneous polyarteritis nodosa, which may be a streptococcus-related disease, is also often treated with prophylactic penicillin.[749] In Wegener granulomatosis, treatment with trimethoprim-sulfamethoxazole may prevent disease relapses.[750]

Studies in rheumatoid arthritis have suggested a role for synthetic tetracycline antibiotics.[751] In early disease, minocycline was more effective than placebo[752] or hydroxychloroquine.[753] The mechanism of action may depend more on the biochemical than on the antimicrobial effect of these agents.[754] Antibiotics do not seem to be effective in enteric reactive arthritis, but they may have a role in urogenital reactive arthritis.[755] Although a small pilot study suggested that minocycline might be effective in systemic sclerosis,[756] a later study refuted those findings.[757]

Biological Therapies

Intravenous Immunoglobulin

Intravenous immunoglobulin (IVIG) is prepared from pooled human plasma. Its effectiveness in the treatment of Kawasaki disease[758] has encouraged its use in many other childhood rheumatic diseases including JDM[759-762] and systemic-onset JRA,[763] although placebo-controlled randomized trials did not show benefit in either systemic-onset or polyarticular-onset JRA.[764,765] There are also many anecdotal reports of improvements in patients with SLE, systemic vasculitides, and autoimmune neuropathies.[766] IVIG has a good safety record, but anaphylactoid reaction is a risk. Other potential side effects include myalgia, fever, and headache during the infusion and aseptic meningitis 24 to 48 hours afterward.[767] Current preparation protocols purify the product so that it is free from contamination with human immunodeficiency virus (HIV), hepatitis C virus, and other known viruses, but there is a risk of transmission of as-yet-unidentified pathogens. Guidelines for IVIG administration are presented in Table 6–21.

The mechanisms whereby IVIG exerts its therapeutic effect are unclear and may differ in different situations. Several reviews have addressed these issues in detail.[766,768-770] Potential mechanisms include (1) modulation of expression and function of Fc receptors; (2) inhibition of complement activation and function of the membrane attack complex; (3) inhibition of cytokine production and function; (4) generation of anti-idiotype antibodies, reducing the production of pathogenic autoantibodies; (5) regulation of cell growth; and (6) effects on the activation, differentiation, and effector functions of dendritic, T, and B cells.[771]

The action of IVIG may be mediated by specific antibodies that neutralize an as-yet-unknown causative agent, such as a virus. IVIG contains antiidiotype antibodies that may bind to the idiotype of an antibody involved in the pathogenesis of the disease.[772] Such antiidiotype antibodies have been shown to suppress autoimmune disease in animal models.[773] Antibodies to inflammatory mediators, including cytokines, may also have important therapeutic roles. The rapid defervescence that occurs after IVIG administration in Kawasaki disease suggests that ILs, particularly IL-1 and IL-6, are removed from the circulation or neutralized, or that their production is stopped by some constituent of the IVIG. Normal serum is known to contain antibodies to IL-1α,[774] IL-6,[775] TNF-α,[776] IFN-α2b, and IFN-γ.[777] Normalization of T cell number and function has also occurred after administration of IVIG.[778] IVIG can neutralize superantigens, which may be involved in Kawasaki disease.[779] Another mechanism of action whereby IVIG might exert its beneficial antiinflammatory effects is a reduction in the expression of adhesion molecules.

Specific Biological Agents

Elucidation of some basic mechanisms involved in inflammatory arthritis has resulted in an understanding of many of the cellular and molecular mechanisms that participate in inflammatory states. Specific biological agents have been developed that can target one or several steps involved in the immune response (Table 6–21). Strategies for intervention (adapted from Wallis and associates[780]) can be grouped as follows:

- Tolerance induction
- Inhibition of MHC, antigen, and T cell receptor interaction
- Inhibition of cellular function and cell-cell interaction
- Interference with cytokines
- Apoptosis

INDUCTION OF TOLERANCE

Autoreactive T cells that escape thymic deletion during ontogeny can be deleted by at least two peripheral mechanisms of tolerance.[781] If the T cells interact with antigen, but are not activated, T cell dormancy, or anergy, develops. If T helper type 2 cells have the same T cell receptor as the autoreactive clone, cytokines with an antiinflammatory profile are released and can suppress an antigen-specific T helper type 1 cell response. This is the principle behind attempts to achieve oral tolerance to an antigen. Reactive T helper type 2 cells can leave the gut and migrate to sites in which the antigen may be localized and are stimulated to release antiinflammatory cytokines, mediating local immunosuppression. Trials of oral administration of type II collagen have been attempted because of the high incidence of autoimmunity to type II collagen in adult rheumatoid arthritis (and in approximately 25% of children with JRA) and the success of this

Table 6–21

Summary of biologicals

Biological Agent	Molecule	Target	C/H; IV/SC	Indication/Other Use	Dose	Major Toxicity	Comments
Etanercept	TNFRII/FcIgG1	TNF-α, TNF-β	H; SC	RA, PsA, Ps, AS, JIA	0.8 mg/kg q wk, maximum 50 mg	rTB, rFungal, lymphoma, MS	With or without MTX
Adalimumab	mAb to TNF-α	TNF-α	H; SC	RA, PsA, Ps, AS, JIA, CD, UC/uveitis	15-30 mg/kg—20 mg q 2 wk; >30 mg/kg—40 mg q 2 wk	rTB, rFungal, lymphoma, MS	With or without MTX
Infliximab	mAb to TNF-α	TNF-α	C; IV	RA, PsA, Ps, AS, JIA, IBD/uveitis	6-10 mg/kg q 2 wk–2 mo	Infusion reactions, rTB, rFungal, lymphoma, MS	With MTX, premedicate with corticosteroid, acetaminophen, antihistamine
Golimumab	mAb to TNF-α	TNF-α	H; SC	RA, PsA, AS	50 mg q mo (adult dose)	rTB, rFungal, lymphoma, MS	With MTX
Certolizumab pegol	Pegylated mAb to TNF-α	TNF-α	H; SC	CD, RA	400 mg initially, wk 2 and 4, then 200 mg q 2 wk or 400 mg q 4 wk (adult doses)	rTB, rFungal, lymphoma, MS	With or without MTX
Anakinra	IL-1Ra	IL-1	H; SC	RA/sJIA	1 mg/kg, maximum 100 mg daily	Injection site reactions	Do not use with other biologicals
Rilonacept	IL-1R/IL-1AcP/IgG1	IL-1	H; SC	CAPS/sJIA	4.4 mg/kg (maximum 320 mg) loading dose, then 2.2 mg/kg q wk (maximum 160 mg)	Injection site reactions	Do not use with other biologicals
Canakinumab	mAb to IL-1	IL-1	H; SC	CAPS/sJIA	150 mg q 8 wk (adult dose)	Injection site reactions	Do not use with other biologicals, studies underway in sJIA
Abatacept	CTLA4-Ig	CD80/86	H; IV	RA/JIA	<75 kg—10 mg/kg wk 0, 2, 4, then q 4 wk; 75-100 kg—750 mg; >100 kg—1000 mg	Injection site reactions	Do not use with other biologicals
Rituximab	mAb to CD20	B cells	C; IV	RA/RF + JIA	375-500 mg/m² IV q wk × 2 doses up to 1g adult dose 1gIVq wk × 2doses	Infusion reactions, progressive multifocal encephalopathy	With MTX, premedicate with glucocorticoid, acetaminophen, antihistamine
Tocilizumab	mAb to IL-6R	IL-6	IV		8 mg/kg/dose q 2 weeks, if <30kg 12 mg/kg/dose	Infusion reactions, cytopenia, increased liver transaminases, hypercholesterolemia	Can be given with methotrexate

AS, ankylosing spondylitis; C, chimeric; CAPS, cryopyrin-associated periodic syndrome; CD, Crohn Disease; H, humanized; IBD, inflammatory bowel disease; IV, intravenous infusion; JIA, juvenile idiopathic arthritis, polyarticular course; mAb, monoclonal antibody; MTX, methotrexate; Ps, psoriasis; PsA, psoriatic arthritis; RA, rheumatoid arthritis; RF, rheumatoid factor; rFungal, reactivated fungal infection; rTB, reactivated tuberculosis; SC, subcutaneous injection; sJIA, systemic-onset JIA; UC, ulcerative colitis.

approach in various animal models of arthritis in which type II collagen autoimmunity occurred.[782] Studies in humans have shown varying results, but results seem to be better when lower doses of collagen are administered.[783] In an open trial involving 10 patients with JRA who were treated with type II chick collagen, 8 responded; no adverse effects were observed.[784] With the advances that have occurred with other therapies, there have been no further studies in this area.

LJP-394 (Abetimus). LJP-394 (abetimus sodium) is a molecule consisting of double-stranded DNA (ds-DNA) epitopes that crosslink anti–ds-DNA antibodies in solution or on cell surfaces. In rodents, LJP-394 seems to induce B cell tolerance by crosslinking anti–ds-DNA surface immunoglobulin receptors on B cells, leading to B cell anergy or apoptosis. Five prospective clinical studies in patients with SLE have shown that abetimus can reduce circulating anti–ds-DNA antibody levels without causing generalized immunosuppression.[785,786]

A randomized, double-blind, placebo-controlled trial was performed to examine whether abetimus prevents or delays renal flares in patients with SLE and previous renal disease.[787] Although the number of renal flares and the time of flares did not differ between the two groups, the time to institute "aggressive treatment" with corticosteroid or cyclophosphamide (or both) was longer, and the number of aggressive treatment courses were fewer in the abetimus group. Because there was a significant reduction in the titer of anti–ds-DNA antibodies and a concomitant, although not significant, increase in the serum complement levels especially in patients with high-affinity anti–ds-DNA antibodies, a second randomized, placebo-controlled study in patients with high-affinity antibodies for the oligonucleotide epitope did not show efficacy.[788]

INHIBITION OF MAJOR HISTOCOMPATIBILITY COMPLEX, ANTIGEN, AND T CELL RECEPTOR INTERACTION

The immune response is driven by the processing and presenting of an antigenic peptide by an antigen-presenting cell to a specific T cell receptor in the context of a specific MHC molecule. Any component of this trimolecular complex could theoretically be targeted for biological modulation. If the initiating antigen were known, an immunization program could be developed to prevent disease, and this is the principle behind oral tolerance (see earlier discussion). T cell receptor vaccines may be one way to prevent or reduce activity of synovial inflammation, as shown in animal models. This strategy would work only if specific variable region (V_β) subtypes could be shown to predominate in synovitis and did not change over time. Early studies in patients with rheumatoid arthritis who were vaccinated with several V_β subtypes show promise and are continuing.[789] Progress has been made using this approach in experimental allergic encephalomyelitis and multiple sclerosis.[790] Data in children with JRA and spondyloarthropathies suggest that this approach may have some merit.[791] Another possible route of attack is to block the MHC site by anti-MHC antibodies.

INHIBITION OF CELLULAR FUNCTION AND CELL-CELL INTERACTION

T cells play a central role in initiating the rheumatoid process in adult disease and in JRA, but their role in continuing to drive the inflammatory process is less clear. Results of early studies using monoclonal T cell–depleting antibodies were disappointing. Initial clinical improvements, if they occurred at all, were short-lived or were associated with profound lymphopenia, precluding further treatment.[792,793] These included studies with anti-CD7 monoclonal antibodies (mAbs); CD-5 plus (immunotoxin composed of murine anti-CD5 mAbs conjugated to the toxin ricin);[794] alemtuzumab (Campath) (humanized α-CDw52 mAb);[795,796] and cM-T412, an anti-CD4 mAb.[797,798]

Possible explanations for the lack of efficacy in these studies are that T cells are not crucial for the perpetuation of synovitis; that the specific T cells targeted by mAbs are not the ones involved in synovitis; that targets are too nonspecific; and that synovial T cells are not affected, even though peripheral T cells may be.[799] One placebo-controlled trial in adults with rheumatoid arthritis treated with nondepleting anti-CD4 mAbs showed some efficacy, but unacceptable CD4 lymphopenia and rash precluded further study.[800] Generation of the immune response involves not only antigen processing and T cell receptor and MHC interactions, but also interactions between molecules expressed on the surface of T cells and on antigen-presenting cells and various adhesion molecules and their companion receptors.

CTLA-4Ig (Abatacept). To activate resting T cells, two molecular signals are required: (1) the interaction of the T cell receptor with processed peptide, presented in the appropriate MHC setting, and (2) interaction of CD28 on T cells with CD80/86 on the surface of the antigen-presenting cell. There is another high-affinity receptor, cytotoxic T lymphocyte–associated antigen-4 (CTLA-4), which can also bind to CD80/86, with a higher avidity than CD28, preventing the second signal required for T cell activation. Abatacept is a fully human, soluble fusion protein composed of the extracellular domain of CTLA-4 and the Fc component of IgG1 selectively inhibiting a costimulatory signal necessary for full T cell activation.[801] By binding to CD28, it can prevent T cell activation. Initial studies in adults with rheumatoid arthritis showed improvement compared with placebo alone[802] and when used together with MTX compared with MTX alone in patients who had an inadequate response to MTX.[803,804]

In an international, multicenter prospective study of 190 subjects with polyarticular-course JIA using a design similar to ones used in the pivotal etanercept and adalimumab trials in JIA, response rates in the open-label phase were 76% in biological-naïve subjects and 39% in subjects who received prior biological therapy. Response rates were similar among all of the subtypes of JIA. In the double-blind withdrawal phase, flares of arthritis occurred in 33 of 62 (53%) patients who were given placebo and 12 of 60 (20%) patients given abatacept (P = .0003). Adverse events were recorded in 37 abatacept recipients (62%) and 34 (55%) placebo recipients (P = .47); there were no serious adverse events in the abatacept group. Abatacept was shown to be effective and generally well tolerated in this trial. It is the first agent to show efficacy in a prospective clinical trial of numerous JIA subjects who had failed previous biological therapy. Although it is difficult to compare results of separate trials, it seems that abatacept is effective, although maximal effect may be achieved a few weeks later, compared with anti-TNF agents.[805] Abatacept is approved by the FDA for use in polyarticular JIA. Guidelines for its use in children are presented in Table 6–22.

Rituximab. Rituximab is a chimeric monoclonal mouse-human antibody that is reactive with the B cell CD20 receptor, which is present on pre-B and mature B cells, but not on stem cells or plasma cells.[806] It is effective in the treatment of relapsed Hodgkin B cell lymphoma. Rituximab exerts its effect by removing B cells from the circulation by antibody-dependent and complement-dependent cellular cytotoxicity and by the induction of apoptosis of B cells. Although the antibody-producing plasma cells are not removed from the circulation, B cells that may act as antigen-presenting cells produce cytokines, and infiltrate tissues are removed for a prolonged period. Memory B cells, which are also responsible for antibody production, may be removed as well.

Rituximab is theoretically beneficial in diseases in which autoantibodies may be pathogenetically important. This was observed first in patients with idiopathic thrombocytopenic purpura[807] and more recently in various other autoimmune diseases. In lymphoma, the usual dose is 375 mg/m^2 administered weekly for four infusions; B cells are reduced dramatically for 6 to 9 months. Alternative dosing in rheumatoid arthritis is 1000 mg intravenously in two doses 2 weeks apart. Rituximab induced a profound depletion of all peripheral blood B

cell populations in patients with rheumatoid arthritis. Repopulation occurred mainly with naïve mature and immature B cells. Patients whose rheumatoid arthritis relapsed on return of B cells tended to show repopulation with higher numbers of memory B cells.[808] Although disease manifestations may return later, coincident with the reappearance of B cells, baseline medications may be tapered during this period.

In a multicenter, randomized, double-blind, placebo-controlled phase III trial in adults with rheumatoid arthritis, a single course of rituximab (two infusions of 1000 mg intravenously each, given 2 weeks apart) with concomitant MTX therapy provided clinically meaningful improvements in disease activity in patients with active, long-standing rheumatoid arthritis who had an inadequate response to one or more anti-TNF therapies.[809] There are many reports of small numbers of adults with dermatomyositis who seem to have responded to rituximab infusions.[810-816] Rituximab is also effective in selected cases of treatment-refractory antineutrophil cytoplasmic autoantibody–associated vasculitis.[817]

Recommendations for use of rituximab in children are presented in Table 6–23; these are based primarily on adult data. Only a limited amount of information about use of rituximab in children is available. Binstadt and colleagues[818] reported on a series of four children with undiagnosed autoimmune illnesses who received rituximab treatment after failure of multiple other agents noting improvement in their neurological manifestations. Nadirs of IgG levels were seen at 4 to 6 months, and three of the four patients required immunoglobulin replacement therapy.

Leandro and associates[819] reported on improvement in five of six patients with SLE treated with a combination of two rituximab infusions of 500 mg, two infusions of 750 mg of cyclophosphamide, and high-dose oral

---

Table 6–22

Guidelines for use of abatacept in the treatment of juvenile idiopathic arthritis

Dose

10 mg/kg for patient's <75 kg (100 mg maximum); 75-100 kg - 75 mg, >100 kg - 1000 mg administered intravenously over ½ hr on weeks 0, 2, 4 then every 4 week.

No premedication is necessary.

Can be given with or without methotrexate intravenously over 30 min on week 0, 2, 4 then every 4 week.

Clinical Monitoring

Document absence of latent or active tuberculosis before starting

Improvement should be seen by the third to fourth dose, but may be delayed

Monitor every 1-2 mo initially, then every 3-6 mo, depending on course

Hold if suspected bacterial infection or varicella

Laboratory Monitoring

CBC with WBC count, differential, and platelet count; AST, ALT, albumin every 4-12 wk

ALT, alanine aminotransferase; AST, aspartate aminotransferase; CBC, complete blood count; WBC, white blood cell.

Table 6–23

Guidelines for use of rituximab

Dose

375-500 mg/m^2 (maximum 1000 mg) intravenously on weeks 0, 2 at 50 mg/hr initially*

If no infusion reaction occurs, escalate dose at 50-mg/hr increments every 30 min to maximum of 400 mg/hr. If first infusion was tolerated well, subsequent infusions can be given over a shorter time with an initial rate of 100 mg/hr and 100-mg/hr increments every 30 min

Premedicate with methylprednisolone 100 mg intravenously 30 min before infusion

Clinical Monitoring

Improvement should be seen within 1 mo of initial infusion

Monitor every 1-2 mo initially, then every 3 mo depending on course

Laboratory Monitoring

Check B cell numbers before and 1 mo after infusion

Quantitative immunoglobulins every 3 mo

*El-Hallak M, Binstadt BA, Leichtner AM, et al. Clinical effects and safety of rituximab for treatment of refractory pediatric autoimmune disease. J Pediatr 2007, 150: 376-82.

corticosteroids. In another study, 11 girls with severe SLE, including 8 girls with class IV or V lupus nephritis, 2 girls with severe autoimmune cytopenia, and 1 girl with antiprothrombin antibody with severe hemorrhage, were treated with 2 to 12 intravenous infusions of rituximab (350 to 450 mg/m²/infusion), with corticosteroids. Depletion of B cells paralleled remission in seven of eight patients. Severe adverse events were seen including two patients with septicemia and four patients with severe hematological toxicity. The authors concluded that rituximab was effective, but were very concerned about the incidence of severe adverse events.[820] Improvement in clinical activity scores, ds-DNA antibodies, renal function, and proteinuria occurred in 18 patients with SLE treated with rituximab, but some patients required repeated courses, and one died of endocarditis.[821]

Side effects are rare and include flushing and itching, usually with the first dose. These manifestations are probably allergic in nature and may be alleviated with pretreatment with an antihistamine and corticosteroids. Reduced levels of immunoglobulins for prolonged periods seemed to be more common and significant in children than in adults and may require immunoglobulin replacement therapy. Of patients, 33% may develop antichimeric antibodies after treatment, and these antibodies are associated with lower serum levels of rituximab at 2 months and less effective B cell depletion.[822] Patients must be observed closely for development of viral infections because infections with parvovirus, varicella-zoster virus, cytomegalovirus, and enterovirus have been reported to develop after rituximab therapy.

After two patients with progressive multifocal leukoencephalopathy after treatment with rituximab were reported, a systematic review identified 52 patients with underlying lymphoproliferative disorders, who developed progressive multifocal leukoencephalopathy after treatment with rituximab and other agents (2 patients with SLE, 1 patient with rheumatoid arthritis, 1 patient with an idiopathic autoimmune pancytopenia, and 1 patient with immune thrombocytopenia). Other treatments included hematopoietic stem cell transplantation (7 patients), purine analogues (26 patients), or alkylating agents (39 patients). One patient with an autoimmune hemolytic anemia developed progressive multifocal leukoencephalopathy after treatment with corticosteroids and rituximab, and one patient with an autoimmune pancytopenia developed progressive multifocal leukoencephalopathy after treatment with corticosteroids, azathioprine, and rituximab. Median time from last rituximab dose to progressive multifocal leukoencephalopathy diagnosis was 5.5 months.[823] These data tend to implicate the other treatments as the cause of progressive multifocal leukoencephalopathy, rather than rituximab alone, but further study is necessary.

Belimumab. Belimumab is a human neutralizing mAb against B lymphocyte–stimulating factor (also known as B lymphocyte stimulator (BLyS).[824] BLyS, a member of the TNF ligand superfamily, is synthesized as a 285-amino acid type II membrane protein and exists in membrane and cleaved 152-amino acid soluble forms. Expressed on monocytes, macrophages, and monocyte-derived dendritic cells, BLyS is upregulated in response to IFN-γ and IL-10, enhancing B cell proliferation and immunoglobulin secretion. Belimumab binds with high affinity to BLyS and inhibits binding of BLyS to its three receptors, inhibiting BLyS-induced proliferations of B cells. BLyS seems to be involved in the pathogenesis of B cell–mediated autoimmune diseases.[825] Relative safety and improvement in anti–ds-DNA antibody titers were shown in select SLE patients.[826,827]

INTERFERENCE WITH CYTOKINES

The biological effects of T cell–derived and monocyte-derived cytokines can explain much of the clinical syndrome of synovitis and the systemic manifestations associated with JRA.[828-830] Cytokines are crucial in perpetuating and damping the immune response, and they are important targets for therapeutic manipulation.

A great deal of evidence supports the role of TNF-α in the initiation and perpetuation of the rheumatoid process. Children with JRA have high levels of TNF-α in the synovial fluid and peripheral circulation.[828,831] Studies in adults have shown that high levels of TNF-α in synovial fluid are associated with bone erosions. Animal studies and early studies in adults showed convincingly that blocking TNF improved symptoms of inflammatory arthritis. Subsequent studies showed that these agents may be dramatically beneficial, not only in reducing disease activity, but also in improving function and slowing, and perhaps reversing, structural damage. Anti-TNF agents currently in use or under study in children are etanercept, infliximab, and adalimumab.

Etanercept. Etanercept is a fully human, dimeric protein containing the extracellular domain of the human p75 TNF receptor fused to the Fc region of human IgG₁ (Fig. 6–20 [online only]). It is produced with the use of recombinant DNA technology. By binding to TNF-α in the circulation, etanercept prevents the interaction of TNF-α with its cell surface receptor, preventing cell activation and perpetuation of the inflammatory cascade. It can also modulate biological responses that are mediated by TNF, such as expression of adhesion molecules, serum concentration of MMPs, and cytokines.[831] Although soluble forms of the TNF-α receptor occur naturally, they are generally inadequate to block TNF activity in systemic inflammatory disorders. The dimeric form of the TNF-α receptor is much more efficient at binding TNF because it binds at a much greater affinity (50 to 1000 times higher) than that of the naturally occurring form. Etanercept also binds lymphotoxin (formerly TNF-β).[832] When administered subcutaneously, its half-life is approximately 4 days. In adults with rheumatoid arthritis, steady-state concentrations are achieved in about 2 weeks.[831]

Etanercept has been used extensively in children with JRA since the initial report of its effectiveness in 2000.[833] It is currently indicated for children who have had an inadequate response to MTX or who have not tolerated it and still have polyarticular disease. The initial study by Lovell and colleagues,[833] a large case series report by Quartier and coworkers,[834] open-label studies,[835-837] and observational registries[834,838] suggest that approximately 70% of children have an initial response to etanercept.

The response is usually dramatic, occurs by the third or fourth injection, and is associated with a dramatic reduction in active joint count and markers of inflammation.

A French study reported that only 39% of patients had a sustained improvement of 30% or more by 12 months.[834] In a large study of nearly 600 subjects, sustained improvement and relative safety were shown over 3 years.[839] Continuous use for 8 years also seems to be safe.[840] The results in children with systemic-onset JRA do not seem to be nearly as promising.[841-844] Improvements in physical function,[845] quality of life,[846] and growth;[847,848] slowing of radiographic progression;[849,850] and cost-effectiveness[851] have been shown. Long-term continuous treatment for 10 years seems to be safe with little evidence of tachyphylaxis.[840,852,853] Guidelines for use of etanercept are shown in Table 6–24.

To date, etanercept has been very well tolerated. A placebo-controlled study showed an increase in symptoms of upper respiratory tract infection and injection site reactions, although these were generally mild[854] and may be treated with topical corticosteroids. Postmarketing studies have reported a variety of unusual side effects, however; most importantly, patients must be closely monitored for systemic infection. This includes bacterial infection, viral infection such as varicella with or without superimposed bacterial infection, and granulomatous infection. Although these are more common in elderly patients, physicians must be attuned to their development in any age group. Two patients in the pivotal trial developed aseptic meningitis secondary to varicella zoster, prompting the recommendation that patients with JIA, if possible, be brought up-to-date with all immunizations in agreement with current immunization guidelines before starting etanercept. Patients with a significant exposure to varicella virus should temporarily discontinue etanercept and be considered for prophylaxis with varicella zoster immune globulin. Live virus vaccination is contraindicated, but concurrent MTX and etanercept did not seem to decrease the rate of seroconversion to MMR vaccination.[855]

Various other side effects have been noted. Although rare enough to be the subject of case reports, there does seem to be an association between treatment with etanercept and the development of vasculitic skin rash[856] and systemic[857] or drug-induced lupus.[858] The associations with pancytopenia and aplastic anemia are less clear.[859] One case of diabetes mellitus after etanercept treatment was reported in a child with JRA.[860] Changes in mood and weight gain have also been noted.[834] Autoimmune hepatitis,[861] thymic enlargement,[862] sterile cholecystitis,[863] tuberculous uveitis,[864] and macrophage activation syndrome[865] have been reported in association with etanercept treatment.

There are conflicting data regarding whether etanercept is effective in the treatment of JIA-associated or idiopathic uveitis.[866-873] mAbs to TNF seem to be more effective (see later) than etanercept for the treatment of uveitis.

Infliximab. Infliximab is a chimeric IgG_1 anti–TNF-α antibody consisting of a mouse antibody and the constant region of the human antibody.[874] It was the first anti-TNF agent that was shown to be effective in patients with rheumatoid arthritis[875,876] and is effective in patients with Crohn Disease. In contrast to etanercept, it binds not only to soluble TNF-α, but also to membrane-bound TNF-α, leading to antibody-dependent and complement-dependent cytotoxicity. It seems to be more efficacious in granulomatous inflammatory disorders (e.g., sarcoidosis), but also seems to be associated with more risk of development of granulomatous opportunistic infections (see later discussion).

Administration of infliximab is via the intravenous route (Table 6–25). Dose and frequency vary with the clinical response. Initial doses in adults usually start at

---

Table 6–24

Guidelines for use of etanercept in the treatment of juvenile idiopathic arthritis

Dose

0.4 mg/kg twice weekly or 0.8 mg/kg/wk subcutaneously
Maximum 50 mg/wk

Clinical Monitoring

Document absence of latent or active tuberculosis before starting
Improvement should be seen by the third or fourth dose
Monitor every 1-2 mo initially, then every 3-6 mo depending on course
Hold if suspected bacterial infection or varicella

Laboratory Monitoring

CBC with WBC count, differential, and platelet count; AST, ALT, albumin every 4-12 wk

ALT, alanine aminotransferase; AST, aspartate aminotransferase; CBC, complete blood count; WBC, white blood cell.

Table 6–25

Guidelines for use of infliximab in the treatment of juvenile idiopathic arthritis

Dose

6-10 mg/kg infusion over approximately 2 hr on wk 0, 2, 6, then every 4-8 wk thereafter, depending on course; dose may be increased up to 10 mg/kg
Start at 10 mL/hr for 15 min, double rate every 15 min until 160 mL/hr for 30 min, then 250 mL/hr until finished
Consider premedication with diphenhydramine, acetaminophen

Clinical Monitoring

Document absence of latent or active tuberculosis before starting
Improvement should be seen by the third or fourth dose
Monitor every 1-2 mo initially, then every 3-6 mo depending on course
Hold if suspected bacterial infection, varicella, or hepatitis B infection

Laboratory Monitoring

CBC with WBC count, differential, and platelet count; AST, ALT, albumin every 4-12 wk

ALT, alanine aminotransferase; AST, aspartate aminotransferase; CBC, complete blood count; WBC, white blood cell.

3 mg/kg and are given at time 0, at 2 weeks, at 6 weeks, and then every 8 weeks depending on clinical response. Doses often require escalation, and doses of 20 mg/kg have been used occasionally in children.[877] Alternatively, the length of time between infusions can be shortened. Administration with MTX is recommended to prevent the development of antiinfliximab antibodies, which seem to correlate with infusion reactions and accelerated clearance of infliximab.[874] It is uncertain, however, that these antibodies actually reduce the effectiveness. Similar to etanercept, combination treatment with MTX seems to improve the response to infliximab in patients with rheumatoid arthritis.[878]

Improvement in signs and symptoms, quality of life, and physical function and prevention of progression of radiological damage in adult rheumatoid arthritis has been shown.[878,880] Infliximab may improve the radiological status without improving the clinical status of disease.[879,880]

Infliximab has been shown to be effective in adults with ankylosing spondylitis,[881] with improvement in work productivity and workday loss,[880] improvement in MRI evidence of spinal inflammation,[882,883] and preliminary evidence of slowing of progression on plain radiograph.[882] A larger study failed to show an effect on radiographic progression in ankylosing spondylitis.[883] Almost all patients relapsed (mean time to relapse 17.5 weeks) after discontinuation.[882]

Infliximab has been found to improve arthritis, psoriasis, dactylitis, and enthesitis in adults with psoriatic arthritis that had been resistant to DMARD therapy,[883,884] with associated improvement in physical function and quality of life,[886] work productivity, and workday loss.[886] Prevention of radiographic progression has been shown as well.[886,887]

Ruperto and Lovell[888] reported the results of a randomized, double-blind, placebo-controlled trial of infliximab in polyarticular-course JRA. The clearance of the drug was more rapid in children with JRA than was observed in adults with rheumatoid arthritis, resulting in lower trough levels before the next dose. Infliximab was generally well tolerated, but the safety profile of 3 mg/kg of infliximab seemed less favorable than 6 mg/kg of infliximab, with more frequent occurrences of serious adverse events, infusion reactions, antibodies to infliximab, and newly induced antinuclear antibodies and antibodies to ds-DNA observed with the 3 mg/kg dose, perhaps related to the lower trough levels in the 3 mg/kg group.[889]

Treatment with infliximab reduced the serum concentrations of IL-6, myeloperoxidase, and soluble adhesion molecules intercellular adhesion molecule-1 and E-selectin. TNF-α levels tended to increase, whereas the concentrations of endogenous TNF antagonists (soluble TNF receptor type I and soluble TNF receptor type II) were reduced.[890] There is accumulating (uncontrolled) evidence that infliximab is effective in the treatment of idiopathic and JIA-related acute and chronic uveitis.[869,891-893]

Infection remains the major concern with the use of infliximab. Many more cases of tuberculosis have been reported in patients treated with infliximab than in patients treated with etanercept, probably because of the destabilization of previously formed granulomas.[894]

Other infections that have occurred with greater than expected frequency include histoplasmosis, coccidioidomycosis, and listeriosis.[874] One case of optic neuritis has been reported in a child.[895] IgA and IgM anti–ds-DNA antibodies can occur with infliximab therapy,[896] but only 1 in 156 patients with antibodies developed a clinical syndrome of SLE.[897] In addition to the side effects noted with etanercept, infusion reactions ranging from mild allergic reactions to anaphylactic reactions may occur, more commonly on the second or third infusions. Infliximab must be administered under close observation. In addition to treatment of JRA, infliximab may be beneficial in other autoimmune diseases, including vasculitis,[898] Kawasaki disease,[899] sarcoidosis,[900,901] uveitis,[902] SAPHO (synovitis, acne, pustulosis, hyperostosis, osteitis) syndrome,[903] chronic recurrent multifocal osteomyelitis,[904] Blau syndrome,[905] and Behçet disease.[906]

Golimumab. Golimumab is a recombinant human IgG mAb to TNF-α. The constant regions of the heavy and light chains of this mAb are identical in amino acid sequence to the corresponding constant regions of the human-mouse chimeric mAb infliximab. In contrast to infliximab, the heavy and light variable regions are of human sequence. The recommended dosage is 50 mg subcutaneously once a month in combination with MTX. The FDA approved golimumab in 2009 for the treatment of moderately to severely active adult rheumatoid arthritis, active psoriatic arthritis, and active ankylosing spondylitis.[907,908] The median half-life increased with intravenous dose from 6.6 days in a group given 0.1 mg/kg to 19.3 days in a group given 10 mg/kg.[909]

In the pivotal trial, subjects were randomly assigned into four groups: MTX plus placebo, golimumab 100 mg plus placebo, golimumab 50 mg plus MTX, or golimumab 100 mg plus MTX.[907] Serious adverse events occurred in 2.3%, 3.8%, 5.6%, and 9%. Serious infections occurred in 0.8%, 0.8%, 2.2%, and 5.6%. One patient died after developing nausea, diarrhea, ileus, aspiration pneumonia, and sepsis. The most frequent adverse events were infection and injection site reaction. Antinuclear antibodies were observed in 12.2% of groups 3 and 4 combined and in 14.9% of group 1, but the group 2 rate was significantly higher (29.3%), perhaps related to the higher dose of golimumab or the absence of MTX. Antibodies to golimumab were observed in 2.1% of the subjects and were not significantly associated with decreased efficacy or injection site reaction. There are no published pediatric data to date.

Adalimumab. Adalimumab is a recombinant human IgG$_1$ mAb that acts in a similar fashion to infliximab and golimumab by binding to TNF within the circulation and on the cell surface.[910] It may result in cell lysis in the presence of complement. Adalimumab is administered subcutaneously with a half-life of approximately 2 weeks. Recommended dosing in adults is 40 mg every second week. As with other anti-TNF agents, the results are seen quickly, but the dose may need to be given once a week for sustained improvement. Injection site reactions can be problematic. In trials in adults with rheumatoid arthritis, adalimumab was shown to be more effective than MTX, in terms of disease activity, function-related and health-related quality of life, and ability to limit structural damage.[910] Adalimumab can be added safely to MTX with increased efficacy.[911] Adalimumab has been found to be effective in adults with psoriatic arthritis[913] and for the spinal and sacroiliac manifestations of ankylosing spondylitis.[914-916]

A pivotal study resulted in FDA approval for polyarticular JIA and provided the evidence for recommended usage (Table 6–26). In a randomized, double-blind, placebo-controlled withdrawal study, 171 patients with active polyarticular-course JRA underwent stratification according to MTX use and received 24 mg/m^2 of adalimumab (maximum dose 40 mg) subcutaneously every other week for 16 weeks.[917] Serious adverse events possibly related to adalimumab occurred in 14 patients; 7 were serious infections (bronchopneumonia, herpes simplex virus infection, pharyngitis, pneumonia, viral infection, and two cases of herpes zoster). Treatment was discontinued in 12 patients because of adverse events. No deaths, malignant conditions, opportunistic infections, tuberculosis, demyelinating diseases, or lupuslike reactions occurred. Of patients, 16% had at least one positive test for antiadalimumab antibodies (6% on MTX; 26% not on MTX). Development of antiadalimumab antibodies did not affect incidence of serious adverse events.

There are some preliminary data to suggest that adalimumab is effective in uveitis.[918] Patients with improved activity were younger and had shorter disease duration.[919]

Certolizumab Pegol. Certolizumab pegol is a pegylated humanized F(ab′)$_2$ fragment of an anti–TNF-α mAb that binds TNF-α. Pegylation increases its half-life. It has a higher affinity for TNF-α; is devoid of the Fc portion of the antibody; and does not induce complement activation, antibody-dependent cellular cytotoxicity, or apoptosis.[920] The efficacy and safety of certolizumab pegol in active rheumatoid arthritis has been assessed in three phase III, multicenter, randomized, double-blind, placebo-controlled clinical trials.[921-923] In the most recent study of 619 subjects, certolizumab pegol plus MTX was more efficacious than placebo plus MTX, rapidly and significantly improving signs and symptoms of rheumatoid arthritis, improving physical function, and slowing radiographic progression. The dose was 200 mg or 400 mg subcutaneously every 2 weeks. Five patients developed tuberculosis.

Common Issues with Anti–Tumor Necrosis Factor Agents. With increasing use of anti-TNF agents, many common concerns have arisen, one of which is the increased risk of infection, particularly tuberculosis and fungal infections, including histoplasmosis.[924-927] Before starting treatment with any of these agents, the following approach is recommended. Patients should be screened for the presence of latent tuberculosis with a tuberculosis skin test. A chest radiograph is probably unnecessary unless the PPD result is positive. If the skin test is positive, a thorough investigation of the patient and family for active tuberculosis must be undertaken, and the patient must receive appropriate treatment. If the investigations are negative, the patient should be given isoniazid (INH) for 9 months. Treatment with anti-TNF agents may be initiated 1 month after starting isoniazid.[928]

The FDA advises close monitoring of patients for signs and symptoms of potential fungal infection, especially in endemic areas, during and after treatment with anti-TNF drugs. Patients in whom fever, malaise, weight loss, sweats, cough, dyspnea, pulmonary infiltrates on chest radiographs, or serious systemic illness develops should undergo a complete diagnostic workup appropriate for immunocompromised patients. If possible, the decision to initiate empirical antifungal therapy in at-risk symptomatic patients should be made in conjunction with an infectious diseases specialist, taking into account the risk for severe infection and the risks of antifungal therapy. TNF inhibitors should be withheld for serious infection or sepsis. Anti-TNF treatment should not be used in patients with active infection and should be discontinued in the case of a serious infection. Mild upper respiratory tract infections are not a reason to stop anti-TNF agents.

Concern remains regarding the development of malignancy, particularly lymphoma.[927] Patients must be observed closely for the occurrence of malignancies. Any association is difficult to decipher, however, because of the known increased incidence of malignancy in patients with rheumatoid arthritis.[859] Using the Swedish Biologic Registry of 6604 patients with rheumatoid arthritis treated with anti-TNF agents, 26 malignant lymphomas were observed during 26,981 person-years of follow-up, which corresponded to a relative risk of 1.35 (95% CI 0.82 to 2.11) compared with patients with rheumatoid arthritis who did not receive anti-TNF agents (336 lymphomas during 365,026 person-years), and 2.72 (95% CI 1.82 to 4.08) versus the general population comparator (1568 lymphomas during 3,355,849 person-years).[929] The FDA is particularly concerned that postmarketing cases of aggressive and fatal hepatosplenic T cell lymphomas, a rare type of T cell lymphoma, have been reported in patients receiving anti-TNF agents. Most

---

Table 6–26

Guidelines for use of adalimumab in the treatment of juvenile idiopathic arthritis

Dose
15-30 kg: 20 mg subcutaneously every 2nd wk
>30 kg: 40 mg subcutaneously every 2nd wk
Can be given with or without methotrexate

Clinical Monitoring
Document absence of latent or active tuberculosis before starting
Improvement should be seen by the second or third dose
Monitor every 1-2 mo initially, then every 3-6 mo depending on course
Hold if suspected bacterial infection, varicella exposure or infection, hepatitis B virus infection

Laboratory Monitoring
CBC with WBC count, differential, and platelet count; AST, ALT, albumin every 4-12 wk

ALT, alanine aminotransferase; AST, aspartate aminotransferase; CBC, complete blood count; WBC, white blood cell.

cases occurred in patients receiving infliximab for Crohn disease or ulcerative colitis who had received concomitant treatment with azathioprine or mercaptopurine; most involved adolescent boys and young men.

The FDA analyzed information from manufacturers of TNF inhibitors approved for use in children (etanercept, infliximab, adalimumab).[930] The FDA investigators identified 48 cases of malignancies in children and adolescents. They estimated that 14,837 children received infliximab, 9200 received etanercept, and 2636 received adalimumab during the studied period. Approximately half of the malignancies were lymphomas. Others included leukemia, melanoma, and solid organ cancers. Of the 48 cases, there were 11 deaths (including 9 from hepatosplenic T cell lymphoma and 1 from T cell lymphoma). The FDA noted that the reported rates for malignancy were higher with infliximab than expected rates, but acknowledged that the primary use of infliximab was for inflammatory bowel disease, as opposed to etanercept, the primary use of which was for JIA. The FDA investigators also noted that 88% of cases were in patients taking other immunosuppressive medications, such as azathioprine, mercaptopurine, and MTX. The FDA concluded there is an increased risk of malignancy with TNF inhibitor exposure, but could not characterize the strength of the association or definitively assign a causal relationship.

Similar concerns exist for the development of demyelinating syndromes, especially multiple sclerosis, with anti-TNF therapy. Early postmarketing studies suggested that demyelinating syndromes, including multiple sclerosis, might be more common in patients treated with etanercept. Another TNF antagonist, lenercept, is used to treat patients with multiple sclerosis, and patients taking active drugs had exacerbations.[931] Patients with JRA have developed demyelinating syndromes, as have adults with rheumatoid arthritis.[932] Guillain-Barré syndrome developed in 15 patients identified from the FDA database.[933] In children, four cases of optic neuritis have been reported.[934] Large studies have failed to show an occurrence greater than what would have been expected, however.[935] Patients with previous demyelinating syndromes should not be treated with TNF antagonists, and patients with a strong family history should be observed carefully for the development of symptoms that may be suggestive of demyelination.

The development of leukocytoclastic vasculitis had been reported in 35 patients; the disease resolved in most patients after discontinuation of anti-TNF therapy.[936] As with most safety signals from postmarketing surveillance, it is difficult to know whether or not these cases are related to anti-TNF therapy, concomitant therapy, the underlying diseases, or demographics of the patients being treated, but caution is required when considering offering this therapy to candidate patients. Finally, trials have been performed to block TNF in patients with congestive heart failure; neither infliximab nor etanercept was effective, and these agents may have even worsened the congestive heart failure.[937] These agents might exacerbate or even induce congestive heart failure in patients with no previous risk factors.[938]

No specific laboratory monitoring seems to be required routinely for any of these agents. Although the induction of antinuclear antibodies is common (approximately 15% of patients), screening for them is necessary only if suspicion of a developing autoimmune disease (e.g., drug-induced lupus) is raised. Guidelines developed for adults suggest withholding biological DMARDs for at least 1 week before and after surgery.[939] No specific recommendations regarding the use of biological DMARDs during pregnancy or breastfeeding were made because of conflicting evidence.

Anakinra. IL-1 plays a prominent role in rheumatoid arthritis by stimulating synoviocytes and chondrocytes to produce small inflammatory mediators (e.g., prostaglandins) and MMPs that lead to cartilage destruction and bone erosions. IL-1 also increases the expression of RANK ligand, leading to osteoclast differentiation and activation, and bone destruction. It exerts its effect by binding to IL-1 receptor and through cell signaling and production of these various molecules and cytokines. IL-1 receptor antagonist (IL-1Ra), or anakinra, is a naturally occurring, acute-phase antiinflammatory protein, part of the IL-1 supergene family.[940]

IL-1Ra is the most important physiological regulator of IL-1-induced activity. By binding to the IL-1 receptor on cell surfaces, it prevents the interaction of the receptor with IL-1 and subsequent cell signaling. An imbalance between IL-1 and IL-1Ra can lead to uncontrolled inflammation.

Anakinra is a human recombinant form of IL-1Ra that is produced by recombinant technology in *Escherichia coli*. Its short half-life of 4 to 6 hours (when dosed at 1 to 2 mg/kg in adults with rheumatoid arthritis[940]) requires daily subcutaneous injection. Several studies showed improvement in ACR-20, ACR-50, and ACR-70 scores versus placebo at 12 and 24 weeks.[907] Although the improvements have not been as dramatic as improvements reported with anti-TNF agents, they do offer another option for treatment.

In a study by Cohen and associates[941] of combination therapy with MTX in patients with rheumatoid arthritis, there was an increasing response to anakinra, and the response occurred by 2 to 4 weeks. The response seemed to be sustained (at least four of six patients improved) in a dose-dependent fashion, and improvement seemed to continue beyond 24 weeks. Anakinra also seems to halt[942] and perhaps even repair bone destruction as viewed radiologically.[943] Dramatic responses to anakinra in systemic-onset JIA, Muckle-Wells syndrome, familial cold autoinflammatory syndrome, and neonatal-onset multisystem inflammatory disease provide evidence for pediatric use (Table 6–27), and provide evidence that this group of disorders are IL-1 driven and autoinflammatory in nature (see later).

Adverse events generally have not been serious. The most common adverse events are injection site reactions, which tend to occur within the first 4 weeks and are rare later. They consist of rash, erythema, and pruritus, and may be relieved with ice packs and application of topical corticosteroid. They are rarely severe enough to stop treatment. Although serious infections (pneumonia, cellulitis) were more common compared with placebo, no deaths from infection have been reported, and,

Table 6–27

Guidelines for use of anakinra in the treatment of systemic juvenile idiopathic arthritis

Dose

1 mg/kg subcutaneously daily (maximum 100 mg)[913]

Safe to use with methotrexate, but should not be combined with TNF inhibitors

Clinical Monitoring

Although not associated with reactivation of latent tuberculosis, documenting a negative PPD tuberculin test before initiation is recommended

Improvement most often occurs within 2 wk

Monitor every monthly initially, then quarterly

Laboratory Monitoring

Neutrophil count before initiating, monthly for 3 mo, then quarterly

PPD, purified protein derivative; TNF, tumor necrosis factor.

in contrast to anti-TNF agents, opportunistic infections have not occurred in the studies to date. It seems safe to use MTX with anakinra,[941] but etanercept does not seem to add benefit to anakinra, and there was concern about the increased infections, particularly pneumonia, with this combination in patients with rheumatoid arthritis.[944]

A small series showed that patients who had failed to respond to anti-TNF agents generally also did poorly with anakinra.[945] In a randomized, placebo-controlled, withdrawal study of the safety and preliminary efficacy of the IL-1Ra anakinra in patients with polyarticular-course JRA, 86 patients entered a 12-week open-label run-in phase (1 mg/kg anakinra daily, ≤100 mg/day). Of responders, 50 entered the 16-week randomized phase of the study, and 44 entered a 12-month open-label extension. Because of low enrollment, the primary end point was changed from efficacy to safety. The incidence and nature of adverse events were similar across all study phases, with the exception of injection site reactions, which were mild to moderate and decreased with time. Anakinra produced a nonsignificant ($P = .11$) reduction in disease flares compared with placebo. When normalized to a dose of 1 mg/kg, anakinra plasma concentrations were similar to values in adult patients with rheumatoid arthritis. In the open-label phase, there seemed to be an unusually high number of responders among the 15 subjects in the study with systemic onset (73% [systemic] versus 55% [pauciarticular and polyarticular]).[946]

Verbsky and White[947] reported two patients with systemic-onset JIA and response to anakinra. Subsequently, Pascual and associates[948,949] reported that after treatment with anakinra, clinical remission occurred in 7 of 13 patients, and a partial response in 2 of 13 patients with systemic-onset JIA was associated with a reversal of gene expression signatures in peripheral blood cells and leukocytes. Seven patients with MTX and etanercept-resistant, systemic-onset JRA treated with anakinra were reported from five separate centers.[950] Most patients improved within 2 weeks and showed a sustained response, which included a reduction in the number of active joints, an improvement in the laboratory values, and a reduction in the requirement for prednisone. Similarly, four children with MTX and etanercept-resistant, systemic-onset JRA were reported from a single center.[951] All four showed improvement of at least 30% after 1 and 2 months of anakinra at a dose of 1 mg/kg/day. Side effects were mild and did not require discontinuation from therapy.

Since these initial reports of response to IL-1 inhibition among patients with systemic-onset JIA, there have been numerous subsequent reports in children and in adults with Still's Disease.[952,953] In one report of 22 patients treated, 10 with dramatic responses seemed to be distinguished by certain clinical features. In a retrospective case series of 35 patients, there were decreases in large joint arthritis counts, but not small joint counts, and greater decreases in sedimentation rates in patients on high-dose versus low-dose anakinra. Fever and rash in all patients resolved. One patient developed macrophage activation syndrome, and another patient developed Epstein-Barr virus infection. One patient who developed visceral leishmaniasis with treatment was reported.[954]

Two patients with neonatal-onset multisystem inflammatory disease had prolonged responses of greater than 1 year to anakinra.[955] Another similar case was described.[956] In a larger study, anakinra markedly improved clinical and laboratory manifestations in all 18 patients studied with neonatal-onset multisystem inflammatory disease, with or without *CIAS1* mutations.[957] Hearing improvement in four patients with Muckle-Wells syndrome was reported.[958-961] Anakinra controlled inflammatory flares in another three patients.[962] Anakinra was also rapidly and remarkably effective in the newly described autoinflammatory syndrome DIRA (deficiency of the IL-1Ra).[963]

Rilonacept. Rilonacept (also known as IL-1 Trap) is a fully human dimeric fusion protein that incorporates the extracellular domains of the IL-1 receptor components required for IL-1 signaling (IL-1 receptor type I and IL-1 receptor accessory protein), linked to the Fc portion of IgG1.[964] It has a half-life of approximately 1 week and blocks IL-1 signaling by acting as a soluble decoy receptor preventing its interaction with cell surface receptors. In two consecutive phase III studies of 47 adults with cryopyrin-associated periodic syndrome including familial cold autoinflammatory syndrome and Muckle-Wells syndrome (one a 6 week randomized double-blind, placebo-controlled trial, and the other a 9-week single-blind withdrawal study), rilonacept at a dose of 160 mg was shown to provide marked and lasting improvement in the clinical signs and symptoms of cryopyrin-associated periodic syndrome and normalized serum amyloid A levels (Table 6–28).[965]

One serious adverse event (worsening sciatica) was not considered to be related to treatment during the trial, but one elderly patient died after developing sinusitis and *Streptococcus pneumoniae* meningitis. Injection site reactions were reported in 48% of the rilonacept group and 13% of the placebo group. Antirilonacept antibodies, which did not seem to affect efficacy or safety profile, developed in 43% of patients. Increases in total cholesterol, low-density lipoprotein cholesterol, high-density lipoprotein cholesterol, and triglycerides were

Table 6–28

Guidelines for use of rilonacept in cryopyrin-associated periodic syndrome or systemic juvenile idiopathic arthritis

Dose

Initiate treatment with loading dose of 4.4 mg/kg (maximum 320 mg) delivered as one or two subcutaneous injections with a maximum single-injection volume of 2cc. If initial dose is given as two injections, they should be at different sites

Continue dosing at 2.2 mg/kg (maximum 160 mg) once weekly

Do not give in combination with TNF inhibitors

Clinical Monitoring

Clinical response is often rapid, sometimes after the first dose

Laboratory Monitoring

Serum lipid monitoring after 2-3 mo of therapy (consider use of lipid-lowering medication if cholesterol or triglycerides or both are elevated)

TNF, tumor necrosis factor.

seen after 6 weeks of open-label therapy. In a smaller study, all five patients with familial cold autoinflammatory syndrome benefited from treatment.[966]

Preliminary data regarding rilonacept treatment in 21 patients with systemic-onset JIA enrolled in a double-blind, placebo-controlled study were presented.[967] Two doses, 2.2 mg/kg/wk (maximum 160 mg) and 4.4 mg/kg/wk (maximum 320 mg), were studied. Data from an open-label phase are published. Improvement in all six of the ACR Pediatric core set was found. Discontinuations were due to loss of efficacy or to worsening pancytopenia, mood alteration, and macrophage activation syndrome. Seven of the 21 subjects had previously received but inadequately responded to anakinra.

Canakinumab. Canakinumab is a fully human anti–IL-1β mAb that selectively blocks IL-1β and has no cross-reactivity with other characterized IL-1β family members, including IL-1α and IL-1Ra. Its long half-life of 30 days permitted every-8-week dosing in a three-part, 48-week, double-blind, placebo-controlled randomized withdrawal study in 35 patients with cryopyrin-associated periodic syndrome.[968-969] The dose range was 2 mg/kg for patients weighing 40 kg or less to 150 mg for patients weighing greater than 40 kg. In the open-label phase, 34 of 35 patients had a complete response; 31 entered the randomized withdrawal phase. Flares occurred in 13 of 16 patients in the placebo group and no patients in the canakinumab group. Two patients had serious adverse events (lower urinary tract infection, vertigo with closed-angle glaucoma). There was an increase in the rate of suspected infections in the withdrawal phase in the canakinumab group compared with the placebo group. No serious infections or immunogenicity against canakinumab was detected.

Interleukin-6 Inhibitor: Tocilizumab. IL-6 seems to be an important potential target, particularly in the treatment of systemic-onset JIA. There is ample evidence that IL-6

is central to the many clinical and laboratory manifestations of this disease. An imbalance between IL-6 and its soluble receptor can lead to increased IL-6 binding on cell surfaces with its receptor, binding gp130, on the cell membrane, leading to intracellular signaling and resulting cytokine production and release.[970] Elegant studies have produced evidence that levels of IL-6 correlate with spikes of fever, thrombocytosis, and joint involvement,[971] and in mice transgenic for IL-6, growth restriction is observed.[972] Neutralization of IL-6 would be expected to be very beneficial.

Tocilizumab is a genetically engineered, humanized, mAb to the IL-6 receptor that is produced by grafting the complementarity-determining region of mouse antihuman IL-6 receptor antibody to human IgG1.[970,973] Tocilizumab competes with the soluble and the membrane-bound IL-6 receptor; the latter prevents cell signaling. Studies in animals showed that tocilizumab reduces joint inflammation in collagen arthritis.[974] Tocilizumab is effective in treating adult rheumatoid arthritis,[975] and case reports have documented efficacy in adult-onset Still's Disease[976] and Castleman disease.[977] The suggested dose is 8 mg/kg biweekly intravenously, tailored as necessary. The half life after the third dose of 8 mg/kg biweekly reached approximately 10 days.[973]

A series of large placebo-controlled clinical trials in adult rheumatoid arthritis showed efficacy versus placebo,[978] superior efficacy to MTX,[979] efficacy in subjects refractory to TNF inhibitors,[980] superior efficacy of tocilizumab in combination with DMARD compared with DMARD alone,[981] and slowing of radiographic progression.[982] Additionally, the results of a 5-year long-term, open-label extension safety study in 143 patients were reported:[983] 32 (22%) withdrew from the study because of adverse events, 1 because of unsatisfactory response, and 14 because of the patient's request or other reasons. The rate of serious adverse events was 27.5 events per 100 patient-years, with 5.7 serious infections per 100 patient-years, based on a total tocilizumab exposure of 612 patient-years.

The results of a preliminary study from Japan were reported, in which 11 children with systemic-onset JIA were treated with tocilizumab in a dose-escalation trial, depending on the initial response to a dose of 2 mg/kg, to a maximum dose of 8 mg/kg. Three patients received 2 mg/kg, five received 4 mg/kg, and three received 8 mg/kg, with a 70% JIA core set response in 33.3%, 60%, and 100%. No children withdrew because of adverse events or disease flare.[984] In a published study, 18 white patients with systemic-onset JIA were treated with a single intravenous infusion of 2 mg/kg, 4 mg/kg, or 8 mg/kg of tocilizumab. No evidence of dose-limiting toxicity was observed, and there were no dose-limiting safety issues. Clinical and laboratory responses were observed by 48 hours after infusion, and these improvements continued well after serum tocilizumab was undetectable. Eleven patients achieved ACR Pediatric–30 definition of improvement criteria; 8 achieved ACR Pediatric–50 improvement, which persisted for 8 weeks.[985]

In a randomized, placebo-controlled, withdrawal study in Japan, 56 children were given three doses of tocilizumab, 8 mg/kg, every 2 weeks during a 6-week open-label lead-in phase. Patients achieving an ACR Pediatric–30 response with a C-reactive protein of less than 5 mg/L were randomly assigned to receive placebo or to continue tocilizumab treatment for 12 weeks or until withdrawal for rescue medication in the double-blind phase. Patients responding to tocilizumab and needing further treatment were enrolled in an open-label extension phase for at least 48 weeks. At the end of the open-label lead-in phase, ACR Pediatric–30, ACR Pediatric–50, and ACR Pediatric–70 responses were achieved by 51 (91%), 48 (86%), and 38 (68%) patients.

There were 43 patients who continued to the double-blind phase; 4 (17%) of 23 patients in the placebo group maintained response compared with 16 (80%) of 20 in the tocilizumab group (P < .0001). By week 48 of the open-label extension phase, ACR Pediatric–30, ACR Pediatric–50, and ACR Pediatric–70 responses were achieved by 47 (98%), 45 (94%), and 43 (90%) of 48 patients. Growth improved and corticosteroids were withdrawn in three patients and reduced in the fourth, and tocilizumab was able to be discontinued in two children after 3 years.

Serious adverse events in the open-label run-in and blinded withdrawal phases were anaphylactoid reaction in a patient who tested negative for IgE-type antitocilizumab antibodies (but who had allergic reactions to aspirin and infliximab), and GI hemorrhage from diffuse acute or chronic colonic ulceration in a patient with chronic diarrhea and rectal bleeding. One patient developed infectious mononucleosis, hepatitis, and neutropenia. Another developed herpes zoster while on placebo. No cases of reactivated tuberculosis occurred. Mild infusion reactions occurred in 10 patients; IgE antibodies were noted in 4. In the extension phase, 13 serious adverse events occurred, including bronchitis, gastroenteritis, and anaphylactoid reaction. Mild increases of alanine aminotransferase (12 subjects) and aspartate aminotransferase (8 subjects) were reported. A large, multinational trial is under way.

APOPTOSIS

Apoptosis (programmed cell death) is a process whereby normal tissue growth is maintained and controlled by the expression of oncogenes. Inflammatory cytokines in the synovial fluid of patients with rheumatoid arthritis upregulate the expression of apoptosis factors, but apoptosis per se seems to be defective,[986] possibly because of a defect in the interaction between the oncogene Fas and its ligand. Strategies to correct defective apoptosis include monoclonal anti-Fas antibodies and administration of Fas ligand; this approach may be amenable to gene therapy (see later discussion).

Combination Therapies

In the past, clinicians were reluctant to use combinations of DMARDs for arthritis because of concerns about increased toxicity of agents with similar toxicity profiles. Numerous factors support the use of combination therapies, however. In adult rheumatoid arthritis, single agents seem to lose efficacy over time;[987] these agents rarely induce sustained long-term remissions. An increased appreciation of the long-term morbidity of rheumatoid arthritis and JRA supports a more aggressive approach

---

Table 6–29

Combination therapies reported to be effective in the treatment of rheumatoid arthritis and juvenile idiopathic arthritis

Sulfasalazine, methotrexate, and hydroxychloroquine[988]

Methotrexate and cyclosporin[724,989]

Methotrexate and leflunomide[376,376a,376b]

Chloroquine and methotrexate[990]

Prednisolone, methotrexate, and sulfasalazine[991,992]

Leflunomide and infliximab[993]

Biological therapy combined with methotrexate[874,911,923,923a, 941,993,994,996]

IV methylprednisolone, IV cyclophosphamide, and methotrexate[559,561]

IV, intravenous.

---

to medical management (Table 6–29).[145] A better understanding of the mechanisms of action of these agents and well-designed studies of combination therapy in adults that showed efficacy without a significant increase in toxicity support the use of this approach. In adult rheumatoid arthritis, studies have shown the efficacy of triple therapy with sulfasalazine, MTX, and hydroxychloroquine versus any two of these drugs alone;[988] MTX and cyclosporine versus MTX or placebo;[724,989] chloroquine and MTX versus MTX;[990] and prednisolone, MTX, and sulfasalazine versus sulfasalazine alone (COBRA trial).[991,992] It has been suggested that the combination of leflunomide and infliximab may also be effective.[993] In addition, the improvement noted with biological therapy can be enhanced by combining it with MTX,[878,911,994,995,996] and the combination of etanercept and MTX may slow structural damage, opening the door to potential long-term remission (TEMPO trial).[996] One combination of the biological agents anakinra and etanercept was no more effective, however, than either agent alone and was more toxic.[997]

In JRA, combination therapy has included intravenous methylprednisolone, intravenous cyclophosphamide, and MTX.[559,561] In addition, MTX is usually used together with either etanercept or infliximab with no increase in toxicity.[816,834,847,998] Combination therapy would seem particularly appropriate in cases of severe systemic-onset JRA. Important questions remaining to be answered include which patients are most at risk for long-term damage and most likely to benefit from combination therapy; whether therapy should be started in combination, or medication should be added only after a partial inadequate response; and whether full or reduced doses of each agent should be used.

Gene Therapy

The successes seen with biological therapy have supported a potential role for gene therapy in patients with arthritis. Strategies include systemic, local, or facilitated local (the ability to target multiple diseased joints selectively by a single parenteral injection) therapy,[999] each of which might avoid the costs and inconvenience of ongoing therapy. Ideally, children with the worst prognoses would be targeted for study. These patients would most likely require systemic rather than local therapy, however, and progress with systemic gene therapy has been slowest. Local or facilitated local therapy might be ideal for oligoarticular JRA when its safety is established.[1000]

Many different types of candidate transgenes have been suggested, including transgenes encoding cytokine antagonists, immunomodulators, antiangiogenic factors, apoptotic agents, antioxidants, inhibitors of mitosis, and molecules that modulate cell signaling and the activities of transcription factors.[999,1001,1002] Proof-of-principle has been shown in animal models of rheumatoid arthritis, Sjögren syndrome, and SLE.[999,1003] Transgenes used in humans with arthritis include IL-1Ra, HSV-tk, TNFR:Fc fusion protein, and transforming growth factor-β.[999] Numerous high-profile deaths in human trials, including one in an arthritis gene therapy trial, have resulted in a more cautious approach by funding agencies and industry, slowing progress. Similar to stem cell transplantation, there are widespread concerns about safety of gene therapy and many people question the use of gene therapy to treat nongenetic nonlethal diseases.[999]

High-Dose Immunotherapy with Transplantation

Cures of adjuvant arthritis in animal models by either syngeneic[1004] or autologous bone marrow transplantation,[1005] together with "experiments in nature" in which patients with rheumatoid arthritis who underwent bone marrow transplantation for other disorders were noted to experience an improvement in their rheumatoid arthritis, have paved the way for new approaches to the treatment of autoimmune disease (i.e., autologous transplantation). The principles behind this treatment are that high-dose myeloablative therapy destroys the autoreactive clones that initiate the autoimmune process, and the marrow can be repopulated with a naïve population of stem cells.[1006] As the immune system redevelops after transplantation, immune cells may become "tolerized" to the putative antigens that are involved in the autoimmune process. Allogeneic matched bone marrow transplantation for patients with RF-positive rheumatoid arthritis and associated aplastic anemia has led to remission of the arthritis. The length of the remission varied from 1 to 13 years.[1007,1008]

Allogeneic bone marrow transplantation carries a significant risk of mortality (15% to 35%) and development of graft-versus-host disease. The use of an autologous transplant, from either marrow or peripheral blood stem cells (autologous stem cell transplantation [ASCT]), reduces the mortality from the procedure to 1% to 5% and is not associated with graft-versus-host disease. High-dose immunotherapy with ASCT has become a preferred method that has been used in treating several autoimmune diseases.

Initial studies in patients with autoimmune diseases and associated malignancies who underwent ASCT showed recurrence of disease within 5 weeks to 1 year.[1009] In these initial studies, the "retransplanted" stem cells were not manipulated in either a positive way (selection for CD34+ stem cells) or a negative way (removal of T cells with potential autoreactivity). Relapses may also occur

because (1) the putative autoantigens responsible for the disease were not eliminated; (2) the HLA status of the host did not change, and a predisposition to select arthritogenic peptides and a limited number of T cell developmental pathways persists; and (3) autoreactive T cells were not completely eliminated before transplantation.

Preliminary studies of ASCT have been described in children with JRA and scleroderma, with excellent outcomes in most, but not all, studies.[1010-1012] An initial mortality rate of 14% raised significant concerns despite remarkable improvement in some patients.[1013]

Wulffraat and associates[1014] reported their experience with 31 patients with polyarticular-course JIA (25 with systemic-onset, 6 with polyarticular-onset) treated with ASCT from eight different European pediatric transplantation centers. Bone marrow cells were transfused in 23 cases and peripheral stem cells, after harvesting with cyclophosphamide (2 g/m^2) and granulocyte colony-stimulating factor, were transfused in 8 cases. T cells were selected for CD34 stem cells by either negative or positive selection techniques. Conditioning included 5 days of antithymocyte antiglobulin on days −9 through −6 and cyclophosphamide (50 mg/kg) on days −5 through −2; low-dose total-body irradiation was given to 21 patients on day −1. Frozen stem cells were thawed and infused on day 0. The neutrophil and platelet counts returned to normal by day 35. In vitro mitogenic T cell responses normalized within 6 to 18 months, and T cell counts were normal by 5 to 9 months.

Seventeen patients had a drug-free period of 8 to 60 months. Mild relapses, which were easy to control, occurred in seven patients. Four patients had no response to ASCT at all, and three patients died—two with macrophage activation syndrome (one induced by EBV) and one with disseminated toxoplasmosis. Catch-up growth was seen in younger children, but not in older children or in children with long disease duration. All patients developed chills, fever, and malaise during the infusion of antithymocyte antiglobulin. In addition to the two patients who died of infection-related causes, infectious complications were common (varicella zoster in seven patients, atypical mycobacteria in one patient, and *Legionella* pneumonia in one patient).

In a more detailed report, 34 children with polyarticular-course JIA (29 with systemic-onset, 5 with polyarticular-onset) in nine different European transplant centers were reported.[1015] Clinical follow-up was 12 to 60 months. Of 34 patients with a follow-up of 12 to 60 months, 18 (53%) achieved complete drug-free remission. Seven of these patients had previously failed treatment with anti-TNF agents. Six of the 34 patients (18%) showed a partial response (30% to 70% improvement), and 7 (21%) were resistant to ASCT. Infectious complications were common. There were three cases of transplant-related mortality (9%), and two cases of disease-related mortality (6%). The authors recommended that future protocols include elimination of total-body irradiation from the conditioning regimen, and prophylactic administration of antiviral drugs and intravenous immunoglobulins until there is a normal CD4+ T cell count, to lessen toxicity.

A cohort of 22 children with polyarticular-course JIA (18 with systemic-onset, 4 with polyarticular-onset) in three centers, representing a subgroup of the afore-mentioned subjects available for long-term follow up, were shown to have delayed recovery (>6 months) of CD4+CD45RA+ naïve T cells, thought to be responsible for the infectious and macrophage activation syndrome complications.[1016] Five patients relapsed up to 7 years after ASCT. Four new patients who were treated with a fludarabin-containing regimen instead of low-dose total-body irradiation had drug-free remission 4 to 5 years later.[1017] Additionally, two patients undergoing alloge-neic transplant with HLA-matched family donors were with 1- to 2-year follow-up.[1017]

In another study, seven children in the United Kingdom initially showed dramatic clinical response, and in four children this response was sustained allowing withdrawal of immunosuppressive and antiinflammatory treatment, significant catch-up growth, and immense improvement of the quality of life during 5 to 8 years of follow-up.[1018] Two patients relapsed within 1 to 12 months, and one died 4 months after transplant. Complications included fatal adenovirus reactivation, hematophagocytic syndrome secondary to EBV, and another hematophagocytic syndrome secondary to cytomegalovirus.

ASCT has been shown to alter laboratory abnormalities that reflect the immunological process, including perforin expression,[1014] expression of myeloid-related proteins (MRP8/MRP14),[1019] and synovial cellularity and cytokine expression.[1020] Encouraging reports from the use of ASCT in patients with SLE[1021-1022] and systemic sclerosis[1023] have led to more than 700 patients (50 children) with autoimmune disease undergoing ASCT,[1024] mostly patients with systemic sclerosis (scleroderma), multiple sclerosis, rheumatoid arthritis, JIA, and SLE. A smaller number of patients have received an allogeneic transplant. The authors observed that overall treatment-related mortality of 7% has since decreased, with no further cases being reported in systemic sclerosis or multiple sclerosis in the last 3 years of follow-up as of the time of the report. This improvement is thought to be due to more careful patient selection. Although ASCT has not been curative in patients with rheumatoid arthritis, the disease seems easier to control with DMARDs after the procedure.[1025]

Many questions remain regarding this treatment and the crucial variables in the protocols. The intensive immunotherapy required (high-dose cyclophosphamide with or without irradiation with or without antithymocyte globulin) may itself result in disease remission, as described in several cases of aplastic anemia and SLE.[1026,1027] It is unclear whether irradiation is necessary, particularly because it may significantly increase the risk of malignancy; it did not seem to improve the outcome in the 31 patients described by Wulffraat and associates.[1014] A protocol that includes fludarabine to spare the need for irradiation seems promising.[1017] It is likely that manipulation of the "graft" is required before reinfusion. The number of stem cells required must be defined. Other preconditioning regimens may be more effective.[1028] Multipotent mesenchymal stromal cells obtained from the bone marrow and expanded ex vivo are immune privileged and apparently of low toxicity, and are thought to provide a positive immunomodulatory effect and may be incorporated into future protocols.[1024]

If ASCT is ultimately proven to be relatively safe and effective, patient selection will be crucial to its success. Patients should be chosen whose disease can be predicted to have a severe outcome, but who are not yet at the stage of severe, irreversible damage. The development of prognostic markers is crucial for proper selection of candidates. The ethical issues of attempting a procedure with a mortality rate of at least 5% in children with chronic diseases but much lower predicted mortality rates are monumental.[1029] The long-term risk of immunosuppression is significant, and safer ways to provide immunosuppression need to be developed.

PAIN

Many children have pain either as a primary problem (see Chapter 11) or as a component of their rheumatic disease.[1030] Various adjunctive medications may be effective to help in the management of these patients.

Antidepressants

Amitriptyline is a tricyclic antidepressant that also inhibits reuptake of serotonin and norepinephrine. In a large metaanalysis of six clinical randomized controlled trials in adult fibromyalgia, amitriptyline, 25 mg/day, was found to have a therapeutic response compared with placebo in the short-term in the domains of pain, sleep, fatigue, and overall patient and investigator impression, but not tender points.[1031] Poor metabolizers have reduced debrisoquin hydrolase activity resulting in higher plasma concentrations at usual doses. This enzyme is also inhibited by numerous drugs, including other antidepressants, phenothiazines, and antiarrhythmics. Cimetidine is reported to reduce hepatic metabolism through another mechanism. For treating pain in children, it is recommended to start at 0.1 mg/kg at bedtime and titrate to a final dose of 0.5 to 2 mg/kg (maximum dose 25 to 50 mg) over 2 weeks.

Duloxetine and milnacipran are selective serotonin and norepinephrine reuptake inhibitors that have analgesic effects by increasing the activity of descending noradrenergic antinociceptive pathways in the brain and spinal cord; both are approved by the FDA for the treatment of fibromyalgia in adults.[1032-1034] Milnacipran has a higher affinity for the norepinephrine transporter than duloxetine and may be more effective than duloxetine for fatigue and difficulty concentrating. Common adverse events for both agents are somnolence, nausea, and decreased appetite.[1035,1036] They are excreted primarily in the urine in the conjugated form. The dose of milnacipran in adults is 100 mg daily, divided into two doses, and for duloxetine is 60 mg once daily, but some authors recommend starting at lower doses initially and gradually increasing the dose to the recommended levels.[1034]

All serotonin-activating medications can increase the risk of bleeding, suicidal tendencies, or both, and should be used with caution in patients at risk for these complications. Children and adolescents should be closely observed for suicidality, especially during the initial few months of therapy or with dose changes.

Neuroleptics

Pregabalin is an $\alpha_2\delta$-calcium channel antagonist that limits the neuronal release of excitatory neurotransmitters, with anxiolytic and analgesic activity with a capability to improve slow wave sleep. It is approved by the FDA for treatment of fibromyalgia in adults.[1037,1038] Adverse effects include dizziness, somnolence, weight gain, and peripheral edema.[1039] The approved dose is 150 to 225 mg divided into two doses daily, but some authors recommend starting at 25 to 75 mg as a single daily dose with an evening meal.[1034] It should be discontinued gradually because sudden discontinuation may precipitate seizures in susceptible individuals. Gabapentin is an older drug with the same mechanism of action and seems to be effective in the treatment of fibromyalgia as well.

REFERENCES

6. P.M. Brooks, R.O. Day, Nonsteroidal antiinflammatory drugs–differences and similarities, N. Engl. J. Med. 324 (24) (1991) 1716–1725.
31. K.J. Skeith, F. Jamali, Clinical pharmacokinetics of drugs used in juvenile arthritis, Clin. Pharmacokinet. 21 (2) (1991) 129–149.
33. T.G. Wells, M.E. Mortensen, et al., Comparison of the pharmacokinetics of naproxen tablets and suspension in children, J. Clin. Pharmacol. 34 (1) (1994) 30–33.
36. L.L. Dupuis, G. Koren, A. Shore, E.D. Silverman, R.M. Laxer, Methotrexate-nonsteroidal antiinflammatory drug interaction in children with arthritis, J. Rheumatol. 17 (1990) 1469–1473.
43. K.S. Barron, D.A. Person, et al., The toxicity of nonsteroidal antiinflammatory drugs in juvenile rheumatoid arthritis, J. Rheumatol. 9 (1) (1982) 149–155.
48. D.J. Lovell, E.H. Giannini, et al., Time course of response to nonsteroidal antiinflammatory drugs in juvenile rheumatoid arthritis, Arthritis Rheum. 27 (12) (1984) 1433–1437.
50. S. Goodman, P. Howard, et al., An open label study to establish dosing recommendations for nabumetone in juvenile rheumatoid arthritis, J. Rheumatol. 30 (4) (2003) 829–831.
51. M.A. Rapoff, J. Belmont, et al., Prevention of nonadherence to nonsteroidal anti-inflammatory medications for newly diagnosed patients with juvenile rheumatoid arthritis, Health Psychol. 21 (6) (2002) 620–623.
52. T. Kroll, J.H. Barlow, et al., Treatment adherence in juvenile rheumatoid arthritis–a review, Scand. J. Rheumatol. 28 (1) (1999) 10–18.
59. J. Zhang, E.L. Ding, et al., Adverse effects of cyclooxygenase 2 inhibitors on renal and arrhythmia events: meta-analysis of randomized trials, JAMA 296 (13) (2006) 1619–1632.
60. P.A. Konstantinopoulos, D.F. Lehmann, The cardiovascular toxicity of selective and nonselective cyclooxygenase inhibitors: comparisons, contrasts, and aspirin confounding, J. Clin. Pharmacol. 45 (7) (2005) 742–750.
61. M.C. Hochberg, COX-2: Where are we in 2003? - Be strong and resolute: continue to use COX-2 selective inhibitors at recommended dosages in appropriate patients, Arthritis Res. Ther. 5 (1) (2003) 28–31.
62. M.M. Wolfe, D.R. Lichtenstein, et al., Gastrointestinal toxicity of nonsteroidal antiinflammatory drugs, N. Engl. J. Med. 340 (24) (1999) 1888–1899.
68. G.F. Keenan, E.H. Giannini, et al., Clinically significant gastropathy associated with nonsteroidal antiinflammatory drug use in children with juvenile rheumatoid arthritis, J. Rheumatol. 22 (6) (1995) 1149–1151.
69. C.M. Duffy, M. Gibbon, et al., Non-steroidal antiinflammatory drug-induced gastrointestinal toxicity in a practice-based cohort of children with juvenile rheumatoid arthritis, J. Rheumatol. 27 (Suppl. 58) (2000) 73.
70. M. Ashorn, P. Verronen, et al., Upper endoscopic findings in children with active juvenile chronic arthritis, Acta. Paediatr. 92 (5) (2003) 558–561.
82. M. Gazarian, M. Berkovitch, et al., Experience with misoprostol therapy for NSAID gastropathy in children, Ann. Rheum. Dis. 54 (4) (1995) 277–280.
87. S. Sawhney, P. Woo, et al., Macrophage activation syndrome: a potentially fatal complication of rheumatic disorders, Arch. Dis. Child 85 (5) (2001) 421–426.
88. J.L. Stephan, I. Kone-Paut, et al., Reactive haemophagocytic syndrome in children with inflammatory disorders: a retrospective study of 24 patients, Rheumatology (Oxford) 40 (11) (2001) 1285–1292.
89. D.M. Clive, J.S. Stoff, Renal syndromes associated with nonsteroidal antiinflammatory drugs, N. Engl. J. Med. 310 (9) (1984) 563–572.
99. H.M. Haftel, J.M. Mitchell, et al., Incidence of renal toxicity from anti-inflammatory medications in a pediatric rheumatology population: role of routine screening of urine, J. Rheumatol. 27 (Syppl. 58) (2000) 73.
104. M.E. De Broe, M.M. Elseviers, Analgesic nephropathy, N. Engl. J. Med. 338 (7) (1998) 446–452.
116. B.A. Lang, L.A. Finlayson, Naproxen-induced pseudoporphyria in patients with juvenile rheumatoid arthritis, J. Pediatr. 124 (4) (1994) 639–642.
118. B. De Silva, L. Banney, et al., Pseudoporphyria and nonsteroidal antiinflammatory agents in children with juvenile idiopathic arthritis, Pediatr. Dermatol. 17 (6) (2000) 480–483.
119. S. Mehta, B. Lang, Long-term followup of naproxen-induced pseudoporphyria in juvenile rheumatoid arthritis, Arthritis Rheum. 42 (10) (1999) 2252–2254.
120. S.G. Schad, A. Kraus, et al., Early onset pauciarticular arthritis is the major risk factor for naproxen-induced pseudoporphyria in juvenile idiopathic arthritis, Arthritis Res. Ther. 9 (1) (2007) R10.
146. C.D. Rose, B.H. Singsen, et al., Safety and efficacy of methotrexate therapy for juvenile rheumatoid arthritis, J. Pediatr. 117 (4) (1990) 653–659.
156. E.S. Chan, B.N. Cronstein, Molecular action of methotrexate in inflammatory diseases, Arthritis Res. 4 (4) (2002) 266–273.
158. A. Ravelli, G. Di Fuccia, M. Molinaro, et al., Plasma levels after oral methotrexate in children with juvenile rheumatoid arthritis, J. Rheumatol. 20 (1993) 1573–1577.
162. L.L. Dupuis, G. Koren, Influence of food on the bioavailability of oral methotrexate in children, J. Rheumatol. 22 (8) (1995) 1570–1573.
168. C.A. Wallace, D.D. Sherry, A practical approach to avoidance of methotrexate toxicity, J. Rheumatol. 22 (6) (1995) 1009–1012.
172. E. Kimura, S. Oga, et al., Comparative study of the pharmacokinetics of MTX in juvenile idiopathic arthritis patients receiving long-term MTX monotherapy or MTX plus chloroquine, J. Clin. Pharm. Ther. 32 (6) (2007) 579–584.
173. J. Haapasaari, H. Kautiainen, et al., Hydroxychloroquine does not decrease serum methotrexate concentrations in children with juvenile idiopathic arthritis, Arthritis Rheum. 52 (5) (2005) 1621–1622.
175. T. Takken, J. Van Der Net, et al., Methotrexate for treating juvenile idiopathic arthritis, Cochrane Database System Rev. 4, 2001.
184. A. Ravelli, G. Ballardini, et al., Methotrexate therapy in refractory pediatric onset systemic lupus erythematosus, J. Rheumatol. 25 (3) (1998) 572–575.
190. A.H. Weiss, C.A. Wallace, et al., Methotrexate for resistant chronic uveitis in children with juvenile rheumatoid arthritis, J. Pediatr. 133 (2) (1998) 266–268.
193. K. Alsufyani, O. Ortiz-Alvarez, et al., The role of subcutaneous administration of methotrexate in children with juvenile idiopathic arthritis who have failed oral methotrexate, J. Rheumatol. 31 (1) (2004) 179–182.
200. P. Hunt, C. Rose, et al., Long-term safety and efficacy of methotrexate in juvenile rheumatoid arthritis, Arthritis Rheum. 36 (1993) S61.
201. A.E. van Ede, R.F.J.M. Laan, H.J. Blom, et al., Methotrexate in rheumatoid arthritis: an update with focus on mechanisms involved in toxicity, Semin. Arthritis Rheum. 27 (1998) 277–292.
212. P.J. Hashkes, W.F. Balistreri, et al., The relationship of hepatotoxic risk factors and liver histology in methotrexate therapy for juvenile rheumatoid arthritis, J. Pediatr. 134 (1) (1999) 47–52.

214. S. Kugathasan, A.J. Newman, et al., Liver biopsy findings in patients with juvenile rheumatoid arthritis receiving long-term, weekly methotrexate therapy, J. Pediatr. 128 (1) (1996) 149–151.

215. P.J. Hashkes, W.F. Balistreri, et al., The long-term effect of methotrexate therapy on the liver in patients with juvenile rheumatoid arthritis, Arthritis Rheum. 40 (12) (1997) 2226–2234.

229. O.W. Kamel, M. van de Rijn, et al., Lymphoid neoplasms in patients with rheumatoid arthritis and dermatomyositis: frequency of Epstein-Barr virus and other features associated with immunosuppression, Hum. Pathol. 25 (7) (1994) 638–643.

237. A.G. Cleary, H. McDowell, et al., Polyarticular juvenile idiopathic arthritis treated with methotrexate complicated by the development of non-Hodgkin's lymphoma, Arch. Dis. Child 86 (1) (2002) 47–49.

239. J. Takeyama, A. Sato, et al., Epstein-Barr virus associated Hodgkin lymphoma in a 9-year-old girl receiving long-term methotrexate therapy for juvenile idiopathic arthritis, J. Pediatr. Hematol. Oncol. 28 (9) (2006) 622–624.

248. M.A. Muzaffer, R. Schneider, et al., Accelerated nodulosis during methotrexate therapy for juvenile rheumatoid arthritis, J. Pediatr. 128 (5 Pt 1) (1996) 698–700.

250. A. van der Meer, N.M. Wulffraat, et al., Psychological side effects of MTX treatment in juvenile idiopathic arthritis: a pilot study, Clin. Exp. Rheumatol. 25 (3) (2007) 480–485.

257. M.E. Lloyd, M. Carr, et al., The effects of methotrexate on pregnancy, fertility and lactation, Qjm. 92 (10) (1999) 551–563.

259. M. Ostensen, F. Forger, Management of RA medications in pregnant patients, Nat. Rev. Rheumatol. 5 (7) (2009) 382–390.

264. Z. Ortiz, B. Shea, et al., The efficacy of folic acid and folinic acid in reducing methotrexate gastrointestinal toxicity in rheumatoid arthritis. A metaanalysis of randomized controlled trials, J. Rheumatol. 25 (1) (1998) 36–43.

292. M.F. Marmor, New American Academy of Ophthalmology recommendations on screening for hydroxychloroquine retinopathy, Arthritis Rheum. 48 (6) (2003) 1764.

296. M.F. Marmor, Hydroxychloroquine at the recommended dose (< or = 6.5 mg/kg/day) is safe for the retina in patients with rheumatoid arthritis and systemic lupus erythematosus, Clin. Exp. Rheumatol. 22 (2) (2004) 143–144.

306. M.A. van Rossum, T.J. Fiselier, et al., Sulfasalazine in the treatment of juvenile chronic arthritis: a randomized, double-blind, placebo-controlled, multicenter study. Dutch Juvenile Chronic Arthritis Study Group, Arthritis Rheum. 41 (5) (1998) 808–816.

310. C.D. Brooks, Sulfasalazine for the management of juvenile rheumatoid arthritis, J. Rheumatol. 28 (4) (2001) 845–853.

311. R. Burgos-Vargas, J. Vazquez-Mellado, et al., A 26 week randomised, double blind, placebo controlled exploratory study of sulfasalazine in juvenile onset spondyloarthropathies, Ann. Rheum. Dis. 61 (10) (2002) 941–942.

366. B. Rozman, Clinical pharmacokinetics of leflunomide, Clin. Pharmacokinet. 41 (6) (2002) 421–430.

367. E. Silverman, R. Mouy, et al., Leflunomide or methotrexate for juvenile rheumatoid arthritis, N. Engl. J. Med. 352 (16) (2005) 1655–1666.

376a. T. Antony, V.M. Jose, B.J. Paul, T. Thomas, Efficacy and safety of leflunomide alone and in combination with methotrexate in the treatment of refractory rheumatoid arthritis, Indian J. Med. Sci. 60 (2006) 318–326.

376b. S.S. Lee, Y.W. Park, J.J. Park, et al., Combination treatment with leflunomide and methotrexate for patients with active rheumatoid arthritis, Scand. J. Rheumatol. 38 (2009) 11–14.

377. R.L. Brent, Teratogen update: reproductive risks of leflunomide (Arava); a pyrimidine synthesis inhibitor: counseling women taking leflunomide before or during pregnancy and men taking leflunomide who are contemplating fathering a child, Teratology 63 (2) (2001) 106–112.

389. D. Zemer, A. Livneh, et al., Long-term colchicine treatment in children with familial Mediterranean fever, Arthritis Rheum. 34 (8) (1991) 973–977.

417. S. Ochonisky, J. Verroust, et al., Thalidomide neuropathy incidence and clinico-electrophysiologic findings in 42 patients, Arch. Dermatol. 130 (1) (1994) 66–69.

466. Z. Punthakee, L. Legault, et al., Prednisolone in the treatment of adrenal insufficiency: a re-evaluation of relative potency, J. Pediatr. 143 (3) (2003) 402–405.

469. H.G. Morris, J.R. Jorgensen, et al., Metabolic effects of human growth hormone in corticosteroid-treated children, J. Clin. Invest. 47 (3) (1968) 436–451.

472. S. Bechtold, P. Ripperger, et al., Growth hormone improves height in patients with juvenile idiopathic arthritis: 4-year data of a controlled study, J. Pediatr. 143 (4) (2003) 512–519.

502. M.S. Klein-Gitelman, L.M. Pachman, Intravenous corticosteroids: adverse reactions are more variable than expected in children, J. Rheumatol. 25 (10) (1998) 1995–2002.

503. N.T. Ilowite, P. Samuel, et al., Dyslipoproteinemia in pediatric systemic lupus erythematosus, Arthritis Rheum. 31 (7) (1988) 859–863.

505. M. Gazarian, B.M. Feldman, et al., Assessment of myocardial perfusion and function in childhood systemic lupus erythematosus, J. Pediatr. 132 (1) (1998) 109–116.

526. J. Homik, M.E. Suarez-Almazor, et al., Calcium and vitamin D for corticosteroid-induced osteoporosis, Cochrane Database Syst. Rev. (2) (2000) CD000952.

537. L.M. Ward, A.E. Denker, et al., Single-dose pharmacokinetics and tolerability of alendronate 35- and 70-milligram tablets in children and adolescents with osteogenesis imperfecta type I, J. Clin. Endocrinol. Metab. 90 (7) (2005) 4051–4056.

541. L.A. DiMeglio, M. Peacock, Two-year clinical trial of oral alendronate versus intravenous pamidronate in children with osteogenesis imperfecta, J. Bone Miner Res. 21 (1) (2006) 132–140.

544. M.L. Bianchi, R. Cimaz, et al., Efficacy and safety of alendronate for the treatment of osteoporosis in diffuse connective tissue diseases in children: a prospective multicenter study, Arthritis Rheum. 43 (9) (2000) 1960–1966.

546. Y.N. Inoue, Shimojo, et al., Efficacy of intravenous alendronate for the treatment of glucocorticoid-induced osteoporosis In children with autoimmune diseases, Clin. Rheumatol. 27 (7) (2008) 909–912.

547. R. Cimaz, M. Gattorno, et al., Changes in markers of bone turnover and inflammatory variables during alendronate therapy in pediatric patients with rheumatic diseases, J. Rheumatol. 29 (8) (2002) 1786–1792.

548. D.I. Shulman, M.R. Palmert, et al., Adrenal insufficiency: still a cause of morbidity and death in childhood, Pediatrics 119 (2) (2007) e484–e494.

553. M. Salem, R.E. Tainsh Jr., et al., Perioperative glucocorticoid coverage. A reassessment 42 years after emergence of a problem, Ann. Surg. 219 (4) (1994) 416–425.

582. H. Derendorf, H. Mollmann, et al., Pharmacokinetics and pharmacodynamics of glucocorticoid suspensions after intra-articular administration, Clin. Pharmacol. Ther. 39 (3) (1986) 313–317.

583. F. Zulian, G. Martini, et al., Comparison of intra-articular triamcinolone hexacetonide and triamcinolone acetonide in oligoarticular juvenile idiopathic arthritis, Rheumatology (Oxford) 42 (10) (2003) 1254–1259.

584. B.A. Eberhard, M.C. Sison, B.S. Gottlieb, N.T. Ilowite, Comparison of the intraarticular effectiveness of triamcinolone hexacetonide and triamcinolone acetonide in treatment of juvenile rheumatoid arthritis, J. Rheumatol. 31 (2004) 2507–2512.

608. H.L. McLeod, C. Siva, The thiopurine S-methyltransferase gene locus – implications for clinical pharmacogenomics, Pharmacogenomics 3 (1) (2002) 89–98.

631. W.M. Bennett, Immunosuppression with mycophenolic acid: one size does not fit all, J. Am. Soc. Nephrol. 14 (2003) 2414–2416.

632. M. Roland, C. Barbet, Mycophenolate mofetil in patients with systemic lupus erythematosus: a prospective pharmacokinetic study, Lupus 18 (5) (2009) 441–447.

657. M. Haubitz, F. Bohnenstengel, et al., Cyclophosphamide pharmacokinetics and dose requirements in patients with renal insufficiency, Kidney Int. 61 (4) (2002) 1495–1501.

673. M. Haubitz, S. Schellong, et al., Intravenous pulse administration of cyclophosphamide versus daily oral treatment in patients with antineutrophil cytoplasmic antibody-associated vasculitis and renal involvement: a prospective, randomized study, Arthritis Rheum. 41 (10) (1998) 1835–1844.

676. S. Pendse, E. Ginsburg, et al., Strategies for preservation of ovarian and testicular function after immunosuppression, Am. J. Kidney Dis. 43 (5) (2004) 772–781.

728. V. Gerloni, R. Cimaz, M. Gattinara, et al., Efficacy and safety profile of cyclosporin A in the treatment of juvenile chronic (idiopathic) arthritis: results of a 10-year prospective study, Rheumatology (Oxf.) 40 (2001) 907–913.

733. H. Tanaka, K. Tsugawa, et al., Treatment of difficult cases of systemic-onset juvenile idiopathic arthritis with tacrolimus, Eur. J. Pediatr. 166 (10) (2007) 1053–1055.

736. A. Ravelli, C. Moretti, F. Temporini, et al., Combination therapy with methotrexate and cyclosporine A in juvenile idiopathic arthritis, Clin. Exp. Rheumatol. 20 (2002) 569–572.

737. L.W. Fu, L.Y. Yang, et al., Clinical efficacy of cyclosporin a neoral in the treatment of paediatric lupus nephritis with heavy proteinuria, Br. J. Rheumatol. 37 (2) (1998) 217–221.

741. L.L. Ioannides-Demos, N. Christophidis, P. Ryan, et al., Dosing implications of a clinical interaction between grapefruit juice and cyclosporine and metabolite concentrations in patients with autoimmune diseases, J. Rheumatol. 24 (1997) 49–54.

743. S.B. Cohen, T.T. Cheng, et al., Evaluation of the efficacy and safety of papapimod, a p38 MAP kinase inhibitor, in a double-blind, methotrexate-controlled study of patients with active rheumatoid arthritis, Arthritis Rheum. 60 (2) (2009) 335–344.

744. T.H. Page, M. Smolinska, J. Gillespie, A.M. Urbaniak, B.M. Foxwell, Tyrosine kinases and inflammatory signalling, Curr. Mol. Med. 9 (2009) 69–85.

758. R.M. Oates-Whitehead, J.H. Baumer, L. Haines, Intravenous immunoglobulin for the treatment of Kawasaki disease in children, Cochrane Database Syst. Rev. 4 (2003) CD004000.

759. B.A. Lang, R.M. Laxer, G. Murphy, et al., Treatment of dermatomyositis with intravenous gammaglobulin, Am. J. Med. 91 (1991) 169–172.

764. E.D. Silverman, G.D. Cawkwell, D.J. Lovell, et al., Intravenous immunoglobulin in the treatment of systemic juvenile rheumatoid arthritis: a randomized placebo controlled trial. Pediatr. Rheumatol. Collaborative Study Group, J. Rheumatol. 21 (1994) 2353–2358.

770. S. Siberil, S. Elluru, et al., Intravenous immunoglobulins in autoimmune and inflammatory diseases: a mechanistic perspective, Ann. N. Y. Acad. Sci. 1110 (2007) 497–506.

771. V.S. Negi, S. Elluru, et al., Intravenous immunoglobulin: an update on the clinical use and mechanisms of action, J. Clin. Immunol. 27 (3) (2007) 233–245.

806. J.C. Edwards, M.J. Leandro, G. Cambridge, B lymphocyte depletion therapy with rituximab in rheumatoid arthritis, Rheum. Dis. Clin. North Am. 30 (2004) 393–403.

808. M.J. Leandro, G. Cambridge, et al., Reconstitution of peripheral blood B cells after depletion with rituximab in patients with rheumatoid arthritis, Arthritis Rheum. 54 (2) (2006) 613–620.

810. S.M. Sultan, K.P. Ng, et al., Clinical outcome following B cell depletion therapy in eight patients with refractory idiopathic inflammatory myopathy, Clin. Exp. Rheumatol. 26 (5) (2008) 887–893.

813. T.D. Levine, Rituximab in the treatment of dermatomyositis: an open-label pilot study, Arthritis Rheum. 52 (2) (2005) 601–607.

814. A. Thatayatikom, A.J. White, Rituximab: a promising therapy in systemic lupus erythematosus, Autoimmun. Rev. 5 (1) (2006) 18–24.

815. M.A. Cooper, D.L. Willingham, et al., Rituximab for the treatment of juvenile dermatomyositis: a report of four pediatric patients, Arthritis Rheum. 56 (9) (2007) 3107–3111.

821. O. Nwobi, C.L. Abitbol, et al., Rituximab therapy for juvenile-onset systemic lupus erythematosus, Pediatr. Nephrol. 23 (3) (2008) 413–419.

823. K.R. Carson, A.M. Evens, et al., Progressive multifocal leukoencephalopathy after rituximab therapy in HIV-negative patients: a report of 57 cases from the Research on Adverse Drug Events and Reports project, Blood 113 (20) (2009) 4834–4840.

826. D.J. Wallace, W. Stohl, et al., A phase II, randomized, double-blind, placebo-controlled, dose-ranging study of belimumab in patients with active systemic lupus erythematosus, Arthritis Rheum. 61 (9) (2009) 1168–1178.

833. D.J. Lovell, E.H. Giannini, A. Reiff, et al., Etanercept in children with polyarticular juvenile rheumatoid arthritis. Pediatric Rheumatology Collaborative Study Group, N. Engl. J. Med. 16 (2000) 763–769.

839. E.H. Giannini, N.T. Ilowite, et al., Long-term safety and effectiveness of etanercept in children with selected categories of juvenile idiopathic arthritis, Arthritis Rheum. 60 (9) (2009) 2794–2804.

855. S. Borte, U.G. Liebert, et al., Efficacy of measles, mumps and rubella revaccination in children with juvenile idiopathic arthritis treated with methotrexate and etanercept, Rheumatology (Oxford) 48 (2) (2009) 144–148.

859. J.J. Cush, Safety overview of new disease-modifying antirheumatic drugs, Rheum. Dis. Clin. North Am. 30 (2004) 237–255.

889. N.T. Ilowite, Update on biologics in juvenile idiopathic arthritis, Curr. Opin. Rheumatol. 20 (5) (2008) 613–618.

890. T. Levalampi, V. Honkanen, et al., Effects of infliximab on cytokines, myeloperoxidase, and soluble adhesion molecules in patients with juvenile idiopathic arthritis, Scand. J. Rheumatol. 36 (3) (2007) 189–193.

894. F. Wolfe, K. Michaud, J. Anderson, K. Urbansky, Tuberculosis infection in patients with rheumatoid arthritis and the effect of infliximab therapy, Arthritis Rheum. 50 (2004) 372–379.

907. E.C. Keystone, M.C. Genovese, et al., Golimumab, a human antibody to tumour necrosis factor {alpha} given by monthly subcutaneous injections, in active rheumatoid arthritis despite methotrexate therapy: the GO-FORWARD Study, Ann. Rheum. Dis. 68 (6) (2009) 789–796.

908. A. Kavanaugh, I. McInnes, et al., Golimumab, a new human tumor necrosis factor alpha antibody, administered every four weeks as a subcutaneous injection in psoriatic arthritis: Twenty-four-week efficacy and safety results of a randomized, placebo-controlled study, Arthritis Rheum. 60 (4) (2009) 976–986.

910. E. Keystone, B. Haraoui, Adalimumab therapy in rheumatoid arthritis, Rheum. Dis. Clin. North Am. 30 (2) (2004) 349–364. vii.

921. E. Keystone, D. Heijde, D. Mason Jr., et al., Certolizumab pegol plus methotrexate is significantly more effective than placebo plus methotrexate in active rheumatoid arthritis: findings of a fifty-two-week, phase III, multicenter, randomized, double-blind, placebo-controlled, parallel-group study, Arthritis Rheum. 58 (2008) 3319–3329.

922. R. Fleischmann, J. Vencovsky, et al., Efficacy and safety of certolizumab pegol monotherapy every 4 weeks in patients with rheumatoid arthritis failing previous disease-modifying antirheumatic therapy: the FAST4WARD study, Ann. Rheum. Dis. 68 (6) (2009) 805–811.

923. J. Smolen, R.B. Landewe, Efficacy and safety of certolizumab pegol plus methotrexate in active rheumatoid arthritis: the RAPID 2 study. A randomised controlled trial, Ann. Rheum. Dis. 68 (6) (2009) 797–804.

929. J. Askling, E. Baecklund, et al., Anti-tumour necrosis factor therapy in rheumatoid arthritis and risk of malignant lymphomas: relative risks and time trends in the Swedish Biologics Register, Ann. Rheum. Dis. 68 (5) (2009) 648–653.

930. www.fda.gov/drugs/drug safety/Postmarket Drug Safety Information for Patients and Providers/Drug Safety Information for Health Professionals/ucm174474.htm

931. TNF neutralization in MS: results of a randomized, placebo-controlled multicenter study. The Lenercept Multiple Sclerosis Study Group and The University of British Columbia MS/MRI Analysis Group, Neurology 53 (3) (1999) 457–465.

933. I.S. Shin, A.N. Baer, et al., Guillain-Barre and Miller Fisher syndromes occurring with tumor necrosis factor alpha antagonist therapy, Arthritis Rheum. 54 (5) (2006) 1429–1434.

935. M.D. Magnano, W.H. Robinson, et al., Demyelination and inhibition of tumor necrosis factor (TNF), Clin. Exp. Rheumatol. 22 (5 Suppl. 35) (2004) S134–S140.

937. D. Khanna, M. McMahon, D.E. Furst, Anti-tumor necrosis factor alpha therapy and heart failure: what have we learned and where do we go from here? Arthritis Rheum. 50 (2004) 1040–1050.

939. K.G. Saag, G.G. Teng, N.M. Patkar, et al., American College of Rheumatology 2008 recommendations for the use of nonbiologic and biologic disease-modifying antirheumatic drugs in rheumatoid arthritis, Arthritis Rheum. 59 (2008) 762–784.

940. S.B. Cohen, The use of anakinra, an interleukin-1 receptor antagonist, in the treatment of rheumatoid arthritis, Rheum. Dis. Clin. North Am. 30 (2004) 365–380.

946. N. Ilowite, O. Porras, et al., Anakinra in the treatment of poly-articular-course juvenile rheumatoid arthritis: safety and preliminary efficacy results of a randomized multicenter study, Clin. Rheumatol. 28 (2) (2009) 129–137.

947. J.W. Verbsky, A.J. White, Effective use of the recombinant inter- leukin 1 receptor antagonist anakinra in therapy resistant sys- temic onset juvenile rheumatoid arthritis, J. Rheumatol. 31 (10) (2004) 2071–2075.

950. P.I. Irigoyen, J. Olson, C. Hom, N.T. Ilowite, Treatment of sys- temic onset juvenile rheumatoid arthritis with anakinra, Arthritis Rheum. 40 (2004) S437–S438.

951. M. Henrickson, Efficacy of anakinra in refractory systemic arthritis, Arthritis Rheum. 40 (2004) S438.

956. C. Boschan, O. Witt, et al., Neonatal-onset multisystem inflam- matory disease (NOMID) due to a novel S331R mutation of the CIAS1 gene and response to interleukin-1 receptor antagonist treatment, Am. J. Med. Genet. A 140 (8) (2006) 883–886.

979. G. Jones, A. Sebba, et al., Comparison of tocilizumab monother- apy versus methotrexate monotherapy in patients with moder- ate to severe rheumatoid arthritis: The AMBITION study, Ann. Rheum. Dis. 2009.

983. N. Nishimoto, N. Miyasaka, et al., Long-term safety and effi- cacy of tocilizumab, an anti-interleukin-6 receptor monoclonal antibody, in monotherapy, in patients with rheumatoid arthritis (the STREAM study): evidence of safety and efficacy in a 5-year extension study, Ann. Rheum. Dis. 2008.

984. S. Yokota, T. Miyamae, T. Imagawa, et al., Phase II trial on anti- IL6-receptor antibody for children with systemic-onset juvenile idiopathic arthritis, Arthritis Rheum. 48 (2003) S429.

998. Lahdenne Vahasalo, Infliximab or etanercept in the treatment of children with refractory juvenile idiopathic arthritis: an open label study, Ann. Rheum. Dis. 62 (3) (2003) 245–247.

1000. A.V. Londino, D. Rothman, P.D. Robbins, C.H. Evans, Gene therapy for juvenile rheumatoid arthritis? J. Rheumatol. 27 (Suppl. 58) (2000) 53–55.

1017. N.M. Wulffraat, E.M. van Rooijen, et al., Current perspectives of autologous stem cell transplantation for severe juvenile idio- pathic arthritis, Autoimmunity 41 (8) (2008) 632–638.

1018. M. Abinun, TJ. Flood, AJ. Cant, et al., Autologous T cell depleted haematopoietic stem cell transplantation in children with severe juvenile idiopathic arthritis in the UK (2000-2007). Mol. Immunol. 2009.

1024. J.M. van Laar, A. Tyndall, Adult stem cells in the treatment of autoimmune diseases, Rheumatology. (Oxford) 45 (10) (2006) 1187–1193.

1029. R.M. Laxer, C. Harrison, Bioethical issues in autologous stem cell transplantation in children and adults with arthritis, J. Rheu- matol. 28 (2001) 2147–2150.

1031. B. Nishishinya, G. Urrutia, et al., Amitriptyline in the treatment of fibromyalgia: a systematic review of its efficacy, Rheumatol- ogy (Oxford) 47 (12) (2008) 1741–1746.

1034. C.S. Boomershine, L.J. Crofford, A symptom-based approach to pharmacologic management of fibromyalgia, Nat. Rev. Rheu- matol. 5 (4) (2009) 191–199.

1039. E. Serra, Duloxetine and pregabalin: safe and effective for the long-term treatment of fibromyalgia? Nat. Clin. Pract. Neurol. 4 (11) (2008) 594–595.

Entire reference list is available online at www.expertconsult.com.

Chapter 7

TRIAL DESIGN, MEASUREMENT, AND ANALYSIS OF CLINICAL INVESTIGATIONS

Hermine I. Brunner and Edward H. Giannini

EVIDENCE-BASED MEDICINE AND CLINICAL INVESTIGATION

Today, more than ever, clinicians are encouraged to practice *evidence-based medicine*. That is, the practitioner must be able to access, summarize, and apply information from the literature to day-to-day clinical problems.[1,2] How strong does the evidence need to be before a clinician modifies his or her practice because of new data in a clinical research report? The same question can be asked of any clinical or biomedical investigation, whether or not it applies to clinical practice. The strength of evidence depends on many factors, including the rigor of the study design; the selection of patients and appropriate controls; and the meticulousness and appropriateness with which the data were gathered, analyzed, interpreted, and reported. In addition, the similarity between the patients described in a study and the patients seen by a particular clinician is of utmost importance in determining its relevance.

The reader must be able to judge the quality of the work to determine its overall validity and the acceptability of the conclusions. The mere fact that the work has been published, even in a reputable journal, may not be enough of a benchmark whereby one decides that the work is of superior quality. Outstanding "Users' Guides to the Medical Literature" have now been published in book form,[3] and the reader is encouraged to supplement the discussion in this chapter with the appropriate Guide for a specific topic.

Any student of clinical research must be aware of the sizable obstacles currently facing the clinical research enterprise.[4,5] There seems to be a general consensus among medical scientists, public health policy makers, and the U.S. Congress that the remarkable advances in biotechnology that have been realized during the past 20 years have not translated at an acceptable rate into improved health status for the United States and the world in general. The situation is thought to be worsening as acquisition of basic science knowledge continues to accelerate. Clinical research is viewed as a continuum—beginning from basic biomedical research, progressing to clinical science and knowledge, eventuating in improved health of the public. Two "major transitional blocks" are identified that impede efforts to apply science to better human health in an expeditious fashion.

The first translational block occurs between basic biomedical research and clinical science and knowledge, and the second block occurs between clinical science and knowledge and improved health. Contributing factors to the first block include lack of study participants willing to participate in research, regulatory burden, fragmented infrastructure, incompatible databases, and a lack of qualified investigators. Contributing to the second block are career disincentives, practice limitations, high research costs, and lack of funding. These obstacles should remain foremost in the reader's mind, with the realization that the design and analysis of studies must be grounded in what is reasonable from logistical, practical, ethical, and economic point of view.

U.S. Food and Drug Administration and Critical Path Initiative for Drug Development

An advance to overcoming the above-mentioned obstacles may be seen in the Critical Path Initiative (CPI), which was announced in 2004 by the U.S. Food and Drug Administration (FDA). The CPI is designed to improve the *process* of drug and instrument development, the quality of evidence generated during development, and the eventual outcomes of use of these products in patients.[6] In brief, the CPI aims to overcome the drug development "pipeline problem" by advancing "the lagging science of drug development." The premise of the CPI is that scientific advances, such as sophisticated imaging technologies, genomics, and biomedical informatics, can accelerate the development process and speed clinically useful products down the pipeline, with the collaboration between private and public sectors.[7]

This chapter provides readers with enough clinical, epidemiological, and biostatistical skills to assess the literature critically and to determine independently the "strength of the evidence." It also promotes basic skills that facilitate the design, undertaking, and reporting of clinical research. Although this chapter emphasizes clinical research, many of the concepts discussed here are easily translated to the realm of basic science. Whether working in the laboratory or in the clinic, an investigator must understand basic concepts, such as frequency distributions and statistical inferences.

DEFINITION OF CLINICAL RESEARCH

Academicians have argued for years about exactly what is incorporated in the concept of clinical research. The Nathan Report defines clinical research as "studies of living human subjects, including the laboratory-based development of new forms of technology; studies of the mechanisms of human disease and evaluations of therapeutic interventions (which are known collectively as translational research); clinical trials, outcome studies, and health care research; and epidemiological and behavioral studies."[7] This area of research includes mechanisms of human disease, therapeutic interventions, clinical trials, and the development of new technologies. Human research, as per this definition, excludes in vitro studies that use human tissues, but do not deal directly with patients. Conversely, laboratory or translational research ("bench-to-bedside"), provided that the identity of the patients from whom the cells or tissues under study are derived is known, constitutes clinical research.

The National Institutes of Health (NIH) considers behavioral studies as a category of clinical research. This class of studies is not considered in this chapter. For special emphasis, this chapter considers clinical trials separately from epidemiological studies (see page 134).

GENERAL TERMINOLOGY AND BASIC CONCEPTS ASSOCIATED WITH CLINICAL STUDIES

To be conversant in clinical study designs and methodology, one needs a working knowledge of the vocabulary and basic concepts relevant to the various approaches. Readers must attempt to generalize the use of common terms from one type of study to the next. For example, "exposure" may mean that the subject was exposed to cigarette smoke in a retrospective case-comparison study, exposed to a drug in a clinical trial, or exposed to a particular mutation in a genetic study.

All clinical investigations may be divided broadly into observational or experimental studies. In observational studies, there is no artificial manipulation of any factor that is to be assessed in the study, and there is no active manipulation of the patient. In observational studies, the subjects have received the "etiological" agent by mechanisms other than active assignment or randomization. Examples of such mechanisms are self-imposed exposure (personal habits or nutritional patterns), prescription by a physician, atmospheric pollutants, and occupational toxins. Observational studies may be either retrospective or prospective. *Retrospective* implies that the data already exist and are retrieved using a systematic approach, but missing data are not retrievable or cannot be verified. In *prospective* observational studies, a cohort is observed prospectively through time, and data are gathered on an ongoing basis. In this case, missing data may possibly be retrieved for purposes of the study, and standardized methods of data verification can be employed. *Experimental studies* are studies in which the investigator artificially manipulates study factors or subjects, such as therapeutic regimen, or some other parameter. In experimental studies, the subjects are observed prospectively, some active maneuver is conducted, and the results of this maneuver are then observed.

Hypothesis-Generating versus Hypothesis-Testing Studies

The design of a clinical investigation depends on whether the study intends to generate hypotheses to be tested in future studies or to test specific hypotheses for which the investigator has some existing evidence to support the belief that they are true or not true. Hypothesis-generating studies are considered *exploratory*; studies that are designed as tests of hypotheses, for which there are preliminary data, are often called *pivotal* or *confirmatory* studies. A single study may have confirmatory and exploratory aspects. Each type of study has distinct advantages and disadvantages. The design chosen is always deeply influenced by reality—what is economically, logistically, ethically, and scientifically possible.

A common exercise used by methodologists is to design the best theoretical experiment to answer the question being posed, without regard to time, money, ethics, patient availability, or anything else that could cause a lessening in the quality of the study; a related approach is known as the *infinite data set*.[8] Realizing that there is no such thing as the perfect clinical study, the designer eliminates the most unrealistic "requirement." For example, it is not likely that one can enroll 300 patients with scleroderma who would agree to the possibility of being randomly assigned to a placebo for 1 year. The study is compromised further and further by reality until one arrives at what can be done in consideration of all the issues. If the resulting study design and its protocol are unacceptable scientifically, perhaps the question cannot (and should not) be answered. The decision to pursue or not to pursue the "compromised" study, based in reality, is one of the most difficult in the entire research process. One's rights as a clinical investigator are the exact opposite of one's constitutional rights as a citizen: the investigator (or the study) may be considered guilty (of anything and everything) until proven innocent by appropriate design and analytical technique.

Main Objectives, Process Objectives, Hypotheses, and Long-Term Goals

The first challenge after identifying a clinical question to be addressed is to establish clearly the main (or primary) objectives and the secondary objectives. *Objectives* are statements as to what the investigators plan to learn or accomplish by conducting the study. *Process objectives* follow the main objectives; they are the procedures that must be completed to meet the main objectives.

Hypotheses are then developed. *Hypotheses* are formal statements that declare what the investigator will test and then either reject or fail to reject, using appropriate statistical techniques. Exploratory (hypothesis-generating) studies may not state hypotheses a priori. Such studies frequently allow the data to drive the hypotheses to be tested in the data-exploration phase. Finally, longer term goals are stated. Often, these goals are to be met only after the main objectives of the current projects are complete. They frequently give a hint as to what future direction the research may take. Clinical research proposals often misstate hypotheses or mix main objectives (specific aims) with process objectives.

The following example may assist the reader in formulating each of these elements of a research proposal: Suppose the question is, "Does the selective cyclooxygenase-2 inhibitor, celecoxib, produce fewer gastrointestinal (GI) adverse effects in children with juvenile idiopathic arthritis (JIA) than naproxen when each drug is given in antiinflammatory doses for a period of 3 months?" The objectives are typically written nonjudgmentally and are more informal in their language than the hypotheses. A primary objective for this project could be, "To determine the incidence of GI side effects among patients with JIA treated for 3 months with celecoxib compared with naproxen." Equally acceptable (but less distinguished from the statement of hypothesis) is, "To test the hypothesis that celecoxib produces fewer GI side effects than naproxen in children with JIA." A secondary objective could be, "To determine the incidence of GI events requiring pharmacological intervention in the two groups and compare the differences." "To enroll 250 patients with JIA in a clinical trial in which one-half are randomly assigned to celecoxib and one-half to naproxen" would be the *process objective*—one of the necessary steps that will be carried out to meet the main objective.

Even large studies typically have only one or two main objectives and accompanying hypotheses. Usually, the *null hypothesis* (H_0) is that the treatments are not different with regard to the primary outcome. H_0 can be stated as, "There is no difference in the incidence of GI side effects among patients treated with naproxen compared with patients treated with celecoxib." The alternative hypothesis (H_a) is, "There is a difference in the incidence of GI adverse drug effects." As stated, the H_a does not specify whether there are more or fewer GI effects with celecoxib. This is a two-tailed hypothesis. A one-tailed hypothesis could be stated as follows: "Patients with JIA treated with celecoxib will have a lower incidence of GI adverse drug effects than patients treated with naproxen." This hypothesis sounds, however, as if the investigator is not interested in testing to see whether celecoxib produces more GI effects, just less. For this reason, the usual approach is to use two-tailed hypotheses, at least in early studies when the direction of the difference (if any) is unknown.

The choice of a one-tailed as opposed to a two-tailed hypothesis influences the statistical interpretation of the data, as discussed later. A secondary null hypothesis in this example might be, "There is no difference in the incidence of GI adverse drug events that require pharmacological intervention among patients with JIA treated with celecoxib compared with patients treated with naproxen." Finally, the longer term goal of the research in this example is not, "To complete the study in a 5-year time frame," but rather, "To provide information on the long-term safety and effectiveness of antiinflammatory medications when used in children with JIA."

EPIDEMIOLOGICAL STUDIES

Clinical epidemiology is a medical science that studies the distribution and determinants of disease frequency in human populations to understand why some people contract a disease and others do not. Epidemiology, combined with biostatistics, makes up the basic tools of the clinical investigator. Epidemiological methods can be used to answer questions in the following categories.

Descriptive Epidemiology

Studies in descriptive epidemiology typically concern themselves with patterns of disease occurrence with respect to person, place, or time. Descriptive epidemiological studies serve as hypothesis-generating studies for studies of causation, much the same way as small exploratory clinical trials serve as preliminary studies for therapeutic confirmatory trials. The *person variable* is concerned with who experiences the disease. A basic tenet is that the disease does not occur at random, but is more likely to develop in some people than in others. Personal factors of potential importance include age, sex, race, ethnicity, socioeconomic status, existing morbidity, health habits, genetics, and epigenetics. (The last refers to heritable alterations in gene expression caused by mechanisms other than changes in DNA sequence.) The *place factor* is concerned with where the disease develops. Variation in place of occurrence can be evaluated at the local, regional, or international level. The *time variable* is concerned with variation in the occurrence of disease in time and its seasonality or periodicity.

A hypothetical example of a descriptive epidemiological study is the investigation of a group of workers in a factory who have what is suspected to be environmentally acquired lupus. The epidemiologist would investigate the detailed characteristics of the workers to determine whether there are patterns among the workers who do and do not have lupus. Do all types of workers (management through hourly manufacturing employees) show the same rate of disease development? Are people living close to the factory or its effluent affected? Systematic investigation of the patterns of disease allows a more precise hypothesis of causation, particularly if some exposure or dose level is found to be more strongly associated with the illness.

Frequency of Disease Occurrence

The frequency of disease occurrence is an important aspect of understanding a disease process. It can be measured in numerous ways. *Prevalence* is the total number of existing cases in a defined population at risk of developing a disease either at a point in time or during some time period (see later). Mathematically, prevalence is equal to the number of existing cases divided by the number of persons in the population at risk of developing the disease. Persons with the disease are subtracted from the denominator because they are no longer at risk of developing it. Prevalence is expressed in different ways: as a proportion (0 to 1), as a percentage (0 to 100), or by actual numbers using a convenient denominator (e.g., cases per 1000 children). Prevalence should be distinguished from a simple, absolute number of cases, which has no denominator.

Point prevalence is the number of new and old cases in a defined population at a given "instant" in time. Hospital epidemiologists frequently are asked to estimate the point prevalence of nosocomial infections among current inpatients. The epidemiologist counts all the confirmed and suspected cases of hospital-acquired infections within the hospital on a given day and divides this total by the census for that day to obtain the point prevalence. *Period prevalence* is the number of new and old cases that exist in a defined population during a given time period (e.g., 1 year).

Incidence is the rate at which newly diagnosed cases develop over time in a population. Mathematically, incidence is equal to the number of new cases (numerator) divided by the number of persons at risk in the population multiplied by the time (duration) of observation (denominator). This rate is expressed in units of cases/person-time. Incidence is related to the concept of risk, defined as the proportion of unaffected individuals who, on average, contract the disease over a specific period. Risk is equal to the number of new cases divided by the number of persons at risk. Risk has no units and can have values between 0 (no new occurrences) and 1 (the entire population becomes affected during the risk period). Epidemiological theory states that incidence is best estimated from prospective studies; prevalence may be calculated by prospective or retrospective approaches.

Prognosis refers to the possible outcomes of a disease and the frequency with which they can be expected to occur. Prognostic factors need not cause the outcome, but must merely be associated with an outcome strongly enough to predict it. Prognosis is narrower in focus and more short term in aspect than the consequences of disease and treatment that are considered in the field of outcomes research. The six most frequently measured outcomes in outcomes research are known as the six *D*s: death, disease, disability, discomfort, dissatisfaction, and dollars. Many studies of prognosis are cohort studies that prospectively monitor large numbers of patients to determine eventual clinical events and then look for certain prognostic factors for the events. At present and in the past, the estimation of prognosis has largely concentrated on clinical variables. Studies of prognosis in JIA have included the sex of the patient, the age at onset, and a variety of clinical and laboratory variables to estimate outcome.[9-11]

Genetics, genomics, and microarrays to study RNA expression (and the accompanying new technologies of informatics and computational medicine) are being investigated more intensely to delineate their ability to predict outcome.[12-19] Pharmacogenetics is a way to determine the probability of response or adverse reaction to certain drugs. An example in rheumatology may be thiomethyl purine transferase enzyme testing before azathioprine therapy.[20]

Etiology of Disease

In his presidential address to the Royal Society of Medicine in January 1965, Hill gave his now famous speech entitled, "The Environment and Disease: Association or Causation."[21] Hill described what have become known as *Koch's postulates for epidemiologists*. These postulates describe what evidence must be present to establish a factor as being causally linked to a disease and include the following:

- *Strength of the association*: How strong is the association between the factor and the outcome? For example, how significant is the probability (*P*) value of the association between dietary intake of calcium and bone mineral density among children with JIA?
- *Consistency of the association*: Does the association between factor and disease persist from one study to the next, even if variations in study design and samples of patients vary substantially?
- *Specificity of the association*: Is the association limited to specific alleles and types of disease, with little association between the alleles and other diseases? As the study of causation has advanced, including genetic risk, the issue of specificity is considered less important than it previously was.
- *Temporal correctness*: Did the exposure to the factor occur before the disease? Temporal correctness becomes more difficult to establish in diseases with extended time intervals between exposure and the onset of clinical manifestations of the disease.
- *Biological gradient*: Is there a dose-response relationship between the factor and the disease? Does increasing the dose or time of exposure to cyclophosphamide result in a subsequent increase in frequency of malignancy?
- *Biological plausibility*: Does the association make sense with what is currently understood about the disease and its pathogenesis?
- *Experiment*: Does the association hold up under experimental conditions? If one reduces the dose or time of exposure to cyclophosphamide, is there a corresponding decrease in the frequency of malignancy?

No single study can prove indisputably that a potential etiological factor causes a disease, complication, or adverse event. The accumulating body of knowledge concerning factor and disease, or (to generalize the terms) treatment and outcome, finally allows the medical community to state that evidence is sufficient to prove a causal link between the two.

An important concept in the study of disease etiology is *relative risk*. The relative risk (also risk ratio) can be defined as the risk of developing a disease among the members of one group (e.g., boys) compared with another group (e.g., girls). Relative risk can range from zero to infinity and has no units. A relative risk of "1" means that there is no difference in risk between the groups. A relative risk greater than "1" means increased risk, and a relative risk less than "1" indicates decreased risk (protection). In pediatric rheumatology, the concept of risk is used frequently to specify increased or decreased risk of disease associated with certain genetic markers. A risk ratio used frequently in genetic studies is lambda, indicating familial aggregation of cases and, indirectly, genetic risk. An example is lambda$_{sibling}$ (λ_s), calculated as the prevalence of a disorder in biological siblings of individuals with the disease divided by the prevalence of the disease in the general population. The λ_s for systemic lupus erythematosus (SLE) has been estimated to be 30, meaning that a sibling of an individual with SLE is 30 times more likely to develop SLE than a member of the general population.[22] *LOD scores (logarithm of odds)* are statistics distinct from λ_s and are commonly used to estimate genetic linkage in families between generic traits, or biomarkers, and genetic traits, or more than one biomarker.

Table 7–1 presents terms that are relevant to risk and shows how each may be calculated using a 2 × 2 contingency table. Disease state (present or absent) is considered the dependent variable and is usually placed in the columns (x-axis). The risk factor (positive or negative) is considered the independent variable and is usually placed in the rows (y-axis). The relative risk is calculated differently from the *odds ratio*, although in medicine the two are frequently used synonymously. More correctly, relative risk is calculated from incidence studies, whereas odds ratios are calculated from retrospective studies.

Diagnosis of Disease and Classification Criteria

The diagnosis of disease, as it applies to epidemiology, refers to the performance of screening and diagnostic tests used in populations, rather than the process of differential diagnosis of individual patients. Classification criteria typically employ a set of "core variables" fashioned into an algorithm. Examples include criteria for flare of JIA,

criteria for improvement in juvenile idiopathic myopathies and lupus, and preliminary criteria for clinical remission in JIA.[23-26]

Validity of a Diagnostic or Screening Test or Criteria

The validity of a diagnostic or screening test or set of criteria involves various parameters, as shown in Table 7–2. The table typically is constructed with the presence or absence of disease as the column labels (i.e., x-axis) and the test results as the row labels (i.e., y-axis). The patients in row 1, column 1, are called true positives; patients in row 1, column 2, are false positives; patients in row 2, column 1, are false negatives; and patients in row 2, column 2, are true negatives. *Sensitivity, specificity, positive* and *negative predictive values, false-positive* and *false-negative rates,* and *reliability* are terms used to describe the validity of a screening test.

A widely used tool that allows one to compare visually the performance of a set of different criteria, or different cut points for a diagnostic or screening test, is known as the *receiver operating characteristic (ROC) curve* (Fig. 7–1). First used in industrial engineering, an ROC curve is a plot of the true-positive rate against the false-positive rate—sensitivity on the y-axis and (1 – specificity) on the x-axis. The overall quality of a test can be summarized by the *area under the ROC curve,* which ranges between 0 and 1. The larger the area under the ROC curve of a test is, the more accurately the test predicts the disease, in terms of sensitivity and specificity. An ROC curve provides information about several parameters: It shows the tradeoff between sensitivity and specificity for different criteria or cut points; the nearer the curve follows the left upper corner of the ROC space, the more accurate the test is. Conversely, the closer the curve approaches to the 45-degree diagonal of the ROC space, the less accurate the test is. Tests with an area of 0.5 or lower are no better than chance to predict whether the disease is present or not and should not be ordered by clinicians. ROC

Table 7–1		
Terms associated with risk factors and disease		
Risk Factor	**Disease Present**	**Disease Absent**
Positive	a	b
Negative	c	d
The 2 × 2 table may be used to calculate associations between the risk factor and the disease		
Term	**Calculation**	**Meaning**
Incidence	(a + c) /(a + b + c + d)	Number of new cases among those at risk
Absolute risk	—	Synonymous with incidence
Attributable risk	[a /(a + b)] – [c /(c + d)]	Incidence among those with the risk factor *minus* incidence among those without the risk factor (sometimes expressed as a percentage of the incidence rate among those with the risk factor)
Relative risk	(a /[a + b]) ÷ (c /[c + d])	Incidence among those exposed *divided by* incidence among those not exposed
Odds ratio	(a × d) /(b × c)	Approximation to the relative risk used in retrospective studies
Case exposure rate	a /(a + c)	Among those *with* the disease, the proportion who had the risk factor
Control exposure rate	b /(b + d)	Among those *without* the disease, the proportion who had the risk factor

Table 7–2

Estimating the validity of a diagnostic test

Test Result	Disease Present	Disease Absent
Positive	True positive (TP)	False positive (FP)
Negative	False negative (FN)	True negative (TN)

The 2 × 2 table may be used calculate measures of the test's validity

Term	Calculation	Meaning
Sensitivity	TP /(TP + FN)	Proportion (or percentage) of persons *with* the disease who test *positive*
Specificity	TN /(TN + FP)	Proportion (or percentage) of persons *without* the disease who test *negative*
Positive predictive value	TP /(TP + FP)	Proportion (or percentage) of persons who test positive who *have* the disease
False-positive rate	FP /(TP + FP)	Proportion (or percentage) of persons who test positive who *do not have* the disease
Negative predictive value	TN /(TN + FN)	Proportion (or percentage) of persons who test negative who *do not have* the disease
False-negative rate	FN /(TN + FN)	Proportion (or percentage) of persons who test negative who *have* the disease
Reliability (also called reproducibility)	—	The ability of a test to yield the same result on retesting

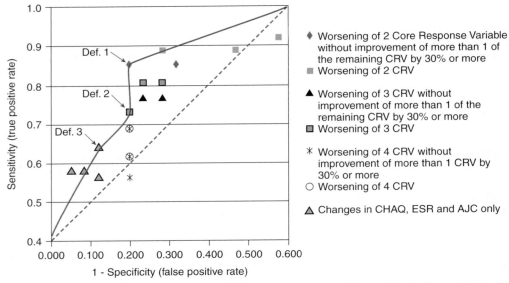

FIGURE 7–1 The receiver operating characteristic (ROC) curve, a plot of the true-positive rate versus false-positive rate (i.e., sensitivity on the *y*-axis, and 1 minus specificity on the *x*-axis). Sensitivity and specificity range between 0 and 1 (or 0% and 100%). ROCs allow one to observe the tradeoff between sensitivity and specificity at various cut points of a diagnostic test. Tests of a certain outcome (disease) with ROC curves that are 45-degree diagonals have an area under the ROC curve of 0.5. These tests are not useful for predicting the outcome (diagnosing the disease). (Modified from Brunner HI, et al: Preliminary definition of disease flare in juvenile rheumatoid arthritis, *J Rheumatol* 29:1058-1064, 2002.) AJC, active joint count; CHAQ, childhood health assessment questionnaire; CRV, core response variable; ESR, erythrocyte sedimentation rate.

analysis is now commonly used in the rheumatology literature to assess the quality of new criteria, diagnostic tests, or predictive tests.[27-29]

Epidemiological Study Designs Aimed at Establishment of Associations and Cause-Effect Relationships

Case-Controlled Retrospective Study

One of the most common types of study designs used to establish an association, or a cause-effect relationship, is an observational case-controlled retrospective study. The term *case-comparison* is now frequently used because the studies are not controlled in the usual sense. In this setting, patients who have the disease are compared with patients who do not have the disease, and data documenting prior exposure to some agent are ascertained retrospectively. The most frequent statistic to come from this type of study is the *odds ratio* (see Table 7–1). The odds ratio is a fairly good estimate of the relative risk, provided that the disease is rare. Patients included in the study are often identified from a search of medical records or a disease registry. There are no standard guidelines for selection of control subjects. The choice of an appropriate control group is crucial, however, to allow for the correct inferences to be made with respect to the importance of a prior exposure. Controls are chosen with the intent to adjust for person, socioeconomic, or environmental factors that may influence the development of a disease besides the "exposure" whose importance is being assessed by the case-control study. Federal and international guidelines in the selection of proper control groups exist.[30,31]

Advantages of case-controlled studies include efficiency, low cost, quick results, and low risk to study subjects. There are several disadvantages of case-controlled studies, however. The temporal relationship of exposure and disease may be obscured. Historical information may be incomplete, inaccurate, or not verifiable; a detailed study of mechanisms of disease is often impossible; and if the study is not well done, results may be biased. Adjustment for covariates is often impossible.

Prospective Cohort Study

The observational approach that most closely resembles an experiment is the prospective cohort study. In this study, a population is defined from which the sample is drawn. Exposure to some factor is established, and subjects are categorized as having been either "exposed" or "not exposed" to a factor thought to contribute risk of some outcome. Each of the two cohorts is monitored prospectively to observe whether the outcome develops. Relative risk is the statistic most commonly used in describing this study. The identification of exposed persons presents several problems. The first is to identify the exposed persons correctly and measure the degree of exposure. This may be done by selecting subjects with some type of unusual occupational or environmental exposure. Another method is selecting subjects who are available and suitable for the needed investigation or selecting subjects who offer some special resource that facilitates the study, such as members of a health plan, or a combination of all these factors.

The advantages of a prospective observational cohort study are that a clear temporal relationship between exposure and disease is established, and the study may yield information about the length of induction (incubation) of the disease. Relative risk can be estimated directly. The design facilitates the study of rare exposures and allows calculation of rates of disease occurrence.

The disadvantages of cohort studies include the potential for loss to follow-up or alteration of behavior because of the long follow-up time that may be necessary. Cohort studies are not particularly good for rare diseases when the outcome is onset of the disease. Detailed studies of the mechanisms of the disease typically are impossible in cohort studies.

A rheumatological example of a cohort study designed to detect disease causation is the study by Inman and associates,[32] who prospectively observed a cohort of persons "exposed" to *Salmonella typhimurium* infection to determine whether reactive arthritis developed. Prospective cohorts also are useful in pediatric rheumatology when the aim is to identify risk factors for development of certain complications or outcomes in a group of children who, typically, have the same disease but vary in predictor or risk variables.[9,33-35]

HEALTH SERVICES RESEARCH

The field of health services research (HSR) was created in the 1960s. Since that time, HSR has evolved to encompass multiple disciplinary perspectives, including methods from cognate disciplines such as economics, statistics, political science, and sociology, and many other schools of thought. The field has also developed new models and techniques to address research questions in specialized areas of inquiry, such as patient safety and access to care. HSR can be defined as the multidisciplinary field of scientific investigation that studies how social factors, financing systems, organizational structures and processes, health technologies, and personal behaviors affect access to health care, the quality and cost of health care, and ultimately individual health and well-being. Research domains are individuals, families, organizations, institutions, communities, and populations.[36]

HSR uses a multitude of methods and techniques, and in the following section the ones commonly or increasingly used in pediatric rheumatology are summarized. A comprehensive list can be found at http://www.hsrmethods.org. Among the key methods of HSR are *systematic reviews,* which are a summary of the literature that uses explicit methods to perform a thorough literature search and critical appraisal of individual studies to identify valid and applicable evidence. Systematic reviews summarize the existing evidence and identify gaps in the current knowledge and are often considered the prerequisite for metaanalyses, which provides a quantitative summary of empirical findings derived from research studies with related hypotheses. The Cochrane Collaboration is an international not-for-profit and independent organization dedicated to making up-to-date, accurate information about the effects of health care readily available worldwide. It produces and disseminates systematic reviews of health care interventions and promotes the search for evidence in the form of clinical trials and other studies of interventions (http://www.cochrane.org).[37]

Metaanalysis is a statistical procedure for synthesizing quantitative results from different studies. Metaanalysis can be used to overcome problems of reduced statistical power of smaller studies, making it a powerful analytical technique. The standard estimates derived by metaanalytic methods are combined probability and average effect size for a set of studies, the stability of these results, and the factors associated with differential treatment outcomes. Common potential shortcomings of metaanalyses that need consideration when performing or interpreting their results include a nonbiased selection of studies; consideration of data quality; their potential conceptual, methodological, and statistical flaws; a possible lack of independence among the studies; and differences in the outcomes reported. Despite these potential shortcomings, metaanalysis is a valid approach to overcome issues of reduced power because of a small study population. Important metaanalyses that have influenced medical decisions in rheumatology include those of the cyclooxygenase-2 inhibitor rofecoxib, which ultimately led to the withdrawal of the product from the market.[38]

Decision analysis is another HSR method that is aimed at supporting evidence-based medical decision making under conditions of imperfect knowledge. Decision analysis is a means of making complicated medical decisions by including all of the factors that could possibly affect the outcome. Decision analysis uses the form of a decision tree as a diagrammatic representation of the possible outcomes and events that are considered in the decision analytical model. Decision analysis itself includes outlining the problem, laying out the options and possible outcomes in explicit detail, assessing the probabilities and values of each outcome, and selecting the "best choice."

Cost-effectiveness analyses are special types of decision analyses that address questions of treatment cost in conjunction with health outcomes. Cost-effectiveness analyses are often done to assess whether the additional costs of new medications are worth paying by the society. A value often mentioned is the *incremental cost-effectiveness ratio (ICER)*, which compares the differences between the costs and health outcomes of two alternative medications and is generally described as the additional cost per additional health outcome. The ICER numerator includes the differences in medication costs, averted disease costs, or averted productivity losses, if applicable. Similarly, the ICER denominator is the difference in health outcomes. Examples of the use of decision analytical tools for supporting rheumatological treatment decision making include how to treat best a child with monarticular JIA,[39] and the cost-effectiveness analysis of the use of biological agents for the treatment of rheumatoid arthritis.[31]

Outcomes research is part of HSR and designed to evaluate the impact of health care on health or economic outcomes. Large population-level data sets are often used to conduct outcomes research, although primary data collection is sometimes conducted. Where large data sets are used, these are often gleaned from administrative or financial data, which may not be ideal for research purposes. Outcomes research includes *pharmacovigilance* (i.e., the process of detecting, assessing, understanding, and preventing adverse effects of approved drugs), and data from postmarketing reports, including adverse drug event reports, are used.

HSR also includes treatment *guideline and benchmark development* to standardize therapies and obtain quality parameters for treatment effectiveness. Other key areas of HSR research are the development and validation of classification and response of disease outcome measures. Clinicians know that not all patients who are diagnosed with rheumatic diseases really have them. Determining whether patients truly have improved, and by how much their disease changes, may also be difficult. Classification criteria allow clinical researchers to recruit patients with similar diseases (e.g., rheumatoid arthritis or SLE) into studies. Response criteria help to determine whether treatments really work (i.e., whether they actually produce clinically important improvement). As the science of clinical research advances, we must update our standards for considering classification and response criteria. Disease outcome measures allow the comparison of patients in a standardized fashion.

Details of how to develop and validate classification and response criteria and outcome measures in terms of their reliability, validity, and diagnostic accuracy can be found elsewhere.[3,40,41]

PATIENT-ORIENTED RESEARCH

The NIH definition of clinical research groups four categories of investigation under the major heading of patient-oriented research: mechanisms of human disease, therapeutic interventions, clinical trials, and development of new technologies. This chapter emphasizes clinical trial classification and methods. Many of the concepts and much of the terminology presented herein can be generalized to the conduct of clinical studies in any of these four areas of clinical research.

Regulatory Affairs and Clinical Trials: Useful Guidelines

For simplicity, the generic term *drug* is used in the following discussions. It should be considered synonymous with any medicinal product, vaccine, or biologic agent. The principles discussed can also apply to interventional procedures such as surgery and radiotherapy. Clinical epidemiologists are frequently concerned with evaluating the effectiveness and safety of new therapies.

Before discussing patient-oriented research, a brief introduction into basic terminology associated with regulatory affairs and associated activities is essential. The Code of Federal Regulations of the FDA, and in particular Title 21 (Food and Drug), is the most relevant to clinical researchers. Regulatory activities for clinical research are described in the *Good Clinical Practice (GCP)* guidance developed by the *International Conference on Harmonisation of Technical Requirements for Registration of Pharmaceuticals for Human Use (ICH)*. The ICH GCPs represent an international quality standard that various regulatory agencies around the world can transpose into regulations for conducting clinical research. The GCPs include guidelines for human rights protection and how clinical trials should be conducted, and define the responsibilities and roles of clinical investigators and sponsors. Links to relevant guidance documents for clinical researchers can be found most quickly at the website of the FDA[42] and the website of the ICH.[43]

Numerous other useful FDA and ICH guidance documents are in the literature and should be consulted for a more detailed explanation of the principles outlined here. Of particular relevance to pediatric rheumatologists is the FDA document entitled, "Guidance for Industry: Clinical Development Programs for Drugs, Devices and Biological Products for the Treatment of Rheumatoid Arthritis."[44] This document summarizes the position of the FDA on what clinical development programs should consist of, and it provides a framework for conducting studies used to obtain regulatory agency approval of therapies for rheumatoid arthritis or JIA.

Classification of Clinical Trials by Initiator, INDs, NDAs, and BLAs

Before general and specific considerations for individual trials can be discussed, an understanding of the various systems of classification of clinical trials is essential. Clinical trials may be initiated either by industry or by an individual investigator. Trials that are part of a clinical development program and conducted under a sponsor's (pharmaceutical company's) *investigational new drug* (IND) submission are usually initiated by industry. Trials undertaken under a sponsor's IND are used frequently by the sponsor in its submission to obtain approval for a new drug, known in the United States and elsewhere as *a new drug application* (NDA). If the NDA is approved by the regulatory agency, the drug may be marketed and labeled for the specific indication (i.e., disease or conditions) stated in the NDA. If the new agent is a biotechnology-derived pharmaceutical, such as a monoclonal antibody, the company files a Biologic License Application (BLA), which is analogous to an NDA for conventional drugs.

Investigator-initiated protocols are typically, but not always, conducted after the drug has been approved for market. The main objective of investigator-initiated protocols may be new dosage regimens or use in diseases other than that for which the drug has obtained an indication. Many such trials are exploratory rather than confirmatory. Funding for investigator-initiated protocols in pediatric rheumatology has come from the NIH, the FDA, manufacturers, foundations, and the European Union.

Classification of Clinical Trials by Phase

Clinical drug development programs are often described as consisting of four temporal phases, numbered I through IV. This system of classification, despite its shortcomings, is perhaps the one most commonly used today by the pharmaceutical industry and by regulatory agencies (Fig. 7–2).[45]

Phase I

Phase I studies are human pharmacology trials whose overall aim is to establish preliminary safety and tolerability of the dose range expected to be needed for later clinical studies and to determine adverse drug effects that can be expected. Studies in this phase include single-dose and multiple-dose administration schedules and have one or more of the following aspects.

PHARMACOKINETICS

Pharmacokinetics studies typically determine the drug's absorption, distribution, metabolism, and excretion pathways. Pharmacokinetics may progress throughout a

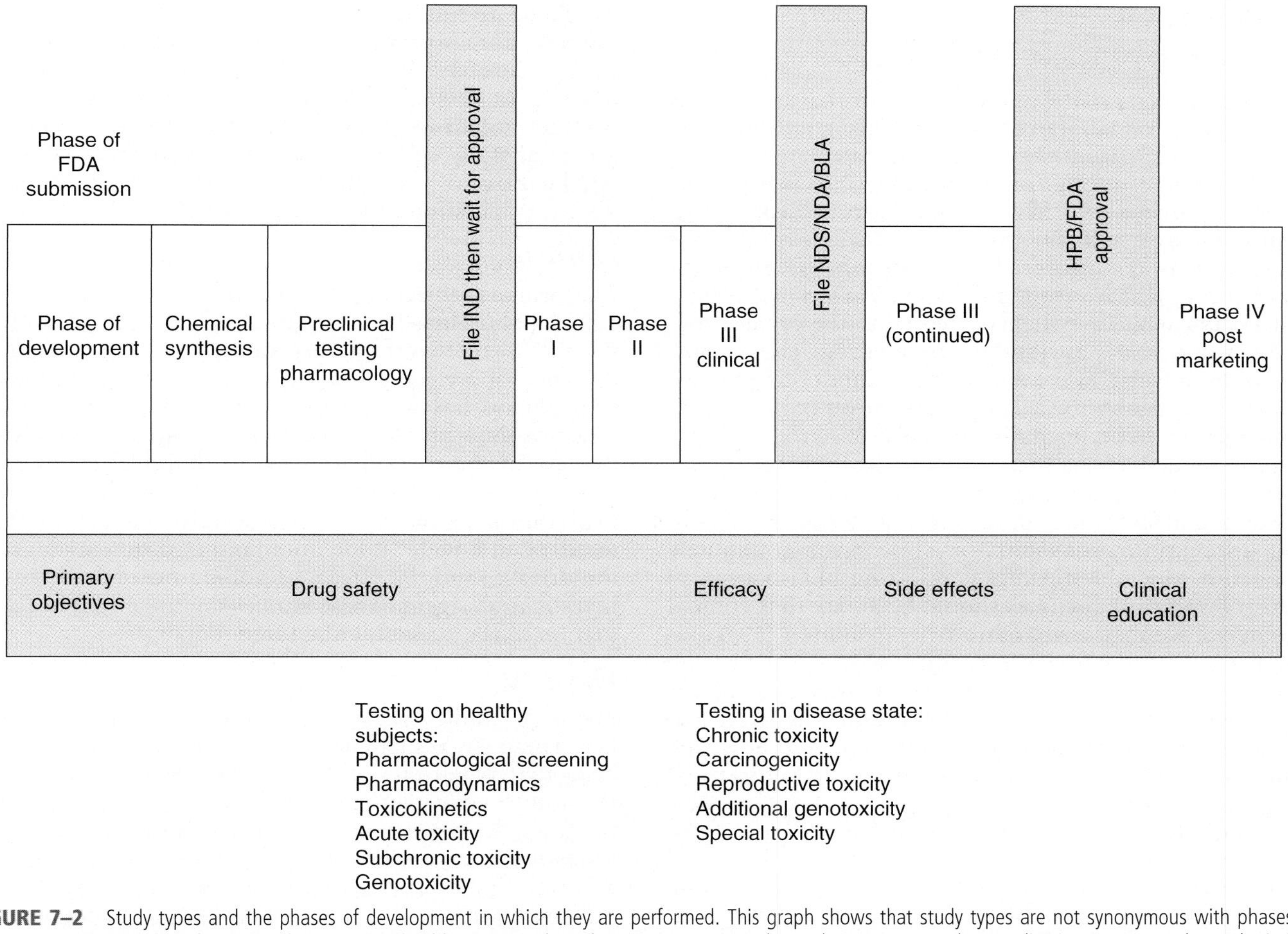

FIGURE 7–2 Study types and the phases of development in which they are performed. This graph shows that study types are not synonymous with phases of development. BLA, biologic license application; HPB, health protection branch; IND, investigational new drug; NDA, new drug application; NDS, new drug submission.

clinical development program and be assessed in separate studies or as part of larger trials to determine efficacy and safety. These studies are necessary to assess the clearance of the drug and to anticipate possible accumulation of the drug or its metabolites and the potential for drug-drug interactions. Assessing pharmacokinetics in subpopulations, such as those with impaired renal function or hepatic failure, is another important aspect of this phase of studies. Pharmacokinetics data are usually expressed using the following terms:[46]

- *Area under the time-concentration curve* (AUC, or AUC_{0-24} if done over a 24-hour period) is a measure of the total amount of drug absorbed; it is frequently estimated after the drug has reached steady-state levels.
- *Peak concentration* (C_{max}) is the maximum concentration reached at a particular dosage.
- *Time to peak concentration* (T_{max}) is used together with C_{max} to measure the rate of absorption.
- *Cumulative percentage of drug recovered* ($A_c\%$) usually relates to urine data and is the cumulative amount of drug recovered over a specific period (e.g., 24 hours) divided by the initial dose.
- *Elimination (or terminal) half-life* ($t_{(1/2)}$) is a measure of how long it takes to clear a drug from the system; it can be estimated by dividing 0.693 by the absolute value of the slope of the terminal linear phase of the concentration profile plotted on a semilog scale.

ESTIMATION OF INITIAL SAFETY AND TOLERABILITY

Drug safety refers to the frequency of adverse drug effects (i.e., physical or laboratory toxicity that could possibly be related to the drug) that are treatment emergent—that is, they emerge during treatment and were not present before treatment, or they become worse during treatment compared with the pretreatment state. An *adverse drug effect* is distinguished from an *adverse event* (or experience), which refers to any untoward experience that occurs while a patient is receiving the medication, whether or not it is attributable to the drug. The seriousness of an adverse event dictates how quickly it must be reported to regulatory agencies and to others who may have ongoing experimental protocols. A *serious adverse event* is defined as one that results in death, is life-threatening, requires inpatient hospitalization or prolongation of existing hospitalization, results in persistent or significant disability or incapacity, or is a congenital anomaly or birth defect. Investigators conducting pharmaceutical industry–sponsored studies should be aware that companies may have their own, more strict definition of serious adverse events. The term *severity* is distinguished from *serious* in that *severity* refers to the intensity of a specific event, whereas *serious* refers to the outcome or consequences of the event. *Drug tolerability* refers to how well subjects are able to tolerate overt adverse drug effects.

ASSESSMENT OF PHARMACODYNAMICS

Pharmacodynamics is the study of the physiological effects of drugs on the body and the mechanisms of drug action. These studies also typically observe the relationship of drug blood levels to clinical response or to adverse drug events. They may provide early estimates of drug activity and potential efficacy, and they help to establish the dosage regimen used in later phases of drug development.

EARLY ASSESSMENT OF DRUG ACTIVITY

Although early assessment of drug activity is not part of human pharmacology, phase I studies also may determine preliminary efficacy in terms of secondary variables that may be confirmed in later studies.

Phase II

Phase II studies are the earliest attempt to establish efficacy in the intended patient population. Many are called therapeutic exploratory studies and form the basis for later trials. The hypotheses may be less well defined than in later studies, and they may be data driven. The designs are flexible so that changes can be made as the data accumulate.

These studies may use a variety of different types of study design, including comparisons with baseline status or concurrent controls. In these studies, the eligibility criteria are typically very narrow, leading to a homogeneous population that is carefully monitored for safety. Further studies may establish the drug's safety and efficacy in a broader population after it is determined that a drug does have activity. These studies may also aim to determine more exactly the doses and regimens for later studies. Phase II studies may use dose-escalation designs to estimate dose response, which may be confirmed in later studies. In phase II, doses of the drug are typically, but not always, less than the highest doses used in phase I. Another important goal of phase II studies is to determine potential study end points, therapeutic regimens (including the use of concurrent medications), and subsets of the disease population (mild versus severe).

Phase III

The primary objective of phase III studies is to confirm a therapeutic benefit. The most typical kind of study is the therapeutic confirmatory study, which provides firm evidence of an agent's efficacy and safety. This type of trial always has a predefined hypothesis that is tested. These studies also estimate (with substantial precision) the size of the treatment effect attributable to the drug. Also incorporated in phase III development are further exploration of the dose-response relationship, study of the drug in a wider population and in different stages of the disease, and the effects of adding other drugs to the investigatory agent. These studies continue to add information to the accumulating safety database.

Phase IV

Phase IV studies begin after the drug reaches the market. These studies extend the prior demonstration of the drug's safety, efficacy, and dose. The most frequent phase IV study is one of therapeutic use, which goes beyond the prior demonstration of the drug's safety and efficacy. These studies show how the drug performs when used in the everyday setting, by patients who may have comorbid conditions or are taking a host of concurrent medications or both. Phase IV postmarketing surveillance and pharmacovigilance studies aim to accumulate longer term safety data from large numbers of subjects followed for extended periods, even after the drug has been discontinued in the patient. An example of the importance of postmarketing surveillance studies is the discovery of the association between rofecoxib use and increased risk of cardiac events. The FDA has published a guidance document for designers of surveillance and vigilance studies.[47]

INVESTIGATIONS IN SPECIAL POPULATIONS

Investigations in children typically are conducted after considerable data have been gathered in an adult population with a similar disease. If clinical development includes children, it is usually appropriate to start with older children before extending the studies to younger children. The exception to the "adults first" rule is when a medication is developed to treat a condition that occurs only in childhood.

The development and testing of drugs for children are far from satisfactory; many drugs used to treat children are licensed for use only in adults, drugs are often unavailable in formats suitable for children, and clinical trials involving children raise complex ethical issues. The use of adult products at lower doses or on a less frequent basis may pose risks to children, as may the use of unlicensed and off-label medicines.[48]

Two U.S. federal acts now mandate that drugs initially developed for use in adults be studied and labeled for children. The *Pediatric Research Equity Act (PREA)* of 2007 (referred to formerly as the Pediatric Rule) requires manufacturers to assess the safety and effectiveness of a drug or biological product in children if the disease for which the drug was developed in adults also occurs in children. The *Best Pharmaceuticals for Children Act (BPCA)* of 2007 provides manufacturers with pediatric exclusivity incentives, provides process for "off patent" drug development, and requires pediatric study results be incorporated into labeling. For special issues relevant to trials in children, the reader is referred to the FDA guidance document on pediatric research.[49]

Similar legislation was introduced by the European Medicines Agency (EMEA) in 2007.[50] To obtain the right to market their medications for use in adults within the European Union, companies are now required to study medicines in pediatric subjects and develop age-appropriate formulations. A Pediatric Committee, based at the EMEA, is responsible for agreement of the *Pediatric Investigation Plan (PIP)* with the companies. The PIP contains a full proposal of all the studies and their timings necessary to support the pediatric use of an individual product. As a reward or incentive for conducting these studies, companies are entitled to extensions of patent protection and market exclusivity.

Classification of Clinical Trials by Objective

The ICH believes that the classification system based on phases of development is inadequate and proposes an alternative classification system based on the objectives of the study. Clearly stated primary and secondary objectives and hypotheses form the backbone around which every clinical trial is developed. These all should be clearly stated in the protocol and study report.

Population

The specific population to be studied is delineated by the inclusion/exclusion criteria. The development of these eligibility criteria is a formidable task. Developers of trials must attempt to reach a compromise between limiting the heterogeneity of the sample and not making the criteria so strict that recruitment of eligible subjects becomes untenable or threatens to restrict the generalizability of results.

The heterogeneity of the patient population that would be allowed to enroll in the trial is influenced by the phase of development. Early, exploratory studies are often concerned with whether a drug has any effect whatsoever. In these trials, one may use a very narrow subgroup of the total patient population for which the agent may eventually be labeled. Later phase, confirmatory trials typically relax the eligibility criteria to allow for a broader, more heterogeneous sample of the target population. Still, if the criteria for enrollment are too broad, interpretation of treatment effects becomes difficult.

Design

The study's phase, objectives, ethics, and feasibility influence the specific design of a trial. New designs have appeared in recent years that reduce the time during which children receive placebo or a known inferior medication.[51,52] More than one type of design may be used to answer the same question. If the same results and conclusions are reached regardless of the design and analysis used, the results are said to show *robustness*. Although a study may be designed as being "pivotal," it is rare that any single trial establishes incontrovertible evidence of an agent's clinical worth.

Comparative and Noncomparative Studies

Trials may be classified as either comparative or noncomparative studies. A comparative study implies that some type of comparison is made between the drug under investigation at a particular dosage level and a placebo, another dosage level of the investigational drug, or an active comparator (an existing drug known to be effective for the specific condition). Noncomparative trials involve no such comparisons with the investigational agent. Studies that compare the agent with placebo or an active comparator are called *controlled studies*. For a discussion and guidance on the proper selection of a control group, the reader is referred to a guidance document by the FDA.[53] Studies that involve dose escalation or that compare the pharmacokinetics and pharmacodynamics for differing dosage levels of the same drug are not considered controlled in the usual sense.

Open Studies

The early human pharmacology studies in the first phase of development and the postmarketing surveillance (phase IV) studies are usually *open label*, meaning that everyone involved with the study, including the patient and the physician, knows what the patient is receiving. Studies that occur in phases II and III may have an open-label extension phase, during which patients who took part in the comparative phase receive the investigational drug openly for an extended period. The chief purpose is to gather longer term safety and efficacy data. Investigator-initiated protocols may also be open if the intent is simply to gather additional information about an agent in another disease or at a dosage level other than that indicated in the label. As one would expect, the possibility of bias in interpretation of safety and efficacy information with open studies is much greater than with blinded studies. Open studies may be randomized to ensure that subject populations are similar in test and control groups.

Blinded Comparative Studies

Beginning either in late phase I or early phase II, blinded, controlled (comparative) studies are performed. *Blinding* refers to the masking of individuals involved in the assessment of the patient and, in some situations, of the data analyst. The purpose of blinding is to prevent identification of the treatment until any opportunity for bias has passed. These biases include (but are not limited to) decisions about whether to enroll a patient, allocation of patients, clinical assessment of end points, and approaches to data analysis and interpretation. Designs in which the assessor and the patient are blinded are called *double-blind designs*. Designs in which only the patient or only the assessor is blinded to the treatment are called *single-blind designs*. Studies should attempt to maintain blinding until the final patient has completed the study, although this has proved difficult in certain pediatric studies of severe diseases. Clinical studies in humans typically have a steering committee to provide oversight of the trial and a data safety and monitoring plan to provide ongoing monitoring. In large trials and in trials that are more than minimal risk, the data safety and monitoring plan often includes the formation of a data safety and monitoring board, which meets regularly to assess trial safety, progress, and quality.

To perform their charges, committee members may observe results of the trial categorized into groups of patients—that is, the committee members are aware of which group a patient is in, but unaware of which intervention that group is receiving. The committee members are said to be group unblinded, whereas the investigators remain totally blinded.

BLIND ASSESSOR

Certain studies present challenges to the maintenance of blinding because blinding is either unethical or impractical. Surgical versus nonsurgical interventions prevent the patient and the surgeon from being blinded because they know whether surgery was performed. In this situation, a blind assessor may be used to evaluate the patient's condition. The blind assessor may be a physician, nurse, or other health professional who evaluates the patient's response to treatment, but is unaware of the treatment being given.

DOUBLE-DUMMY DESIGN TO MAINTAIN BLINDING

Another situation in which blinding of the patient is difficult is when the dosage administration regimen is different for two drugs being compared. An example in rheumatology is the comparison of methotrexate (administered once weekly) versus hydroxychloroquine (administered once daily). In this case, the double-dummy design can be a useful way to maintain the blind. In the example mentioned, patients who are to receive methotrexate take active methotrexate once per week and dummy hydroxychloroquine each day, whereas patients who are to receive hydroxychloroquine receive active hydroxychloroquine each day and dummy methotrexate once per week. Double-dummy designs are limited by ethical issues involving repeated infusions or other aggressive means of delivering the "dummy" agent.

Randomization

The purpose of randomization is to introduce a deliberate element of chance into patient assignment to the treatment groups. Randomization reduces (but does not eliminate) the chance of an unequal distribution of known or unknown prognostic factors among the treatment groups. It also reduces possible bias in the selection and allocation of subjects.

Many randomization schemes are currently employed. The simplest form of randomization is unrestricted. Patients are assigned to one of two or more treatment groups by a sequential list of treatments. The list of treatments is known as the randomization schedule. Blocked randomization is commonly used to ensure that equal numbers of patients are placed in each treatment group (Table 7–3). Note in Table 7–3 that the assignment to groups is not sequential, but when the block is full an equal number of patients will have been enrolled into each group.

If the blocks are too small, there is a risk of unblinding. As an extreme example, suppose blocks were only two cells large for a study that planned to compare two drugs. If a clinical investigator knew the block size, enrolled only two patients, and became aware of what drug one of the patients was receiving through an adverse drug effect, then he or she would automatically know what drug the other patient was receiving. If the blocks are too large, they may not be completely filled, increasing the likelihood of unequal assignment to the groups.

Table 7–3

Example of a randomization schedule (nonstratified, blocks of 8)*

	Patient Number			
Randomization Block 1				
Treatment A	1	2	6	8
Treatment B	3	4	5	7
Randomization Block 2				
Treatment A	12	13	14	15
Treatment B	9	10	11	16

*The first patient entering the study receives treatment A, the second receives treatment A, the third receives treatment B, and so on. The sequence of assignments is random. When the block is full, equal numbers of patients have been enrolled into each treatment group. After block 1 is full, the assignment moves to block 2.

In more recent pediatric rheumatology studies involving two groups, block sizes of six to eight have been used. Clinical investigators are never made aware of block size during the trial.

Blocks may also be stratified by some prognostic factor to ensure equal distribution of the factor among the treatment groups. In multicenter trials, randomization may be stratified by center, such that each center has its own set of blocks. This tends to produce equal numbers of patients in each group at individual centers. In pediatric rheumatology, stratification by center is frequently impossible because only small numbers of patients are enrolled at each center. If a multicenter trial uses only one randomization schedule for all centers, whether it is unrestricted or stratified, the study is said to be randomized across all centers. Typically, a central coordinating center takes responsibility for giving all centers randomization numbers. The use of more than two stratification factors is rare. Such designs are logistically difficult and do little to achieve a balance of prognostic factors.

Typically, the data safety and monitoring board checks whether randomization is achieving balance of important prognostic factors while the trial is continuing. If imbalance of one (or at the most two) prognostic factors is found, the randomization scheme may be altered to achieve more balanced groups. This is known as *adaptive randomization.*

Design Configurations of Comparative Studies

Design configurations refer to treatment group assignments after initial randomization (i.e., whether or not patients remain in the same treatment group throughout the study). All of these configurations may be open, blinded, or both.

Randomized controlled trials (RCTs) are comparative designs in which subjects are randomly allocated to two or more specific treatment groups. The comparator may be placebo or an existing therapy that is to be compared with a newly developed active agent. Phase II and early phase III designs often employ a placebo, whereas late phase III and phase IV studies employ an active comparator. RCTs may be open, single blind, or double blind. In open studies, it is crucial that random allocation to a treatment group be done before knowledge of which treatment the subject is to receive. Various design configurations may employ the basic RCT approach, including parallel, crossover, blinded withdrawal, factorial, and group-sequential studies.

If patients remain in the same group to which they are initially assigned, the study is known as a *parallel group design.* In *crossover designs,* patients switch from one treatment to the next, often in a randomized manner, and each acts as his or her own control for purposes of analysis. The crossover design in the trial must be distinguished from the frequently used open-label extension phase (discussed earlier), in which all patients receive the active drug. *Factorial designs* allow for study of the interaction of two treatments that are likely to be used in combination. The simplest factorial design is a 2 × 2 design in which patients are assigned to receive drug *A* only, drug *B* only, both drug *A* and drug *B*, or neither drug *A* nor drug *B*. Factorial designs are also used to study dose

response when two agents are used together. Group sequential designs are particularly well suited to interim analyses. This design implies that the various treatment groups are evaluated for safety and efficacy at periodic intervals during the trial to determine whether the trial should continue or be stopped because of safety or efficacy concerns. Other comparative designs, whose basic approaches are evident from their names, include dose-escalation and fixed-dose, dose-response trials.

A design used to study etanercept in the treatment of polyarticular JIA is the *blinded withdrawal design.*[51] In this approach, all patients receive active medication long enough to establish whether patients respond (according to a standard definition). Patients who are not classified as "responders" after the prescribed time period are discontinued from the study and classified as therapeutic failures. Patients who respond are randomly assigned either (1) to be withdrawn blindly from active medication and given placebo or (2) to continue to receive active medication but in a blind manner. A common phenomenon in blinded withdrawal studies is a mild flare of disease among patients who continue to receive (blinded) active medication after randomization. This is called the *reverse placebo effect* because it is the reverse of the beneficial effect that often is observed in patients who are blindly randomly assigned to placebo. The primary outcome after randomization can be time to flare or percentage who flare (according to a standard definition).

A design that has gained widespread acceptance in oncology and is now being used in pediatric rheumatology is the *open randomized, actively controlled trial.* Patients are randomly assigned to one of two or more treatment arms, all of which are active. The trial is open, and, in general, no additional trial procedures or visits other than routine care are required. These trials have numerous advantages, but also substantial disadvantages. These trials tend to be more "user friendly" than studies that are part of a clinical development program. Perhaps their biggest advantage is that they are inexpensive to conduct because third-party payers may be billed for the procedures. They are not used to seek a new label or indication for an agent, and they are considered exploratory.

N-OF-1 DESIGN

The N-of-1 approach repeatedly and randomly crosses over individual patients from one therapy to the next. The randomization scheme may be *A, B, B, A, A, B.* A current pediatric rheumatology example is the N-of-1 study in JIA by Huber and colleagues.[54] Data from numerous N-of-1 trials in individuals may be combined to increase the sample size, but this is fraught with difficulties and sources of potential bias. These studies are considered exploratory and are hampered in rheumatic and other diseases by the carryover effects of the treatment, natural fluctuations of the disease state unrelated to therapy, and logistical problems. Reviews of the usefulness and pitfalls of N-of-1 studies have been published.[55,56]

Intent of Comparative Studies

The type of comparison that one intends to carry out must be decided on before the protocol can be developed. Major types of comparisons include trials to show superiority, trials to show equivalence, trials to show noninferiority, and trials to show dose-response relationship. All comparative trials must possess *assay sensitivity*, defined as the ability of a study to distinguish between active and inactive treatments.[57]

Trials to show *superiority* are perhaps the most frequent type of comparative studies. They are designed to show superiority of the investigative agent compared with either placebo or an active comparator or to show a dose-response relationship. In pediatric rheumatology, placebo-controlled studies have become more difficult, because some existing agents are clearly better than placebo. In such situations, the use of a placebo design is considered unethical, and an active comparator is substituted.

Trials to show *equivalence* do not aim to show superiority, but rather equivalence (either biological or clinical). They intend to show that the difference in response to two or more treatment approaches is clinically unimportant. For equivalence trials, the usual statistical approach is to use two-sided confidence intervals (CIs) (explained later). Equivalence is inferred if the entire CI of the true treatment difference falls within the equivalence margins. Stated another way, a statistical test of inference that results in a nonsignificant P value (i.e., no difference between the test drug and the active comparator) is not enough to conclude that the two agents are equivalent.

Trials to show *noninferiority* are similar to equivalence trials, but the question is asked in only one direction (i.e., whether the investigative agent is no worse than the standard therapy). In this case, a one-tailed CI is used to infer noninferiority. A simple one-sided test of the null hypothesis (H_0) that finds "no difference" between the treatments is insufficient to make conclusions about noninferiority.

The latter two trial types can be difficult to design, and sample size requirements are often much higher than for superiority trials. This is particularly true in active control equivalence or noninferiority trials that do not use placebo or that do not use multiple doses of the new drug.[57] The lack of internal validity makes external validation necessary. Active comparators should be chosen that have been shown through convincing, confirmatory trials to be efficacious in the particular condition. The same response variables should be used in the equivalence or noninferiority trials that were used in the confirmatory trials of the active comparator, and equivalence margins should be clinically sound. Trials to show dose-response relationships occur throughout the development phase of a drug and may have numerous objectives, including confirmation of efficacy, establishment of the dose-response curve, estimation of the most appropriate starting dose, strategies for dose adjustment, and estimation of the maximum dose.

Ethical Requirement for Clinical Equipoise in Comparative Studies

Clinical equipoise refers to the equality regarding probability of benefit that must exist between two or more groups being compared in a study. This probability of benefit is derived from existing, scientifically valid evidence of the effectiveness of the agents being tested, and

not from anecdotal or "gut" feelings. In other words, an investigator may ethically enroll patients into a comparative trial if there is a lack of convincing evidence of superiority of one of the agents, or if there is reasonable doubt in the medical community about the clinical utility of the agents. The requirement of clinical equipoise is often mistakenly interpreted as making any placebo-controlled study unethical. Ongoing debate in the literature of the ethics of placebo-controlled trials, particularly in children, is much too extensive to discuss in detail here.[57-59] Excellent arguments for when placebo trials are appropriate have been presented by Freedman and colleagues.[60-62] According to these authors, five conditions in which a placebo control may be used are as follows:

- There is no standard treatment.
- Standard treatment is no better than placebo.
- Standard treatment is placebo.
- The net therapeutic advantage of standard treatment has been called into question by new evidence.
- Effective treatment exists, but is unavailable because of cost or short supply.

The final arbiter is always the Human Subjects or Ethics Committee.

Conducting the Clinical Trial

With the advent and widespread use of independent for-profit clinical research organizations and site management organizations, the quality of clinical trial conduct has increased substantially. Academic research organizations appeared in the 1990s. Although not typically involved in the day-to-day operations of the trial, academic research organizations provide the basic scientific and theoretical background for the trial. These functions may include biological justification for the selection of the particular therapy, identification of biological and clinical response variables, development of the protocol, interpretation of the results, and final report preparation.

Pediatric rheumatology clinical trials, with few exceptions, are multicentered approaches. This term implies that multiple clinical investigative sites are used to enroll enough patients to meet statistical power requirements. A coordinating center is responsible for coordinating almost all trial activities. The role of the coordinating center is determined in part by whether a clinical research organization is used, and whether the trial is part of a clinical development program or an investigator-initiated protocol. Site monitoring may be a function of the coordinating center or the clinical research organization. During visits to clinical sites, site monitors—known throughout industry as clinical research associates—verify the data on the case report forms against source documentation (i.e., original reports from the laboratory and clinical records). Data collection (or capture) is moving to "paperless coordinating centers." Before the widespread use of electronic communication, almost all data were collected during the site-monitoring visit, or forms were mailed or faxed to the coordinating center or directly to the sponsor. Use of e-mail and electronic entry of data is increasing. The electronic age has drastically reduced the number of patients entered into trials who do not meet the eligibility criteria and the amount of inappropriate, incorrect, or missing data.

The coordinating center may or may not be distinct from the data coordinating center, which takes on the overall development of electronic case report forms, programming, quality assurance procedures, data collation, and data storage. The data coordinating center typically prepares the data for ongoing monitoring and final analysis. *Data collation* refers to the reorganization of the raw data from the case report forms to summary tables and spreadsheets. This step is necessary before data analysis can be performed and facilitates the review of safety and efficacy data by the data safety and monitoring board. The data safety and monitoring board is charged with, among other items, determining whether the trial should continue unchanged, be modified, or be stopped early because of safety or efficacy concerns.

Data Analysis Plan

The role of the statistician begins with planning of the study and power estimations. At a minimum, the statistical considerations document includes the following items:

1. Whether descriptive statistics, statistical inference, or both will play a role in the analysis
2. Identification of the primary and secondary response (outcome) variables
3. Calculation of sample size, including assumptions that will be used to justify the sample size, which include the α and β error levels, the difference that one wishes to detect as statistically significant, and how the variance estimate will be obtained
4. How the various analysis sets of patients to be used in the analysis will be formed, including the plan for handling dropouts, noncompliant patients, and other sets of patients who do not complete the protocol as written
5. Which statistical tests of inference will be used and the justification for their use
6. Plans for adjustment of *P* values based on the number of secondary hypotheses to be tested
7. Statement of which aspects of the analysis plan are expected to generate confirmatory data and which are exploratory, including plans for any subgroup analyses
8. Plans for handling covariates
9. The data management and statistical analysis software that will be used

Plans for exploratory studies may not be as formal as plans for confirmatory trials because the former permit the use of data-driven hypotheses to be tested. That is, data exploration is encouraged in exploratory, hypothesis-generating, nonpivotal trials. A single study may have confirmatory and exploratory aspects. Most of these items are discussed later (see "Understanding and Describing Data" and "Statistical Tests of Inference Commonly Used in Clinical Investigations"); others are self-explanatory. Items 2 and 4 require further attention here.

Primary and Secondary Response Variables

Response variables are defined as outcomes that will be used as the main evidence of the treatment effect of the investigational drug. *Treatment effect* is defined as an effect that is expected to result from a therapy. In comparative trials, the treatment effect of interest is a comparison of two or more agents. Treatment effect is distinguished from *effect size* (effect size is a measure of the strength of the relationship between two variables), which is a measure of the responsiveness (sensitivity to change) of the outcome variable and is defined mathematically as the mean change of the variable among the patient groups divided by the standard deviation (SD) of the baseline score. A related term is the *standardized response mean,* which is the mean change in a variable's score from baseline to the follow-up visit, divided by the SD of this change.[63] In studies designed primarily to observe safety and tolerability of an agent, the "response" variable relates to adverse events or treatment-emergent adverse drug effects, rather than to efficacy.

The choice of primary response variables largely depends on the objectives of the trial and should reflect clinically relevant effects. Secondary response variables are usually (but not always) associated with the exploratory nature of the study. *Surrogate end-points* are outcomes that are intended to relate to a clinically important end-point, but do not in themselves measure a clinical benefit. The use of biological surrogate end points in rheumatology as primary outcomes is suspect. For example, a decrease in some targeted T cell type may not produce clinical benefit even though the desired biological effect was achieved.

A frequently encountered problem in rheumatology is that of multiplicity (i.e., the use of multiple primary end-points with repeated statistical testing). To avoid this problem, the use of composite variables has become popular. This strategy involves the integration or combining of multiple relevant variables into a single variable, using a predefined algorithm. Three examples of composite variables are the American College of Rheumatology (ACR) 20 (ACR-20)[64] and the Disease Activity Score[65] for use in trials of adults with rheumatoid arthritis, and the ACR Pediatric-30 for use in trials of children with JIA.[66] Each attempts to categorize patients dichotomously as improved or not improved, using a core set of variables assembled into an algorithm. Composite variables avoid the multiplicity problem without requiring adjustment of the type I error level (described later) owing to multiple hypothesis testing.

Response Variables Based on Claims Allowed

The claims that the FDA allows for antirheumatic and antiinflammatory therapies for rheumatoid arthritis and JIA include reduction in signs and symptoms, major clinical response, complete clinical response, remission, prevention of disability, and prevention of structural damage.[44] The *reduction in signs and symptoms claim* is usually the first to be granted for marketing approval. This claim is typically established in trials of at least 6 months' duration, unless the product belongs to an already well-characterized pharmacological class, in which case trials of 3 months' duration are sufficient to establish efficacy for signs and symptoms. For trials in adults, the FDA recommends that ACR-20 criteria be used. In pediatric rheumatology, the FDA suggests that ACR Pediatric-30 be used for JIA.

The *major clinical response claim* is awarded to agents that are able to show a response at the ACR-70 level, rather than the 20% improvement needed for a signs and symptoms claim. This claim is based on statistically significant improvement response rates by the ACR-70 definition compared with background therapy in a randomized controlled group. Trial duration should be a minimum of 7 months for an agent that is expected to have a rapid onset of action and longer for agents with less rapid effects.

The *complete clinical response* claim is granted to a drug that produces a remission for at least 6 continuous months by the ACR-20 criteria and by radiographic arrest. Complete clinical response indicates that the patient is in remission, but is still taking antirheumatic drugs. Typically, trials for a complete clinical response last a minimum of 1 year.

Remission is defined as continuation of the same result after all antirheumatic drugs have been withdrawn. The remission claim is granted if remission by the ACR definition and radiographic arrest (no radiographic progression by the method of Larsen and colleagues[67] or by the modified method of Sharp and associates[68]) are maintained over a continuous 6-month period while the patient is off all antirheumatic therapy. A drug need not be a cure to be awarded a remission claim. A remission claim can be granted even if the patient relapses after 6 months or more of remission. Trials aimed at a remission claim should be at least 1 year in duration. Wallace and colleagues[26] developed a preliminary definition of clinical remission for use in JIA.

The *prevention of disability claim* is granted to drugs for which the primary outcome is a functional ability measure, such as the Childhood Health Assessment Questionnaire or the Arthritis Impact Measurements Scale. In addition, the full effect of JIA on a patient is not captured without the use of a more general health-related measure of quality of life. For this reason, data from a validated measure such as the Medical Outcome Study Short-Form Health Survey (SF-36),[69] the Childhood Health Questionnaire, or the Pediatric Quality of Life Inventory Scales (PedsQL)[70] should also be gathered, and the patient's condition should not worsen on these measures over the duration of the trial.

The *prevention of structural damage* claim is granted to drugs that exhibit either a slowing of radiographic progression or the prevention of new erosions shown by radiography or other measurement tools such as magnetic resonance imaging (MRI). These trials should be at least 1 year in duration.

Other clinical efficacy response variables are possible, and in pediatric rheumatology the ACR Pediatric-30 is likely to be inappropriate for the study of rheumatic conditions of childhood other than JIA. Whatever variables are chosen, they must possess a host of validity characteristics, including responsiveness (sensitivity to change within the trial's duration), face (clinical sensibility), content (comprehensiveness), construct (biological sensibility, or how the variable is hypothesized to behave compared with how it does behave), and criterion (does it agree with the gold standard, if one exists) validity.[71] In addition, variables should be reproducible (reliability) and, if more than one variable is chosen, nonredundant with one another.

Analysis Sets (Patients)

Not all patients who enter a trial complete the protocol as it is written. The analysis plan must state how subjects who drop out, are noncompliant, or in some other manner do not follow the protocol specifications will be handled. The formation of analysis sets should be aimed at minimizing bias and avoiding an increase in the possibility of an erroneous conclusion that a difference is present between groups when it is not (type I error, described later). The *per-protocol set* (also called valid cases set, efficacy sample, or evaluable subjects sample) comprises subjects who closely follow and complete the protocol. In practice, consideration of only the per-protocol set results in the loss of valuable information from patients who perhaps completed most of the study or had only one or two minor protocol deviations related to concurrent medication. The *full-analysis set* is also used for the primary analysis. The full-analysis set refers to the intent-to-treat approach and is derived from all randomized patients, including patients who dropped out early or had protocol deviations.

Historically, the *intent-to-treat* analysis meant that all patients, whether they dropped out, were noncompliant, or otherwise deviated from the written protocol, were evaluated for outcome at the time that they would have had their last visit (because one intended to treat them until then). The concept is embodied in the brief saying, "Once randomized, analyzed." This approach results in the introduction of substantial bias, however, and is problematic in rheumatology and other specialties in which patients, once off trial, are lost to follow-up and receive various other medications and procedures. It is now common to use a modified intent-to-treat analysis, the *last-observation-carried-forward* approach. This technique involves using the last value obtained for a response variable (no matter when in the trial it was measured) as if it were measured at the scheduled final visit. In this way, the data from noncompleters who were exposed to the drug long enough to experience treatment effects (if any) can be combined with the data from the per-protocol set.

UNDERSTANDING AND DESCRIBING DATA

In any type of clinical investigation, the investigators collect data and want to be able to summarize, interpret, and convey it to other parties. To do this, it is important to understand how measurements are made, how data can be displayed, and how the types of data determine the appropriate statistical test. The types of measurements (variables) determine which statistical test to use.

Scales of Measurement: Categorical, Ordinal, and Continuous Data

The scale or level of data has important implications for how information is displayed and summarized. All data may be classified into one of the following measurement scales: categorical, ordinal, or continuous (numerical).

Nominal or Categorical Variables

For categorical (qualitative) variables, sometimes called nominal variables (i.e., "in name only"), each subject can be placed into one of the categories. Variables with two possible outcomes, such as "yes/no" or "male/female," are called dichotomous. Categorical variables are categorized in terms of proportions or percentages (i.e., the study population was 75% female and 25% male). The best ways to display categorical data include contingency tables and bar charts.

Ordinal Variables

On an ordinal scale, the variables used have an inherent order. Subjects can be placed in "ranked" or "ordered" categories. Examples of ordinal variables include the severity scores of swelling (0 to 3+), Apgar scores, and tumor staging. Order exists among the categories, but the difference between adjacent categories is not uniform throughout the scale. Ordinal variables are best summarized using percentages and proportions. The entire set of data measured as an ordinal scale may be summarized by a median value.

Interval or Continuous Variables

Continuous variables are observations in which the differences between numbers have meaning on a numerical scale. These are quantitative measures. Examples are age, height, weight, blood pressure, survival time, and laboratory values such as serum creatinine. Although interval variables all have meaning on a numerical scale, differing degrees of precision are required for different types of studies. Age in a study of adults may be estimated to the closest year; in children, age may have to be estimated to the closest month, and in neonates, to the closest day or hour. Means and SDs (discussed later) are used to summarize continuous variables.

When to Convert Higher Levels of Data to Lower Levels

As a rule, one should work with the highest level of data possible because of increased quantitative precision and because parametric statistics are generally more powerful than nonparametric equivalents (see later discussion). There are times, however, when numerical data should be converted to ordinal or nominal data before further analyses are conducted. Situations in which "lowering" the level of data may be appropriate include the following:

- In a multicenter study in which different methods are used to generate a numerical value (e.g., the antinuclear antibody titer when different substrates are used). In this situation, one may be forced to "dichotomize" patient results, describing them as simply "normal" or "elevated," and conduct the analysis using statistics appropriate for a nominal, rather than a continuous, variable.
- If the experimenter suspects measurement error in the data. An example is adherence with a prescribed drug dosage or with a clinical trial or physical therapy program. It may be necessary to divide the patients dichotomously and classify each as "compliant" or "noncompliant."
- If reliability (reproducibility) of the measurement tool is unknown or likely to be poor. In pediatrics, the reliability of measurement on visual analogue scales is suspected to be low in young children. Rather than reading the result in centimeters from the left side of the scale, investigators frequently place a grid that is divided into 10 equal segments over the visual analogue scale line and read the result as a whole number from 0 to 10. This effectively converts a continuous variable to an ordinal level outcome.

Concepts Related to Measurement of Variables: Validity, Variability, and Bias

In clinical research, not all patients treated identically experience an identical response. This is known as the *variability* that is common to virtually all human experimentation. Certain important terms are associated with describing how this variability may have arisen. In some situations, its sources can be minimized or eliminated altogether. Variability is sometimes called error. *Error* may be broadly classified into nonrandom and random error. *Nonrandom error is also called bias* or systematic error. It results in a lack of validity of a measure and influences the accuracy of the measure. Validity generally is equated with accuracy. *Random error* refers to imprecision. The different types of random error and systematic error are graphically shown in Figure 7–3.

Potential Sources of Variability in Measurement of Individuals

Variability may arise among individuals from numerous factors, including diurnal variation; changes related to factors such as age, diet, and exercise; and environmental factors, such as season or temperature. Variability may also arise from measurement characteristics, including poor calibration, inherent lack of precision of the

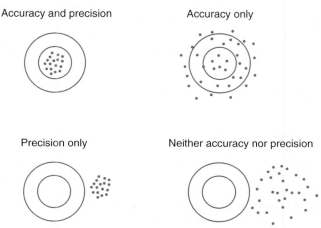

Accuracy and precision

Accuracy only

Precision only

Neither accuracy nor precision

FIGURE 7–3 Combinations of accuracy and precision in describing a continuous variable. Accuracy is impaired by bias or systematic error; precision is impaired by random error.

instrument, or reading or recording errors of the information provided.

External versus Internal Validity

External validity may be equated with generalizability of the study results. It determines the population settings to which measurement and treatment variables can be generalized. *Internal validity* refers to how valid the conclusions are within the patient sample studied; it is a basic minimum requirement without which any study is not interpretable. The question of external validity is meaningless without first establishing whether the study is internally valid. Both types of validity are important. They may be at odds, however, in that study design features that increase one may tend to decrease the other.

Bias

Sources of bias that may occur in clinical studies include selection, measurement, unacceptability, confounding, recall, referral, volunteer, withdrawal, attention, investigator, and verification, among others. To complicate matters further, the same type of bias may be known by different names or be a subset of some other bias (see later discussion). Many are self-explanatory. A few of the more important types of bias are discussed here.[72] *Selection bias* is the distortion of study effects resulting from the sampling of subjects and includes volunteer bias, nonresponse bias, and bias resulting from loss to follow-up. Another subtype of selection bias is referred to as *detection bias*.

Measurement bias (also information bias) is distortion of the study effect resulting from inaccurate determination of the study variables (either exposure or disease). Measurement bias may be divided into nondifferential and differential misclassification. Nondifferential information bias can occur if the exposure is not accurately assessed. This type of bias may occur in occupational research if job titles are used as a surrogate for exposure status. Another form of nondifferential measurement bias is *unacceptableness bias*, in which the exposure may be underreported by patients if it is unacceptable behavior. This is likely to have an impact on all subjects, not just subjects with the disease of interest. *Differential misclassification bias* includes recall bias, in which the recall of information about exposure is influenced by whether the person has the disease (i.e., cases may have more accurate memory of events leading to disease than controls who have no disease). *Interview bias* can occur if the circumstances under which different groups of subjects are interviewed are incompatible. These circumstances include time from exposure to interview, setting of the interview, person doing the interview, manner in which questions are asked (prompting), and whether the subject has knowledge of the research hypothesis. Case-control studies are particularly vulnerable to information bias.

Confounding bias is a distortion of the study effect that results from mixing of the exposure associated with the disease with the effects of one or more extraneous variables. An extraneous variable that wholly or partially accounts for the apparent effect of the exposure or that masks an underlying true association is called a confounder. Examples of confounding are (1) an apparent association between an exposure and a disease that may be due to another variable, and (2) an apparent lack of association between exposure and disease that results from failure to control for the effect of some other factor. Brunner and colleagues[73] present an example of confounding bias in pediatric rheumatology. These investigators attempted to identify risk factors for damage in childhood-onset SLE. An association was found between damage and disease duration, indicating a possible (and logical) cause-effect relationship between the two. When the data were corrected for the confounder disease activity over time, disease duration disappeared as a predictor of damage.

To assess the possibility of confounding, the standard technique of stratifying the data by the potential confounder may be used. One looks for an association between the exposure (as a possible causal factor) and the disease; then one compares the subjects who have the confounder with subjects who do not to see whether an association exists. Another common method is to use *Mantel-Haenszel procedures* to calculate an overall relative risk in which the results from each stratum are weighted by the sample size of the stratum.[74] Only established risk factors for the disease should be investigated as potential confounders. In brief, these can be dealt with in the design of the study (i.e., by matching) or by stratification or multivariate analysis (see later discussion).

Propensity Scoring

The results of observational studies in which random allocation to treatment is not done may be *confounded by indication*. This means that more ill patients receive the more aggressive of the available therapies, making conclusion of which therapy is better difficult. Stated another way, the patient groups may not be similar enough at baseline in regard to important covariates that may influence outcome. Propensity scoring attempts to quantitate how similar patients are at baseline in regard to these covariates. It establishes the likelihood that a patient receives a treatment, based on pretreatment covariates. Each patient receives a propensity score and then is matched to similar patients, and outcomes are compared among treatment groups, controlling for the score. An example of the use of propensity scores in pediatric rheumatology is the study by Seshadri and associates[75] of the use of aggressive corticosteroid in juvenile dermatomyositis.

Describing Data and the Frequency Distribution of Continuous Variables

Descriptive statistics are commonly used to represent individual data points graphically or to summarize groups of data, regardless of the data level. Many exploratory and epidemiological studies use only descriptive statistics, rather than inferential statistics (tests of hypotheses). Graphs such as dose-response curves represent descriptive statistics. *Rates* and *ratios* are commonly used in epidemiological studies to describe disease frequency and distribution. A *rate* (or proportion) implies that the numerator is part of the denominator and is usually associated with a time element (e.g., an annual case-fatality rate of 11/120 implies that the 11 deaths came from the total of 120 cases). The numerator of a ratio is not part of the denominator (e.g., the female/male ratio among patients with oligoarticular-onset JIA is 6:1).

Statisticians employ many types of distributions for describing and analyzing data. These include the binomial (Bernoulli), geometric, chi-square, Poisson, t, and F distributions, among others. The frequency distribution of continuous variables is most commonly referred to in the medical literature and is the only distribution discussed in detail in this chapter. Its parameters form the basis of much of the descriptive statistics used in the reporting of data from clinical investigations.

A frequency distribution of a continuous variable is simply an x-y plot of the possible values that a variable can take on (x-axis) versus the number of observations having the particular values (y-axis). If the frequency distribution is normally distributed, it is called a gaussian distribution (Fig. 7–4).

Measures of Central Tendency, Skewness, and Kurtosis

Every distribution of continuous variables has an arithmetic mean (average), which is calculated by adding the observations and dividing the sum by the number of observations. The median of any distribution is the centermost value. If the distribution has an even number of observations (i.e., there is no center value), the median is calculated by averaging the two most center values. The median is also the 50th percentile. The mode is the most frequently observed value. The *mean, median,* and *mode* all are called measures of central tendency. A distribution has only one mean and one median, but numerous modes are possible; this leads to forms such as *bimodal* and *multimodal* distributions.

In a normal distribution, the mean, median, and mode are all the same value. Figure 7–5 shows the effect of positive skewing on the measures of central tendency. The *skewness* is said to be positive because there are too many observations in the upper (shaded) tail (i.e., toward the right side of the distribution). This type of skewing typically occurs in distributions that have a fixed lower boundary, but no upper boundary (e.g., results of liver function tests). *Negative skewing* is the mirror image and has the opposite effect on central tendency measures. An example is the age at onset of disease among patients with oligoarticular JIA. Kurtosis is a measure of the peakedness of a distribution.

Measures of Spread or Variation

The frequency distribution of continuous variables can be described by its mean and its SD. The SD is a measure of the spread of values. Abbreviations in common use for the mean include $\bar{x}$ for the sample mean and μ for the underlying population mean from which the sample was drawn. The SD in a formula is designated s for the sample SD and σ for the population SD; it is the square root of the variance of the distribution. Variance is calculated by subtracting the mean from each of the individual values in the distribution, squaring the differences (to eliminate the negative sign), summing the squares, and dividing the result by the number of observations minus 1. The sample variance is abbreviated s^2, and the variance of the population from which the sample was drawn is σ^2.

If a frequency distribution is normally distributed, the distance ±1 SD from the mean includes 68.3% of the observations, ±2 SD includes 95.8% of the observations, and ±3 SD includes 99.7% of the values. Actual distributions from clinical investigations may include more or fewer of the observations at the SD cut points than these theoretical percentages indicate.

Z Scores: Placing a Single Value within a Distribution of Values

Frequently, clinical investigators find it useful to locate exactly where an individual patient's value for some variable lies within a distribution of values. Because the normal distribution depends on two parameters, the mean and the SD, there is an infinite number of normal curves, based on the variable being measured. All tables of the normal distribution are for the distribution described by a mean of 0 and SD of 1. Any variable with a mean not

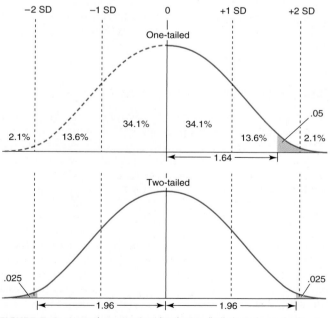

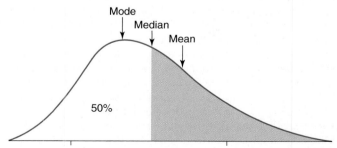

FIGURE 7–4   Normal or gaussian distribution (bell-shaped curve), showing the approximate percentage of observations expected to be found within 1 and 2 standard deviations (SD) from the mean value. Also note the critical values for one-tailed and two-tailed tests of hypotheses.

FIGURE 7–5   Effect of positive skewing on the location of the mean, median, and mode. (The mean and median are skewed to the right.) The effect of negative skewing is the mirror image of this figure.

equal to 0 and SD equal to 1 must be rescaled so that these parameters are met. The solution is to convert the variable to a standard normal variable, Z (also called a standard normal deviate).

In a clinical trial of calcium supplementation in post-pubertal girls with JIA, eligibility criteria may include the requirement that the patient's bone mineral content (by dual-energy x-ray absorptiometry) must be less than 1.5 SD below the mean of the normal population. A Z score can be calculated by subtracting the population mean from the measured value in the individual and dividing the result by the SD of the population: $Z = (x_i - \mu)/\sigma$, where x_i is the individual's value. One may transform the Z scale back to the original scale. If the population mean is 2143 g, and the population SD is 308 g, a patient whose bone mineral content is less than 1681 g (i.e., 2143 – [308 × 1.5] respecting the negative direction) qualifies for the study with regard to this eligibility criterion. A Z score also can be calculated using the sample mean and SD. In addition, two means can be compared to determine whether they are statistically significant via the Z test if the sample size is large. Any continuous numerical variable can be converted to the Z scale.

Standard Error of the Mean

The standard error of the mean (SEM) represents a different concept from the SD. Mathematically, it is expressed as $SEM = SD/\sqrt{n}$, where n is the sample size. Because samples drawn from an underlying population do not each produce the same mean value (but tend to cluster around the same value), one must calculate the range of where the true (unknown) population mean lies. From the formula, it can be seen that the greater the n (i.e., the larger the denominator), the smaller the SEM. The SEM gives the clinical investigator an idea of how "tightly" the estimated mean from the sample represents the true, underlying mean. Investigators often ask statisticians what should be plotted when presenting the data as a mean and its accompanying measure of variability, the SD or SEM. Because the SEM is always less than the SD, investigators tend to plot it rather than SD. A rule of thumb is that the SD should be used when comparing values from individual subjects with a population distribution. The SEM is used when plotting mean values of two groups of subjects.

Confidence Intervals

As stated earlier, the SD encompasses the variability of individual observations, and the SEM indicates the variability of means. The mean ± 1.96 SD estimates the range of values within which 95% of the observations from subjects can be expected to fall (see Fig. 7–4). Similarly, the mean ± 1.96 SEM estimates the range in which 95% of the means of repeated samples from the same population should fall. If the mean and the SEM are known, 95% CIs can easily be estimated. These limits indicate the range of values within which the investigator is 95% sure that the true mean of the underlying population lies. One can easily calculate any CI level (e.g., 90% CI, 99% CI) by using the critical values that cut off specific areas of the curve. CIs are frequently used in addition to statistical hypothesis testing. They can be calculated for the

chi-square test, the t test, regression, and various other tests of statistical inference.

Describing Nonnormal or Nonparametric Distributions

Not all parameters used to describe normal distributions are helpful when one is attempting to describe distributions that are nongaussian (i.e., do not follow a bell-shaped curve or reasonable approximation). Although the median, mode, and range (described earlier) are helpful, the mean and SD may be quite meaningless in this situation. A commonly used method is to group the ranked values in a nonnormal distribution into quartiles, which are similar to percentiles, but with only four categories: Q1 = 25%, Q2 = 50%, Q3 = 75%, and Q4 = 100%. The spread, or dispersion, of a nonnormal distribution is described in terms of the interquartile range. This is the difference between the highest value in the third quartile (i.e., the 75th percentile) and the highest value in the first quartile (i.e., the 25th percentile).

STATISTICAL TESTS OF INFERENCE COMMONLY USED IN CLINICAL INVESTIGATIONS

This section does not attempt to describe comprehensively the myriad statistical procedures that are readily available to the clinical investigator through such computer programs as Statistical Analysis System (SAS), the Statistical Package for Social Sciences (SPSS), or Bayesian Inference Using Gibbs Sampling (BUGS) for bayesian analysis. Rather, a basic introduction to statistical concepts is provided, followed by a description of the inferential and other procedures found most commonly in the literature. Formulas are not stressed, because virtually all statistical procedures are now conducted with the use of computer programs. The reader is referred to Table 7–4 for a short summary of what type of test is most appropriate in which setting.[76]

Basic Concepts Relevant to Analysis

Statistical approaches may be divided into frequentist methods and bayesian approaches. Frequentist methods refer to P values and CIs, which can be interpreted as the frequency of specific outcomes from the same experimental situation if it is repeated many times. That is, what are the chances of this outcome (and outcomes even more extreme) if one repeats the experiment many times? Bayesian analysis permits a calculation of the probability that a treatment is superior according to the observed data and prior knowledge. It begins with a posterior probability distribution for some parameter, which is derived from the data, and a prior probability distribution for that parameter. The posterior distribution is used as the basis for statistical inference.[77] This chapter emphasizes the frequentist school because most statistics in today's literature follow frequentist rather than bayesian theory. For more details on bayesian analysis the reader is referred to a popular textbook.[78]

Table 7–4

Summary of statistical tests

No. Dependent Variables	No. Independent Variables	Type of Dependent Variable	Type of Independent Variable	Measure	Test
1	0 (1 sample)	Continuous normal	Not applicable (none)	Mean	One-sample *t*-test
		Continuous non-normal		Median	One-sample median
		Categorical		Proportions	Chi-square goodness-of-fit, binomial test
	1 (2 independent samples)	Normal	2 categories	Mean	2 independent sample *t*-test
		Nonnormal		Medians	Mann-Whitney, Wilcoxon rank sum test
		Categorical		Proportions	
	0 (1 sample measured twice *or* 1 (2 matched samples)	Normal	Not applicable/categorical	Means	Paired *t*-test
		Nonnormal		Medians	Wilcoxon signed ranks test
		Categorical		Proportions	McNemar, chi-square test
	1 (≥3 populations)	Normal	Categorical	Means	One-way ANOVA
		Nonnormal		Medians	Kruskal-Wallis
		Categorical		Proportions	Chi-square test
	≥2 (e.g., 2-way ANOVA)	Normal	Categorical	Means	Factorial ANOVA
		Nonnormal		Medians	Friedman test
		Categorical		Proportions	Log-linear, logistic regression
	0 (1 sample measured ≥3 times)	Normal	Not applicable	Means	Repeated measures ANOVA
	1	Normal	Continuous		Correlation simple linear regression
					Nonparametric correlation
		Nonnormal	Categorical or continuous		Logistical regression
		Categorical	Continuous		Discriminant analysis
	≥2	Normal	Continuous		Multiple linear regression
		Nonnormal			
		Categorical			Logistical regression
		Normal	Mixed categorical and continuous		Analysis of covariance general linear models, general estimation equations (regression)
		Nonnormal			
		Categorical			Logistical regression
2	≥2	Normal	Categorical		MANOVA
≥2	≥2	Normal	Continuous		Multivariate multiple linear regression
2 sets of 2 more	0	Normal	Not applicable		Canonical correlation
≥2	0	Normal	Not applicable		Factor analysis

ANOVA, analysis of variance; MANOVA, multivariate analysis of variance.

The types of variables in the study and the number of variables studied determine the choice of the appropriate statistical approach. The first step is to determine which variables are independent (predictor or explanatory) variables and which are dependent (outcome or response) variables. An independent variable is the parameter that is the explanatory factor or thought to be the cause. A dependent variable is one whose value is the outcome in the study or the response or is thought to be the effect.

The second step is to determine the measurement scale of the variable: categorical (nominal), ordinal (ranked), or continuous (interval) numeric, definitions for which were provided earlier. The third step is to determine whether the study observations are independent of each other.

In the design of a clinical study, one must determine whether the groups to be compared are independent or paired. Samples in which the values of one group cannot be predicted from the values of the other group are said to consist of independent groups. In other words, the patient group and the control group represent different individuals, rather than the same individual measured at two different times. With paired (matched) groups, the values of one group may be predicted from values of the other. In a paired experiment, a patient may be measured before and after therapy, in which case the patient acts as her or his own control, or a patient may be paired with another individual who has been matched with respect to all of the independent variables (e.g., age, duration of disease) that may affect the dependent variable (response). In animal studies, in which genetically identical animals are frequently used in research, paired experiments are the rule. In human clinical studies, it is rare that two groups can be matched for all of the independent variables that may influence the outcome variable. An investigator may wish to match the groups as closely as possible, to eliminate bias, but still treat the groups as if they were independent, improving the overall quality of the experimental design, as described earlier.

The nature and distribution of the values of the variables also determine whether parametric or nonparametric tests can be used. The use of a parametric test is based on certain assumptions. The major assumption is that the variable of interest follows a *normal distribution*. It may be possible to transform variables that are not normally distributed. This technique expresses the values of observations on another scale, such as a natural log scale. This may allow the use of parametric statistical tests when the actual values obtained in the study do not follow a normal distribution. Another alternative is to use a nonparametric test. Nonparametric methods are based on weaker assumptions in that they do not assume a normal distribution or equality of variance between the different groups. There are nonparametric procedures for most statistical needs, but because they are not based on the assumption of normality, nonparametric tests are more conservative. They are also less powerful (i.e., less able to reject the null hypothesis when it is false) than their parametric counterparts.

Two Types of Statistical Error and P Values

Type I error is the probability of rejecting a null hypothesis when it is true—that is, concluding that there is a difference when there is none. It is abbreviated as α (alpha error) and set by the investigator at a certain level, commonly at 0.05. The P value is the calculated type I error level based on the data; it is defined as the likelihood that a difference at least as large as the observed difference could have occurred by chance alone. It is analogous to a false-positive result in diagnostic tests (discussed earlier). P values that are larger than the predefined type I error are called *not statistically significant*; values at or below the preset type I error are called *statistically significant*.

The debate about when and how to adjust P values to deal with the issue of multiplicity, or multiple hypothesis testing, seems far from resolved; a spirited debate continues, particularly in new technologies, such as microarray data.[79,80] When one is conducting exploratory studies not aimed at establishing definite cause-effect relationships, P values need not be corrected for fear of missing a possible true association or difference. False-positive results

can be discarded later in confirmatory, pivotal studies. In confirmatory studies aimed at adding pivotal evidence to a cause-effect relationship, there is no need to correct the P value for the main test of hypothesis (i.e., that on which sample size was based). Results of secondary, exploratory hypotheses should present uncorrected and corrected P values, however. An alternative to correcting the P value is to set α lower (e.g., at 0.01 instead of 0.05) in anticipation of conducting multiple hypothesis testing.

There are numerous techniques for correcting P values for multiple comparisons; the most widely used is the Bonferroni correction. To adjust a P value using the Bonferroni correction, the P value obtained is multiplied by the number of statistical tests. A P value of 0.05 obtained in a series of 10 tests of hypotheses becomes (0.05×10), or 0.5. Alternatively, when the experiment is designed, the α error level can be divided by the number of anticipated tests (in the example, $0.05 \div 10 = 0.005$), with values of P value greater than this level referred to as nonsignificant.

Type II error is the probability of failing to reject a false null hypothesis in favor of the alternative hypothesis—that is, concluding that there is no difference when there is a difference. It is commonly abbreviated as β (beta error) and is equivalent to the false-negative rate. Table 7–5 summarizes of the types of decision errors, illustrating the concepts of the null hypothesis and α and β errors.

Traditionally, type I error levels are set lower than type II error levels (e.g., 0.05 for type I and 0.2 for type II). In other words, the experimenter is more willing to make a type II error than a type I error. The conventional rationale for this approach is that type I errors are more serious because they can result in the abandonment of an established, beneficial therapy in favor of a new therapy when no such change is warranted.

Power, the ability of a statistical test to identify a true difference if one exists, is expressed mathematically as ($1 - \beta$). It is a consideration in the design of an experiment because the power of the test is affected by the sample size. The distribution of the test statistic is divided into two areas: acceptance and rejection. These concepts are graphically shown in Figure 7–6. If the null hypothesis is rejected, one concludes that the evidence supports a significant difference between the groups. If the null hypothesis is not rejected, one concludes that there is no such difference. The lower the P value, the higher the level of significance.

Sample Size

The estimation of sample size requires considerable statistical skill and knowledge of the underlying basic assumptions being made by the investigator. It involves some guesswork, and the resulting calculation may not always yield the correct sample size needed to answer a specific

Table 7–5		
Outcome of study		
True Situation	**Accept H_0**	**Reject H_0**
H_0	Correct	Type I error
H_a	Type II error	Correct

H_0, null hypothesis; H_a, alternative hypothesis.

question. This problem occurs when the investigator's assumptions do not hold true for the sample that is actually enrolled in the study. Sample size should always be calculated during the development of the clinical investigative protocol.

Sample size is most frequently calculated with the use of computer programs, based on specific assumptions including an estimate of the magnitude of effect (i.e., how much difference can one expect between a control group and a treated group in terms of the primary outcome), the desired type I error level (usually 0.05), and the type II (β) error level (i.e., 1 – power). To calculate the sample size

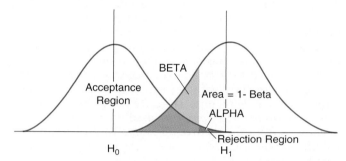

FIGURE 7–6 Theoretical visual representation of acceptance and rejection regions, alpha (α) and beta (β) error regions, and power. There are four possibilities when one compares the means (or other summary descriptors of a distribution of values) of two (or more) populations or samples. (1) One may correctly conclude that there is no difference between the two means (i.e., correctly accept, or fail to reject, the null hypothesis [H_0] of no difference). In this case, the mean of the treated group would fall within the distribution on the left anywhere in the acceptance region (*white*), but not in the rejection region (*black*) and also not in the stippled region (β). This implies that the second mean arose from a population having the same underlying mean as the population that gave rise to the first mean, and the experimenter correctly recognized this situation. (2) One may correctly conclude that there is a difference between the two means (i.e., correctly reject H_0 in favor of the alternative hypothesis [H_1 or H_a] that there is a difference between the two means). In this case, the mean of the treated group would fall within the rejection region (*black*) or farther to the right. This implies that the second mean arose from a population with a different underlying mean from that of the population that gave rise to the first mean, and the experimenter correctly recognized this fact. (3) The investigator may incorrectly conclude that there is a difference between the two means when there is not a difference (i.e., incorrectly reject H_0 in favor of H_1 when it should not be rejected). In this case, the value of the second mean happened to fall into the rejection, or α region, even though it arose from the same population as the first mean. This is known as a type I error, and its probability of occurrence is based on the α error level set by the experimenter—how much chance is one willing to take of concluding that there is a difference when there is not? This determines the size or area of the rejection region. A type I error implies that the second mean arose from a population with the same mean as the population that gave rise to the first mean, but the experimenter failed to recognize this fact because the second mean fell far out in the tail of the distribution, as shown in the graph. (4) The investigator may incorrectly conclude that there is no difference between two means when there is a difference (i.e., incorrectly accept, or fail to reject, H_0 when it is actually false). In this case, the second mean fell somewhere in the β region, leading the experimenter to believe, incorrectly, that the second mean came from the same population that gave rise to the first mean. This is known as a type II error, and its probability of occurrence is based on where the experimenter sets the power (1 – β error level) of a test. Power determines the size of the β area on the graph and is usually heavily dependent on sample size. A type II error implies that the second mean arose from a population with a different mean from that of the population that gave rise to the first mean, but that the experimenter failed to recognize this fact because the second mean fell close to the first mean (i.e., in the β region).

needed for a parametric test, such as the t test, one must also estimate the variance in the variable of interest. The variance estimate may come from published data or from a pilot study that was designed to assess preliminarily the question under consideration.

Because many sample size calculations result in the requirement of an unrealistic number of patients, the statistician is often asked to find ways to decrease the number of patients needed. Sample size may be decreased by increasing the acceptable type I error level, by increasing the acceptable type II error level, by increasing the size of difference required to detect a statistically significant difference (which should also be clinically relevant), and by choosing an outcome variable with a smaller amount of variance. The most common ways to do this include improving the precision of the measurements of the outcome variable, training investigators, using better equipment, and repeatedly measuring the outcome.

Post Hoc Power Analysis

In the event that an investigation yields nonsignificant differences, the concern is that the investigator has committed a type II error. One option to address this situation is the calculation of the sample size that would be necessary to find the observed difference statistically significant. Another option is the calculation of the size of the difference one could detect as statistically significant with sufficient power (e.g., 80%), given the sample size and variance obtained in the study; this is termed the *minimum detectable difference*. If the minimum detectable difference is much larger than would be considered clinically significant, the investigator may conclude that the investigation did not include a sufficient number of patients to detect a clinically meaningful difference as statistically significant. If the minimum detectable difference is smaller than the difference that is considered clinically *important*, the test was adequately powered, and the investigator may conclude that there is no difference between the samples.

Confidence Intervals (Limits) on Statistical Tests of Inference

CIs are frequently calculated for a statistical hypothesis test. They may be calculated for the t test, chi-square test, analysis of variance, regression, and most other tests of inference. A 95% CI is a range of values within which, the experimenter believes, there is a 95% probability that the true underlying (unknown) mean (or difference in means) lies. The most frequently reported CI is at the 95% level. The confidence limits are related to the P value. If one calculates the CI of a test that compares two means or difference in means, and zero is within the range of the 95% CI, the statistical test (P value) should not be significant because there is some probability that the true difference between the two means is zero.

Statistical versus Clinical versus Biological Significance

An important concept that is frequently overlooked is that a statistically significant difference may not indicate clinical significance. Particularly if the sample size is large, many tests may result in a statistically significant finding when there is a relatively small degree of clinically significant difference between the two groups. Biological significance, compared with statistical significance, has come into the forefront with the testing of new immune response modifiers (biologic agents).

One-Sample Tests

Statistical hypothesis testing may be completed on studies involving one or more groups. The most frequent approach to analyzing data from a clinical investigation that involves only one group is to compare that group with a known population or expected value.

Binomial Test of Proportions

Perhaps the most frequently used test for comparing one sample with a known population is the binomial test. This test asks the question, "What is the probability of x number of successes in N independent trials, given that the probability of success on any one trial is y?" The binomial test has limited applicability in describing the statistical probability that a therapy is beneficial because the odds of success typically are unknown. In pediatric rheumatology, the question may be, "What is the probability that 50 patients with JIA treated with methotrexate will experience improvement as determined by a given index or measure?" The problem is that one is typically unsure of the exact probability of a success in a single-arm independent trial. In some situations, the probability of success is arbitrarily given the value of 0.5 (i.e., 50% chance), and the binomial test is done either to confirm or to fail to confirm that level of probability of success.

Goodness-of-Fit Chi-Square Test

The goodness-of-fit chi-square test is related to the Pearson chi-square test (discussed later), in which observed proportions are compared with expected values. The goodness-of-fit chi-square test can be used to test the significance of a single proportion or of a theoretical model, such as the mode of inheritance of a gene. A reference population is often used to obtain the expected values. Suppose the frequency of an allele that is thought to produce risk for polyarticular JIA is known to be 2 in 100 in the general population. The observed frequency of the allele in a sample of patients with polyarticular JIA is found to be 10 in 100, however. To assess whether this much deviation from the expected value is significant, the goodness-of-fit chi-square test can be used.

One-Sample t Test

When a statistical inference is desired on a single mean, the one-sample t test may be used. The test is similar to the Student t test for comparing two means, described later. If one wishes to determine whether the mean height of 9- to 10-year-old girls with SLE is significantly less than that of the general population of 9- to 10-year-old girls, a one-sample t test would be appropriate.

Two-Sample Tests

The two-sample test to be used is determined by the level of the data and by certain other assumptions, as defined later.

Chi-Square Test with One Degree of Freedom

For categorical (nominal) data and ordinal data with very few ranks, the most frequently used hypothesis test is the Pearson chi-square (χ^2) test. This nonparametric statistical test of inference is for assessing the association between the two variables. It is most commonly performed on contingency tables such as a 2×2 cross-tabulation, which has one degree of freedom (1 df). The significance of the resulting chi-square statistic is determined from a table of critical values.

There are several useful points to remember about the interpretation of this statistic. For chi-square with 1 df (i.e., 2×2 tables), the statistic becomes significant at the 0.05 level if the χ^2 value is 3.841 or greater, and the larger the chi-square value, the more significant it is. Most tables of critical values report two-tailed probabilities; the P value is divided by 2 to find the one-tailed probabilities. Chi-square analysis with greater than 1 df (i.e., tables larger than 2×2) requires larger values to be significant; *Yates continuity correction* is used to compensate for deviations from the theoretical (smooth) probability distribution if the total N assessed in the contingency tables is less than 40.

Fisher Exact Test

The Fisher exact test is used as a replacement for the chi-square test when the expected frequency of one or more cells is less than 5. This test is commonly used in studies in which one or more events are rare.

McNemar Test

The chi-square test assumes independence of the cells, as noted earlier. Experimental designs exist for observing categorical outcomes more than once in the same patient. The McNemar test (also known as the paired or matched chi-square) provides a way of testing the hypotheses in such designs. An example for the use of this statistic may be to test two different concentrations of an analgesic lotion that are given to 51 patients in sequence. The null hypothesis is that the proportion of patients who experience relief when they apply analgesic lotion 1 is the same as the proportion of patients who experience relief when they apply lotion 2. Alternatively, the McNemar test would be used when comparing the effects of the two analgesic lotions in two groups of patients that are matched for independent variables that may influence the dependent variable (i.e., the proportion of patients with pain relief).

Mantel-Haenszel Chi-Square Test

The Mantel-Haenszel chi-square test is known as a stratified chi-square test and is frequently used to detect confounding variables. The procedure involves breaking the contingency table into various strata and then calculating an overall relative risk, with the results from each stratum being weighted by the sample size of the stratum.

Common Errors with Chi-Square Tests

Perhaps because of its frequent use, the chi-square test is often employed or interpreted inappropriately. Common mistakes include unnecessary conversion of continuous or ordinal level data to categorical data to use the chi-square test, nonindependence of the cells in the table (an exception is when McNemar chi-square test is used); use of the chi-square rather than Fisher exact test when expected cell frequencies are lower than 5; and confusion of statistical significance by chi-square values with clinical or biological importance.

Student t Test

What the chi-square test is to categorical data, the *t* test is to continuous data. This test is used for comparing two sample means from either independent or matched samples. The matched *t* test is more efficient (i.e., more powerful) than the Student *t* test for independent groups.

Nonparametric Tests

The *t* tests described earlier are parametric tests. That is, they make assumptions about the underlying distributions, including normality and equality of variances between groups. The *t* test is a very robust test; it is still valid even if its assumptions are substantially violated. If the violations are severe, the investigator may transform the data using either natural logarithms (described earlier) or nonparametric tests. Nonparametric tests ignore the magnitude of differences between values taken on by the variables and work with ranks; no assumptions are made about the distribution of the data. For two-group comparisons, either the Mann-Whitney *U* test is used for independent data or the Wilcoxon signed rank test is used for paired data.

K-Sample Tests

Clinical investigations involving more than two samples (groups) require that modifications be made to the analysis plan to accommodate the need for multiple comparisons.

Chi-Square Test with More than One Degree of Freedom

When categorical data are analyzed, there may be more than two categories for one or both variables (i.e., the table may be larger than 2 × 2). If the chi-square test statistic is found to be significant in a table larger than 2 × 2, it is frequently difficult to determine which proportions were different. One must attempt either to collapse the number of cells in the table or break the table up into several smaller tables. This may require adjustment of the resulting *P* values because of multiple comparisons. The degrees of freedom of contingency tables larger than 2 × 2 are equal to the number of rows minus 1 plus the number of columns minus 1.

Analysis of Variance

ONE-WAY ANALYSIS OF VARIANCE

The use of repeated *t* tests to detect differences among more than two means is considered unacceptable because the resulting *P* value does not accurately describe the chance one has taken of committing a type I error. The one-way analysis of variance (ANOVA) is used for the purpose of comparing more than two sample means.

ANOVA divides the total variance among all subjects into two portions: the amount of variance that is a result of the difference between the groups of subjects, and the amount of variance that results from differences within each group. The ratio of the amount between and the amount within each group is known as the *F ratio*. The corresponding test of significance is known as the *F test*. If statistical significance is achieved, the investigator must go one step further. The significance may have arisen because just two means were different from one another, or perhaps all the means were different from one another. To determine exactly which means were different, tests must accommodate the fact that multiple comparisons are being made. This is determined by applying a multiple comparison. Commonly used multiple comparison tests include Tukey honest significant difference test, the Newman-Keuls test, Scheffé multiple contrasts test, and, if one wishes to make multiple comparisons to only one group, Dunnett test.

MULTIWAY ANALYSIS OF VARIANCE

ANOVA procedures have an additional capability that can increase the efficiency of analyses when one wishes to compare the influence of two or more independent variables on one dependent variable simultaneously. Suppose one wished to test the effects of methotrexate and a physical therapy program on the disease status of a group of patients with polyarticular JIA. One could carry out two separate studies, conduct *t* tests for treatment effects on the methotrexate-treated patients and the physical therapy–treated patients, and compare each with placebo or no physical therapy. This approach requires substantial numbers of patients to meet sample-size requirements for each study. A two-way ANOVA factorial design could make much more efficient use of the available subjects, however, and provide information about the interaction (effect modification) between methotrexate and physical therapy. In this situation, patients could be randomly assigned to both treatments, yielding four groups (methotrexate alone, physical therapy alone, methotrexate and physical therapy, and neither methotrexate nor physical therapy). In addition to providing information about the effect of each treatment alone (i.e., the two main effects), a two-way ANOVA factorial design examines the effect of the interaction between the two treatments. ANOVA techniques can be extended to three-way, four-way, and beyond, provided that the sample size is large enough.

REPEATED MEASURES ANALYSIS OF VARIANCE

Repeated measures ANOVA tests the equality of means among various groups when all subjects are measured for the dependent variable under numerous conditions or levels of the independent variables. Use of the standard ANOVA is inappropriate because it does not account for the correlation between repeated measures of the same variable. It is used frequently in longitudinal research when subjects are measured repeatedly in regard to some outcome. This technique also is useful when there is a large amount of variance among subjects in a group, and when recruitment to a study is difficult because it improves the study's efficiency because each subject is measured under all conditions.

NONPARAMETRIC ANALYSIS OF VARIANCE

ANOVA procedures discussed to this point are parametric tests and, as such, make various assumptions about the underlying distribution. If these assumptions are substantially violated, the nonparametric equivalent of ANOVA, the Kruskal-Wallis test, can be used. This test is subject to the same sample-size limitations as the chi-square test. If the sample size in any group is less than 5, one must use the Fisher exact test and exact probabilities, as described earlier.

Correlation and Regression

One of the most important measures of statistical correlation is the *Pearson product-moment correlation*. This statistic is appropriate for estimating the relationship between two variables, *x* and *y*, both of which are measured along a continuous scale. Correlation is a two-way model that does not require assumptions of causality. The correlation (r) can range between –1 and +1. The magnitude of the correlation shows the strength of the relationship between the two variables. The larger the absolute value of the correlation, the more strongly associated are *x* and *y*. In the extreme, where r = +1 or –1, all the data values fall perfectly on a straight line. The sign of the correlation indicates the direction of the relationship. A positive sign means that the two variables are directly related (i.e., they tend to increase or decrease together). A negative sign for r indicates that the two variables are inversely related (i.e., the value of one tends to decrease as that of the other increases). Correlation assumes that the joint distribution of *x* and *y* is bivariate normal; that is, their joint probability distribution must be normal. If this assumption is violated substantially, the nonparametric *Spearman rank correlation*, which yields a Spearman rho (r_s), is used. Because Spearman rank correlation deals with ranks, it can be used with continuous variables that violate assumptions and with ordinal data.

Pearson and Spearman correlation coefficients can be interpreted as follows: Variables are unrelated if the r (or r_s) is less than 0.2, values between 0.2 and 0.4 represent weak correlations, and values between 0.41 and 0.6 represent moderate correlations. Coefficients larger than 0.8 constitute strong correlations between the *x* and *y* variables tested.

Regression is a one-way model in which predictor or explanatory independent (*x*) variables are thought to affect the dependent outcome (*y*) variables, but not vice versa. In simple regression models (i.e., models that include only a single predictor), and in multiple regression models, the direction of the effects must be prespecified. The simple linear regression equation is y = a + bx, where *a* is the intercept and *b* is the beta coefficient (or slope). By using various values of *x* in the equation, the predicted value of *y* for a given *x* can be determined. Simple regression models serve as building blocks for the larger, more complex, and more realistic models, including polynomial regression models and structural equation models.

Multiple Linear Regression

The technique whereby a multitude of independent variables (e.g., x_1, x_2, x_3) can be simultaneously investigated for their influence on a continuous dependent variable (*y*) is known as multiple linear regression. The method models the dependent variable as a linear function of all the (k) independent variables. That is,

$$y = a + b_1x_1 + b_2x_2 + b_3x_3 + \cdots + b_kx_k$$

This method is particularly helpful in evaluating extraneous variables as possible confounders of the linear relationship between two continuous variables. In other words, linear regression permits the investigator to assess the separate unconfounded effects of several independent variables on a single dependent variable. The x_i terms can be continuous or categorical variables. The b_i (beta coefficients) terms are the regression coefficients. Each b_i is "corrected" simultaneously for the linear relationship between its associated x_i and all the other x_i's and for the linear relationship between the other x_i's and *y*. An overall r^2 value is calculated for the model. It represents the percentage of the total variance of *y* that is accounted for by the linear relationship with all the x_i's. A common mistake is to refer to multiple linear regression as a multivariate technique; technically it is not because it deals with multiple independent variables, rather than multiple dependent variables.

Multiple Logistic Regression

Multiple logistic regression is distinguished from multiple linear regression in that the outcome variable (dependent variables) is dichotomous (e.g., diseased or not diseased). Its aim is the same as that of all model-building techniques: to derive the best-fitting, most parsimonious (smallest or most efficient), and biologically reasonable model to describe the relationship between an outcome and a set of predictors. Here, the independent variables are called *covariates*. Importantly, in multiple logistic regression, the predictor variables may be of any data level (categorical, ordinal, or continuous). A major use of this technique is to examine a series of predictor variables to determine those that best predict a certain outcome. A pediatric rheumatology example of the use of this technique can be found in the article by Ruperto and associates,[11] in which predictor variables that are measurable during the very early stages of JIA (e.g., number of active joints during the first 6 months of illness, erythrocyte sedimentation rate [ESR]) were tested to determine their relative predictive ability for either a favorable or a less favorable outcome (i.e., a dichotomous dependent variable) at least 5 years later.

Analysis of Covariance

Analysis of covariance (ANCOVA) combines the principles of ANOVA with the principles of regression. A chief advantage of this technique is that, in contrast to ANOVA, the independent variables can be of any data level. ANCOVA is often used to adjust for initial (baseline) differences between or among groups. In other words, one of its chief purposes is to eliminate systematic bias. Suppose two groups of patients had unequal numbers of swollen joints at baseline (even though the study may have been randomized). The initial number of swollen joints is used as the covariate. ANCOVA adjusts the posttreatment means of the groups to what they would have been if all groups had started out equally on the covariate.

The other purpose of ANCOVA is to reduce the within-group (or error) variances, making the test more efficient (powerful). Suppose a clinical trial investigates the effect on the ESR of a biological agent and an active comparator. Subjects are randomly assigned to receive one or the other treatment, and the change in ESR is observed. Within each treatment group, there is considerable variation in ESR, reflecting individual differences among patients in the degree of active inflammation. In other words, ESR and active inflammation are covarying (covariates). If one could statistically remove this part of the within-group variability by allowing the degree of inflammation to be the covariate in the analysis, a smaller error term would result, and the test would gain power. ANCOVA provides a method to do this. ANCOVA provides a method for adjusting for differences at baseline between groups and reduces the amount of variation within groups that is caused by covariates, increasing power and capability to detect differences.

Survival Analysis

Survival (life table) analysis was developed primarily for the study of how long a particular cohort of subjects survives. The term *survival* is now used in a broader sense for data that involve time to a certain event, such as time to failure of a drug or time before remission.[25] There are two basic types of life table analysis: the fixed-interval (actuarial) model and the Kaplan-Meier survival analysis. The latter is used much more frequently in medicine than the former. In actuarial analysis, the lengths of each interval shown on the *x*-axis all are equal (e.g., 1 year). This is the technique used by life insurance companies to estimate the probability of a person's surviving to a certain age. In the Kaplan-Meier approach, the end of an interval is demarcated by an event. The horizontal components of the lines are unequal, as they are in the actuarial technique. An example of the actuarial method in pediatric rheumatology can be found in a study by Giannini and colleagues[81] of the time to occurrence of eye disease among patients with certain major histocompatibility complex alleles. An example of the Kaplan-Meier approach can be found in the study by Lovell and associates,[51] in which time to failure in subjects given placebo was compared with time to failure in subjects given etanercept. Methods exist for comparing the difference of the life table graphs; the most frequently used is the generalized Wilcoxon test. Figure 7–7 is a graphic representation of a comparison between the characteristic lines of an actuarial model and a Kaplan-Meier analysis. Lee and Wang[82] provide an outstanding reference for survival analysis techniques.

Measures of Agreement Among and Within Raters

It is often necessary to express in statistical terms how well various raters agree with one another (interrater agreement) or with themselves (intrarater agreement). These are commonly referred to as *measures of reliability* or *reproducibility*. Lack of agreement, either among or within raters, indicates that the values for the measure are nonreliable or nonreproducible. This has dire consequences for the interpretation of the results and for statistical interpretation. Various tests exist for expressing the degree of agreement between and within raters.

The most frequently used test to express rater agreement when the outcome is dichotomous is the kappa test ratio (known also as Cohen kappa, or $\varkappa$). The $\varkappa$ scores range between 0 and 1 and are often expressed as percentages: less than 20% is considered negligible agreement; 20% to 40%, minimal; 40% to 60%, fair; 60% to 80%, good; and greater than 80%, excellent.[83] Data with three or more categories (i.e., ordinal data) require the use of the more complex weighted kappa test; *Kendall W*, or *coefficient of concordance*, can also be used. W values range from 0, which indicates poor agreement, to +1, which indicates perfect agreement among all raters.

Intraclass Correlation

If more than two raters are to be compared for reliability, the intraclass correlation coefficients are more appropriate than conducting repeated two-way comparisons between pairs of raters (there is a correction for correlation between raters that becomes apparent when the range of measurement is large). Intraclass correlation coefficients evaluate the level of agreement among all raters, and the measures (scores) must be parametric in nature. The coefficient represents the amount of agreement: 1 is perfect

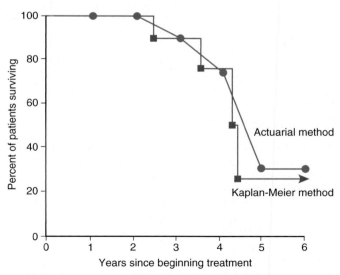

FIGURE 7–7 Comparison of the Kaplan-Meier and actuarial survival curves, showing a theoretical example of the percentage of patients surviving after 0 to 6 years of treatment. (Modified from Kramer MS: *Clinical epidemiology and biostatistics: a primer for clinical investigators and decision-makers,* Berlin, 1988, Springer-Verlag.)

agreement, and 0 is no agreement. Conversely, ANOVA on the matrix produces an F value (described previously) and tells the investigator whether the raters are significantly different from one another.[84]

Multivariate Analyses

This section provides a basic concept of multivariate statistics and an overview of the more popular and increasingly used multivariate tests. Interested readers are referred to the text by Stevens[85] for in-depth discussions of the concepts and tests involved. Multivariate analysis deals with the statistical analysis of data collected on more than one dependent variable. These variables may be correlated with each other, and their statistical dependence is often taken into account when analyzing such data. This consideration of statistical dependence makes multivariate analysis different in approach and considerably more complex than the corresponding univariate analysis, when there is only one response variable under consideration.

The response variables considered are often described as *random variables*, and because their dependence is one of the things to be accounted for in the analyses, these response variables are often described by their joint probability distribution. Multivariate normal distribution is one of the most frequently made distributional assumptions for the analysis of multivariate data. If possible, any such consideration should ideally be dictated by the particular context. Also in many cases, such as when the data are collected on a nominal or ordinal scales, multivariate normality may not be an appropriate or even viable assumption. In the real world, most data collection schemes or designed experiments result in multivariate data. An example of such situations is a new drug that is to be compared with a control for its effectiveness. Two different groups of patients are assigned to each of the two treatments, and they are observed weekly for next 2 months. The periodic measurements on the same patient exhibit dependence, and the basic problem is multivariate in nature. If the measurements on various possible side effects of the drugs are also considered, the subsequent analysis has to be done under several carefully chosen models.

A rule of thumb is that there should be at least 10 subjects for each dependent variable investigated in the study. A study in which the subject/variable ratio is smaller is likely to be unreliable.

Hotelling T[2] Test

Just as the *t* test is used when one wishes to compare one dependent variable in two different groups, The Hotelling T^2 test is used when there are two groups with multiple dependent variables. The process involves the comparisons of the vectors of the means in the treated group and in the control group. So-called discriminant function analysis (described subsequently) is used to determine which variables are contributing the most to the significant finding.

Multivariate Analysis of Variance

Just as the ANOVA was used for the comparison of more than two means, so too is the multivariate analysis of variance (MANOVA), rather than the Hotelling

T^2, used in situations with more than two groups and multiple dependent variables. Its use, instead of separate univariate ANOVAs, is related to accounting for intercorrelations among the dependent variables. Group means and within-group variability must be computed for each dependent variable. There are numerous ways to calculate whether there a significant differences between groups, the most common of which is *Wilk lambda*. As with the Hotelling T^2, significance can arise from one or several of the variables.

Discriminant Function Analysis

Discriminant function analysis is MANOVA reversed. In MANOVA, the independent variables are the groups, and the dependent variables are the predictors. In discriminant function analysis, the independent variables are the predictors, and the dependent variables are the groups. As previously mentioned, discriminant function analysis is usually used to predict membership in naturally occurring groups. It answers the question: Can a combination of variables be used to predict group membership? Usually, several variables are included in a study to see which ones contribute to the discrimination between groups. Discriminant function analysis is broken into a two-step process: One first performs the multivariate test, and, if statistically significant, proceeds to see which of the variables have significantly different means across the groups.

Classification Tree Analysis

Classification and Regression Tree (CART) is a method of data mining. In these tree structures, CART is related to discriminant analysis. The tree end points represent classifications, and branches represent conjunctions of features that lead to the classifications. CART trees need to be discriminated from decision analysis trees constructed to help with making decisions. CART allows for *recursive partitioning* iteratively, and selects variables that split the sample into progressively purer groups. It has a theoretical advantage over techniques such as logistic regression, in that the structure of the classes in relation to the predictor variables is not assumed—that is, different combinations of the predictor variables may identify subgroups. An example for the use of CART analysis may be the attempted development of new classification criteria for psoriatic arthritis.[86]

Factor Analysis

Factor analysis is used for data exploration to reveal patterns of interrelationships among variables that are not readily apparent, for confirmation of hypotheses, and for reducing the number of variables to a manageable level. In situations involving many different observations concerning the same patient or groups of patients, factor analysis can be used to determine whether it is possible that some of these observations are a result of just a few underlying factors. That is, the correlation among many dependent variables may be explained by some underlying factor or factors. The fact that a young boy is experiencing swollen joints, a rash, intermittent fevers, and a decrease in hemoglobin with an increase in white blood cell count is a result of underlying factors: He is experiencing the onset of systemic JIA, and pathological processes are occurring in his hematopoietic system.

When groups of patients are studied, the symptoms tend to "load" on the underlying factors differentially. Factor loading is expressed in a factor loading matrix, in which each row of the matrix is a variable, and each column is a factor. Such a matrix examines how highly each variable correlates with, or loads on, each factor. Each variable may load onto one or more variables. Next, one must decide which factors are most important to keep and which can be discarded as not contributing enough to the explanation of the variables. This is done by calculating an *eigenvalue*, which is the amount of variance in the data that is explained by a particular factor. The procedure to this point is called *principal component analysis*. Additional steps in factor analysis include rotation of axes to determine which are general factors (most variables load significantly on them) and which are bipolar factors (some variables load positively and some load negatively on them). Factorial complexity is determined by observing how many variables load significantly onto two or more factors.

Multivariate Analysis of Covariance

The multivariate analysis of covariance (MANCOVA) is an extension of univariate ANCOVA in which group means at follow-up are adjusted for differences at baseline, and within-group variance is reduced by removing variation caused by covariates. The objective of MANCOVA is to determine whether several groups differ on a set of dependent variables after the follow-up means have been adjusted for any initial differences on the covariates at baseline.

Item Response Theory and Rasch Analysis

Item response theory (IRT), also known as *latent trait theory*, is used for statistical analysis and the development of outcome measures. Among other things, the purpose of IRT is to provide a framework for evaluating how well questionnaires or outcome measures work, and how well individual questions that are part of the questionnaire work. A special type of IRT is the so-called *Rasch analysis*, which has been used in recent years to assess the usefulness of common rheumatology outcome measures.[87-89] Questionnaires or outcome measures developed by and adhering to IRT or Rasch principles function like a common ruler and can be used to describe accurately within-patient and between-patient differences and change over time.

JUDGING THE QUALITY OF A REPORT CLINICAL INVESTIGATION

The most helpful and up-to-date series of guides to the reader of clinical reports was published in the *Journal of the American Medical Association*. These "Users' Guides to the Medical Literature," subsequently published in book form,[3] provide logical checklists of questions for readers attempting to weigh the evidence from many different types of clinical studies.[3] In brief, each Guide asks three basic questions:

- Are the results of the study valid?
- What were the results?
- Will the results help me in caring for my patients?

Practical examples from everyday clinical situations are used to illustrate how one determines the answer and eventually weighs the evidence from the report. Because not all epidemiological studies deal with patients, judging the quality of an epidemiological investigation requires an approach that is similar to but separate from judging clinical investigations.

Judging the Evidence from a Clinical Trial and the CONSORT Statement

Although the above-cited Users' Guides contain information for judging clinical trials, more detailed guides are available. In 1995, a group of medical journal editors, clinical epidemiologists, and statisticians developed a consensus statement about how randomized controlled trials should be reported—the Consolidated Standards of Reporting Trials (CONSORT) statement. Since the previous edition of this text, the statement has been revised,[90] and a study has been done to determine its impact on reporting of trials.[91,92] The statement contains a checklist of 21 items that deal chiefly with methods, results, and discussion. It identifies key pieces of information necessary to evaluate the internal and external validity of a report. A flow diagram is also recommended; using a two-group, parallel design, randomized, controlled trial as an example, it provides a graphic display of allocation and status of patients throughout the trial. Some modification of the statement's recommendations is usually necessary because of differences in study design. Overall, it provides an outstanding template, however, on which to formulate or judge the report of a clinical trial. Guidelines for determining authorship of articles that are generally accepted by editors of medical journals have now been published.[93]

REFERENCES

1. Evidence-based medicine, a new approach to teaching the practice of medicine, JAMA. 268 (1992) 2420–2425.
2. H.I. Brunner, E.H. Giannini, Evidence-based medicine in pediatric rheumatology, Clin. Exp. Rheumatol. 18 (2000) 407–414.
3. G. Guyatt, Users' guides to the medical literature: essentials of evidence-based clinical practice, second ed., McGraw-Hill Medical, New York, 2008.
6. J. Woodcock, R. Woosley, The FDA critical path initiative and its influence on new drug development, Annu. Rev. Med. 59 (2008) 1–12.
8. L.E. Moses, Statistical concepts fundamental to investigations, N. Engl. J. Med. 312 (1985) 890–897.
11. N. Ruperto, A. Ravelli, J.E. Levinson, et al., Long-term health outcomes and quality of life in American and Italian inception cohorts of patients with juvenile rheumatoid arthritis, II: early predictors of outcome, J. Rheumatol. 24 (1997) 952–958.
21. A.B. Hill, The environment and disease: association or causation? Proc. R. Soc. Med. 58 (1965) 295–300.
26. C.A. Wallace, N. Ruperto, E. Giannini, Preliminary criteria for clinical remission for select categories of juvenile idiopathic arthritis, J. Rheumatol. 31 (2004) 2290–2294.

29. S. Magni-Manzoni, N. Ruperto, A. Pistorio, et al., Development and validation of a preliminary definition of minimal disease activity in patients with juvenile idiopathic arthritis, Arthritis Rheum. 59 (2008) 1120–1127.

31. U.S. Food and Drug Administration: E10 choice of control group and related issues in clinical trials (website). http://www.fda.gov/Regulatory Information/Guidances/ucm129459.htm. Accessed June 30, 2009.

37. A. Levin, The Cochrane Collaboration, Ann. Intern. Med. 135 (2001) 309–312.

40. J.A. Singh, D.H. Solomon, M. Dougados, et al., Development of classification and response criteria for rheumatic diseases, Arthritis Rheum. 55 (2006) 348–352.

44. U.S. Food and Drug Administration: Clinical Development Programs for Drugs, Devices, and Biological Products for the Treatment of Rheumatoid Arthritis (RA) (website). http://www.fda.gov/downloads/Drugs/GuidanceComplianceRegulatoryInformation/Guidances/ucm071579.pdf. Accessed June 30, 2009.

45. R. Temple, Current definitions of phases of investigation and the role of the FDA in the conduct of clinical trials, Am. Heart. J. 139 (2000) S133–S135.

56. P.M. Peloso, Are individual patient trials (n-of-1 trials) in rheumatology worth the extra effort? J. Rheumatol. 31 (2004) 8–11.

57. R. Temple, S.S. Ellenberg, Placebo-controlled trials and active-control trials in the evaluation of new treatments, part 1: ethical and scientific issues, Ann. Intern. Med. 133 (2000) 455–463.

58. A.J. Vickers, A.J. de Craen, Why use placebos in clinical trials? A narrative review of the methodological literature, J. Clin. Epidemiol. 53 (2000) 157–161.

59. E.J. Emanuel, F.G. Miller, The ethics of placebo-controlled trials—a middle ground, N. Engl. J. Med. 345 (2001) 915–919.

60. B. Freedman, K.C. Glass, C. Weijer, Placebo orthodoxy in clinical research, II: ethical, legal, and regulatory myths, J. Law. Med. Ethics. 24 (1996) 252–259.

61. B. Freedman, Placebo-controlled trials and the logic of clinical purpose, IRB. 12 (1990) 1–6.

63. P.R. Fortin, G. Stucki, J.N. Katz, Measuring relevant change: an emerging challenge in rheumatologic clinical trials, Arthritis Rheum. 38 (1995) 1027–1030.

66. E.H. Giannini, N. Ruperto, A. Ravelli, et al., Preliminary definition of improvement in juvenile arthritis, Arthritis Rheum. 40 (1997) 1202–1209.

72. D.L. Sackett, Bias in analytic research, J. Chronic. Dis. 32 (1979) 51–63.

76. Services UAT: What Statistical Analysis Should I Use? (website). http://www.ats.ucla.edu/stat/spss/whatstat/. Accessed June 30, 2009.

90. D. Moher, K.F. Schulz, D.G. Altman, The CONSORT statement: revised recommendations for improving the quality of reports of parallel-group randomized trials, Ann. Intern. Med. 134 (2001) 657–662.

91. D. Moher, K.F. Schulz, D.G. Altman, The CONSORT statement: revised recommendations for improving the quality of reports of parallel-group randomised trials, Clin. Oral. Invest. 7 (2003) 2–7.

Entire reference list is available online at www.expertconsult.com.

Chapter 8

ASSESSMENT OF HEALTH STATUS, FUNCTION, AND QUALITY OF LIFE OUTCOMES

Ciarán M. Duffy and Brian M. Feldman

Pediatric rheumatic diseases influence many, if not all, aspects of a child's life—not only physical, but also social,[1] emotional,[2] educational, and economic.[3] The impact of pediatric rheumatic disease is not only on the child, but extends to the entire family.[4] Conversely, the family's functioning can have a significant impact on the outcome of the child's illness.[4] This chapter describes the instruments that have been developed to assess this web of influence in a quantitative fashion and specifically focuses on the measurement of functional status and quality of life (QoL), with an emphasis on measures developed or used for juvenile idiopathic arthritis (JIA). Some brief discussion is included on measures in use for systemic lupus erythematosus (SLE) and juvenile dermatomyositis (JDM). Table 8–1 presents a glossary of terms pertinent to assessment of outcomes.

BACKGROUND

Why Quality of Life Is Measured

Today, most pediatric rheumatic diseases are not fatal. They affect children and their families by interfering with normal health, however, and they may have an impact on the enjoyment of life. Many of these diseases are not curable; in situations in which there is no cure, it is important to know that our treatments, at least, make our patients feel better.[5] In the field of rheumatology, QoL has gained wide popularity because it has been shown to measure outcomes that are of direct interest and importance to patients, to provide effective measurements of patient status, to be predictive of patient outcome, and to produce reliable and effective measures of treatment impact.[6-9]

Concepts of Structure and Function, Activity Limitation, Participation Restriction, Health, and Quality of Life

The terms used to describe the consequences of chronic health conditions have been unclear and overlapping.[10] For this reason, the World Health Organization (WHO) developed the International Classification of Functioning and Health (ICF). The ICF provides a common vocabulary for the consequences of disease.[11,12] This work followed from the WHO description of health as a biopsychosocial construct[13] and the definition of QoL as an "individual's perceptions of their position in life in the context of the culture and value systems in which they live and in relation to their goals, expectations, standards and concerns."[14] The ICF framework is particularly applicable to rheumatic diseases.[15-19]

According to the ICF model (Fig. 8–1), a health condition affects an individual in three domains—structures and functions (anatomy and physiology), activities (e.g., activities of daily living), and social participation. Each of these domains affects the others. For example, JIA might lead to muscle atrophy, weakness, cartilage erosion, joint contracture, and pain (structure and function domain). In addition, a child with JIA may not be allowed by his or her parents to run and play (activities domain) and not be allowed by his or her teacher to participate in school games (participation domain). In this example, joint pain, weakness, and contracture may also limit the ability to run, and this inability to run may be another reason why the child cannot participate in school games.

In the ICF model, each of the domains may be affected by personal factors and by environmental factors. Given the same level of anatomic and physiologic damage, one child may be unable to attend school, whereas another more highly motivated child may be trying out for the basketball team. An example of environmental modification is a wheelchair-bound child who may be unable to participate in a school dance unless a ramp or other accessibility modifications are made.

QoL—which had been considered an additional domain in older models of health outcomes[20]—is not defined in the ICF model. It is a term used ubiquitously in daily language. The term was originally applied by sociologists to try to determine the effect of material affluence on people's lives. This sociological approach was developed in the United States during World War II. The concept broadened so that it eventually included education, social welfare, economics, and industrial

Table 8–1

Glossary of commonly used terms

Ceiling effect	Situation in which the highest score on an instrument does not represent the best status a subject can have; patients with the highest score can still improve more
Content validity	Extent to which items in the instrument comprehensively assess the domain of interest
Convergent validity	Correlation of instrument scores to accepted but not gold standard parameters measuring the same domain
Criterion validity	Degree to which a measure correlates with a gold standard; such a standard does not exist for quality of life
Discriminant instrument	Designed to differentiate most effectively among groups of people
Domain or dimension	Area of behavior or experience that is being measured
Evaluative instrument	Designed to detect most effectively change in the status of a person over time
Face validity	Estimation of whether an instrument appears to be measuring what it is intended to measure: does it look reasonable? (seldom quantitated)
Floor effects	Situation in which the lowest possible score on an instrument does not represent the worst status a subject can have; patients with the worst score can still deteriorate further
Generalizability	Extent to which an instrument can yield accurate and reliable results when used in circumstances or subjects different from those in which it was originally validated; for example, able to be used in varying socioeconomic, ethnic, and geographical disease types or disease severity
Patient preference	Instruments designed so that each individual selects the parameters on the instrument that are most important to him or her
Predictive validity	Extent to which a score on an instrument at one point predicts patient outcome at a later time
Reliability	Extent to which a measuring procedure yields the same results on repeated trials if all the conditions remain unchanged
Responsiveness (sensitivity to change)	Extent to which scores on an instrument given at different times in the same subject (or subjects) will change if there is a true change in the status of the subject
Surrogate or proxy reporter	Someone who answers on behalf of another and reports what he or she thinks the subject would answer for himself or herself (e.g., parent reporting for a child)

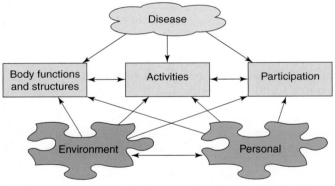

FIGURE 8–1 International Classification of Functioning and Health (ICF).

growth.[21] This broad societal approach was also incorporated into questionnaires that were developed to assess the status of an individual within this broad framework of concern.

Many of these areas of concern or domains, although important to an individual, are well outside the influence of disease and health care interventions. Also, QoL is considered to be a highly subjective construct, one that can be determined only by an affected individual based on the individual's own goals and expectations[10,22] and the individual's personal evaluation of his or her current situation in many domains of life.[23,24] For this reason, other terminology was developed to describe QoL, e.g., health-related quality of life (HRQoL), life satisfaction, self-esteem, well-being, general health, functional status, and life adjustment.[21]

The earliest published uses of the term *HRQoL* date from the early 1980s.[25,26] At that time, it was appreciated that medical interventions might only rarely have an impact on overall QoL. Another term was needed because, among other reasons, QoL became a reason for registration of new medications. HRQoL has been the term used most often. Tools purporting to measure HRQoL mostly measure symptoms (i.e., according to the patient) related to the ICF domains of structure and function, activities, and participation, and value these symptoms according to normative expectations (i.e., values of groups of individuals rather than one individual).[10,27-29] HRQoL can be defined as patient-reported "perceptions of health."[30]

For the purpose of this chapter, discussion of QoL is mostly restricted to HRQoL. HRQoL is a complex concept that contains numerous subcomponents. Experts differ as to what constitutes HRQoL, and consequently various instruments have been developed to measure it. These instruments may be divided into generic and disease-specific measures.[27] Generic HRQoL measures are measures that purport to be broadly equal across different types and severity of disease, across different medical treatments or health interventions, and across different demographic or cultural subgroups. They are designed to capture aspects of health and disease that cross broad diagnostic categories and social or demographic subgroups. Disease-specific HRQoL measurements are designed to assess specific diseases or patient populations; such instruments are usually more responsive to changes in individual subject status. The last 25 years have seen the development and validation of various instruments to measure the various ICF domains and generic and disease-specific HRQoL. These instruments were first developed in adult rheumatology, but in the last 20 years tools specifically designed to be used in pediatric rheumatic diseases have been developed.

Hierarchy of Outcomes

The ICF framework can be used to structure a hierarchy of outcomes. The first level of outcome assessment is within the domain of structure and function. Measures of so-called disease activity fit in this domain. Disease activity is the aspect of outcome assessment that has been the traditional focus of trials in rheumatology. Disease activity measures include parameters most familiar to clinicians, such as joint counts, morning stiffness, and erythrocyte sedimentation rate. The major drawback to measures in this area is that they are not directly what the patient is interested in. Measures of disease activity are still widely used in clinical trials, however, because inhibition of the disease process or activity is an essential component of an effective therapeutic intervention (especially for pharmacological interventions). At this time, measurement of disease activity is a necessary but insufficient approach to measuring patient outcome. When the performance characteristics of the traditional disease activity measures used in rheumatology were scientifically assessed, many instruments were found to be unreliable, redundant, insensitive to change, or not correlated with long-term patient outcome.[7] For example, even experienced clinicians often disagree when assessing joint count.[31,32]

The next level up the hierarchy is the measurement of activity and activity limitation and social participation. This domain reflects physical function and disability and social handicaps. The focus here is on measuring the ability of the person to perform physical activities of daily life, such as dressing, walking, climbing stairs, and self-care, and to participate meaningfully in society. This is an area of more relevance to the patient. Several instruments have been developed and validated to quantify functional ability in patients with JIA. These are discussed in greater detail later. In addition, most HRQoL instruments measure aspects of activity and participation. Measures at this level are in accordance with the view of the WHO that health is a state of physical, mental, and social well-being.[33] Disease-specific HRQoL measures, such as the Health Assessment Questionnaire (HAQ)[7] and the Arthritis Impact Measurement Scale (AIMS),[34] were developed to incorporate the broad WHO concept of health but by addressing areas that are affected by rheumatic disease. HAQ includes questions addressing mortality, functional status, physical discomfort, psychological discomfort, treatment side-effects, and economic impact.[7] Despite concerns regarding the ability to measure QoL in children,[35] major advances have been made in the development and validation of disease-specific HRQoL tools for children with rheumatic diseases. These instruments are discussed later.

The highest level in the hierarchy is the measurement of overall QoL. Overall QoL is affected by many life issues and events that do not clearly relate to health.[24] According to the WHO, QoL "...reflects the view that quality of life refers to a subjective evaluation, which is embedded in a cultural, social, and environmental context. (As such, quality of life, cannot be equated simply with the terms 'health status,' 'life style,' 'life satisfaction,' 'mental state' or 'well-being')."[36]

Because a QoL measure "...focuses upon respondents' 'perceived' quality of life, it is not expected to provide a means of measuring in any detailed fashion symptoms, diseases or conditions, nor disability as objectively judged, but rather the perceived effects of disease and health interventions on the individual's quality of life. [It] is, therefore, an assessment of a multi-dimensional concept incorporating the individual's perception of health status, psycho-social status and other aspects of life."[36]

Although QoL can be measured,[37] it is unclear how its measurement can contribute to health care. With this in mind, the development of a core set of measures for application in clinical trials in pediatric rheumatic diseases (JIA,[38] SLE,[39-41] and JDM[39,42-44]) has been extremely important. These core sets incorporate the types of instruments already alluded to, but focus mainly on the measurement of disease activity (Table 8–2).

PROCESS OF INSTRUMENT DEVELOPMENT

The development and validation process for activity limitation assessment or HRQoL instruments has been well established,[45] but for most health care providers the terminology and statistical approaches are unfamiliar. The development of a new instrument is labor intensive, requires sequential studies, entails input from a wide range of individuals, and needs frequent revisions of the original tool before completion. More than 20 iterations were required in the development of HAQ.[7] The developmental process for two of the functional assessment tools validated for children with JIA each required 3 to 5 years of work.[46-49] Given the broader scope of content, HRQoL instruments for JIA have taken at least as long.[50-52] The process used to develop and validate health measurement questionnaires has been described in textbooks[53] and published articles,[54] and several articles have described thoroughly the steps used for instruments specifically focused on children with rheumatic diseases.[50,55]

A key question to be addressed by anyone who is considering developing a new survey instrument or questionnaire is whether there is truly a need. At this time, there are hundreds of validated questionnaires, and review of the literature may reveal one that could serve the purpose. Researchers tend to magnify the deficiencies of existing measures and significantly underestimate the effort required to develop an adequate new measure.[53] There are several compendia of measuring scales. If one or more existent scales are found, these scales need to be evaluated. If the conclusion is that no existent questionnaire is satisfactory, much work awaits the brave souls who choose to develop a new tool (Table 8–3). The rest of this

Table 8–2

Core set measures and the definition of improvement of disease activity for juvenile idiopathic arthritis (JIA), systemic lupus erythematosus (SLE), and juvenile dermatomyositis (JDM)

JIA	SLE	JDM (PRINTO)	JDM (IMACS)
Core Set	Core Set	Core Set	Core Set
Physician Global Assessment	Physician Global Assessment	Physician Global Assessment	Physician Global Assessment
Patient/parent global assessment	Patient/parent global assessment	Patient/parent global assessment	Patient/parent global assessment
Active Joint Count	Global Disease Activity Tool (ECLAM, SLEDAI, SLAM)	Global Disease Activity (Disease Activity Status)	—
Joints with limited range of motion	—	Muscle strength (manual muscle testing or CMAS)	Muscle strength (manual muscle testing)
Acute phase reactant (ESR or CRP)	Renal involvement (24-hr proteinuria)	Muscle enzymes (CK, LDH, AST, ALT, aldolase)	Muscle enzymes (at least 2 of CK, LDH, AST, ALT, aldolase)
HRQoL or measure of physical function (e.g., CHAQ)	—	Functional ability (e.g., CMAS or CHAQ)	Functional ability (e.g., CMAS or CHAQ)
	HRQoL (CHQ–Physical Summary Score		—
—	—	—	Extramuscular disease
Definition of Improvement	Definition of Improvement	Definition of Improvement	Definition of Improvement
≥30% improvement in 3 of 6 measures with no more than 1 showing >30% worsening	≥50% improvement in 2 of 5 measures with no more than 1 showing >30% worsening	See text page 166	≥20% improvement in 3 of 6 measures with no more than 2 showing ≥20% worsening (muscle strength excluded)

IMACS, International Myositis Assessment and Clinical Studies group; PRINTO, Pediatric Rheumatology International Trials Organization
Data from Giannini et al, [38], Ruperto et al,[39-41,44] Rider et al.[42,43]

Table 8–3

Comparison of properties of the instruments used for juvenile rheumatoid arthritis*

Parameter	CHAQ[†]	JAFAR	JASI	JAQQ	CAHP	QoMLQ	CHQ	Peds QL
Reliability	Strong[‡]	Strong	Strong	Strong	Moderate	Strong	Strong	Strong
Validity	Strong	Strong	Strong	Strong	Moderate	Strong	Strong	Strong
Responsiveness	Moderate	Weak	Moderate	Very strong	NA	Strong	Moderate	Strong
Discriminative ability	Moderate	Moderate	Strong	Strong	Moderate	NA	Moderate	Strong
Applicable to a wide range	Very strong	No	No	Very strong	Moderate	Strong	Strong	Very strong
Applicable to a heterogeneous population	Very strong	Strong	No	Very strong	NA	NA	Very strong	Strong
Measures physical function	Moderate	Moderate	Very strong	Strong	Strong	No	Moderate	Moderate
Measures health-related quality of life	No	No	No	Strong	Strong	Strong	Strong	Strong
Measures pain	Moderate	Moderate	No	Strong	No	No	Moderate	Moderate
Tested widely	Very strong	Moderate	No	Strong	No	No	Strong	Strong
Easy to use	Strong	Strong	No	Strong	No	Very strong	Moderate	Strong

*Although most instruments have been developed using patients defined as having juvenile rheumatoid arthritis based on the criteria of the American College of Rheumatology, they are probably equally applicable to patients defined by the International League of Associations for Rheumatology as having juvenile idiopathic arthritis.

†CAHP, Childhood Arthritis Health Profile; CHAQ, Childhood Health Assessment Questionnaire; CHQ, Child Health Questionnaire; JAFAR, Juvenile Arthritis Functional Assessment Report; JASI, Juvenile Arthritis Self-report Index; JAQQ, Juvenile Arthritis Quality of Life Questionnaire; Peds QL, Pediatric Quality of Life Inventory; QoMLQ, Quality of My Life Questionnaire.

‡No, property absent; Weak, property present but weak; Moderate, property present and moderately strong; Strong, property present and strong; Very strong, property present and very strong; NA, not applicable.

chapter describes the various tools available in pediatric rheumatology. For a more complete description of these instruments, the reader is referred to the instruments themselves or to published reviews.[9,56,57]

BACKGROUND ON AVAILABLE INSTRUMENTS FOR CHILDHOOD RHEUMATIC DISEASES

As discussed already, there is an increasing need to incorporate estimates of physical, social, and mental functioning into health assessment, particularly in the assessment of chronic diseases,[10,27,58,59] in an attempt to provide an all-encompassing measure of HRQoL. HRQoL not only includes health status and physical functioning, but should also attempt to incorporate some part of the patient's own perception of what particular aspects of life affect him or her significantly and to what extent this is influenced by the disease.[10] These concerns have been considered in the development of measurement tools for adult rheumatic diseases[34,60,61] and have been shown to be reliable, valid, and responsive in various conditions.[62-67] They are now believed to be required for inclusion in clinical trials.[68,69]

Since 1986, various groups have attempted to develop the definitive measure for application in JIA. The length of time involved suggests that this is a complex task. The ideal instrument should be practical and easy to use; should be capable of completion by the parent or the child within a short time; should measure activity limitation and participation restriction; should, as suggested by Singsen,[70] measure psychological and social function, including school, family, and behavioral issues; and should include a measurement of pain (Table 8–4). None of the instruments developed to date meets all of these criteria. Each instrument has unique characteristics that make it distinct, however, and each one may have different indications for use. In the following sections, each instrument is discussed with an emphasis on its development, its measurement properties, and the settings in which it might be used.

Most instruments developed to date for childhood rheumatic diseases have their application in JIA (Table 8–5). Some instruments have been developed or have been modified for use in other pediatric rheumatic diseases such as SLE or JDM. The most relevant measures are discussed here with an emphasis on those applicable to JIA.

INSTRUMENTS FOR JUVENILE IDIOPATHIC ARTHRITIS

Disease-specific measures of functional status developed for JIA include Childhood Arthritis Impact Measurement Scales (CHAIMS),[71] Childhood Health Assessment Questionnaire (CHAQ),[47] Juvenile Arthritis Functional Assessment Scale (JAFAS) and Report (JAFAR),[48] and Juvenile Arthritis Self-report Index (JASI).[55,72] Disease-specific measures of HRQoL include Juvenile Arthritis Quality of Life Questionnaire (JAQQ)[50] and Childhood Arthritis Health Profile (CAHP).[51,52] More recently, there has been a greater focus on the use of generic instruments to assess HRQoL in children with JIA. Such measures include Quality of My Life Questionnaire (QoMLQ),[73] Child Health Questionnaire (CHQ),[74] and Pediatric Quality of Life Inventory (Peds QL)[75] (Table 8–5). All of these instruments are discussed briefly here, and Table 8–3 summarizes their comparative properties.

Childhood Arthritis Impact Measurement Scales

CHAIMS was the first disease-specific measure developed for JIA.[71] This was a modification of the AIMS.[34] Its measurement properties were poor, however, except for the pain dimension, and, as a result, it has not had widespread use.

Childhood Health Assessment Questionnaire

CHAQ[47] was derived from the adult HAQ.[7,60] It comprises two indices, Disability and Discomfort. The Disability Index assesses function in eight areas—dressing and grooming, arising, eating, walking, hygiene, reach, grip, and activities—distributed among a total of 30 items. In each functional area, there is at least one question that is relevant to children of all ages. Each question is rated on

---

Table 8–4

Required properties of the ideal instrument for juvenile idiopathic arthritis

Reliable
Valid
Responsive (sensitive to change)
Discriminative ability
Easy to use and score
Applicable to wide age range and to heterogeneous population
Measures physical function comprehensively
Measures health-related quality of life (including psychosocial functioning) comprehensively

---

Table 8–5

Instruments developed for and used in juvenile rheumatoid arthritis

Measures of Physical Function
Childhood Health Assessment Questionnaire (CHAQ)
Juvenile Arthritis Assessment Scale (JAFAS) and Report (JAFAR)
Juvenile Arthritis Self-Report Index (JASI)

Measures of Health-related Quality of Life
Juvenile Arthritis Quality of Life Questionnaire (JAQQ)
Childhood Arthritis Health Profile (CAHP)
Quality of My Life Questionnaire (QoMLQ)
Childhood Health Questionnaire (CHQ)
Pediatric Quality of Life Inventory Scales (Peds QL)

a 4-point scale of difficulty in performance, scored from 0 to 3. The Disability Index is calculated as the mean of the eight functional areas. Discomfort is determined by the presence of pain, as measured by a 100-mm visual analogue scale (VAS). In addition, a 100-mm VAS measures patient or parent global assessment of arthritis.

In the original validation study, mean scores for patients were 0.84 for the Disability Index and 0.82 for the Discomfort Index. Reliability was very good. Convergent validity was also very good, with excellent correlations with Steinbrocker's functional class, active joint count, disease activity index, and degree of morning stiffness. Mean scores for parents and children were not significantly different from one another and were highly correlated, suggesting that parents can reliably report for their children. CHAQ was completed by parents in all cases and by children 8 years and older in a mean of 10 minutes. Responsiveness was established later.[76]

CHAQ has been shown to be a useful instrument for outcome evaluation in longitudinal studies.[77-91] It has also been used in a variety of settings, translated into many different languages and undergone modifications in attempts to improve it while still maintaining excellent reliability, validity, and parent-child correlations.[92-106] One study emphasized the importance of considering disease duration of the population under study because correlations of other measures with CHAQ were progressively higher as disease duration increased.[106] Although one study suggested that it had poor responsiveness,[107] good responsiveness has been shown in other studies, including several longitudinal studies of etanercept.[108-112] Several studies have shown its usefulness in the evaluation of rehabilitative interventions.[113-118] Other studies suggest that it is highly predictive of the presence of significant pain,[119,120] and to be highly predictive of short-term outcomes in a large cohort of Canadian children.[121] Scores of 0.13, 0.63, and 1.75 represent mild, mild to moderate, and moderate disability,[122] whereas the minimum clinically important change score (MCID) for improvement is −0.188 and for deterioration is +0.125.[123] Although CHAQ does not measure psychosocial function in its present form, an earlier version showed reasonable measurement properties in this domain.[124] A digital form developed and validated in a Dutch population was declared to be user-friendly.[125]

CHAQ has excellent reliability and validity and reasonable responsiveness. It also has good discriminative properties, can be administered to children of all ages, and is of great use in the clinical setting for long-term follow-up of children with JIA. It is valuable for longitudinal studies and clinical trials and has become the preferred measure in both settings. Some attempts have been undertaken to modify it, but the original version is still used in most studies.

Juvenile Arthritis Functional Assessment Scale and Report

Juvenile Arthritis Functional Assessment Scale (JAFAS)[126] is an observer-based scale, whereas Juvenile Arthritis Functional Assessment Report (JAFAR)[46] is completed by the patient or parent. Items for both instruments were derived from the AIMS, HAQ, and McMaster Health Index Questionnaire.[127]

JAFAS requires standardized simple equipment and can be administered in about 10 minutes by a health professional who times the child's performance on 10 physical tasks. Good reliability and convergent validity have been shown. The major limitation of JAFAS is the requirement of a trained observer and standardized equipment.

JAFAR comprises one dimension and contains 23 items that assess ability to perform physical tasks in children older than 7 years on a 3-point scale scored from 0 to 2; the score range is 0 to 46, with the lower score indicating better function. Two separate versions are available, one for the child (JAFAR-C) and one for the parents (JAFAR-P). Reliability is good for both versions. Construct validity is also good, with predictable correlations among JAFAR-C, JAFAR-P, JAFAS, and pain, and moderate correlations with measures of disease activity. Similar measurement properties were found in an English study.[128] A Dutch translation of JAFAR also showed good measurement properties.[95] Responsiveness was shown in a small trial of intravenous immunoglobulin in polyarticular JIA.[129] JAFAR has also proved to be a useful measure of functional ability in studies on osteopenia[130,131] and sleep disturbance[132] in JIA.

JAFAR has excellent reliability and validity, but limited responsiveness. It cannot be administered to children younger than 7 years, and this prohibits its use in children with early onset of JIA. Nonetheless, it is a practical instrument that is useful in the clinical setting and in the longitudinal follow-up of most children with JIA.

Juvenile Arthritis Self-Report Index

JASI[55] was developed with a specific focus on physical activity in children older than 8 years with JIA. Its emphasis is on responsiveness, and it is aimed primarily at evaluation of rehabilitation interventions. Through a detailed process, as suggested by Kirshner and Guyatt,[54] an instrument with 100 items, distributed in five categories of physical function (self-care, domestic, mobility, school, and extracurricular), was developed. The score range is from 0 to 100, with higher scores indicating better function. A 7-point ordinal scale of difficulty in performing tasks was included. In a secondary component, JASI Part 2, patients identify up to five tasks that are most problematic, and these tasks are evaluated on sequential follow-up. This maneuver makes this component of JASI potentially more responsive and patient specific.

In a validation study, JASI was shown to have good measurement properties.[72] It was completed for the most part by the patients in a mean time of 49.8 minutes (including 10 minutes of instruction). The mean JASI Part 1 score for the group was 78.2 (range 20 to 100), suggesting overall excellent function. There was reasonable spread of scores, suggesting that JASI has discriminative ability. Reliability was shown with excellent intraclass correlations. Construct validity was established by demonstration of predicted correlations with other measures used. In a subsample of patients, level of agreement was good between JASI scores and observation of performance of tasks by a therapist. JASI Part 2 was also reliable, but less so.

JASI has been developed in a meticulous fashion, resulting in excellent reliability and validity. Data for JASI Part 2 suggest that it is responsive, although further data are needed to establish this property clearly. It cannot be administered to children younger than 8 years, however, and this prohibits its use in children with early onset of JIA. Also, because it is comprehensive, it takes a long time to complete, and this may make it less attractive for routine clinical use. Nonetheless, JASI is a comprehensive instrument with excellent measurement properties whose greatest value is probably as a research tool for longitudinal studies or to help identify specific goals in a rehabilitation setting.

Juvenile Arthritis Quality of Life Questionnaire

JAQQ[50] was developed by following standard principles of item generation.[54] The parents of 91 patients with JIA were interviewed to generate items. For children 9 years and older, parents and children were interviewed separately, a process that demonstrated a very high level of agreement between patients and parents over a wide array of perceived difficulties.[133] Additional items on psychosocial function were added by the incorporation of a previously developed psychosocial instrument.[134]

Generated items were subsequently reduced by application of scores assigned by patients, parents, and a panel of experts and categorized into four dimensions—gross motor function, fine motor function, psychosocial function, and general symptoms—each with approximately 20 items. A 1-to-7-point ordinal scale of frequency of difficulty with the particular item in question was applied, with higher scores indicating worse function. Respondents score all items and are asked to identify up to five items in each dimension with which they are having difficulty; they may also volunteer their own items for each dimension. The mean score for the five highest scoring items in each dimension is computed as the Dimension Score (range 1 to 7); Total JAQQ Score is computed as the mean of the four Dimension Scores (range 1 to 7).

This version of JAQQ was completed by 30 patients in 20 minutes initially, and then in 5 minutes on retesting 5 weeks later, showing good construct validity, with moderate correlations with measures of disease activity and excellent correlations with pain. Correlations for the psychosocial dimension were smaller, as predicted, being best with pain. Responsiveness was shown by correlations of change scores, which were moderate with sum of joint severity score and physician global assessment of change, and excellent with pain. Responsiveness was also shown by the ability of JAQQ to discriminate among patients based on physician global assessment of change.

After this initial study, the item number was reduced to 74—gross motor function, 17 items; fine motor function, 16 items; psychosocial function, 22 items; and general symptoms, 19 items. A pain dimension, added as a supplement to JAQQ, included a 100-mm VAS, a 5-point ordinal scale, and, for children younger than 10 years, a 5-point happy/sad face model.[135] Face and content validity of this version was confirmed by 20 pediatric rheumatologists and therapists. Construct validity and responsiveness were established.[136] Responsiveness was established further before and a mean of 8 weeks after the start of new drug therapy.[137] Responsiveness was also shown to be maintained over time[138] and to be at least as good as responsiveness of CHAQ, CHQ, or Peds QL.[139] Enhancement of responsiveness was shown by a reduction in the number of items scored, and in this study MCID was shown to be 0.35.[140]

JAQQ has been translated into several languages and has been shown to maintain its measurement properties in several different cultural settings.[141-143] In an English study of adolescents with JIA, and JAQQ was shown to have excellent reliability and validity.[143] In a further study, the same group showed improvement in JAQQ scores, with excellent responsiveness, after the introduction of a transitional care program.[144] A high level of agreement between the perception of children with JIA and their parents concerning HRQoL was shown in a Canadian study.[145] Another more recent Canadian study showed that JAQQ was highly predictive of several short-term outcomes in a large cohort of children with JIA.[121]

JAQQ has been developed in a detailed fashion, resulting in excellent reliability, validity, and responsiveness. It can be administered to children of all ages and disease onset types in a reasonable time with minimal assistance, and it can be scored quickly by hand; this makes it practical for use in the clinical setting. More recent data show that it is highly predictive of short-term outcomes, highlighting its value for longitudinal studies.

Childhood Arthritis Health Profile

CAHP[51] is a parent report that is self-administered and consists of three modules—generic health status measures, JIA-specific health status measures, and patient characteristics. Three functional scales—gross motor function, fine motor function, and role activities (play, family, friends)—were determined for the JIA-specific scales. Internal reliability was shown by good interitem correlations within scales and minimal item scale variation. Correlation coefficients for the JIA-specific scales with one another ranged from 0.84 to 0.97, whereas those for the generic functioning scales were 0.73, showing validity of these scales and further suggesting that the JIA-specific scales provide additional information beyond that of the generic functioning scales. In a follow-up report,[52] the discriminative ability of CAHP was demonstrated. CAHP is a promising instrument, but as yet too few data have been published to determine its usefulness.

Quality of My Life Questionnaire

QoMLQ was developed in an attempt to distinguish between difficulties resulting from the disease itself and difficulties that are more generic.[73] It comprises two separate 100-mm VAS, anchored with the descriptors "worst" and "best," that direct respondents to indicate their "quality of life," in aspects caused by the disease itself (HRQoL) and those caused by overall difficulties not directly related to the disease (QoL). This approach showed the importance of distinguishing between these factors because clear differences were noted among respondents between the two scales.

In a further study[37] that included 131 parent-child pairs, there was a high level of agreement between parents and children for QoL and moderate agreement for HRQoL. In this study, there were good correlations for components with pain and disease severity, establishing its convergent construct validity. Also, MCID for improvement in QoL and HRQoL were 7 mm and 11 mm, and for deterioration were −33 mm and −38 mm, providing the opportunity for clinicians to interpret changes in score.

QoMLQ is a short and easy-to-use generic instrument that has been shown to be highly reliable and valid. Given these qualities, it is likely to see more widespread use.

In further work from the same group, a novel approach was used in attempting to measure the gap between one's current situation and one's expectations, in some respects an extension of the work alluded to earlier. Contemporary measures of QoL tend not to take this "gap" into consideration. This study attempted to measure these gaps for a whole series of domains in children with rheumatic diseases. The result was the development of a measure with 72 items distributed among 5-gap scales (GapS). The GapS is currently undergoing further development.[24]

Child Health Questionnaire

CHQ[74] is a generic instrument that comprises numerous different forms. The form used most commonly in children with JIA is the Parent Form 50 (PF 50), which contains 50 items distributed in several dimensions— global health, physical activities, everyday activities, pain, behavior, well-being, self-esteem, general health, and family. These sections are complemented by general questions about the child and the caregiver. Two separate scores can be computed that estimate physical and psychosocial function; both are scored from 0 to 100, with the higher score indicating better function.

In a study of short-term outcome in 116 children with JIA observed for less than 2.5 years, Selvaag and colleagues[146] showed poorer physical status but minimal psychological impairment in JIA patients relative to controls using CHQ. Numerous studies from the Pediatric Rheumatology International Trials Organization (PRINTO), which has validated CHQ for use in 32 languages,[99] disagree with this, however. In one study that included 6639 participants (one half had JIA, and one half were healthy), mean scores for physical and psychosocial summary scores were significantly lower for JIA patients relative to controls.[147] In a further study that included three distinct geographical regions (Eastern Europe, Western Europe, and Latin America), determinants of poor HRQoL were similar across all regions, with physical well-being affected by the level of disability and psychosocial well-being affected by the intensity of pain.[148] CHQ was used in combination with CHAQ in a trial of methotrexate, where it was shown to be highly responsive[109]; this was further confirmed in the follow-up of the same study group.[149] One study suggested, however, that

JAQQ may be at least as responsive as CHQ for studies in JIA.[139] Because of its generalizability, CHQ has become the preferred measure of QoL for JIA trials.

Pediatric Quality of Life Inventory

Peds QL is a modular instrument designed to measure HRQoL in children and adolescents 2 to 18 years old.[75] It contains a generic core integrated with a disease-specific core. The generic core has undergone various iterations, the most recent of which, the Peds QL 4.0 Generic Core Scales, contains 23 items distributed in four scales—physical, emotional, social, and school functioning. The Peds QL 3.0 Rheumatology Module contains 22 disease-specific items distributed in five scales (pain, daily activities, treatment, worry, and communication). It is completed by children and their parents and consists of developmentally appropriate forms for varying age groups. When it is completed separately, parent-child concordance has been shown to be good. The module takes approximately 15 minutes to complete. Each item is scored on a 5-point scale (0 to 4), with a higher score indicating worse function. A mean Scale Score is computed based on the number of items scored. This score is extrapolated in a reverse fashion to a scale of 0 to 100, with a higher score indicating better function. Total Scale Scores are computed as the mean across all items scored in that scale. This process is the same for the Generic Core Scale and the Rheumatology Module.

This instrument was shown to have excellent reliability, validity, and responsiveness in a study of 271 children with various rheumatic diseases, 91 of whom had JIA, and their parents.[150] Reliability varied with the age of the child, being less for younger children. Reliability was also not as good for the Rheumatology Module.

Lower HRQoL, as exemplified by lower Peds QL generic and rheumatology module scores, was noted in one study, despite minimal symptoms or little or no disease activity,[151] whereas another study showed significantly reduced scores in children with polyarticular JIA, particularly in fatigue scores.[152] A further study showed lower Peds QL scores for Medicaid patients even when correcting for health care use and degree of disease activity.[153]

Responsiveness has not been tested in a trial setting. Nonetheless, this instrument represents an important addition to the pool of outcome measures available for use in JIA, and further studies are being followed with interest.

Composite Disease Activity Scores for Juvenile Idiopathic Arthritis

American College of Rheumatology (ACR) JIA core set and pediatric response criteria focus on change in disease state and assess improvement or deterioration in disease activity. Individually, these measures are incomplete, however. A composite disease activity score for JIA, Juvenile Arthritis Disease Activity Score (JADAS), has been developed.[154] JADAS includes four of the measures included in the core set—active joint count, physician's global assessment of disease activity, patient and parent global assessment of overall well-being, and erythrocyte sedimentation rate. Joint count is modified based on evaluation of 10, 27, or 71 joints in three different versions of the instrument. JADAS has been shown to have good measurement properties, including responsiveness, and is a very useful addition.

INSTRUMENTS AVAILABLE FOR USE IN RHEUMATIC DISEASES OTHER THAN JUVENILE IDIOPATHIC ARTHRITIS

There has been considerable recent international effort to develop appropriate measures for use in JDM and SLE in adults and children. This effort has culminated in the development of measures of disease activity and damage[155] and a core set of measures for childhood-onset and adult-onset diseases.[156,157] The core set for JDM was conducted simultaneously with a similar effort for juvenile SLE (see Table 8–2).[157]

Through an initial survey of 267 physicians worldwide, followed by a nominal group technique process, 37 response variables for JDM were examined. Ultimately, a core set for JDM was arrived at comprising six measures (see Table 8–2). This instrument has undergone validation testing in an attempt to define improvement in the core set.[158] Such improvement is defined as a minimum of 15% improvement in the domains of muscle strength and physical function, a minimum of 20% improvement for physician and patient global assessments and overall global assessment, and a minimum of 30% improvement in muscle enzymes. To complement this core set, which focuses predominantly on myositis, a measure has been developed to measure activity of the skin in JDM—Cutaneous Assessment Tool (CAT).[159] This tool has excellent measurement properties, which have been maintained even with a modification of the scoring method.[160]

In addition to the core set and CAT, a specific outcome measure has been developed to assess physical function in JDM—Childhood Myositis Assessment Scale (CMAS).[161] This is a therapist-administered assessment of muscle strength, endurance, and function with excellent measurement properties. It is scored on a scale of 0 to 52, based on the ability of the child to perform specific tasks scored by an observer. CMAS has been shown to have outstanding intra-observer and inter-observer reliability. It has been shown to have good validity and good correlations with manual muscle testing.

CHAQ has also been validated for use in JDM patients. It was shown to have excellent test-retest reliability, validity, and responsiveness[162-165] and to be valuable as a measure of outcome.[163] CHQ was used in combination with CHAQ in a study of 272 children with JDM.[166] It performed well and showed that there was a significant reduction in HRQoL as evidenced by decreased physical and psychosocial summary scores.

As a component of the initiative discussed for JDM, a similar effort was conducted for juvenile SLE.[157] In this component of the study, 41 response variables were tested. Ultimately, measures of disease activity were those depicted (see Table 8–2) and included specific SLE immunological tests and renal function measures and physician and parent/patient global assessments, an overall global assessment, a measure of growth and development, and a measure of HRQoL (most likely CHQ, but this has not been finalized). Brunner and associates[167] previously validated the Systemic Lupus Erythematosus Disease Activity Index (SLEDAI) for juvenile SLE and in a more recent study showed the responsiveness of European Consensus Lupus Activity Measurement (ECLAM) for juvenile SLE, suggesting that it might be more sensitive than SLEDAI in this population.[168] Two studies described the extent of damage in juvenile SLE[169,170] using Systemic Lupus International Collaborating Clinics (SLICC)/ACR Damage Index. A Canadian study showed reduced fitness, increasing fatigue, and reduced HRQoL, measured by CHQ, in a group of 15 adolescents with SLE.[171] Neither fatigue nor fitness correlated with disease activity, disease damage, or HRQoL, however. Similar findings were observed in 24 children using Peds QL.[172]

Finally, a new instrument to measure HRQoL in SLE has been developed—Simple Measure of the Impact of Lupus Erythematosus in Youngsters (SMILEY).[173] It contains four domains—effect on self, limitations, social, and burden of SLE—that address patient perceptions of HRQoL. In the initial validation study, SMILEY was shown to have excellent reliability and validity and is currently undergoing further study.

CONCLUSION

In this chapter, we have highlighted the ICF framework (see Fig. 8–1) as suggested by WHO and have illustrated how it might be used to structure a hierarchy of outcomes. The first level of outcome assessment is within the domain of structure and function. Measures of so-called disease activity, of which there are many, fit in this domain. Measures such as active joint count are often of most interest to the treating physician. The next level up the hierarchy is the measurement of activity and activity limitation and social participation. This level reflects physical function and disability and social handicaps. This area is usually of most relevance to the patient. Measurement in this area includes measures of HRQoL. The highest level in this hierarchy is the measurement of overall QoL. Overall QoL is affected by many life issues and events that do not relate only to health, but are of greater societal interest. Although measures have been developed that apply to all three levels, measurement of QoL has proved most difficult, and although it can be measured, it is unclear how its measurement can contribute to health care. For this reason, the greatest focus of clinicians has been on measures of disease activity and HRQoL.

Measures of disease activity have been discussed briefly for JIA, JDM, and SLE. The major development has been the adoption of a core set of measures for each of these diseases (see Table 8–2). The development of a composite score, JADAS, for JIA, and a measure of skin disease activity, CAT, for JDM have been important additions.

We have focused our attention on measures of HRQoL with a particular emphasis on JIA. The properties of these various instruments were compared (see Table 8–3). They differ significantly from one another and have been developed with different objectives in mind, so that each has unique qualities. Four measures—CHAIMS, CHAQ, JAFAR, and JASI—have a specific focus on physical function, whereas the others—JAQQ, CAHP, QoMLQ, CHQ, and Peds QL—attempt to measure HRQoL in addition to physical function. QoMLQ also attempts to measure QoL. Of these various measures, CHAQ and CHQ are most widely used, and their measurement properties are excellent. JAQQ, Peds QL, and QoMLQ are also excellent measures, however, and these are being used increasingly. Because they contribute measurement over a broader domain and are relatively easy to use, they may prove to be superior over time.

Attempts to develop better measures for JDM and SLE continue. Further study of CMAS is ongoing, and there has been increasing study of established measures such as CHAQ and CHQ for JDM. Ongoing work continues to evaluate adult SLE measures in children with SLE and studies that included CHQ and PedsQL. The addition of a specific HRQoL for childhood SLE—SMILEY— has been important, and further work on it is ongoing.

The past several years have been a very exciting and active time of research. Ongoing research will add to our knowledge and understanding of this complex process of measurement, not only in JIA, but also in other pediatric rheumatic diseases.

REFERENCES

5. C. Eiser, R. Morse, The measurement of quality of life in children: past and future perspectives, J. Dev. Behav. Pediatr. 22 (2001) 248–256.
6. P. Tugwell, C. Bombardier, W.W. Buchanan, et al., Methotrexate in rheumatoid arthritis: impact on quality of life assessed by traditional standard-item and individualized patient preference health status questionnaires, Arch. Intern. Med. 150 (1990) 59–62.
9. C.M. Duffy, Measurement of health status, functional status, and quality of life in children with juvenile idiopathic arthritis: clinical science for the paediatrician, Rheum. Dis. Clin. North Am. 33 (2007) 389–402.
10. T.M. Gill, A.R. Feinstein, A critical appraisal of the quality of Quality of Life measurements, JAMA 272 (1994) 619–626.
11. World Health Organization, ICF beginner's guide, WHO, Geneva, 2002 http://www.who.int/classifications/icf/training/icfbeginnersguide.pdf.
16. G. Stucki, A. Cieza, The International Classification of Functioning, Disability and Health (ICF) in physical and rehabilitation medicine, Eur. J. Phys. Rehabil. Med. 44 (2008) 299–302.
18. G. Stucki, T. Ewert, How to assess the impact of arthritis on the individual patient: the WHO ICF, Ann. Rheum. Dis. 64 (2005) 664–668.
19. M. Weigl, A. Cieza, P. Cantista, et al., Determinants of disability in chronic musculoskeletal health conditions: a literature review, Eur. J. Phys. Rehabil. Med. 44 (2008) 67–79.
24. G.W. Gong, M. Barrera, J. Beyene, et al., The Gap Study (GapS) interview—developing a process to determine the meaning and determinants of quality of life in children with arthritis and rheumatic disease, Clin. Exp. Rheumatol. 25 (2007) 486–493.
27. G.H. Guyatt, J.O. Sander, V. Van Zanten, et al., Measuring quality of life in clinical trials: a taxonomy and review, Can. Med. Assoc. J. 140 (1989) 1441–1448.
28. G.H. Guyatt, D.H. Feeny, D.L. Patrick, Measuring health-related quality of life, Ann. Intern. Med. 118 (1993) 622–629.
29. G.H. Guyatt, Insights and limitations from health-related quality-of-life research, J. Gen. Intern. Med. 12 (1997) 720–721.
30. M.A. Testa, D.C. Simonson, Assessment of quality-of-life outcomes, N. Engl. J. Med. 334 (1996) 835–840.
38. E.H. Giannini, R. Ruperto, A. Ravelli, Paediatric Rheumatology International Trials Organization (PRINTO): Preliminary definition of improvement in juvenile arthritis, Arthritis Rheum. 40 (1997) 1202–1209.
47. G. Singh, B.H. Athreya, J.F. Fries, et al., Measurement of health status in children with juvenile rheumatoid arthritis, Arthritis Rheum. 37 (1994) 1761–1769.
48. D.J. Lovell, Newer functional outcome measurements in juvenile rheumatoid arthritis: a progress report, J. Rheumatol. 19 (suppl 33) (1992) 28–31.
50. C.M. Duffy, L. Arsenault, K.N. Watanabe Duffy, et al., The Juvenile Arthritis Quality of Life Questionnaire: development of a new responsive index for juvenile rheumatoid arthritis and juvenile spondyloarthritides, J. Rheumatol. 24 (1997) 738–746.
54. B. Kirshner, G. Guyatt, A methodologic framework for assessing health indices, J. Chron. Dis. 38 (1985) 27–36.
55. V.F. Wright, M. Law, V. Crombie, et al., Development of a self-report functional status index for juvenile rheumatoid arthritis, J. Rheumatol. 21 (1994) 536–544.
59. A.R. Feinstein, B.R. Josephy, C.K. Wells, Scientific and clinical problems in indexes of functional disability, Ann. Intern. Med. 105 (1986) 413–420.
61. P. Tugwell, C. Bombardier, W.W. Buchanan, et al., The MAC-TAR patient preference questionnaire: an individualized functional priority approach for assessing improvement in clinical trials in rheumatoid arthritis, J. Rheumatol. 14 (1987) 446–451.
72. V.F. Wright, J. Longo Kimber, M. Law, et al., The Juvenile Arthritis Functional Status Index (JASI): a validation study, J. Rheumatol. 23 (1996) 1066–1079.
73. B.M. Feldman, B. Grundland, L. McCullough, et al., Distinction of quality of life, health-related quality of life, and health status in children referred for rheumatology care, J. Rheumatol. 27 (2000) 226–233.
74. J.M. Landgraf, L. Abetz, J.E. Ware, Child Health Questionnaire (CHQ): a user's manual, The Health Institute, New England Medical Center, Boston, 1996.
75. J.W. Varni, M. Seid, C.A. Rode, The Peds QL: measurement model for the Pediatric Quality of Life Inventory, Med. Care 37 (1999) 126–139.
77. B. Andersson Gare, A. Fasth, Wiklund I: Measurement of functional status in juvenile chronic arthritis: evaluation of a Swedish version of the Childhood Health Assessment Questionnaire, Clin. Exp. Rheumatol. 11 (1993) 569–576.
79. N. Ruperto, A. Ravelli, J.E. Levison, et al., Long term health outcomes and quality of life in American and Italian inception cohorts of patients with juvenile rheumatoid arthritis, II. early predictors of outcome, J. Rheumatol. 24 (1997) 952–958.
80. K. Minden, U. Kiessling, J. Listing, et al., Prognosis of patients with juvenile chronic arthritis and juvenile spondyloarthropathy, J. Rheumatol. 27 (2000) 2256–2263.
82. M. Zak, F.K. Pedersen, Juvenile chronic arthritis into adulthood: a long-term follow up study, Rheumatology 39 (2000) 198–204.
84. L.R. Spiegel, R. Schneider, B.A. Lang, et al., Early predictors of poor functional outcome in systemic onset juvenile rheumatoid arthritis: a multicentre cohort study, Arthritis Rheum. 43 (2000) 2402–2409.
85. K. Oen, P. Malleson, D. Cabral, et al., Disease course and outcome of juvenile rheumatoid arthritis in a multicentre cohort, J. Rheumatol. 29 (2002) 1989–1999.
86. F. Fantini, V. Gerloni, M. Gattinara, et al., Remission in juvenile chronic arthritis: a cohort study of 683 consecutive cases with a mean 10 year follow up, J. Rheumatol. 30 (2003) 579–584.
89. S. Bowyer, P.A. Roettcher, G.C. Higgins, et al., Health status of patients with juvenile rheumatoid arthritis at 1 and 5 years after diagnosis, J. Rheumatol. 30 (2003) 394–400.
90. K. Oen, P. Malleson, D. Cabral, et al., Early predictors of long-term outcome in patients with juvenile rheumatoid arthritis: subset-specific correlations, J. Rheumatol. 30 (2003) 585–593.
91. S. Magni-Manzoni, A. Pistorio, E. Labo, et al., A longitudinal analysis of physical functional disability over the course of juvenile idiopathic arthritis, Ann. Rheum. Dis. 67 (2008) 1159–1164.
99. N. Ruperto, A. Ravelli, A. Pistorio, et al., Cross-cultural adaptation and psychometric evaluation of the Childhood Health Assessment Questionnaire (CHAQ) and the Child Health Questionnaire (CHQ) in 32 countries, Clin. Exp. Rheumatol. 19 (suppl 23) (2001) S1–S9.
119. C. Sallfors, L.R. Hallberg, A. Fasth, Gender and age differences in pain, coping and health status among children with chronic arthritis, Clin. Exp. Rheumatol. 21 (2003) 785–793.

120. K. Oen, M. Reed, P. Malleson, et al., Radiologic outcome and its relationship to functional disability in juvenile rheumatoid arthritis, J. Rheumatol. 30 (2003) 832–840.

121. K. Oen, L. Tucker, A.M. Huber, C.M. Duffy, Predictors of early inactive disease in a juvenile idiopathic arthritis cohort: results of a Canadian multicenter, prospective inception cohort study, Arthritis Rheum. 61 (2009) 1077–1086.

122. H. Dempster, M. Porepa, N. Young, B.M, Feldman, et al., The clinical meaning of functional outcome scores in children with juvenile arthritis, Arthritis Rheum. 44 (2001) 1768–1774.

123. H.I. Brunner, M.S. Klein-Gittelman, M.J. Miller, et al., Minimal clinically important differences of The Childhood Health Assessment Questionnarie, J. Rheumatol. 32 (2005) 150–161.

125. L.M. Geerdink, F.H. Prince, C.W. Looman, et al., Development of a digital Childhood Health Assessment Questionnaire for systemic monitoring of disease activity in daily practice, Rheumatology 48 (2009) 858–863.

126. D.J. Lovell, S. Howe, S. Shear, et al., Development of a disability measurement tool for juvenile rheumatoid arthritis, Arthritis Rheum. 32 (1989) 1390–1395.

133. C.M. Duffy, L. Arsenault, K.N. Duffy, Level of agreement between parents and children in rating dysfunction in juvenile rheumatoid arthritis and juvenile spondyloarthritides, J. Rheumatol. 20 (1993) 2134–2139.

143. K.L. Shaw, T.R. Southwood, C.M. Duffy, et al., Health-related quality of life in adolescents with juvenile idiopathic arthritis, Arthritis Rheum. 55 (2006) 199–207.

144. J.E. McDonagh, T.R. Southwood, K.L. Shaw, The impact of a co-ordinated transitional care program on adolescents with juvenile idiopathic arthritis, Rheumatology 46 (2007) 161–168.

145. K.T. April, D.E. Feldman, R.W. Platt, C.M. Duffy, et al., Comparison between children with juvenile idiopathic arthritis and their parents concerning perceived quality of life, Qual. Life Res. 15 (2006) 655–661.

147. S. Oliveira, A. Ravelli, A. Pistorio, et al., Proxy-reported health-related quality of life of patients with juvenile idiopathic arthritis: the Pediatric Rheumatology International Trials Organization multinational quality of life cohort study, Arthritis Rheum. 57 (2007) 35–43.

150. J.W. Varni, M. Seid, T. Smith Knight, et al., The Peds QL in Pediatric Rheumatology: reliability, validity and responsiveness of the Pediatric Quality of Life Inventory Generic Core Scales and Rheumatology Module, Arthritis Rheum. 46 (2002) 714–725.

153. H.I. Brunner, J. Taylor, M.T. Britto, et al., Differences in disease outcomes between Medicaid and privately insured children: possible health disparities in juvenile rheumatoid arthritis, Arthritis Rheum. 55 (2006) 378–384.

157. N. Ruperto, A. Ravelli, K.J. Murray, et al., Preliminary core set of measures for disease activity and damage assessment in juvenile systemic lupus erythematosus and juvenile dermatomyositis, Rheumatology 42 (2003) 1452–1459.

158. L. Rider, E.H. Giannini, M. Harris-Love, et al., Defining clinical improvement in adult and juvenile myositis, J. Rheumatol. 30 (2003) 603–617.

159. A.M. Huber, E.M. Dugan, P.A. Lachenbruch, et al., Preliminary validation and clinical meaning of the Cutaneous Assessment Tool (CAT) in juvenile dermatomyositis, Arthritis Rheum. 59 (2008) 214–221.

160. A.M. Huber, P.A. Lachenbruch, E.M. Dugan, et al., Alternative scoring of the Cutaneous Assessment Tool in juvenile dermatomyositis: results using abbreviated formats, Arthritis Rheum. 59 (2008) 352–356.

161. D.J. Lovell, C.B. Lindsley, R.M. Rennebohm, et al., Development of validated disease activity and damage indices for the juvenile idiopathic inflammatory myopathies, II: the Childhood Myositis Assessment Scale (CMAS): a quantitative tool for the evaluation of muscle function. The Juvenile Dermatomyositis Disease Activity Collaborative Study Group, Arthritis Rheum. 42 (1999) 2213–2219.

164. A.M. Huber, J.E. Hicks, P.A. Lachenbruch, et al., Validation of the Childhood Health Assessment Questionnaire in the juvenile idiopathic myopathies, J. Rheumatol. 28 (2001) 1106–1111.

167. H.I. Brunner, B.M. Feldman, C. Bombardier, et al., Sensitivity of the systemic lupus erythematosus disease activity index, British Isles Lupus Assessment Group Index, and systemic lupus activity measure in the evaluation of clinical change in childhood-onset systemic lupus erythematosus, Arthritis Rheum. 42 (1999) 1354.

171. K.M. Houghton, L.B. Tucker, J.E. Potts, D.C McKenzie, et al., Fitness, fatigue, disease activity, and quality of life in pediatric lupus, Arthritis Rheum. 59 (2008) 537–545.

172. L.N. Moorthy, M.J. Harrison, M. Peterson, et al., Relationship of quality of life and physical function measures with disease activity in children with systemic lupus erythematosus, Lupus 14 (2005) 280–287.

Entire reference list is available online at www.expertconsult.com.

Chapter 9

MANAGING CHILDREN WITH RHEUMATIC DISEASES

Balu H. Athreya and Carol B. Lindsley

Rheumatic diseases are chronic, multisystem diseases characterized by an unpredictable course with periods of exacerbation and remission. Care of affected children requires consultations with medical and surgical specialists. Many of these disorders cause muscle weakness and joint contractures with functional disabilities requiring the services of physical and occupational therapists, counselors, and social service agencies (Table 9–1). Treatment of these diseases with anti-inflammatory agents, immunosuppressive agents, and biological immune modulators is discussed in various chapters dealing with individual disease categories. This chapter discusses general principles of management, such as team care, compliance, school attendance, and transition to adult care. A small section on immunization is also included. Physical and occupational therapy and rehabilitation will be dealt with in Chapter 12.

There are multiple dimensions to the effects of chronic illness on children and on members of their families.[1] Several early studies suggested that chronic illness has a negative impact on psychosocial development,[1,2] family,[3] school life,[4] and family finances.[5,6] Studies focusing on children with rheumatic diseases growing up before the availability of modern drugs showed that 30% to 50% entered adult life with active disease.[7,8] Severe disability was common in this young adult population with decreased physical functions, poor health perception, and pain.[9,10] All of the psychosocial and physical problems assume greater importance when such children reach adolescence[11] or when they grow up to be adults with continuing disease activity.[12,13]

The current approach to early treatment, which uses immune modulators and intra-articular glucocorticoids, has resulted in reduced incidence of severe deformities. However, in one recent study conducted after the introduction of the newer therapies, persistent disease activity and impaired functioning were still seen frequently.[14]

Earlier observations of poor outcome for children with rheumatic diseases have not been substantiated in recent studies. Even studies that emphasized the negative impacts of growing up with juvenile rheumatoid arthritis (JRA) (or Juvenile idiopathic arthritis [JIA]) showed that many of these patients completed college, worked full time, and raised children.[9,12,13,15] Recent well-designed studies seem to indicate that JRA is not necessarily a psychosocial stressor, and families of children with JRA are, in general, resilient.[16,17] Patients with JRA growing into early adulthood were shown to be able to earn a living, live independently, and have a stable spousal relationship, although patients with active disease had poor health-related quality of life in the physical component.[18] Some of these children do suffer disabilities, have reduced function and employment status and decreased social acceptance,[19] and have overall adjustment problems and internalization of symptoms.[20] For all of these reasons, a program of care for children with rheumatic diseases should plan for the whole child and the future and should be comprehensive (i.e., family-centered, community-based, coordinated, and cost-effective) (Table 9–2).[21]

Current research suggests that planning for care of these children should be based on new concepts of disablement, should be evidence-based, and should be individualized. New concepts of the "disablement" process include four distinct constructs: active pathology, impairment, functional limitation, and disability.[22] Each of these stages offers potential for intervention. In addition, there may be other factors, such as coping skills, access to care, economics, and the family's psychosocial climate,

---

Table 9–1

Components of the management of rheumatic diseases in children

Medical and surgical management

Family-centered, community-based, coordinated care (school, outreach)

Psychosocial management (social services, mental health services, financial)

Musculoskeletal rehabilitation (physical therapy, occupational therapy, orthopaedics)

Well-child care issues (growth and development, nutrition, immunization, anticipatory guidance)

Continuity of care

Cost-effective care

Table 9–2

Steps in implementing family-centered, community-based care

Recognizing the pivotal roles of the child and the family in the planning of care

Developing resources in the community where the child lives

Recognizing parents and professionals as equals in a partnership of care

Empowering the family with information through education and support

Encouraging pediatricians to assume a greater role in case coordination, become knowledgeable about available local resources, and work with community agencies

Increasing communication among disciplines and between patients and health professionals

Breaking barriers to the development of such a system

Table 9–3

Risk and resilience

Risk factors	Resilience factors
Severity of disease and disability	Family's ability to solve problems
Degree of functional independence	Social support
Daily hassles and struggles	Coping skills

From Wallender JL, Varni VW: Adjustment in children with chronic physical disorders: programmatic research on a disability-stress coping module. In La Greca AM, Siegel LJ, Wallender JL et al, editors: *Stress and coping in child health,* New York, 1991, Guilford.

that contribute to the disablement process and therefore are appropriate targets for intervention. The newer International Classification of Function, Disability and Health (ICF) includes external factors such as physical, social and attitudinal that impact on disability and impairment.[23] Newer tools for the evaluation of disability include items to measure body function and structure, activities and participation, and environmental and personal factors.[24] Based on this conceptual framework, specific tools have been developed for use in specific conditions such as rheumatoid arthritis and osteoarthritis[25] and for use in children (ICF-CY).[26]

Based on their well-designed study, Noll and colleagues suggested that "randomly occurring, challenging life events do not alter the child's potential for inclusive fitness by denigrating their social status or emotional well-being."[27] Therefore, it is important to know why some patients and families are vulnerable to functional and psychosocial disabilities and others are not.[16,17] One concept to explain this difference in vulnerability focuses on risk factors that tend to push children with chronic illness and their families to dysfunction and disability and resilience factors that tend to give them more stability.[28,29] The relative predominance of risk factors or resilience factors influences outcomes (Table 9–3).

Therefore, in planning for the care of these children, emphasis should be on the child and the family, and efforts should be aimed not only at controlling the disease and managing the current problems, but also at planning for the future. Steps should be taken to improve the resilience of patients and families through better education to cope with the vicissitudes of these diseases, improved social and peer support for the children and their parents, and education in stress management to help them cope better with their disease and disability.

Accurate diagnosis is the first step. Rheumatic diseases may be acute and explosive in onset, or they may evolve over a period of months and years. Only one organ system may be affected, or several systems may be involved. They may mimic several other inflammatory and noninflammatory diseases. It may not be possible to place an accurate diagnostic label at first, and yet life-threatening complications and functional disabili-

TEAM CARE

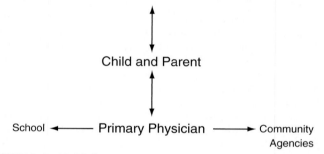

FIGURE 9–1   Model of team care.

ties may have to be managed. Great skill and patience are required to support the families in managing their problems in the face of uncertainties in diagnosis and prognosis. Therein reside the challenges and pleasures of rheumatology.

Expertise should be the cornerstone of the care of children with rheumatic diseases. Comprehensive treatment centers should be based in tertiary-care academic centers. The treatment team (Fig. 9–1) should consist of a pediatric rheumatologist, a nurse specialist, physical and occupational therapists, a social worker, and a psychologist, all working with the child's primary care physician. Consultations with an orthopaedic surgeon, ophthalmologist, nutritionist, and dentist should be available when required. Team care is expensive and is not required for every child, particularly with the recent advances in medical management. However, these services should be available when needed.

The child and family should be the central focus of the team. The roles of the primary care physician and the rheumatologist are listed in Table 9–4. Effective communication between the primary care physician and the specialist, and the availability of one contact person at the tertiary center, are the other essential requirements for comprehensive care.[30] Specially trained nurses have fulfilled the contact function effectively in many pediatric rheumatology centers.[31]

Table 9–4

Role of physicians in the care management team

The Primary physician	Pediatric rheumatologist
Care of intercurrent illness	Overall management of the rheumatic disorder
Immunization	Detailed guidelines and directions for the management of a specific problem
Developmental issues	Ongoing medical explanation for the management decisions
Anticipatory guidance	Minor counseling
Working with the community agencies	Physical therapy/occupational therapy
Working with the school system	Monitoring for drug toxicity
	Referral to other subspecialty

PATIENT EDUCATION

Children with rheumatic diseases and their parents require education on several issues. These issues are discussed in detail in several publications. The mode of teaching has to vary to suit the needs and skills of parents. Language barriers, cultural backgrounds, and literacy issues must be kept in mind before such programs are organized. Education about the disease, medications, adverse effects of medications, and therapy programs should take place both individually by the pediatric rheumatologist and in parent support groups. The belief system of the family should be explored, and all doubts and questions should be addressed. Information required by parents varies with the time that has passed since diagnosis. It also depends on the developmental needs of the child. Therefore, education must be individualized.[32]

Information is easily available on the Internet. However, families need help to receive information from reliable sources, such as the Arthritis Foundation (http://www. arthritis.org), and they need assistance with interpretation of the information gathered.

COUNSELING

A trusting relationship is the most important requirement for effective counseling. To be trusted, one must be trustworthy. Open, honest communication with the child and the parents is a major component of this relationship.

Collecting information about a child's illness, behavior, and family dynamics may require many visits and observations. Deep, empathic listening is the first step. One must listen to what the child and family say and observe what they do. Nonverbal cues must be attended to.

As physicians, we are trained to look for and diagnose weaknesses in the person and the system. In addition, we should look for strengths in the patient, family, and the community. It is important to know the strengths so that we can build on them while finding ways to compensate for the weaknesses. This strength may lie in the extended family, an interested schoolteacher, or a loving

grandparent. Some families grow in strength in the presence of adversity. Factors that contribute to successful coping should be supported and encouraged.[28,33] Referral to a clinical psychologist may be needed.

Children with physical disabilities and deformities and children who look different because of a rash or steroid therapy are bound to feel different and self-conscious. Physical disability and fluctuation in disease activity may make it difficult for these children to participate in social and family activities. Emphasizing what they can do and planning activities in which they can participate should help their sense of self-worth and morale. There should be alternative plans and backup arrangements. Involvement of siblings, friends, and classmates in helping a disabled child during activities should help create a successful experience for everyone.

ADHERENCE (COMPLIANCE)

Children with chronic illness soon become tired of taking medicines day after day with no end in sight. They often ask why they have to do mindless exercises that do not appear to help them in any way. Therefore, compliance with medication and therapy programs becomes a major issue for children with chronic diseases.[34] The word "compliance" implies that the physician gives orders and the patient obeys. But the ideal situation is an informed patient who chooses to follow the treatment prescribed by a trusted physician after being convinced of the benefits and made aware of the consequences of not following the treatment. In other words, the patient chooses to adhere to the prescribed program. In pediatrics, one must consider the child, the parent, and the care-giver to make sure the treatment plan is followed. Patient and parent education and incorporation of the needs of family members in the planning process are essential. Listening to the specific needs of a child and family and incorporating them into the plan, as well as designing a plan that accounts for the stresses and strengths of the family and their cultural values, increases the likelihood of the plan being followed. Factors that affect adherence and strategies to enhance adherence are listed in Tables 9–5 and 9–6.

SIBLING ISSUES

Stress related to living with chronic illness affects every member of the family, including siblings. The role of siblings and their impact on the developmental needs of the patient may vary with the age and cognitive level of siblings, their perception of the child with chronic illness, parental attitudes, and the demands placed on unaffected siblings.[35] Feelings may range from guilt (that siblings are responsible for the sick child in some magical way), to fear of catching the illness, to embarrassment.[36]

Siblings may resent the extra time and attention given to the affected child and perceived favoritism in matters of discipline. Realistically, parents may not be able to provide adequate time to satisfy the developmental needs of the siblings. This is a problem for single parents in particular.

Table 9–5

Factors that influence adherence

Cognitive/emotional (e.g., limited ability to understand, depression)
Behavioral (e.g., defiance, adolescent independence)
Cultural (e.g., alternative concepts of disease model)
Social and family issues (e.g., unstable family)
Disease-related (e.g., chronicity)
Medication-related (e.g., side effects)
Organizational (e.g., appointments in the clinic)
Economics (e.g., cost of visit)

From Kroll T, Barlow JH, Shaw K: Treatment adherence in juvenile rheumatoid arthritis: a review, *Scand J Rheumatol* 28:10-18, 1999.

Table 9–6

Strategies to facilitate and promote adherence

Informational handouts
Cues and reminders
Positive feedback
Discipline
Steps to minimize discomfort and inconvenience
Dealing effectively with complaints
Monitoring disease process for changes

Adapted from Rapoff M: Compliance with treatment regimens for pediatric rheumatic diseases, *Arthritis Care Res* 3:40-47, 1989.

Table 9–7

Approaches to siblings of children with chronic illness

Include siblings in clinic visits.
Talk with siblings and explore their needs.
Determine the perception of the siblings on the impact of the illness on family members.
Help them deal with their friends' questions.
Encourage and enlist sibling participation in developing care plans.
Conduct sibling group discussions at local and national support groups.

Table 9–8

Related school services needed by chronically ill children

Administration of medications
Implementation of medical procedures
Emergency preparations
Schedule modifications
Modified physical education
Transportation
Building accessibility
Toileting/lifting assistance: support therapies
Physical therapy
Occupational therapy
Speech and language therapy
Counseling services (school, career, personal)

Data from Walker DK, Jacobs FH: Chronically ill children in schools. In Hobbs N, Perrin J, editors: The constant shadow: issues in chronic childhood illness in America, San Francisco, 1984, Jossey-Bass. Modified from Walker DK: Care of chronically ill children in schools, *Pediatr Clin North Am* 31: 221, 1984.

Depending on the parental demands, some siblings may take an important role in the medical treatment of the affected child (such as reminding about medications and helping with therapy); others may be protected from this role by their parents. Some siblings may take a more protective role in school and outside the home.

Disease severity, parental functioning, family stress, and family support systems are some of the determinants of the effects of chronic illness on siblings. In spite of ambivalent feelings, siblings of children with arthritis function well in life[37] and can be a great source of extra support, both at home and at school. It is important to evaluate the needs of siblings in caring for children with chronic illness and to help support their needs.[38] Some ideas to reduce the negative impact on siblings are given in Table 9–7.

SCHOOL ISSUES

Rheumatic diseases in general do not affect the ability of the child to learn and think, except for conditions that affect the central nervous system, such as systemic lupus erythematosus (SLE) or due to the side effects of drugs. Children with arthritis can and should attend school except in special circumstances. However, the school system often must institute several adaptations to the standardized schedule.[4] In the United States, children with chronic illness and disabilities must be educated in the "least restrictive environment." Individualized education plans have to be formulated at the parent's request, and there are strong "due process" requirements.[39]

Depending on the medical condition and the disability, one or more of the "related school services" listed in Table 9–8 may need to be provided for children with special health care needs to ensure proper educational opportunities.[40] In the newer definitions of disability, participation in daily and community life activities is recognized as an explicit component of health.[23-26]

Special school services are important components of community-based services. They provide physical adaptations in schools for handicapped access, elevators, classes on the same floor, and a duplicate set of books. Transportation, school counseling, nutrition, adaptive physical education, and homebound instruction are some of the other services that may be needed.[4,40]

Many common concerns expressed by children and parents in relation to school, as well as suggested solutions, are given in Table 9–9. The nurse can provide an individualized checklist for parents; this list can be shared with the school nurse or teacher. School nurses are some of the best advocates for children with disabilities

Table 9–9

Common school concerns for students with rheumatic diseases

Difficulty	Strategy
Inactivity, stiffness due to prolonged sitting	Sit at side or back of room to allow walking around without disturbing class
	Change position every 20 minutes
	Ask to be assigned jobs that require walking (e.g., collect papers)
Climbing stairs or walking long distances	Request elevator permit
	Schedule classes to decrease walking and climbing
	Request extra time getting from classes
	Use wheelchair if needed
Carrying books or cafeteria tray	Keep two sets of books: one in class, one at home
	Have a buddy help carry books
	Get a backpack or shoulder bag for books
	Determine cafeteria assistance plan (helper, reserved seat, wheeled cart)
Getting up from desk	Request an easel-top desk or special chair
Handwriting (slow, messy, painful)	Use "fat" pen/pencil, crayons
	Use felt-tip pen
	Stretch hands every 10 minutes
	Use tape recorder for note-taking
	Photocopy classmate's notes
	Use computer for reports
	Request alternative to timed tests (oral test, extra time, computer)
	Educate teacher (messy writing may be unavoidable at times)
Shoulder movement and dressing	Wear loose-fitting clothing
	Wear clothes with Velcro closures
	Get adaptive equipment from occupational therapist
Reaching locker	Modify locker or request alternative storage place
	Use lockers with key locks instead of dials
Raising hand	Devise alternative signaling method

From *Raising a child with arthritis: a parent's guide.* Atlanta, 1998, Arthritis Foundation.

and special needs. Well-informed school nurses can work with teachers and physical education instructors to make appropriate modifications within the school. Therefore, communication between the tertiary center staff members (particularly the nurse) and the school nurse is essential. In addition, special educational programs for school nurses are very useful. It is important to recognize that teachers and parents tend to emphasize issues related to activities of daily living as limiting school life, whereas children themselves rate peer acceptance and self-concept as more important.[41] Therefore, these children need more help with peer support and better coping skills.

Finally, if a child is considering vocational training or college after high school, early planning is essential. This planning should start at the beginning of secondary school at the very latest. One of the author's successful "graduates" wrote a checklist in preparation for her entry into college (Table 9–10). In addition to those listed, adequate rest is crucial to optimal function.

TRANSITION

Growing up through adolescence into young adult life is a major task for any child. This time becomes a challenge for children with chronic illness and their

Table 9–10

Rheumatic diseases and planning for college

Visit the college before choosing in order to evaluate the walking distances between buildings, stairs, and elevators and for general accessibility.

Know the different climate changes (e.g., if you feel better in the summer, you may want to pick a campus with a warm climate). Also, climate changes can cause flare-ups or increased stiffness.

It is always good to get to know a local doctor in your college area or health service before troubles occur, so that he or she knows your past history and can help you right away if there are any problems.

If you have the chance to pick your own schedule during your first year, make sure you give yourself enough time to get from one class to another (e.g., if you have to walk to buildings from one end of campus to the other).

Also try not to overburden yourself with classes and too many credit hours—there will always be bad days, so expect them.

If you are not a morning person or if you are a "night owl," schedule your classes in the afternoon.

And always—no matter how "bad" the food is—eat as regularly as possible: breakfast, lunch, and dinner. It helps in the long run, even if your stomach does not feel so at the time.

Take extra medicine with you at the start of school and give yourself time to find the nearest pharmacy.

parents.[11] Adolescents with chronic diseases have to be encouraged gradually to take control of their disease management. This requires preparation of the family and child before adolescence. Preparation of these children requires attention to independent living skills and self-advocacy. Both physicians and parents have to let go of the child in a sensitive and gradual way. The parent has to trust, and the child must prove that he or she can be trusted to take care of ongoing management and needs. Adolescent support groups with professional leadership may be helpful.

Transition to adult care is a process that should start when a child reaches adolescence.[11,42,43] This requires planning and coordination with participation from the patients, family, the pediatric service, and the adult service. It should be comprehensive and responsive to the needs of the patient.[43] Some of the subjects that should be addressed individually or in group sessions are preparing for college, sexuality, alcohol and drugs, and vocational planning. The young person will need training in self-management, communication, and decision making.

FINANCIAL ISSUES

Children with chronic illness account for a large proportion of health care expenditures in the United States.[6,44] For instance, families of children with rheumatic diseases may spend hundreds to thousands of unreimbursed dollars out of pocket per year,[3,5,6] not including time lost from work. In the current competitive environment, children with chronic illness and disabilities are particularly vulnerable. The high cost that goes with chronic illness, and the pressures to cut costs, may make it difficult to provide adequate and appropriate care for children with chronic illness and disabilities.[44] In the United States, families need to be educated about various types of coverage and how to work with health maintenance organizations and insurance companies. Families need to learn about child welfare systems and social security benefits. They also have to learn to work with their school systems. Parents must be advocates for their children and learn both their own rights and responsibilities and those of their children.[39] Both parents and physicians need to work through the political process to bring about changes in financing of medical care that will ensure access to appropriate services for all children with disabilities.[45]

NUTRITION

Nutritional abnormalities affect a significant number of children with rheumatic diseases.[46,47] Factors that contribute to these abnormalities include metabolic effects of inflammation, physical inactivity, reduced energy intake and effects of drugs used to treat these diseases. In addition, both patients and physicians have always wondered about the relationship between diet and arthritis based on two observations: fasting has been shown to have anti-inflammatory effects, at least in the short term, and rare patients have been shown to develop arthritis associated with food sensitivity.[47]

Patients and parents are also influenced by the publicity for alternative and complementary medicine, because scientific medicine cannot promise a cure for rheumatic diseases. Therefore, the following questions are raised often: 1. Can specific food items aggravate or precipitate symptoms of arthritis? 2. If so, what food items should be avoided in the diet? 3. What is the role of dietary supplements, special diets, and an elimination diet?

The physician's main goal should be to control inflammation as rapidly as possible and thus minimize the nutritional abnormalities. The child should be maintained on a well-balanced, healthy diet with adequate vitamins and minerals and should be encouraged to be as physically active as possible. The physician also has to counsel parents on the proper role of nutrition and educate them on fad diets and dietary supplements.

Physicians have to teach parents that at present there is no specific dietary recommendation for the treatment of rheumatic diseases based on evidence. There are no data to recommend an elimination diet, although rare patients may exhibit altered immune response to items such as milk. Moreover, an elimination diet should be tried only under strict medical supervision, because there is a danger of precipitating malnutrition and deficiency diseases. Megavitamins and macrobiotic diets should be avoided.

Evidence-based advice should include supplemental calcium and vitamin D, particularly for children on glucocorticoid therapy, folic acid for children on methotrexate, salt restriction and potassium supplementation for children on long-term glucocorticoid therapy, and supplemental iron with or without vitamin C for children with anemia of chronic illness.[48,49]

In previous decades, the main dietary focus for patients with arthritis was increasing caloric consumption. However, as new therapies have been developed, the number of patients with insufficient caloric intake has declined. Today, childhood obesity is becoming an important issue in children with arthritis. Increased body weight adds increased stress on the weight-bearing joints. An individualized weight management plan and consultation with a dietitian are indicated for some patients. Programs that include exercise along with dietary restriction are more likely to be successful. Obesity is often a family problem, and successfully controlling it requires family participation.

In addition, children with rheumatic diseases on chronic glucocorticoid therapy are at increased risk for accelerated atherosclerosis. Therefore, the American Heart Association places children with chronic inflammatory diseases in Tier II in their algorithm for cardiovascular risk reduction.[50] According to this algorithm, all children in this tier should be screened for additional risk factors. The screens include obtaining history of early coronary heart disease in the family and amount of physical activity, measurement of blood pressure, body mass index, and fasting blood sugar, and lipid profile. On the basis of this screening, patients may have to be referred to a dietitian or other specialists for further management.

UNCONVENTIONAL REMEDIES

Practitioners of scientific, evidence-based medicine truthfully acknowledge that the etiology of rheumatic diseases is not yet known and a cure cannot be assured. Therefore, it is easy for parents to believe those who promise miracles. This is also the age of alternative medicine.[51,52] There are pressures from well-meaning friends and relatives to try unproven remedies widely advertised in newspapers and on the Internet.

The use of alternative and complementary methods of treatment is increasing even among children although detailed analysis of available studies do not show any benefit or only limited benefit.[52] One of them is clearly dangerous, particularly in children with arthritis (cervical manipulation).

It is safe to assume that many parents have tried or are trying one or more unconventional remedies. This is particularly true of parents who use such remedies themselves and those who grew up in other cultures. It is better to keep an open and noncritical relationship with patients and their family members so that they feel comfortable talking about these remedies. It is important for pediatric rheumatologists to be aware of the currently available alternative remedies, so they can provide proper guidance when patients ask about such methods. This is an opportunity to educate parents on the conduct of scientific studies and to explain to them the difference between controlled trials and testimonials. It is better to let them try some remedies that are innocuous (acupuncture), caution about some potentially dangerous treatments (e.g., megavitamins, cervical manipulation), and refuse to be part of certain other approaches (e.g., bee-sting therapy). It is always wise not to make parents feel guilty or ashamed and allow room for them to come back without losing face and feeling humiliated.

GOALS OF REHABILITATION

The overall goals of rehabilitation are to maximize function, to prevent deformities, and to help a child achieve developmental milestones—physical, psychosocial, emotional, educational, and vocational. The concept is to help the child and family lead as normal a life as possible. Goals must be set in collaboration with the parents and the child. One has to account for the needs of the family, their strengths and weaknesses, their economic and human resources, their coping styles, and their cultural values. The child's developmental level and interests also must be acknowledged. These will be discussed in Chapter 12.

IMMUNIZATION

There are two major questions related to immunization and rheumatic diseases. First, is there any relationship between immunization and onset or exacerbation of these diseases? Second, what are the recommendations for children with rheumatic diseases who are taking immune modulators and the newer biological agents?

Although some reports suggest that immunization may exacerbate or initiate an arthritic or vasculitic disorder,[53-55]

other studies do not support this association.[56,57] Recent studies in adults and children receiving immune modulators and the newer biologicals showed no exacerbation of the basic diseases following immunization with inactivated influenza virus vaccine.[57-59] Although there are variations in response between patients on methotrexate as compared with those on tumor necrosis factor inhibitors, there is overall good response to immunization with influenza vaccine. Therefore, it appears that the benefits of yearly immunization of adults and children with rheumatic diseases against influenza far outweigh any risk in most situations.[58,60]

Children receiving chronic salicylate therapy and all children with SLE, dermatomyositis with significant muscle weakness, systemic scleroderma with cardiopulmonary or renal disease, or systemic vasculitis may benefit from a yearly influenza virus (inactivated virus) vaccination. Studies also indicate that patients taking glucocorticoids and immunosuppressive drugs respond to influenza vaccine,[57,61] and pneumococcal vaccine[58] with adequate antibody titers. Children with SLE and splenic hypofunction should receive the pneumococcal vaccine.[62] However, such immunization should not give rise to a false sense of security, because immunity is not guaranteed.

Ideally, children should have received the routine recommended immunizations and the antibody status confirmed before the start of immunosuppressive therapies and biological immune modulators. It is best to advise families to keep the regular schedule of immunizations while cautioning them about the possibility of a flare-up. There are, however, a few special circumstances, exceptions, and precautions:

1. *Active Disease:* Children with severe, active rheumatic disease should not receive any immunization.
2. *Varicella-Zoster (VZV):* Varicella can be a major problem for children receiving immunosuppressive therapy, glucocorticoids, methotrexate, and/or biological agents. For all of these children, suggested management strategy for the prevention of is given in Table 9–11. Ideally, the antibody level against VZV should be known before the start of therapy. Varicella and other live virus and bacterial vaccines are generally contraindicated in children taking glucocorticoids in doses of 2 mg/kg/day of prednisone or its equivalent, to a total of 20 mg/day of prednisone or equivalent for children who weigh more than 10 kg when given for longer than 14 days.[63] For children receiving smaller doses, the risk/benefit

---

Table 9–11

Varicella prevention strategy for children taking glucocorticoids, immunosuppressives, and biological agents

Document successful vaccination in the past; measure serum antibody level.

If seronegative (susceptible), immunize with varicella vaccine 3 weeks before starting therapy.

Susceptible children exposed to varicella should receive varicella-zoster immunoglobulin within 72 hr after exposure.

If chicken pox develops, treat with oral or parenteral acyclovir depending on severity and spread. Stop Enbrel and methotrexate temporarily, but continue glucocorticoids.

ratio must be assessed. Salicylate should not be used for at least 6 weeks after varicella vaccine administration. The potential for Reye syndrome in children treated with salicylates in association with varicella or influenza has been widely discussed.[64]

3. *Children on Immunosuppressive Therapy and on biological immune modulators*
Children undergoing immunosuppressive therapy, receiving biological immune modulators, or undergoing glucocorticoid therapy should not receive any live virus or bacterial vaccine. If glucocorticoids and cytotoxic drugs have been stopped, live virus vaccines may be given after a minimum of 3 months. It is also important to remember that the new nasal spray vaccine for influenza contains live virus and is therefore contraindicated in immuno-compromised patients and their contacts. Only the inactivated parenteral form of the influenza vaccine should be used. Recommendations made by the Committee on Infectious Diseases of the American Academy of Pediatrics should be followed for children.[63] The British Society of Rheumatology recommends the use of influenza A, meningococcus C, *Haemophilus* b, hepatitis B, and tetanus toxoid but warns that the response may be suboptimal.[60]

4. Children receiving intravenous immunoglobulin should wait for at least 3 months after the last dose to ensure an adequate immune response.[65]

APPENDIX 9-1

RESOURCES FOR FURTHER INFORMATION ON RHEUMATIC DISEASES FOR PATIENTS AND PARENTS

ORGANIZATIONS

1. American Juvenile Arthritis Organization—Arthritis Foundation
1330 W. Peachtree Street
Atlanta, G.A 30309, USA
www.arthritis.org/communities/juvenile_arthritis
2. Lupus Foundation of America, Inc.
2000 L Street NW, Suite 710
Washington, DC 20036, USA
http://www.lupus.org
3. Scleroderma Foundation
300 Rosewood Drive, Suite 105
Danvers, MA 01923, USA
http://www.scleroderma.org
4. Spondylitis Association of America
14827 Ventura Boulevard, Suite 119
PO Box 5872
Sherman Oaks, CA 91403, USA
http://www.spondylitis.org
5. The Family Village
Waisman Center
University of Wisconsin-Madison
1500 Highland Avenue
Madison, WI 53705-2280, USA
http://www.familyvillage.wisc.edu (a great Web site for information on all chronic diseases and rare syndromes)
6. National Dissemination Center for Children with Disabilities
PO Box 1492
Washington, DC 20013, USA
http://www.nichcy.org
7. Canadian Association for Adolescent Health
Section médecine de l'adolescence
Sainte-Justine Hospital
7th floor, 2nd bloc
3175 Côte Sainte-Catherine
Montreal QC H3T 1C5, CANADA
http://www.acsa-caah.ca/pdf/ang/on_trac.pdf

MONOGRAPHS/BOOKS

1. Huff C: *Raising a child with arthritis, revised and updated: a parent's guide: from infancy to young adulthood.* Atlanta, 2008, Arthritis Foundation.
2. Lehman TJA: *A parent's guide to rheumatic disease in children.* New York, 2008, Oxford University Press.

REFERENCES

1. N. Hobbs, J.M. Perrin, Issues in the care of children with chronic illness: a source book on problems, services and policies, Jossey-Bass, San Francisco, 1985.
2. I.B. Pless, C. Power, C.S. Peckham, Long-term psychosocial sequelae of chronic physical disorders in childhood, Pediatrics 91 (1993) 1131–1136.
3. M.C. McCormick, M.M. Stemmler, B.H. Athreya, The impact of childhood rheumatic diseases on the family, Arthritis Rheum. 29 (1986) 872–879.
4. D.A. Lovell, B.H. Athreya, H.M. Emery, et al., School attendance and patterns, special services and special needs in pediatric patients with rheumatic diseases, Arthritis Care Res. 3 (1990) 196.
5. S.H. Allaire, B.S. DeNardo, I.S. Szer, et al., The economic impact of juvenile rheumatoid arthritis, J. Rheumatol. 19 (1992) 952–955.
6. P.W. Newacheck, W.R. Taylor, Childhood chronic illness: prevalence, severity, and impact, Am. J. Public Health 82 (1992) 364–371.
7. B.A. Gare, A. Fasth, The natural history of juvenile chronic arthritis: a population based cohort study. II: Outcome, J. Rheumatol. 22 (1995) 308–319.
8. C.A. Wallace, J.E. Levinson, Juvenile rheumatoid arthritis: outcome and treatment for the 1990s, Rheum. Dis. Clin. North Am. 17 (1991) 891–905.
9. L.S. Peterson, T. Mason, A.M. Nelson, et al., Psychosocial outcomes and health status of adults who have had juvenile rheumatoid arthritis: a controlled, population-based study, Arthritis Rheum. 40 (1997) 2235–2240.
10. J.C. Packham, M.A. Hall, Long-term follow-up of 246 adults with juvenile idiopathic arthritis: functional outcome, Rheumatology 41 (2002) 1428–1435.
11. P. Rettig, B.H. Athreya, Leaving home: preparing the adolescent with arthritis for coping with independence and the adult rheumatology world, in: D. Isenberg, J.J. Miller (Eds.), Adolescent rheumatology, Martin Dunitz, London, 1998.
12. J.C. Packham, M.A. Hall, Long-term follow-up of 246 adults with juvenile idiopathic arthritis: education and employment, Rheumatology 41 (2002) 1436–1439.
13. J.C. Packham, M.A. Hall, Long-term follow-up of 246 adults with juvenile idiopathic arthritis: social function, relationships and sexual activity, Rheumatology 41 (2002) 1440–1443.

14. N. Solari, S. Viola, A. Pistorio, et al., Assessing current outcomes of Juvenile Idiopathic Arthritis A Cross-sectional Study in a tertiary center sample, Arthritis Rheum. 59 (2008) 1571–1579.

15. J.J. Miller, 3rd: Psychosocial factors related to rheumatic diseases in childhood, J. Rheumatol. 20 (Suppl. 38) (1993) 1–11.

16. D.K. Routh, Commentary: juvenile rheumatoid arthritis as a stressor, J. Pediatr. Psychol. 28 (2003) 41–43.

17. L.M. Dahlquist, Commentary: are children with JRA and their families at risk or resilient? J. Pediatr. Psychol. 28 (2003) 43–46.

18. M. Arkela-Kautiainen, J. Haapasaari, H. Kautiainen, et al., Favorable social functioning and health related quality of life of patients with JIA in early adulthood, Ann. Rheum. Dis. 64 (2005) 875–880.

19. J. Reiter-Purtill, C.A. Gerhardt, K. Vannatta, et al., A controlled longitudinal study of the social functioning of children with JRA, J. Pediatr. Psychol. 28 (2003) 17–28.

20. J.S. LeBovidge, J.V. Lavigne, G.R. Donenberg, et al., Psychological adjustment of children and adolescents with chronic arthritis: a meta-analytic review, J. Pediatr. Psychol. 28 (2003) 29–39.

21. E.J. Brewer Jr., M. McPherson, P.R. Magrab, et al., Family-centered, community-based, coordinated care for children with special healthcare needs, Pediatrics 83 (1989) 1055–1060.

22. J. van der Net, A.B. Prakken, P.J. Helders, et al., Correlates of disablement in juvenile chronic arthritis: a cross-sectional study, Br. J. Rheumatol. 35 (1996) 91–100.

23. L.I. Iezzoni, V.A. Freedman, Turning of the disability tide: the importance of definitions, JAMA. 299 (2008) 332–334.

24. WHO ICF, International classification of functioning, disability and health, World Health Organization, Geneva, 2001.

25. G Stucki, A Cieza, The international classification of functioning, disability and health (ICF) core sets for rheumatoid arthritis: a way to specify function, Ann. Rheum. Dis. 63 (Suppl. 2) (2004) ii 40–ii45.

26. World Health Organization -WHO Workgroup for Developmental Version of ICF for Children and Youth, International classification of functioning, disability and health—version for children and youth ICF-CY, World Health Organization, Geneva, 2007.

27. R.B. Noll, K. Kozlowski, C. Gerhardt, et al., Social, emotional, and behavioral functioning of children with juvenile rheumatoid arthritis, Arthritis Rheum. 43 (2000) 1387–1396.

28. R.T. von Weiss, M.A. Rapoff, J.W. Varni, et al., Daily hassles and social support as predictors of adjustment in children with pediatric rheumatic diseases, J. Pediatr. Psychol. 27 (2002) 155–165.

29. J.L. Wallender, V.W. Varni, Adjustment in children with chronic physical disorders: programmatic research on a disability-stress coping module, in: A.M. La Greca, L.J. Siegel, J.L. Wallender, C.E. Walker (Eds.), Stress and coping in child health, Guilford, New York, 1991.

30. F.A. Mervyn, "They get this training but they don't know how you feel." National Fund for Research into Crippling Diseases, Horsham, UK, 1975.

31. B.H. Athreya, Regionalized arthritis resources, Arthritis Rheum. 20 (Suppl) (1977) 604.

32. I.M. Rosenstock, V.J. Strecher, M.H. Becker, Social learning theory and the Health Belief Model, Health Educ. Q. 15 (1988) 1751–1783.

33. J.D. Akikusa, R.C. Allen, Reducing the impact of rheumatic diseases in childhood, Best Pract. Res. Clin. Rheumatol. 16 (2002) 333–345.

34. T. Kroll, J.H. Barlow, K. Shaw, Treatment adherence in juvenile rheumatoid arthritis: a review, Scand. J. Rheumatol. 28 (1999) 10–18.

35. A.M. Gallo, B.J. Breitmayer, K.A. Knafl, et al., Stigma in childhood chronic illness: a well sibling perspective, Pediatr. Nurs. 17 (1991) 21–25.

36. A. Birenbaum, On managing a courtesy stigma, J. Health Soc. Behav. 11 (1970) 196.

37. D. Daniels, J.J. Miller 3rd, A.G. Billings, et al., Psychosocial functioning of siblings of children with rheumatic disease, J. Pediatr. 109 (1986) 379–383.

38. P.D. Williams, A.R. Williams, J.C. Graff, et al., A community-based intervention for siblings and parents of children with chronic illness or disability: the ISEE study, J. Pediatr. 143 (2003) 386–393.

39. J.T. Cassidy, C.B. Lindsley, Legal rights of children with musculoskeletal disabilities, Bull. Rheum. Dis. 45 (1996) 1–5.

40. C.H. Spencer, R.Z. Fife, C.E. Rabinovich, The school experience of children with arthritis: coping in the 1990s and transition into adulthood, Pediatr. Clin. North Am. 42 (1995) 1285–1298.

41. J. Taylor, M.H. Passo, V.L. Champion, School problems and teacher responsibilities in juvenile rheumatoid arthritis, J. Sch. Health 57 (1987) 186–190.

42. P.H. White, Success on the road to adulthood: issues and hurdles for adolescents with disabilities, Rheum. Dis. Clin. North Am. 23 (1997) 697–707.

43. J.E. McDonagh, Young people first, juvenile idiopathic arthritis second: transition care in rheumatology, Arthritis Rheum. 59 (2008) 1162–1170.

44. J.M. Neff, G. Anderson, Protecting children with chronic illness in a competitive marketplace, JAMA. 274 (1995) 1866–1869.

45. American Academy of Pediatrics, Committee on Children with Disabilities: Managed care and children with special health care needs: a subject review, Pediatrics 102 (1998) 657–660.

46. A.G. Cleary, G.A. Lancaster, F. Annan, et al., Nutritional impairment in juvenile idiopathic arthritis, Rheumatology (Oxford) 43 (2004) 1569–1573.

47. C.J. Henderson, R.S. Panush, Diet, dietary supplements and nutritional therapy in rheumatic diseases, Rheum. Dis. Cl. N. Am. 25 (1999) 937–968.

48. R.H. Martin, The role of nutrition and diet in rheumatoid arthritis, Proc. Nutrition Soc. 57 (1998) 231–234m.

49. D.J. Lovell, D. Glass, J Ranz, A randomized clinical trial of calcium supplementation to increase bone mineral density in children with Juvenile Rheumatoid Arthritis, Arthritis Rheum. 54 (2006) 2235–2242.

50. W. Kavey R-E, V. Allada, S.R. Daniels, et al., Cardiovascular risk reduction in high-risk pediatric patients: a scientific statement from the American Heart Association Expert Panel on Population and Prevention Science: the Council on Cardiovascular Disease in the Young, Epidemiology and Prevention, Nutrition, Physical Activity and Metabolism, High Blood Pressure Research, Cardiovascular Nursing and the Kidney in Heart Disease; and the Interdisciplinary Working Group on Quality of Care and Outcomes Research; endorsed by the American Academy of Pediatrics, Circulation 114 (2006) 2710–2738.

51. K.J. Kemper, S. Vohra, R. Walls, et al., The use of complementary and alternative medicine in pediatrics, Pediatrics 122 (2008) 1374–1386.

52. S. Singh, E. Ernst, Trick or treatment, Norton, New York, 2008.

53. C.M. Benjamin, G.C. Chew, A.J. Silman, Joint and limb symptoms in children after immunisation with measles, mumps, and rubella vaccine, BMJ. 304 (1992) 1075–1078.

54. C.J. Castresana-Isla, G. Herrera-Martinez, J. Vega-Molina, Erythema nodosum and Takayasu's arteritis after immunization with plasma derived hepatitis B vaccine, J. Rheumatol. 20 (1993) 1417–1418.

55. R. Mader, A. Narendran, J. Lewtas, et al., Systemic vasculitis following influenza vaccination: report of 3 cases and literature review, J. Rheumatol. 20 (1993) 1429–1431.

56. P. Ray, S. Black, H. Shinefield, et al., Risk of chronic arthropathy among women after rubella vaccination. Vaccine Safety Datalink Team, JAMA. 278 (1997) 551–556.

57. P.N. Malleson, J.L. Tekano, D.W. Scheifele, et al., Influenza immunization in children with chronic arthritis: a prospective study, J. Rheumatol. 20 (1993) 1769–1773.

58. R. Ravikumar, J. Anolik, John Looney R: Vaccine responses in patients with rheumatoid arthritis, Current Rheumatology Reports 9 (2007) 407–415.

59. P. Mamula, J.E. Markowitz, D.A. Piccoli, et al., Immune response to influenza vaccine in pediatric patients with inflammatory bowel disease, Clin. Gastroenterol Hepatol. 5 (2007) 851–856 (e publication).

60. K. Davies, P. Woo, British Paediatric Rheumatology Group: Immunization in rheumatic diseases of childhood: an audit of the clinical practice of British Paediatric Rheumatology Group members and a review of the evidence, Rheumatology 41 (2002) 937–941.

61. C.L. Park, A.L. Frank, M. Sullivan, et al., Influenza vaccination of children during acute asthma exacerbation and concurrent prednisone therapy, Pediatrics 98 (1996) 196–200.

62. R.N. Lipnick, J. Karsh, N.I. Stahl, et al., Pneumococcal immunization in patients with systemic lupus erythematosus treated with immunosuppressives, J. Rheumatol. 12 (1985) 1118–1121.

63. Report of the Committee on Infectious Diseases, American Academy of Pediatrics, second ed., Elk Grove Village, IL, 2006.

64. E.S. Hurwitz, M.J. Barrett, D. Bregman, et al., Public Health Service study of Reye's syndrome and medications: report of the main study, JAMA. 257 (1987) 1905–1911.

65. A.H. Rowley, S.T. Shulman, Current therapy for acute Kawasaki syndrome, J. Pediatr. 118 (1991) 987–991.

Chapter 10

RADIOLOGIC INVESTIGATION OF PEDIATRIC RHEUMATIC DISEASES

Paul Babyn and Andrea Schwarz Doria

Imaging often plays a key role in establishing the presence, severity, and extent of joint disease and can also help monitor for disease complications, exclude other diagnoses, and assess treatment response. Imaging can now provide early diagnosis and visualization of inflammatory abnormalities including synovitis and osteochondral damage. This chapter provides an approach to the radiologic investigation of the child with juvenile idiopathic arthritis. The distinct advantages and disadvantages of the available imaging modalities are initially reviewed as this forms the basis for rational imaging evaluation (Table 10–1).[1-3]

A variety of imaging modalities aid in the assessment and diagnosis of a multitude of other inflammatory disorders, as well as their complications. Examples include the use of angiography for the vasculitides, high-resolution chest computerized tomography scans for the lung disease of systemic sclerosis, and magnetic resonance imaging for the inflammatory myopathies. These and other techniques are covered in the disease-related chapters.

AVAILABLE IMAGING MODALITIES

Radiography

Radiography remains the initial and most commonly used means used to evaluate joint abnormalities. Radiography is typically used for assessment of symptomatic and often contralateral joints. Intraarticular soft tissue components have very similar radiographic density and cannot be clearly differentiated from each other or from adjacent muscles, fascia, tendons, ligaments, nerves, or vessels by radiography. Displacement of adjacent periarticular fat deposits help determine joint effusions of the elbow, knee, and ankle. However, the relationship of these radiolucent fat stripes in other joints is more complex, making accurate determination of joint effusions—for example, about the hip and shoulder—more difficult radiographically.

In neonates and young children, radiography demonstrates wide apparent joint spaces representing immature unossified epiphyses. These chondroepiphyses will eventually ossify, reducing the apparent joint space to the thickness of the opposing layers of articular cartilage and any intervening joint fluid.

Occasionally, intraarticular gas can be seen as a normal finding, but it can also be seen following infection, trauma, or invasive procedure. Radiographically, normal intraarticular gas appears as an intraarticular crescentic lucency and is caused by sudden lowering of intraarticular pressure by muscle pulls or external traction (Fig. 10–1). In the presence of a significant joint effusion, this phenomenon cannot normally be produced; however, its presence cannot be relied upon to exclude effusion. Intraarticular gas can also be identified with sonography or magnetic resonance imaging (MRI). On MRI, intraarticular gas may simulate meniscal tears, intraarticular loose bodies, or chondrocalcinosis.

Although radiography should be used initially in evaluation of joints, the introduction of the crosssectional imaging techniques has provided a significant improvement in anatomical delineation and diagnosis.

Sonography

Recent advances in sonography, including better transducers and more pediatric musculoskeletal experience, have stimulated increased use of this modality in assessment of pediatric joint disease. Sonography is ideal for assessing the pediatric musculoskeletal system, largely because of its ability to visualize intraarticular structures such as cartilage and thickened synovium without the need for radiation (Fig. 10–2). Sonography is very sensitive in detecting joint effusion, particularly in the hip and shoulder, where plain films are insensitive. It can also be used to guide joint aspiration or injection (Fig. 10–3).[4] Intraarticular masses may also be detected with sonography, although their appearance is often nonspecific. Tendons and ligaments can be assessed with higher frequency transducers.[5] Normal tendons have an echogenic fibrillar appearance on ultrasound. Fluid within the synovial sheath appears as an anechoic halo surrounding the tendon while synovial thickening appears as a hypoechoic thickening around the tendon (Fig. 10–4). Vascular anatomy can be assessed by combining sonography with Doppler effects. Synovial hyperemia, for example, leads to increased Doppler signal. Sonography can also be used

Table 10–1

Commonly used imaging modalities

Conventional radiography

Traditional standard for assessment of established joint damage including bone erosions, joint space narrowing, joint subluxation, misalignment, or ankylosis

Advantages: low cost, high availability, helpful in differential diagnosis, reasonable reproducibility, validated assessment methods

Disadvantages: Not sensitive in detecting early bone disease or soft tissue manifestations, projectional superimposition, use of ionizing radiation

Ultrasound

Ultrasound can assess joint effusion and synovitis by detecting synovial thickening of inflamed joints, bursas, or tendon sheaths. Vascularity can be assessed with Doppler sonography. Follow-up studies have shown improvement in ultrasound measures of synovitis following successful treatment.

Ultrasound can be used to guide punctures of joints, bursas, and tendon sheaths, improving the success rates of diagnostic or therapeutic aspirations.

Advantages: Noninvasive, relatively low cost, lack of ionizing radiation, ability to visualize both inflammatory and destructive disease manifestations, easy repeatability, possibility of examining several joint regions at one session, potential for guiding interventions

Disadvantages: Not all joint areas are accessible, operator dependence, time for examination

Magnetic Resonance Imaging

MRI directly visualizes both inflammatory and destructive aspects of arthritic disease. It has potential for accurate monitoring of treatment efficacy. Allows assessment of all structures in arthritic disease including synovial membrane, intraarticular and extraarticular fluid collections, cartilage, bone erosions and edema, ligaments, tendons, tendon sheaths

Advantages: Multiplanar tomographic imaging, excellent soft tissue contrast, lack of ionizing radiation. It is more sensitive than clinical and radiographic examination for detection of inflammatory soft tissue changes and early bone changes.

Disadvantages: Potential allergic contrast reactions, higher cost/lower availability compared with radiography, longer examination times, and evaluation of only a few joints per session, possible need for sedation.

MRI and/or ultrasound can be used in evaluation of suspected but not definite inflammatory joint disease to determine presence of synovitis, tenosynovitis, enthesitis, or bone erosions. Both may be helpful in verifying inflammatory disease response to therapy or choosing appropriate follow-up.

Compiled from Lamer S, Sebag GH: MRI and ultrasound in children with juvenile chronic arthritis, *Eur J Radiol* 33:85-93, 2000; Daldrup-Link HE, Steinbach L: MRI imaging of pediatric arthritis, *Magn Reson Imaging Clin N Am* 17:3 451-467, 2009; Grassi W, Filippucci E, Busilacchi P et al: Musculoskeletal ultrasound, *Best Pract Res Clin Rheumatol* 18:813-826, 2004; Ostergaard M, Duer A, Ejbjerg B et al: Magnetic resonance imaging of peripheral joints in rheumatic diseases, *Best Pract Res Clin Rheumatol* 18:861-879. 2004; Ostergaard M, Ejbjerg B, Szkudlarek M et al: Imaging in early rheumatoid arthritis: roles of magnetic resonance imaging, ultrasonography, conventional radiography and computed tomography, *Best Pract Res Clin Rheumatol* 19:91-116, 2005.

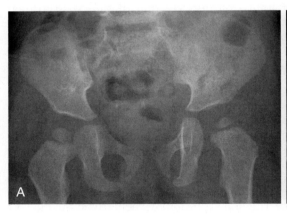 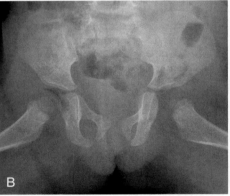

FIGURE 10–1 Two-year-old girl with left developmental hip dysplasia. **A,** Small ossification centers and wide apparent joint space from unossified epiphyseal cartilage. **B,** Normal intraarticular gas seen from traction during frog-leg radiography. The smaller ossification center of the left hip compared with the normal right hip in this child reflects underlying left developmental hip dysplasia.

to assess for other periarticular soft tissue abnormalities including popliteal cysts or other soft tissue masses.

Computed Tomography

Multidetector computed tomography (CT) scanners generate detailed high-resolution images of bone and can be used to evaluate the joint space and detect adjacent bone abnormalities including tarsal coalitions, bone erosions, subchondral cysts, or primary osseous lesions such as osteoid osteoma. Current-generation CT scanners are fast, and

sedation is generally not required for all but the youngest patients. Intravenous contrast may be required for soft tissue assessment. Because MRI now provides better soft tissue contrast without need for radiation, CT is primarily used to provide detailed assessment of osseous structures.

Magnetic Resonance Imaging

Magnetic resonance imaging provides exquisite multiplanar images with superb tissue contrast. It can define vascular anatomy, often without the need for intravenous

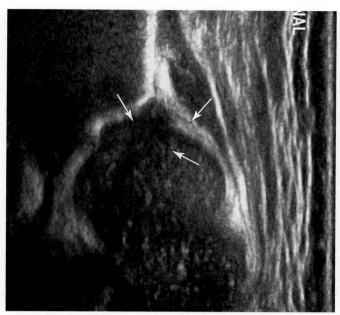

FIGURE 10–2 Normal hip sonogram in a 1-month-old boy with entirely cartilaginous femoral head. The image has been rotated for ease of visualization. The acetabular labrum composed of fibrocartilage is echogenic *(upper right arrow of figure)* on sonography. The hyaline cartilage of the acetabulum is not echogenic *(upper left arrow)*. The cartilaginous femoral head and the internal vessels identified within the femoral head are normal *(lower arrow)*.

contrast. However, high cost, limited availability, and the frequent need for sedation have limited its more widespread use. It is the best modality to examine all joint components (perhaps excepting cortical bone) including bone marrow, hyaline and fibrocartilage, ligaments, menisci, synovium and joint capsule, joint fluid, and the unossified cartilaginous skeleton.[6]

MRI provides multiplanar evaluation with a combination of available imaging sequences—including T1- and fast spin echo T2–weighted sequences, gradient echo sequences, and postcontrast studies—all tailored to the specific clinical problem.[7-9] Three-dimensional (3D) sequences can also be obtained, making it possible to reformat images in any desired plane.[10] Cartilaginous structures, including the growth plate, are well seen with gradient-recalled echo techniques or fat-suppressed fast proton density sequences. Gadolinium-enhanced MRI imaging can help differentiate physeal from unossified epiphyseal cartilage and can visualize normal vessels present within the chondroepiphysis.[11] MRI is very helpful in detecting synovial abnormalities within the joint.[12] The normal synovium appears as a thin line on MRI with minimal enhancement following contrast administration (Fig. 10–5). MRI can be used to assess changes in the synovium as a result of therapy.[13] A small amount of joint fluid may normally be seen with MRI.

Pannus is seen as masses of low to intermediate signal intensity on T1- and T2-weighted sequences with contrast enhancement following gadolinium infusion. Subchondral cysts and bone erosions appear as low-signal areas on T1 sequences.[7]

Additionally, MRI can be used to demonstrate muscle pathology, typically demonstrating nonuniform increased

signal intensity on T2-weighted images and normal signal on T1-weighted images. These findings are not specific but may help in selection of a biopsy site.

A number of novel MRI techniques are under evaluation for improved assessment of synovial, cartilaginous, or osseous abnormalities. These MRI techniques include diffusion-weighted and perfusion imaging, delayed gadolinium-enhanced cartilage imaging, and T2 quantification. Diffusion-weighted imaging evaluates the translational movement (Brownian motion) of water molecules that occurs in all tissues. Alteration of normal diffusion can occur in some diseases, including infection, inflammation, and infarction. Perfusion imaging assesses blood flow using intravenously administered paramagnetic contrast agents and may be helpful in characterizing ischemic or hyperemic areas. Potential uses of this technique include recognition of epiphyseal ischemia and quantification and monitoring of synovial inflammation.

Delayed gadolinium-enhanced MRI cartilage imaging (dGEMRIC) is a sensitive technique for assessing cartilage proteoglycan content using the negative charge of the intravenously administered paramagnetic MRI contrast agent. The contrast agent distributes into cartilage inversely to the fixed-charge density of negatively charged glycosaminoglycan. T1 relaxation time in the presence of gadolinium agent is approximately linearly related to the glycosaminoglycan content. dGEMRIC may be used to assess early cartilage injury with depletion of glycosaminoglycans. Cartilage assessment can also be provided by mapping T2 relaxation time measurements. These may help characterize the structural integrity of the cartilaginous tissue and quantitatively assess the degree of cartilage degeneration.

Arthrography

Currently, arthrography is rarely indicated. Intraarticular contrast injection may, however, be combined with CT or (now more frequently) with MRI to better delineate joint detail including the evaluation of intraarticular loose bodies or labral tears within the shoulder or hip joint.

Bone Scintigraphy

Bone scintigraphy can help differentiate osseous causes of joint pain from other causes, including synovial, neuromuscular, or periarticular soft tissue disorders. Bone scintigraphy has been used to assess whether an osseous lesion is solitary or multifocal and can reveal increased activity across the joint in arthritis or infection. Specialized adjuncts to routine scintigraphic imaging include magnification scintigraphy, single photon–emission computed tomography, or more recently, positron emission tomography CT.[14] Dual energy x-ray absorptiometry (DEXA) scanning is used in assessment of bone density.

Radiographic Features of Joint Disease

A variety of radiographic features can be encountered with joint disease. Specific joint findings will depend on the underlying abnormality, chronicity of disease, and response to therapy. Potential radiographic features that

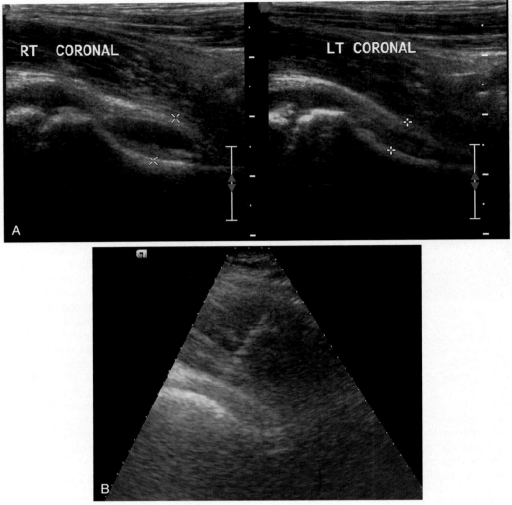

FIGURE 10–3   Ultrasound performed for question of hip joint effusion. **A,** A right hip effusion with widened joint space *(x-x)* compared with normal left hip. **B,** Needle placement under ultrasound guidance.

can be encountered are listed in Table 10–2. A systematic approach to interpretation of any joint imaging is highly recommended. This will ensure that the salient radiographic features are considered. One popular approach is the ABCDs of joint disease, where one assesses joint *Alignment, Bone* density and other bone changes, *Cartilage* loss, *Distribution* of joint disease (whether monoarticular, oligoarticular, or polyarticular), and *Soft* tissue abnormalities. The application of this approach to juvenile idiopathic arthritis is shown in Table 10–3.

INFLAMMATORY ARTHRITIS

Juvenile Idiopathic Arthritis

In juvenile idiopathic arthritis (JIA), synovial infiltration by inflammatory cells leads to synovial proliferation and thickening, increased secretion of synovial fluid, and pannus formation. Inflammatory changes can also involve the synovial sheaths of tendons and bursae, which can give rise to periostitis. With prolonged inflammation, more extensive joint changes, including cartilage

destruction, bone erosions, and joint malalignment, are often present.

Radiography

Radiographs of symptomatic areas should be obtained at initial presentation to exclude other differential diagnoses and assist in diagnosis. The earliest abnormalities include soft tissue swelling, osteopenia, and effusions; periosteal reaction may occasionally be seen. These changes, however, are not always present. Radiography is often of limited value because inflamed soft tissues are not well discriminated from adjacent normal soft tissues. Typically the osteopenia is initially periarticular, becoming more diffuse with time. Osteopenia is typically seen with infectious or inflammatory arthritides and also in Charcot joints. It may be subtle and better recognized by comparing to the contralateral (if unaffected) extremity (Fig. 10–6). With longstanding disease there may be uniform bone loss with a thin cortex. Uncommonly a linear subphyseal demineralization can be observed, but this is more often seen in leukemia (Fig. 10–7).[15]

Joint effusions are encountered commonly and can be seen in inflammatory or in noninflammatory joint disease.

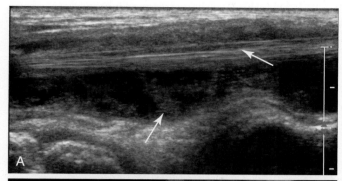

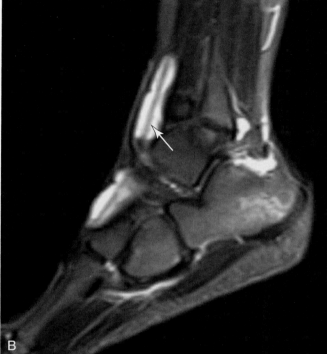

FIGURE 10–4 **A,** Longitudinal sonogram showing extensive tenosynovitis. *Upper arrow* demarcates the tendon with hypoechoic fluid and synovial proliferation *(lower arrow).* **B,** Corresponding sagittal T2-weighted MRI with *arrow* showing the tendon surrounded by high signal fluid.

Signs of knee effusions include fullness in the suprapatellar region, best seen on the lateral view. In the elbow, knee, and ankle, there is displacement of adjacent fat lines and fat pads.

Periosteal reaction, when present, is commonly seen in the phalanges, metacarpals, and metatarsals but can also occur in the long bones.

Joint space narrowing may be caused by cartilage loss. In JIA, the joint space narrowing is usually uniform. Chondrolysis can also be seen in slipped capital femoral epiphysis, with joint infection, or following joint surgery.

Joint space narrowing and bone erosions are later radiographic findings typically noted two or more years after disease onset. However, in some patients with rheumatoid factor–positive polyarthritis or systemic arthritis, early erosive disease can occur.

Bone erosions are typically located at joint margins in the bare areas but may also occur at tendinous insertions. Bone erosions can also be seen in sepsis, especially with chronic infections, or in hemophilia as a result of intraosseous hemorrhage. Growth of granulation tissue into bone can also give rise to an erosive appearance. Pigmented villonodular synovitis may cause well-marginated erosions on both sides of the joint, often with preserved joint width and bone density. Large erosions can be seen in the Camptodactyly-Arthropathy-Coxa Vara-Pericarditis (CACP) syndrome.[16]

Deformity of the fingers, whether with boutonniere or swan neck deformity, can be seen in a variety of disorders including JIA, CACP syndrome, or systemic lupus erythematosus (SLE). Enlarged or irregular epiphyseal ossification centers can be seen in hemophilia, JIA, and tuberculosis arthritis. Atlantoaxial subluxation may be noted in JIA, the arthropathy of Down syndrome, dysostosis multiplex, and SLE.

Changes in bone growth and maturation, with changes in the normal size of ossification centers and alteration of normal bone modeling, can be seen in JIA but also in joint infections and hemophilia. Enlargement of ossification centers, contour irregularity, and squaring (typically of the patella) can also be seen, as well as trabecular changes. Tibiotalar slant can also be noted in JIA.

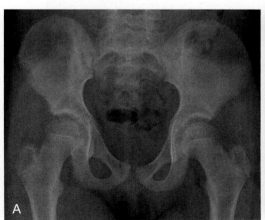

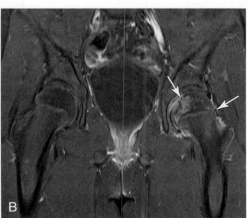

FIGURE 10–5 **A,** Pelvic radiograph of a 10-year-old girl with left hip pain following a fall. No abnormality is identified on plain film. **B,** Coronal T1-weighted fat-suppressed image following contrast administration with mild synovial thickening of left hip and abnormal femoral head enhancement *(arrows).* The right hip is normal.

Table 10–2

Radiographic features of joint disease

Osteopenia
Joint effusion
Joint space narrowing with focal or diffuse cartilage thinning
Bone erosions, subchondral cysts, and bone resorption
Changes in size of ossification centers
Subchondral sclerosis and osteophyte formation
Periosteal new bone formation
Malalignment, subluxation, dislocation
Joint ankylosis
Joint disorganization and destruction
Soft-tissue swelling, atrophy and calcification
Spinal manifestations

Data from Johnson K, Gardner-Medwin J: Childhood arthritis: classification and radiology, *Clin Radiol* 57:47-58, 2002.

Table 10–3

Radiographic features of juvenile idiopathic arthritis

Alignment
Atlantoaxial subluxation
Coxa valga or varus
Finger deformities including boutonniere or swan neck deformity
Knee valgus
Hallux valgus

Bone density
Juxtaarticular osteoporosis
Diffuse osteoporosis (late)
Metaphyseal lucent band (rarely)
Periosteal reaction adjacent to affected small joints

Cartilage and joint spaces
Erosions (late), may appear corticated
Cartilage space narrowing (late)
Ankylosis (especially spine, wrists)

Distribution
Monoarticular, oligoarticular, or polyarticular

Growth abnormalities

Affected small bones are shorter than normal
Overgrowth (lengthening) of affected long bones
Advanced maturation of affected epiphyses
Large epiphyses
Micrognathia (may have mandibular notching)
Protrusio acetabuli
Small fused cervical vertebrae
Angular carpal bones
Square patella
Intercondylar notch widening (also a feature of hemophilia)

Soft tissues
Effusions and joint distension
Nodules
Periarticular calcification (probably due to corticosteroid injections)

Data from Johnson K, Gardner-Medwin J: Childhood arthritis: classification and radiology, *Clin Radiol* 57:47-58, 2002.

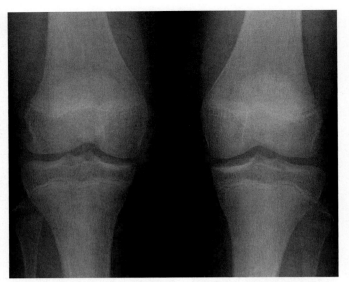

FIGURE 10–6 Frontal radiograph of both knees which shows subtle demineralization of the right knee.

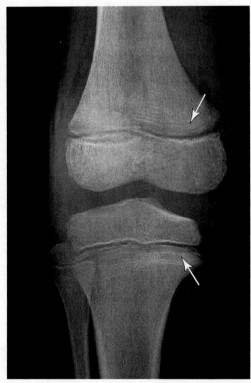

FIGURE 10–7 Frontal knee radiograph of a child with several weeks of knee pain initially suspected of having juvenile inflammatory arthritis. Note linear subphyseal lucency *(arrows)*, which suggested leukemia which was confirmed by bone marrow biopsy.

Late sequelae of JIA include epiphyseal deformity, abnormal angular carpal bones (Fig. 10–8), widening of the intercondylar notch of knees, and premature fusion of the growth plate with brachydactyly. Growth disturbances are more frequent if disease onset is early. Joint space narrowing as well as osseous erosions are usually late manifestations. At the hip, protrusio acetabuli,

FIGURE 10–8 Unilateral carpal arthritis with marked involvement on the left. Note the joint space narrowing, carpal bone erosions and irregularity, and overall demineralization.

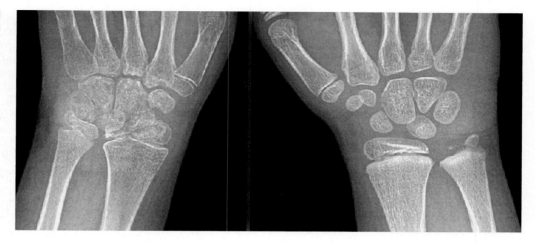

FIGURE 10–9 Three-year-old girl with persistent effusion and knee pain for 1 month. Moderate suprapatellar joint effusion is present on lateral radiograph (A) Fat-suppressed T1-weighted axial MRI image joint effusion post intravenous administration of contrast (B) shows low signal effusion and moderate uniform synovial thickening and synovitis.

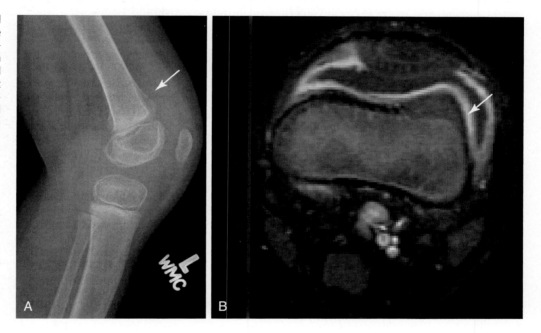

premature degenerative changes, coxa magna, and coxa valga can be seen. Joint space loss can progress to ankylosis, particularly in the apophyseal joints of the cervical spine and wrist. Ankylosis can also be rarely seen, however, in larger joints, including the hips. Subluxation of the joints, especially at the wrist, may be evident, and atlantoaxial subluxation may also occur. Growth disturbance of the temporomandibular joint (TMJ) may lead to micrognathia and temporomandibular disk abnormality.

Sonography

In JIA, sonography is more sensitive than conventional radiography and clinical assessment but inferior to MRI. Doppler sonography may assist in evaluating the activity of synovitis. Sonographic guidance can also be used for joint aspiration or injection.

Magnetic Resonance Imaging

Without contrast, proliferating synovium on MRI appears as thickened synovium of intermediate soft tissue density on T1- and T2-weighted sequences. It may have slightly higher signal intensity than adjacent fluid on unenhanced T1-weighted images. Pannus appears as thickened intermediate to dark signal intensity on T2-weighted images and is best seen when outlined by bright signal joint fluid. Its variable signal intensity reflects the relative amount of fibrous tissue and hemosiderin. Intravenous administration of gadolinium-based contrast agents improves visualization of thickened synovium, especially with use of fat suppression techniques (Fig. 10–9). Proliferating synovium appears as enhancing linear, villous, or nodular tissue. Images should be obtained immediately after contrast injection because diffusion of contrast material from the synovium into joint fluid occurs over time. Hypervascular inflamed pannus enhances significantly, whereas fibrous inactive pannus shows much less enhancement. Quantitative techniques have been developed for synovial volume. MRI is more sensitive than clinical evaluation in detecting some specific joint involvement—including the TMJ, which often demonstrates inflammatory change in the absence of clinical symptoms.

The development of a variety of fast-imaging methods with increased signal-to-noise ratio provides greater cartilage–synovial fluid contrast and has improved the MRI evaluation of cartilage morphology. Fat-suppressed three-dimensional spoiled gradient-recalled echo imaging provides excellent contrast because cartilage is of bright signal compared with adjacent structures. Other sequences that are valuable in cartilage assessment include driven equilibrium Fourier transform, dual-echo steady-state imaging, Dixon water-fat separation technique, and steady-state free precession.

Hemosiderin deposition can occur in JIA but is more frequently seen in other disorders, including pigmented villonodular synovitis, hemophilic arthropathy, synovial hemangioma, and posttraumatic synovitis.[17-19] Gradient echo sequences are most sensitive in detecting hemosiderin deposition within the synovium with signal loss occurring due to increased magnetic susceptibility.

Hemosiderin-containing synovitis appears very low in signal (black) on all MRI sequences, and this is accentuated on gradient-echo sequences (Fig. 10–10).

With prolonged synovial inflammation well-defined intraarticular nodules termed "rice bodies" may be present. Rice bodies likely arise from detached fragments of hypertrophied synovial villi. On MRI, rice bodies have dark signal on T2-weighted images owing to their fibrous tissue composition and are associated with joint effusion, synovial hypertrophy, and synovial enhancement after gadolinium administration (Fig. 10–11). Rice bodies may develop in JIA and also in tuberculosis.[20]

Because cartilage is one of the earliest sites of damage in JIA, this is an important area to be evaluated with MRI. Cartilage is of bright signal on both fast-spin echo and fat-suppressed proton density sequences, with hyaline cartilage having the highest intensity. Articular cartilage should be assessed for areas of altered signal, thinning,

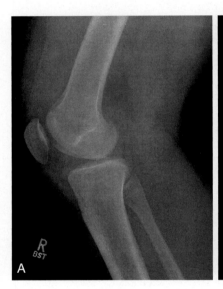
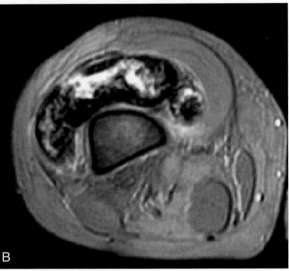

FIGURE 10–10 Fourteen-year-old boy with right knee swelling for one year. **A,** Lateral knee radiograph shows suprapatellar joint effusion. **B,** Axial gradient-echo MRI image showing low–signal intensity margins of suprapatellar bursa due to pigmented villonodular synovitis and hemosiderin deposition.

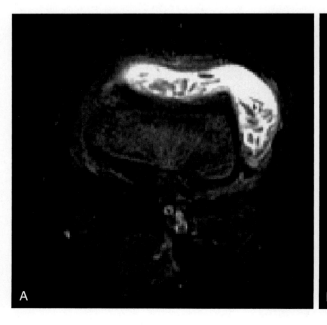
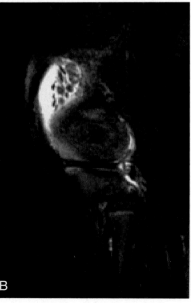

FIGURE 10–11 Axial and sagittal fat-suppressed T2-weighted MR images showing moderate joint effusion and multiple intraarticular low signal intensity rice bodies.

erosions, or deep cartilage loss that may extend to the subchondral bone (Fig. 10–12).

Imaging in the Assessment of Response to Therapy

Once therapy has begun for patients with JIA, imaging can be a helpful adjunct, along with clinical and laboratory parameters, to assess disease activity and response to therapy. To date, several studies have looked at radiographic changes before and after initiation of therapy. Recent studies have used CT and/or MRI to describe joint changes and have also begun to use more quantitative measures of disease activity, including measurement of synovial volume.

Radiography

Radiography can be helpful in monitoring for the presence of joint distension, epiphyseal overgrowth, osteopenia, joint space narrowing, erosions, subchondral cysts, and periostitis. Sparling and colleagues[21] showed that intraarticular therapy was able to prevent further radiographically detectable joint damage over time. A smaller study using radiography, sonography, and MRI[22] showed that, following the injection of intraarticular triamcinolone hexacetonide (TH), radiography was the best method to use to demonstrate epiphyseal overgrowth and osteopenia.

Carpal length is another parameter that has been used in follow-up. Carpal length is defined as the radio-metacarpal length plotted against the length of the second metacarpal bone on a chart with normal growth carpal scores, as described by Poznanski and colleagues.[23] The values are compared before and after treatment with an increase in carpal length (a positive change) indicating improvement. Three studies have shown improvements in carpal length in clinical responders to methotrexate[24,25] and etanercept.[26] Improved carpal length may be due to halting of the disease process along with possible articular cartilage regeneration in these growing children.

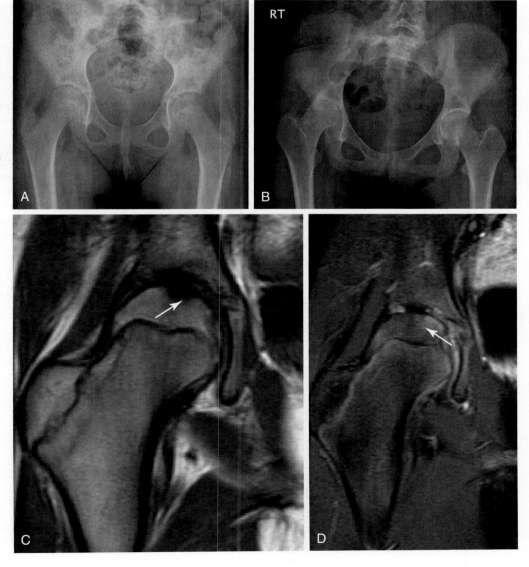

FIGURE 10–12 A child with systemic juvenile arthritis. **A,** Initial pelvic radiograph at 9 years of age with minimal decrease in hip joint width on right. **B,** several years from initial with further progression, including joint space loss, femoral and acetabular irregularity, and sclerosis. Pelvis MRI was obtained at the age of 13 for question of avascular necrosis. Coronal MRI images show joint space narrowing, focal abnormal femoral signal intensity with increased enhancement post contrast in keeping with avascular necrosis. Coronal T1 **C,** Post contrast fat-suppressed T1 **D.**

Sonography

Sonography can be a valuable tool in the assessment of disease activity because it is noninvasive, allows for a rapid examination, does not require sedation, and is cost-effective. Eich and colleagues used ultrasound to determine the presence of effusion, pannus, popliteal cysts, and lymphadenopathy in 10 children with JIA affecting 15 joints (11 knee and 4 hip joints) before and after intraarticular therapy and concluded that ultrasound was as sensitive as MRI in demonstrating joint effusion and/or pannus, but differentiation between the two was difficult, particularly in the hip joint.

Computed Tomography

In one study of the TMJ, CT was used to assess disease activity before and after therapy. Ringold and colleagues studied arthritis of the TMJ in 25 children who underwent intraarticular steroid injection with either triamcinolone acetonide or TH.[27] Twenty five patients underwent 74 total injections with a mean follow-up of 26 months (range: 5 to 52 months). The most common findings on baseline CT were joint space narrowing, erosions, and condylar flattening. Overall, 10 of 15 patients showed worsening radiologic changes, 3 showed stable changes, and 2 showed improvement. The authors commented that poor outcome was likely a result of selection bias, because only 15 of 25 patients underwent posttreatment imaging.

Magnetic Resonance Imaging

MRI is now the modality of choice to document changes before and after therapy. MRI can be used to monitor cartilage and bone erosions, effusion, pannus, and synovial volumes.[10] Huppertz and colleagues examined 21 children with arthritis of the knees and ankles who received intraarticular injection with TH.[28] MRI imaging was done immediately before the injection and at a median period of 49 days and 13 months after injection. Before therapy, MRI showed effusion with a median thickness of 11 mm and increased synovial enhancement signal in all 21 cases. These authors showed that intraarticular steroid therapy has a long-lasting beneficial effect, with suppression of synovial inflammation and reversion of pannus formation. Similarly, Niedel and colleagues assessed joint changes in 50 children undergoing 67 hip injections using unenhanced and gadolinium-enhanced MRI.[29] Joints that continued to demonstrate synovitis after injection had more significant radiographic deterioration than those with minimal

postinjection synovitis. These findings demonstrate that TH is able to reduce joint synovitis and effusion.[21]

Researchers have recently begun to use MRI to quantify synovial volumes and disease activity.[30,31] Using this approach, Graham and colleagues[30] imaged the small joints of the hands and wrists of 10 JIA patients at baseline, 6 weeks and 3 months after starting therapy.[32,33] The authors demonstrated that total synovial volume averaged 3.7 ml (range: 2.3 to 12.4) at initial examination and 2.2 ml at final examination. Synovial volume calculated from MRI correlated well with total hand swelling score and total number of active joints at each time point. Workie and colleagues looked at the utility of quantitative dynamic–contrast-enhanced MRI based on pharmacokinetic (PK) modeling to evaluate disease activity in the knee.[34] The authors demonstrated that PK parameters and synovial volumes were significantly decreased at 12 months after intraarticular steroid therapy, however improvement in synovial volume appeared to lag behind dynamic parameters, reflecting delay or subclinical synovitis. The authors postulated that patients who exhibit improvement in PK parameters but have an elevated synovial volume may have less active synovial inflammation and a more inactive fibrotic synovium. Thus, dynamic PK parameters may be able to provide additional information concerning disease activity.

Of all the imaging modalities, MRI has been shown to be the most sensitive modality in the assessment of TMJ arthritis in children (Fig. 10–13). Cahill and colleagues injected TMJ joints in 15 children with JIA and performed MRI scans 6 to 12 months after injection.[35] Joint changes (effusion, meniscal abnormalities, and loss of normal joint space) and bone changes (erosions and mandibular condyle abnormalities) were present in all joints before injection. Follow-up imaging showed improvement in 11 of 15 patients. The authors found good correlation between lack of acute findings on MRI and improvement in clinical findings and proposed their grading scheme as a useful tool for future trials.

A critical appraisal of radiologic scoring systems for assessment of juvenile idiopathic arthritis is discussed in the paper by Doria.[36]

Complications and Side Effects of Joint Injections

The most common radiographic finding postinjection is intraarticular calcification. This can resolve or persist for some time (Fig. 10–14). It typically does not impair

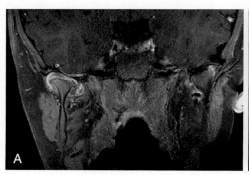 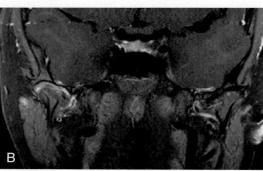

FIGURE 10–13 T2-weighted coronal MRI images of the TMJ joint in a 6-year-old female patient with JIA before and after intraarticular steroid injection. **A,** Increased synovial enhancement of the right TMJ before injection. **B,** Mild decrease in synovial enhancement 1 year after the injection.

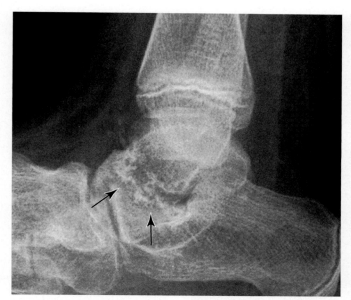

FIGURE 10–14 An x-ray image of the subtalar joint in an 11-year-old female patient with JIA. Note the extensive periarticular calcification *(black arrows)*, which developed after the child underwent intraarticular joint injection.

joint function. Damage to cartilage during the procedure is a potential complication but was not found when specifically looked for.[28,37] It is a difficult to know whether other postinjection changes reflect the underlying severity of the disease or the effects of the local treatment.[21] A summary of complications associated with joint injections is shown in Table 10–4.

Appendicular Skeleton

Radiography typically shows asymmetrical involvement of the large joints of the lower limb (i.e., hip, ankle, knee, and tarsal joints). The interphalangeal joint of the hallux is also frequently involved. Radiographs may be normal initially or can demonstrate soft tissue swelling, effusion, ossification and epiphyseal overgrowth, erosions, osteopenia, joint space narrowing, or rarely fusion. Bone erosions may be associated with irregular bone apposition at joint margins referred to as "whiskering." With hip involvement, these proliferative changes are noted at the junction of the femoral head and neck. Dactylitis may be seen with soft tissue swelling and periosteal reaction along the shaft of metacarpals, metatarsals, or phalanges.

Enthesitis can involve the calcaneous and tibial tuberosity with soft tissue swelling at tendon insertions, localized osteopenia, and bone erosion and/or spur formation, particularly at the site of insertion of the Achilles tendon into the calcaneus, plantar aponeurosis, or patella. Periostitis may also be seen (Fig. 10–15).

Enthesitis-related Arthritis

Radiographic findings of enthesitis-related arthritis and other spondyloarthropathies are similar to those encountered in other forms of JIA, with the exception of sacroiliitis and enthesitis, which are more specific for spondyloarthropathy (Table 10–5).[38,39]

Table 10–4

Summary of complications associated with joint injections

Common
Subcutaneous atrophy
Intraarticular or periarticular calcifications
Crystal-induced synovitis

Uncommon
Cushingoid effects
Small patella
Intraarticular tibial bony spur
Patellar osteochondritis dissecans
Avascular necrosis of the distal radial and femoral epiphysis

Data from Job-Deslandre C, Menkes CJ: Complications of intra-articular injections of triamcinolone hexacetonide in chronic arthritis in children *Clin Exp Rheumatol* 8:413-416, 1990; Huppertz HI, Tschammler A, Schwab KO et al: Intraarticular corticosteroids for chronic arthritis in children: efficacy and effects on cartilage and growth, *J Pediatr* 127:317-321 1995.

Table 10–5

Radiographic features of enthesitis-related arthritis and spondyloarthropathies

Peripheral joints
Asymmetrical involvement of large lower limb joints
Involvement of interphalanged joint of the hallux
New bone at the margins of erosions
Affected joints—show swelling, effusion, epiphyseal overgrowth, erosions, osteopenia, cartilage space narrowing, and rarely fusion
Dactylitis—swelling and periosteal new bone of fingers or toes
Periosteal new bone—e.g., metatarsals, proximal femur
Entheses
Especially tibial tubercle and posterior aspect of calcaneus
Swelling, erosion, new bone formation
Sacroiliitis
Radiographic changes generally delayed until late teens
Asymmetrical involvement may occur early, then become symmetrical
Erosions occur first on the iliac side of sacroiliac joint
"Pseudowidening" occurs due to erosion
Sclerosis and finally ankylosis develop

Data from Azouz EM, Duffy CM: Juvenile spondyloarthropathies: clinical manifestations and medical imaging, *Skeletal Radiol* 24:399-408, 1995; Jacobs JC, Berdon WE, Johnson AD et al: HLA-B27–associated spondyloarthritis and enthesopathy in childhood: clinical, pathologic, and radiographic observations in 58 patients, *J Pediatr* 100:521-528, 1982.

Sonography

On sonography, enthesitis may show loss of the normal fibrillar echotexture of the tendon and irregular fusiform thickening.[40] Doppler sonography can be used to assess low-velocity flow in small synovial vessels.[41] D'Agostino and colleagues reported response to treatment with infliximab in young adults presenting with inflammatory heel pain.[42] Using Doppler sonography Tse and colleagues also demonstrated the ability of color Doppler

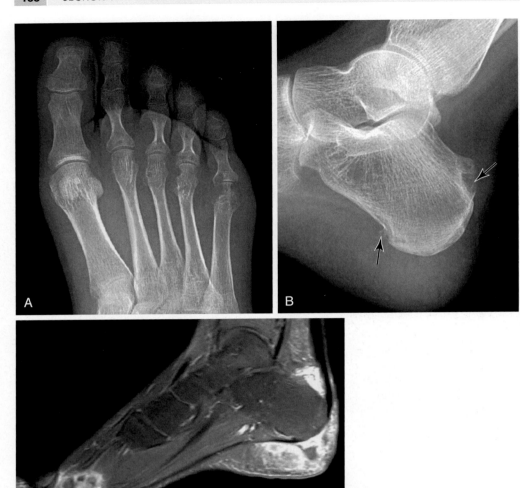

FIGURE 10–15   Seventeen-year-old woman with juvenile enthesitis–related arthritis. **A,** The forefoot shows joint space narrowing and extensive bone erosions involving multiple metatarsophalangeal joints, especially the fifth metatarsophalangeal joint. **B,** Erosions are also noted in the hindfoot at the insertion of the plantar fascia and calcaneal tendons. **C,** Sagittal contrast-enhanced fat-suppressed T1-weighted image with intense enhancement adjacent to the calcaneal tendon, heel, and metatarsophalangeal joint.

sonography to show improvement in increased vascularity at the cortical bone insertion of enthesis and along the adjacent synovium in children with spondyloarthropathy, suggesting that this technique may add valuable information to gray-scale sonography.[43]

Magnetic Resonance Imaging

With MRI one may see bone marrow edema, tenosynovitis, granulation tissue, or cortical erosion at the site of enthesitis.[9]

Axial Skeleton

In early enthesitis related arthritis (ERA) changes in the spine and sacroiliac joints are generally not seen until the latter part of the second decade or even adulthood. There may be localized osteitis, erosions, and sclerosis—particularly at the vertebral margins. Syndesmophytes and atlantoaxial subluxation are rarely seen in children.

Radiographs may demonstrate unilateral or bilateral sacroiliitis with indistinct articular margins (also known as *pseudowidening*), erosions, and reactive sclerosis, particularly on the iliac side of the joint. Radiography shows asymmetrical sacroiliac joint space widening initially, but eventually the classic bilateral symmetrical joint involvement can be seen with joint space narrowing and ankylosis. Radiographic evaluation of the sacroiliac joints is often especially difficult in teenagers. Diffuse osteopenia of the pelvic bones is also seen as a late change.

Magnetic Resonance Imaging

MRI can demonstrate early inflammatory changes in the sacroiliac joints and spine and is especially sensitive for evaluation of subchondral bone marrow edema not shown on other types of imaging (Fig. 10–16).[44] The administration of gadolinium-DTPA chelates improves the detection of early sacroiliitis. On MRI, periarticular low signal may be seen on T1-weighted images with high signal on T2-weighted images from inflammatory changes in bone marrow. Low signal on both sequences will be seen with bone sclerosis. MRI may also demonstrate erosions in articular cartilage.[44] Evaluation of more widespread anatomical assessment, including whole-body MRI, is currently underway and appears useful at least in demonstrating the presence of multiple sites of enthesitis-related disease.

FIGURE 10–16 Eleven-year-old boy with enthesitis-related arthritis. **A,** MRI showed bilateral hip joint effusions and abnormal bone signal adjacent to the left sacroiliac joint and left greater trochanter *(arrows)*. Coronal T1-weighted image shows low signal *(arrows in a)*. **B,** coronal short-tau inversion recovery image shows increased signal intensity in these regions.

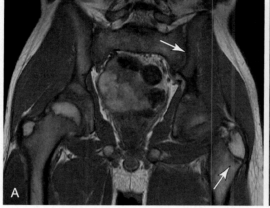
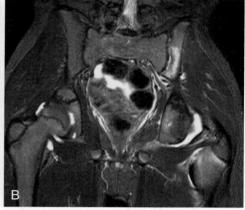

FIGURE 10–17 Fourteen-year-old boy with arthritis and longstanding history of limping and abnormal gait. **A,** pelvic radiograph showing sclerosis adjacent to the sacroiliac joints; **B,** finding confirmed on MRI with multiple erosions evident.

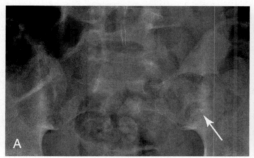
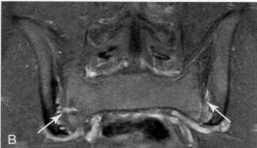

Computed Tomography

Sacroiliitis may be demonstrated on either CT or MRI at an earlier stage compared with radiography (Fig. 10–17). CT scan of the sacroiliac joints is useful in demonstrating sclerosis or erosive disease not evident on radiographs. Although MRI is preferable, if CT is used angled scans through the sacroiliac joint should be used to lower the radiation dose.

Scintigraphy

Bone scintigraphy can overcome the difficulty in recognizing early unilateral sacroiliac abnormalities on radiography. However, there is normally a higher concentration of physiological activity in pediatric sacroiliac joints. Mild to moderate increases in the radioisotope uptake, especially when bilateral, may make assessment difficult. Asymmetric uptake is more common in childhood spondyloarthropathies other than juvenile ankylosing spondylitis.

Radiography

Psoriatic Arthritis

Radiographs obtained in the initial phase of the disease may be normal or show juxtaarticular osteoporosis. Characteristic radiographic features of psoriatic arthritis include asymmetric involvement, sausage digits, joint erosions, joint space narrowing, bony proliferation

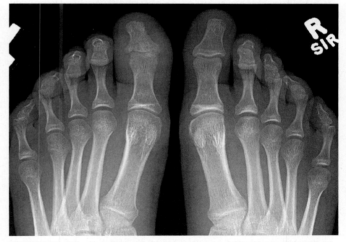

FIGURE 10–18 Dactylitis of the left great toe in child with psoriatic arthritis. There is diffuse soft tissue swelling of the digit along with narrowing of the first metatarsophalangeal joint and interphalangeal joint. Irregularity of the base of the distal phalanx is present.

(including periarticular and shaft periostitis enthesitis), osteolysis (including "pencil-in-cup" deformity), acroosteolysis, spur formation, and ankylosis. The bone erosions tend to be larger and more asymmetric than those seen in JIA; however, generally the radiographic features may be indistinguishable from those of other forms of subtypes. The characteristic changes seen at the distal interphalangeal joints are uncommon in children (Fig. 10–18).

Sonography

Sonography may also be a useful tool in the assessment of psoriasis. Sonography with Doppler evaluation is more sensitive than clinical examination for detection of abnormalities in the hands and wrists, along with calcaneal enthesitis of adults with psoriatic arthritis, and is a reliable tool for assessment of joint response to therapy with biologic agents.

Magnetic Resonance Imaging

In psoriatic arthritis, MRI demonstrates erosive changes, joint space narrowing, ligament disruption, and tenosynovitis. Sausage digits are seen in patients with psoriatic arthritis and reactive arthritis. These swollen fingers or toes result from tenosynovitis, soft tissue edema, and synovial proliferation.[45] MRI may also be used to evaluate the responsiveness of therapy, as can be noted by a significant reduction in gadolinium uptake following treatment with infliximab.[46,47]

Axial Skeleton

Sacroiliitis and vertebral involvement typically manifest later on during the progression of the disease. The sacroiliitis of juvenile psoriatic arthritis is usually asymmetric and resembles that of reactive arthritis. Syndesmophytes, paraspinal calcification and atlantoaxial subluxation are rare in children.

CT may be useful in assessing spine disease, but has little role in the assessment of peripheral joints. Previous studies have shown that CT is as accurate as MRI for assessment of erosions in the sacroiliac joints but is not as affective for identifying synovial inflammation. CT can be used guide sacroiliac joint injection.[46]

Acknowledgment

The authors would like to acknowledge the contributions of Nasir A. Khan, medical student, University of Toronto.

REFERENCES

1. P. Babyn, A.S. Doria, Radiologic investigation of rheumatic diseases, Pediatr. Clin. North Am. 52 (2005) 373–411, vi.
2. E. Azouz, M: Juvenile idiopathic arthritis: how can the radiologist help the clinician? Pediatr. Radiol. 38 (suppl. 3) (2008) S403–408.
3. T. Southwood, Juvenile idiopathic arthritis: clinically relevant imaging in diagnosis and monitoring, Pediatr. Radiol. 38 (suppl. 3) (2008) S395–402.
4. M. Backhaus, Ultrasound and structural changes in inflammatory arthritis: synovitis and tenosynovitis, Ann. N Y Acad. Sci. 1154 (2009) 139–151.
5. M. Ruhoy, K.L. Tucker, R.G. McCauley, et al., Hypertrophic bursopathy of the subacromial-subdeltoid bursa in juvenile rheumatoid arthritis: sonographic appearance, Pediatr. Radiol. 26 (1996) 353–355.
6. P.C. Khanna, M.M. Thapa, The growing skeleton: MR imaging appearances of developing cartilage, Magn. Reson. Imaging. Clin. North Am. 17 (2009) 411–421.
7. V.M. Gylys-Morin, MR imaging of pediatric musculoskeletal inflammatory and infectious disorders, Magn. Reson. Imaging. Clin. North Am. 6 (1998) 537–559.
8. S. Lamer, G.H. Sebag, MRI and ultrasound in children with juvenile chronic arthritis, Eur. J. Radiol. 33 (2000) 85–93.
9. H.E. Daldrup-Link, L. Steinbach, MRI imaging of pediatric arthritis, Magn. Reson. Imaging. Clin. North Am. 17 (2009). 451–467.
10. H. Cakmakci, A. Kovanlikaya, E. Unsal, et al., Short-term follow-up of the juvenile rheumatoid knee with fat-saturated 3D MRI, Pediatr. Radiol. 31 (2001) 189–195.
11. T. Laor, D. Jaramillo, MRI imaging insights into skeletal maturation: what is normal? Radiology 250 (2009) 28–38.
12. F.M. McQueen, The MRI view of synovitis and tenosynovitis in inflammatory arthritis: implications for diagnosis and management, Ann. N. Y. Acad. Sci. 1154 (2009) 21–34.
13. M. Ostergaard, M. Stoltenberg, P. Gicteon, et al., Changes in synovial membrane and joint effusion volumes after intraarticular methylprednisolone. Quantitative assessment of inflammatory and destructive changes in arthritis by MRI, J. Rheumatol. 23 (1996) 1151–1161.
14. A. Shammas, Nuclear medicine imaging of the pediatric musculoskeletal system, Semin. Musculoskelet. Radiol. 13 (2009) 159–180.
15. I. Spilberg, G.J. Meyer, The arthritis of leukemia, Arthritis Rheum. 15 (1972) 630–635.
16. R.M. Laxer, B.J. Cameron, D. Chaisson, et al., The camptodactyly-arthropathy-pericarditis syndrome: case report and literature review, Arthritis Rheum. 29(3) (1986). 439–444.
17. A. Cotten, R.M. Flipo, B. Herbaux, et al., Synovial haemangioma of the knee: a frequently misdiagnosed lesion, Skeletal Radiol. 24 (1995) 257–261.
18. D.J. Sartoris, D. Resnick, The radiographic differential diagnosis of juvenile chronic arthritis, Aust. Paediat. J. 23 (1987) 273–275.
19. S.M. Bravo, C.S. Winalski, B.N. Weissman, et al., Pigmented villonodular synovitis, Radiol. Clin. North Am. 34 (1996) 311–326.
20. C. Chung, B.D. Coley, L.C. Martin, et al., Rice bodies in juvenile rheumatoid arthritis, Am. J. Roentgenol. 170 (1998) 698–700.
21. M. Sparling, P. Malleson, B. Wood, et al., Radiographic followup of joints injected with triamcinolone hexacetonide for the management of childhood arthritis, Arthritis Rheum. 33 (1990) 821–826.
22. G.F. Eich, F. Halle, J. Hodler, et al., Juvenile chronic arthritis: imaging of the knees and hips before and after intraarticular steroid injection, Pediatr. Radiol. 24 (1994) 558–563.
23. A.K. Poznanski, R.J. Hernandez, K.E. Guire, et al., Carpal length in children—a useful measurement in the diagnosis of rheumatoid arthritis and some congenital malformation syndromes, Radiology 129 (1978) 661–668.
24. L. Harel, L. Wagner-Weiner, A.K. Poznanski, et al., Effects of methotrexate on radiologic progression in juvenile rheumatoid arthritis, Arthritis Rheum. 36 (1993) 1370–1374.
25. A. Ravelli, S. Viola, B. Ramenghi, et al., Radiologic progression in patients with juvenile chronic arthritis treated with methotrexate, J. Pediatr. 133 (1998) 262–265.
26. S. Nielsen, N. Ruperto, V. Gerloni, et al., Preliminary evidence that etanercept may reduce radiographic progression in juvenile idiopathic arthritis, Clin. Exp. Rheumatol. 26 (2008) 688–692.
27. S. Ringold, T.R. Torgerson, M.A. Egbert, et al., Intraarticular corticosteroid injections of the temporomandibular joint in juvenile idiopathic arthritis, J. Rheumatol. 35 (2008) 1157–1164.
28. H.I. Huppertz, W.A. Kaiser, Serial magnetic resonance imaging in juvenile dermatomyositis–delayed normalization, Rheumatol. Int. 14 (1994) 127–129.
29. J. Neidel, M. Boehnke, R.M. Küster, et al., The efficacy and safety of intraarticular corticosteroid therapy for coxitis in juvenile rheumatoid arthritis, Arthritis Rheum. 46 (2002) 1620–1628.
30. T.B. Graham, T. Laor, B.J. Dardzinski, et al., Quantitative magnetic resonance imaging of the hands and wrists of children with juvenile rheumatoid arthritis, J. Rheumatol. 32 (2005) 1811–1820.
31. A. Kuseler, T.K. Pedersen, T. Herlin, et al., Contrast enhanced magnetic resonance imaging as a method to diagnose early inflammatory changes in the temporomandibular joint in children with juvenile chronic arthritis, J. Rheumatol. 25 (1998) 1406–1412.
32. T.B. Graham, J.S. Blebea, V. Gylys-Morin, et al., Magnetic resonance imaging in juvenile rheumatoid arthritis, Semin. Arthritis Rheum. 27 (1997) 161–168.
33. J.W. Graham, W. Jan, MRI and the brain in systemic lupus erythematosus, Lupus 12 (2003) 891–896.
34. D.W. Workie, T.B. Graham, T. Laor, et al., Quantitative MRI characterization of disease activity in the knee in children with juvenile idiopathic arthritis: a longitudinal pilot study, Pediatr. Radiol. 37 (2007) 535–543.

35. A.M. Cahill, K.M. Baskin, Kaye RD, et al., CT-guided percutaneous steroid injection for management of inflammatory arthropathy of the temporomandibular joint in children, Am. J. Roentgenol. 188 Jan (2001) 182–186.

36. A.S. Doria, P.S. Babyn, B. Feldman, et al., A critical appraisal of radiographic scoring systems for assessment of juvenile idiopathic arthritis, Pediatr. Radiol. 36 (2006) 759–772.

37. H.I. Huppertz, A. Tschammler, Horwitz AE, et al., Intraarticular corticosteroids for chronic arthritis in children: efficacy and effects on cartilage and growth, J. Pediatr. 127 (1995) 317–321.

38. J.C. Jacobs, W.E. Berdon, A.D. Johnston, et al., HLA-B27-associated spondyloarthritis and enthesopathy in childhood: clinical, pathologic, and radiographic observations in 58 patients, J. Pediatr. 100 (1982) 521–528.

39. A.M. Prieur, Spondyloarthropathies in childhood, Baillieres Clin. Rheumatol. 12 (1998) 287–307.

40. P.V. Balint, D. Kane, H. Wilson, et al., Ultrasonography of entheseal insertions in the lower limb in spondyloarthropathy, Ann. Rheum. Dis. 61 (2002) 905–910.

41. M. Kamel, H. Eid, R. Mansour, et al., Ultrasound detection of heel enthesitis: a comparison with magnetic resonance imaging, J. Rheumatol. 30 (2003) 774–778.

42. M.A. D'Agostino, R. Said-Nahal, C. Hacquard-Bouder, et al., Assessment of peripheral enthesitis in the spondyloarthropathies by ultrasonography combined with power Doppler: a cross-sectional study, Arthritis Rheum. 48(2) (2003) 523–533.

43. S.M. Tse, R.M. Laxer, P.S. Babyn, A.S. Doria, Radiologic improvement of juvenile idiopathic: arthritis-enthesitis-related arthritis following anti-tumor necrosis factor-alpha blockade with etanercept. J. Rheumatol. 33 (2006) 1186-1188.

44. M. Bollow, J. Braun, T. Biedermann, et al., Use of contrast-enhanced MRI imaging to detect sacroiliitis in children, Skeletal Radiol. 27 (1998) 606–616.

45. E.Y. Lee, R.P. Sundel, S. Kim, et al., MRI findings of juvenile psoriatic arthritis, Skeletal Radiol. 37 (2008) 987–996.

46. S. Weckbach, S. Schewe, H.J. Michaely, et al., Whole-body MRI imaging in psoriatic arthritis: additional value for therapeutic decision making, Eur. J. Radiol. 2009, epub ahead of print.

Chapter 11

PAIN

Michael A. Rapoff and Carol B. Lindsley

Chronic or intermittent pain is a primary symptom of many pediatric rheumatic diseases, especially arthritis. Patients often report mild to moderate pain.[1-4] About 25% to 30% report moderate to severe pain,[5,6] and most children with arthritis report at least some pain lasting from 30 minutes to 24 hours a day, with a mean of 4.3 hours per day.[7] A 2-month daily diary study showed that children with arthritis report pain on an average of 73% of the days, with the majority (76%) reporting pain on more than 60% of the days.[8] A 2-week electronic pain diary study showed that adolescents with arthritis reported, on average, mild pain intensity, whereas 9.2% reported no pain, and 17.1% reported pain on every diary entry.[9] About 60% of children with juvenile rheumatoid arthritis (JRA) report joint pain at disease onset, 50% report pain at 1-year follow-up, and 40% continue to report pain 5 years later.[10] Moreover, adults who as children were diagnosed with JRA report significantly more pain, fatigue, and disability than gender-matched healthy controls.[11] Thus, pain is a significant problem for some children with JRA and presumably JIA (juvenile idiopathic arthritis) that persists into adulthood and is associated with greater disability. Pain affects multiple areas of their lives, and its effect is not fully explained by disease activity alone.

The purpose of this chapter is to: 1) outline a biobehavioral model of pain, including nociceptive, emotional, cognitive, and behavioral aspects of arthritis-related pain and implications for treatment based on the model; 2) review cognitive-behavioral treatments for chronic pain, including arthritis-related pain; and 3) describe measures of pain.

BIOBEHAVIORAL MODEL OF PAIN

A comprehensive understanding of pain and its treatment requires a multidimensional approach that goes beyond nociceptive activity associated with the disease. A model that acknowledges this complexity of pain is needed as a foundation for development of effective pharmacological and nonpharmacological treatments. The most widely accepted definition of pain ("an unpleasant sensory and emotional experience associated with actual or potential tissue damage") views it as simultaneously a physiological and psychological experience.[12] Beginning with the *gate control* theory of pain,[13] researchers have advanced a biobehavioral model focused on the unique and interactive components of nociceptive activity, emotions, cognitions, and behavior.[14,15]

Nociceptive Activity. *Nociception* describes the physiological, anatomical, and chemical properties of the nervous system that contribute to the perception of pain.[16] Noxious mechanical, thermal, or chemical stimuli generate neuronal impulses conducted along peripheral (afferent) nerve fibers that synapse in the dorsal horn circuitry of the spinal cord and project to the thalamus and cortex via the spinothalamic tract. Neural projections also descend from the brain and synapse with neurons in the spinal cord (Fig. 11–1). The dorsal horn circuitry is an important site within the central nervous system, where modulation (excitatory or inhibitory) of neuronal impulses takes place. The inhibition of spinal nociceptive transmission can diminish the experience of pain, as when endogenous opioids (such as endorphins) are released during stress and produce analgesic effects.[16,17] This descending pain modulation system, first proposed in the gate control theory of pain,[13] provides a neurochemical and anatomical basis for considering the pain-enhancing or pain-inhibiting effects of psychological factors, such as cognitions and emotions.[16,17] Nociceptors may be modality specific or polymodal (respond to multiple types of stimuli). Activation occurs only with intense, potentially damaging stimuli and generally there is no spontaneous activity.[18] The cell bodies of the afferent nociceptive fibers are in the dorsal root ganglia and terminate over several spinal segments in the dorsal horn of the spinal cord.[19]

In rheumatic disease–related pain, nociceptive afferents in the joint are located in the joint capsule and ligaments, bone, periosteum, articular fat pads, and perivascular sites.[16] They are activated by joint motion or any noxious movement or stimuli such as inflammation or injury. Two nociceptive neuropeptide neurons dominate: the isolectin-positive and the calcitonin gene-related peptide-containing neurons. Both spatial and temporal summation in a population of nerve fibers results in the sensation of pain and correlates with the magnitude.[20] The enhanced pain associated with arthritis is probably due to the response of joint afferents to the mechanical and heat stimulation present during inflammation and chemical mediators of joint inflammation, such as prostaglandins, which sensitize joint afferent fibers.[21] This inflammation-induced sensitization of articular afferents likely contributes to hyperalgesia, an

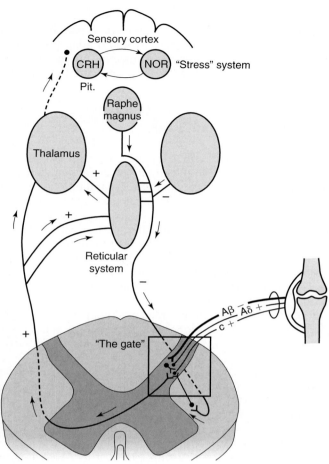

FIGURE 11–1 Diagram showing overview of pain pathways from the peripheral sensory nerves to the cerebral cortex. CRH, corticotropin-releasing hormone; NOR, norepinephrine.

increased response to stimuli that are typically painful, and allodynia, pain due to stimuli, which do not typically provoke pain.[22] Also, studies of experimentally induced pain found reduced pain threshold in inflamed and noninflamed joints of children with active arthritis and to a lesser degree in the joints of children in remission.[23-25] The persistence of lowered pain threshold, even after nociceptive input to the joint might be expected to cease, suggests a role for long-lasting structural and functional changes or "neuroplastic alterations" due to "central sensitization."[26,27] Thus, peripheral and central sensitization mechanisms may be operative in arthritis-related pain.

Emotions. Pain is an emotional, as well as a sensory, experience.[28-31] There is strong correlational support for the link between negative emotions, particularly anxiety and depression, and increased pain intensity and interference in the lives of children with JRA.[1-5,8,32,33] Also, daily stressful events and negative mood have been linked to increased pain, stiffness, and fatigue in children with JRA.[34] Although causality studies examining the link between emotional distress and pain have yet to be conducted, emotional distress and pain may share common etiological factors, are reciprocally linked, and can occur concurrently.[28,35] Increased anxiety can induce muscle tension, thereby directly inducing or exacerbating musculoskeletal pain, or increased pain can induce anxiety about future prognosis or interference

with life activities. Also, substance P, a neuropeptide, has been implicated in the pathophysiology of inflammatory disease, depression and anxiety, and pain, thus possibly sharing a common mediating factor.[36]

Cognitions. Cognitive factors refer to how people attend (or not) to pain and how they evaluate their pain experience. The focus in the pain literature has been on maladaptive rather than adaptive thinking. Cognitive processing of pain can be maladaptive in at least two ways: (1) people can fail to attend to information or fail to generate self-talk that might be helpful in coping with pain, or (2) people can engage in dysfunctional thinking that leads to maladaptive coping and greater pain (such as wishful or catastrophic thinking). Catastrophizing may be the most "toxic" type of dysfunctional thinking related to pain.[37,38] Catastrophizing is thought to include three components: (1) rumination (preoccupation with pain-related thoughts); (2) magnification (exaggeration of the threat value of pain); and (3) helplessness (adopting a helpless orientation to cope with pain).[38]

Several studies have investigated cognitive coping strategies in children with arthritis. Studies in Denmark have found that catastrophizing is associated with higher pain intensity during a cold pressor paradigm[39] and clinically over a 3-week period.[40] Reid and colleagues[41] found that "emotion-focused avoidance" coping (catastrophizing and expressing negative emotions) was associated with greater pain intensity, pain duration, and anxiety. Varni and colleagues[42] found that "cognitive self-instruction" (primarily wishful thinking) was related to greater emotional distress and that "cognitive refocusing" (engaging in activities as a distraction from pain) was related to less pain intensity and emotional distress. Another study found that "pain control and rational thinking" (controlling and decreasing pain while avoiding catastrophizing) predicted lower pain intensity.[6]

Behaviors. When children are in pain, they exhibit a wide variety of pain behaviors, such as limping, grimacing, crying, resting, or asking for medication. How others respond to these pain behaviors can be adaptive or maladaptive for the child experiencing pain. Pain behaviors such as guarding and malpositioning of affected joints may be maladaptive for children with arthritis. Caregivers' responses to children's pain-related behaviors may also be maladaptive, such as when parents allow children to avoid attending school, resulting in low academic performance and missed opportunities for social interactions. Conversely, if children engage in "well" behaviors (e.g., positive coping strategies) and parents reinforce adaptive behaviors, children would be expected to experience less pain and disability from pain. This operant behavioral perspective is well supported in the pediatric pain literature, mostly with respect to chronic abdominal pain or headache.[43] For instance, one study found that children with JRA who reported resting more and withdrawing from activities showed higher levels of pain and emotional distress.[42] Another study found that children with JRA who engaged in "approach" coping (including talking to a friend or family member about how they felt) showed less functional disability.[41]

Treatment Implications. A biobehavioral model of pain would suggest a number of treatment options.[15] Early identification and aggressive pharmacological treatment of chronic arthritis could lead to enhanced pain relief and improved function, both short term and long term, via a reduction in peripheral and central sensitization mechanisms. Adequate control of the inflammatory disease is of utmost importance in the overall approach to pain management. Adherence to effective pharmacological therapies (see Chapter 6) can be less than optimal, and strategies for improving and maintaining adherence need to be routinely implemented in pediatric rheumatology practice.[44]

There are neurochemical mechanisms that suggest the value of nonpharmacological therapies in the treatment of arthritis-related pain, such as cooling and resting inflamed joints (to control nociceptive inputs and avoid peripheral sensitization) and relaxation or other psychological treatments to control pain by influencing "central" mechanisms.[26]

Psychological interventions that reduce negative emotional states would be expected to directly or indirectly reduce pain intensity and pain interference. Helping children to manage disease-related stressors (e.g., relaxation and problem-solving techniques) should result in concomitant reductions in negative emotions and pain. Enlisting the social support and reinforcement of family and friends should foster greater participation in social and recreational activities by patients, thereby reducing emotional distress and preoccupation with pain and suffering. Psychopharmacological agents (such as the serotonin-specific reuptake inhibitors, or SSRIs) could help reduce depression and pain through common biological pathways.

For children who are not "mindful" or fail to attend to their thoughts about pain, increasing their awareness of these thoughts (by using "thought diaries" to record thoughts when their pain is bothersome) may be a useful first step in learning to cope with their pain. However, without additional coping strategies, just making children mindful of their pain-related thoughts could lead to nonadaptive thinking.

Cognitive "restructuring" may be helpful in countering nonadaptive thinking about pain. This involves having children identify negative thoughts (e.g., "I can't do anything to make my pain better."), challenge or question these thoughts, and substitute more helpful thoughts (e.g., "I can distract myself or do relaxation exercises to reduce my pain."). There may be a role for distraction in the management of pain, such as encouraging children to engage in behaviors that divert their attention from their pain. Imagery techniques (e.g., vividly imagining a relaxing place or experience) combined with relaxation exercises are often helpful in diverting attention from pain and reducing muscle tension, thereby reducing pain.

Parents are important role models for their children and need to be made aware of how they cope with their own pain (such as headaches) and thereby influence how their children cope with pain. One may need to directly assist parents in learning more adaptive strategies for coping with pain so they can model these strategies for their children (e.g., not avoid responsibilities because of pain and use effective medical or psychological therapies to control pain). Providers also need to teach family members (especially parents) and friends to respond in adaptive ways

to children's pain behaviors. This would include avoiding being overly solicitous and attentive to pain behaviors and, instead, reinforcing alternative and adaptive coping strategies. Children require assistance in finding ways (in spite of their pain) to do what they want and need to do.

COGNITIVE-BEHAVIORAL TREATMENTS FOR PAIN

Cognitive-behavioral therapy (CBT) approaches to chronic pediatric pain typically involve teaching children to use deep breathing, guided imagery, and relaxation and to replace maladaptive thinking (such as catastrophizing) with adaptive thinking (such as focusing on what can be done to control pain and encouraging oneself to engage in more effective coping). Parents are taught to encourage their children to stay as active as possible and to engage in positive coping. Parents are also taught to avoid reinforcing pain behaviors (such as allowing children to avoid school or other responsibilities). A CBT approach, in conjunction with standard pharmacological treatments, is consistent with the biobehavioral model of pain and is empirically supported as a treatment for chronic pediatric pain.[45-47]

Two published studies have tested CBT for children with JRA. Lavine and colleagues[48] used a multiple baseline design with 8 children with JRA to evaluate a six-session treatment that included relaxation and biofeedback training. They showed significant reductions in pain intensity and pain-related behaviors at follow-up. Walco and colleagues[49] used a single-group pre-posttest design with 13 children with JRA to evaluate an eight-session treatment that included progressive muscle relaxation, deep breathing, and guided imagery. Parents were seen for two sessions to review how they could reinforce "well" behaviors and avoid reinforcing pain behaviors. There were significant reductions in pain intensity at immediate follow-up as well as maintenance of gains at 6-month and 12-month follow-ups. Although these studies are promising, they involved small samples and no control or alternative treatment comparison groups. There is a need for well-controlled, multisite pain intervention trials for children and adolescents with arthritis.

PAIN MEASURES

As with adults, self-report measures of pain are considered the gold standard for assessing pain intensity, duration, and location in children 3 years of age and older.[50] The most widely used and validated self-report measure of pain for patients with JRA is the Pediatric Pain Questionnaire (PPQ) developed by Varni and colleagues.[51] The PPQ contains a visual analog scale (VAS), which is a 10-cm horizontal line, anchored with descriptors "not hurting" or "no pain" and "hurting a whole lot" or "severe pain." The patient makes a vertical line on the VAS for present pain and the VAS for worst pain for the previous week (Fig. 11–2). The PPQ also contains a body gender-neutral outline that shows the front and back sides of the body. There are four boxes underneath

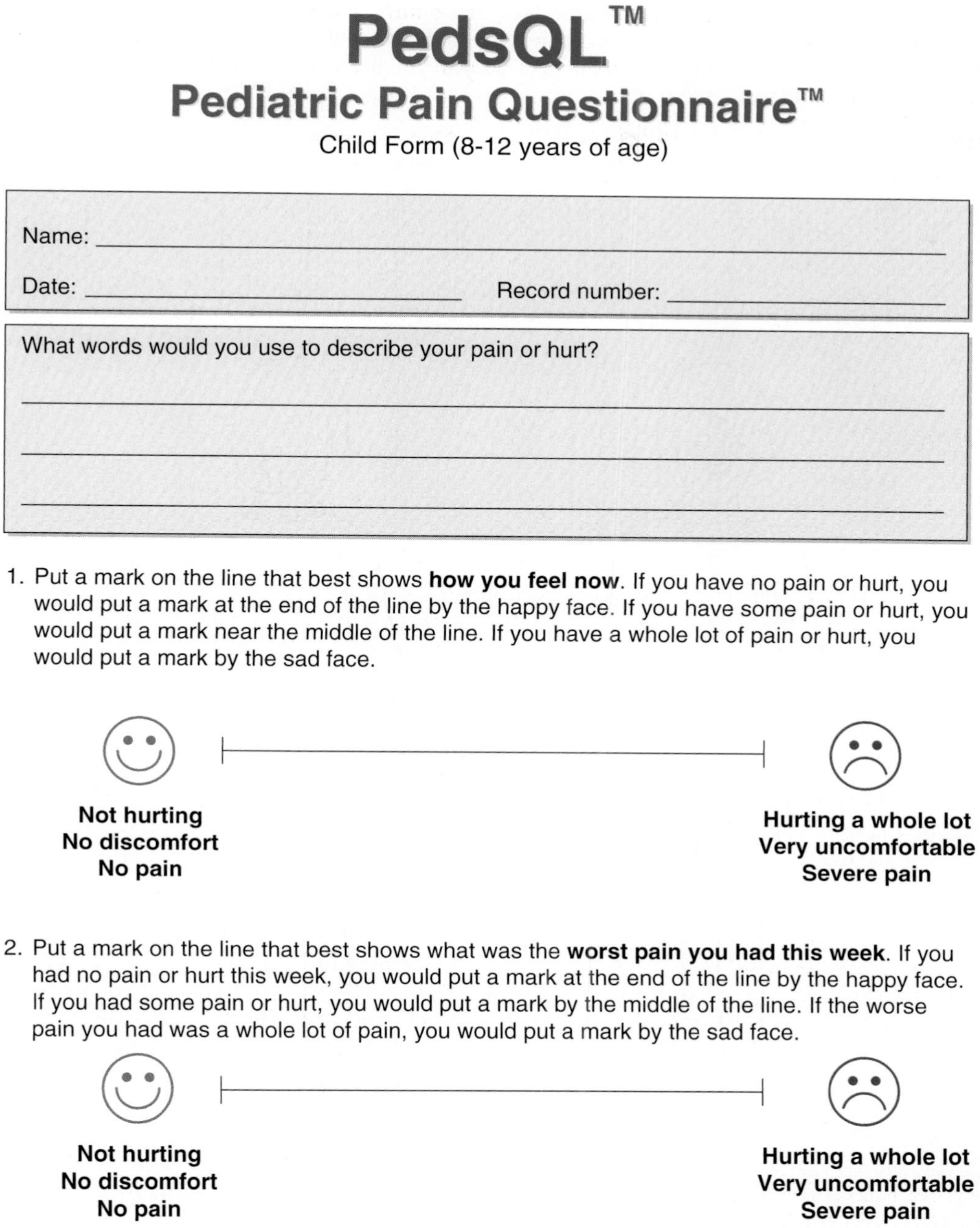

PedsQL™
Pediatric Pain Questionnaire™
Child Form (8-12 years of age)

Name: _____

Date: _____   Record number: _____

What words would you use to describe your pain or hurt?

_____

_____

_____

1. Put a mark on the line that best shows **how you feel now**. If you have no pain or hurt, you would put a mark at the end of the line by the happy face. If you have some pain or hurt, you would put a mark near the middle of the line. If you have a whole lot of pain or hurt, you would put a mark by the sad face.

Not hurting
No discomfort
No pain

Hurting a whole lot
Very uncomfortable
Severe pain

2. Put a mark on the line that best shows what was the **worst pain you had this week**. If you had no pain or hurt this week, you would put a mark at the end of the line by the happy face. If you had some pain or hurt, you would put a mark by the middle of the line. If the worse pain you had was a whole lot of pain, you would put a mark by the sad face.

Not hurting
No discomfort
No pain

Hurting a whole lot
Very uncomfortable
Severe pain

FIGURE 11–2 Pediatric Pain Questionnaire VAS (Adapted from Varni JW, Thompson KL, Hanson V: The Varni/Thompson Pediatric Pain Questionnaire. I. Chronic musculoskeletal pain in juvenile rheumatoid arthritis, *Pain* 28:27-38, 1987.)

descriptive categories of pain intensity ("none, mild, moderate, severe"). Patients are given a standard set of eight colors. From these they select colors to match pain intensities (coloring the four boxes with selected colors) and they apply these colors to the appropriate place on the body outline with the color intensity match (Fig. 11–3). Children younger than 7 years will usually need to be read instructions for completing the PPQ.[52] The PPQ VAS is useful in documenting the intensity of pain, and the body outline allows patients to localize their pain, as well as rate its intensity.

Investigators should consider using electronic pain measures (such as e-diaries), rather than pencil and paper ones, because electronic measures have been validated with patients with arthritis, they are feasible, and they result in fewer errors and omissions compared with paper ones.[9,50,53]

Observational measures of pain behaviors need to be further developed for children with arthritis, particularly those children who are preverbal or have limited verbal capacity.[54] Jaworski and colleagues have developed an observational measure for patients with JRA.[55] This measure contains six pain behaviors (guarding, bracing, active rubbing, rigidity, single flexing, and multiple flexing) that are coded by observers viewing a videotape of a 10-minute session during which children perform a

Pick the colors that mean **No hurt, A little hurt, More hurt,** and **A lot of hurt** to you and color in the boxes. Now, using these colors, color in the body to show how you feel. Where you have no hurt, use the **No hurt** color to color in your body. If you have hurt or pain, use the color that tells how much hurt you have.

No pain No hurt	Mild pain A little hurt	Moderate pain More hurt	Severe pain A lot of hurt

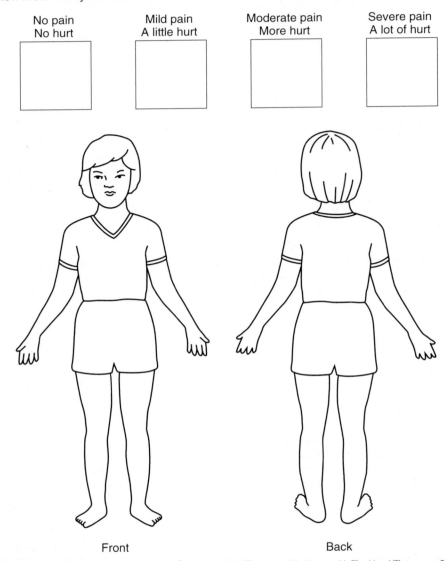

Front   Back

FIGURE 11–3   Pediatric Pain Questionnaire Body Outline (Adapted from Varni JW, Thompson KL, Hanson V: The Varni/Thompson Pediatric Pain Questionnaire. I. Chronic musculoskeletal pain in juvenile rheumatoid arthritis, *Pain* 28:27-38, 1987.)

series of maneuvers including sitting, walking, standing, and reclining in a standardized sequence. This measure has been found to be reliable and valid, but it requires fairly extensive training of observers and has been used in only one study thus far.[52] Observational measures can supplement self-report measures and document functional limitations.

REFERENCES

1. R.A. Gragg, M.A. Rapoff, M.B. Danovsky, et al., Assessing chronic musculoskeletal pain associated with rheumatic disease: further validation of the Pediatric Pain Questionnaire, J. Pediatr. Psychol. 21 (1996) 237–250.
2. K.J. Hagglund, L.M. Schopp, K.R. Alberts, et al., Predicting pain among children with juvenile rheumatoid arthritis, Arthritis Care Res. 8 (1995) 36–42.
3. K.L. Thompson, J.W. Varni, V. Hanson, Comprehensive assessment of pain in juvenile rheumatoid arthritis: an empirical model, J. Pediatr. Psychol. 12 (1987) 241–255.
4. J.W. Varni, M.A. Rapoff, S.A. Waldron, et al., Chronic pain and emotional distress in children and adolescents, J. Dev. Behav. Pediatr. 17 (1996) 154–161.
5. C.K. Ross, J.V. Lavigne, J.R. Hayford, et al., Validity of reported pain as a measure of clinical state in juvenile rheumatoid arthritis, Ann. Rheum. Dis. 48 (1989) 817–819.
6. L.E. Schanberg, J.C. Lefebvre, F.J. Keefe, et al., Pain coping and the pain experience in children with juvenile chronic arthritis, Pain 73 (1997) 181–189.
7. B. Benestad, O. Vinje, M.B. Veierød, et al., Quantitative and qualitative assessments of pain in children with juvenile chronic arthritis based on the Norwegian version of the Pediatric Pain Questionnaire, Scand. J. Rheumatol. 25 (1996) 293–299.
8. L.E. Schanberg, K.K. Anthony, K.M. Gil, et al., Daily pain and symptoms in children with polyarticular arthritis, Arthritis Rheum. 48 (2003) 1390–1397.

9. J.N. Stinson, B.J. Stevens, B.M. Feldman, et al., Construct validity of a multidimensional electronic pain diary for adolescents with arthritis, Pain 136 (2008) 281–292.

10. D.J. Lovell, G.W. Walco, Pain associated with juvenile rheumatoid arthritis, Pediatr. Clin. North Am. 36 (1989) 1015–1027.

11. L.S. Peterson, T. Mason, A.M. Nelson, et al., Psychosocial outcomes and health status of adults who have had juvenile rheumatoid arthritis, Arthritis Rheum. 40 (1997) 2235–2240.

12. International Association for the Study of Pain, Pain terms: a list with definitions and notes on usage: recommended by the IASP subcommittee on taxonomy, Pain 6 (1979) 249–252.

13. R. Melzack, P.D. Wall, Pain and mechanisms: a new theory, Science 150 (1965) 971–979.

14. R.J. Gatchel, Y.B. Peng, M.L. Peters, et al., Psychol. Bull. 133 (2007) 581–624.

15. M.A. Rapoff, C.B. Lindsley, The pain puzzle: a visual and conceptual metaphor for understanding and treating pain in pediatric rheumatic disease, J. Rheumatol. 58 (suppl.) (2000) 29–33.

16. A. Randich, Neural substrates of pain and analgesia, Arthritis Care Res. 6 (1993) 171–177.

17. McGrath PA: Pain in children: nature, assessment and treatment, Guilford, New York, 1990.

18. H.G. Schaible, B.D. Grubb, Afferent and spinal mechanisms of joint pain, Pain 55 (1993) 5–54.

19. H.G. Schaible, R.F. Schmidt, Effects of an experimental arthritis on the sensory properties of fine articular afferent units, J. Neurophysiol. 54 (1985) 1109–1122.

20. D.T. Felson, The sources of pain in knee osteoarthritis, Curr. Opin. Rheum. 17 (2005) 624–629.

21. R.A. Meyer, J.N. Campbell, S.N. Raja, Peripheral neural mechanisms of nociception, in: P.D. Wall, R. Melzack (Eds.), Textbook of pain, third ed., Churchill Livingstone, Edinburgh, 1994.

22. J. Levine, Y. Taiwo, Inflammatory pain, in: P.D. Wall, R. Melzack (Eds.), Textbook of pain, third ed., Churchill Livingstone, Edinburgh, 1994.

23. J.A. Hogeweg, A.C.J. Huygen, C. De Jong-De Vos Van Steenwijk, et al., The pain threshold in juvenile chronic arthritis, Br. J. Rheumatol. 34 (1995) 61–67.

24. J.A. Hogeweg, W. Kuis, R.A.B. Oostendorp, et al., General and segmental reduced pain thresholds in juvenile chronic arthritis, Pain 62 (1995) 11–17.

25. M. Thastum, R. Zachariae, M. Schøler, et al., Cold pressor pain: comparing responses of juvenile arthritis patients and their parents, Scand. J. Rheumatol. 26 (1997) 272–279.

26. W. Kuis, C.J. Heijnen, J.A. Hogeweg, et al., How painful is juvenile chronic arthritis? Arch. Dis. Child 77 (1997) 451–453.

27. T.J. Coderre, J. Katz, Peripheral and central hyperexcitability: differential signs and symptoms in persistent pain, Behav. Brain Sci. 20 (1997) 404–419.

28. S.M. Banks, R.D. Kerns, Explaining high rates of depression in chronic pain: a diathesis-stress framework, Psychol. Bull. 119 (1996) 95–110.

29. J.W. Burns, P.J. Quartana, S. Bruehl, Anger inhibition and pain: conceptualizations, evidence, and new directions, J. Behav. Med. 31 (2008) 259–279.

30. L.C. Campbell, D.J. Clauw, F.J. Keefe, Persistent pain and depression: a biopsychosocial perspective, Biol. Psychiatry 54 (2003) 399–409.

31. C.R. Chapman, The psychophysiology of pain, in: J.D. Loser (Ed.), Bonica's management of pain, third ed., Lippincott, Williams, & Wilkins, Philadelphia, 2001.

32. A.L. Hoff, T.M. Palermo, M. Schluchter, et al., Longitudinal relationships of depressive symptoms to pain intensity and functional disability among children with disease-related pain, J. Pediatr. Psychol. 31 (2006) 1046–1056.

33. J.W. Varni, M.A. Rapoff, S.A. Waldron, et al., Effects of perceived stress on pediatric chronic pain, J. Behav. Med. 19 (1996) 515–528.

34. L.E. Schanberg, M.J. Sandstrom, K. Starr, et al., The relationship of daily mood and stressful events to symptoms in juvenile rheumatic disease, Arthritis Care Res. 13 (2000) 33–41.

35. A. Gamsa, Is emotional disturbance a precipitator or a consequence of chronic pain? Pain 42 (1990) 183–195.

36. M.A. Rosenkranz, Substance P at the nexus of mind and body in chronic inflammation and affective disorders, Psychol. Bull. 133 (2007) 1007–1037.

37. F.J. Keefe, M.E. Rumble, C.D. Scipio, et al., Psychological aspects of persistent pain: current state of the science, J. Pain 5 (2004) 195–211.

38. M.J.L. Sullivan, S.R. Bishop, J. Pivik, The Pain Catastrophizing Scale: development and validation, Psychol. Assess. 7 (1995) 524–532.

39. M. Thastum, R. Zachariae, M. Schøler, et al., A Danish adaptation of the Pain Coping Questionnaire for children: preliminary data concerning reliability and validity, Acta. Paediatrica. 88 (1998) 132–138.

40. M. Thastum, T. Herlin, R. Zachariae, Relationship of pain-coping strategies and pain-specific beliefs to pain experience in children with juvenile idiopathic arthritis, Arthritis Care Res. 53 (2005) 178–184.

41. G.J. Reid, C.A. Gilbert, P.J. McGrath, The Pain Coping Questionnaire: preliminary validation, Pain 76 (1998) 83–96.

42. J.W. Varni, S.A. Waldron, R.A. Gragg, Development of the Waldron/Varni Pediatric Pain Coping Inventory, Pain 67 (1996) 141–150.

43. L.M. Dahlquist, M.S. Nagel, Chronic and recurrent pain, in: M.C. Roberts, R.G. Steele (Eds.), Handbook of pediatric psychology, fourth ed., Guilford Press, New York, 2009, 153–170.

44. M.A. Rapoff, Adherence to pediatric medical regimens, second ed., Springer, New York, 2010.

45. C. Eccleston, S. Morley, A. Williams, et al., Systematic review of randomized controlled trials of psychological therapy for chronic pain in children and adolescents, with a sub-set meta-analysis of pain relief, Pain 99 (2002) 157–165.

46. E.W. Holden, M.M. Deichmann, J.D. Levy, Empirically supported treatments in pediatric psychology: recurrent pediatric headache, J. Pediatr. Psychol. 24 (1999) 91–109.

47. D.M. Janicke, J.W. Finney, Empirically supported treatments in pediatric psychology: recurrent abdominal pain, J. Pediatr. Psychol. 24 (1999) 115–127.

48. J.V. Lavigne, C.K. Ross, S.L. Berry, et al., Evaluation of a psychological treatment package for treating pain in juvenile rheumatoid arthritis, Arthritis Care Res. 5 (1992) 101–110.

49. G.A. Walco, J.W. Varni, N.T. Ilowite, Cognitive behavioral pain management in children with juvenile rheumatoid arthritis, Pediatrics 89 (1992) 1075–1079.

50. J.N. Stinson, G.C. Petroz, G. Tait, et al., e-Ouch: Usability testing of an electronic chronic pain diary for adolescents with arthritis, Clin. J. Pain 22 (2006) 295–305.

51. J.W. Varni, K.L. Thompson, V. Hanson, The Varni/Thompson Pediatric Pain Questionnaire. I. Chronic musculoskeletal pain in juvenile rheumatoid arthritis, Pain 28 (1987) 27–38.

52. M.A. Rapoff, Pediatric measures of pain: the Pain Behavior Observation Method, Pain Coping Questionnaire (PCQ), and Pediatric Pain Questionnaire (PPQ), Arthritis Care Res. 49 (2003) S90–S95.

53. T.M. Palermo, D. Valenzuela, P.P. Stork, A randomized trial of electronic versus paper pain diaries in children: impact on compliance, accuracy, and acceptability, Pain 107 (2004) 213–219.

54. C.L. von Baeyer, L.J. Spagrud, Systematic review of observational (behavioral) measures of pain for children and adolescents aged 3 to 18 years, Pain 127 (2007) 140–150.

55. T.M. Jaworski, L.A. Bradley, L.W. Heck, et al., Development of an observation method for assessing pain behaviors in children with juvenile rheumatoid arthritis, Arthritis Rheum. 38 (1995) 1142–1151.

Chapter 12

OCCUPATIONAL AND PHYSICAL THERAPY FOR CHILDHOOD RHEUMATIC DISEASES

Gay Kuchta and Iris Davidson

Because of the chronic and multisystem nature of rheumatic diseases in childhood, optimal care requires early and ongoing intervention by an interdisciplinary team of health professionals, including occupational and physical therapists.[1-5] As the medical management of rheumatic diseases has evolved, the spectrum of problems dealt with by therapists has changed dramatically. The earlier concentration on management of major joint contractures, muscle weakness, or mobility challenges has been augmented by increased attention to function in all spheres: physical, emotional, social, and educational. Furthermore, the scope of the diagnostic challenges presented to the therapist now includes the entire range of childhood rheumatic diseases.

Insofar as is possible, therapy is based on evidence. Very often the limited information from studies in childhood rheumatic diseases must be supplemented by information in adult populations with similar diseases and by personal experience.[6] The management team members must work closely with each other and with the child and family in a way that recognizes cultural norms and developmental stages.

INDICATIONS FOR REFERRAL TO A THERAPIST

Ideally, the therapist's initial assessment and management of the patient should take place at the time of diagnosis. Periodic re-evaluations occur throughout the disease course as indicated and should continue even during disease remission, since restrictions of function often persist beyond the stage of active disease.

Specific indications prompting referral to a therapist include symptoms of active disease such as pain, stiffness, and fatigue, as well as changes in function or participation in social or school activities (Table 12-1). Information that will maximize the effectiveness of a referral to physiotherapy or occupational therapy includes the child's diagnosis, the extent of systemic involvement, comorbidities, medications, and planned medical interventions, as outlined in Table 12-2.

SYMPTOM ASSESSMENT AND MANAGEMENT

Many symptoms that impact on the child's function are common to all rheumatic diseases. The timing of symptom management is determined by (Table 12-3) disease, its stage, and the degree to which it is controlled. As outlined in Table 12-4, the intervention goals in early disease are to minimize symptoms; as the disease is controlled, the goals and interventions change to maximize and normalize function.

Pain

Pain is the primary issue leading children and their families to seek medical attention.[7,8] Unresolved pain is the reason the great majority of patients seek complementary and alternative medicines.[9] Although very young children with oligoarthritis frequently do not report pain, children with polyarticular juvenile idiopathic arthritis (JIA) recorded pain on 70% of days, and 50% of those with connective tissue diseases noted the presence of pain within the week prior to questioning.[10] Pain impacts on the quality of life in any disease and even a small decrease (1 cm) in the visual analogue pain scale is correlated with a significant improvement in quality of life.[11] The impact of chronic pain is illustrated in Figure 12–1 and ranges from sleep disturbance to joint contractures and psychosocial-educational disturbances.

In the assessment of pain, it is important to determine and record the parameters of the child's pain (i.e., location, duration, intensity, frequency, quality, history and functional impact on self-care, play, school and psychosocial development). Developmentally appropriate outcome measures[12-16] are used as required. Recognition of pain behaviors is important, especially in those children who report no pain verbally. Social aggression, withdrawal from usual social or physical activities, irritability, or abnormal movement patterns can all indicate the presence of pain. The impact of pain on movement, posture, and development of gross and fine motor milestones should also be noted.

Table 12-1

Reasons to refer to occupational and physical therapy

Physician Triggers for Referral	OT/PT Response to Referral Will Include
Active disease Morning stiffness Avoidance of activity because of pain or weakness Overwhelming fatigue Restrictions or asymmetric movement of any musculoskeletal area Marked mood or behavior change, especially isolation from peers Regression of age-appropriate developmental behaviors Growth abnormalities Reduced school attendance or output (>10 days absence in the past 4 months including medical appointments) Change in quality of sleep Inability to do normal activities in a timely manner	• Assess and manage pain • Assess and manage impairments • Assess and manage functional restrictions • Develop consistent, reliable measures of change in range, muscle strength, and function over time • Evaluate and teach coping skills • Reinforce education of disease process and management • Education on the need and safety of physical activity • Teach ergonomics • Provide vocational counseling • Provide ongoing patient/family support • Facilitate integration into school/community • Advocate for the child with the family and community

Table 12-2

Baseline Information for the Therapists

Information	Reason

The Diagnosis	• To integrate pathophysiology of the condition, the long-term outcome, pattern of disease, and progression
	• To plan realistic assessment/treatment in both disciplines
	  • safe exercise techniques
	  • functional implications inherent in diagnosis
	• To educate the child and family appropriately
	• To report back to the physician on disease flares or emerging new symptoms

Systemic involvement • skin • musculoskeletal • cardiovascular • central nervous system • eyes	• When multiple disciplines are involved, integrate therapy times with necessary appointments • Watch for inconsistent disease progression • Consider safety in progression of therapy • Integrate the impact into the functional assessment and treatment planning
Planned medical interventions • medication changes • aspirate and inject joint • imaging • referrals to other disciplines	• Educate the family and provide resources • Identify phobias and communicate to team members • Facilitate planning around interventions and school attendance • Optimize timing of OT/PT interventions
Comorbidities • physical • psychiatric • developmental	• Learn of and communicate with other teams, caregivers, or school personnel • Reduce duplication of services
Current medications	• Assess compliance and educate on role of medications in long-term outcome • Look for possible side effects and report to physician or nurse • Know when to expect a therapeutic response
Red flags for therapy interventions • multiple system involvement • social history • implications of recent imaging or lab test results	• Activity restrictions imposed by other subspecialists (e.g., cardiologist) • Impaired vision • Psychiatric conditions • Guardianship issues with restricted access • Extended family rheumatology issues • Bony changes that would impact on therapy • Severe anemia that impacts on function and exercise

Adapted from Kuchta G, Davidson I, editors: Occupational and Physical therapy for children with rheumatic diseases, Oxford, 2008, Radcliffe.

Teaching children age-appropriate nonpharmacological pain-modifying techniques increases their sense of control over their pain and decreases the overall pain experience.[8] Techniques that the child and family can utilize at home are the most useful. These techniques treat pain through peripheral, spinal segmental, supraspinal, and cortical pathways. General techniques such as use of thermal modalities, splinting, pacing activities, and joint protection are particularly suited for home. Heat and cold both reduce pain temporarily. For hot, swollen joints, application of ice over the affected joint until it is erythematous and numb is the usual recommendation. Gentle heat is more effective in reducing muscle spasm and morning stiffness. Superficial joints in the hands and feet respond better to contrast baths, in which the painful part is alternately submerged in hot and cold

Table 12–3

Functional implications of physical findings (upper extremity)

Joint	Physical findings	Functional implications
TMJ	• Unilateral or bilateral TMJ crepitus or pain, resulting in diminished or asymmetric mouth opening and dental malocclusion (open anterior overbite in bilateral disease • Asymmetric mandibular growth or bilateral undergrowth	• Pain and difficulty biting or chewing • Poor dental hygiene • Sleep disturbance due to pain • Difficulty in intubation for anesthetics • Compromised nutrition • Altered body image with social implications
C Spine	• Range of motion (ROM) decreased in extension (ext) >side flexion (SF)> rotation (rot)> flexion (flex) • Loss of kyphosis and increased lordosis on attempted upward gaze • Atlantoaxial subluxation (rarely symptomatic)	• Impacts on dressing, sleep, school activities (writing, keyboarding, reading, floor sitting, sports, driving, recreation) • No contact sports permitted when C1 and C2 subluxation present • Intubation can be difficult
T Spine and L Spine	• Poor posture • Limited motion • Marked increase or decrease in thoracic kyphosis +/- scoliosis • Limited thoracic and lumber flexion	• Pain secondary to poor body positioning and mechanics • Abnormal gait • Limited sitting and standing tolerance impact school and leisure activities • Poor sleep
Shoulder Excessive scapular rotation	• Restricted range leading to adaptive posture or movement patterns secondary to involvement in either glenohumeral, acromioclavicular or sternoclavicular joints • Weakness/atrophy of rotator cuff muscles and scapular stabilizers	• Donning clothes over head, jackets, bra closures, back packs restricted. • Washing/ arranging hair difficult • Sleep disturbance due to increased pain in side lying • Any activities which transmit body weight through the joint e.g. climbing frames, crawling, gymnastics, being lifted up by the arms will be impacted • Physical education (PE)/ sports which require upper extremity (UE) use will be compromised

water. Thermal modalities need to be used with caution and the body's response carefully monitored. Compromised circulation or sensation may contraindicate their use. With rheumatic disease–related Raynaud phenomenon, inappropriate use of thermal modalities can result in tissue damage. Detailed information on the therapeutic intervention and safety issues can be found in the references.[17-19] Massage by a parent or caregiver reduces muscle tension, which can contribute to pain. Massage is particularly useful to desensitize the affected area in children who have both inflammatory disease and a chronic regional pain syndrome. Neural stretches may also be used at home to reduce pain but have not been studied in children with rheumatic diseases.

Table 12-3—cont'd

Functional implications of physical findings (upper extremity)

Joint	Physical findings	Functional implications
Elbow	• Flexion deformity (FD) reduces functional length of the arm • Loss of ext. and supination most common • Reduced flexion range has the most impact on function • Substitutions by surrounding joints compensate for reduced ROM	• All hand to face activities can be affected (e.g. eating, dental hygiene) • Writing endurance commonly reduced • Carrying even light weights increases pain • Opening doors esp. heavy fire or washroom doors is difficult • Perineal care may be impacted; rarely discussed
Wrists	• Note direction of deviation (ulnar or radial are possible) • Compensatory deviations at the metacarpal phalangeal (MCP) joints • Hypo- or hypermobility in either row of carpal bones • Restricted range • Pain at the end of range • Note abnormal movement patterns	• Most common source of UE disability • Major cause of school issues at all grade levels • Gross and fine motor milestone delay in young children • All sustained UE activities can be affected especially when the dominant side is involved. • Grip strength is usually reduced due to wrist posture and pain issues
Hands	• Reduced web space (carpo-metacarpal CMC joint of the thumb restricted) • Thumb interphalangeal joint (IP) hypermobility • Reduced tuck and fist positions • MCP flexion loss is common • Proximal interphalangeal joint (PIP) and Distal IP extension loss is common • Boutonnière deformity can occur early • Flexor tendon nodules /trigger finger • Tenodesis	• Thumb instability impacts on prehension in tripod pinch (eg buttons, pen or scissors) • Grasp of large object compromised by CMC restrictions • Trigger finger pain leads to avoidance and UE faulty movement patterns • Delayed developmental milestones if child is unable to explore environment • Reduced dexterity and power impacts activities of daily living and self care • Hand function restrictions have a great impact on school • Hand pain and joint gelling are common causes of sleep disturbance • Perineal care is often impacted (seldom reported) • Intimacy can be impacted for teens

Continued

Specific techniques such as cognitive-behavioral, biofeedback, and electrical modalities can be used on an individual basis as needed. They are only appropriate in older or cognitively competent children who can report responses reliably. Transcutaneous electrical nerve stimulation (TENS) used several times a week, or even daily, is useful in treating children with complex regional pain syndromes or localized inflammatory pain. Units can be purchased or rented and parents can be taught to use this technique safely at home. Benefit is established within two treatments, and response becomes increasingly prolonged in those children in whom it is effective. Therapist-applied interferential stimulation is effective in treating pain as well. Because both interferential therapy and TENS stimulate the same neural pathways, their use is determined by availability and therapist choice. There is mounting evidence[20] for the use of low-level lasers for the reduction of pain and morning stiffness in adults with inflammatory disease but none in children. Cognitive-behavioral techniques such as breathing, progressive relaxation,

Table 12–3—cont'd

Functional implications of physical findings (lower extremity)

Joint	Physical findings	Functional implications
Hip	• Loss of extension and internal rotation are most common • Positive Trendelenburg or gluteus medius limp secondary to muscle weakness • Pain on weight bearing • Gait abnormalities	• Compensatory lumbar lordosis with pain • Short stride length, • Reduced sitting and walking tolerance • Difficulty climbing stairs • Lower extremity (LE) dressing difficulties • Getting on and off the toilet increases pain • Sitting cross legged for story time or assembly is difficult • Restricted sexual activity for teens • Impact on ability to continue, sports, dance, recreational activities • Increased fatigue
Knee Leg length changes	• Loss of hyperextension • Loss of full flexion • Muscle weakness and wasting • Patellar malalignment • Abnormal gait • Enthesitis • Long bone over-growth common in JIA • Undergrowth common in linear scleroderma • Scoliosis due to asymmetry of lower extremity (LE) • Changes in posture	• Altered range in adjacent joints • Inability to squat or sit on heels, kneel at school or places of worship • Floor sitting, stairs, rising from ground all difficult • Prolonged sitting in class, movies, airplanes or car is painful. • Difficulty rising due to joint gelling • Self care related to toileting and showering can be unsafe • Leg length discrepancy > $\frac{1}{8}$" is significant requiring a shoe raise • Increased energy expenditure
Ankle	• Reduced dorsiflexion > plantar flexion • Tight Achilles tendon • Enthesitis • Tendon sheath inflammation • Muscle wasting • Abnormal gait	• Changes in foot progression angle (in-toe or out-toe) • Shortened stride length • Decreased power for activities such as hopping, jumping and running • Descending stairs difficult, abnormal patterns common • Early heel rise or no heel strike

visualization, and thought stopping can be used anywhere by the child to gain control over pain. Studies have shown these techniques to be very effective for children with JIA,[21,22] but the authors have found it useful for children with connective tissue diseases (CTD) and chronic pain syndromes as well.

Education regarding the child's pain and guidelines on how to respond need to be disseminated beyond the family to the school-based team and sport/leisure activity coaches. Children are encouraged to continue to participate to the best of their ability and to use changes in their pain levels to indicate when they should temporarily withdraw. Most children are the best judges of their physical limitations, and their decisions should be respected, with

few exceptions. Activity restrictions imposed because of co-morbidities must be adhered to. In the child with JIA, radiographic evidence of cervical instability precludes participation in contact sports.

Even after disease control is achieved and pain is no longer a problem, abnormal movement patterns and postures that developed secondary to pain often persist and require a formal retraining program. Often patients' confidence in their body's ability to respond to physical demands may be compromised. The young child may need encouragement to engage in normal behaviors such as jumping and climbing. Persistent pain that inhibits function requires reconsideration of the etiology and therapeutic approach.

Table 12-3—cont'd

Functional implications of physical findings (lower extremity)

Joint	Physical findings	Functional implications
Subtalar	• Decreased inversion or eversion • Spontaneous fusion	• Ambulation difficulties on uneven ground (snow, mud or grass) • Reflex righting mechanism painful and difficult (child falls easily, teens feel vulnerable in crowds) • Inefficient gait patterns increase energy expenditure
Foot and toes	• Decreased pronation/supination (in conjunction with subtalar motion restriction) • Enthesitis • Decreased extension of MTP1 • Toe deformities (hammer, cock up) • Dactylitis • Tarsitis	• Ambulation difficulties on uneven ground due to mid foot restriction and pain • Restricted toe off causes decreased stride length on opposite side • Reduces standing tolerance • Avoidance of hopping and running • Antalgic gait • Unable to squat on extended toes
General growth retardation in boy age 12	• Multiple joint restrictions • Pain limiting motion • Reduced energy for sustained activity • Delayed puberty	• Many difficulties with independence in self care, work or leisure • Restricted mobility • Problems with peer pressure, teasing and social isolation • Limited vocational choices • Interventions in problem solving and coping are required

Fatigue

All rheumatic diseases of childhood are associated with fatigue.[23,24] Some of the common causes are uncontrolled disease resulting in anemia, pain, nonrestorative sleep,[25,26] antalgic movement patterns requiring increased energy expenditure,[27] depression, and marked weight gain secondary to corticosteroids. Fatigue is often a silent problem that is poorly recognized but has a major impact on quality of life. The relationship between fatigue, fitness levels, and endurance in rheumatic diseases is not clear.[23] Fatigue issues need to be dealt with early in those children with a diagnosis of systemic lupus erythematosus (SLE), mixed connective tissue disease, juvenile dermatomyositis (JDM), or vasculitis because it is often a presenting complaint.

Fatigue can be assessed in a number of ways. Older children can score their fatigue on a verbal or visual analogue scale or compare their own energy level to that of their peers or to their pre-illness level. The Kids Fatigue Scale[23,28] is an adapted measurement tool used with children aged 6 to 16. Causes of fatigue can be determined by assessing sleep patterns, looking for abnormal movement patterns or postures, determining endurance for specific activities, and measuring muscle strength. An ergonomic assessment of the home and classroom may indicate environmental contributors to fatigue.

Management of fatigue requires discussion with the child, family, and, when appropriate, the school. An understanding of the impact of fatigue on the child's ability to cope with educational demands will aid the school in adapting demands for academic and athletic participation. Ergonomic issues such as the weight of books carried in a backpack, inappropriate seating, multiple flights of stairs, and long distances required to move from class to class all contribute to fatigue. This in turn has a negative impact on the child's mood and ability to concentrate. Other issues such as the amount of repetition included in homework assignments and concurrent deadlines also need discussion. The basic concepts of time management and pacing high- and low-energy activities are introduced to help the child achieve functional goals.

Table 12–4

Rheumatic disease intervention

Uncontrolled Disease Goal: Minimize Symptoms	Controlled Disease Goal: Maximize Function	Clinical Remission Goal: Normal Function	Ongoing Chronic Disease Goal: Optimize Function Within Limitations

• Direct assessment to patient's stated problems
• Provide frequent reassessment to monitor changes
• Teach pain management and coping skills (esp. with JIA)
• Teach fatigue management (esp. with CTD)
• Maintain range, strength, and muscle length using exercises, splinting, and positioning
• Reinforce education on disease management
• Intervene at school with all diagnoses
• Provide adaptive devices as indicated
• Teach sleep hygiene
• OT/PT interventions minimal until disease under some control
	• Full assessment to identify and monitor persisting deficits and their impact on the body mechanics
	• Modify pain and fatigue management techniques
	• Improve function
	• Increase range, muscle strength and length
	• Increase participation in family, school, and leisure activities
	• Improve exercise tolerance and balance
	• Introduce the concepts of self-image and self-efficacy to child and family
	• Review and monitor necessary school interventions
	• Teach coping skills such as time management and pacing activities
	• Review understanding of disease management as child matures
	• Interventions reviewed every 4-12 weeks
	• Focus for majority is a home program
	• "Hands on" interventions (i.e., serial casting) may require 3 appointments/wk
	• Occasionally intensive inpatient rehabilitation needed
		• Semiannual to annual full assessment to determine persistent physical and psychosocial sequelae of previous issues.
		• Focus on:
		  • Abnormal movement patterns
		  • Mechanical malalignments
		  • Risk-taking behaviors
		  • Physical and psychological developmental milestones
		• Promote physical and emotional independence
		• Work on fine motor control, balance, endurance, power
		• Integration /participation in activities and community
		• Coping strategies for Raynaud phenomenon taught
		• Reinforce self-image as healthy individual
		• Encourage healthy life choices
			• Full assessments with disease flares
			• Annual assessment to monitor deficits
			• Assess and plan for preoperative and post operative interventions
			• Address changing pain patterns
			• Adaptations to the environment at home and school
			• Effective adaptive movement patterns
			• Teach use of mobility aids
			• Problem-solving to maintain independence and participation in self-care, leisure, and work
			• Teach coping skills such as CBT
			• Vocational assessment
			• Provide documentation for financial support

CBT, cognitive-behavioral therapy; *CTD*, connective tissue diseases; *JIA*, juvenile idiopathic arthritis.

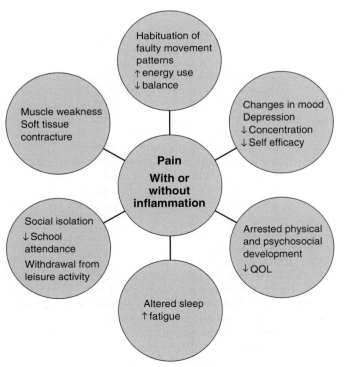

FIGURE 12–1 Impact of pain.

Underlying issues that contribute to fatigue such as pain, poor aerobic fitness, abnormal body mechanics, and poor sleep hygiene must be addressed together with healthy lifestyle coaching.

Nonrestorative Sleep

Sleep disturbances are common in all rheumatic diseases, at every age and during all disease phases.[29]

In the assessment of sleep[17] it is important to know the family norms around sleep times and sleeping arrangements. In the older child and adolescent, inappropriate bed times and arising times are common, particularly in the child with a pain amplification syndrome. Age-appropriate bedtimes should be encouraged. The interval between bedtime and onset of sleep and the reasons for delay in sleep onset should be determined. The frequency of sleep disruption and the child's subjective evaluation of the quality of sleep should be recorded. Daytime sleepiness and frequency and duration of naps should be monitored and can indicate a high fatigue level or poor quality sleep at night. The child's sleeping environment and prebedtime activities may contribute to sleep disruptions. Corticosteroids, particularly when given at suppertime or later, frequently interfere with sound sleep. Depth of sleep can be negatively impacted by the use of night-time splints.

Activities in the bedroom should be limited to those conducive to initiation of sleep. Bedroom activities that promote restlessness or anxiety (such as doing homework, playing on the computer, or watching television) should be discouraged. Avoidance of foods containing high levels of sugar or caffeine and limitation of exercise close to bedtime may aid initiation of sleep. In general, vigorous aerobic exercise should be avoided within 2 hours of bedtime. Alterations in the physical environment, such as maintaining a comfortable room temperature and exploring variations in type and weight of bedcovers and types and styles of pillows, may make it easier for the child to fall asleep. Judicious use of pillows to decrease weight bearing through painful joints can decrease pain and improve quality of sleep. If the child shares the bedroom with others, noise issues and bedtime rituals need to be examined. Cognitive-behavioral techniques similar to those used for pain may be required to reduce anxiety and stress, which can make sleep initiation difficult. Improving sleep patterns is a gradual and prolonged process, often requiring at least a month.[30,31]

Decreased Range of Motion

Restrictions in joint range of motion may reflect intrinsic joint inflammation (increased intraarticular fluid, synovial hypertrophy, pain) or tendon or muscle shortening.[32] In children with severe, longstanding JIA, joints may become subluxed or ankylosed, resulting in limitation or absence of joint motion. In disorders such as scleroderma, tightening of the periarticular soft tissues leads to joint range restriction. In juvenile dermatomyositis, muscle atrophy and disuse may limit functional range of motion.

Passive range of motion of all affected joints should be assessed using a goniometer in order to obtain consistent, precise, and reproducible measurements.[33] Active range should also be recorded when it differs significantly from passive range—for example, when a quadriceps lag exists. Particular attention should be paid to the tenodesis effect of muscles that cross two joints, such as the gastrocnemius. If the muscle is on stretch when joint range is measured, a false "joint restriction" may be recorded. During function, a joint may be used within a restricted range due to limitations imposed on it by the overlying short muscles. Normal range of motion varies considerably with age and with each individual, and without knowledge of the normal ranges in each child, the development of minor restrictions can easily be overlooked. Up to 34% of the pediatric population is hypermobile,[34,35] and a decrease in hypermobility may be an important indicator of joint restriction. Functional range requirements are related to age. Attention to the quality of movement and the use of compensatory movement patterns is integral to a range assessment. Abnormal motions such as wrist or knee deviation should also be documented.

A full assessment should be done initially and then at intervals determined by the rate of evolution of the disease and the child's response to therapy. The initial assessment not only defines the extent of the restriction but establishes a baseline for purposes of comparison.

Techniques to improve joint range include active and passive stretching, mobilization, serial casting, and splinting. Most range deficits can be resolved with a specific, active home exercise program. To maximize adherence, this should not exceed 10 minutes per day. Improvements are evident in 4 to 8 weeks. Muscle strength in the newly acquired range must be improved to maintain gains. In mildly active or inactive joints, passive stretching at end range and mobilizations are effective. In children with joint restrictions that persist in spite of adequate active exercise and passive stretching, intraarticular corticosteroid injection followed immediately by serial casting in a position of maximal extension should be considered. This technique is most effective for contractures at the knees, wrists, elbows, fingers, and ankles. Casts are generally changed every 48 hours until a functional range is achieved. (i.e., 0° knee extension, 60° wrist extension, 10° ankle dorsiflexion). A bivalved cylindrical cast is worn as a night splint until passive and active ranges are equal. This goal can be obtained in as little as 48 hours or may take as long as 6 months to achieve in longstanding deformities. A long-term range and muscle-strengthening exercise program is necessary to maintain the gains in range of motion.[36] The authors have had success using muscle stimulation in end range or referring patients to orthopedics for tendon lengthening or botox injection when serial casting has been ineffective. Respecting the child's pain during these interventions improves adherence to the prescribed program and produces faster results.[37] Adaptations to joint restrictions (e.g., rocker bars on shoes, reaching aids) may be required either as a temporary measure during early or acute disease or as a permanent intervention for end-stage damaged joints.

Decreased range of motion secondary to muscle shortening is evident when muscles such as extensor digitorum and gastrocnemius cross two or more joints. This is particularly important in children with JDM and scleroderma. Muscles can shorten as a result of the disease process, adaption secondary to long-term range loss, abnormal posture or movement patterns, or muscle imbalances. Three 30-second stretches done daily for 2 to 3 weeks should improve adaptive shortening. Daytime splinting in the stretched position for tenodesis can prevent progression of the deformity.

Muscle Weakness

Muscle weakness in children with rheumatic disease may result from muscle tissue disease, pain, disuse, abnormal use, or develop secondary to adjacent joint inflammation. It is a particularly serious problem in children with juvenile dermatomyositis, in which muscle weakness may be severe and prolonged.

Muscle strength should be assessed in all muscle groups. In children with dermatomyositis, muscle weakness is predominantly proximal and usually symmetrical. These children may also have weakness of the muscles of respiration and swallowing and will require specialized assessments. In children with inflammatory joint disease, weakness is usually restricted to muscles impacted by affected joints. In children with systemic sclerosis, weakness of the musculature of the hands may be most evident. To obtain reliable, reproducible measures of muscle strength that can be compared over time, it is essential that standardized procedures be used by an experienced examiner. Attention to specific limb positions stipulated in many muscle-testing methods is essential to ensure reproducibility of results. A 5- or 10-point scale for manual muscle testing is the most commonly used, but it is subjective.[38] More objective testing devices, such as dynamometers, modified sphygmomanometers, or vigorometers, have age-appropriate norms.[39-42] Functional muscle tests such as the Childhood Myositis Assessment Scale,[43,44] are also age-dependent. The greatest variable affecting all methods of muscle strength assessment is the child's motivation to exert maximum effort. Degree of effort should be recorded if less than maximum is suspected. Loss of muscle bulk is not always consistent with muscle weakness. In very young children with JIA and others with CTD, full strength often returns but normal bulk frequently does not.

Aerobic exercise capacity is reduced in children with rheumatic diseases when compared with their peers. The gold standard of aerobic capacity assessments is the measurement of maximal oxygen consumption (VO_2 peak) while on a treadmill or ergonometric bicycle. This method is not widely available, however, and the 6- or 9-minute walk, which tests the distance a child can walk in the prescribed time, is the most commonly used clinical test.[47,48] After the baseline is defined, children with diminished exercise capacity are instructed to slowly increase the frequency, intensity, type, and duration of moderate to vigorous physical activities. Frequently, a supervised gym program is required to initiate change. Ongoing improvement and maintenance will require a lifestyle change that is supported by the family.[49] Anaerobic capacity has been shown to be significantly reduced in children with JIA and CTD.[50,51] Anaerobic capacity can be measured by various clinical tests such as the Muscle Power Sprint test,[52-54] but improvement of anaerobic capacity following an exercise intervention has not been demonstrated in a pediatric rheumatology population.

Assessment of self-care, activities of daily living, and school and leisure activities is required to evaluate the extent of the impact of weakness. Muscle weakness not only has a direct impact on the ability to participate in activities but may affect self-efficacy. The effort required to keep up can lead to discouragement and mood changes, which in turn can lead to withdrawal from activities.[55] Muscle weakness contributes to fatigue, altered balance and reduced endurance, and vulnerability to physical trauma. For example, teens with significant muscle weakness negotiating crowded high school hallways are at particular risk for injury. At school, unnecessary physical demands on the child with muscle weakness such as stair climbing and book carrying should be minimized. The use of computers with voice recognition and predictive software may be important for the child with significant upper extremity weakness. On rare occasions, mobility aids may be required for generalized weakness.

Physical education teachers and sports coaches should be taught to recognize the fluctuating nature of the symptoms of many rheumatic diseases and the impact of muscle weakness on the child's ability to participate in athletic activities. Subtle strength deficits are particularly evident during endurance activities. Children should be encouraged to participate in physical education activities to the extent of their abilities but be allowed to modify or be excused from participation in activities that are beyond their limits at that time. Exercise programs to address specific as well as generalized weakness include a variety of isometric, isotonic, isokinetic, concentric, and eccentric contractions. Muscle strengthening is started as soon as possible. Pain control will improve effective contractions. In children with JDM, the use of early gentle strengthening with no evidence of detrimental effect is supported by recent literature.[56] Because of the characteristic pattern of muscle weakness in JDM, emphasis is placed on improving core musculature. Neuromuscular electrical stimulation in combination with voluntary contractions may be beneficial in retraining very weak muscles in older children. With all strengthening exercises, muscle substitution and pain should be avoided. Once muscle strength has been regained, re-integration into functional patterns is introduced. Ongoing monitoring is required.

Decreased Function

Normal function can be defined globally as the individual's ability to successfully perform self-care and participate in work or school and leisure activities. Optimal function depends on both physical and psychological health. Disruption in either sphere will result in impairment, restrictions, or disability. Culture and age-appropriate development determine the norms.

Poor School Attendance and Performance

A primary measure of function in a child with a rheumatic disease is school attendance. School absenteeism has a significant impact on academic achievement[57] and is a significant problem for children with rheumatic diseases. School issues are the most common stressors for families, even greater than medication side effects.[58] The most common symptoms impacting attendance are pain, fatigue, disrupted sleep, poor concentration, drug side effects (such as weight gain and nausea), and limited mobility. Factors related to treatment (medical and therapy appointments, drug administration) also contribute to school absences. Physical factors that may affect school attendance and participation include the need for transportation to and from school, the physical environment of the school, and any impediments to access to classrooms, washrooms, activity centers, and recreation facilities.

Early involvement with the school establishes an ongoing collaborative consultation with the staff to alert them to potential issues. Children with systemic connective tissue diseases or with pain amplification syndromes are at particular risk for prolonged school absences. Subsequent re-entry to school may be difficult and may be complicated by fatigue or by altered body image due to disability or drug side effects. An altered physical appearance can also lead to bullying or exclusion. Many children benefit from having an individual education plan early in their disease because it allows the staff to be more flexible (e.g., give the child access to the elevator, an extra set of texts, or the use of a laptop computer). Therapists are frequently required to provide documentation to support these changes.

The school staff's understanding of the child's physical and psychological challenges and awareness of safety issues (such as fracture risk in children with osteoporosis, need for limitation of sun exposure in children with SLE or JDM, and avoidance of cold in children with Raynaud phenomenon) should be assessed. If the child is required to take medications during school hours, discussion with the teachers is necessary, and a plan for the safe storage and administration of medications should be put in place. Teachers frequently identify a change in the child's ability to concentrate. This may reflect the effects of pain, or be a side effect of medications such as corticosteroids and nonsteroidal antiinflammatory agents. In children with SLE who have a high risk of neuropsychiatric syndromes, a change in ability to concentrate may also indicate a change in disease activity.[59] A marked change in concentration should be communicated to the rheumatologist. Therapists can teach coping skills to minimize the impact, but a formal psychoeducational assessment is often useful to identify specific problem areas. Early identification and understanding of concentration issues permit adaptation of the child's school routine and promote the teachers' understanding of the problem

Restricted Self-Care

Self-care refers to the age-appropriate activities such as eating, dressing, hygiene, cooking, household chores, and shopping. Pain, as well as decreased muscle strength, limited joint range, impaired balance, and reduced endurance, affects the ability of the child to engage in self-care activities. In children with inflammatory joint disease, morning stiffness affect the duration of self-care routines. The timing of medications can make a significant impact on ease of morning self-care activities. A hot shower or bath on first awakening may reduce morning stiffness. Additional pain medication may also be of benefit.

In addition to a careful history from the child and parent, observation of the child engaging in self-care activities is very useful in determining the degree of difficulty. Validated outcome measurement tools such as the Children's Health Assessment Questionnaire, Juvenile Arthritis Functional Assessment Report, Juvenile Arthritis Functional Assessment Scale, and Juvenile Arthritis Functional Status Index[60] are useful in quantifying self-care limitations and allowing comparisons over time.[17] However, these measures are not always sensitive to individual patient restrictions (see Chapter 8).

Interventions to improve self-care include decreasing restrictions of range, muscle strength, balance, or endurance and providing alternative techniques or aides and adaptations. Adherence to exercises is better if improvement impacts on functional abilities that are important to the child.

Inability to Maintain Leisure Activities

Play is the work of childhood and its value to children's physical and psychological development cannot be underestimated.[61] Play activities can be divided into three broad categories: quiet recreation, active recreation, and socialization.[62] History should be taken to explore all three categories.

Children with rheumatic disease have a variety of barriers to play and leisure activities either directly or indirectly related to their disease. Play and leisure activities are often restricted by pain, decreased range of motion, fatigue, and the time limitations imposed by medical appointments and exercise programs. Discussion with the family and child about the importance of balance between work and play is an ongoing part of therapy. Long-term restrictions to play and leisure can lead to arrested skill acquisition and development. It may be necessary to advocate on behalf of the child with coaches, teachers, and the family to facilitate the child's continued involvement in valued activities. Therapeutic interventions such as exercises should enhance play and leisure activities, not replace them. Conversely, play and sport do not eliminate the need for a targeted exercise program.

Decreased Mobility

Impaired mobility results from deficits in one or more of six dimensions: flexibility, strength, accuracy, speed, adaptability, and endurance.[63,64] A thorough assessment of each dimension takes into account physical, social, psychological, and environmental factors. Treatment is driven by assessment findings (Table 12–5). Persistent abnormal posture and movement patterns require a retraining program. Lower limb retraining is particularly effective when carried out in a warm pool. The warmth and buoyancy decreases pain and improves flexibility, allowing more normal movement patterns to occur. Splints and orthotics are used to protect, restore, or improve function by reducing pain from the inflammatory process, supporting joints, or correcting alignment. In adults, persistent malalignment is associated with the early onset of secondary osteoarthritis,[65] and it seems likely that this is also true in children.

The need for splinting has diminished dramatically in recent years because of earlier disease control. Well-designed prefabricated splints are less expensive than custom-made splints and are often more acceptable to teens as their peers associate them with sports injuries. Splints are usually required only on a temporary basis during flares. However, custom-made splints are better when long-term use is required. Foot orthoses must be used in conjunction with good supportive running shoes, because the heel counter of the shoe provides 50% of the efficacy of the orthotic.[66]

EFFECTS OF UVEITIS ON FUNCTION

Children with JIA are susceptible to uveitis, which may lead to impaired vision. Treatment of uveitis usually requires the use of topical corticosteroids, sometimes as

Table 12–5

Functional assessment of decreased mobility

Upper Extremity	Lower Extremity
• Weight-bearing on flat palms • Reaching above head with elbows extended • Reaching the back of head and behind the back • Holding a pen/pencil and writing for 5 minutes pain free • Cutting with a knife and fork • Lifting and pouring from a large pitcher into a glass • Picking up and holding several coins and receiving change • Putting on a backpack • Donning and doffing a T-shirt, shoes, and socks	• Walking a minimum of 50 ft (6- 9 minutes is preferred) • Running a minimum of 50 feet • Hopping on one foot or two, depending on age • Tiptoe walking • Heel walking • Climbing at minimum of 16 stairs • Squatting with buttocks touching heels • Floor sitting and rising • Donning and doffing shoes and socks

Activities are:
• Observed and discussed
• Sustained for a functional length of time

Look for:
• Activities limited by pain
• Completed in a timely manner (e.g., walking in time to cross a major road that has traffic lights)
• Compensations secondary to loss of flexibility or strength
  • e.g., LE—Gower sign, Trendelenburg, foot pivoting on the stair edge
  • e.g., UE—weight-bearing through MCPs rather than through a flat palm
• Quality of movement (i.e., coordination on stairs and hopping)
• Balance
• Speed of motion
• Accuracy in fine and gross motor activities

LE, lower extremity; *MCPs*, metacarpophalangeal joints; *UE*, upper extremity.

frequently as hourly, which may prevent the child from attending school and interfere with the parents' ability to attend work. Restricted vision will impair safe mobility, may lead to poor school performance and social isolation, and precipitate disruptive behavior at school or home. Attention to the effects of impaired vision on function may identify problems that require referral to a team specialized in vision loss at school or in a health care facility.[67]

Long-Term Considerations

Education

Ongoing education of the child and family underpins all treatment programs and is the domain of practice of all team members. Families often have misconceptions about rheumatic diseases and face a barrage of advice from well-meaning, but ill-informed friends and relatives. Direction to good information sources available on the world-wide web helps the child and parents make informed choices about therapy (see, for example, www.printo. it; www.printo.it/pediatric-rheumatology/; www.kidswi tharthritis.org; www.arthritis.org; www.niams.nih.gov; www.arthritis.ca; www.rheumatology.org.au). It is important that the advice provided by all members of the team be consistent and given in lay language.[68] Education has been shown to improve family coping and reduce stress.[69] In addition to reinforcing general education, therapists provide specific information on occupational and physical therapy interventions.

Transition

Transition is defined as the "purposeful, planned movement of adolescents and young adults with chronic physical and mental conditions from a child-centered to adult oriented health care system."[70] The timing of transition is determined by the local health care system and can occur at various times from 13 to 18 years of age. The skills necessary for a successful transition are introduced at diagnosis and updated as the child matures.[71]

The goal of transition is to help the child or young adult become more independent in managing health care needs and to assume adult roles such as a student, worker, friend, parent, partner, and homemaker. Assessment of physical status and performance of activities of daily living with the goal of independent living is critical at this age. Educational and vocational goals should be identified. Specific assessments such as driver training or vocational aptitude skills are arranged as needed.[72] Documentation of physical limitations and their functional impact may be required to obtain financial assistance for postsecondary education. During adolescence, parental supervision of treatment is slowly withdrawn, and the responsibility for care is shifted to the young adult. Adherence to recommendations in this stage is variable and compromised by the child's need for autonomy. Parental anxiety about their child's emerging autonomy must be addressed, the therapist often acting as an advocate for the child within the family. Sexuality issues are best addressed by the team member with whom the adolescent is most comfortable. Adolescents have identified continuity of staffing as an important issue for them during the period of transition.[73]

A retreat or camp experience can be a powerful learning milieu for both patients and staff. Staff experience firsthand what it is like to live with a rheumatic disease. In this setting, campers can witness positive coping skills modeled by both peer counselors and young adults with similar diagnoses and shared experiences. Transition skills are a focus of the camp, and activities integrate education and fun. Campers report feeling less isolated following attendance at a camp as they form new valued friendships. Knowledge of their disease has been shown to improve significantly as a result of the experience.[74,75]

End-Stage Disease

In children with JIA who have joint damage (end-stage disease), pain is one of the major residual problems requiring occupational and physical therapy. It is frequently due to secondary osteoarthritis exacerbated by flares of continuing inflammation. All pain techniques should be reviewed. Splinting for pain is most useful at this stage of the disease. Uncontrolled pain with loss of function is an indication for surgical intervention, especially joint replacement. Joint replacement is very seldom required in children or adolescents, but when indicated it is essential that the patient be psychologically, and physically prepared for the procedure. Preoperatively, the patient should become familiar with the postoperative protocol and learn skills such as the use of walking aids or one-handed self-care devices as needed. Occasionally, in order to prepare the child for the rigors of postoperative care, intensive preoperative therapy is required. For example, upper body strength and range may need improvement to allow for effective crutch-walking postoperatively. A coordinated plan between the surgical and rehabilitation teams is necessary to ensure best results.[76] An intensive postoperative therapy program is often required to maximize the benefits of the surgical intervention.

Despite end-stage disease, children should be expected to progress developmentally towards independent living. To this end, the use of accommodative splinting, compensatory movement patterns to overcome the effects of permanent deformities, adaptive equipment, power mobility, and modifications to the home environment or arrangement of housing designated for people with disabilities should be considered.

Social isolation can be a major problem for the young adult with limited mobility. The ability to drive a car can enhance community access. A driving assessment, driving instruction, and possession of a pass for designated parking areas may be appropriate. For others, public transportation passes, power mobility or the acquisition of an *assist* or *seeing eye* dog will improve mobility within the community. A major aim of the rehabilitative process at this stage is to foster independent living. The therapist should coach patients to advocate for themselves, so they are socially and psychologically capable of living independently. Connecting adolescents with others who have overcome similar issues is often helpful. This can be done through social groups or exchange of email addresses following consent from both children and their families. Interventions should be patient driven, time limited, and goal oriented to optimize long-term function. The focus should be on the child's abilities rather than disabilities.

SUMMARY

Recent changes in medical management have led to a paradigm shift in focus for physical and occupational therapy. However, recent long-term outcome studies,[55,77-81] show that, despite marked improvements in disease control, children continue to report sub-optimal health-related quality of life. This important area is a major focus of occupational and physical therapy.[82,83]

REFERENCES

1. J.D. Akikusa, R.C. Allen, Reducing the impact of rheumatic diseases in childhood, Best Pract. Res. Clin. Rheumatol. 16 (2002) 333–345.
5. P.N. Malleson, in: I.S. in Szer, Y. Kimura, P.N. Malleson, T.R. Southwood (Eds.), Arthritis in Children and Adolescents, Oxford University Press, 2006, 301–302.
6. S. Klepper, Exercise and fitness in children with arthritis: Evidence of benefits for exercise and physical activity, Arthritis Care Res. 49 (2003) 435–443.
7. K.K. Anthony, L.E. Schanberg, Pain in children with arthritis: A review of the current literature, Arthritis Care Res. 49 (2003) 272–279.
8. P.N. Malleson, K. Oen, D.A. Cabral, et al., Predictors of pain in children with established juvenile rheumatoid arthritis, Arthritis Care Res. 51 (2004) 222–227.
9. D.E. Feldman, C. Duffy, M. De Civita, et al., Factors associated with the use of complimentary and alternate medicine in juvenile idiopathic arthritis, Arthritis Care Res. 51 (2004) 527–532.
10. L.E. Schanberg, K.K. Anthony, K.M. Gil, et al., Daily pain and symptoms in children with polyarticular Arthritis, Arthritis Rheum. 48 (2003) 1390–1397.
11. S. Dhanani, J. Quenneville, M. Perron, et al., Minimal difference in pain associated with change in quality of life in children with rheumatic disease, Arthritis Care Res. 47 (2002) 501–505.
13. D. Bieri, R.A. Reeve, G.D. Champion, et al., The faces pain scale for self assessment of the severity of pain experienced in children: development, initial validation, and preliminary investigation for ratio scale properties, Pain 41 (1990) 139–150.
14. C.L. Hicks, C.L. von Baeyer, P. Spafford, et al., The faces Pain scale-Revised: Towards a common metric in pediatric pain management, Pain 93 (2001) 173–183.
15. J.W. Varni, K.L. Thompson, V. Hanson, The Varni/Thompson Pediatric Pain Questionnaire. 1. Chronic musculoskeletal pain in juvenile rheumatoid arthritis, Pain 28 (1987) 27–38.
17. G. Kuchta, I. Davidson, Occupational and physical therapy for children with rheumatic diseases, Radcliffe Press, Oxford UK, 2008.
21. G.A. Walco, J.W. Varne, N.T. Ilowite, Cognitive-behavioral pain management in children with juvenile rheumatoid arthritis, Pediatrics 89 (6) (1992) 1075–1079.
23. K.M. Houghton, L.B. Tucker, J.E. Potts, et al., Fitness, fatigue, disease activity, and quality of life in pediatric lupus, Arthritis Care and Res. 59 (2008) 534–537.
25. G. Zamir, J. Press, A. Tal, A. Tarasiuk, Sleep fragmentation in children with juvenile rheumatoid arthritis, J. Rheumatol. 25 (1998) 1191–1197.
26. B.J. Bloom, J.A. Owens, M. McGuinn, et al., Sleep and its relationship to pain, dysfunction and disease activity in juvenile rheumatoid arthritis, J. Rheumatol. 29 (2002) 169–173.
27. O. Bar-Or, Pathophysiological factors which limit the exercise capacity of the sick child, Med. Sci. Sports Exer. 18 (1986) 276–282.
29. C.M. Passarelli, S. Roizenblatt, C.A. Len, et al., A case-control sleep study in children with polyarticular juvenile rheumatoid arthritis, J. Rheumatol. 33 (2006) 796–802.
30. www.sleepfoundation.org, Accessed, April 2010.
31. www.sleepeducation.com, Accessed, April 2010.
32. E. Demirkaya, L. Ozcakar, T. Turker, et al., Musculoskeletal sonography in juvenile systemic lupus erythematosus, Arthritis Care and Res. 61 (2009) 58–60.
36. W. Barden, D. Brooks, Ayling- Campos A, Physical therapy management of the subluxed wrist in children with arthritis, Physical Therapy 75 (1995) 879–885.
39. E.A. Beenakker, J.H. van der Hoeven, J.M. Fock, et al., Reference values of maximum isometric muscle force obtained in 270 children aged 4-16 years by hand held dynamometry, Discord. 11 (2001) 441–446.

40. W. Dunn, Grip strength of children aged 3-7 years using a modified sphygmomanometer: comparison of typical children and children with rheumatic disorders, AJOT 47 (1992) 421–428.

41. V. Mathiowetz, D.M. Wiemer, S.M. federman, Grip and pinch strength norms for 6 to 19 year-old, Am. J. Occup. Ther. 40 (1986) 705–711.

43. D.J. Lovell, C.B. Lindsley, R.M. Rennebohm, et al., Development of validated disease activity and damage indices for the juvenile idiopathic inflammatory myopathies II. The Childhood Myositis Assessment Scale (CMAS): A quantitative tool for the evaluation of muscle function, Arthritis Rheum. 42 (1999) 2213–2219.

44. R.M. Rennebohm, K. Jones, A.M. Huber, et al., Normal scores for nine maneuvers of the childhood myositis assessment scale, Arthritis Care Res. 51 (2004) 365–370.

45. T. Takken, N. Spermon, P.J.M. Hekders, et al., Aerobic exercise capacity in patients with juvenile dermatomyositis, J. Rheumatol. 30 (2003) 1075–1080.

47. E. Paap, J. van der Net, P.J.M. Helders, et al., Physiologic response of the six-minute walk test in children with juvenile idiopathic arthritis, Arthritis Care Res. 53 (2005) 351–356.

49. O.T.H.M. Lelieveld, W. Armbrust, M.A. van Leeuwen, et al., Physical activity in adolescents with Juvenile idiopathic arthritis, Arthritis Care Res. 59 (2008) 1379–1384.

50. O.T.H.M. Lelieveld, M. van Brussel, T. Takken, et al., Aerobic, and Anaerobic Exercise Capacity in Adolescents with Juvenile Idiopathic Arthritis, Arthritis Care Res. 57 (2007) 898–904.

54. T. Takken, J. van der Net, P. Helders, The reliability of an aerobic and an anaerobic exercise tolerance test in patients with juvenile onset dermatomyositis, J. Rheumatol. 32 (2005) 734–739.

55. K.L. Shaw, T.R. Southwood, C.M. Duffy, et al., Health related Quality of life in adolescents with Juvenile idiopathic Arthritis. British Society of Paediatric and Adolescent Rheumatology, Children's Chronic Arthritis Association, Lady Hoare trust for physically disabled children, Arthritis Care Res. 55 (2006) 199–207.

56. S.M. Maillard, R. Jones, C.M. Owens, et al., Quantitative assessment of the effects of a single exercise session on muscles in Juvenile dermatomyositis, Arthritis Care Res. 53 (2005) 558–564.

58. P.J. Degotardi, T.A. Revenson, N.T. Ilowite, Family-level coping in juvenile rheumatoid arthritis: Assessing the utility of a quantitative family interview, Arthritis Care Res. 12 (1999) 314–323.

59. W.L. Sibbitt Jr., J.R. Brandt, C.R. Johnson, et al., The incidence and prevalence of neuropsychiatric syndromes in pediatric onset lupus erythematosus, J. Rheumatol. 29 (2002) 1536–1542.

61. J. Hackett, Perceptions of play and leisure in junior school aged children with juvenile idiopathic arthritis: What are the implications for Occupational Therapy, Br. J. Occupational Ther. 66 (2003) 303–310.

67. www.uveitis.org, July 3, 2010.

68. S. Cavallo, D.E. Feldman, B. Swaine, et al., Is parental coping associated with quality of life in juvenile idiopathic arthritis? Pediatr. Rheumatol. 7 (2009) 7.

71. J.E. McDonagh, Young People first, juvenile idiopathic arthritis second: Transition care in rheumatology, Arthritis Care Res. 8 (2008) 1162–1170.

72. L.B. Tucker, D.A. Cabral, Transition of the adolescent patient with rheumatic disease: issues to consider, Pediarti. Clin. North America 52 (2005) 641–652.

74. K.J. Hagglund, N.M. Doyle, D.L. Clay, et al., A family retreat as a comprehensive intervention for children with arthritis and their families, Arthritis Care Res. 9 (1996) 35–41.

76. G. Kuchta, I. Davidson, Physiotherapy and Occupational therapy In: Arthritis in Children and Adolescents, Oxford University Press, Oxford, 2006 381-391.

77. M. Seid, L. Opipari, B. Huang, et al., Disease control and health-related quality of life in juvenile idiopathic arthritis, Arthritis Care Res. 61 (2009) 393–399.

78. H. Foster, N. Marshall, A. Myers, et al., Outcomes in adults with juvenile idiopathic arthritis: A quality of life study, Arthritis Rheum. 48 (2003) 767–775.

79. P. Woo, Systemic juvenile idiopathic arthritis: diagnosis, management, and outcome, Nature Clin. Prac. Rheumatol. 2 (2006) 28–34.

80. N. Ruperto, S. Buratti, C. Duarte-Salazar, et al., Health-related quality of life in juvenile-onset systemic lupus erythematosus and its relationship to disease activity and damage, Arthritis Care Res. 51 (2004) 458–464.

81. M.T. Apaz, C. Saad-Magalhaes, A. Pistorio, et al., Health related quality of life of patients with juvenile dermatomyositis: Results from the Paediatric Rheumatology International Trials Organisation Multinational Quality of life Cohort study, Arthritis Care Res. 61 (2009) 509–517.

83. A.O. Hersh, E. von Scheven, J. Yazdanny, et al., Differences in long-term activity and treatment of adults with childhood onset and adult onset systemic lupus erythematosus, Arthritis Care Res. 61 (2009) 13–20.

Entire reference list is available online at www.expertconsult.com.

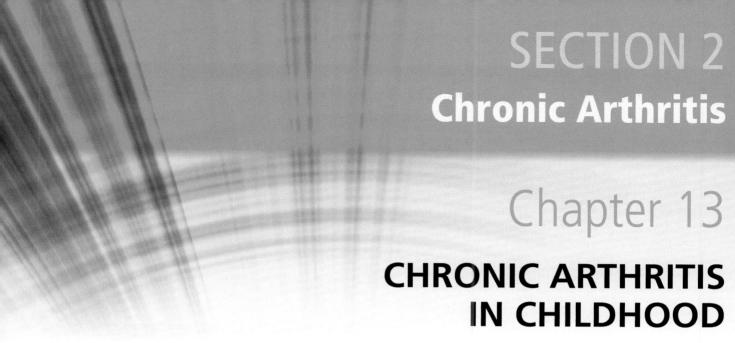

Chapter 13

CHRONIC ARTHRITIS IN CHILDHOOD

Ross E. Petty and James T. Cassidy

Chronic arthritis, the most common chronic rheumatic disease of childhood, is one of the more frequent chronic illnesses of children and an important cause of short- and long-term disability.

It is not a single disease, but a group of related, genetically heterogeneous, phenotypically diverse immunoinflammatory disorders affecting joints and other structures, possibly activated by contact with an external antigen or antigens. Since its introduction in 1994, the term *Juvenile Idiopathic Arthritis* (JIA) has largely supplanted the terms *Juvenile Chronic Arthritis* (JCA) and *Juvenile Rheumatoid Arthritis* (JRA). However, it is necessary to understand the older classifications in order to interpret the literature on the subject. The intent of this chapter is to provide a general introduction to JIA. Each subtype of disease is discussed in separate chapters.

CLASSIFICATIONS OF CHRONIC CHILDHOOD ARTHRITIS

Chronic arthritis in childhood is a complex area of study, not least because of inconsistencies of definition and terminology. In the 1970s, two sets of criteria were proposed to classify chronic arthritis in childhood: those for JRA, developed and validated by a committee of the American College of Rheumatology (ACR),[1] and those for JCA, published by the European League Against Rheumatism (EULAR).[2] Inconsistencies between these two classifications were confusing, and a classification proposed by the Pediatric Task Force of the International League of Associations for Rheumatology (ILAR)[3] sought to provide an internationally agreed system of definitions to further the study of childhood arthritis These three classifications are compared in Table 13–1. Problems in applying all of these criteria include the necessity to exclude other

diseases for which there are no validated diagnostic or classification criteria for children, and the fact that all three were based only on populations of northern European derivation.

ACR Criteria for Classification of Juvenile Rheumatoid Arthritis

The ACR criteria have been widely used, validated, and revised (Table 13–2),[1,4-6] but they are applicable primarily to white North American children. They define the age limit in children, the duration of disease necessary for a diagnosis, and the characteristics of the arthritis. The requirement that age at onset of arthritis be less than 16 years was a criterion based more on practice patterns than on age-related biological variation in disease. Furthermore, although persistent objective arthritis in one or more joints for 6 weeks was sufficient for diagnosis, a disease duration of at least 6 months was required before the onset type could be determined (unless characteristic systemic features were present).

The type of onset is defined by a constellation of clinical signs present during the first 6 months of illness. Oligoarticular onset is defined as arthritis in four or fewer joints. Polyarticular onset is defined as arthritis in five or more joints. In determination of the onset type, each joint is counted separately, except for the joints of the cervical spine, carpus, and tarsus; each of these structures is counted as one joint. Systemic-onset JRA is characterized by a daily (quotidian or intermittent) fever spiking to greater than 39° C for at least 2 weeks in association with arthritis of one or more joints. Most children with systemic-onset disease also have a characteristic rash, and many have other evidence of extraarticular involvement, such as lymphadenopathy, hepatosplenomegaly, or pericarditis. Nine course subtypes were identified during long-term follow-up.

Table 13–1

Comparison of EULAR, ACR, and ILAR criteria for classification of chronic arthritis of childhood

Characteristic	ACR	EULAR	ILAR
Onset types	3	6	6
Course subtypes	9	None	1
Age at onset of arthritis	<16 yr	<16 yr	<16 yr
Duration of arthritis	= 6 wk	= 3 mo	= 6 wk
Includes JAS	No	Yes	Yes
Includes JPsA	No	Yes	Yes
Includes inflammatory bowel disease	No	Yes	Yes
Other diseases excluded	Yes	Yes	Yes

ACR, American College of Rheumatology; *EULAR,* European League Against Rheumatism; *ILAR,* International League of Associations for Rheumatology; *JAS,* juvenile ankylosing spondylitis; *JPsA,* juvenile psoriatic arthritis.

Table 13–2

Criteria for the classification of juvenile rheumatoid arthritis

1. Age at onset <16 yr
2. Arthritis (swelling or effusion, or presence of two or more of the following signs: limitation of range of motion, tenderness or pain on motion, and increased heat) in one or more joints
3. Duration of disease 6 wk or longer
4. Onset type defined by type of disease in first 6 mo:
   a. Polyarthritis: ≥5 inflamed joints
   b. Oligoarthritis (pauciarticular disease): <5 inflamed joints
   c. Systemic-onset: arthritis with characteristic fever
5. Exclusion of other forms of juvenile arthritis

Modified from Cassidy JT, Levinson JE, Bass JC et al: A study of classification criteria for a diagnosis of juvenile rheumatoid arthritis, *Arthritis Rheum* 29:274-281,1986.

Table 13–3

Criteria for a diagnosis of juvenile chronic arthritis

1. Age at onset <16 yr
2. Arthritis in one or more joints
3. Duration of disease 3 mo or longer
4. Type defined by characteristics at onset:
   a. Pauciarticular: <5 joints
   b. Polyarticular: >4 joints, rheumatoid factor negative
   c. Systemic: arthritis with characteristic fever
   d. Juvenile rheumatoid arthritis: >4 joints, rheumatoid factor positive
   e. Juvenile ankylosing spondylitis
   f. Juvenile psoriatic arthritis

From EULAR Bulletin 4: *Nomenclature and classification of arthritis in children,* 1977, Basel, National Zeitung AG,.

Table 13–4

Proposed classification criteria for juvenile idiopathic arthritis: Durban, 1997

1. Systemic
2. Oligoarthritis
   a. Persistent
   b. Extended
3. Polyarthritis (rheumatoid factor negative)
4. Polyarthritis (rheumatoid factor positive)
5. Psoriatic arthritis
6. Enthesitis-related arthritis
7. Undifferentiated arthritis
   a. Fits no other category
   b. Fits more than one category

From Petty RE, Southwood TR, Baum J et al: Revision of the proposed classification criteria for juvenile idiopathic arthritis: Durban, 1997, *J Rheumatol* 25:199-1994, 1998.

EULAR Criteria for the Classification of Juvenile Chronic Arthritis

In 1977, at the EULAR conference on the Care of Rheumatic Children in Oslo, the term *juvenile chronic arthritis* was proposed for the heterogeneous group of disorders that present as chronic arthritis in childhood (Table 13–3).[2] These criteria differ from the ACR criteria in three ways: (1) Arthritis must have been present for at least 3 months; (2) juvenile ankylosing spondylitis (JAS), psoriatic arthropathy, and arthropathies associated with inflammatory bowel disease are included; (3) the term *juvenile rheumatoid arthritis* is applied only to children with arthritis and rheumatoid factor (RF) seropositivity, although no definition of RF seropositivity is provided.

ILAR Criteria for the Classification of Juvenile Idiopathic Arthritis

In 1993, the Pediatric Standing Committee of ILAR proposed a classification of the idiopathic arthritides of childhood (Table 13–4). This classification[3] and its subsequent revisions (Durban, Edmonton)[7-9] were developed with the aim of achieving homogeneity within disease categories. The designation *undifferentiated arthritis* includes conditions that, for whatever reason, either do not meet criteria for any other category or meet criteria for more than one category. These criteria have been subject to a number of studies comparing them with other criteria.[10-26] They were intended to be modified as new evidence for pathogenesis became available.

For the student of pediatric rheumatology, differences in nomenclature require that care be taken in interpreting the literature, because the terms JRA, JCA, and JIA are often incorrectly used as if they were interchangeable and synonymous. This dilemma has been the subject of several publications.[27-30]

HISTORICAL REVIEW

In the first published documentation of inflammatory polyarthritis in childhood in 1864, Cornil[31] described a 29-year-old woman who had had chronic inflammatory arthritis since the age of 12 years. Diamant-Berger[32] reviewed the subject in 1890 and included 35 previously published cases and 3 of his own. He described an acute onset of disease, the predominant involvement of large joints, a course characterized by exacerbations and remissions, frequent disturbances of normal growth, and a generally good prognosis.

George Frederic Still presented the classic description of chronic childhood arthritis in 1897,[33] while he was a medical registrar at the Hospital for Sick Children, Great Ormond Street, London. He pointed out that the disease almost always began before the second dentition, was more frequent in girls, and was usually of insidious onset. Still observed that there was often no articular pain and that children exhibited a marked tendency to early contracture and muscle atrophy. The cervical spine was affected in the majority of cases, often during the early stages of the disease. The acute onset of disease in 12 patients who had lymphadenopathy, splenomegaly, and fever was described in detail. Pleuritis and pericarditis were common, although rash was not noted. Still suggested that childhood arthritis might have a different etiology from that of rheumatoid arthritis or might include more than one disease. This classic description is an outstanding example of bedside observation. Today, the term *Still's disease* is most often used to describe the adult onset (beyond the age of 16 years) of this acute systemic arthritis. French authors have often used the term *syndrome de Chauffard-Still* for chronic arthritis with lymphadenopathy and splenomegaly. In 1901, Hirschsprung[34] confirmed the observations that a chronic articular disease was associated with lymphadenopathy and splenomegaly in young children and also noted the occurrence of hepatomegaly. In 1939, Atkinson[35] reviewed 118 cases of Still's disease, 86 of whom had severe arthritis, lymphadenopathy, and splenomegaly. Others found a much lower proportion of children with this systemic form of the disease.[36,37]

Recognition that chronic arthritis in children differed from that in adults took some time. As late as 1957, in a textbook edited by Short, Bauer, and Reynolds, it was stated that "We adopted the generally accepted principle that rheumatoid arthritis is the same disease in adults and children with certain minor differences"[38] It is now generally acknowledged that chronic arthritis in children differs clinically, often genetically, and possibly pathogenically from adult rheumatoid arthritis, with the exception of rheumatoid factor–positive polyarthritis, which is very similar to adult rheumatoid arthritis.

The interested reader is referred to a number of case series of historic importance.[39-47] These publications reported what, today, would be considered largely untreated patients and serve as a reminder of the serious potential long- and short-term effects of childhood arthritis, including death in 7%[42] to 9%.[43]

EPIDEMIOLOGY

Chronic arthritis in children is not rare, but the true frequency is not known. It appears to be worldwide in distribution, but the reported incidence and prevalence vary considerably throughout the world.[48,49] This may reflect the ethnicity, immunogenetic susceptibility, and environmental influences of the population under study,[50,51] or may result from underreporting in the developing world, where data are very sparse. There is little evidence to indicate that the incidence in Asia or Africa differs substantially from that in Europe, North America, or Australia, from where most studies of incidence and prevalence have been reported. Published studies are summarized in Table 13–5. Of note, population-based studies (Group I) report the highest disease frequency, and those with the most complete clinical evaluations[52,53] report the highest prevalence of all. Importantly, there are no studies from Africa, and only one small study from Asia.

In a review of published studies, Oen and Cheang[54] noted that reported prevalence was higher for population-based studies and for data from North America.

Incidence and Prevalence

Reported annual incidence rates of chronic childhood arthritis have ranged from less than 1 per 100,000 in Japan to more than 20 per 100,000 in Norway (Table 13–5).[48,52-74] Almost all of these reports were clinic-based studies from Europe or North America, and all but four used the ACR or EULAR criteria.

Prevalence rates for chronic arthritis in childhood have ranged from fewer than 10 per 100,000 in France[61] to 400 per 100,000 in an Australian study.[53] Most have been clinic or hospital based, and most have used the ACR or EULAR criteria. In the report of Danner and colleagues,[75] the ILAR criteria were used in a hospital- or clinic-based population and demonstrated a prevalence of 19.8 cases per 100,000 children under 16 years of age. The difference between referred and community-based study populations in determining prevalence is emphasized by the survey by Manners and Diepeveen,[53] in which a prevalence of 400 per 100,000 was found based on a physical examination by a pediatric rheumatologist of each of the 2241 12-year old Australian school children included in the survey. Although this prevalence is considerably higher than that reported in most other studies, Mielants and colleagues[52] found a prevalence of 167 per 100,000 in a similar study of Belgian children. The results of these two community-based reports, when compared to the clinic- or practitioner-based studies, suggest that a substantial proportion of children with chronic arthritis are not brought to medical attention. Estimates of the global frequency of JIA are shown in Table 13–6. Using a range of reference data from European, North American, or Australian studies, an estimated 1.7 to 8.4 million children in the world have arthritis, mostly undiagnosed.

Clearly, musculoskeletal pain is not uncommon in children and far exceeds the prevalence of inflammatory arthritis.[76] Published data are difficult to compare because of varying referral patterns, the heterogeneity of the disease, its evolution over time, differences in classification criteria, dissimilarity of source populations, and variable case ascertainment.[50] Substantial geographical and ethnic differences are present in regard to age at onset, relative frequencies of onset types, and immunological markers.

Table 13–5

Studies of the incidence and prevalence of chronic childhood arthritis

Authors (ref. no.)	Origin	Year	Diagnostic Criteria	Incidence (per 100,000 Children/yr)	Prevalence (per 100,000 Children)
Towner et al (58)	USA	1983	EULAR, ACR	83.7-113.4	10.8-13.9
Peterson et al (68)	USA	1996	ACR	86.1-94	11.7
Mielants et al (52)	Belgium	1993	EULAR	167	—
Andersson Gäre (50)	Sweden	1994	EULAR	86.3	10.9
Manners & Diepeveen (53)	Australia	1996	EULAR	400	—
Kaipiainen-Seppanen & Savolainen (66)	Finland	1996	ACR	—	14
Ozen et al (70)	Turkey	1998	EULAR	64	—
Kiessling et al (73)	Germany	1998	EULAR	20	3.5
Gewanter et al (59)	USA	1983	ACR	16-43	—
Kunnamo et al (60)	Finland	1986	ACR	—	18.2
Prieur et al (61)	France	1987	EULAR	8-10	1.3-1.9
Arguedas et al (72)	Costa Rica	1998	EULAR	31.4	6.8
Laaksonen (54)	Finland	1966	English	75-100	6-8
Bywaters (56)	UK	1968	English	60-70	—
Sullivan et al (57)	USA	1975	ACR	65	9.2
Rosenberg (62)	Canada	1990	ACR	39.7	5-8
Denardo et al (64)	USA	1994	ACR	—	4
Oen et al (55)	Canada	1995	ACR	32	5
Malleson et al (65)	Canada	1996	ACR	40	8
Symmonds et al (67)	UK	1996	EULAR	—	10
Fujikawa & Okuni (69)	Japan	1997	ACR	—	0.83
Moe & Rygg (71)	Norway	1998	EULAR	148.1	22.6

ACR, American College of Rheumatology; *EULAR,* European League Against Rheumatism.

Table 13–6

Estimates of the incidence and prevalence of JIA in childhood

UNICEF Region	Pop. < 18 yr	Incidence	Prevalence
East Asia/Pacific	567,000,000	29,484-56,700	487,620-2,268,000
South Asia	536,000,000	27,872-53,600	444,880-2,144,000
Industrialized	225,000,000	11,700-22,500	186,750-900,000
Latin America	190,000,000	9880-19,000	157,000-760,000
Eastern Europe	138,000,000	7176-13,800	114,540-552,000
West/Central Africa	151,000,000	750-15,000	125,330-604,000
East/Southern Africa	147,000,000	7644-14,700	122,010-588,000
TOTAL	2,105,000,000	109,456-210,300	1,747,150-8,420,000

UNICEF Regions
Incidence ranges based on prevalence ranges estimates of 83/100,000[52,58] and 400/100,000[53]

Proportions of JIA Subtypes

In Europe and North America, it clear that oligoarthritis is the most common subtype, accounting for approximately 50% of patients in most large series. RF-positive polyarthritis is least common. There is considerable variation in the reported relative proportions of the other types. In India, and Asia, oligoarthritis appears to be much less frequently recognized.

Age at Onset

Arthritis was arbitrarily defined beginning before the age of 16 years. Onset before 6 months of age is distinctly unusual; however, the age at onset is often quite early, with the highest frequency occurring between 1 and 3 years of age.[53,57,77] Quite distinct distributions of age at disease onset characterize each subset. (See Chapters 14 to 18)

Sex Ratio

In North and South America, Europe, and Australasia, twice as many girls as boys are affected. Marked differences in this ratio are apparent in the different onset types. In reports from parts of Asia, however, boys predominate. Whether this reflects biological or cultural differences is not clear.

Geographical and Racial Distribution

The incidence and prevalence data outlined previously were derived primarily from American or northern European white populations. There are few comparable data for other geographical or racial groups.[94,78,79] Nonetheless, suggestions of racial disparity in frequency exist.[48,80-83]

Lower frequencies of JRA have been reported in children of Japanese, Filipino, or Samoan origin than in white children living in Hawaii.[84] The incidence of JRA in Japan was reported to be low (0.83 per 100,000),[85] and chronic arthritis may be less common in Americans of Chinese ancestry than in American white children,[78] but there is a paucity of data describing these children. Studies from Asia are minimal, but reports from India have most often noted a higher frequency of polyarthritis, compared with oligoarthritis or systemic-onset disease.[86-88]

Schwartz and colleagues[87] concluded that the proportion of African-American children with JRA in a referral clinic population in the United States was consistent with their representation in the population served. However, there was a striking underrepresentation of this ethnic group in young children with oligoarticular and polyarticular onsets. Some reports suggest that chronic arthritis in children and adults is less frequent in African than in European populations; in Nigeria, however, the proportion of all patients with onset of chronic inflammatory arthritis in childhood may be somewhat higher.[82,83]

Saurenmann and colleagues[89] compared the frequencies of JIA in children of differing ethnic origin in a multiethnic hospital-based cohort of more than 1000 children in Toronto. They noted that children of African or Asian origin were underrepresented overall in comparison with their proportion of the healthy population. Children of European origin were more likely to have extended oligoarthritis or psoriatic arthritis than other ethnic groups. Those of Asian origin were more likely to have enthesitis-related arthritis (ERA), and those of African origin were more susceptible to RF-positive polyarticular disease.

An analysis of white and Western Canadian Indian children suggests that, although the overall frequency of chronic arthritis in aboriginal children is not higher than that for the white population, the frequency of human leukocyte antigen (HLA)–B27–associated arthritis is appreciably higher in the aboriginal group.[90] However, Oen and colleagues[91] noted a high overall incidence of the disorder (23.6 per 100,000), in addition to a high frequency of seronegative spondyloarthropathies, in Inuit children of northern Canada. The data reported by Boyer and associates[92] suggest that the incidence of RF-seropositive polyarthritis is increased in southeast Alaskan Yupik Eskimo children. The numbers of patients in these studies are small, however, and conclusions with respect to actual incidence and prevalence of chronic arthritis in these groups are tentative.

ETIOLOGY AND PATHOGENESIS

The etiology is unknown, although it is almost certainly multifactorial, and probably differs from one onset type to another. Systemic arthritis is characterized neither by the presence of autoantibodies nor a strong genetic predisposition and may be more appropriately considered to be an autoinflammatory disease. Autoantibodies are common in oligoarthritis (antinuclear antibodies), and RF-positive polyarthritis (IgM rheumatoid factor). In these disorders it seems likely that the humoral immune system is central to the pathogenesis of the disease. Paradoxically, immunodeficiency states such as selective IgA deficiency and hypogammaglobulinemia are statistically more frequent in children with chronic arthritis than in the general population (Chapter 42). In contrast, ERA, RF-negative polyarthritis, and to some extent psoriatic arthritis have less tendency to autoantibody formation but have strong association with polymorphisms at the histocompatibility locus. That genetic factors are only part of the puzzle is demonstrated by the fact that familial arthritis is very rare, although not unknown. The fundamental pathological process is chronic inflammation, in which the immune system plays a critical role, although not necessarily an autoimmune one (Chapters 3 and 4).

In all subtypes, products of activated T cells and macrophages are involved in pathogenesis, and as yet undetected genetic or immunological factors probably play key roles.

Environmental influences have received little attention. One study alleged that breastfeeding has a protective effect on the development of the disorder,[93] especially in oligoarticular disease; however, a strong relationship was not confirmed in another investigation.[94] Maternal smoking during pregnancy has been reported to be a risk factor for the development of arthritis in the first 7 years of life, especially in girls.[95]

In addition to polygenic genetic predispositions, disordered immune responses, and putative environmental triggers, any theory of pathogenesis must account for a number of factors: the clinical heterogeneity of the disease; the much higher prevalence of oligoarthritis, polyarthritis, and psoriatic arthritis in girls, and the strikingly higher incidence of ERA in boys; the narrow peak ages at onset for some types such as oligoarthritis, in contrast to the absence of a peak age at onset for systemic disease; and the association of extraarticular complications such as uveitis in certain disease subsets. There may be multiple etiological events, or the disorder may result from a single pathogenic vector with diverse clinical patterns evolving from interactions with the host. It may be postulated that an environmental agent affecting a child with a particular genetic predisposition, at a point of vulnerability—defined by age, intercurrent illness, prior antigenic experience, trauma, hormonal abnormalities, psychological stress or immunological maturity—results in a clinical disorder. It is necessary to consider differing sets of conditions for development of each onset type and course subtype.

Immunopathogenic Mechanisms

A number of observations contribute to the hypothesis that the immune system is intimately involved in pathogenesis. First, there is abundant evidence of altered immunity, abnormal immunoregulation, cytokine production, and polymorphisms of genes involved in the immune response.[96-101] Second, there is an association between specific immunodeficiencies and rheumatic diseases, including chronic arthritis (see Chapter 42). Third, there is a close relationship between immune reactivity and inflammation, the hallmark of arthritis. Whether it is principally an immunogenetically determined disorder or an antigen-driven immunological response is uncertain. The topics of immunopathogenesis and inflammation are discussed in detail in Chapters 3 and 4.

Innate Immunity

The importance of the innate immune system is beginning to be recognized (see Chapter 3).[102,103] That neutrophils have an important role in synovitis is not surprising, considering their abundance in inflamed synovial fluid. Enzymes contained in neutrophil granules cause direct damage to connective tissue structures. Uncontrolled activation of polymorphonuclear leukocytes appears to be central to the ongoing inflammation of polyarticular disease.[104]

Frosch and colleagues[105] have described a strong association between systemic disease and myeloid-related proteins (MRP) 8 and 14, produced by both neutrophils and monocytes. Frosch et al[106] reported that children with pauciarticular JRA had very high synovial fluid and serum levels of MRP 8 and 14. These proteins are ligands for the Toll-like receptor (TLR) 4. TLRs recognize preserved microbial elements (lipopolysaccharide) but also factors of host origin that are present in inflamed joints: members of the heat shock protein family,[22,60,70,96] high-mobility group 1 (HMG-1), hyaluronan, and fibronectin.[107] Foell and colleagues[108] found increases in a related protein, S100, that correlated well with disease activity. Levels were elevated in cases of oligoarticular and polyarticular disease but most extremely elevated in those of systemic disease. Levels in synovial fluid were approximately 10 times higher than those in serum. MRP8, MRP14, and S100 are proinflammatory mediators. These studies indicate the importance of neutrophils in pathogenesis. Studies by Jarvis and colleagues[104] using gene array technology demonstrated the upregulation of genes associated with neutrophil function in systemic and polyarticular arthritis.

Dysregulated interleukin-1 (IL-1) β has been implicated in the pathogenesis of systemic disease.[109] Furthermore, genetic polymorphisms of the IL-1 β gene associated with systemic disease appear to contribute to susceptibility to this disease.[110] There are complex interconnections between the innate and adaptive immune systems (see Chapter 4).

Adaptive Immunity

B-lymphocyte numbers are normal to increased, and polyclonal B-cell activation is reflected in the hypergammaglobulinemia present in many children with arthritis, depending on onset type, at least partly reflecting the nonspecific inflammatory response.

Autoantibodies

Autoantibodies to nuclear, immunoglobulin, and other antigens are common in sera of children with arthritis. There is no evidence, however, that they participate directly in disease pathogenesis, and they may result from a response to epitopes expressed or produced as a result of inflammation and tissue damage. Among these autoimmune phenomena are antibodies to histones;[111-117] antineutrophil cytoplasmic antibodies;[118-120] antiperinuclear, antikeratin, and anti-RA33 antibodies;[121-123] anticardiolipin antibodies;[115,124-126] and the DEK oncoprotein (possibly associated with interferon-γ [IFN-γ]).[127] Antibodies to HMG proteins[128] are increased in JRA to a defined epitope on HMG-17,[129,130] and in oligoarticular disease to an HMG-2 protein.[131,132] Autoimmunity to types I, II, and IV collagens have been demonstrated in some studies.[133-135] Immunity to cartilage link protein has been noted.[136] Immunoglobulin A (IgA) antigliadin antibodies have been described[137] but are not predictive of celiac disease in JCA.[138] Anticyclic citrullinated peptide antibodies have been reported, especially in RF-seropositive disease,[139] but less frequently than in adults with RA.[140]

Levels of circulating immune complexes parallel activity of the arthritis and systemic features.[141-143] Complement activation is also reflected in levels of fragment Bb of the alternative pathway and C4d, which correlate with circulating immune complexes and clinical activity of the disease.[144,145] The immune complexes identified in synovial fluid also vary in size, composition, ability to activate complement, and potential for induction of proinflammatory cytokine secretion.[111]

T Lymphocytes and Cytokine Profiles

Wouters and colleagues have studied the distribution of T lymphocytes in the peripheral blood of patients with oligoarticular, polyarticular or systemic JIA compared with age-matched healthy controls.[146] Total peripheral blood lymphocyte numbers, and numbers of CD3+, CD4+, and CD8+ cells were normal in all types of disease. The frequency of activated T cells (expressing CD57, and CD16/56.) was increased in the oligoarticular and polyarticular subtypes. Those with systemic disease had marked decrease in the numbers of natural killer cells.

Discrepancies have been observed in the frequencies of markers of T-cell activation: Tac or IL-2 receptor expression was found to be normal,[147,148] HLA-D related (DR) antigens normal[148,149] or increased,[150] and very-late–activation antigen increased only in children with active disease.[148] Although many of these studies suggest a global T-cell regulatory defect, their results may have been influenced by therapy. Massa and colleagues[151] found that treatment with methotrexate (MTX) led to a decrease in CD4+2 CD8+ and γ/δ T-cell numbers.

CD4+ T cells are the predominant infiltrating cell in the inflamed synovium of children. Synovial fluid T cells appeared to be similar in type and responsiveness to those in peripheral blood in some studies,[147] but in others CD4+ T cells were decreased in synovial fluid but increased in synovial tissue.[152] Selective recruitment of

T cells expressing CCR5 and CXCR3 has been reported.[153] In most instances, T cells from the synovial fluid or membrane had increased expression of activation markers.[147,153] Studies of Scola and colleagues[154] indicated that cytokine expression patterns were typical of a type I bias.

Murray and colleagues[155] studied synovial T-cell infiltrates in 17 children and found that the level of T-cell activation (CD3$^+$ IL-2R$^+$) was significantly higher in oligoarthritis (especially for CD8$^+$ cells) and that the CD4/CD8 ratio was lower. A subsequent study of the immunohistological patterns of expression of synovial Th1 and Th2 cells found increased secretion of IL-4.[156] Clonotypical restriction has been reported.[157] Patterns of expression of TNF-α and -β and their receptors and other cytokines have also been studied.[156,158,159] Ozen and colleagues[160] observed a marked Th1 response in synovial fluid mononuclear cells in 4 of 5 children by immunofluorescent identification of intracellular cytokines through flow cytometric analysis (increased IFN-γ in addition to IL-4). The chemokine receptor CCR4 has been linked to a similar increase in the IL-4/IFN ratio.[161] Coculture with heat-shock protein (HSP) 60 produced only a slight increase in IFN-γ products in the one synovial fluid sample tested. A recent report indicated that synovial dendritic cells express the receptor activator for NF-κB (RANK).[162]

Gattorno and colleagues[163] investigated the pattern of cytokine production in T-cell clones from synovial fluid mononuclear cells in five children with oligoarthritis. Large amounts of IFN-γ were produced with a predominant Th1/Th0 pattern. Raziuddin and coworkers[164] found a mixed Th-cell response in stimulated peripheral blood mononuclear cells in systemic-onset disease. Studies of single nucleotide polymorphisms have confirmed different genetic influences in systemic-onset disease for IL-6[165,166] and macrophage migration inhibitory factor (MIF).[167,168] Similar studies in oligoarthritis have focused on TNF haplotypes.[169] Synovial cytokine levels differ in children with JRA compared with adults with RA.[170] TNF-α G → A –238 and –308 polymorphisms may define outcomes in subtypes of chronic arthritis in children.[171]

Speculations on pathogenesis have centered on the possibility that there are disordered interactions between type 1 (Th1) and type 2 (Th2) helper T cells (see Chapter 3).[172,173]. A number of excellent reviews have been published.[98,101,174,175] TNF-α (Th1) and its soluble receptors and IL-6 (Th2) occupy a central role in pathogenesis[176] and provide a rationale for current therapeutic studies.[177] MIF is increased in concentration in the vascular compartment of children with arthritis. This abnormality is directly related to excess transmission of a promoter haplotype that increases susceptibility to chronic inflammation.[178]

T-Cell Receptor Polymorphism

Abnormalities of T cell receptor (TCR) peptide chains are reported. Oligoclonal selection of the TCR chain is more characteristic of synovial fluid and tissues than peripheral blood.[179,180] Maksymowych and associates[181] confirmed a high frequency of the TCR allele

TCR-Vβ6.1 among HLA-DQA*0101–positive children. A subsequent report identified this TCR null allele as a risk factor for a polyarticular course in children with early-onset oligoarticular disease positive for DQA1*0101.[182] This association was not confirmed in a study from Norway,[183] nor did Nepom and coworkers[184] identify TCR polymorphism in their studies of oligoarticular-onset JRA. In the report of Thompson and colleagues,[180] TCR-Vβ8 was clonally expanded in children with polyarticular disease and TCR-Vβ20 was increased in oligoarthritis.

Hormonal Factors

The often striking differences in sex ratio, as well as the characteristic preadolescent or postadolescent peaks in incidence of specific categories of childhood arthritis, suggest that reproductive hormones may play important roles in pathogenesis.[185,186] In a study by Khalkhali-Ellis and colleagues,[187] androgen levels in children with chronic arthritis and in aged-matched controls were similar for progesterone and dehydroepiandrosterone (DHEA). However, in prepubertal patients, 17β-estradiol was undetectable, and the concentration of the sulfated conjugate of DHEA was significantly less than in controls. Testosterone was lower in the synovial fluid than in matched serum; patients with the lowest synovial fluid levels were those with disease of the longest duration. Therefore, low androgen levels may contribute to pathogenesis because they exert a protective effect against cartilage degradation.[188]

A number of studies have identified an interesting association of elevated serum prolactin levels in chronic arthritis and in systemic lupus erythematosus (SLE) (see Chapter 21). Prolactin is produced by cells of the anterior pituitary and other cells, including lymphocytes; in addition to its endocrine effects, prolactin enhances cell proliferation and survival.[189] Levels were increased in children with chronic arthritis and antinuclear antibody (ANA) seropositivity.[185,190,191] The prolactin concentration correlated with levels of IL-6 and with a chronic course of the disease. Both glucocorticoids and hydroxychloroquine inhibit prolactin secretion.[186]

Infection

That infections can cause arthritis in children is not in doubt. Arthritis after viral infections is probably common, although it is usually self-limited. The subject of infection and arthritis is thoroughly reviewed in Chapters 37-40.

Postvaccination arthritis has been described after routine immunizations,[192] and after measles-mumps-rubella vaccine, a chronic arthropathy was documented in one study, predominantly in females.[193]

Arthritis in children has also been linked to perinatal infection with the influenza virus A2H2N2.[194,195] This unique epidemiological study raised the possibility of delayed expression of disease resulting from a presumed intrauterine or neonatal viral infection. A tenuous link between chronic arthritis and parvovirus B19 has also been noted.[196-199] Parvovirus DNA was found in 48% of children with arthritis, but not in controls, although IgG antibodies were found in both groups, suggesting a possible role of *persistent* virus in pathogenesis of arthritis.[200] In another study, IgM antibodies to parvovirus B19 were demonstrated in significantly more children with arthritis, compared with those with acute self-limited arthritis or in a healthy control population.[199] Chronic arthritis (especially RF-negative polyarthritis, spondyloarthritis, and oligoarthritis) has been described in children with human immunodeficiency virus infections.[201] The cyclical pattern of incidence of chronic arthritis documented from 1979 to 1992 in Manitoba by Oen and colleagues[55] correlated with the occurrence of infections to *Mycoplasma pneumoniae*.

Humoral and cellular immune responses to highly conserved bacterial HSPs are present in children with chronic arthritis.[202-208] HSPs have been demonstrated in the serum and synovial fluid.[205,207,208] Van Eden and colleagues[209] postulated that reactive T cells are part of the normal immune repertoire for TCR V-gene products; self-HSPs and bacterial HSPs may trigger this response. In 13 of 15 children with oligoarthritis, T-lymphocyte proliferative responses to HSP 60 were detected an average of 12 weeks before remission of the inflammatory disease.[205,210] Spontaneous remission was characterized by CD30+ T cells directed to HSP 60.[211] Albani and associates[208,212] demonstrated immune responses to the dnaJ HSP from *Escherichia coli*, especially in children with polyarticular disease. This protein has five amino acids that are homologous with those in the binding groove of DRB1, which in itself is increased in frequency in these children. Therefore, molecular mimicry may play a role in pathogenesis.[213-215] Despite this circumstantial evidence, a direct link between infection and chronic childhood arthritis has remained elusive.

Psychological Factors

It is well documented that psychological stress is particularly common in families of children with arthritis.[215,216] Psychological factors inherent in the family and child affect their adaptation to chronic illness but are unlikely to have played a role in the causation of the disease. Some studies suggest that susceptibility to arthritis is associated with dysregulation of the autonomic nervous system that leads to lack of an appropriate response of the child's immune system to stimuli[217] and may be influenced by neuroendocrine gene polymorphisms.[218]

Physical Trauma

Chronic arthritis has been reported by parents to follow minor physical trauma to an extremity. Such trauma may serve as a localizing factor, or it may simply call attention to an already inflamed and weakened joint. Benign hypermobility and the rare syndrome of congenital insensitivity to pain are both associated with trauma and may predispose to joint inflammation. The fact that certain joints (e.g., the knee) are frequently affected could be interpreted to suggest that trauma associated with

weight-bearing in the young child is a factor in initiating chronic inflammation.

Animal Models of Inflammatory Joint Disease

The study of animal models of human disease provides clues about etiology, but these models are, at best, approximations of human disease. Fundamental differences in etiology and pathogenesis almost certainly exist and may be difficult to recognize. In spite of these limitations, and because of the obvious difficulties involved in direct study of human rheumatic diseases, various spontaneous and induced models of disease in animals have been the focus of a number of studies and may be relevant to human diseases.

Adjuvant Disease

Intradermal injection of complete Freund adjuvant (mineral oil, detergent, and *Mycobacterium butyricum*) into the footpad of susceptible strains of rats results in the development of a chronic polyarthritis, sometimes accompanied by lesions of the skin and auricular cartilages and an anterior uveitis.[91,219,220] This disease is adoptively transferable by T lymphocytes, and the model may be manipulated by T-cell clones capable of inducing, preventing, or ameliorating the disease.[221,222] Antibody appears to have no significant role in pathogenesis. The course of adjuvant arthritis may be intermittent or chronic, resulting in tissue destruction with calcification and ankylosis of joints. The arthritogenic component of the adjuvant is a peptidoglycan dimer, muramyl dipeptide.[223]

Polyarthritis Induced by Type II Collagen

Native type II collagen in incomplete Freund adjuvant induces chronic polyarthritis in certain strains of rats and mice.[224,225] The disease can be passively transferred with specific antibody to type II collagen,[225] although cell-mediated immunity is also important[226]

Arthritis Induced by Infectious Agents

Erysipelothrix rhusiopathiae and *Mycoplasma* are each capable of inducing arthritis in domestic pigs,[227] and *Mycoplasma* species are arthritogenic in many other species, including the rabbit, cow, goat, sheep, mouse, chicken, and turkey.[228] Spontaneous infection with *Chlamydia psittaci* causes polyarthritis in lambs.[229] Reovirus causes synovitis in chicks.[230] Caprine arthritis is caused by infection with a retrovirus.[231]

A disease resembling rheumatoid arthritis spontaneously occurs in dogs[232] and MRL/l mice.[233]

Transgenic Mice

The NSE/hIL-6 transgenic mouse overexpresses IL-6 and is characterized by stunted growth.[234] Levels of insulinlike growth factor (IGF)–binding protein 3 are decreased and result in a decreased association of IGF-I in the 150-kD ternary complex secondary to increased clearance of the IGF-I. The TNF-α-transgenic mouse has been studied for the development of bone disease[235] and arthritis.[236]

GENETIC BACKGROUND

Familial Chronic Arthritis in Children

Familial chronic arthritis is uncommon, and multigeneration cases are rarely recognized. Over a 10-year period, an American registry identified 200 sets of siblings with JRA, of whom 21 are twins (13 identical).[237] The sibling recurrence risk (λs) has been estimated at 15.[238] Within any one family, arthritis tends to have the same type of onset, and even the same complication of uveitis.[239] An examination of time of onset of arthritis in families in which two or more children were affected indicated that the interval between onset of arthritis in each pair of siblings varied from 7 months to 11 years. In no instance was disease onset simultaneous, although in most cases the ages at onset were similar. There is no association between birth order and the development of arthritis.[240]

The development of chronic arthritis in twins has been extensively studied.[238,240-243] A concordance rate of 44% was reported in identical twins and one of 4% in dizygotic twins.[244] Studies by Clemens and associates[245] of more than 2000 children with JCA documented a remarkable concordance between siblings for onset of disease, clinical manifestations, and disease course. Ten of 12 sibling pairs who were concordant for type of onset shared two DR antigens; the other two pairs shared one HLA-DR antigen.

A multicenter study reconfirmed these findings in 71 sibling pairs, and in 3 siblings in 3 families, all of whom had chronic arthritis; 94% of these children were white.[238] The mean interval between onset of disease in the siblings was 4.4 years (standard deviation [SD], 4.2 years). More than three-quarters were concordant for onset type, and 79% were concordant for disease course. Among seven sets of twins, the interval between disease onset was shorter (3.3 months), and all were concordant for onset type (6 oligoarthritis, 1 polyarthritis) and course subtype. Uveitis was concordant in only 3 of 16 sibling pairs. There is also an increased prevalence of autoimmunity in these families with JRA.[246] Chronic inflammatory rheumatic diseases are more common in parents of multiple offspring affected by chronic arthritis.[247]

One further association bears attention: the occurrence of JIA and adult RA in the same family. Documentation of this event is scant, and it must be concluded that JIA and RA uncommonly occur in the same family, which is consistent with their different HLA associations. However, Rossen and colleagues[248] studied four families with multiple cases of JRA and RA and concluded from histocompatibility data that susceptibility to arthritis was influenced by a dominant allele with variable penetrance and expressivity. An increased frequency of autoantibodies has been documented in first-degree relatives of children with chronic arthritis.[249]

Genes Associated with Increased Risk of Chronic Childhood Arthritis

The genetic basis is complex and incompletely understood. Possible genetic associations have been reviewed by Phelan and colleagues.[237] It appears that there are at least three well-established genetic risk factors: HLA Class I and Class II genes, the PTPN22 gene, and the IL2RA/CD 25 gene.

Human Leukocyte Antigen Relationships

These complex interactions and age- and sex-specific windows of susceptibility and protection of HLA genes were examined by Murray and colleagues.[250] As an illustration, the population distribution for HLA-DR4 in relation to age at disease onset and sex is depicted in Figure 13–1.

Associations with Class I Antigens

An increased frequency of A2, B27, and B35 alleles has been documented.[250-254] A2 is associated predominantly with early-onset oligoarticular disease in girls.[252] HLA-B27 may confer an age-related risk to oligoarthritis in boys (50% risk at 7.3 years; 80% risk at 11.9 years)[250] and is clearly associated with enthesitis-related arthritis.

Associations with Class II Antigens

Class II genetic associations are more numerous and complex in relation to specific onset types and course subtypes than are the few documented class I specificities.[255] These associations are most obvious in early-onset oligoarthritis (DR 5 and 8) and in RF-seropositive polyarthritis (DR 4). They are more heterogeneous in RF-seronegative polyarthritis and systemic disease.

In addition, an increased frequency of certain class III MHC genes may contribute to susceptibility in some populations[251] but not in others.[256,257]

Associations with Protein Tyrosine Phosphatase N22 (PTPN22)

A missense single nucleotide polymorphism (rs2476601) in the PTPN22 gene has been associated with JIA. The PTPN22*T allele occurred in 15% of JIA patients, compared to 10.3% of controls.[258] The association was strongest with the RF-negative polyarthritis subgroup. The allele was also increased in the oligoarthritis persistent and extended groups but not in the systemic onset group. It has been postulated that the T allele of PTPN22 is associated with decreased ability to downregulate T-lymphocyte activity. This association has also been found in adult rheumatoid arthritis, SLE, and diabetes mellitus.[258]

Association with the Interleukin 2 Receptor Alpha (IL2A/CD25)

Hinks, Ke, and Barton[259] have recently described a strong association of JIA with the rs2104286 polymorphism of the receptor for IL 2, expressed by regulatory T cells and thought to have an important role in the development of autoimmunity. This polymorphism was increased in children with the oligoarthritis subsets, particularly in girls and in ANA-positive patients.

Other Genetic Associations

A number of non-HLA genes, on chromosome 6 or on other chromosomes, may be important in a predisposition to chronic arthritis or in its pathogenesis.[260] A weak

HLA-DR4

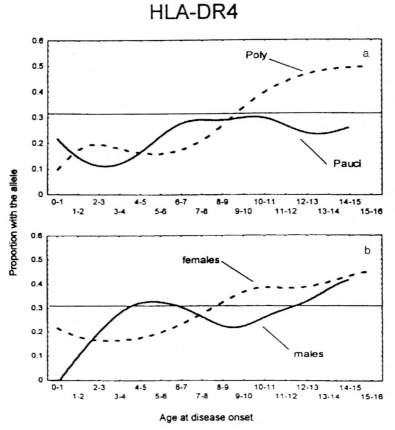

FIGURE 13–1 Proportion of the study population, by disease-onset type (*A*) and by sex (*B*), in each age-at-onset category with the HLA-DR4 allele. The *horizontal line* represents the frequency of the allele in the control group. Pauci, pauciarticular; Polyarticular. (From Murray KJ, Moroldo MB, Donnelly P, et al: Age-specific effects of juvenile rheumatoid arthritis-associated HLA alleles. Arthritis Rheum. 42: 1843-1853, 1999, Copyright © 1999. Wiley-Liss, Inc. Reprinted by permission of Wiley-Liss, Inc., a subsidiary of John Wiley & sons, Inc.)

association with TAP 2B, a polymorphism in a member of the adenosine triphosphate–binding cassette superfamily, is present for early-onset disease.[261] TAP1B may function as an additive susceptibility factor.[262] Interaction with other non-HLA genes such as IL-1A2, a variant of the IL-1α gene, is also possible in early-onset oligoarthritis.[263] The gene for IL-1α, or a gene for which its polymorphism is a marker, may also contribute risk for early-onset disease and uveitis.[263,264] One study suggested that homozygosity of the B allele of the large multifunctional protease 2 (LMP2) proteasome subunit may increase susceptibility to a putative subtype of chronic arthritis that is associated with B27.[265] Associations have also been reported for the LMP7 gene.[266] Polymorphism in the osteoprotegerin gene may correlate with articular erosions and low bone mass (see Chapter 49).[267]

Associations with Other Autoimmune Diseases and Chromosomal Abnormalities

There may also be an association of the various types of onset with genetic and chromosomal abnormalities[268] and with other autoimmune diseases. Most frequently reported is insulin-dependent diabetes mellitus.[269,270] In a referral diabetic clinic population of 200 children, 6 had polyarticular disease and 1 had probable early JAS.[269] A syndrome that includes flexion contractures, short

stature, and skin changes, the so-called Rosenbloom syndrome, may complicate diabetes mellitus and should not be confused with inflammatory joint disease (see Chapter 41). Myasthenia gravis was reported in four children with chronic arthritis.[271] Autoimmune neuromyotonia has also been noted. Autoimmune thyroiditis has also been reported.[272]

Other non-HLA genetic associations have been suggested that might increase a predisposition to disease. Chronic arthritis has been observed in patients with IgA deficiency and with deletion of the short arm of chromosome 18.[273] The phenotypic profile of the chromosome translocation in the velocardiofacial syndrome—del(22q11.2)—includes chronic destructive arthritis, normal numbers of T lymphocytes, and normal or elevated serum immunoglobulins.[274] Turner syndrome has also been identified in a number of patients.[275] In a study of this association,[276] 18 of approximately 500 children with JRA were found to have Turner syndrome. Polyarticular disease was present in 7 who had progressive seronegative arthritis and a 45 XO genotype. It is not entirely clear whether the arthropathy of Down syndrome differs from idiopathic chronic arthritis.[268] In children with Down syndrome and arthritis, the joint disease has often been indistinguishable from polyarticular disease. In some children, the arthritis is more like psoriatic arthritis; and psoriasis is seemingly increased in frequency in trisomy 21. Polyarthritis was reported in a child with partial trisomy 5q, monosomy 2p.[268]

CLINICAL MANIFESTATIONS

Constitutional Signs and Symptoms

Anorexia, weight loss, and growth failure occur in many children. Significant fatigue is rarely a feature of limited articular disease, but it is a common symptom in children with polyarticular or systemic disease, especially at onset and during periods of poor disease control. It may be expressed as an increased sleep requirement, lack of energy, or increased irritability. Night pain may interrupt sleep and contribute to fatigue. Sleep fragmentation may also exacerbate pain as well as fatigue in these children.[277-279] In a recent study, however, Ward and colleagues[280] could not demonstrate a difference between children with arthritis and healthy subjects with respect to sleep characteristics.

Pain and Stiffness

Aspects of pain in children with arthritis have been reviewed by Anthony and Schanberg.[281] It is the rare child who has no pain in the presence of active arthritis. Although a child with chronic arthritis may not complain of pain at rest,[282,283] active or passive motion of a joint elicits pain in the inflamed joint, particularly at the extremes of the range of motion. Pain is usually described as aching or stretching and is of mild-to-moderate severity. In contrast, children with pain-amplification syndromes almost always describe pain as extremely severe (see Chapter 48). Pain elicited by pressure (tenderness) is usually maximal at the joint line, over hypertrophied, inflamed synovium, or at entheses. Bone pain or tenderness is not characteristic of arthritis, and its presence should alert the examiner to the possibility of a malignancy or infection involving bone.[284]

The manner in which a child communicates discomfort or dysfunction varies with developmental stage. The young child may not complain of pain but may alter the manner in which the affected joint is used, assume a posture of guarding the joints, or entirely refuse to use a limb in order to avoid pain. Their expression of pain is thereby physical rather than vocal. In such circumstances, parents report that the child does not appear to be in pain but that he or she limps or reverts to more infantile patterns of movement.

The experience of pain is influenced by many factors, including disease activity, age, sex, pain threshold, family pain culture, and coping strategies. Pain is usually an indicator of the presence of active disease. Ilowite and colleagues determined, however, that disease activity accounted for only 10% of the variance in reported pain scores.[285] The pain threshold, as measured by cold pressor tests, was found to be lower in children with JIA than in controls.[286] The influences of sex and age on pain perception are unclear. Some studies detected no age-related differences in reporting of pain.[287,288] In others, younger children with limited joint disease complained of the most

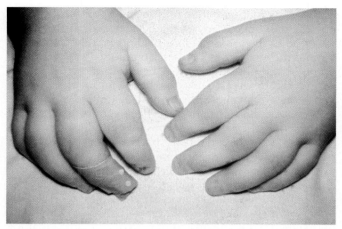

FIGURE 13–2 The joints of the wrists and hands of a 2½-year-old boy with systemic-onset disease are swollen, warm, and painful. The proximal and distal interphalangeal joints are erythematous. There are flexion contractures of the fingers.

severe pain,[289,290] whereas in other studies[282,283] older children reported more pain.

Using a visual analogue scale, Varni and colleagues[291] confirmed that reports of pain by children as young as 5 years of age correlated well with reports made by parents and physicians. It therefore seems reasonable to conclude that children with arthritis experience as much pain as adults when that pain is accurately evaluated in relation to developmental stage.

Both acute and chronic pain in children are often underappreciated and therefore undertreated. Children with chronic arthritis reported pain as a major symptom that affected their daily activities.[282] Pain may be an important component of functional disability. It may limit school attendance, physical activity, and social interactions.[292] Psychological factors in children and their families may significantly affect functioning. Emotional distress in the child and in the mother, as well as the level of family harmony, correlate with a higher degree of reported pain in the child.[293]

Joint stiffness, particularly on arising or after prolonged inactivity, may be described by the child. More often, however, evidence of stiffness is provided by the parent, who describes slowness or awkwardness of the gait, most marked in the morning, which improves with activity or the application of heat to the affected area. The duration of morning stiffness may be an indicator of the degree of joint inflammation. Stiffness lasting less than 5 minutes is of doubtful significance; stiffness lasting more than 30 minutes signifies a considerable level of joint inflammation. The pathophysiology of joint stiffness is unclear.

Characteristics of the Inflamed Joint

The actively inflamed joint exhibits the cardinal signs of inflammation: swelling, pain, heat, loss of function, and sometimes erythema (Figure 13–2).

Swelling of a joint may result from periarticular soft tissue edema, from intraarticular effusion, or from hypertrophy of the synovial membrane. Effusion and hypertrophy of the synovial membrane are common, whereas in arthritis accompanying diseases such as Henoch-Schönlein purpura, periarticular swelling is more prominent. Evidence of increased intraarticular fluid is obtained by visual inspection. Small outpouchings of synovium are not uncommon and are particularly evident at the extensor hood of the proximal interphalangeal (PIP) joints and around the wrist or ankle. Less commonly, synovial cysts occur in the antecubital area or anterior to the shoulder[294] (Figure 13–3). They may be the initial or sole manifestation of chronic arthritis and, if unilateral, may be misinterpreted as a tumor or as deep venous thrombosis. Large synovial cysts are an unusual complication. These may occur in the popliteal space (Baker cyst) (Figure 13–4), rupture into adjacent muscles, and dissect into the calf.[295] This event is characterized by sudden sharp pain and swelling in the calf, followed by crescentic ecchymoses about the malleoli. A normal child may occasionally develop a transient popliteal cyst.[296] Ultrasound imaging, or magnetic resonance imaging (MRI) aids in making the correct diagnosis. In the knee, excess intraarticular fluid can be demonstrated by an increased patellar tap or the presence of a bulge sign. The presence of fine synovial crepitus on movement of the joint through range of motion signifies, in addition, the presence of synovial hypertrophy.

Inflamed joints are often warm but usually not erythematous. In contrast, the joint may be erythematous in septic arthritis or acute rheumatic fever and in some of the other reactive arthritides.

Inflamed joints usually lose range of motion, particularly in extension, although to some extent this depends on which joint is involved. Hyperextension is characteristically the first range to be lost in the cervical spine. Elbows, wrists, metacarpophalangeal and interphalangeal joints usually lose range in extension or hyperextension first, but flexion range is also often diminished. The hallmark of intraarticular hip joint disease is loss of internal rotation. There is loss of hyperextension or extension, and sometimes flexion in the knees. Loss of ankle dorsiflexion, subtalar eversion, and midfoot supination are characteristic. Loss of dorsiflexion of the first metatarsophalangeal joint may be of considerable functional significance.

The Pediatric Gait, Arms, Legs, Spine screen is an excellent tool for the quick evaluation of the child for evidence of musculoskeletal disease. It is most applicable for use by the general physician or pediatrician and does not include the detailed examination that a pediatric rheumatologist would perform.[297]

Distribution of Affected Joints

Any joint may be affected, but large joints are most frequently involved. Small joints of the hands and feet may also be affected, particularly in polyarticular-onset disease. Attention must also be directed to the temporomandibular joint (TMJ) and to the cervical, thoracic, and lumbosacral spine. Disease in the apophyseal joints of the cervical spine occurs at onset in approximately 2% of children and may present as a torticollis.[298] Approximately 60% eventually develop involvement of this area of the axial skeleton. Subluxation of the atlantoaxial joints may occur early, rendering the child at risk for injury in an accident or with attempted intubation before general anesthesia. The sternoclavicular, acromioclavicular, and sternomanubrial joints are infrequently affected. Cricoarytenoid arthritis is unusual but may be responsible for acute airway obstruction.[299] Inflammation of the synovial joints of the middle ear, the incudomalleal and incudostapedial articulations, is rarely appreciated

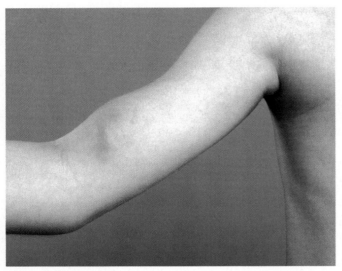

FIGURE 13–3   Brachial synovial cyst. A 6-year-old girl developed this dissecting cyst of her right arm as the first manifestation of chronic arthritis. Later, bilateral effusions developed in both knees.

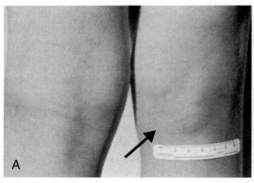
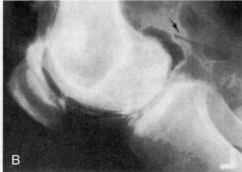

FIGURE 13–4   A, Popliteal cyst or Baker cyst. The cyst was associated with pain at the back of the knee, was somewhat tender, and transilluminated. Aspiration yielded clear yellow fluid of low inflammatory activity. **B,** Arthrogram of a popliteal cyst, with contrast medium outlining the communication *(arrow)* between the synovial space and this dissecting cyst in an 18-year-old boy who had had arthritis since the age of 9 years.

clinically. Tympanometric studies, however, have indicated that subclinical disease may be present in almost two-thirds of children with JRA.[300]

Patterns of joint involvement are often quite characteristic. Thus, symmetrical involvement of large and small joints is typical of RF-positive or RF-negative polyarticular disease. Arthritis predominantly affecting the joints of the lower extremity characterizes ERA and oligoarticular JIA. The presence of hip joint disease rarely occurs in oligoarticular JIA but is not uncommon in ERA. Psoriatic arthritis tends to be somewhat asymmetrical and involves both large and small joints, sometimes including the distal interphalangeal joints.

Tenosynovitis

Tenosynovitis is quite common, but it is generally not a striking or isolated clinical complaint. The most common sites are the extensor tendon sheaths on the dorsum of the hand, the extensor sheaths over the dorsum of the foot, and those of the posterior tibial tendon and the peroneus longus and brevis tendons around the ankle. Triggering or loss of extension of the fingers may result from a stenosing synovitis of the flexor tendon sheaths. Clinically recognized carpal tunnel syndrome is uncommon in children with involvement of the wrists. Tenosynovitis of the superior oblique tendon of the eye may cause pain on upward gaze, sometimes with diplopia, the so-called Brown syndrome.[301,302]

Extraarticular Manifestations

Generalized Abnormalities of Growth and Development

Abnormalities of physical growth and development may complicate chronic arthritis. Linear growth is retarded during periods of active systemic disease.[303] With better disease control, attainable through the use of methotrexate and the biologicals, severe growth retardation is increasingly uncommon.

In a 1987 study of 56 children between the ages of 4 and 18 years who had JRA for more than 1 year, Bacon and White[304] found that the mean height for age was below the 35th percentile for children with polyarticular or systemic-onset disease. Mean weight for age and weight per height were significantly diminished in those with polyarticular disease. In a study published in 1990 of adults who had had arthritis as children, Lovell and colleagues[305] documented growth retardation (height less than 5th percentile) in 50% of children with systemic onset, 11% of those with oligoarticular onset, and 16% of those with polyarticular onset. Glucocorticoid therapy could only partly explain these observations. In a more recent study (2003), a marked decrease in height velocity (–2 SD) was observed in 56% of children with systemic arthritis.[306] In this study, growth retardation was associated with glucocorticoid administration, nutritional status, bone mineral density, and early disease onset. Each of these studies reflects the effect of disease in a population treated in the pre-methotrexate, pre-biologicals era and is an important reminder of the potentially devastating effects of untreated or undertreated JIA on normal growth and development. It is clear that growth suppression is much less severe in contemporary populations of children with arthritis.

The mechanisms of growth suppression in JIA are being elucidated. High levels of proinflammatory cytokines, such as IL6, IL1β, and TNFa, seen in children with active arthritis directly or indirectly influence growth plate chondrocytes and linear bone growth.[307] Levels of growth hormone and IGF-I and -II may be impaired.[308] IGF-I was inversely correlated with IL-6 levels in children with systemic disease.[309]

Localized Growth Disturbances

Localized growth disturbances result from accelerated development of ossification centers of the long bones of an inflamed joint or premature fusion of the physis. During early active disease, development of the ossification centers is accelerated, apparently related to the hyperemia of inflammation and local production of growth factors. The result may be either overgrowth of the affected limb or, ultimately (though much less commonly) premature fusion of the involved epiphyses, resulting in diminished length.

Arthritis of the lower limb, especially of the knee, frequently causes accelerated growth and epiphyseal maturation. If this occurs in one knee only, a discrepancy of leg lengths results. A difference of greater than 1 cm is probably significant, and differences of 5 cm or more occasionally occur. Apparent leg-length inequality may also result from pelvic rotation and scoliosis. As the child grows, inequalities of minimal to moderate degree may disappear, but they persist in up to two-thirds of these children. Whether the long-term result is shortening or lengthening of the affected limb appears to depend considerably on the age of the child—or, more precisely, on the degree of maturation of the skeleton—at the time of the inflammatory insult. If the child is very young and the potential for growth is considerable, the affected limb tends to grow longer. If the disease occurs shortly before the physis would be expected to fuse, shortening of the affected limb is more likely. Significant leg length inequality was reported to occur much less frequently in a setting in which intraarticular corticosteroids were used to treat inflammation.[310]

Micrognathia is a striking example of localized growth retardation (Figure 13–5). Marked alterations of facial morphology (e.g., micrognathia, retrognathia) may result. In a Swedish survey of 70 children, 56% had symptoms (crepitus, pain, difficulty opening the mouth) and 41% had radiographic evidence of TMJ pathology attributable to arthritis.[311] In one patient, the disease began in a TMJ. Another study corroborated the frequency (50%) of TMJ abnormalities and alterations in mandibular growth.[312] Extreme micrognathia is most likely to occur if arthritis begins before 4 years of age.

The mandible ossifies by intramembranous bone production. A number of factors contribute to mandibular growth abnormalities. Pain in a TMJ may inhibit normal masseter muscle development, which in turn retards mandibular bone development, resulting in a shortened mandibular ramus and body. Destruction of the condyle

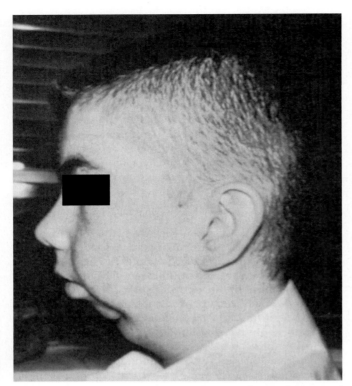

FIGURE 13–5 Arthritis began in this young man at the age of 2 years and pursued an unremitting polyarticular course. Disease of both temporomandibular joints has caused micrognathia and retrognathia with an anterior open underbite.

of the mandible causes further diminution of overall mandibular height. In some children, overgrowth of the condyle may contribute to TMJ dysfunction.[313] Although the stereotypical abnormality is bilateral micrognathia with an anterior open overbite, unilateral TMJ disease is much more common than bilateral disease. It is characterized by mandibular asymmetry; deviation to the affected side on opening of the jaw; difficulty in palpating the affected mandibular condyle; and pain, tenderness, or crepitus of one or both TMJs. In many instances, TMJ arthritis appears to be asymptomatic, although some children report a preference to chew on the unaffected side, experience pain with maximum opening of the mouth, or are aware of clicking or other sounds accompanying movement of the joint. Little is understood about the effect of chronic arthritis on dental caries or periodontal disease.[314]

Sexual Maturation

Puberty and secondary sexual characteristics are often delayed in children with active inflammation.[315] In a group of Italian girls menarche was later than in their mothers or in age-matched normal controls.

Osteopenia

Osteopenia has emerged as a potentially major determinant of functional outcome in young adults who have had chronic arthritis as children.[316-323] Children with chronic arthritis have a diminished bone mass and are at increased risk for fractures in adulthood and for an earlier onset of

osteoporosis.[324-326] An important determinant of future fracture risk is the peak bone mass achieved at the end of skeletal maturation, which is almost complete by the late years of adolescence. Genetic polymorphisms of the vitamin D and calcitonin receptors[327] and the osteoprotegerin gene[267] may play a role in the development of low bone mass. These interrelationships are discussed in Chapter 49.

Fitness

There persists a widespread but unsubstantiated assumption that physical activity in children with arthritis should be limited. Children with arthritis tend to be less physically active than their peers. Lelieveld and colleagues[328] documented limited physical activity in adolescents with JIA compared to their peers, as measured by a 3-day activity diary. Takken and colleagues[329] noted reduced maximal oxygen consumption in children with JIA compared with controls. Lilieveld concluded that adolescents with arthritis had low aerobic and anaerobic fitness levels.[328]

Skin and Subcutaneous Tissue

The classic rash of systemic-onset disease is discussed in Chapter 14. A second cutaneous change, occurring particularly in children with involvement of the hands, is a dark discoloration of the skin over the PIP joints.[330] The presence of this finding may reflect disease chronicity. In children with tender joints, retention keratosis may simulate a pigmented lesion and reflects inability to perform adequate self-care. Nodules occur in a variety of rheumatic diseases in children. Subcutaneous rheumatoid nodules occur in 5% to 10% of children with chronic arthritis, almost always confined to those with polyarthritis (see Chapter 15). Tendon-associated nodules may reflect tenosynovitis, especially in the flexor tendons of the fingers.

Asymmetrical lymphedema of the subcutaneous tissues of one or more extremities has been documented in several children with arthritis.[331-333] The swelling is usually painless and may be somewhat pitting. The cause is unknown, except for its unclarified relationship to inflammation, but does not seem to be related to local obstruction caused by joint swelling. The course is chronic but may improve over several years. Treatment includes the use of pressure stockings or gloves.

Cutaneous vasculitis is very rare and occurs most often in the older child with RF-positive polyarthritis. This type of vessel involvement must be distinguished from benign digital perivasculitis (Figure 13–6), which is more frequent, and may occasionally be associated with vascular calcification seen on radiographs along the course of the digital arteries. The occurrence of Raynaud phenomenon is generally indicative of a connective tissue disease rather than chronic arthritis.

Pityriasis lichenoides et varioliformis acuta (Mucha-Habermann disease) has been recorded in a few children with JRA,[334,335] and may be entirely coincidental.

Muscle Disease

Atrophy and weakness of muscles around inflamed joints is characteristic and is often accompanied by a shortening of the muscles and tendons that results in flexion contractures. Marked atrophy of the vastus medialis muscle

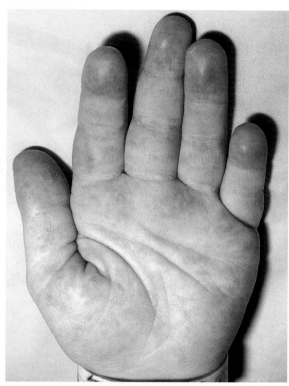

FIGURE 13–6 Punctate erythema of the palms and finger pads was the sole manifestation of benign perivasculitis in this 5-year-old girl with chronic arthritis. The lesions were not raised or tender and disappeared after treatment with nonsteroidal antiinflammatory drugs.

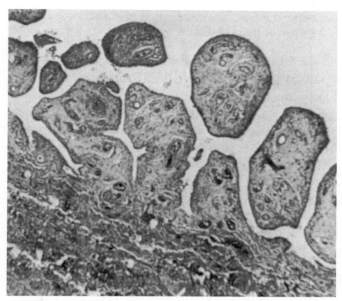

FIGURE 13–7 Photomicrograph of synovial tissue from the knee of a young boy with arthritis. Villous hyperplasia and hypertrophy, edema, proliferation of new blood vessels, and infiltration by mononuclear cells are prominent.

is characteristic of arthritis in the knee. The calf muscles become atrophic when the ankle joint is involved. Sacroiliitis may be associated with severe atrophy of the gluteus maximus and thigh muscles. A nonspecific myositis may account for some of the associated fatigue and muscle weakness. It does not have a characteristic distribution, and histopathological studies are sparse. Data from adults with RA suggest that it is characterized by a perivasculitis and lymphocytic infiltrates (lymphorrhages). Serum levels of muscle enzymes are not increased. A few children with widespread, prolonged, active arthritis develop progressive muscle atrophy that is most severe and persistent if it occurs before 3 years of age.[336]

Characteristic involvement of other systems is generally specific to each subtype of disease and is discussed in those chapters.

PATHOLOGY

The histopathological features of chronic arthritis in children are similar to those described in RA. There is villous hypertrophy and hyperplasia of the synovial lining layer (Figure 13–7). The subsynovial tissues are hyperemic, edematous, and infiltrated with lymphocytes and plasma cells. Vascular endothelial hyperplasia is often prominent. There is a selective accumulation in the synovium of activated T cells, which are clustered around antigen-presenting dendritic cells. Fibrin may be layered onto the superficial surface of the synovium or incorporated

within it. An exuberant synovitis eventually results in progressive erosion and destruction of articular cartilage and, later, of contiguous bone with pannus formation. Rheumatoid nodules and necrotizing vasculitis are rarely, if ever, present in synovial tissue from children with chronic arthritis.

In RA, the primary infiltrating cell is the T lymphocyte, which may be distributed diffusely throughout the synovium or form nodules or germinal centers. CD4+ helper-inducer T cells and CD8+ suppressor-cytotoxic T cells may be present. In addition, macrophages and dendritic cells abound in mature synovitis. In late disease, B lymphocytes and plasma cells producing RF can be demonstrated. Multinucleated giant cells and mast cells are also present. Hyperplasia of synovial lining cells, fibroblasts, and blood vessels leads to the development of papillary fronds. Extension of the inflammatory granulation tissue or pannus that spreads from the synovium and invades the cartilage and bone results in osteolysis, which is visible radiographically as erosion and subchondral cyst formation. Erosions occur preferentially in the "bare" areas of the joint, where bone is not covered by articular cartilage (see Chapter 2). They are irregular but sharply defined. Dissolution of the cartilage (chondrolysis) results from enzymatic digestion by neutral proteases, cathepsin, and collagenase from phagocytic cells of the pannus. Immune complexes may also contribute to chondrolysis. Metaplasia of the granulation tissue may result in the formation of new cartilage, bone, or fibrous tissue, leading to ankylosis. End-stage disease is characterized by deformity, subluxation, and fibrous or bony ankylosis.

Joint destruction usually occurs later in the disease course in childhood than in adulthood, and permanent joint damage is absent in many children even after years of chronic inflammation. Newer studies with MRI are likely to revise the impression of the extent of joint damage in early disease. The greater thickness of juvenile cartilage may offer some protection in this regard. The hyaline cartilage of the hip is destroyed in progressive stages during the course of severe disease, and during healing it may be replaced by a fibrocartilaginous layer. Rice bodies may be present and consist primarily of amorphous fibrous material, fibrin, and small amounts of collagen. Viable cells are incorporated within this matrix and appear more normal than the synovial cells of the inflammatory foci. The majority of these cells resemble type B synovial lining cells, although a few type A cells are also visible. Residual blood vessels in some of these bodies attest to their former attachment to the synovial membrane.

The characteristic rash of systemic disease is characterized by minimal perivascular infiltration of mononuclear cells around capillaries and venules in the subdermal tissues. A neutrophilic perivasculitis resembling that of the rash of rheumatic fever may accompany the more flagrant lesions.

Subcutaneous nodules may be histopathologically typical of rheumatoid nodules, or they may have a looser connective tissue framework resembling that of the nodules of rheumatic fever (see Chapter 40). Classic rheumatoid nodules consist of three distinct zones: a central area of necrosis and granulation tissue, surrounded by a radially arranged palisade of connective tissue cells that, in turn, is enveloped by chronic inflammatory cells. In children, the central area of fibrinoid necrosis and the epithelioid palisades may be absent or less structured.

The serosal lining surfaces of the pleural, pericardial, and peritoneal cavities of the body may exhibit a nonspecific fibrous serositis that is characterized clinically by effusion and pain. Enlargement of the lymph nodes is related to a nonspecific follicular hyperplasia that in rare instances may closely resemble lymphoma. Hepatic abnormalities are characterized by a nonspecific collection of periportal inflammatory cells and hyperplasia of Kupffer cells.

Kruithoff et al. have compared the synovial histopathology in adult rheumatoid arthritis with juvenile spondyloarthropathies, juvenile oligoarthritis, and juvenile polyarthritis.[337] There was broad overlap among these disease categories with the exception of hypervascularity, which was less pronounced in juvenile polyarthritis. The three subtypes displayed the same pronounced lining layer hyperplasia and marked inflammatory cell infiltration with a mixed population of lymphocytes and macrophages. Whereas differences did not reach significance when each group was compared separately, the inflammatory cell infiltration tended to be higher than in adult arthritis and was frequently characterized by numerous plasma cells and the presence of lymphoid aggregates.

LABORATORY EXAMINATION

Although the laboratory may provide support for a diagnosis of chronic arthritis, no laboratory test or combination of studies can confirm the diagnosis. The laboratory can be used to provide evidence of inflammation, to support the clinical diagnosis, to monitor toxicity of therapy, and as a research tool to understand more completely the pathogenesis of the disease.

Hematological Indices

Hematological abnormalities reflect, in a general way, the extent of the inflammatory disease. Children with limited joint disease seldom exhibit any hematological aberrations beyond that of mild anemia. Those with moderately extensive arthritis usually have a normocytic hypochromic anemia. The anemia may be moderately severe with a hemoglobin in the range of 7 to 10 g/dL (70 to 100 g/L) in children with severe, uncontrolled disease. Although the anemia is attributable to chronic disease (low serum iron, low total iron-binding capacity, adequate hemosiderin stores),[338] iron deficiency may also play a role. Plasma iron transport and iron available for erythropoiesis are reduced in systemic disease.

Leukocytosis is common in children with active disease, and leukocyte counts are strikingly high, 30,000 to 50,000 cells/mm^3 (30 to 50 × 10^9/L), in children with systemic-onset disease. Polymorphonuclear leukocytes predominate. The platelet count may rise dramatically in severe involvement; in disease of long standing, thrombocytosis may signal an exacerbation. Thrombocytopenia is rare and may signal an evolution of the disease into SLE, drug toxicity, or the development of macrophage activation syndrome.

The Acute Phase Response

Elements of the acute phase response are often abnormal. The erythrocyte sedimentation rate (ESR) reflects principally the plasma fibrinogen level and is a useful but not totally reliable measure of active disease at onset and during follow-up of a child with arthritis. It is occasionally helpful in monitoring the therapeutic efficacy of a medication program, although the ESR does not necessarily correlate with the articular response to medications.[339] The C-reactive protein (CRP) level may be a more reliable monitor of the inflammatory response; at least it is less often increased in a child in whom no clinical inflammatory disease can be found.

The third component of complement (C3) is often elevated in the sera of children with active disease, acting as an acute phase protein. The activated form of the molecule (C3d) may be increased as well. This observation indicates that the pathogenesis of arthritis in children may include complement-mediated tissue damage.[340] Immune complexes are present in the sera of some children with systemic-onset disease and polyarthritis[122] and in children who are RF seropositive.[141,341] It has been suggested that children with systemic disease might have a defect in antibody-forming capacity or in macrophage function that results in decreased clearance of circulating immune complexes.

Increases in serum levels of the immunoglobulins are correlated with activity of the disease and reflect the acute-phase response. Extreme hypergammaglobulinemia is present in the sickest children and returns toward normal with clinical improvement.

In one study, 37% of 200 children with JRA had hypergammaglobulinemia, defined as a level of 1.96 SD or higher from normal, in at least one immunoglobulin class.[342] In general, persistent hypergammaglobulinemia was an important hallmark of a deteriorating clinical course and poor therapeutic response. Selective IgA deficiency occurred in 4% of the children with JRA. No relation of immunoglobulin concentrations to age at onset or duration of disease was found. In contrast, another study found normal levels of immunoglobulins in 86% to 94% of children with chronic arthritis.[343] Significantly increased concentrations of IgG, IgA, and complement factor C4 were present in children with active disease, whereas elevated IgM levels were characteristic of the disease itself. Marked increases in low–molecular-weight IgM have been described, presumably reflecting a perturbation of intracellular assembly of subunits.[344]

Autoantibodies

Rheumatoid Factors

Classic IgM RFs were first detected by assays relying on the agglutination of IgG-coated latex particles or human or sheep erythrocytes. Most laboratories now use nephelometry or an enzyme-linked immunosorbent assay. RFs of other immunoglobulin isotypes have been reported, but their significance is uncertain. RFs are unusual in a child younger than 7 years of age and are seldom helpful diagnostically at onset of disease.

The diagnostic importance of RF seropositivity in a child with possible chronic arthritis is mitigated by the frequent occurrence of abnormal titers in the other connective tissue diseases of childhood, especially in SLE, and in apparently healthy children. In a study of the diagnostic utility of RF serology in children,[345] RF tests were as likely to be positive in children with diseases other than chronic arthritis as in that disorder (specificity, 326/332 [98%]; sensitivity, 5/105 [4.8%]). As a diagnostic aid, therefore, tests for RFs are of little utility.

RFs are most common in children with later age at onset and polyarticular disease, and in those who are older, have longer disease duration, have subcutaneous rheumatoid nodules or articular erosions, or are in a poorer functional class. They are especially common in the presence of HLA-Dw4 (DRB1*0401) and Dw14 (DRB1*0404) specificities. These observations suggest that RFs might be a result rather than a determining event in children who go on to experience unremitting, disabling disease during the early adult years.

Anticyclic citrullinated peptide (CCP) antibodies are also found in children with RF-positive polyarthritis.[139] Brunner and Sitzmann[346] reported the results of a study of children with JIA, other autoimmune disorders, and healthy children, and found that the incidence of anti-CCP antibodies was not increased in children with arthritis (4.4%), and when present occurred in children with RF-positive polyarthritis. It does not appear that measurement of anti-CCP antibodies adds appreciably to the diagnosis or management.

In the studies of Moore and associates,[347,348] 68% to 75% of children with JRA had "hidden RFs," defined as IgM 19S antiglobulins detected by acid elution of IgM-containing fractions of serum from a gel filtration column. Hidden RFs were found in 59% of children who lacked classic RFs. Titers correlated with activity of the disease and did not differ significantly between those with polyarticular and oligoarticular disease. These studies have focused on North American and European patients. Somewhat lower frequencies have been noted elsewhere.[341]

Antinuclear Antibodies

Tests for ANAs usually use Hep-2 cell lines as substrate. Titers are usually low to moderate. The most common patterns seen by fluorescence microscopy are homogeneous and speckled. Most ANAs are of the IgG class, although antibodies of the IgM and IgA classes are found. The frequency of ANAs is highest in girls of younger age at onset, especially in those with oligoarticular disease, and lowest in older boys and in those with systemic-onset disease. ANAs reach their highest prevalence (65% to 85%) in children who have oligoarthritis and uveitis.[349,350] Therefore, the presence of ANAs supports the diagnosis and is important in identification of children most at risk for chronic uveitis. Persistent ANA seropositivity occurs in healthy children, and in a small but significant group of children with musculoskeletal complaints in whom no autoimmune or rheumatic disease was found.[351-353] Care must therefore be exercised in interpreting the significance of ANA seropositivity in children who do not have objective evidence of arthritis.

The antigenic specificities of ANAs have not been identified. Evaluation of specificities by Western blot with Hep-2 cell nuclei demonstrated extensive heterogeneity of reactivity.[112] Antibodies to double-stranded DNA and the extractable nuclear antigens are not characteristic of JIA.

Plasma Lipids

Dyslipoproteinemia occurs *de novo* in children with chronic arthritis, separate from the effects of glucocorticoids.[354,355] Tselepis and colleagues[356] reported that 14 patients with active arthritis had lower plasma cholesterol and high-density lipoprotein cholesterol levels and higher triglycerides than controls or comparable children with another disease. Plasma platelet-activating factor (PAF) acetylhydrolase activity was also decreased in parallel with the activity of the disease. These low levels of PAF acetylhydrolase activity may have resulted in a loss of antiinflammatory activity, because PAF is a lipid mediator of inflammation. Gonçalves and colleagues[357] found lower levels of both high-density lipoproteins and triglycerides in JIA patients than in controls.

Some of these changes may reflect the effects of treatment.

Synovial Fluid Analysis

Synovial fluid is usually a group II or inflammatory fluid (Table 13–7). The principal cellular constituents are polymorphonuclear neutrophils and mononuclear cells, including lymphoid dendritic cells The leukocyte count does not always correlate with the degree of clinical activity. Very low counts, such as 600 cells/mm³ (0.6 × 10⁹/L), have been observed in fluid from joints clinically involved by intensely active and symptomatic disease. Conversely, counts in the range of septic arthritis, such as 100,000 cells/mm³ (100 × 10⁹/L), have been described in children with otherwise classic disease. Synovial fluid levels of glucose may be low, as in adult RA. Synovial fluid complement levels are not as uniformly depressed as in adult

Table 13–7

Characteristics of synovial fluid in the rheumatic diseases

Group and Condition	Synovial Complement Findings	Color and Clarity	Viscosity	Mucin Clot	WBC Count	PMN (%)	Miscellaneous
Noninflammatory							
Normal	Normal	Yellow and clear	Very high	Good	<200	<25	
Traumatic arthritis	Normal	Xanthochromic and turbid	High	Fair to good	<2,000	<25	Debris
Osteoarthritis	Normal	Yellow and clear	High	Fair to good	1000	<25	
Inflammatory							
Systemic lupus erythematosus	Low ↓	Yellow and clear	Normal	Normal	5000	10	Lupus erythematosus cells
Rheumatic fever	Normal to High ↑	Yellow and cloudy	↓	Fair	5000	10-50	
Chronic arthritis	Normal to High ↑	Yellow and cloudy	↓	Poor	15,000-20,000	75	
Reactive arthritis	High ↑	Yellow and opaque	↓	Poor	20,000	80	
Pyogenic							
Tuberculous arthritis	Normal to High ↑	Yellow-white and cloudy	↓	Poor	25,000	50-60	Acid-fast bacteria
Septic arthritis	High ↑	Serosanguineous and turbid	↓	Poor	50,000-300,000	>75	Low glucose, bacteria

PMN, polymorphonuclear leukocyte; *WBC,* white blood cell.

disease.[358] Rynes and colleagues[359] found intraarticular activation of the classic, but not the alternative, complement pathway in some children. Complement activation products, however, were not detected in the joint fluid of children with oligoarticular disease in the study by Miller and associates.[360] The concentration of glycosaminoglycans in synovial fluid (hyaluronic acid and chondroitin sulfates) is decreased compared with normal controls, accounting for the low viscosity of inflamed synovial fluid.

TREATMENT

Approach to Management

Although chronic arthritis cannot yet be cured, spontaneous remissions fortunately occur in many children, and, in the interim, disease control is often achievable. The goal of therapy should be to induce disease remission, and in the process to control pain and preserve range of motion, muscle strength, and function; to manage systemic complications; and to facilitate normal nutrition, growth, and physical and psychological development (see Chapter 8) (Table 13–8). Along with advances in therapeutics has come a raised expectation for disease control. An "adequate" response is no longer considered to be acceptable under most circumstances. The possibility of absolute control of inflammation is a goal that should be pursued within the constraints of safety and cost. Although the major focus of medical therapy is on the arthritis, other extraarticular complications

Table 13–8

Objectives of the treatment of chronic arthritis in children

Immediate
Relieve discomfort
Preserve function
Prevent deformities
Control inflammation

Long-term
Achieve disease remission
Minimize side effects of disease and treatment
Promote normal growth and development
Rehabilitate
Educate

(e.g., uveitis, serositis, growth retardation, osteopenia) require consideration.

The treatment program should be family centered, community based, and well coordinated. An ideal approach involves a multidisciplinary team that consists of a pediatric rheumatologist, nurse clinician, social worker, physical therapist, occupational therapist, and psychologist. Consultation with a physiatrist, psychiatrist, orthopaedic surgeon, dentist, or nutritionist is often indicated. Regular ophthalmological consultation is mandatory. Because this rheumatic disorder is characterized by chronic or recurrent inflammation of the joints and varying systemic manifestations, the child and family must accept the need for long-term treatment and surveillance. Patient and family education and incorporation of the family's needs into the management program are essential to facilitate optimal compliance and therapeutic benefit.[361] Most children with chronic arthritis require a combination of pharmacological, physical, and psychosocial approaches. A priority in management is to foster normal psychological and social development and participation in peer-group activities. Regular attendance at school is strongly encouraged; only rarely is home instruction justified. The child should also remain in the physical education program at school (if at all possible), if not as a participant then as an involved member of the class assigned to alternative activities; otherwise, the child should be enrolled in adaptive physical education. Children should largely determine their own level of activity. Inappropriate restriction of recess time or peer-group association can be harmful both physically and psychologically. Participation in recreational activities and camps with other children with arthritis is frequently of benefit. Children who attend camps or activities such as those of the Juvenile Arthritis Alliance (www.arthritis.org) realize that they are not the only ones with arthritis, profit from group educational experiences, and have the opportunity to test their limits in a safe, supportive, and understanding environment. Vocational evaluation and advice is appropriate in the adolescent with arthritis.

For the adolescent patient with ongoing active disease requiring management by a rheumatologist, transition to a team including adult and pediatric rheumatologists, nurses, social workers and therapists is an effective way of ensuring continuing care[362] (see Chapter 9).

Pharmacological Management

The systematic approach to pharmacological treatment is to begin with the safest, simplest, and most conservative measures. If this approach proves inadequate, other therapeutic modalities are promptly selected in an orderly progression. It is now realized that the more rapidly inflammation can be controlled, the less likely it is that there will be permanent sequelae. NSAIDs are the mainstay of initial treatment in approximately 75% of patients. Three developments, however, have fundamentally altered the current therapeutic approach beyond that point: Intraarticular glucocorticoids have proved effective in treating joint disease; low-dose MTX has substantially changed the choice of treatment options; and new therapeutic modalities such as the anti-TNFa, anti–IL-1 or anti–IL-6 biologics promise even further improvements in the risk/benefit ratio. Although combination pharmacotherapy is attractive in a child with severe disease for whom more limited regimens have failed, adequate clinical studies of effectiveness and safety are generally lacking. Specific recommendations for therapy are presented in Chapters 14 to 18. A discussion of the pharmacological aspects of these agents is provided in Chapter 6.

It is not usually possible at onset of the disease to predict which children will recover and which will go on to have unremitting disease with lingering disability or enter adulthood with serious functional impairment.[363]

Therefore, the initial therapeutic approach must be vigorous in all children. Furthermore, therapeutic strategies must recognize differences in approaching the different subtypes of onset. Evolution of the disease course and recognition of prognostic indicators will lead to ongoing modifications of the program in keeping with the response of the child.

Evidence of improvement is based on a review of the clinical course, repeated physical examinations, charting of the articular severity index and global responses, and laboratory estimates of inflammation. These evaluations have been systematized in the so-called core set variables.[364] A minimal clinically significant response is an improvement of at least 30% in at least three of the variables, with worsening by no more than 30% in not more than one variable. More demanding criteria require 50% or 70% improvement.[365] A preliminary definition of a disease flare in JRA has also been studied.[366]

It is almost impossible to be confident of the risk/benefit ratio for many of the therapeutic regimens for children with chronic arthritis.[367] The possibility that there may be important differences in the therapeutic efficacy of antirheumatic drugs depending on ethnicity and genetic background has been largely unexplored.[368] Toxicity is often a foremost concern in the long-term use of glucosteroids, immunosuppressive agents, or biologicals. Because of the relative lack of scientific guidance by appropriately designed studies, undertaken in adequate numbers of children with appropriate control of confounding factors such as type of onset and course of the disease, the experience and judgment of the pediatric rheumatologist become very important.

Alternative or complementary therapies, although of no proven benefit, are widely used by children with chronic arthritis. Their use is often fostered by information or misinformation available through the Internet. Parents should be directed to more objective sources of information, such as the Arthritis Foundation's Guide to Alternative Therapies.[369]

As monotherapy, NSAIDs should be continued for at least 3 to 6 months after all evidence of active disease has disappeared. Methotrexate therapy should probably be continued for up to 1 year after a remission has been achieved. One might also consider a different mode of withdrawal, such as decreasing administration to every 2 weeks for a period of time before discontinuation.[370] In combination therapy, a consensus has not developed on withdrawal of medications. Perhaps NSAIDs can be discontinued first along with steroids, MTX tapered next, and then, finally, biologicals stopped. In children, potentially toxic regimens such as prolonged use of glucosteroid and immunosuppressive drugs should be employed only in uncontrolled or life-threatening disease.

Nutrition

The child's overall nutrition, development, and growth are important aspects of long-term management. Assessment of nutritional status should be a component of every patient's evaluation.[371] Growth retardation and impaired bone mineralization almost invariably occur during periods of active disease and are exacerbated by glucocorticoid administration, anorexia, or inanition. Nutritional and vitamin supplementation (Calcium, vitamin D and folic acid) are often indicated. Management of malnutrition is often difficult in the systemically ill, anorectic child. Nocturnal nasogastric feeding has been used to maintain adequate nutrition in such a child.[305] Specific measures to address osteopenia and osteoporosis are reviewed in Chapter 49. Marked microcytic, hypochromic anemia may not be improved by oral iron supplementation, which often adversely affects appetite. Occasionally, a child benefits from intravenous iron administration followed by recombinant erythropoetin.[372]

Henderson and Lovell[373] suggested the use of a four-parameter test to screen for protein-energy malnutrition. The presence of any two of the following abnormalities indicates the need for a detailed nutritional assessment: weight below 5th percentile, weight-for-height index below 80th percentile, arm circumference below 5th percentile, and serum albumin less than 2.8 mg/dL (28 g/L).

Physical and Occupational Therapy

The objectives of physical and occupational therapy are to minimize pain, maintain and restore function, and prevent deformity and disability. These aspects of treatment are critically important in the child's total management program.[374,375] Physical and Occupational Therapy in children with rheumatic diseases are discussed in Chapter 12.

Orthopaedic Surgery

Orthopaedic surgery has an important, but limited, role in management of chronic arthritis in young children. In the older child, however, surgical approaches to joint contractures, dislocations, or joint replacement become important components of therapy, and the orthopaedic surgeon plays an important role at this stage.[376-378] Approaches to some problems, such as limb overgrowth, have not been completely clarified.[379] Fortunately, the use of intraarticular steroid has dramatically reduced the incidence and severity of leg-length inequality.[310]

Synovectomy

The long-term outcome of children with joint disease is not altered by prophylactic synovectomy. However, synovectomy may be useful in some children for relief of mechanical impairment of joint motion related to joint pain or synovial hypertrophy.[380-384] Care must be taken to prevent a postsurgical contracture, and the use of a continuous-motion apparatus has been recommended for this purpose, especially in the young child. Arthroscopic surgery greatly reduces the morbidity associated with synovectomy.[384]

Carl and colleagues[385] reported the results at a mean of 50 months of open hip joint synovectomies in 56 patients with JRA carried out between 1985 and 1997. Synovectomy was performed if, after medical therapy with NSAIDs, systemic glucosteroids and disease modifying antiinflammatory drugs (MTX, sulfasalazine or biologics), the patient had persistent synovitis (demonstrated by ultrasound), pain, joint effusion, and a limitation of range of motion of the hip. The authors concluded that synovectomy allowed significant improvement in hip function (pain, mobility, and ability to walk) in patients with early or late disease, as assessed radiologically by Larsen scores. Five patients required total hip joint replacement at a mean of 39 months after surgery.

Dell'Era and colleagues[386] reported the results of arthroscopic synovectomy at a mean of 5.4 years following surgery in 19 patients (31 knees) with JIA performed between 1990 and 2005. Disease recurred in 67% of those with oligoarthritis, 95% of those with polyarthritis, and in all with psoriatic arthritis. Recurrence occurred most quickly (0.8 years) in those with polyarthritis. Only 26% of these patients had received MTX. Another 26% had received sulfasalazine, and only 2 patients had received an anti-TNF agent. The authors concluded that synovectomy of the knee could be useful to "buy time."

In the studies reported by Carl and colleagues[386] and Del'Era and colleagues,[387] details of prior medical treatment are not provided. It is therefore difficult to assess if synovectomy of the hip or knee has an important role in the management of children treated appropriately with intraarticular steroids and MTX or biologics.

Soft Tissue Surgery

Soft tissue releases, posterior capsulotomy, and tendon lengthening occasionally are useful in a child with a severe contracture of the knee or hip. In other instances, balanced traction is necessary to expedite the treatment of a knee contracture, although this is often difficult to maintain in the young child. Tenosynovectomy may be indicated to reduce the risk of tendon rupture over the dorsum of the wrist or for adhesive flexor tenosynovitis and trigger finger, which sometimes occurs in children who are RF seropositive.

Reconstructive Surgery

Reconstructive surgery has become important in the older patient with marked disability. Total joint prostheses, particularly for the hip or knee, have proved to be of great benefit.[387,388] Usually, surgery is postponed until bone growth has ceased. Other special considerations include the status of the other lower-extremity joints, activity of the rheumatic disease in general, currently unresolved questions concerning wear and longevity of prostheses, and possible lack of adequate motivation for rehabilitation in some patients. Children with upper extremity disease may be further incapacitated either before or after lower-extremity surgery because of difficulty with crutch-walking. Preservation of muscle function in anticipation of surgical intervention requires a rehabilitation program over many years devoted to maintaining muscle strength as near normal as possible.

Counseling the Family

It is of signal importance that the child with arthritis and the parents be educated about the present state of knowledge regarding outcome, and therapy. Counseling should be initiated by the physician at the time of the first visit and reinforced and continued at follow-up by the team. Educational efforts are repeated as needed during the subsequent clinical course, especially in an effort to increase compliance.[389,390]

In management, the first priority, together with initial efforts to control the activity of the disease, is to foster normal psychological and social development. Although some families have had psychologically important disruptions such as divorce, separation, death, or adoption, recent studies indicate that families of children with chronic illnesses are quite functional.[391,392]

It is important to emphasize that coordinated care of the child with a chronic disease requires a team effort. This concept presents problems for newly established clinical services because of the number of personnel who need to be involved in an ideal program in addition to the child, the family, the school, and the community agencies. One study found that, for most children with chronic arthritis, and children with other chronic diseases, basic care was either divided or duplicated, and many aspects of a total supportive program were neglected.[393]

COURSE OF THE DISEASE AND PROGNOSIS

The course of untreated arthritis has probably not changed in the last century. The devastating consequences of prolonged untreated disease are still occasionally encountered in the developed world and are much more common in the developing world. Fortunately, the disease course and outcome continue to change dramatically with appropriate early therapy. This makes all long-term outcome studies of historical, rather than current, importance. To a considerable extent, the outcome with treatment is related to the disease subtype and is discussed in the appropriate chapters. Nonetheless, certain generalizations can be made.

Disease Course

The course of chronic arthritis is especially unpredictable early in the disease, as indicated by the requirement for a 6-month assessment before disease subtype classification can be made. Once established, the course tends to be more predictable and repetitive. After this initial period of observation, it is usually possible to estimate prognosis and therapeutic response on which changes in the management program can be based. It is impossible to predict the eventual disease outcome in any individual child. Furthermore, "outcome" is a complex concept that can be measured in a number of ways[394] (see Chapters 7 and 8).

Functional Disability and Psychosocial Outcome

It had been estimated historically that 70% to 90% of children with chronic arthritis have a satisfactory outcome without serious disability.[395,396] A small percentage (perhaps 5%) develop a recurrence of arthritis as adults.[397,398] Approximately 10% to 20% of children enter adulthood with moderate to severe functional disabilities.[399] Delay in referral and initiation of an acceptable therapeutic program are associated with a poorer functional outcome.

Recent data have been presented on outcome for specific onset types[400-403] and for long-term follow-up from specific referral centers.[396,404-413] The data of Wallace and Levinson[414] documented poorer long-term results than previously recorded (Table 13–9). At 15 to 20 years, 17% of the patients were in Steinbrocker functional class III to IV, and 45% still had active disease (activity of disease was approximately equal for each onset type). For reference the most frequently used functional classification is provided in Table 13-10. Reviews of previous studies of outcome have been published.[363,415] A study by Ruperto and colleagues[416] evaluated long-term outcome in a group of 227 patients from Cincinnati and Pavia. This study examined the effect of specific demographic, clinical, and immunological variables that were present during the first 6 months of the illness. The mean duration of disease at assessment was 15 years (range, 5.3 to 36.1 years). The best predictor of long-term disability was the initial articular severity score. Early hand involvement was also a strong predictor of future disability, pain, and

---

Table 13–9					
Functional outcome of Chronic Arthritis					
		Steinbrocker Class (%)			
Author (ref. no.)	Follow-up (yrs)	I	II	III	IV
Wallace and Levinson (414)	15–20			(17)	
Oen et al (420)	0.5			(2.5)	
Zak and Pedersen (399)	10		6.1	(7.7)	
	26		21.5	(10.8)	
Minden et al (411)	7	49	39	10	2
	17	55	33	11	1

Table 13–10

Functional Classification of patients with Rheumatoid Arthritis.

Class I	Complete functional capacity
Class II	Functional capacity adequate to conduct normal activities despite discomfort or limited mobility
Class III	Functional capacity adequate to perform some activities of usual occupation or self-care
Class IV	Largely or totally incapacitated; bedridden or confined to a wheelchair, permitting little or no self-care

Modified from Steinbrocker O. Traeger CH, Batterman RC. Therapeutic criteria in rheumatoid arthritis. *JAMA* 140: 659-662, 1949

Table 13–11

Functional outcome of juvenile rheumatoid arthritis by the Childhood Health Assessment Questionnaire (CHAQ)

Type of onset (n)	Follow-up (mean yr)	CHAQ score	
		Mean	Range
Systemic (40)	11.6	0.25	0-2.75
Pauciarticular (224)	12.5	0	0-2.13
Polyarticular (RF–) (80)	12.6	0.19	0-2.75
Polyarticular (RF+) (40)	13.9	0.62	0-3.0

RF, rheumatoid factor.
Data from Oen K, Malleson PN, Cabral DA et al: Early predictors of long-term outcome in patients with juvenile rheumatoid arthritis: subset-specific correlations, *J Rheumatol* 30: 585-593, 2003.

impaired well-being. ANA seropositivity was associated with less disability. This study confirmed that quality-of-life scores are much more difficult to forecast because of the multiple domains that are functioning in this type of outcome. Extensions of this study[416] indicated that long-term outcome, based on quality-of-life scales and health assessment questionnaires, was favorable in most patients 5 years or more after onset of symptoms.[417,418]

The Childhood Health Assessment Questionnaire (CHAQ) has been evaluated for measurement of health status in early and late disease.[419] Oen and colleagues[420] surveyed early predictors of long-term outcome on the CHAQ in 392 patients with JRA (of 652 eligible), including 327 white patients, who were 8 years of age or older and had a minimum of 5 years of follow-up. The most significant early predictors were age at onset and being male. In addition to the results in Table 13–11, worse disability was observed for systemic onset in males, less disability in patients with RF-negative disease, and a shorter duration of activity in RF-positive polyarthritis. ANA seropositivity in oligoarthritis was associated with a longer duration of activity, as was a younger age at onset. The RA shared epitope was associated with less disability in systemic disease. A subsequent report examined radiologic outcome in children from the same clinics.[421]

More recently, investigators have attempted to avoid the confounding factors of referral-based and clinic follow-up by primarily basing their outcome studies on population surveys. Data from the U.S. Pediatric Rheumatology Disease Registry[416] in 703 patients observed between 1992 and 1997, before the era of biological therapy, indicated that more than 25% of those with polyarthritis, and almost one half of those with systemic onset, had functional limitations affecting school activities. Joint space damage on radiographs was evident at 5 years in two-thirds of the polyarticular and systemic-onset groups. Some investigators have also taken the approach recommended by the World Health Organization in 1980 to examine functional adaptation in relation to impairment (based on organ disease), disability (related to personal quality of life),[422] and handicap (related to society's perception of the functioning ability of the individual).[423]

A study by Peterson and colleagues[424] evaluated the physical and psychosocial impacts of disease in a population-based cohort of 44 adults who had experienced onset of the disease during childhood. Controls (n=102) were age- and sex-matched. Average follow-up was 24.7 years, and mean age was 34 years. The patients had greater disability, more body pain, increased fatigue, poorer health perception, and decreased physical functioning along with lower rates of employment and lower levels of exercise compared with the control group. On the other hand, educational achievement, annual income, health insurance status, and rates of pregnancy and childbirth were similar to those of the controls. Active disease was present in 66%, and 16% were under regular medical care for their arthritis. This study concluded that adults who had had chronic arthritis developed long-term physical and psychosocial impairments that have been often ignored in the evaluation of functional outcome.

Many of the same outcomes and prognostic factors were identified in a study by Flato and colleagues of 268 patients with JRA who were monitored for a median of 14.9 years (range, 11.7 to 25.1 years).[425] Another study from Norway[426] included 53 patients with arthritis and 19 with juvenile spondyloarthropathy. Forty-three (60%) of the 72 patients were in a remission at the time of the study, and 60% reported no disability. This study and subsequent reports[425,427] supported the conclusion that long-term outcome was more favorable than previously reported, perhaps related to less bias of admission to the study and the early use of more aggressive therapeutic regimens. This group of investigators had previously indicated that poor psychosocial functioning in 22% of the patients on follow-up was associated with premorbid psychosocial dysfunction, chronic family difficulties, and major life events.[427] They also confirmed that approximately 19% of the patients were still suffering from chronic pain without evidence of active arthritis.[428] It is also the impression of the authors, and of others,[429] that a chronic pain syndrome may persist in these patients well after their arthritis has remitted.

A number of studies of adaptation to chronic illnesses in children have been completed recently.[391,392,429-432] Studies of adaptation have been limited by assumptions that disease groups of chronic illnesses are homogeneous and that comprehensive adaptation models involve both risk factors and resistance factors within the child and family. In one study,[391] 107 children with JRA, 114 with insulin-dependent diabetes mellitus, and 88 healthy controls were evaluated every 6 months for 2 years. Differences were observed between mothers and fathers with regard to dependent variables of depression, anxiety, somatization, strain at work, days of work loss due to child's illness, and extent to which the illness interfered with leisure time in the family. Married mothers missed more work than fathers but demonstrated less overall functional impairment. Single mothers did not differ from married mothers or fathers. The dependent variables—particularly those related to depression, anxiety, and strain at work—decreased for all parents during the two years of observation. Premorbid diagnostic groups were associated with maternal depression and paternal distress in passive coping. Parental depression and distress were associated with the child's behavior, complaints of pain, and ability to deal with anger and disappointment. Anger level and anger expression styles were highly associated with depression.[433] Children who turned their anger inward were most likely to report depression. The child's functioning did not appear to be related to the clinical diagnostic group. Trajectories within the child's and family's adaptations could be identified independent of the diagnostic groups.[392] This and other studies have concluded that interventions to ameliorate parental distress have beneficial effects on child behavior and on parental reactions to that behavior and the chronic illness.[293,434-436]

Transition of the child to young-adult vocational planning, and eventually a place in adult life, have been the subject of a number of studies. Excellent summaries are contained in several publications.[362,437-441]

Death

In early studies of chronic arthritis in children, the overall death rate was 1% to 4%.[442,443] The disease-associated death rate is now perhaps less than 1% in Europe and less than 0.3% in North America. This mortality represents, however, a fourfold to fourteenfold increase compared with standardized rates. In a study from England,[444] the standardized mortality ratio was 3.4 for males (95% CI, 2.0 to 5.5) and 5.1 for females (95% CI, 3.2 to 7.8). The majority of the deaths in Europe were previously related to the development of amyloidosis;[445] in the United States, deaths occurred predominantly in children with systemic-onset disease and in many cases were related to infection. Infections were associated in the early studies with glucocorticoid therapy and are currently less often fatal.

The major causes of death in 46 children observed by Bywaters at Taplow[446,447] were renal failure (which in one half of the children was associated with amyloidosis) and infections. At the 15-year evaluation, excess mortality was identified in girls who developed arthritis early in life and the frequency of amyloidosis had risen to 7.4%. It was rarely observed as early as 1 year after onset but could develop as late as 23 years after, most commonly in children with systemic disease. Spontaneous remissions occurred. Even in Europe, amyloidosis as a complication of chronic arthritis appears to be on the decline, with a decreasing number of deaths[448]; however, a recent series from Turkey reported a frequency of 10%.[449]

Amyloidosis refers to the tissue deposition of the fibrillar protein amyloid.[450] Secondary amyloidosis occurs as a complication of chronic inflammatory conditions such as arthritis or infection and in diseases such as familial Mediterranean fever. It is characterized clinically by proteinuria and the nephrotic syndrome, diarrhea, hepatosplenomegaly, or unexplained anemia in a child with profound hypergammaglobulinemia. Amyloidosis may be preceded by marked elevations of CRP, an acute phase reactant that is similar in structure to serum amyloid A (SAA) protein.[451] SAA protein responds as an acute phase reactant and is increased in concentration in children with active disease. Although no HLA associations have been confirmed in children who develop amyloidosis,[452] a genetic marker for the amyloid P component was identified in one study by restriction fragment length polymorphism.[453] Diagnosis is confirmed by examination of tissue sections stained by Congo red dye. Under the polarizing microscope, amyloid deposits assume a green color that is virtually pathognomonic.[454] Rectal submucosa is the most frequently recommended biopsy site; renal biopsy may be hazardous because of an increased tendency toward bleeding. Radionuclide imaging using radioiodinated autologous serum amyloid P is a noninvasive technique for diagnosis and monitoring.[455]

BURDEN OF DISEASE

The economic burden of any disease including JIA is difficult to measure precisely and depends to some extent on the medical care delivery system. The unreimbursed cost to the family of a child with a chronic rheumatic disease per year is considerable.[456] Allaire and colleagues[456] estimated annual direct medical costs per patient with JRA in the United States in 1992 at $7905. Three recent studies of burden of disease in countries with some form of universal prepaid health care indicate that not only is there is considerable cost in the first year after diagnosis, but that this cost continues into adulthood, especially in those with ongoing active disease.

Minden and colleagues[457] studied the economic costs in 215 German patients an average of 17 years after disease onset, using clinical records, a structured interview and questionnaires. Direct costs (health care [including physician], hospital, and drug costs) accounted for 45% of the total cost. Indirect costs (sick leave, work disability, lost productivity in older patients) accounted for 55%. The authors estimated that the mean annual cost was 3500 Euros. The economic burden was greatest in those with active RF-positive polyarthritis (€ 17,000) and extended oligoarthritis (€ 11,000), and lowest in those with active ERA (€ 1500) and persistent oligoarthritis (€ 2700). Costs were higher in those with active disease than in those in whom the disease was in remission.

Bernatsky and colleagues[458] studied economic burden of disease in 155 Canadian children (mean age 10 years) with arthritis, and 181 children (mean age 10.5 years) with other, mainly non-chronic disorders). The annual direct cost medical care, hospitalization, drugs) was estimated to be Canadian $3,002 in children with arthritis and Canadian $1,315 in the comparison group. In a subgroup analysis of children with another chronic disease (asthma), the annual direct cost was much less (Canadian $1,300) than for children with arthritis. The economic burden was highest in children with active arthritis.

Thornton and colleagues[459] studied the economic burden in 297 children in the first year of diagnosis in the United Kingdom. Mean annual economic cost was £1649 (SD £1093, range £401 to £6967). Costs were highest for those with ERA, extended oligoarthritis or systemic disease.

PERSPECTIVE

In spite of new insights into causation and considerable advances in treatment, chronic arthritis remains an important cause of chronic pain and disability in childhood. Particularly when considering heroic pharmacological therapy, one should remember that the disease is often self-limited, albeit after years of activity, and is seldom fatal. On the other hand, undue delay in instituting advanced treatment that may be effective can result in irretrievable damage to joints and other organs and impaired skeletal maturation. The art of medicine is at least as important as its science in guiding the pediatric rheumatologist's planning of a therapeutic approach. An important factor working in favor of the program of management is the child's unceasing potential for growth. To a large extent, it is this intrinsic endowment for future physical and psychological development that enables so much to be accomplished in most children. Even so, much work remains in clarifying the nature and management of these diseases and their complications.

REFERENCES

1. E.J. Brewer, J.C. Bass, J.T. Cassidy, Criteria for the classification of juvenile rheumatoid arthritis, Bull. Rheum. Dis. 23 (1972) 712–719.
2. European League Against Rheumatism, EULAR Bulletin no. 4: nomenclature and classification of arthritis in children, National Zeitung AG, Basel, 1977.
9. R.E. Petty, T.R. Southwood, P. Manners, et al., International League of Associations for Rheumatology classification of juvenile idiopathic arthritis, second revision, Edmonton, 2001 J. Rheumatol. 31 (2004) 390–392.
33. G.F. Still, On a form of chronic joint disease in children, Med. Chirurg. Trans. 80 (1897) 47.
49. K. Oen, Comparative epidemiology of the rheumatic diseases in children, Curr. Opin. Rheumatol. 12 (2000) 410–414.
50. G.B. Andersson, Juvenile arthritis—who gets it, where and when? A review of current data on incidence and prevalence, Clin. Exp. Rheumatol. 17 (1999) 367–374.
52. H. Mielants, E.M. Veys, M. Maertens, et al., Prevalence of inflammatory rheumatic diseases in an adolescent urban student population, age 12 to 18, in Belgium, Clin. Exp. Rheumatol. 11 (1993) 563–567.
53. P.J. Manners, D.A. Diepeveen, Prevalence of juvenile chronic arthritis in a population of 12-year-old children in urban Australia, Pediatrics 98 (1996) 84–90.
65. P.N. Malleson, M.Y. Fung, A.M. Rosenberg, The incidence of pediatric rheumatic diseases: results from the Canadian Pediatric Rheumatology Association Disease Registry, J. Rheumatol. 23 (1996) 1981–1987.
67. D.P. Symmons, M. Jones, J. Osborne, et al., Pediatric rheumatology in the United Kingdom: data from the British Pediatric Rheumatology Group National Diagnostic Register, J. Rheumatol. 23 (1996) 1975–1980.
89. R.K. Sauernmann, J.B. Rose, P. Tyrell, et al., Epidemiology of juvenile idiopathic arthritis in a multiethnic cohort, Arthritis Rheum. 56 (2007) 1974–1984.
98. F. De Benedetti, A. Ravelli, A. Martini, Cytokines in juvenile rheumatoid arthritis, Curr. Opin. Rheumatol. 9 (1997) 428–433.
101. P. Woo, Cytokines and juvenile idiopathic arthritis, Curr. Rheumatol. Rep. 4 (2002) 452–457.
108. D. Foell, J. Roth, Proinflammatory S100 proteins in arthritis and autoimmune disease, Arthritis Rheum. 50 (2004) 3762–3771.
109. V. Pascual, F. Allantaz, E. Arce, et al., Role of interleukin 1 (IL-1) in the pathogenesis of systemic onset juvenile idiopathic arthritis, and clinical response to IL-1 blockade, J. Exp. Med. 201 (2005) 1479–1486.
140. T. Avcin, R. Cimaz, F. Falcini, et al., Prevalence and clinical significance of anti-cyclic citrullinated peptide antibodies in juvenile idiopathic arthritis, Ann. Rheum. Dis. 61 (2002) 608–611.
159. M.A. Muzaffer, J.M. Dayer, B.M. Feldman, et al., Differences in the profiles of circulating levels of soluble tumor necrosis factor receptors and interleukin 1 receptor antagonist reflect the heterogeneity of the subgroups of juvenile rheumatoid arthritis, J. Rheumatol. 29 (2002) 1071–1078.
208. B. Prakken, W. Kuis, W. Van Eden, et al., Heat shock proteins in juvenile idiopathic arthritis: keys for understanding remitting arthritis and candidate antigens for immune therapy, Curr. Rheumatol. Rep. 4 (2002) 466–473.
215. S. Albani, Infection and molecular mimicry in autoimmune diseases of childhood, Clin. Exp. Rheumatol. 12 (Suppl. 10) (1994) S35–S41.
237. J.D. Phelan, S.D. Thompson, D.N. Glass, Susceptibility to JRA/JIA: complementing general autoimmune and arthritis traits, Genes Immun. 7 (2006) 1–10.
250. K.J. Murray, M.B. Moroldo, P. Donnelly, et al., Age-specific effects of juvenile rheumatoid arthritis-associated HLA alleles, Arthritis Rheum. 42 (1999) 1843–1853.
255. W. Thomson, J.H. Barrett, R. Donn, et al., Juvenile idiopathic arthritis classified by the ILAR criteria: HLA associations in UK patients, Rheumatology (Oxf) 41 (2002) 1183–1189.
258. A. Hinks, A. Barton, S. John, et al., Association between PTPN22 and rheumatoid arthritis and juvenile idiopathic arthritis in a UK population, Arthritis Rheum. 52 (2005) 1694–1699.
259. A. Hinks, X. Ke, A. Barton, et al., Association of the IL2RA CD25 gene with juvenile idiopathic arthritis, Arthritis Rheum. 60 (2009) 251–257.
281. K.K. Anthony, L.E. Schanberg, Assessment and management of pain syndromes and arthritis pain in children and adolescents, Rheum. Dis. Clin. North Am. 33 (2007) 625–660.
290. P.N. Malleson, K. Oen, D.A. Cabral, et al., Predictors of pain in children with established juvenile rheumatoid arthritis, Arthritis Rheum. 51 (2004) 222–227.
297. H.E. Foster, L.J. Kay, M. Friswell, et al., Musculoskeletal screening examination (pGALS) for school age children based on the adult GALS screen, Arthritis Rheum. 55 (2006) 709–716.
328. O.T. Lelieveld, W. Armbrust, M.A. Van Leeuwen, et al., Physical activity in adolescents with juvenile idiopathic arthritis, Arthritis Rheum. 59 (2008) 1379–1384.
337. E. Kruithof, V. Van den Bossche, L. De Ryke, et al., Distinct synovial histopathologic characteristics of juvenile onset spondyloarthritis and other forms of juvenile idiopathic arthritis, Arthritis Rheum. 54 (2006) 2594–2604.
352. D.A. Cabral, R.E. Petty, M. Fung, et al., Persistent antinuclear antibodies in children without identifiable inflammatory rheumatic or autoimmune disease, Pediatrics 89 (1992) 441–444.
354. N.T. Ilowite, P. Samuel, L. Beseler, et al., Dyslipoproteinemia in juvenile rheumatoid arthritis, J. Pediatr. 114 (1989) 823–826.
362. L.B. Ilowite, D.A. Cabral, Transition of the adolescent patient with rheumatic disease: issues to consider, Ped. Clin. North Am. 52 (2005) 641–652.
364. E.H. Giannini, N. Ruperto, A. Ravelli, et al., Preliminary definition of improvement in juvenile arthritis, Arthritis Rheum. 40 (1997) 1202–1209.
366. H.I. Brunner, D.J. Lovell, B.K. Finck, et al., Preliminary definition of disease flare in juvenile rheumatoid arthritis, J. Rheumatol. 29 (2002) 1058–1064.
375. G. Kuchta, I. Davidson, Occupational and Physical Therapy for Children with Rheumatic Diseases, Radcliffe, Oxford (2009).
385. H.-D. Carl, A. Schraml, B. Swoboda, et al., Synovectomy of the hip in patients with juvenile rheumatoid arthritis, J. Bone Joint Surg. 89 (2007) 1986–1992.
386. L. Dell'Era, R. Facchini, F. Corona, Knee synovectomy in children with juvenile idiopathic arthritis, J. Ped. Ortho. B. 17 (2008) 128–130.

394. H. Dempster, M. Porepa, N. Young, et al., The clinical meaning of functional outcome scores in children with juvenile arthritis, Arthritis Rheum. 44 (2001) 1768–1774.

396. F. Fantini, V. Gerloni, M. Gattinara, et al., Remission in juvenile chronic arthritis: a cohort study of 683 consecutive cases with a mean 10 year followup, J. Rheumatol. 30 (2003) 579–584.

400. K. Oen, P.N. Malleson, D.A. Cabral, et al., Early predictors of longterm outcome in patients with juvenile rheumatoid arthritis: subset-specific correlations, J. Rheumatol. 30 (2003) 585–593.

401. S. Guillaume, A.M. Prieur, J. Coste, et al., Long-term outcome and prognosis in oligoarticular-onset juvenile idiopathic arthritis, Arthritis Rheum. 43 (2000) 1858–1865.

403. L.R. Spiegel, R. Schneider, B.A. Lang, et al., Early predictors of poor functional outcome in systemic-onset juvenile rheumatoid arthritis: a multicenter cohort study, Arthritis Rheum 43 (2000) 2402–2409.

407. J.C. Packham, M.A. Hall, Long-term follow-up of 246 adults with juvenile idiopathic arthritis: functional outcome, Rheumatology (Oxf) 41 (2002) 1428–1435.

411. K. Minden, M. Niewerth, J. Listing, et al., Long-term outcome in patients with juvenile idiopathic arthritis, Arthritis Rheum. 46 (2002) 2392–2401.

420. K. Oen, P.N. Malleson, D.A. Cabral, et al., Disease course and outcome of juvenile rheumatoid arthritis in a multicenter cohort, J. Rheumatol. 29 (2002) 1989–1999.

421. K. Oen, M. Reed, P.N. Malleson, et al., Radiologic outcome and its relationship to functional disability in juvenile rheumatoid arthritis, J. Rheumatol. 30 (2003) 832–840.

444. E. Thomas, D.P. Symmons, D.H. Brewster, et al., National study of cause-specific mortality in rheumatoid arthritis, juvenile chronic arthritis, and other rheumatic conditions: a 20 year followup study, J. Rheumatol. 30 (2003) 958–965.

457. K. Minden, M. Niewerth, J. Listing, et al., Burden and cost of illness in children with juvenile idiopathic arthritis, Ann. Rheum. Dis. 63 (2004) 836–842.

458. S. Bernatsky, C. Duffy, P. Malleson, et al., Economic impact of juvenile idiopathic arthritis, Arthritis Care Res. 57 (2007) 44–48.

459. J. Thornton, M. Lunt, D.M. Ashcroft, et al., Costing juvenile idiopathic arthritis: examining patient based costs during the first year after diagnosis, Rheumatology (Oxf.) 47 (2008) 985–990.

Entire reference list is available online at www.expertconsult.com.

Chapter 14

SYSTEMIC JUVENILE IDIOPATHIC ARTHRITIS

Fabrizio De Benedetti and Rayfel Schneider

Systemic arthritis is one of the most perplexing diseases of childhood. The onset can be quite nonspecific and may suggest bacterial or viral infection, malignancy, or another inflammatory disease. The evolution of the disease eventually makes the diagnosis, which is entirely clinical, evident. For almost a century, this disorder bore the name *Still's disease,* in recognition of its early description by George Frederic Still.[1]

DEFINITION AND CLASSIFICATION

This disease—defined as *systemic arthritis* by the International League of Associations for Rheumatology (ILAR) classification of juvenile idiopathic arthritis (JIA),[2] *systemic-onset juvenile rheumatoid arthritis* (JRA) by the American College of Rheumatology classification, or *systemic-onset juvenile chronic arthritis* by the European League Against Rheumatism classification—is unique among the chronic arthritides of childhood in several ways. In particular, the range and severity of characteristic extraarticular features mark this disease as a systemic illness with joint inflammation that ranges from mild to severe.

Diagnosis of systemic arthritis by the ILAR criteria requires the presence of arthritis and a documented quotidian fever of at least 2 weeks' duration, plus one of the following: typical rash, generalized lymphadenopathy, enlargement of liver or spleen, or serositis. Criteria and exclusions are shown in Table 14–1.

EPIDEMIOLOGY

Among the various JIA subtypes included in the ILAR classification, systemic arthritis accounts for 5% to 15% of children with JIA seen in North America and Europe. Systemic JIA (s-JIA) is found worldwide. The exact prevalence of the disease is not known. Some population-based studies are available from Europe showing an annual incidence for systemic arthritis between 0.3 and 0.8 cases per 100,000 children under 16 years of age.[3-7] At least in Europe, incidence appears to be higher in northernmost countries compared with Southern European countries. In Asia, s-JIA may account for a greater proportion of all childhood arthritis: in India and in Japan 25% and 50%, respectively, of JIA appears to be systemic arthritis.[8,9]

Most studies indicate no definite peak age at onset of systemic arthritis.[10-13] In a recent large multicenter study, there was a broad peak of onset between 1 and 5 years.[14] It occasionally manifests before 1 year of age, and it also occurs in adolescence and adulthood. Children of both sexes are affected with approximately equal frequency.

Although an earlier study documented a marked seasonal variation in 28 children over a 10-year period, with no patients having disease onset in the winter months,[11] subsequent studies in Canada and Israel failed to find clear evidence for seasonal variation.[10,13]

ETIOLOGY AND PATHOGENESIS

Although the onset resembles an infectious disease, s-JIA has not been consistently associated with any pathogen. Its low frequency in family members and the absence of a consistent seasonality of onset indicate that, if an infectious agent is involved in its etiology, it is only one of several factors.

Autoantibodies and autoreactive T cells are not features of s-JIA. Moreover, in contrast to classic diseases, genetic associations with human leukocyte antigen (HLA) class I or II alleles are not present. On the contrary, a vast body of evidence points to the involvement of cells and cytokines of the innate immune response, suggesting that s-JIA may be considered an autoinflammatory disease.

Genetic Background

Systemic JIA is rarely familial, with only a few sibling pairs having been reported.[15] Earlier studies showing the association of s-JIA with different HLA alleles have not been replicated,[16] in contrast with other subtypes of JIA, where multiple replicates of disease association with HLA have been reported. At present, the best defined association is with the G variant of a promoter polymorphism

Table 14-1

Systemic juvenile idiopathic arthritis: International League of Associations for Rheumatology (ILAR) diagnostic criteria

Arthritis in any number of joints together with a fever of at least 2 weeks' duration that is documented to be daily (quotidian) for at least 3 days and is accompanied by one or more of the following:
- Evanescent rash
- Generalized lymphadenopathy
- Enlargement of liver or spleen
- Serositis

Exclusions:
- Psoriasis or a history of psoriasis in the patient or a first-degree relative
- Arthritis in an HLA B27-positive male beginning after the sixth birthday
- Ankylosing spondylitis, enthesitis-related arthritis, sacroiliitis with inflammatory bowel disease, Reiter syndrome, or acute anterior uveitis—or a history of one of these disorders in a first-degree relative
- The presence of IgM RF on at least two occasions at least 3 mo apart

HLA, human leukocyte antigen; *IgM,* immunoglobulin M.

of the interleukin (IL)-6 genes, which has been confirmed as a susceptibility gene for s-JIA in family studies in a multicenter setting.[14,17] This promoter polymorphism affects IL-6 production, with the G allele being associated with higher IL-6 expression. Other studies support the association of s-JIA with proinflammatory cytokine gene polymorphisms. The –308 G→A polymorphism of the TNF-α promoter, which is related to high production of TNF-α, has been reported to be associated with systemic JRA in Japanese,[18] but no replication studies on large Caucasian patients populations are available. A functional promoter polymorphism of the macrophage migration inhibitory factor (MIF) promoter (–173 G→C) has been associated with s-JIA and with JIA as a whole.[19-21] More recently, a comprehensive study of polymorphisms in the IL-1 and IL-1 receptor loci showed association of noncoding polymorphisms in the genes of IL-1 receptor type II, IL-1α, and IL-1 receptor antagonist.[22] It is therefore tempting to speculate that the interactions of these polymorphisms, possibly combined with others yet to be identified, broadly predispose patients to mount a more vigorous inflammatory response to environmental stimuli, such as infectious agents.

Pathogenesis and Cytokines

Although the pathogenesis of s-JIA still requires considerable clarification, there is substantial evidence of a dysregulated innate immune response with consequent increased production of inflammatory cytokines. Studies on gene expression profiles in blood cells support this hypothesis. The most recent one, in untreated patients during the early phase of the disease, showed over-representation of genes of the IL-6 and TLR/IL-1R pathways.[23] Moreover, gene pathways related to natural killer cells or T cells

were downregulated.[23] These findings are similar to what is found in patients with septic shock, again pointing to innate immune activation. Previous studies on gene expression profiles have, at least in part, shown comparable data. However, direct comparison is hampered by the fact that earlier studies used samples from patients treated with various immunosuppressive drugs.[24-27] A study in Japan has also recently shown a downregulation of genes encoded by mitochondrial DNA and involved in oxidative phosphorylation.[25] This finding suggests mitochondrial damage in sJIA; however, the link with innate immune activation remains to be established. These studies provide a wealth of mechanistic information that may lead to a better molecular definition of s-JIA.

From a practical point of view, it is generally believed that prominent innate immunity activation results in elevated levels of several inflammatory cytokines. These include IL-1, IL-6, IL-7, IL-8, IL-18, macrophage inhibitory factor (MIF), and tumor necrosis factor (TNF).[28-34] Using a multiplex approach for the measurement of up to 30 cytokines in JIA patients and subsequent cluster analysis, it was recently shown that patients with s-JIA cluster together and can be distinguished from patients with oligoarticular or polyarticular JIA, again pointing to specific molecular mechanisms sustaining inflammation in s-JIA.[35] The role of each one of these mediators is far from being clarified.

TNF-α levels, as well as levels of the two soluble TNF receptors, are increased in systemic s-JIA.[31,34,36,37] TNF-α levels do not correlate with elevations of temperature.[34,38] Although in vivo production of TNF is increased, the clinical response to TNF blockade of patients with s-JIA is limited compared with that in other JIA subtypes (see Treatment). This observation suggests that TNF does not play a major role in s-JIA and that a different cytokine network and/or hierarchy is present.

A vast body of evidence supports a major role of increased IL-6 production in mediating signs and symptoms of s-JIA.[39] IL-6 is markedly elevated in the blood and synovial fluid.[31,34,40-42] The IL-6 level increases just before fever spikes and correlates with the systemic features of the disease, arthritis, and increase in acute phase reactants.[34,38,40] In vitro studies have documented increased production of IL-6 by peripheral blood mononuclear cells (PBMC) from patients with s-JIA.[43] In addition to the involvement of IL-6 in animal models of arthritis,[44] several data support a role for prominent IL-6 production in the limitation of growth, systemic osteoporosis, thrombocytosis, and microcytic anemia seen in this disease.[40,45-47]

Studies on serum and synovial fluid levels of IL-1β in s-JIA have yielded controversial results. This may be due to technical difficulties in measuring IL-1β levels reliably. Sera from patients with active s-JIA induced expression of IL-1β in PBMC from healthy controls,[27,48] as well as expression of some IL-1β–inducible genes.[27] Other studies have failed to identify an IL-1β signature in PBMC from patients with active s-JIA.[49,50] A careful study of inflammasome and subsequent caspase 1 activation and IL-1β secretion by PBMC of patients with s-JIA failed to find in vitro abnormalities.[51] Even if data on the production of IL-1β in s-JIA are controversial and the molecular and cellular mechanism(s) are not clarified, the administration of the IL-1 receptor antagonist anakinra resulted in a marked clinical benefit in approximately one-half of the patients with s-JIA (see Treatment), leading to the conclusion that IL-1β may be involved in the pathogenesis of s-JIA. Recent data on the myeloid-related protein 8 (MRP-8) and MRP-14 complex provide a possible molecular basis for increased inflammatory cytokine production, particularly of IL-1β, in s-JIA. MRP-8/MRP-14 levels are markedly elevated in the serum of active s-JIA patients.[52] The MRP-8/MRP-14 complex, an endogenous ligand for Toll-like receptor 4, induces inflammatory cytokines and, on endothelial cells, a pro-thrombotic proinflammatory state.[53,54] A recent report showed that neutralization of MRP-8/MRP-14 inhibited the stimulatory effect of s-JIA sera on IL-1β production,[48] suggesting that MRP-8/MRP-14 may be at least one of the factors involved.

CLINICAL MANIFESTATIONS

Children with systemic arthritis are usually very ill at the time the diagnosis is made. They are fatigued, anemic, febrile, in pain, and frequently have lost weight. These features of the disease predominate early in the course and may overshadow the arthritis. A recent study documented the frequency of initial clinical features in 136 children with systemic-onset JRA.[55] The most common features were fever (98%), arthritis (88%) and rash (81%). Only 39% had lymphadenopathy, 10% had pericarditis, and fewer had hepatosplenomegaly. The high frequency of extraarticular manifestations emphasizes the systemic nature of this disease.

Approximately 10% of patients have onset of s-JIA with severe systemic involvement that may precede development of overt arthritis by weeks, months, or, rarely, years. The interval between onset of systemic signs and appearance of arthritis may be as long as 10 years. The presence of arthritis must be confirmed, however, before a diagnosis of JIA can be considered definite. It is extremely rare for fever to first manifest after the development of arthritis.

Musculoskeletal Disease

Arthritis

Any number of joints can be affected at onset of or during the disease course, but monoarthritis is uncommon and the course is characteristically polyarticular. The knees, wrists, and ankles are most commonly involved, but cervical spine and hip disease, as well as inflammation of the small joints of the hands and the temporomandibular joint, occur in more than one-half of the patients. At onset of the systemic features, the joint disease may be minimal, but usually it increases in severity over weeks or months. In some children, the joint disease is a severe polyarthritis that is very resistant to treatment and eventually results in significant disability. Joint damage sometimes ensues rapidly with joint space loss, erosions, and even ankylosis occurring within the first 2 years of onset. In others, it is less severe and eventually goes into clinical remission. Severe destructive polyarticular arthritis has been reported in approximately one-third of patients after a mean follow-up of 5 years.[56]

Tenosynovitis and Synovial Cysts

Tenosynovitis is frequently seen in children with a polyarticular course. The most common sites involved are the extensor tendon sheaths on the dorsum of the hand, the finger flexor tendon sheaths, the extensor sheaths over the dorsum of the foot, and those of the posterior tibial tendon and the peroneus longus and brevis tendons around the ankle. Occasionally, stenosing tenosynovitis results in trigger finger or loss of interphalangeal joint extension. Tenosynovitis of the superior oblique tendon may cause Brown syndrome. Some children develop synovial cysts that communicate with shoulder, elbow, wrist, or knee joints.

Myalgia and Myositis

Myalgias are common during periods of active systemic inflammation and may be more painful than the arthritis. Myositis with muscle pain and tenderness, elevation of muscle enzymes, and typical magnetic resonance imaging abnormalities have been reported.[57]

Systemic Disease

Fever

The temperature rises to 39° C or higher on a daily or twice-daily basis, with a rapid return to baseline or below the baseline (Fig. 14–1). This quotidian pattern is highly suggestive of the diagnosis of JIA, although very early in the course of the disease the classic quotidian fever may not be apparent, and the pattern may be indistinguishable from that of sepsis. In these children, a more typical fever pattern may be seen after treatment with nonsteroidal antiinflammatory drugs (NSAIDs) is initiated. The fever may occur at any time of the day but is characteristically present in the late afternoon to evening in conjunction with the rash. The temperature may be subnormal in the morning. Chills are frequent at the time of the fever, but rigors are rare. These children are often quite ill while febrile but may be surprisingly well during the rest of the day. Hyperpyrexia, a temperature higher than 40.5° C, is rare. The fever must be present for at least 2 weeks to fulfill the diagnostic criteria, but it usually lasts for several months, recurs with flares of disease, and occasionally persists for years.

Rash

The intermittent fever is almost always accompanied by a classic rash that consists of discrete, erythematous macules 2 to 5 mm in size that may appear in linear streaks (Fig. 14–2).[58] This rash is usually described as being salmon pink, but very early in the disease it may be more erythematous, although never purpuric. It most commonly occurs on the trunk and proximal extremities but may develop on the face, palms, or soles. The macules are often surrounded by a zone of pallor, and larger lesions develop central clearing. The rash tends to be migratory and is strikingly evanescent in any one area.

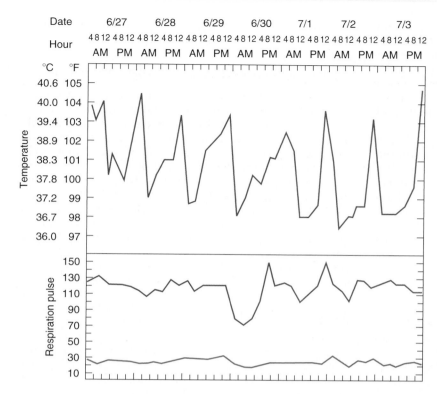

FIGURE 14-1 Intermittent fever of systemic JIA in a 3-year-old girl. The fever spikes usually occurred daily in the late evening to early morning (quotidian pattern), returned to normal or below normal, and were accompanied by severe malaise, tachycardia, and rash.

Individual lesions disappear within a few hours and leave no residua. The rash may be much more persistent in children who are systemically very ill, and it may reappear with each systemic exacerbation. Individual lesions may be elicited by rubbing or scratching the skin (the *Koebner phenomenon* or *isomorphic response*) or by a hot bath or psychological stress. The rash is sometimes pruritic,[59] particularly in older patients, and may be indistinguishable from urticaria. Prominent urticarial eruptions in association with fever and arthralgias are seen in some autoinflammatory syndromes that resemble systemic JIA, or adult-onset Still's disease,[60] raising questions about the specificity of the systemic arthritis rash.

Cardiac Disease

Pericarditis

The overall prevalence of pericardial involvement in JRA is estimated at 3% to 9%.[61,62] Pericarditis and pericardial effusions occur almost exclusively in systemic disease.[62-67] Pericarditis tends to occur in the older child, but it is not related to sex, age at onset, or severity of joint disease.[63] It may precede development of arthritis or occur at any time during the course of the disease, usually accompanied by a systemic exacerbation. Episodes typically persist for 1 to 8 weeks. Most pericardial effusions are asymptomatic, although some children have dyspnea or precordial pain that is exacerbated by lying supine and may be referred to the back, shoulders, or neck. Examination may document diminished heart sounds, tachycardia, cardiomegaly, and a pericardial friction rub, usually at the left lower sternal border.[66] In many cases, pericardial effusions develop insidiously, are not accompanied by obvious

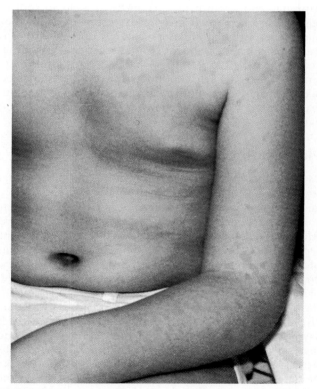

FIGURE 14-2 Typical rash of systemic-onset disease in a 3-year-old boy. The rash is salmon-colored, macular, and nonpruritic. Individual lesions are transient, occur in crops over the trunk and extremities, and may occur in a linear distribution (Koebner phenomenon) after minor trauma such as a scratch.

cardiomegaly or typical electrocardiographic changes (low voltage, ST-segment elevation, T-wave inversion), and escape recognition except by echocardiography.[64] In a study from Los Angeles,[64] an effusion or pericardial thickening was present in 36% of patients, and 81% of children who had active systemic manifestations at the time of the study had abnormal echocardiographic findings. In more than one-half of these patients, pericarditis would not have been diagnosed without echocardiography. Tamponade is a rare, but serious complication that requires urgent drainage of pericardial fluid. It is characterized by venous distention, hepatomegaly, peripheral edema, pulsus paradoxus and an enlarged cardiac silhouette on chest radiography. Chronic constrictive pericarditis is very rare.[65,68,69] In general, children with pericarditis do not fare worse than others in outcome. This complication should not necessarily be regarded as a poor prognostic sign, although pericarditis is frequently present in children with JRA at necropsy.[63,66]

Myocarditis

Myocarditis is much less common than pericarditis and may result in cardiomegaly and congestive heart failure.[70,71] In three cases reported by Miller and French,[70] failure occurred in the absence of overt pericardial effusions in children with severe active systemic disease. Goldenberg and colleagues[62] reported four children with systemic JRA complicated by perimyocarditis and two with myocarditis in a retrospective study of 172 children with JRA.

Endocarditis

Although endocarditis in the context of systemic inflammatory disease should prompt exclusion of acute rheumatic fever, valvular disease, seemingly unrelated to other causes, has been documented in at least two individuals with systemic JRA.[72,73] These patients had onset of systemic arthritis in early childhood, but aortic insufficiency was not diagnosed until years later. A good outcome was reported after placement of a prosthetic valve in one patient.

Pleuropulmonary Disease

Parenchymal pulmonary disease is rare, but diffuse interstitial fibrosis occurs in a small number of children[74-77] and may precede other evidence of JIA.[78-80] Athreya and colleagues[75] noted interstitial disease in 8 of 191 children with JRA, all of whom had a systemic onset. Another report detailed pathological findings in a child who died of pulmonary fibrosis.[74] Pulmonary function studies in 16 children with JRA documented abnormalities in 10 of them.[80] In some children, such abnormalities may be the result of respiratory muscle weakness.[81,82] Pleural effusions may occur with pericarditis, or they may be asymptomatic and be detected only as incidental findings on chest radiographs. One child has been reported with primary pulmonary hypertension.[83] Although pulmonary interstitial and intra-alveolar cholesterol granulomas have been reported in only one patient,[84] we have seen two additional patients who developed lipoid pneumonia diagnosed by lung biopsies. These three patients had severe refractory systemic disease and all developed

respiratory failure, resulting in death (two patients) or lung transplantation (one patient).

Lymphadenopathy and Splenomegaly

Enlargements of lymph nodes and spleen may occur alone or together and are characteristic of systemic JIA. Marked symmetrical lymphadenopathy is particularly common in the anterior cervical, axillary, and inguinal areas and may suggest the diagnosis of lymphoma. The enlarged lymph nodes are typically nontender, firm, and mobile. Tender lymphadenopathy may reflect necrotizing lymphadenitis associated with Kikuchi disease.[85] Mesenteric lymphadenopathy can cause abdominal pain or distention and may lead to the erroneous diagnosis of an acute surgical abdomen. Splenomegaly usually is most prominent within the first years after onset. The degree of splenomegaly may be extreme (Fig. 14-3), but it has not been associated with Felty syndrome (splenic neutropenia) in children with systemic JIA.

Hepatic Disease

Hepatomegaly is less common than splenomegaly. Moderate to marked enlargement of the liver is often associated with only mild derangement of functional studies and relatively nonspecific histopathological changes.[86] This type of liver disease is most evident at onset and usually diminishes with time. Chronic liver disease does not occur. Massive enlargement of the liver is usually accompanied by abdominal distention and pain. Progressive hepatomegaly is characteristic of secondary amyloidosis.

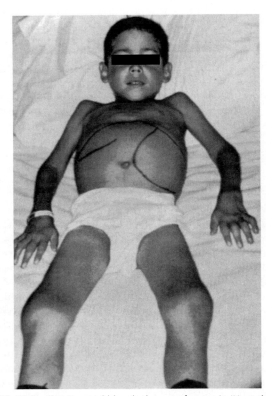

FIGURE 14-3 This 8-year-old boy had onset of systemic JIA at the age of 4 years. There is symmetrical large and small joint arthritis. Note the axillary lymphadenopathy and marked hepatosplenomegaly.

Unexplained acute yellow atrophy has been recorded.[87] Occasionally, a fatty liver is associated with glucocorticoid administration. Elevated transaminases occur in approximately 25% of patients at presentation[55] and may also occur with treatment with NSAIDs (see Chapter 6). A rare, and apparently benign, transient elevation of serum alkaline phosphatase has been observed in several children with JRA.[88,89] This abnormality presumably does not result from hepatotoxicity, although it may be confused with it. Reye syndrome occasionally occurred in children treated with aspirin.[90] Intercurrent infection with varicella or influenza appears to precipitate this serious complication (see Chapter 6).

Central Nervous System Disease

Acute neurological events are rare in children with systemic JIA and adult-onset Still's disease but may carry a significant mortality risk. Deaths have been reported with noninfectious meningitis with neutrophilic cerebrospinal fluid pleocytosis[91-94] and cerebral edema associated with the rapid development of hyponatremia, most likely the result of inappropriate antidiuretic hormone secretion.[95] Children with fever and vomiting appear to be most at risk of developing this latter complication and should be carefully monitored with regard to fluid balances and serum electrolytes and should not receive hypotonic intravenous fluid solutions. Encephalopathy, seizures, and intracranial hemorrhages have been reported with macrophage activation syndrome (MAS), complicating systemic JIA.[96] Some patients develop benign raised intracranial pressure, perhaps as a result of chronic corticosteroid use or related to other medications. Epidural lipomatosis causing spinal cord compression has been reported in two patients.[97]

Nasal Septal Perforation

Nasal septal perforation has been reported in three patients from a single center.[98] These patients had a severe, refractory disease course, and one had leukocytoclastic skin vasculitis at the time the nasal septal perforation was identified.

Macrophage Activation Syndrome

The most devastating complication of systemic JIA, macrophage activation syndrome (MAS), bears close resemblance to secondary hemophagocytic lymphohistiocytosis (HLH) and is associated with serious morbidity and sometimes death. It is characterized by prominent activation of T cells and macrophages leading to an overwhelming systemic inflammatory response. MAS may be somewhat more common in boys, and it is most strongly associated with systemic JIA occurring in at least 7% during the disease course,[99] although many more patients present with incomplete clinical and laboratory features of the syndrome. It has been reported, albeit rarely, in a number of other rheumatic diseases including polyarthritis, adult-onset Still's disease, systemic lupus erythematosus and Kawasaki disease.[100-103] A detailed description of clinical picture of MAS and of its pathophysiology is provided in chapter 45.

MAS often follows an infection, particularly by members of the herpesvirus family, including Epstein-Barr virus.[99-104]

Table 14–2

The main clinical and laboratory features of macrophage activation syndrome

Clinical	Laboratory
Unremitting fever	Fall in ESR
Bruising, purpura, and mucosal bleeding	Fall in WBC and platelet counts
Enlarged lymph nodes, liver, spleen	Elevated ferritin
Liver dysfunction (jaundice, liver failure)	Elevated liver enzymes and LDH
CNS involvement (disorientation, seizures)	Elevated triglycerides
Multiple organ failure	Fall in fibrinogen and elevated D-dimers. Prolonged PT and PTT
	Bone marrow hemophagocytosis

ALT, alanine aminotransferase; *AST*, aspartate aminotransferase; *ESR*, erythrocyte sedimentation rate; *LDH*, lactic dehydrogenase; *PT*, prothrombin time; *PTT*, partial thromboplastin time; *WBC*, white blood cell count.

Early reports noted the onset of MAS after changes in medications, particularly the institution of treatment with a gold compound, sulfasalazine, nonsteroidal anti-inflammatory drug (NSAID), hydroxychloquine, or D-penicillamine.[105-107] More recently, it was suggested that methotrexate and etanercept might trigger the syndrome.[108-110] Considering the wide array of pharmacologic agents that have been reported to be associated with MAS, it seems likely that these events were coincidental, occurring in a child who was susceptible to MAS and who required additional therapy for uncontrolled systemic JIA.

MAS most often occurs during periods of active disease, but has been reported to occur at the time of disease onset,[100,101] at any time during the disease course, including, albeit rarely, during periods of disease remission. It is characterized clinically by the rapid development of an unremitting fever, hepatosplenomegaly, lymphadenopathy, hepatic dysfunction (sometimes with jaundice and liver failure), encephalopathy, purpura, bruising, and mucosal bleeding.[96,104,111,112] More severely affected patients develop multi-organ involvement that may progress to respiratory distress, renal failure, disorientation, seizures, reduced level of consciousness, hypotension and shock.

Laboratory studies indicate the presence of hematocytopenias, especially thrombocytopenia. Normal or even elevated neutrophil counts may be seen in the early stages. Typically, liver enzyme, LDH, triglyceride, and ferritin levels are elevated, sometimes with extreme hyperferritinemia > 10,000 µg/l and serum albumin is low. The prothrombin time (PT) and the partial thromboplastin time (PTT) are prolonged, and blood levels of the vitamin K-dependent clotting factors are decreased. Markedly elevated levels of d-dimers are present in the plasma. The erythrocyte sedimentation rate (ESR) may drop sharply and remain paradoxically low in association with hypofibrinogenemia induced by consumptive coagulopathy and disseminated intravascular coagulation, but CRP is typically elevated. Hematuria and proteinuria may progress to acute renal failure requiring dialysis. Cerebrospinal fluid may show pleocytosis and

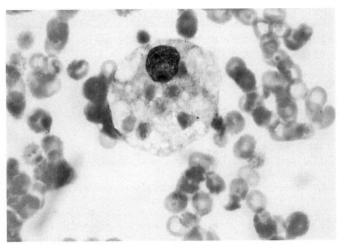

FIGURE 14-4 Bone marrow aspiration demonstrating phagocytosis of erythrocytes and platelets by a histiocyte in a child with macrophage activation syndrome.

an elevated protein concentration, but is often difficult to obtain because of the risk of bleeding associated with the coagulopathy. The demonstration of prominent phagocytosis of other hematopoietic cells by macrophages in the bone marrow or other tissues such as lymph nodes, liver or spleen is diagnostic (Fig. 14–4), but florid MAS may occur in the absence of demonstrated tissue hemophagocytosis in up to 15% of the patients. Mild tissue hemophagocytosis may be seen without MAS.[113] Table 14–2 summarizes the main clinical and laboratory features of MAS. Some of these laboratory abnormalities, typically less prominent, occur in children with systemic JIA even in the absence of MAS.

Prompt diagnosis of MAS in patients with s-JIA is necessary to initiate treatment as quickly as possible. The guidelines for the diagnosis of HLH[114] have not been validated for the diagnosis of MAS. Strict application of these guidelines may in fact result in unnecessary delays in the diagnosis and treatment of MAS and increased morbidity and mortality. Careful and frequent monitoring of the clinical and laboratory trends is much more important than the absolute laboratory test values. Since patients with active s-JIA typically have marked elevation of WBCs, neutrophils, platelets and fibrinogen, sudden and sustained reductions of these, in association with other clinical and laboratory features of MAS suggest the diagnosis even in the absence of more profound cytopenias and hyofibrinogenemia. Preliminary criteria for the diagnosis of MAS have recently been suggested by Ravelli, but not yet validated.[115] These include a combination of clinical features (central nervous system dysfunction, hemorrhages and hepatomegaly) and laboratory features (platelets $\leq 262 \times 10^9/l$, AST > 59 U/l, WBC $\leq 4 \times 10^9/l$ and fibrinogen ≤ 2.5 g/l. MAS must be differentiated from active systemic disease and from viral infections and medication toxicities that can result in hematocytopenias and elevated transaminase levels.

Treatment

MAS must be treated vigorously and rapidly because of the extreme morbidity and high fatality rates. One approach has been to use intravenous methylprednisolone pulse therapy,[96,99,102,111] although some patients are glucocorticoid resistant and require additional treatment. There are inconsistent reports of the efficacy of intravenous immunoglobulin, which may be more effective if administered early in the course of MAS.[116] Several reports describe the rapid resolution of features of MAS with cyclosporine over the course of a few days,[117-119] leading some to consider oral or intravenous cyclosporine a first-line agent. Careful monitoring for cyclosporine toxicity is required, especially when it is administered intravenously. For rapidly progressive disease with multiorgan involvement, early treatment with the combination of systemic corticosteroids, cyclosporine and etoposide, as recommended in the HLH-2004 protocol, may be effective.[114] The HLH-2004 protocol as well as other potential approaches with ATG and biologicals are discussed in chapter 45.

Amyloidosis

Secondary amyloidosis as a complication of JIA is exceedingly rare in North America but has been reported in earlier studies in 5% to 7% of children with chronic arthritis in Europe[120,121] and in 10% in a Turkish series from the 1990s.[122] It is seen most commonly in children with systemic arthritis. Even in Europe, amyloidosis as a complication of chronic arthritis is on the decline, with a decreasing number of deaths.[122-125] A recent report of 24 children in Finland with JIA-associated amyloidosis, diagnosed over a 30-year period, identified no new cases from 1991 to 2005.[126] Although no HLA associations have been confirmed in children who develop amyloidosis,[127] a genetic marker for amyloid P component was identified.[128] Rectal submucosa is the most frequently recommended biopsy site; renal biopsy can be hazardous because of an increased tendency toward bleeding. Radionuclide imaging using radioiodinated autologous serum amyloid P is a noninvasive technique for diagnosis and monitoring of amyloidosis.[129]

The major causes of death in 46 children with arthritis monitored by Bywaters at Taplow[130] were renal failure (which in one-half of the children was associated with amyloidosis) and infections. At the 15-year evaluation, excess mortality was identified in girls who had onset of arthritis early in life. After 15 years of arthritis, the frequency of amyloidosis had risen to 7.4% among children with arthritis in the United Kingdom.[121] It was rarely observed as early as 1 year after onset of the arthritis but could develop as late as 23 years after onset. Spontaneous remissions occurred. The outcome of JIA-associated amyloidosis in the Finnish series was also poor, with a mortality rate of 42% and renal insufficiency or renal transplantation required in 25% of survivors, after a mean follow-up of 15 years.[131] Amyloidosis is typically accompanied by elevated levels of serum amyloid-A (SAA) and inflammatory markers such as CRP. Control of the underlying disease is critical in treating amyloidosis, and the potential to induce regression of amyloid deposits and improve the function of affected organs has been related to lowering levels of SAA.[132] Treatment with chlorambucil improved survival in JIA-associated amyloidosis,[124] and more recently treatment with TNF-α inhibitors[133] and anti-IL6 receptor antibody[134] has been reported to result in regression of amyloidosis in some patients.

DIAGNOSIS AND DIFFERENTIAL DIAGNOSIS

The diagnosis of systemic arthritis is clinical, and it is a diagnosis of exclusion. In its fully developed state, the clinical characteristics are quite diagnostic. In particular, the presence of a classic rash and quotidian fever indicate the likelihood of this diagnosis. The ILAR criteria emphasize the importance of both the arthritis and the fever to the diagnosis and require that fever be present for two weeks and documented to be quotidian for 72 hours.

Differential Diagnosis

The differential diagnosis of suspected systemic JIA may be difficult, especially at onset or early in the course of the disease, when the child may have a high, spiking fever and evidence of systemic inflammation but no arthritis and no specific sign or symptom that allows a definitive diagnosis.[135] In such children, the possibilities of malignancy, inflammatory bowel disease, vasculitis such as polyarteritis nodosa, or other connective tissue diseases such as systemic lupus erythematosus should be considered (Table 14–3). Children with systemic-onset disease may be thought to have an acute infectious disease or septicemia. Infectious mononucleosis and other viral illnesses may mimic the disease, but for the most part the arthropathies that occur secondary to viral infections are transient. Documenting the presence of arthritis or a typical rash helps to establish the diagnosis. Laboratory test results reflect significant systemic inflammation, but are not specific. In many instances, the diagnosis is one of exclusion until a full complement of characteristic abnormalities has been observed, a process that can take several months or possibly years. When the constellation of clinical and laboratory findings is not typical for the diagnosis of systemic arthritis, more extensive investigations, including imaging of the chest and abdomen, examination of bone marrow, and biopsies of lymph nodes or affected organs may be necessary. It is very important to exclude the expanding spectrum of autoinflammatory syndromes (see Chapter 43). Although these are rare, they can have clinical and laboratory features that closely mimic systemic arthritis. Some of these syndromes may begin at an earlier age than systemic arthritis, may have a shorter duration of each fever episode, and may be accompanied by arthralgia or arthritis. Tumor necrosis factor receptor–associated periodic syndrome may manifest with recurrent fever for several weeks, rash, arthralgia or arthritis, and myalgia.[136] Among the cryopyrin-associated periodic syndromes, chronic inflammatory neurological and articular syndrome frequently manifests in early infancy and the neurological and ophthalmological features may be prominent. Muckle-Wells syndrome, however, often presents with fever, urticarial rash, and sometimes arthritis, with the later development of hearing loss. Genetic testing can be helpful in identifying these syndromes but may not be completely sensitive.

Table 14–3

Differential diagnosis of systemic juvenile idiopathic arthritis

Infections
- Bacterial endocarditis
- Acute rheumatic fever
- Cat scratch disease (Bartonella)
- Lyme disease (Borrelia burgdorferi)
- Brucellosis
- Mycoplasma
- Many others

Malignancy

Rheumatic and inflammatory diseases:
- Systemic lupus erythematosus
- Dermatomyositis
- Polyarteritis nodosa
- Kawasaki disease
- Serum sickness
- Sarcoidosis
- Castleman disease

Inflammatory bowel disease

Autoinflammatory syndromes
- Familial Mediterranean fever
- Mevalonate kinase deficiency (mevalonic aciduria and hyperimmunoglobulin D syndrome)
- Periodic fever, aphthous stomatitis, pharyngitis, and adenitis (PFAPA)
- TNF receptor–associated periodic syndrome (TRAPS)
- Muckle-Wells syndrome
- Familial cold autoinflammatory syndrome
- Chronic infantile neurological cutaneous and articular syndrome (CINCA)

Fever in children with infectious diseases is of the septic type. It is more hectic, spikes less predictably, and usually does not repetitively return to baseline each day, as does the fever of JIA, and the child remains ill even during a relatively afebrile interval. A sustained or remittent fever is characteristic of acute rheumatic fever and should respond dramatically to NSAIDs. Although many children with systemic JIA have isolated pericarditis, a pericardial effusion with evidence of endocarditis such as a diastolic murmur suggests a diagnosis of rheumatic fever or bacterial endocarditis. Onset of rheumatic fever in the developed countries of the world typically occurs in children between the ages of 5 and 15 years (see Chapter 40). The arthritis is characteristically acute and painful, migratory, and asymmetrical, involving the peripheral joints without sequelae. The initial episode usually lasts no longer than 6 weeks but may persist for as long as 3 months. Evidence of a prior infection with β-hemolytic group A streptococci is present; however, the antistreptolysin O titer may be chronically increased to a moderate degree in one-third of children with JIA as a manifestation of inflammation rather than evidence of recent streptococcal infection.[137] In acute rheumatic fever, a rise or fall in antistreptolysin O titer should be documented.

Adult-onset Still's Disease

Adult-onset Still's disease was first reported in 1942. It may manifest in either sex as fever of unknown origin. Hallmarks of adult-onset Still's disease are similar to those of childhood-onset disease,[138-141] but sore throat is a more common symptom than in systemic JIA. There is a similar association with MAS and hyperferritinemia, and a very low proportion of glycosylated ferritin has been reported in both adult-onset Still's disease and reactive HLH.[142-144] Bywaters[139] described 14 young women with characteristic features of Still's disease, including fever, rash, polyarthritis, and an elevated ESR. In a National Institutes of Health study, all of the patients were men, and one-half were actually experiencing an exacerbation of arthritis after a long remission of systemic disease that began in childhood.[138] Characteristic radiographic changes (e.g., pericapitate involvement) have been described.[145]

PATHOLOGY

The rash of JRA is one of the most characteristic clinical hallmarks of the disease. It is characterized by minimal perivascular infiltration of mononuclear cells around capillaries and venules in the subdermal tissues.[58] A neutrophilic perivasculitis resembling that of the rash of rheumatic fever may accompany the more flagrant lesions.

The serosal lining surfaces of the pleural, pericardial, and peritoneal cavities of the body may exhibit nonspecific fibrous serositis, which is characterized clinically by effusion and pain. Enlargement of the lymph nodes is related to a nonspecific follicular hyperplasia that in rare instances may closely resemble lymphoma. Hepatic abnormalities are characterized by a nonspecific collection of periportal inflammatory cells and hyperplasia of Kupffer cells. Synovitis does not differ histologically from that seen in other types of JIA (see Chapter 13).

LABORATORY EXAMINATION

Indicators of inflammation are usually striking in active systemic JIA. The WBC is often higher than 30,000 to 50,000 cells/mm^3 (30 to 50 × 10^9/L), with a predominance of polymorphonuclear leukocytes. The platelet count is usually elevated, sometimes to more than 1,000,000/mm^3 (1000 × 10^9/L), although rarely thrombocytopenia occurs early in the disease course.[146] Hemoglobin in the range of 7 to 10 g/dL (70 to 100 g/L) is usual, and occasionally it is even lower. Erythrocytes are characteristically hypochromic but can be normocytic or microcytic. Erythroid aplasia has been reported.[147,148] The ESR is usually very high, except in patients with MAS, in whom it may be normal. C-reactive protein is elevated, and ferritin levels are often very high, reflecting the extent of inflammatory disease. Moderately elevated ferritin and D-Dimers, usually accompanied by high fibrinogen, can be seen in the presence of active systemic inflammation, but the clinician must be vigilant for early features of MAS. If the ESR and fibrinogen are noted to suddenly or even steadily decrease, despite other prominent features of inflammation, MAS may be evolving.

Polyclonal elevation of immunoglobulin levels characterizes the immune response, but autoantibodies such as rheumatoid factors and antinuclear antibodies are uncommon. Complement levels are usually increased as part of the acute-phase response, and increased levels of complement activation products have been reported.[149]

Synovial fluid analysis confirms the presence of an inflammatory arthritis, with cell counts in the range of 10,000 to 40,000/mm^3, predominantly polymorphonuclear leukocytes. When there is marked systemic inflammation, synovial fluid white cell counts can rise to the 100,000/mm^3 range, mimicking those seen in septic arthritis.

The laboratory profile, although supportive of the diagnosis, is nonspecific and can be seen in other infectious and inflammatory conditions. Recently, a marker of granulocyte activation, S100A12, was reported to be significantly elevated in patients with systemic JIA, with a sensitivity of 66% and a specificity of 94% to distinguish between systemic JIA and infections.[150] Serum concentrations of MRP-8/MRP-14 have been reported to be useful in differentiating systemic JIA from infections and possibly other causes of systemic inflammation.[48]

RADIOLOGICAL EXAMINATION

Radiographs demonstrate bone and soft tissue changes in a high proportion of children with systemic JIA. In addition, growth abnormalities may be marked, and generalized delay in bone age is a frequent observation. Juxta-articular osteoporosis indicates the effect of active arthritis. In a study of 30 children with systemic JRA, Oen and colleagues[151] found that radiographs performed within the first 2 years of disease revealed joint space narrowing in 30%, erosions in 35%, and growth abnormalities in 10%. These early changes, which have also been shown to correlate with thrombocytosis and persistently active systemic symptoms in the first 6 months from onset,[56] were most frequently seen in wrist, hip, and shoulder radiographs. In later radiographs (a median of 6.4 years after onset), joint space narrowing was demonstrated in 39%, erosions in 63%, and growth abnormalities in 25%. Changes in the cervical spine and hips were most common in late radiographs. Ankylosis, especially involving the wrist and apophyseal joints of the cervical spine, is seen in severe, refractory disease (see Chapter 10).[152]

TREATMENT

Approach to Management

The child with s-JIA is often acutely ill and may require hospitalization for initial management. In addition to medications to minimize joint inflammation, attention must be directed to the diagnosis and management of extraarticular manifestations. Careful assessment of pulmonary and cardiac status, the severity of anemia, and the possibility of MAS are all parts of the initial evaluation.

The general principles of management, outlined in Chapters 6 and 9, should be applied to the management of systemic JIA. It is important to note that, while several controlled clinical trials have been performed in JIA, very few have been specifically designed to evaluate efficacy in s-JIA. Although evidence-based information regarding treatment of s-JIA is therefore largely lacking, some controlled trials have recently been initiated.

It is often appropriate to use an NSAID as initial therapy, both to aid in control of the systemic inflammatory features (e.g., fever) and to modulate joint pain and inflammation. Because systemic features seldom respond satisfactorily to NSAIDs alone, if the diagnosis is firmly established, the early use of glucocorticoids is indicated. Intravenous methylprednisolone (30 mg/kg/day to a maximum of 1 g/day on 1 to 3 consecutive days) is effective in controlling systemic and articular features of the disease, but the effect is often short-lived. Therefore, oral prednisone (1 to 2 mg/kg/day to a maximum of 60 mg/day in one or more doses) is often necessary. Tapering glucocorticoids to a minimum acceptable dose, or withdrawing them, may be extremely difficult in patients with severe s-JIA but should be a major goal in order to minimize the side effects of long-term treatment with these drugs. If the number of joints with resistant inflammation is small, intraarticular triamcinolone hexacetonide may be very effective and multiple intraarticular injections should be considered, even for those with many active joints. However, benefits from intraarticular corticosteroid injections may be less durable than they are for other subtypes of JIA,[153] especially if performed when the systemic disease is very active.

Disease-modifying antirheumatic drugs have been traditionally used in patients with s-JIA, with the goal of sparing glucocorticoids, but their efficacy is usually limited. Although most of the evidence is provided by uncontrolled studies, biologic agents that inhibit the three pivotal inflammatory cytokines (TNF, IL-1 and IL-6) have already changed the approach to the treatment of s-JIA. Although some patients may respond very favorably to anti-TNF agents, TNF inhibition in s-JIA is not as effective as in other JIA subtypes, and there is little evidence for its effectiveness for systemic symptoms. Therefore, TNF inhibition may not be considered the first-line biological approach in patients with persistently active s-JIA. There is accumulating evidence that inhibition of IL-1 or IL-6 is highly efficacious in a significant number of patients with persistent s-JIA, with improvements seen in both systemic symptoms and arthritis. The long-term benefits of these approaches still need to be determined. More importantly, the interplay between IL-6 and IL-1 in the pathogenesis of s-JIA still needs to be clarified. Hopefully, mechanistic studies may help to identify predictors of response to either IL-1 or IL-6 inhibition, allowing a personalized approach to treatment. When exactly to introduce a treatment with a biologic is not yet clear. Early introduction may limit steroid toxicity.

Pharmacological Therapy

Anti-TNF Agents

In the original multicenter clinical trial of etanercept, there were 22 patients with systemic arthritis who were refractory or intolerant to methotrexate.[154] In the double-blind phase of this trial, 7 of 8 patients (88%) receiving placebo flared, compared with 4 of 9 (44%) receiving etanercept. The frequency of flare was much lower in children with polyarticular JIA (21%). In the 2-year follow-up study,[155] an ACR30 response occurred in 59%, a pediatric ACR30 response in 53%, and a pediatric ACR70 response in 47%. Published data from three different national registries of JIA patients on etanercept showed a significantly higher rate of treatment failure (i.e., failure to achieve an ACR30 response) and of flares during treatment in patients with s-JIA compared to other JIA onset types.[156-158] The proportion of patients that continued etanercept after 2 years was approximately 40% in s-JIA compared to more than 80% in non–s-JIA.[157] A multicenter survey on 82 s-JIA patients treated with etanercept in the Unites States showed an excellent response in approximately one-third of the patients.[159] Anecdotally, infliximab or adalimumab have been reported to be effective in some children with systemic JIA, even if they have failed to respond to etanercept. Studies of the efficacy of infliximab or adalimumab in s-JIA have not been reported, and no data are available on the patients with systemic onset and polyarticular-course enrolled in the two published pivotal controlled trials.[160,161] Recently published experience from a single center in South America reported that, of 45 s-JIA patients treated with various TNF inhibitors, approximately one-fourth reached clinical remission; half of them flared in the subsequent year.[162]

Anti–IL6 Receptor

The only available IL-6 inhibitor is tocilizumab (TCZ), a humanized anti–IL-6 receptor antibody. Two small phase I and II studies with TCZ in s-JIA reported a prompt improvement in clinical and laboratory parameters.[163,164] Following these, a phase III, withdrawal design, study of TCZ in 56 patients with s-JIA has been performed in Japan.[165] Approximately two-thirds of the patients reached an ACR30 response at the end of the 6-week open phase. Following randomization to continuing TCZ or switching to placebo, TCZ was clearly superior to placebo in maintaining clinical and biological (CRP <1.5 mg/dL) response. At the end of the subsequent 48-week open phase extension, approximately 90% of the patients were still taking TCZ, with the great majority of them (90%) having achieved an ACR70 response. In this trial, TCZ was administered at 8 mg/kg every 2 weeks, but the optimal dose and frequency of TCZ has not been determined. A placebo-controlled trial is ongoing at present, with a different dosing regimen for children with a lower body weight.

Anti–IL-1 treatment

Following an initial observation of a very favorable response to IL-1 inhibition with anakinra in two patients with treatment resistant s-JIA,[166] several publications have reported on the response of s-JIA patients to anakinra. The drug is usually administered at a dose of 1-2 mg/kg/day. No controlled trial has been published. A rather prompt effect of anakinra on systemic features and laboratory measures of inflammation has been observed in a large proportion of patients (from 50% to 90% in the different reports),[27,51,167-169] but anakinra appears to be less effective for arthritis. In one of the largest reported series, an ACR50 response was observed only in 25% of the patients,[168] whereas in another large series, a complete response was observed in approximately 40% of the patients.[51] Overall, up to one-half of the patients with s-JIA appear to respond promptly to anakinra, and at least some may indeed reach clinical remission. Preliminary results of treatment with canakinumab, a fully humanized monoclonal antibody to IL-1β, are promising,[170] and a controlled trial is under way.

Methotrexate

In children with s-JIA, the response rate to methotrexate is not as high as it is for oligoarthritis or polyarthritis, and there is no evidence that it is efficacious for the systemic features. In a placebo-controlled study, there was no significant difference in ACR30 response rate, systemic feature score, ESR, or CRP between those children who received oral methotrexate and those who received placebo.[171]

Intravenous Immunoglobulin

Intravenous immunoglobulin (IVIg) has been used to treat systemic JIA, although the evidence supporting its use is limited. In small, uncontrolled trials, IVIg was found to be useful for systemic features but not consistently effective for arthritis.[172-175] A controlled, randomized trial of IVIg in children with systemic-onset diseases indicated that the drug had little benefit compared with placebo.[176] However, the results were considered inconclusive because of the small sample size. The place of IVIg, therefore, remains unclear, but it may be considered in a child with active systemic manifestations that have not responded to NSAIDs and glucocorticoids. The usual dose is 1-2 g/kg/day administered every 2-4 weeks for a period of at least 6 months. Shorter courses may be used for acute refractory systemic features of the disease.

Cyclosporine-A

Cyclosporine-A has also been reported to be useful in systemic aspects of the disease. In an open, prospective study, the most dramatic response was rapid disappearance of fever in 52% of the patients. The effects on joint inflammation were less impressive, although a reduction of at least 50% in the number of active joints was observed in one-third of the patients after 3 months of therapy.[177] Toxicity to cyclosporine led to discontinuation in one-quarter of the patients, and an additional 50% discontinued the drug because of disease flare or inefficacy. In a more recent multicenter open study, of 184 patients with s-JIA who started cyclosporine-A, only 74 were still taking the drug at the last follow-up visit. Of these, only 5% achieved a complete clinical response, 30% had mild disease activity, but 65% had moderate or severe disease activity.[178]

Thalidomide

Some reports support the use of thalidomide in children with treatment-resistant systemic JIA. A multicenter retrospective review of experience in 13 children with treatment-resistant s-JIA provides evidence that this drug may have a role.[179] All patients received thalidomide in a dose of 3 to 5 mg/kg/day. Improvement in active joint count, required prednisone dose, and inflammatory indices were seen by 6 months, with 10 of the 13 patients obtaining an ACR50 response; in the 5 patients who were monitored for 24 months, the improvement appeared to be sustained. Three additional patients with systemic JIA unresponsive to etanercept and with a subsequent favorable response to thalidomide have also been reported.[180]

Autologous Stem Cell Transplantation

Most children with rheumatic diseases who have received autologous stem cell transplantation (ASCT) have had s-JIA. Long-term follow-up data have been published by the Utrecht group and, more recently, also by a United Kingdom multicenter study.[181,182] Drug-free complete remission was obtained in 4 out of the 7 patients in the United Kingdom study and in 8 of the 22 patients in the Dutch study. Significant mortality was, however, reported by both groups (1 of 7 in the United Kingdom and 4 of 22 in the Netherlands). Fatal MAS appears to be the major complication. Following the initial observation of the MAS cases, the original protocol has been modified to avoid profound T cell depletion and to ensure better control of systemic disease before and after transplantation. Total body irradiation has not been used in the most recently transplanted patients. Following these modifications, no ASCT deaths were observed. Given the promising results with the novel biologics, currently ASCT should be considered only in those children who have failed anti–IL-1 and anti–IL-6 treatments.

COURSE OF THE DISEASE AND PROGNOSIS

The acute manifestations of systemic JIA are variable in duration and last from weeks to months. Systemic features such as fever, rash, and pericarditis tend to subside during the initial months to years of the disease (2 to 5 years) but may recur in conjunction with exacerbations of the arthritis. About 40% of the children with systemic JIA follow a monocyclic disease course and eventually recover almost completely, after a variable period. A small proportion of children have a polycyclic course characterized by recurrent episodes of active disease interrupted by periods of remission without medications. Studies over the last 30 years have consistently shown that more than one-half of the children with systemic JIA have a persistent disease course.[183-186] This has resulted in progressive involvement of more and more joints and moderate to severe functional disability in some studies[56,187,188] but not in others.[189] Those who follow a severe, protracted course may have profound morbidity secondary to long-term treatment with systemic glucocorticoids. The eventual functional outcome in these children depends more on the number of joints involved and on continuing activity than on the nature of the systemic disease.[185] The persistence of systemic symptoms without arthritis is unusual and is seldom a cause of permanent disability. In the Cincinnati series, 48% of children with systemic JRA still had active arthritis 10 years later.[190] More recent studies have reported remission in only approximately one-third of patients.[184,191-193]

The most important early predictors of destructive arthritis are polyarthritis, thrombocytosis, persistent fever, or the need for systemic corticosteroids in the first

6 months after disease onset.[56,187,194,195] Persistently elevated levels of fibrin D-Dimer may be associated with poor joint and functional outcomes.[196] Early hip arthritis may also be associated with a worse outcome. Male sex has been reported to correlate with worse disability in children with systemic disease,[197] but this has not been consistent. A polymorphism of the MIF gene is the first genetic predictor of poor outcome in systemic JIA to be identified. The MIF-173*C allele results in higher serum and synovial fluid levels of MIF and is associated with poor response to glucocorticoid treatment, persistently active disease, and poor outcome.[19] It remains to be determined whether treatment with newer biologic agents will result in better outcomes for children with this disease.

In early studies of JRA, the death rate was 2% to 4%.[198,199] The disease-associated death rate is now perhaps less than 1% in Europe and less than 0.5% in North America. The majority of the deaths associated with JRA in Europe were related to amyloidosis; in the United States, deaths occurred predominantly in children with systemic arthritis and, in many cases, were related to infections associated with glucocorticoid therapy. MAS remains a serious and potentially fatal threat. Deaths have rarely been reported as a result of neurological and cardiac complications and lipoid pneumonia.

REFERENCES

2. R.E. Petty, T.R. Southwood, P. Manners, et al., International League of Associations for Rheumatology classification of juvenile idiopathic arthritis: second revision, Edmonton, 2001, J. Rheumatol. 31 (2004) 390–392.
14. E.M. Ogilvie, M.S. Fife, S.D. Thompson, et al., The -174G allele of the interleukin-6 gene confers susceptibility to systemic arthritis in children: a multicenter study using simplex and multiplex juvenile idiopathic arthritis families, Arthritis Rheum. 48 (2003) 3202–3206.
19. F. De Benedetti, C. Meazza, M. Vivarelli, et al., Functional and prognostic relevance of the -173 polymorphism of the macrophage migration inhibitory factor gene in systemic-onset juvenile idiopathic arthritis, Arthritis Rheum. 48 (2003) 1398–1407.
23. M.G. Barnes, A.A. Grom, S.D. Thompson, et al., Subtype-specific peripheral blood gene expression profiles in recent-onset juvenile idiopathic arthritis, Arthritis Rheum. 60 (2009) 2102–2112.
32. W. de Jager, E.P. Hoppenreijs, N.M. Wulffraat, et al., Blood and synovial fluid cytokine signatures in patients with juvenile idiopathic arthritis: a cross-sectional study, Ann. Rheum. Dis. 66 (2007) 589–598.
39. F. de Benedetti, Martini: Targeting the interleukin-6 receptor: a new treatment for systemic juvenile idiopathic arthritis? Arthritis Rheum. 52 (2005) 687–693.
46. F. De Benedetti, N. Rucci, A. Del Fattore, et al., Impaired skeletal development in interleukin-6-transgenic mice: a model for the impact of chronic inflammation on the growing skeletal system, Arthritis Rheum. 54 (2006) 3551–3563.
48. M. Frosch, M. Ahlmann, T. Vogl, et al., The myeloid-related proteins 8 and 14 complex, a novel ligand of toll-like receptor 4, and interleukin-1beta form a positive feedback mechanism in systemic-onset juvenile idiopathic arthritis, Arthritis. Rheum. 60 (2009) 883–891.
51. M. Gattorno, A. Piccini, D. Lasiglie, et al., The pattern of response to anti-interleukin-1 treatment distinguishes two subsets of patients with systemic-onset juvenile idiopathic arthritis, Arthritis Rheum. 58 (2008) 1505–1515.
55. E.M. Behrens, T. Beukelman, L. Gallo, et al., Evaluation of the presentation of systemic onset juvenile rheumatoid arthritis: data from the Pennsylvania Systemic Onset Juvenile Arthritis Registry (PASOJAR), J. Rheumatol. 35 (2008) 343–348.

56. R. Schneider, B.A. Lang, B.J. Reilly, et al., Prognostic indicators of joint destruction in systemic-onset juvenile rheumatoid arthritis, J. Pediatr. 120 (1992) 200–205.
58. E.G. Bywaters, I.C. Isdale, The rash of rheumatoid arthritis and Still's disease, Q. J. Med. 25 (1956) 377–387.
59. J. Schaller, R.J. Wedgwood, Pruritus associated with the rash of juvenile rheumatoid arthritis, Pediatrics 45 (1970) 296–298.
62. J. Goldenberg, M.B. Ferraz, A.P. Pessoa, et al., Symptomatic cardiac involvement in juvenile rheumatoid arthriti, Int. J. Cardiol. 34 (1992) 57–62.
73. J. Heyd, J. Glaser, Early occurrence of aortic valve regurgitation in a youth with systemic-onset juvenile rheumatoid arthritis, Am. J. Med. 89 (1990) 123–124.
75. B.H. Athreya, R.A. Doughty, M. Bookspan, et al., Pulmonary manifestations of juvenile rheumatoid arthritis. A report of eight cases and review, Clin. Chest Med. 1 (1980) 361–374.
84. R. Schultz, J. Mattila, M. Gappa, et al., Development of progressive pulmonary interstitial and intra-alveolar cholesterol granulomas (PICG) associated with therapy-resistant chronic systemic juvenile arthritis (CJA), Pediatr. Pulmonol. 32 (2001) 397–402.
86. J. Schaller, B. Beckwith, R.J. Wedgwood, Hepatic involvement in juvenile rheumatoid arthritis, J. Pediatr. 77 (1970) 203–210.
93. A. Ohta, M. Yamaguchi, T. Tsunematsu, et al., Adult Still's disease: a multicenter survey of Japanese patients, J. Rheumatol. 17 (1990) 1058–1063.
94. F. Tabak, M. Tanverdi, R. Ozaras, et al., Neutrophilic pleocytosis in cerebrospinal fluid: adult-onset Still's disease, Intern. Med. 42 (2003) 1039–1041.
98. T. Avcin, E.D. Silverman, V. Forte, et al., Nasal septal perforation: a novel clinical manifestation of systemic juvenile idiopathic arthritis/adult onset Still's disease, J. Rheumatol. 32 (2005) 2429–2431.
99. S. Sawhney, P. Woo, K.J. Murray, Macrophage activation syndrome: a potentially fatal complication of rheumatic disorders, Arch. Dis. Child 85 (2001) 421–426.
102. J.L. Stephan, I. Kone-Paut, C. Galambrun, et al., Reactive haemophagocytic syndrome in children with inflammatory disorders: a retrospective study of 24 patients, Rheumatology (Oxford) 40 (2001) 1285–1292.
114. J.I. Henter, A. Horne, M. Arico, et al., HLH-2004: Diagnostic and therapeutic guidelines for hemophagocytic lymphohistiocytosis, Pediatr. Blood Cancer 48 (2007) 124–131.
115. A. Ravelli, S. Magni-Manzoni, A. Pistorio, et al., Preliminary diagnostic guidelines for macrophage activation syndrome complicating systemic juvenile idiopathic arthritis, J. Pediatr. 146 (2005) 598–604.
117. R. Mouy, J.L. Stephan, P. Pillet, et al., Efficacy of cyclosporine A in the treatment of macrophage activation syndrome in juvenile arthritis: report of five cases, J. Pediatr. 129 (1996) 750–754.
123. B.M. Ansell, Chlorambucil therapy in juvenile chronic arthritis (juvenile idiopathic arthritis, J. Rheumatol. 26 (1999) 765–766.
131. K. Immonen, A. Savolainen, H. Kautiainen, et al., Longterm outcome of amyloidosis associated with juvenile idiopathic arthritis, J. Rheumatol. 35 (2008) 907–912.
133. J.E. Gottenberg, F. Merle-Vincent, F. Bentaberry, et al., Anti-tumor necrosis factor alpha therapy in fifteen patients with AA amyloidosis secondary to inflammatory arthritides: a followup report of tolerability and efficacy, Arthritis Rheum. 48 (2003) 2019–2024.
134. Y. Okuda, K. Takasugi, Successful use of a humanized anti-interleukin-6 receptor antibody, tocilizumab, to treat amyloid A amyloidosis complicating juvenile idiopathic arthritis, Arthritis. Rheum. 54 (2006) 2997–3000.
136. A. Manki, R. Nishikomori, M. Nakata-Hizume, et al., Tumor necrosis factor receptor-associated periodic syndrome mimicking systemic juvenile idiopathic arthritis, Allergol. Int. 55 (2006) 337–341.
150. H. Wittkowski, M. Frosch, N. Wulffraat, et al., S100A12 is a novel molecular marker differentiating systemic-onset juvenile idiopathic arthritis from other causes of fever of unknown origin, Arthritis Rheum. 58 (2008) 3924–3931.
151. K. Oen, M. Reed, P.N. Malleson, et al., Radiologic outcome and its relationship to functional disability in juvenile rheumatoid arthritis, J. Rheumatol. 30 (2003) 832–840.

158. P. Quartier, P. Taupin, F. Bourdeaut, et al., Efficacy of etanercept for the treatment of juvenile idiopathic arthritis according to the onset type, Arthritis Rheum. 48 (2003) 1093–1101.

159. Y. Kimura, P. Pinho, G. Walco, et al., Etanercept treatment in patients with refractory systemic onset juvenile rheumatoid arthritis, J. Rheumatol. 32 (2005) 935–942.

165. S. Yokota, T. Imagawa, M. Mori, et al., Efficacy and safety of tocilizumab in patients with systemic-onset juvenile idiopathic arthritis: a randomised, double-blind, placebo-controlled, withdrawal phase III trial, Lancet 371 (2008) 998–1006.

168. T. Lequerre, P. Quartier, D. Rosellini, et al., Interleukin-1 receptor antagonist (anakinra) treatment in patients with systemic-onset juvenile idiopathic arthritis or adult onset Still disease: preliminary experience in France, Ann. Rheum. Dis. 67 (2008) 302–308.

171. P. Woo, T.R. Southwood, A.M. Prieur, et al., Randomized, placebo-controlled, crossover trial of low-dose oral methotrexate in children with extended oligoarticular or systemic arthritisy, Arthritis Rheum. 43 (2000) 1849–1857.

176. E.D. Silverman, G.D. Cawkwell, D.J. Lovell, et al., Intravenous immunoglobulin in the treatment of systemic juvenile rheumatoid arthritis: a randomized placebo controlled trial, Pediatric Rheumatology Collaborative Study Groupy, J. Rheumatol. 21 (1994) 2353–2358.

179. T.J. Lehman, S.J. Schechter, R.P. Sundel, et al., Thalidomide for severe systemic onset juvenile rheumatoid arthritis: a multicenter study, J. Pediatr. 145 (2004) 856–857.

181. M. Abinun, T.J. Flood, A.J. Cant, et al., Autologous T cell depleted haematopoietic stem cell transplantation in children with severe juvenile idiopathic arthritis in the UK (2000-2007), Mol. Immunol. 47 (2009) 46–51.

182. D.M. Brinkman, I.M. de Kleer, R. ten Cate, et al., Autologous stem cell transplantation in children with severe progressive systemic or polyarticular juvenile idiopathic arthritis: long-term follow-up of a prospective clinical trial, Arthritis Rheum. 56 (2007) 2410–2421.

187. L.R. Spiegel, R. Schneider, B.A. Lang, et al., Early predictors of poor functional outcome in systemic-onset juvenile rheumatoid arthritis: a multicenter cohort study, Arthritis Rheum. 43 (2000) 2402–2409.

194. C. Modesto, P. Woo, J. Garcia-Consuegra, et al., Systemic onset juvenile chronic arthritis, polyarticular pattern and hip involvement as markers for a bad prognosis, Clin. Exp. Rheumatol. 19 (2001) 211–217.

195. C. Sandborg, T.H. Holmes, T. Lee, et al., Candidate early predictors for progression to joint damage in systemic juvenile idiopathic arthritis, J. Rheumatol. 33 (2006) 2322–2329.

Entire reference list is available online at www.expertconsult.com.

Chapter 15

POLYARTHRITIS

Alan M. Rosenberg and Kiem G. Oen

DEFINITIONS

Chronic childhood arthritis affecting more than four joints during the first 6 months of disease is defined as polyarthritis.[1,2] In the classification of the International League of Associations for Rheumatology (ILAR),[2] polyarthritis is further categorized as rheumatoid factor (RF) negative if tests for RF are negative, and RF positive if RF is detected on two occasions at least three months apart (Table 15–1). Consequently, this chapter considers RF-negative and RF-positive polyarthritis juvenile idiopathic arthritis (JIA) subsets separately, as distinctive clinical entities.

RHEUMATOID FACTOR–NEGATIVE POLYARTHRITIS

Epidemiology

Polyarthritis accounts for approximately 20% of JIA patients in British and Canadian studies, and of these approximately 85% have negative tests for RF as determined by standard assays.[3,4] Within the polyarthritis subset the proportion that is seronegative for RF varies in accord with population ethnicity.[5-8]

Incidence and Prevalence

Incidence and prevalence data, estimated from population surveys, vary widely as a consequence of differences in case ascertainment, diagnostic and classification criteria applied, accessibility to health care, referral patterns, and genetic and ethnic characteristics of the source population.[9] The incidence of chronic childhood arthritis has been estimated at 7 to 21 per 100,000 in North American and Northern European population-based studies.[10-15] Prevalence rates of 121 to 220 per 100,000 have been reported; metaanalysis has indicated a chronic childhood arthritis prevalence of 132 per 100,000 in population-based studies.[6] Assuming that approximately 20% of the captured populations has polyarthritis and 85% of these are RF negative, the annual incidence and prevalence figures for RF-negative polyarthritis can be estimated to be 1 to 4 per 100,000 and 21 to 37 per 100,000, respectively.

Age at Onset and Sex Ratio

Although the RF-negative polyarthritis JIA subtype can begin at any age before 16, the onset age distribution displays a biphasic tendency, with one peak at 1 to 3 years of age and another encompassing later childhood and adolescence. RF-negative polyarthritis affects girls approximately 4 times more frequently than boys.[3,4] The predominance of females is greater in those with an onset age during the teenage years (female/male ratio 10:1) than in those with a younger onset age (female/male ratio 3:1).

Geographic and Racial Distribution

JIA occurs worldwide but prevalences vary widely among geographical regions. Both RF-negative and RF-positive polyarthritis are overrepresented in some Native North American populations.[6] Among a group of 113 children with polyarthritis from Saskatchewan, Canada, 31 (27.4%) were Native Canadians compared with the general Native Canadian population of 14.9%. Of the 31 children with polyarthritis, 17 (54.8%) were RF negative and 14 (45.2%) were RF positive, indicating a relatively higher proportion of RF-positive polyarthritis in this population than in the nonnative population. Oen and Cheang[6] reported that polyarthritis accounted for a higher proportion of East Indian (61%), and North American Indian (64%) children with chronic arthritis, compared with caucasian children (27%). Saurenmann and colleagues[4] analyzed ethnicity as a risk factor for JIA in a multiethnic cohort. Among 223 children with RF-negative polyarthritis, no significant differences in percentages of European and non-European patients were found. However, the Native Canadian Indian population had a high relative risk (3.2) of developing RF-negative polyarthritis.

Etiology and Pathogenesis

The etiology of polyarthritis is unknown. Like many rheumatic diseases, JIA is believed to have complex origins that include interactions among an array of susceptibility genes and as yet unidentified exogenous factors. Environmental and lifestyle influences have been proposed as factors promoting arthritis in the context of genetic vulnerability. Within the group of RF-negative polyarthritis, variations in clinical characteristics, courses, and outcomes suggest that this JIA class is more heterogeneous

Table 15-1

ILAR criteria for the classification of the polyarthritis JIA subtype

RF-Negative Polyarthritis

Arthritis affecting five or more joints during the first 6 months of disease; a test for RF is negative

Exclusions:

- Psoriasis or a history of psoriasis in the patient or first-degree relative
- Arthritis in an HLA-B27–positive male beginning after the sixth birthday
- Ankylosing spondylitis, enthesitis-related arthritis, sacroiliitis with inflammatory bowel disease, Reiter syndrome, acute anterior uveitis, or a history of one of these disorders in a first-degree relative
- IgM RF on at least two occasions at least 3 months apart
- The presence of systemic JIA in the patient

RF-Positive Polyarthritis

Arthritis affecting five or more joints during the first 6 months of disease; two or more tests for RF at least 3 months apart during the first 6 months of disease are positive

- Psoriasis or a history of psoriasis in the patient or first-degree relative
- Arthritis in an HLA-B27–positive male beginning after the sixth birthday
- Ankylosing spondylitis, enthesitis-related arthritis, sacroiliitis with inflammatory bowel disease, Reiter syndrome, acute anterior uveitis, or a history of one of these disorders in a first-degree relative
- The presence of systemic JIA in the patient

IgM, Immunoglobulin M; *ILAR,* International League of Associations for Rheumatology; *JIA,* juvenile idiopathic arthritis; *RF,* rheumatoid factor

than the collective name suggests. Consequently, within this JIA subset, etiologies and pathogenic processes are likely varied.

As with other JIA subtypes, immune and inflammatory responses that characterize polyarthritis exhibit a predominantly proinflammatory profile during active disease and a regulatory, antiinflammatory profile during inactive disease.[16,17]

No cytokine or chemokine response patterns in either blood or synovial fluid are unique to RF-negative polyarthritis. De Jager and colleagues[16] noted comparable plasma level increases in interleukin (IL)-6 and -12, and chemokine C-C motif ligand (CCL)3, C-X-C motif ligand (CXCL)9, and CXCL10 in a small group of children with RF-negative polyarthritis (10 patients) and oligoarthritis with a polyarticular course (5 patients). In this same group synovial fluid levels of certain cytokines (IL-6 and IL-15) and chemokines (CCL12, CCL3, CCL11, CXCL8 and CXCL9) were higher in synovial fluid than in plasma. Increased levels of IL-17 have been found in seronegative polyarthritis (as well as in enthesitis-related arthritis) and are considered to be of potential pathogenic importance by promoting other proinflammatory cytokines and enhancing matrix metalloproteinases production, leading to cartilage degradation.[18] CCL20 derived from synovial fluid mononuclear cells was increased in children with polyarthritis (including those with extended oligoarticular JIA); the enhanced production was attributed to the hypoxic synovial environment.[19] The hypoxic synovial environmental also has been suggested as a factor that

promotes increases in intraarticular vascular endothelial growth factor and osteopontin, which enhance angiogenesis in synovial tissue in children with RF-negative polyarthritis and extended oligoarthritis JIA subsets.[20]

Genetic Background

Evidence supporting a genetic influence in the pathogenesis of JIA includes ethnic variability in the incidence of certain JIA subsets, female preponderance, increased sibling recurrence rates of the same JIA subtype,[21] and associations with both human leukocyte antigen (HLA) and non-HLA genes.

Human Leukocyte Antigen Genes

Genes both within and outside the major histocompatibility complex (MHC) have been evaluated for their contribution to genetic susceptibility to JIA. The HLA class I A2 allele confers susceptibility in RF-negative polyarthritis, as do the class II alleles DRB1*08, DQAI*04 and DPB1*03.[22] These HLA-related profiles are distinct from those characterizing RF-positive polyarthritis[22] and support the view that children without RF have a discrete disease that is different, at least genetically, from that of children with RF. Furthermore, some of the HLA alleles that confer susceptibility to RF-negative polyarthritis (A2, DRB1*08 and DQA1*04) also confer susceptibility to the oligoarthritis JIA subtype,[22] suggesting that children with RF-negative polyarthritis are more allied genetically with the oligoarthritis JIA subtype than with RF-positive polyarthritis.

Non-HLA Genes

The TRAF1/C5 region located on chromosome 9q33-34 encodes the tumor necrosis factor (TNF) receptor–associated factor 1 and the complement component 5.[23] In RF-negative polyarthritis patients, there is a significant increase in the A allele of a single nucleotide polymorphism (SNP) in the TRAF1/C5 region when compared with controls.[23] Homozygotes for the susceptibility allele (AA) have an odds ratio (OR) of 2.51 (95% CI 1.23 to 5.14) compared with the homozygotes of the protective allele (GG), whereas heterozygotes have an OR of 1.50 (95% CI 0.81 to 2.77). In extended oligoarthritis (defined as the accumulation of more than 4 joints after 6 months from onset) and RF-positive polyarthritis, a trend towards an increased A allele frequency is observed (49% and 50% respectively, versus 41% in controls), suggesting a possible association of the allele with the polyarticular phenotype in general rather than with the RF-negative polyarticular subset specifically.[23]

The protein tyrosine phosphatase, nonreceptor type 22 (PTPN22) gene codes for lymphoid-specific phosphatase, which modulates antibody-mediated T cell activation. A missense SNP in the gene coding for PTPN22 reduces the ability to downregulate T cell activation and has been associated with JIA.[24,25] Among the JIA subsets the strongest association of this SNP is with RF-negative polyarthritis.[25] However, the association of the PTPN22 gene with JIA has not been found consistently,[26,27] possibly a reflection of ethnic differences in the study populations.

The SLC11A1 (solute carrier family 11 member 1) gene regulates macrophage-mediated resistance to certain intracellular pathogens and is associated with susceptibility to certain infectious diseases and possibly, JIA.[28] The SLC11A1 locus appears to exert an independent effect on JIA susceptibility, but in patients with RF-negative polyarthritis the locus appears to have an enhancing effect on disease susceptibility with the HLA-DRB1 locus.[28]

Clinical Manifestations

In children with RF-negative polyarthritis articular disease predominates; extraarticular features are infrequent and are less severe than in those who are RF positive. Variations in onset ages, clinical and serological manifestations, and courses suggest the RF-negative class of polyarthritis comprises at least several different clinical entities. For example, some patients with RF-negative polyarthritis have a young onset age and positive tests for antinuclear antibody (ANA) and uveitis; apart from the number of involved joints, therefore, they are clinically indistinguishable from some patients with the oligoarthritis JIA subtype.

Joint Disease

Onset of arthritis may be acute, but it is more often insidious, with progressive involvement of additional joints. Morning stiffness or gelling after inactivity, indicative of active arthritis, may persist for hours, or occasionally all day. The arthritis may be remittent or indolent. The joints are swollen as a result of synovial hypertrophy and intraarticular fluid and may be warm but are generally not tender or red. Among children with RF-negative polyarthritis knees, wrists and ankles are the most commonly affected joints both at initial presentation and throughout the disease course. Small joint involvement of the hands or feet may occur early or late in the course of the disease; the second and third metacarpophalangeal (MCP) and proximal interphalangeal joints are most commonly affected.[29] The distal interphalangeal joints are seldom affected in children with polyarthritis at onset. The temporomandibular joint (TMJ) is commonly affected in children with a polyarticular disease course regardless of onset subtype; children with the RF-negative polyarthritis are more likely to have TMJ involvement, particularly at long-term follow-up, than those who are RF positive.[30,31] The earlier age at onset, when the TMJ might be more vulnerable to degradation processes, is thought to be the reason for the greater prevalence of involvement in the RF-negative group compared with the RF-positive group.[30,31] Cervical spine involvement is not commonly recognized early in the course of RF-negative polyarthritis either clinically or radiographically.[32] However, reduced range of motion of the cervical spine, particularly loss of extension, can occur later in the course of RF-negative polyarthritis and ankylosis of the apophyseal joints of the second and third vertebrae can be demonstrated radiographically (Fig. 15–1)

In children with RF-negative polyarthritis, the number of affected joints tends to be less and the pattern of involvement more asymmetrical than in RF-positive polyarthritis (Fig. 15–2). In RF-negative disease, involvement of wrists and small joints of the hands is less frequent than in RF-positive disease. Clinical signs of hip

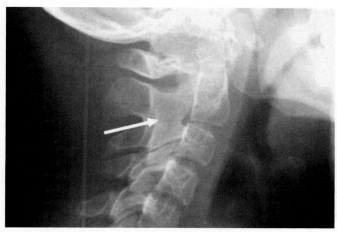

FIGURE 15–1 Lateral radiograph of the cervical spine of a child with RF-negative polyarthritis showing bony ankylosis of the apophyseal joints of the second and third cervical vertebrae.

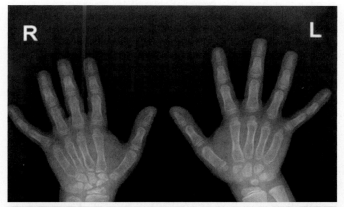

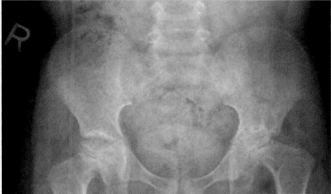

FIGURE 15–2 Radiographs of a child 6 years after onset of RF-negative polyarthritis. Wrist radiographs illustrate distinct asymmetry of involvement with the left wrist displaying strikingly more advanced disease than the right. Marked deterioration of hip joints bilaterally with apparent early ankylosis on the left is noted.

involvement are present in fewer than 20% of children with RF-negative polyarthritis at onset, but progressive radiographic abnormalities of the hip joint become evident with longer term following (Fig. 15–2). Oen and colleagues[32] reported that radiological signs of hip joint involvement (early joint space narrowing and eventual growth abnormalities) were more likely to occur in RF-negative than RF-positive polyarthritis; the tendency for RF-negative polyarthritis to have its onset at a younger age than it does in RF-positive disease might be a factor contributing to the higher prevalence of growth changes in the seronegative group.

In a small subset of RF-negative patients with polyarthritis, clinical signs of joint effusion and synovial hypertrophy are absent, although these children have joint stiffness and progressive joint contractures associated with laboratory indicators of inflammation. These children have been described as having "dry synovitis." Ostrov[33] has proposed preliminary criteria for dry synovitis as follows: Joint pain and stiffness reported in the patient history for at least 3 months, minimal joint effusion, minimally palpable synovial tissue on examination that is associated with morning stiffness for greater than 1 hour, loss of range of motion (with or without contractures) of involved joints detected on physical examination, and improvement in the symptoms and physical findings with appropriate medical treatment. This uncommon subset of polyarthritis can be considered a variant of RF-negative polyarthritis, although it has also been suggested to be a forme fruste of scleroderma.[33] There is insufficient information about dry synovitis to definitively define its prevalence, clinical features, course, and response to treatment.

Systemic Manifestations

Systemic manifestations in children with seronegative polyarthritis are unusual but can include fatigue and growth failure. Low-grade fever seldom occurs.

Fatigue is a common symptom in children with polyarthritis and can be present even in the absence of active joint disease.[34] Ringold and colleagues[35] studied fatigue in 60 children with polyarthritis, of whom 24 (61.2%) were RF negative, using the PedsQL Multidimensional Fatigue Scale, which includes assessment of general fatigue, sleep/rest fatigue, and cognitive fatigue domains. Both children and their parents/proxies reported lower scores in all domains compared with controls.[35] Factors contributing to fatigue can include pain and stress, decreased muscle mass, low aerobic and anaerobic capacity, a higher exercise heart rate, and the presence of anemia.[34,36,37] Ward and colleagues did not find that sleep disturbances contributed to fatigue in a group of 70 children with JIA of whom 40 (50.7%) had the polyarthritis subtype.[38]

Growth disturbances are common in JIA.[39-42] In children with polyarthritis height-for-age Z scores (an expression of the number of standard deviations from the normal mean) may decline in the first several years of disease but tend to return to normal with longer term follow-up.[40] In those children without RF, the negative deviation is less marked and less prolonged than in those with RF, although the difference tends to be significant only with longer disease duration.[40] Low growth velocity tends to correlate with disease severity and activity and with the number of involved joints.[39,41,42]

Extraarticular Manifestations

NODULES

Subcutaneous nodules occur rarely (<1%) in RF-negative polyarthritis. There is insufficient information to know the frequency with which subcutaneous nodules might

eventually develop in the seronegative polyarthritis JIA group.

UVEITIS

After oligoarticular JIA (which accounts for more than one-half of JIA patients affected by uveitis), chronic asymptomatic uveitis is most common in the RF-negative polyarthritis group.[43,44] Approximately 15% of children with RF-negative polyarthritis have uveitis, and children with RF-negative polyarthritis account for approximately 20% of all JIA uveitis patients.[43] Sabri and colleagues[43] reported that 32 of 142 JIA patients with uveitis (22.5%) had RF-negative polyarthritis; none of the children with RF-positive JIA had uveitis. As with the oligoarthritis JIA subgroup, uveitis in RF-negative polyarthritis tends to be associated with younger onset age and a positive test for ANA (see Chapter 20).

CARDIOVASCULAR AND PULMONARY DISEASE

RF-negative polyarthritis is not typically associated with overt cardiovascular pathology. Bharti and colleagues[45] reported that children with arthritis, regardless of onset subtype, had significantly greater left ventricular volumes and other abnormalities suggesting abnormal left ventricular diastolic relaxation. However, patients with polyarticular disease had better diastolic left ventricular filling than did those those with systemic or oligoarticular arthritis.[45] The authors suggest that significantly higher blood pressure and heart rates in juvenile arthritis might account for the observed diastolic functional changes. They also speculate that subclinical diastolic dysfunction observed in children with juvenile arthritis might portend overt cardiovascular disease later in life. Knook and colleagues[46] demonstrated lower 1-second forced vital capacity and peak expiratory flows in a group of 31 children with chronic arthritis. of whom more than two-thirds had RF-negative polyarthritis. These abnormalities were attributable to impairment in respiratory muscle strength rather than intrinsic restrictive or obstructive lung disease.[46]

Differential Diagnosis

The differential diagnosis for a child with polyarthritis includes other rheumatic diseases, infection, other inflammatory conditions, malignancies, and metabolic and genetic disorders.

Rheumatic Diseases

The onset of polyarthritis in a girl later in childhood or during adolescence should suggest the possible diagnosis of systemic lupus erythematosus (SLE) (see Chapter 21). The arthritis of SLE may mimic that of JIA, although it is nonerosive and less likely to be deforming; the presence of other clinical hallmarks and a positive test for anti–double-stranded DNA antibodies establishes the diagnosis of SLE. SLE may develop years after the initial diagnosis of RF-negative polyarticular JIA.[47]

The differential diagnosis of RF-negative polyarthritis also includes enthesitis-related arthritis (ERA) (see Chapter 17). Predominant involvement of large joints of the lower extremities and the presence of enthesitis supports the diagnosis of ERA, although enthesitis can occur, albeit uncommonly, in other types of JIA.[48]

Scleroderma begins insidiously with joint contractures of the small joints of the hands, mimicking features of polyarthritis but ordinarily without associated signs of intraarticular swelling. Arthritis may occur in childhood dermatomyositis but can be distinguished from JIA by clinical manifestations such as rash and muscle weakness.

Infections

Septic arthritis affecting multiple joints is unusual; only 3% of the 65 children with septic arthritis reported by Al Saadi and colleagues[49] had more than one involved joint. Elwood and colleagues[50] reported the case of a child with longstanding polyarthritis who, while receiving immunosuppressive therapy for treatment of her arthritis, developed multifocal septic arthritis due to group A beta-hemolytic streptococcal infection. Lyme disease may be polyarticular, but it can usually be differentiated from RF-negative polyarthritis by its intermittent pattern of arthritis activity and the accompanying cutaneous, neurological, and cardiac abnormalities (see Chapter 39). Arthritis caused by *Neisseria gonorrhoeae* may have an early migratory polyarticular phase.[51]

Reactive polyarthritis in response to infection in the respiratory, gastrointestinal, or genitourinary tracts can ordinarily be distinguished from JIA polyarthritis by a limited duration of the disease and associated clinical manifestations[52,53] (see Chapter 39). Group A beta-hemolytic streptococcal throat infection can be associated with acute, painful, nonerosive, migratory polyarthritis (see Chapter 40).

Malignancy

Malignant infiltration of bone or synovium can mimic polyarthritis, although in most instances the malignant focus is in juxtaarticular bone rather than in the joint. (see Chapter 46). However, joint swelling can occur in acute lymphoblastic leukemia as a result of leukemic infiltration of the synovium. Involvement in malignancy tends to be oligoarticular rather than polyarticular.[54] In addition to the systemic manifestations of malignancy, there may be moderate to severe anemia or elevation of an ESR that is out of keeping with other features of their disease.

Other Inflammatory Conditions

Arthritis associated with inflammatory bowel disease (see Chapter 19), or sarcoidosis (see Chapter 35) should be considered in the differential diagnosis of RF-negative polyarthritis. Sickle cell disease in the very young child causes diffuse, symmetrical swelling of the hands and feet (hand-foot syndrome) that may mimic true arthritis (see Chapter 41). Hypermobility syndromes, mucopolysaccharidoses, familial hypertrophic synovitis,[55,56] familial arthritis and camptodactyly,[57] familial osteochondritis dissecans,[58] Stickler syndrome,[59] velocardiofacial syndrome,[60] Turner syndrome,[61] and relapsing polychondritis[62] are rare causes of disease that may suggest a diagnosis of polyarticular JIA.

Laboratory Examination

The laboratory provides evidence of inflammation, is useful in excluding other diagnoses, and is important in classification, prognostication, and guiding therapy.

Indicators of Inflammation

Children with polyarthritis typically have moderate elevations of ESR and C-reactive protein. Many have elevated white blood cell counts and platelet counts and a normocytic hypochromic anemia characteristic of chronic inflammation.

Autoantibodies

RHEUMATOID FACTORS

RFs are antibodies that bind to the CH2 and CH3 domains of the Fc portion of human or animal immunoglobulin (Ig) G (IgG). Customarily, RF is detected by particle agglutination assays such as latex fixation or nephelometric techniques that preferentially detect pentameric IgM RF. Approximately one-third of children with polyarthritis who do not have IgM RF detectable by agglutination methods have IgM RF detected when using a more sensitive enzyme immunoassay (EIA).[63-68] RF detected by either technique is associated with deforming joint disease, joint space narrowing, and joint erosions.[64,69] Furthermore, children with IgM RF-negative polyarthritis, as determined by conventional methods, can have "hidden RFs." The hidden IgM RF is 19S IgM RF, which, because it is bound to IgG in the serum being tested, cannot generate a response in the standard agglutination assay until it is acid eluted from the IgG. Up to 85% of children with polyarticular disease have been reported to have such antibodies, which are associated with active disease.[70-72]

IgA RF, alone or in combination with IgM RF, has been associated with active disease or severe disability in polyarthritis.[64,73] Using EIA, Gilliam and colleagues found IgA RF in 4 of 23 (17.4%) and IgM RF in 9 patients (39.1%) with RF-negative polyarthritis.[64] Both IgA and IgG RFs are associated with joint space narrowing and joint erosions, although the correlation is substantially less than with IgM RF. Application of more sensitive methods, such as EIA, suggests the possibility that some "RF-negative" polyarthritis patients might be more appropriately assigned to the RF-positive polyarthritis category. Anti-citrullinated protein antibodies (ACPA) are found in 0% to 17% of children with RF-negative polyarthritis.[64,74,75]

ANTINUCLEAR ANTIBODIES

ANA are present in approximately one half of children with RF-negative polyarthritis, typically in low to medium titers (1:80 to 1:640).[76,77] In a group of 68 children with RF-negative polyarthritis reported by Ravelli and colleagues, 33 (48.5%) were ANA positive.[77] The group of ANA-positive RF-negative polyarthritis patients was not significantly different from the group with oligoarthritis with respect to age at first presentation, sex ratio, frequency of symmetrical arthritis, or prevalence of uveitis. Furthermore, the number of involved joints with limited range of motion was greater in the ANA-negative group than the ANA-positive group. These observations suggest that ANA positivity, irrespective of JIA onset subtype, distinguishes a relatively homogenous group characterized by early onset, female predominance, asymmetric arthritis, and an increased risk of chronic uveitis. Thus, RF-negative polyarthritis, when associated with a positive ANA test, is more like oligoarticular JIA than is ANA-negative polyarthritis. The antigenic specificities of ANA in JIA are generally unknown.[78] Antibodies to individual histones and to histone-histone and histone-DNA complexes are occasionally, but inconsistently, found.[79]

SYNOVIAL FLUID ANALYSIS

Synovial fluid analysis in RF-negative polyarthritis reveals a nonspecific inflammatory reaction that is not clearly distinguishable from that found in other JIA subtypes. In children with polyarthritis (including those with extended oligoarthritis), polymorphonuclear neutrophil counts in synovial fluid tend to be higher than in persistent oligoarticular disease but not significantly different from counts in systemic JIA or enteroarthritis.[80,81] Cytokine, chemokine, and proteome profiles in synovial fluids are not well enough defined to be of practical clinical utility.[16,19,20,82]

Radiological Examination

In radiographs taken within 2 years after disease onset, joint space narrowing (including decreased joint space, ankylosis, and carpal collapse) was demonstrated in 12% of one group of 39 children.[32] Radiographs (obtained at last follow-up, a median of 6.5 years after onset) showed joint space narrowing in 43%. Erosions and growth abnormalities likewise increased with time (Chapter 10).

Pathology

Although the synovial membrane is the principal site of pathology in JIA, there is little substantive information about the histopathological and immunopathological characteristics of JIA joint tissues. The limited information available suggests that the histological appearance of the synovium is similar for all JIA subtypes, although greater hypervascularity in the polyarthritis group relative to ERA, psoriatic arthritis, and oligoarthritis has been noted.[83]

Treatment

As with all forms of chronic childhood arthritis, RF-negative polyarthritis requires a multifaceted approach to management. The mainstays of treatment include early and judicious use of pharmacotherapy, physical and occupational therapy, and promotion of healthy lifestyles, including optimizing nutrition and physical activity. Achieving and sustaining complete disease control is no longer an unrealistically achievable objective.

Medical Management

Initial treatment with nonsteroidal antiinflammatory drugs (NSAIDs) is appropriate. Naproxen or ibuprofen is most commonly used in North America, but indomethacin is favored by some pediatric rheumatologists in Europe and elsewhere. Some physicians combine initial NSAID therapy with a disease-remitting agent, usually methotrexate. In any event, failure of NSAIDs to control the disease within 6 to 8 weeks should prompt the addition of methotrexate. Methotrexate is usually given by mouth initially, in dosages of 10 to 15 mg/m^2/week. In the absence of an adequate response, the dosage can be increased to 15 to 20 mg/m^2/week, preferably administered subcutaneously. The response to methotrexate is usually excellent.[84-86] For patients unresponsive to or intolerant of methotrexate, leflunomide is an alternate option, although there is insufficient information to evaluate leflunomide's role in RF-negative polyarthritis specifically.[87]

Anti-TNF agents are effective in treating children with polyarthritis who are unresponsive to methotrexate or leflunomide alone, although there is little information to indicate that RF status correlates with responsiveness.[88-94]

Glucocorticoids are important as intraarticular therapy. Breit and colleagues[95] reported a longer median duration of response to intraarticular triamcinolone hexacetonide in children with juvenile chronic arthritis who were RF negative (105 weeks) than in those who were RF positive (63 weeks). Glucocorticoids have a limited role as systemic therapy in polyarthritis, although judicious use of systemic steroids as a bridging agent can be considered until disease-modifying agents begin to have their effect. Drugs such as gold compounds and penicillamine are seldom used since the advent of generally safer and more efficacious pharmacotherapeutic options. Although hydroxychloroquine is at times used in RF-negative polyarthritis as an adjunctive agent, often in combination with methotrexate, there is little evidence to support its efficacy.

Exercise and Physical and Occupational Therapy

There is ample evidence indicating that regular participation in physical activity by children with JIA is beneficial.[96] Although functional impairment generally correlates with the extent and severity of articular disease, poor fitness also occurs even in those with mild symptoms and persists even after disease remission.[36] Both aerobic and anaerobic exercise capacity is decreased in children with polyarthritis compared with oligoarticular disease; those with RF-positive polyarthritis are somewhat more limited than those with RF-negative disease[36] (see Chapter 12).

Notwithstanding the advantages of active exercise, it is important to have a carefully designed passive therapy program. Children tend to function within the range of motion they have, not the range they should be trying to achieve. Focused physical therapy should be instituted as soon as the degree of inflammation subsides sufficiently to facilitate the child's cooperation. Physical therapy aimed at restoration of normal range of motion can be facilitated by pretreatment with an analgesic such as acetaminophen and the application of heat or ice. Major contractures are often more amenable to therapy after intraarticular injection of triamcinolone hexacetonide.

Surgery

The need for surgical management is less common now than in the past as a consequence of more effective medical management. Nonetheless, some children with resistant or untreated disease will require joint replacement of hips, knees or, occasionally, small joints of the hands. Such procedures are seldom needed in childhood, but in adults with long-standing disease of juvenile onset they add greatly to function and quality of life. Prior to surgical procedures, the child with polyarthritis should be thoroughly evaluated for conditions that might increase risk. In polyarthritis, for example, cervical spine and temporomandibular joint involvement pose potential added anesthetic risks, immunosuppression can increase risks of perioperative infection, and poor bone quality can compromise the integrity of joint implants.

Course of the Disease and Prognosis

RF-negative polyarthritis is a chronic disease, lasting years or decades. Oen and colleagues[76] reported that only 25% of 80 children with RF-negative polyarthritis diagnosed between 1977 and 1994 and followed for at least 5 years had gone into remission by age 16 years. Furthermore, children who had not gone into remission by this age were likely to have ongoing active arthritis into their late 20s or early 30s. These data suggest that RF-negative polyarthritis continues to be associated with substantial morbidity and functional disability in most affected children.

RHEUMATOID FACTOR–POSITIVE POLYARTHRITIS

RF-positive polyarthritis is defined by ILAR criteria as arthritis cumulatively affecting 5 or more joints during the first 6 months, in the presence of two positive tests for RF performed at least 3 months apart.[2] In addition, exclusion criteria specified in the ILAR criteria must be applied (see Table 15–1).

The RF-positive polyarthritis subtype of JIA shares a similar clinical phenotype, serology, and immunogenetic profile with that of adult rheumatoid arthritis, and both can occur in the same family. In European populations, approximately 15% of children with polyarthritis are RF positive, representing approximately 3% of the JIA population.

Epidemiology

Incidence and Prevalence

The wide variations in reported incidences of RF-positive polyarthritis probably reflects differences in patient selection and geographical origin contributed to by both genetic and environmental influences.[6,9,97] The reported frequencies of RF-positive polyarthritis range from 51% in a series of Native Canadian Indian children to 17% of East Indian, 14% of African-American, 12.5% of Japanese, 0.2 to 5% of European, and 1% of American children and adolescents with chronic arthritis.[3,8,10,98-104]

There is limited published information about incidence and prevalence rates for the RF-positive polyarthritis onset subtype. Estimated incidence rates of 0.3 to 0.5 per 100,000 person-years at risk have been reported or can be calculated from publications from Europe.[10,11,101,102] In comparison, incidence estimates as high as 12.3 can be calculated from published data for East Coast Alaskan Indian children[105] and 8.1 per 100,000 person-years at risk for Native Canadian Indian children in Manitoba.[106] Similarly, estimates of point prevalence of 0 to 6.7 in Europe and 54 per 100,000 at risk for Manitoba Canadian Indian children can be calculated from published data.[98,103,106,107]

Age at Onset and Sex Ratio

The mean age at juvenile onset of RF-positive polyarthritis is 9 to 11 years; range is 1.5 to 15 years.[8,101,108,109] Affected girls outnumber boys from 4 to 13 to 1 in large series.[4,100,101,108,110,111]

Etiology and Pathogenesis

As with other JIA subtypes, the etiology of RF-positive polyarthritis remains unknown. Whether there is a role of RFs or ACPA is speculation, but in adults these antibodies have been demonstrated years before the onset of overt rheumatoid arthritis,[112-114] suggesting that they may have a pathogenic role. Clinical disease may not occur until ACPA are deposited in synovium, a process that is facilitated by immune complexes formed by RF.[115] There are no comparable data for children. An analogous pathway likely applies to children with RF-positive polyarthritis, but triggers for citrullination may differ in the pediatric population.

Genetic Background

HLA Genes

RF-positive polyarthritis and adult RA share genetic predispositions. HLA antigens account for an estimated one-third of the genetic risk for RA.[116] The shared epitope (SE), a specific sequence present on a number of HLA DR antigens, is associated with increased risk for both adult RA and RF-positive JIA. The SE is found on HLA-DR4 (HLA-DRB1*0401, *0404, *0408, or *0405), DR1 (DRB1*0101), and DR14 (DRB1*1402) alleles.[117]

Population frequencies and particular SE-bearing HLA alleles vary in different ethnic groups. Thus, RF-positive polyarthritis and RA are associated with DR4 (DRB1*04) alleles, mainly DRB1*0401 and *0404, in Caucasian populations with relative risks ranging from 3.2 to 7.2 for the former and 3.8 to 8.9 for the latter.[118-125] The associated allele is DRB1*0405 in Japanese and DRB1*1402 in some North American Native populations.[117,126-128] Double doses of the SE further increase the relative risk of the disease.[123,124]

In some Native North American Indian tribes both DRB1*04 alleles and DRB1*1402 carry the SE and are associated with RA, whereas in other populations the frequency of DRB1*1402 is so high that no significant increase is found in patients with RA.[111,127-129] In Native

Canadian Indian children the situation is more complex because both the SE and DRB1*0901 occurring together as a genotype are associated with RF-positive polyarthritis.[8,130] This dual association supports the suggestion that a greater genetic influence is associated with earlier age at onset.

Population frequencies of the SE tend to correlate with frequencies of RA and RF-positive polyarthritis. For example, the frequency of the SE in Caucasian populations is 27% to 36%, whereas Native North American Indian populations with high incidence and prevalence rates of RA and RF-positive polyarthritis have frequencies of 66% to 98%.[118,122,129,130]

More recently the association of the SE has been found to be limited to ACPA-positive RA.[131,132] ACPA are also associated with DR4, in children with polyarthritis.[74]

Non-HLA genes

Attempts to discover associations of JIA with genes outside the MHC have been hampered by the relative rarity of JIA and its respective subtypes.[22] Detecting gene association requires stratified analyses by JIA subtype because subtype-specific associations may be masked if only the total JIA group is considered. Furthermore, because of differences in population frequencies, cases and controls need to be selected from the same population.

Associations of CTLA-4 genes with both RA and JIA are controversial. The inconsistency in observed associations of CTLA-4 with JIA might relate to the specific SNP studied, population frequencies, patient selection, and lack of power.[22,133] One study found no association between CTLA-4 and JIA in a large cohort of patients as a whole but showed a borderline association with RF-positive polyarthritis.[133] Whole genome scans in JIA have failed to reveal specific associations with RF-positive polyarthritis.[134,135]

Clinical Manifestations

Joint Disease

Upper and lower extremity large and small joints are affected, as well as the cervical spine and TMJs. The thoracic and lumbar spine and sacroiliac joints are spared. Although large joints are commonly involved, the characteristic pattern is symmetrical arthritis affecting the MCP and PIP joints of the hands, the wrists, and the MTP and PIP joints of the feet. In contrast to RF-negative polyarthritis, micrognathia does not usually occur with TMJ involvement because of the later age at onset. Early limited range of motion occurs at the wrists and can eventually progress to more substantial debility and deformity (Fig. 15–3). Deformities that develop at the hands include ulnar drift at the wrists and the MCP joints and boutonnière and swan neck deformities at the fingers (Fig. 15–4). Deformities that develop at the feet include hallux valgus deformity at the first MTP joints, hammertoe, and cock-up toe deformities.

Systemic Manifestations

Fatigue and weight loss may occur with active disease. Fever is rare in RF-positive polyarthritis, and a rash does not occur.

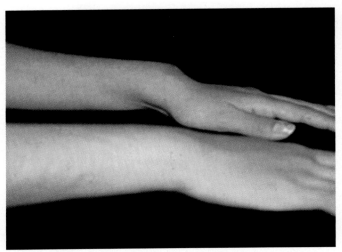

FIGURE 15–3 Subluxation of the left wrist in a child with RF-positive polyarthritis.

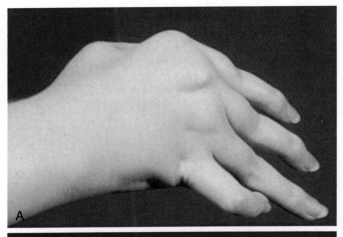

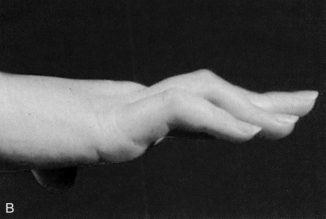

FIGURE 15–4 Hands of children with RF-positive polyarthritis. **A,** swan neck deformities in digits 2, 3, and 4 displaying characteristic extension at the proximal interphalangeal joints and flexion at the distal interphalangeal joints. Ulnar deviation at the metacarpophalangeal joints is also demonstrated. **B,** Boutonnière deformities at digits 4 and 5 displaying characteristic flexion at the proximal interphalangeal joints and extension at the distal interphalangeal joints.

Extraarticular Manifestations

Other than nodules, extraarticular disease manifestations associated with adult RA described below rarely occur in patients with RF-positive polyarthritis onset subtype, whether during childhood, adolescence, or adulthood.

NODULES

The most common extraarticular signs in patients with RF-positive polyarthritis are rheumatoid nodules (Fig. 15–5). In Ansell's series, 30% of patients with polyarticular RF-positive arthritis had rheumatoid nodules during the first year of disease.[136] Nodules often occur distal to the olecranon and at other bony prominences and pressure points, on flexor tendon sheaths, Achilles tendon, and on the soles of the feet. They are firm, mobile, and nontender; however, pressure of the nodule against soft tissues or bone may cause pain. The presence of rheumatoid nodules indicates a poor prognosis. Accelerated nodulosis may occur in patients on methotrexate. In this case the nodules are multiple, develop over a short time, tend to occur on the hands, and regress on discontinuation of methotrexate. This complication has been described in two children with RF-positive polyarthritis and one with systemic JIA.[137,138] Methotrexate-induced nodulosis is associated with minimal discomfort and may stabilize with use of hydroxychloroquine. Nodulosis associated with methotrexate does not necessarily preclude continuation of methotrexate therapy.[137,139]

Rheumatoid nodules must be distinguished from subcutaneous nodules of rheumatic fever, which are smaller, so-called benign rheumatoid nodules that are not associated with chronic arthritis, and from granuloma annulare, which are small nodules arranged in a circular pattern.

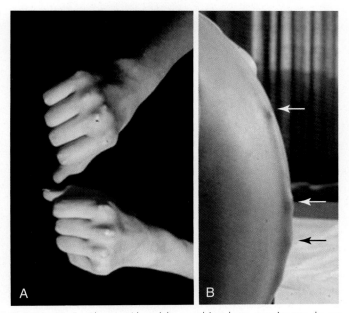

FIGURE 15–5 Rheumatoid nodules overlying bony prominences in an adolescent with RF-positive polyarthritis.

VASCULITIS

Rheumatoid vasculitis is rarely described in RF-positive polyarthritis during childhood or adolescence. In 1978, Ansell noted nailfold and extensive cutaneous vasculitis in several patients during prolonged follow-up.[140] However, the lack of reports of this complication in recent literature may reflect improved therapies for arthritis or less severe disease, as vasculitis in adults with RA tends to occur in those with the most severe disease.

FELTY SYNDROME

Felty syndrome consists of persistent neutropenia, splenomegaly, and RA and is associated with frequent infections. The bone marrow is normocellular, and the mechanism of neutropenia is complex, involving both antigranulocyte antibodies and decreased granulopoiesis.[141] In adults, Felty syndrome occurs in RF-positive patients with long disease duration. It has been reported rarely in adolescents with RF-positive polyarthritis and in adults who had juvenile onset disease.[142,143]

CARDIOVASCULAR AND PULMONARY DISEASE

Valvular heart disease has been reported in at least eight patients with childhood-onset RF-positive polyarthritis.[144-151] Aortic insufficiency is the most common lesion. Patients present with sudden onset of congestive heart failure or may deteriorate suddenly after a variable period of stability following the detection of cardiac murmurs. Valve replacement is almost always required. Cardiac symptoms may start during childhood, adolescence, or adulthood, at intervals varying from 4 to 17 years from onset of JIA. However, pathological murmurs may be detected as early as 1 year after onset. Patients with JIA who have organic cardiac murmurs should be evaluated for valvular insufficiency and monitored carefully.

Pulmonary parenchymal disease, so-called rheumatoid lung, has been reported in seven children with RF-positive polyarthritis.[152-158] Two types of pulmonary involvement have been reported: lymphoid interstitial pneumonitis and bronchiolitis obliterans or bronchiolitis obliterans organizing pneumonia (BOOP). These pulmonary complications may occur during childhood and adolescence or in adulthood. The time interval between the clinical presentation of pulmonary disease and onset of JIA has ranged from 10 years before to 20 years after onset of JIA. Symptoms include tachypnea, dyspnea, a nonproductive cough, and fever. On auscultation crackles and an end-inspiratory squeak are often heard. Diagnosis is based on clinical history and findings, pulmonary function tests, chest radiographs, and high-resolution computed tomography (HRCT). Bronchoalveolar lavage and/or lung biopsy may be necessary. Pulmonary function tests show reduced lung volumes and decreased diffusion capacity. A restrictive pattern is seen when interstitial pneumonitis is present and an obstructive pattern in BOOP. Chest radiographs may be normal or may show interstitial infiltrates. HRCT abnormalities include ground glass changes suggesting inflammation, bronchiectasis, or bronchiolectasis (suggesting BOOP), and honeycombing (suggesting fibrosis). The differential diagnosis includes drug-induced pulmonary toxicity and infection. The prognosis of rheumatoid lung is variable in children and adolescents. Although a few patients have improved with corticosteroid therapy, others have deteriorated despite corticosteroid and immunosuppressive therapy.

Differential Diagnosis

The differential diagnosis of polyarthritis is discussed above. Specific diagnoses to be considered in the context of RF-positive polyarthritis are connective tissue diseases, reactive arthritis, and infections, in which polyarticular arthritis and a positive test for RF may occur concurrently. Among the connective tissue diseases, SLE and overlap syndromes, including mixed connective tissue disease, are diagnostic considerations in the child or adolescent with polyarticular arthritis who has a positive test for RF. RF is positive in 10% to 30% of children with SLE and in approximately two-thirds of children with mixed connective tissue disease. RF may be present in cases of acute rheumatic fever. Tuberculosis and subacute bacterial endocarditis can be associated with arthritis accompanied by a positive test for RF.

Laboratory Investigations

Indicators of Inflammation

These are identical to those in RF-negative polyarthritis discussed earlier.

Autoantibodies

RHEUMATOID FACTOR

The classification of RF-positive polyarthritis is based on the presence of two positive tests for RF performed at least 3 months apart in a patient who has polyarticular joint involvement during the first 6 months of disease.[2] In practice, patients with RF-positive polyarthritis are characterized by persistently positive IgM RF, generally in high titre.

ANTICITRULLINATED PROTEIN ANTIBODIES

In children with JIA only those with polyarthritis onset subtypes have ACPA; however, similar to adults with RA, the concordance with RF positivity is not complete. Although individual series are small (9 to 20 patients), the frequency of ACPA in RF-positive polyarthritis varies from 57% to 90% (mean 73%), and, as discussed earlier, some patients (up to 17%) with RF-negative polyarthritis have positive ACPA tests.[74,75,159-161] As in adults there is an association of ACPA positivity with DR4 and erosions.[74] Currently, it is not clear that testing for ACPA in children with polyarthritis has prognostic value greater than RF.

ANTINUCLEAR ANTIBODIES

Positive tests for ANA have been reported in 80% of children with RF-positive polyarthritis and 57% of those with RF-negative polyarthritis.[76]

SYNOVIAL FLUID ANALYSIS

Synovial fluid analyses from patients with RF-positive polyarthritis show an inflammatory fluid not clearly differentiated from that found in other forms of JIA. Synovial fluid cell counts and proportions of neutrophils may be higher in RF-positive polyarthritis than in those with oligoarticular arthritis.[80]

Radiological Examination

Most information on joint damage in RF-positive polyarthritis comes from a limited number of studies of plain radiographs of patients treated before the introduction of biological therapies. Joint space narrowing and erosions occur within the first 1 to 2 years after onset and are most frequent at the wrists, hands, feet, and shoulders.[32,162] At the wrist, cartilage loss occurs at the proximal wrist joint and in the intercarpal joints, resulting in carpal ankylosis and shortening.[32,163] Both erosions and cartilage loss occur more frequently in RF-positive polyarthritis than in other forms of JIA.[32,164,165] Atlantoaxial subluxation of the cervical spine is more frequent in patients with RF

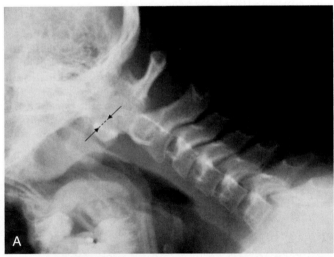
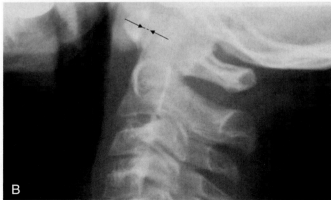

FIGURE 15–6   Flexion **(A)** and extension **(B)** radiographs of the cervical spine of a child with RF-positive polyarthritis. The increased distance between the posterior surface of the anterior arch of the first cervical vertebra and the anterior margin of the odontoid *(arrows)* in flexion suggests mild atlantoaxial subluxation in this patient.

(36% frequency) than in other patients with JRA (16%) (Fig. 15–6)[166] (see Chapter 10).

Pathology

Synovium

Despite similarities in overall appearance, the cellular infiltrates may differ among various types of arthritis. For example, immunohistological examination shows a greater predominance of CD4 T cells over CD8 T cells in polyarticular JRA and RA, compared with oligoarticular JRA and juvenile spondyloarthropathies.[167]

Rheumatoid Nodules

The mature rheumatoid nodule consists of characteristic zones.[168] The innermost zone is a core of necrotic tissue containing cellular material surrounded by fibrinoid, an eosinophilic material composed mainly of fibrin. The next layer is a palisade of radially arranged elongated mononuclear cells, and the outermost connective tissue layer is a vascular region containing a lymphocytic infiltrate. Lymphocytes are found both in a perivascular and/or a diffuse distribution. Immunohistochemical studies have shown that the palisade consists of macrophages and the majority of the lymphocytes are T cells—both CD4 and CD8, in ratios of 1:1 to 3:1.[168-170] B cells and plasma cells are scarce. Dendritic cells are also found in perivascular areas or scattered in the periphery of the nodules but are rare and are not found in close proximity to T cells.[169]

Cardiac Valvular Lesions

Excised aortic valves of children with RF-positive polyarthritis who have aortic insufficiency are grossly thickened.[144,151] Granulomatous, nodular lesions are often present on the valve cusps.[148,150,151] Histological findings include destruction of the normal architecture of the valve, granulomas that are histopathologically similar to rheumatoid nodules, nonspecific inflammatory changes, and fibrosis.[144,146,148,150,151]

Pulmonary Lesions

Lung biopsies of patients with RF-positive polyarthritis who have parenchymal lung disease show typical findings of interstitial pneumonia and bronchiolitis obliterans.[152,153,155-157] In the former the alveolar septa are thickened by a predominantly lymphocytic infiltrate. Lymphoid follicles or germinal centers, plasma cells, and histiocytes are also seen within the septae. Bronchiolitis obliterans is characterized by infiltrates of lymphocytes and plasma cells in the bronchiolar wall, destruction of the respiratory epithelium, occlusion of bronchioles with plugs of inflammatory cells and mucus, and fibrosis and obliteration of bronchioles. In BOOP granulation tissue extends into the alveolar spaces. Chronic interstitial inflammation is seen concurrently with bronchiolitis obliterans or BOOP.[156,157]

Treatment

Aggressive medical treatment of RF-positive polyarthritis is warranted because of its almost uniformly poor prognosis.[88] Children with this disease should be treated with NSAIDs and a disease-modifying antirheumatic drug (DMARD) at the time of diagnosis in the absence of contraindications. Methotrexate or methotrexate in combination with hydroxychloroquine and/or sulfasalazine should be the DMARD of first choice. If there is an inadequate response after 3 months, medications should be escalated. Consideration should be given to a combination of DMARDs or substituting leflunomide for methotrexate. NSAIDs should be used as adjunctive therapy because they can help improve symptoms but do not impact substantially on the disease course. Intraarticular steroid injections should be used, particularly for large, painful joints early in the treatment regimen. Low-dose prednisone, if used at all, should be limited to a bridging period until DMARD therapy becomes effective. Failure to respond adequately despite all these measures over 3 to 6 months is an indication for biologic therapy. As for patients with RF-negative polyarthritis, the total treatment plan includes patient and parent education, physical and occupational therapy, maintenance of physical activities, and optimal nutrition, including calcium and vitamin D. `

Course of the Disease and Prognosis

Mortality

In 1983 Ansell reported an 8% mortality rate among 85 patients with RF-positive polyarthritis.[136] Renal amyloidosis was the cause of death in 2 patients and quadriplegia resulting from cervical spine involvement complicated by infection in another.[136] In a series of 24 patients with JRA and amyloidosis from Finland, the mortality rate 15 years after the diagnosis of amyloidosis was 42%, and the cause of death was renal failure in five, infection in three, leukemia in one, and one had a perioperative death.[171] However, patients who died were not listed by onset subtype. No new case of amyloidosis complicating JIA had been reported since 1991 in Finland, and the complication appears to be increasingly rare worldwide.

More recent data also indicate an increased mortality in patients with JIA.[172,173] In Scotland, the standardized mortality ratio (the ratio of observed to expected deaths), derived from International Classification of Disease codes on hospital records and linkage to national death registers, was 3.39 for males and 5.09 for females with juvenile chronic arthritis.[172] Deaths among patients with musculoskeletal and connective tissue disease are most frequently related to circulatory or respiratory causes, although no details are available. Similarly, in Rochester, Minnesota, a high mortality of 0.27 compared with an expected rate of 0.068 per 100 patient years was calculated for adults with a history of JRA.[173] The causes of death were other autoimmune disorders. No subtype-specific death rates are available in either report.

Remission

Remission is often imprecisely defined, but patients with RF-positive polyarthritis have the lowest remission rates among children with chronic arthritis, varying from no remissions to a 5% frequency of remission, off medications during 8 to 10 years of follow-up.[174-176] However, clinical remission on medications can be achieved in 65% of patients.[176]

Disability

Until recently patients with RF-positive polyarthritis continued to have significant disability. The frequency of patients with severe disability or in Steinbrocker functional class III (capable of limited to few or none of activities of usual occupation or self-care) or IV (incapacitated largely or wholly bedridden, capable of little or no self-care) was 15% in 1976 and 1994 publications and 5% in 2002 after mean or median disease durations of 14 to 20 years.[175,177,178] However, in Childhood Health Assessment Questionnaires,18% of patients had scores of >1.5, reflecting severe disability.[175] These reports originated from pediatric rheumatology centers, where selection bias may be less and follow-up times shorter than in reports from adult rheumatology clinics. For example, in an adult rheumatology clinic, 38% of adult patients with RF-positive polyarthritis since childhood and with a mean disease duration of 28 years were in Steinbrocker Class III or IV, and 53% had a health assessment questionnaire score of >1.5.[179] Whether these poor outcomes will continue as treatment choices improve is a subject requiring continuing investigation.

REFERENCES

2. R.E. Petty, T.R. Southwood, P. Manners, et al., International League of Associations for Rheumatology classification of juvenile idiopathic arthritis: second revision, Edmonton, 2001, J. Rheumatol. 31 (2004) 390–392.
3. N. Adib, K. Hyrich, J. Thornton, et al., Association between duration of symptoms and severity of disease at first presentation to paediatric rheumatology: results from the Childhood Arthritis Prospective Study, Rheumatology (Oxford) 47 (2008) 991–995.
4. R.K. Saurenmann, J.B. Rose, P. Tyrrell, et al., Epidemiology of juvenile idiopathic arthritis in a multiethnic cohort: ethnicity as a risk factor, Arthritis Rheum. 56 (2007) 1974–1984.
5. K. Oen, D.B. Robinson, P. Nickerson, et al., Familial seropositive rheumatoid arthritis in North American Native families: effects of shared epitope and cytokine genotypes, J. Rheumatol. 32 (2005) 983–991.
6. K.G. Oen, M. Cheang, Epidemiology of chronic arthritis in childhood, Semin. Arthritis Rheum. 26 (1996) 575–591.
7. A.M. Rosenberg, R.E. Petty, K.G. Oen, et al., Rheumatic diseases in Western Canadian Indian children, J. Rheumatol. 9 (1982) 589–592.
8. K. Oen, M. Schroeder, K. Jacobson, et al., Juvenile rheumatoid arthritis in a Canadian First Nations (aboriginal) population: onset subtypes and HLA associations, J. Rheumatol. 25 (1998) 783–790.
9. P.J. Manners, C. Bower, Worldwide prevalence of juvenile arthritis why does it vary so much? J. Rheumatol. 29 (2002) 1520–1530.
12. P.N. Malleson, M.Y. Fung, A.M. Rosenberg, The incidence of pediatric rheumatic diseases: results from the Canadian Pediatric Rheumatology Association Disease Registry, J. Rheumatol. 23 (1996) 1981–1987.
13. L.S. Peterson, T. Mason, A.M. Nelson, et al., Juvenile rheumatoid arthritis in Rochester, Minnesota 1960-1993: is the epidemiology changing? Arthritis Rheum. 39 (1996) 1385–1390.
14. A.M. Rosenberg, Longitudinal analysis of a pediatric rheumatology clinic population, J. Rheumatol. 32 (2005) 1992–2001.
15. A.T. Borchers, C. Selmi, G. Cheema, et al., Juvenile idiopathic arthritis, Autoimmun. Rev. 5 (2006) 279–298.
16. W. de Jager, E.P. Hoppenreijs, N.M. Wulffraat, et al., Blood and synovial fluid cytokine signatures in patients with juvenile idiopathic arthritis: a cross-sectional study, Ann. Rheum. Dis. 66 (2007) 589–598.
19. M.C. Bosco, S. Delfino, F. Ferlito, et al., Hypoxic synovial environment and expression of macrophage inflammatory protein 3gamma/CCL20 in juvenile idiopathic arthritis, Arthritis Rheum. 58 (2008) 1833–1838.
20. M.C. Bosco, S. Delfino, F. Ferlito, et al., The hypoxic synovial environment regulates expression of vascular endothelial growth factor and osteopontin in juvenile idiopathic arthritis, J Rheumatol 36 (2009) 1318–1329.
21. M.B. Moroldo, M. Chaudhari, E. Shear, et al., Juvenile rheumatoid arthritis affected sibpairs: extent of clinical phenotype concordance, Arthritis Rheum 50 (2004) 1928–1934.
22. S. Prahalad, D.N. Glass, A comprehensive review of the genetics of juvenile idiopathic arthritis, Pediatr. Rheumatol. Online Journal 6 (2008) 11.
32. K. Oen, M. Reed, P.N. Malleson, et al., Radiologic outcome and its relationship to functional disability in juvenile rheumatoid arthritis, J. Rheumatol. 30 (2003) 832–840.
34. L.E. Schanberg, K.M. Gil, K.K. Anthony, et al., Pain, stiffness, and fatigue in juvenile polyarticular arthritis: contemporaneous stressful events and mood as predictors, Arthritis Rheum. 52 (2005) 1196–1204.
35. S. Ringold, C.A. Wallace, F.P. Rivara, Health-related quality of life, physical function, fatigue, and disease activity in children with established polyarticular juvenile idiopathic arthritis, J. Rheumatol. 36 (2009) 1330–1336.
36. M. van Brussel, O.T. Lelieveld, J. van der Net, et al., Aerobic and anaerobic exercise capacity in children with juvenile idiopathic arthritis, Arthritis Rheum. 57 (2007) 891–897.
37. S.E. Klepper, Exercise in pediatric rheumatic diseases, Curr. Opin. Rheumatol. 20 (2008) 619–624.
38. T.M. Ward, P. Brandt, K. Archbold, et al., Polysomnography and self-reported sleep, pain, fatigue, and anxiety in children with active and inactive juvenile rheumatoid arthritis, J. Pediatr. Psychol. 33 (2008) 232–241.
40. J.J. Liem, A.M. Rosenberg, Growth patterns in juvenile rheumatoid arthritis, Clin. Exp. Rheumatol. 21 (2003) 663–668.
46. L.M. Knook, I.M. de Kleer, C.K. van der Ent, et al., Lung function abnormalities and respiratory muscle weakness in children with juvenile chronic arthritis, Eur. Respir. J. 14 (1999) 529–533.
48. A.M. Rosenberg, R.E. Petty, A syndrome of seronegative enthesopathy and arthropathy in children, Arthritis Rheum. 25 (1982) 1041–1047.
64. B.E. Gilliam, A.K. Chauhan, J.M. Low, et al., Measurement of biomarkers in juvenile idiopathic arthritis patients and their significant association with disease severity: a comparative study, Clin. Exp. Rheumatol. 26 (2008) 492–497.
67. F.T. Saulsbury, Prevalence of IgM, IgA and IgG rheumatoid factors in juvenile rheumatoid arthritis, Clin. Exp. Rheumatol. 8 (1990) 513–517.
75. H.M. Habib, Y.M. Mosaad, H.M. Youssef, Anti-cyclic citrullinated peptide antibodies in patients with juvenile idiopathic arthritis, Immunol. Invest. 37 (2008) 849–857.
76. K. Oen, P.N. Malleson, D.A. Cabral, et al., Early predictors of longterm outcome in patients with juvenile rheumatoid arthritis: subset-specific correlations, J. Rheumatol. 30 (2003) 585–593.
77. A. Ravelli, E. Felici, S. Magni-Manzoni, et al., Patients with antinuclear antibody-positive juvenile idiopathic arthritis constitute a homogeneous subgroup irrespective of the course of joint disease, Arthritis Rheum. 52 (2005) 826–832.
79. R.W. Burlingame, R.L. Rubin, A.M. Rosenberg, Autoantibodies to chromatin components in juvenile rheumatoid arthritis, Arthritis Rheum. 36 (1993) 836–841.
82. D.S. Gibson, S. Blelock, J. Curry, et al., Comparative analysis of synovial fluid and plasma proteomes in juvenile arthritis--proteomic patterns of joint inflammation in early stage disease, J. Proteomics 72 (2009) 656–676.
84. E.H. Giannini, E.J. Brewer, N. Kuzmina, et al., Methotrexate in resistant juvenile rheumatoid arthritis: results of the U.S.A.-U.S.S.R. double-blind, placebo-controlled trial, The Pediatric Rheumatology Collaborative Study Group and: The Cooperative Children's Study Group, N. Engl J. Med. 326 (1992) 1043–1049.
87. E. Silverman, R. Mouy, L. Spiegel, et al., Leflunomide or methotrexate for juvenile rheumatoid arthritis, N. Engl. J. Med. 352 (2005) 1655–1666.
88. P.J. Hashkes, R.M. Laxer, Medical treatment of juvenile idiopathic arthritis, JAMA 294 (2005) 1671–1684.
90. D.J. Lovell, E.H. Giannini, A. Reiff, et al., Long-term efficacy and safety of etanercept in children with polyarticular-course juvenile rheumatoid arthritis: interim results from an ongoing multicenter, open-label, extended-treatment trial, Arthritis Rheum. 48 (2003) 218–226.

94. D.J. Lovell, N. Ruperto, S. Goodman, et al., Adalimumab with or without methotrexate in juvenile rheumatoid arthritis, N. Engl. J. Med. 359 (2008) 810–820.

96. S.E. Klepper, Exercise and fitness in children with arthritis: evidence of benefits for exercise and physical activity, Arthritis Rheum. 49 (2003) 435–443.

104. E.D. Ferucci, D.W. Templin, A.P. Lanier, Rheumatoid arthritis in American Indians and Alaska Natives: a review of the literature, Semin. Arthritis Rheum. 34 (2005) 662–667.

110. S. Bowyer, P. Roettcher, Pediatric rheumatology clinic populations in the United States: results of a 3 year survey: Pediatric Rheumatology Database Research Group, J. Rheumatol. 23 (1996) 1968–1974.

111. K. Oen, H.S. El-Gabalawy, J.M. Canvin, et al., HLA associations of seropositive rheumatoid arthritis in a Cree and Ojibway population, J. Rheumatol. 25 (1998) 2319–2323.

115. F. van Gaalen, A. Ioan-Facsinay, T.W. Huizinga, et al., The devil in the details: the emerging role of anticitrulline autoimmunity in rheumatoid arthritis, J. Immunol. 175 (2005) 5575–5580.

117. J.D. Gorman, L.A. Criswell, The shared epitope and severity of rheumatoid arthritis, Rheum. Dis. Clin. North. Am 28 (2002) 59–78.

123. B.S. Nepom, G.T. Nepom, E. Mickelson, et al., Specific HLA-DR4-associated histocompatibility molecules characterize patients with seropositive juvenile rheumatoid arthritis, J. Clin. Invest. 74 (1984) 287–291.

124. B. Nepom, The immunogenetics of juvenile rheumatoid arthritis, Rheum. Dis. Clin. North Am. 17 (1991) 825–842.

125. R.K. Vehe, A.B. Begovich, B.S. Nepom, HLA susceptibility genes in rheumatoid factor positive juvenile rheumatoid arthritis, J. Rheumatol. (Suppl. 26) (1990) 11–15.

131. L. Klareskog, P. Stolt, K. Lundberg, et al., A new model for an etiology of rheumatoid arthritis: smoking may trigger HLA-DR (shared epitope)-restricted immune reactions to autoantigens modified by citrullination, Arthritis Rheum. 54 (2006) 38–46.

134. A. Hinks, A. Barton, N. Shephard, et al., Identification of a novel susceptibility locus for juvenile idiopathic arthritis by genome-wide association analysis, Arthritis Rheum. 60 (2009) 258–263.

135. S.D. Thompson, M.B. Moroldo, L. Guyer, et al., A genome-wide scan for juvenile rheumatoid arthritis in affected sibpair families provides evidence of linkage, Arthritis Rheum. 50 (2004) 2920–2930.

159. J.M. Low, A.K. Chauhan, D.A. Kietz, et al., Determination of anti-cyclic citrullinated peptide antibodies in the sera of patients with juvenile idiopathic arthritis, J. Rheumatol. 31 (2004) 1829–1833.

160. P. Dewint, I.E. Hoffman, S. Rogge, et al., Effect of age on prevalence of anticitrullinated protein/peptide antibodies in polyarticular juvenile idiopathic arthritis, Rheumatology (Oxford) 45 (2006) 204–208.

163. R.A. Williams, B.M. Ansell, Radiological findings in seropositive juvenile chronic arthritis (juvenile rheumatoid arthritis) with particular reference to progression, Ann. Rheum. Dis. 44 (1985) 685–693.

164. A.M. Selvaag, B. Flato, K. Dale, et al., Radiographic and clinical outcome in early juvenile rheumatoid arthritis and juvenile spondyloarthropathy: a 3-year prospective study, J. Rheumatol. 33 (2006) 1382–1391.

168. M. Ziff, The rheumatoid nodule, Arthritis Rheum. 33 (1990) 761–767.

172. E. Thomas, D.P. Symmons, D.H. Brewster, et al., National study of cause-specific mortality in rheumatoid arthritis, juvenile chronic arthritis, and other rheumatic conditions: a 20 year followup study, J. Rheumatol. 30 (2003) 958–965.

174. F. Fantini, V. Gerloni, M. Gattinara, et al., Remission in juvenile chronic arthritis: a cohort study of 683 consecutive cases with a mean 10 year followup, J. Rheumatol. 30 (2003) 579–584.

175. K. Oen, P.N. Malleson, D.A. Cabral, et al., Disease course and outcome of juvenile rheumatoid arthritis in a multicenter cohort, J. Rheumatol. 29 (2002) 1989–1999.

176. C.A. Wallace, B. Huang, M. Bandeira, et al., Patterns of clinical remission in select categories of juvenile idiopathic arthritis, Arthritis Rheum. 52 (2005) 3554–3562.

179. J.C. Packham, M.A. Hall, Long-term follow-up of 246 adults with juvenile idiopathic arthritis: functional outcome, Rheumatology (Oxford) 41 (2002) 1428–1435.

Entire reference list is available online at www.expertconsult.com.

Chapter 16

OLIGOARTHRITIS

Ross E. Petty and James T. Cassidy

DEFINITION

Oligoarthritis is defined as a chronic inflammatory arthritis of unknown origin that begins before the age of 16 and lasts for at least 6 weeks (Table 16–1).[1] It is further characterized as either persistent (if no more than four joints are affected during the disease course) or extended (if, after the initial 6-month period, the total number of affected joints exceeds four). The ILAR classification also requires that patients who otherwise fulfill these criteria be excluded from the category if they have psoriasis, if there is a family history of psoriasis or a disease associated with the human leukocyte antigen (HLA) allele HLA-B27 in a first-degree relative, if the disease began in a male older than 6 years of age, or if two positive tests for rheumatoid factor (RF) were obtained at least 3 months apart. Such exclusions do not apply to the EULAR criteria for oligoarticular juvenile chronic arthritis[2] or American College of Rheumatology (ACR) criteria for pauciarticular juvenile rheumatoid arthritis[3] (see Chapter 13) (Table 16–1). Oligoarthritis is a distinctly, if not uniquely, pediatric disease, and it is the most commonly diagnosed category of chronic arthritis among children in North America and Europe. In these classifications, the words *oligoarticular* and *pauciarticular* have the same meaning: few joints (<4). Oligoarticular is derived from a Greek root; pauciarticular from a Latin root.

EPIDEMIOLOGY

Oligoarthritis accounts for 50% to 80% of all children with chronic arthritis, at least in North American and European white populations. Oen and Cheang[4] noted that the proportion of all children with chronic arthritis who had oligoarthritis (ACR or EULAR criteria) was higher in North American and European patients (58%) than in East Indian (25%), North American Indian (26%), or other racial groups (31%). A study of a multiethnic cohort of Canadian children with JIA (ILAR criteria) confirmed the relatively low proportion of non-European children with either persistent or extended oligoarticular JIA, compared with children of European ancestry seen in the same clinic.[5] Several reviews of incidence and prevalence studies have been published.[4,6-8]

Incidence

Reports of the incidence of oligoarthritis are difficult to interpret because of the variation in criteria used to classify the patients. Using information from hospitals and community physicians, Andersson-Gare and colleagues[9] determined an annual incidence of oligoarthritis (EULAR criteria) of 7/100,000 children younger than 16 years of age in Sweden. Using the same criteria, a Norwegian study[10] reported a somewhat higher incidence of 11.2/100,000/year. It should be noted that 42% of these children were HLA-B27–positive, strongly suggesting that children with enthesitis-related arthritis (ERA) or juvenile ankylosing spondylitis (JAS) were included in the group. In studies that used the ACR criteria, estimates of the incidence have ranged from less than 1/100,000/year in Japan[11] to more than 18/100,000/year in Finland.[12]

Prevalence

The prevalence of oligoarthritis in reported studies varies greatly depending on the diagnostic criteria used; whether the study was hospital, clinic, or community based; and the geographical location of the study.[7] Using information from hospitals and community physicians, Andersson-Gare and

---

Table 16–1

Classification of oligoarthritis (ILAR criteria)

Arthritis in four or fewer joints during the first 6 mo of disease

Persistent oligoarthritis: Never more than four joints affected

Extended oligoarthritis: More than four joints affected after the first 6 mo of disease

Exclusions:
- Psoriasis or a history of psoriasis in the patient or a first-degree relative
- Arthritis in an HLA-B27 positive male beginning after the sixth birthday
- Ankylosing spondylitis, enthesitis-related arthritis, sacroiliitis with inflammatory bowel disease, Reiter syndrome, or acute anterior uveitis or a history of one of these disorders in a first-degree relative
- Presence of IgM RF on at least two occasions at least 3 mo apart
- Presence of systemic arthritis

HLA, human leukocyte antigen; IgM, immunoglobulin M; ILAR, International League of Associations for Rheumatology; RF, rheumatoid factor.

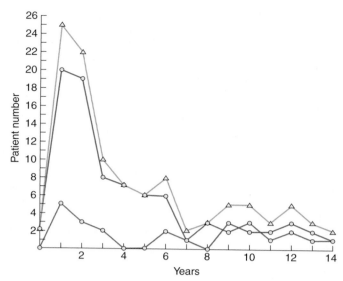

FIGURE 16–1   Age at onset of oligoarticular JRA: total group (-△-), girls (-○-), boys (-△-). (Data from Sullivan DB, Cassidy JT, Petty RE: Pathogenic implications of age of onset in juvenile rheumatoid arthritis, *Arthritis Rheum* 18:251, 1975.)

associates[9] found 146 children with oligoarthritis (EULAR) in a population of 400,600 children younger than 16 years of age, a prevalence of 36/100,000. In the study by Manners and Diepeveen,[13] oligoarthritis fulfilling the EULAR criteria for JCA was found in 9 of 2241 12-year-old school children who were examined by the authors. This prevalence (4/1000) is markedly higher than that reported in other studies but may be closest to reality, because it was community based and verified by physical examination by a pediatric rheumatologist. It is possible that this high prevalence is not representative of the disease worldwide, however.

Age at Onset

Oligoarthritis has a striking age at onset distribution, with a peak incidence between 1 and 2 years of age (Fig. 16–1).[13] A small proportion of children with oligoarthritis have disease onset after this time, but when this occurs it raises the possibility of alternative diagnoses, such as ERA, JAS, psoriatic arthritis, or developing polyarthritis.

Sex Ratio

In North America and Europe, oligoarthritis is predominantly a disease of girls, with a female/male ratio of approximately 3:1. In children with uveitis, the ratio of girls to boys is even higher: 5:1 to 6.6:1.[14-17] In Asia, however, oligoarthritis occurs predominantly in boys, and uveitis is reported to be rare.[18]

GENETICS

Early-onset oligoarthritis, particularly if it is complicated by uveitis, appears to be very uncommon in populations of non-European origin. Oligoarthritis is seldom familial. When sibling pairs both have JRA, however, three quarters are concordant for onset type (most commonly oligoarthritis).[19] It is likely that oligoarthritis, like other types of childhood arthritis, is a multigenic disease (see Chapter 5).

HLA Genes

There are quite characteristic associations of oligoarthritis, or subsets of oligoarthritis, with some HLA genes. The unusual disease association of an A locus antigen, A2, has been reported and confirmed in children with JRA (ACR criteria) in general and in early-onset pauciarticular JRA in girls in particular.[20-22]

An increase in the HLA-B27 allele in early studies was possibly related to inclusion of children with juvenile ankylosing spondylitis (similar to enthesitis-related arthritis of the ILAR classification).[23,24] Later investigations documented inconsistent increases in the frequency of this antigen in subgroups of children with JRA.[24,25] However, B27 may confer an age-related risk for pauciarticular JRA (ACR criteria) in boys (50% risk at 7.3 years; 80% risk at 11.9 years).[21]

Among the class II alleles, the most consistent association has been with the DRB1*08-DQA1*04-DQB1*04 haplotype encoding DR8 and DQ4. These two alleles are in strong linkage disequilibrium, but a recent report showed that it was DR8, not DQ4, that was associated with JIA.[25] DR8, DR5, DR6, DPB1*0201, and certain DQ alleles are also reportedly more frequent in children with early-onset oligoarthritis[21,23,26,27] and in pauciarticular JRA, with relative risks in the range of 2 to 13.[23,26,28-33] Linkage disequilibrium probably accounts for some of the reported associations. The transmission disequilibrium test was used by Moroldo and colleagues[23] to examine linkage and association in 101 white families who had a child with oligoarthritis. DR8 and DR5 (as well as A2, B27, and B35) had significantly higher frequencies of transmission to the affected child; DR4 and DR7 were found less often. These data suggest that these numerous HLA associations partly reflect linkage between the HLA genetic region in children with JRA and a population stratification effect. However, age and sex influenced these effects. Prahalad and colleagues[34] used sibling pairs with arthritis to confirm the linkage of pauciarticular JRA with the HLA-DR region, especially DR8 and DR11. Using restriction fragment length polymorphisms, Morling and colleagues[32] found that children with pauciarticular JRA had increased frequencies of DRB1*08; DRB3*01/02/03 (DRw52); DQA1*0401 and 0501; DQB1*0301; DPA1*0201; and DPB1*02, compared with healthy controls. Both subtypes of DR5 (DR11 and DR12) and DR8 (DRB1*0801) contributed to susceptibility to early-onset oligoarticular disease.[35,36] DR11, DR12, and DR8 haplotypes share similar DQA1 alleles: DQA1*0401, *0501, and *0601.[37,38] These three DQ alleles have a common motif in exon 2 at the 42 to 53 positions, which was present in 86% of children with JCA but in only 36% of controls.[36,37] Haas and colleagues[37] demonstrated that distinct differences in the DQA1 promoter are strongly associated with susceptibility to early-onset disease. Nepom and associates[38] identified a 13-nucleotide region of sequence identity in the first hypervariable region of DR5, DR6, and DR8 alleles, which is a possible "shared epitope" that could be important in antigen recognition.

DR1 and DR4 are present in lower frequency in young girls with persistent pauciarticular JRA and antinuclear antibody (ANA) seropositivity, compared with the normal population.[21] DR1 is a risk factor for extended oligoarthritis as well as for polyarthritis in older children.[39] It is in linkage disequilibrium with DQA*0101, which is associated in one study with progressive erosive disease in children with early-onset pauciarticular JRA and was negatively associated with the presence of uveitis.[40] This DQA gene, although not present in all children with the disease, may be critically important in the development of this onset type.[41] DQA*0101[42] and A2*0101[43] are also binding sites for the 45-kD DEK proto-oncogene. Anti-DEK antibodies are characteristic of oligoarticular-onset disease (78% positive), especially in children who are ANA seropositive and have a history of uveitis, and may negate the regulatory function of the gene,[44] or they may simply be a reflection of autoimmunity.[45] One study associated ANA seropositivity in early-onset disease with DQB1*0603.[46]

Pauciarticular JRA is also associated with DP2 (DPB1*0201),[47-49] which in one study[48] was present in 67% of patients but only 34% of controls. It has been suggested that this DP allele increases the risk conferred by DR alleles but is not sufficient in itself to increase susceptibility to pauciarticular JRA.[50] A number of studies have discussed the role of interactions among alleles at different loci in producing susceptibility to disease.[32,51] Interactions between class I and class II genes led to the hypothesis that at least two genetic loci are involved in the predisposition to oligoarthritis; they have been named JRA 1 and JRA 2.[23,39,40,52-55] A third locus, JRA 3, has been postulated for a DP gene.

In linkage studies, Zeggini and coworkers[22] demonstrated linkage to HLA-A, -B, and -DRB1 in girls with oligoarthritis, with persistent and extended types. They suggested that linkage appeared to be attributable to preferential maternal transmission of these alleles.

Non-HLA Genes

A number of genes involved in antigen presentation or cytokine expression may be important in either a predisposition to JCA or its pathogenesis.[56] A weak association with the transporter-associated protein (TAP) gene TAP2B, a polymorphism in a member of the adenosine triphosphate–binding cassette superfamily, is present in patients with early-onset disease.[57] TAP1B may function as an additive susceptibility factor.[58] One study suggested that homozygosity of the B allele of the LMP2 proteasome subunit may increase susceptibility to a putative subtype of JRA that is associated with B27.[59]

Interaction with other non-HLA genes is also possible; IL-1A2, a variant of the IL-1β gene, is associated with early-onset oligoarthritis.[60] Children with extended oligoarthritis (ILAR criteria) were shown to have a high frequency of the interleukin-1 receptor antagonist gene IL1RN*2; this was also observed, to a lesser extent, in children with ERA.[61] The gene for the cytokine IL-1β, or a gene for which its polymorphism is a marker, may contribute risk for early-onset disease and uveitis.[60,62] A significant increase in IL1RN*2 in Czech patients with JIA, compared with controls, was reported, especially in those with oligoarthritis, ERA, and other categories.[61]

Crawley and colleagues[63] found a decrease in the IL-10 phenotype associated with low IL-10 production in children with arthritis affecting fewer than five joints, compared with those with more than four affected joints. The frequency of the tumor necrosis factor (TNF)α2 microsatellite allele was significantly increased in Latvian children with oligoarticular JCA, and the frequency of TNFα9 was significantly decreased in this population.[64] The TNFα2 allele is associated with high TNF-α production.[65] Zeggini and colleagues reported an increased frequency of the intronic +851 TNF SNP in persistent oligoarticular JIA (odds ratio, 3.86; 95% confidence interval, 1.6 to 9.2).[66] A review of the genetics of JIA has been recently published.[67] Genetic associations are summarized in Table 16–2.

ETIOLOGY AND PATHOGENESIS

The etiology of oligoarthritis is unknown. The narrow age-at-onset profile suggests the possibility of exposure to a ubiquitous environmental agent, possibly a virus, but none has been consistently identified. In a study of six twin pairs with pauciarticular JRA, there was an average of approximately 3 months (range, 0 to 12 months) separating disease onset in each twin, again raising the question of an environmental agent as an initiating event.[68] One study alleged that breastfeeding has a protective effect on the development of JRA,[69] especially oligoarticular disease; however, a strong relationship was not confirmed in another investigation.[70]

Studies of T lymphocytes have yielded conflicting results. Maksymowych and associates[71] reported a high frequency of the T-cell receptor allele TCR-Vβ6.1 among HLA-DQA*0101–positive children. A subsequent report identified this TCR null allele as a risk factor for a polyarticular course in children with early-onset oligoarticular disease positive for DQA1*0101.[72] This association was not confirmed in a Norwegian study,[73] nor did Nepom and coworkers[74] identify TCR polymorphism in their studies of pauciarticular-onset JRA. In the report of Thompson and colleagues,[75] TCR-Vβ8 was clonally expanded in children with polyarticular disease, and TCR-Vβ20 was increased in those with oligoarthritis. Murray and colleagues[76] studied synovial T-cell infiltrates in 17 children (12 with polyarticular and 5 pauciarticular disease) and found that the level of T-cell activation (CD3+ IL-2R+) was significantly higher in oligoarthritis (especially for CD8+ cells) and that the CD4/CD8 ratio was lower. In a subsequent report,[77] these investigators found that IL-4 messenger RNA (mRNA) was more frequently identified in the synovium of children with pauciarticular JRA than in those with polyarticular onset or course. They suggested that the presence of IL-4 mRNA might be important in restricting the disease to an oligoarticular pattern.

The high frequency of autoantibodies to nuclear antigens indicates a break in immunological tolerance,

Table 16–2

Human leukocyte antigen associations in oligoarthritis

HLA Gene	Criteria	Associations	Reference No.
A2	ACR	Young age, female sex	20,21
B27	ACR	Erosion when present with DR8	137
DR 6	ACR	Oligoarthritis	21
DRB1*08	ACR	Oligoarthritis	23
	EULAR	Early onset	35
	ACR	Persistent disease	137
DRB3*01/2/3	ACR	Oligoarthritis	23
DPA*0101	ACR	Progressive erosive disease	40
	ACR	Decreased in uveitis	40
DPA1*0201	ACR	Oligoarthritis	40
DPB1*0201	EULAR	Oligoarthritis	47
	ACR	Oligoarthritis	49
DR 1	ACR	Extended oligoarthritis	39
	ACR	Decreased in persistent oligoarthritis	39
DR 4	ACR	Decreased in oligoarthritis	21
DR11 (DR5)	EULAR	Early onset	35
DR12 (DR5)	EULAR	Early onset	35
DQA1*0401	ACR	Oligoarthritis	23
DQA1*0501	ACR	Oligoarthritis	23
DQB1*0301	ACR	Oligoarthritis	23
DQB1*0603	EULAR	Early onset, ANA positive	46

ACR, American College of Rheumatology; ANA, antinuclear antibody; EULAR, European League Against Rheumatism; HLA, human leukocyte antigen.

but there is no evidence that autoantibodies as such participate in disease pathogenesis. The identity of the specificities of the antigens to which ANAs react in children with oligoarthritis is still largely unknown. Antibodies to an epitope on the high-mobility group (HMG)-17 protein are increased in JRA, and antibodies to an HMG-2 protein are increased in oligoarticular disease.[78,79] A number of studies have identified an interesting association between elevated serum prolactin levels and JRA as well as systemic lupus erythematosus (see Chapter 21). Levels were increased in children with JRA and were associated with ANA seropositivity.[80] Modest hyperprolactinemia was also identified in prepubertal girls who were ANA seropositive and had oligoarthritis.[81,82] The prolactin concentration correlated with levels of IL-6 and with a chronic course of the disease.

Humoral and cellular immune responses to highly conserved bacterial heat shock proteins (HSPs) are present in children with JRA.[83-89] HSPs have been demonstrated in the serum and synovial fluid of children with JRA.[89-93] Van Eden and colleagues[92] postulated that reactive T cells are part of the normal immune repertoire for TCR V-gene products; self-HSPs and bacterial HSPs may trigger this response.[93-95] In 13 of 15 children with oligoarthritis, T-lymphocyte proliferative responses to HSP-60 were detected an average of 12 weeks before remission of the inflammatory disease.[89,90] The investigators hypothesized that induction of tolerance to specific T-cell epitopes of HSP-60 by nasal administration may be a promising route of immunotherapy for childhood arthritis.[96] There is a high frequency of the highly proinflammatory Th17 cells in synovial tissue of children with JIA.[97]

CLINICAL MANIFESTATIONS

The first 6 months of disease is characterized by inflammation in four or fewer joints. These children are not systemically ill, and, except for chronic uveitis, extraarticular manifestations are distinctly unusual. Oligoarthritis in a child is predominantly a disease of the lower extremities. In a study[98] of 64 children with pauciarticular JRA, one or both knees were most commonly affected at disease onset (89%), followed by the ankles (36%). Arthritis affecting small joints of the fingers and toes occurred in only 6% of the children, and arthritis in elbows, hips, wrists, or temporomandibular joints in 3%. Although it is the authors' impression that wrists and small joints of the hands or feet are seldom affected in pauciarticular JRA at onset, others disagree.[99] In at least one half of the reported cases, only a single joint is affected (monarticular onset), usually the knee.[100-102] Uveitis may be present at onset of the disease; it eventually affects up to 20% of children and is usually asymptomatic (see Chapter 21).

DIAGNOSIS

The differential diagnosis depends on a number of factors, including the onset type and pattern of joint involvement, the duration of disease at the time the child is evaluated, and the sex and age of the child. In some instances, oligoarticular JIA is a diagnosis of exclusion.[103,104] In a child with monarthritis of recent onset (i.e., within 72 hours), the differential diagnosis must include septic arthritis, trauma (including nonaccidental trauma resulting in a hemarthrosis), and hematological and oncological disease (including hemophilia, and malignancy) (Table 16–3).[105] If the monarthritis is longstanding, sepsis (except for tuberculosis), trauma, and malignancy are very unlikely. A painful joint effusion of short duration may be caused by trauma, or, rarely in children, it may be associated with an internal structural abnormality such as a discoid meniscus[106] or osteochondritis dissecans (see Chapter 34). The monarthritis of hemophilia results from bleeding into a major joint, which is often initiated by even minor trauma. Recurrent involvement has been described in occult celiac disease.[107,108] Rare causes of chronic monarthritis, such as tuberculosis, sarcoidosis, and villonodular synovitis, should also be considered. A migrating monarthritis, sometimes associated with fever and a rash, has been described in children of Assyrian ancestry.[109] The various forms of idiopathic osteolysis may mimic arthritis of a limited number of joints (e.g., wrists) at onset. Rarely, arthritis has resulted from administration of a drug such as isotretinoin[110,111] or antithyroid medication.[112,113]

Oligoarticular JIA is the most common cause of chronic oligoarthritis, especially in girls younger than 6 years of age. Psoriatic arthritis, which affects large and small joints in an asymmetrical pattern, is also a possibility at this age (see Chapter 18). ERA is a more likely cause of a monarthritis or oligoarthritis of the lower extremities with onset in the older child or adolescent.[114] A diagnosis of oligoarticular JIA or psoriatic arthritis may be substantiated by the demonstration of asymptomatic anterior uveitis by slit-lamp examination, although juvenile sarcoidosis/Blau syndrome also rarely manifests in this way. ANA seropositivity supports the diagnosis of JRA or psoriatic arthritis but may also be found in some healthy children[115] and in some children with noninflammatory musculoskeletal pain.[116] Lyme disease may manifest as an oligoarthritis (see Chapter 38).

In the child with oligoarthritis, the affected joint is swollen and often warm but usually not very painful or tender, and almost never red. The child is not systemically ill. If a joint is acutely painful and erythematous or if the child is febrile, septic arthritis is more likely the correct diagnosis. Immediate joint aspiration is always indicated in such a patient to exclude septic arthritis or osteomyelitis. Needle or arthroscopic synovial biopsy is useful in children with monarthritis in whom granulomatous disease is suspected.[117] Culture and microscopic examination of synovial tissue may be more rewarding in the case of tuberculosis than culture of the fluid only. A negative purified protein derivative skin test virtually excludes the diagnosis of active tuberculosis. Biopsy should not be performed simply to confirm a diagnosis of oligoarthritis.

Arthritis of the hip joint is rare at the onset or during the course of oligoarthritis. In the authors' experience of 145 children with oligoarthritis seen early in their course, only 1 girl had initial involvement of the hip.

Table 16–3

Differential diagnosis of monarthritis

Acute monarthritis
Early rheumatic disease
   Oligoarthritis
   Enthesitis-related arthritis
   Psoriatic arthritis
Arthritis related to infection
   Septic arthritis
   Reactive arthritis
Malignancy
   Leukemia
   Neuroblastoma
Hemophilia
Trauma
Familial Mediterranean fever
Chronic monarthritis
Juvenile idiopathic arthritis
   Oligoarthritis
   Enthesitis-related arthritis
   Juvenile psoriatic arthritis
Villonodular synovitis
Sarcoidosis, Blau syndrome
Tuberculosis
Hemophilia
"Pseudoarthritis" (e.g., hemangioma, synovial chondromatosis, lipoma arborescens)
Some episodic fever syndromes (mevalonate kinase deficiency, chronic infantile neurocutaneous and articular syndrome, or neonatal onset multisystem inflammatory disease)

Onset of apparent arthritis in the hip in a very young child should be considered first to be a septic process or a congenital dislocation.[118] In the older child, osteonecrosis of the femoral head (Legg-Calvé-Perthes disease) is a diagnostic consideration. In the adolescent age group, a slipped capital femoral epiphysis may initially mimic JIA. In older boys, ERA may manifest as unilateral or bilateral hip disease (see Chapter 17). In children with transient synovitis of the hip, pain may be severe, but the process is self-limited, lasting no more than 1 to a few weeks.

LABORATORY EVALUATION

Laboratory indicators of inflammation may be normal in children with oligoarthritis, although mild to moderate elevation of the erythrocyte sedimentation rate (ESR) and elevation of C-reactive protein levels may occur. Hemoglobin levels and white blood cell and platelet counts are usually normal, and the presence of marked abnormalities in these parameters should suggest a diagnosis other than oligoarthritis.

Tests for RF are almost always negative, although, occasionally, children with a single affected joint (often the wrist) have RF. In contrast, tests for ANAs are positive in low titer (1:160) in 65% to 85% of children with oligoarthritis, particularly in girls and in those with uveitis.[119-121] Antibodies to double-stranded DNA and the extractable nuclear antigens are not detectable.

Antibodies that react with citrullinated peptides have rarely been demonstrated in children with oligoarthritis, their frequency depending to some extent on the antigen used.[122,123] Syed and colleagues noted that IgA anti-CCP antibodies were more common than other isotypes in children with JIA.[124] Anticardiolipin antibodies were reported in 18% of children with oligoarthritis (compared with 4% in a healthy population).[125] They do not appear to be associated with intravascular thrombosis, however.

Elevated concentrations of activated C3 (C3c, C3d) were demonstrated in about one third of children with active oligoarthritis (a lower frequency than in children with systemic arthritis or polyarthritis).[126] Circulating immune complexes are not characteristic of oligoarthritis.

Routine synovial fluid analysis does not distinguish one type of JIA from another. The fluid is usually moderately inflammatory, with a cell count of 5 to 20,000 cells/mm³, mostly polymorphs.

RADIOGRAPHIC EVALUATION

The radiographic changes in oligoarthritis are similar to those seen on other kinds of arthritis, although often less severe (see Chapter 10). In a follow-up study[127] of 97 children with pauciarticular JRA, joint space narrowing was present in only 5% of children early in the disease course, increasing to approximately 15% at a median of 6.2 years after disease onset. Erosions were seen in 10% of children with early disease, and in approximately 25% of children 6 years later. Bone overgrowth was more common; it occurred in more than 20% of children early in the disease and slightly more frequently later in the disease course. Not surprisingly, overgrowth was most common at the knee (Figs. 16–2 and 16–3).

Magnetic resonance imaging with gadolinium confirms the presence of synovitis, increased intraarticular fluid, and, occasionally bone marrow edema. Its main utility, however, is in differentiating other causes of joint swelling, particularly in the child with monarthritis.[128]

In a study of 32 children with JIA (including 20 with oligoarthritis), it was demonstrated that ultrasound was able to detect subclinical synovitis in 5.5% of clinically normal joints. The authors point out that application of this technique could result in reclassification of some children with clinical oligoarthritis.[129]

MANAGEMENT

Prompt and accurate diagnosis is essential to the optimal outcome for treatment of oligoarthritis. Because of the subtlety of the signs and symptoms, medical attention

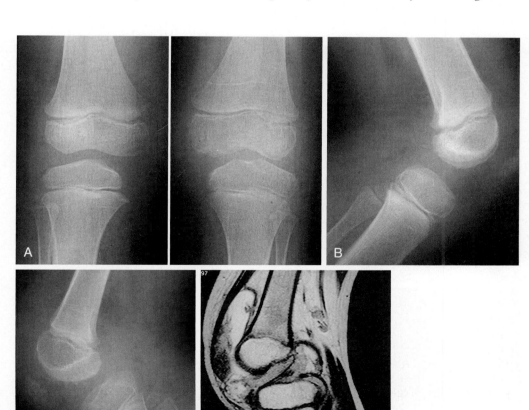

FIGURE 16–2 **A–C,** Anteroposterior and lateral radiographic films of the knees of a 3-year-old girl who developed monarthritis of the left knee at the age of 2 years with an initial flexion contracture of 32 degrees. There is marked joint space narrowing with regional osteoporosis of the left knee and epiphyseal enlargement. **D,** Postgadolinium magnetic resonance imaging sagittal studies of the left knee. There is a large joint effusion with marked inflammatory synovial hypertrophy, demonstrated by enhancement of the pannus throughout all compartments of the joint. There are also thinning and irregularity of the articular cartilage involving the femur, tibia, and patella. There is almost bone-on-bone apposition of the femorotibial articulation. Asymmetrical enlargements of the epiphyses of the left knee are visible, with relative hypoplasia of the menisci.

may not be sought early in the disease course. The aim of therapy should be to achieve total remission of signs and symptoms of joint inflammation. Initial management of oligoarthritis should include careful clinical general and musculoskeletal assessment. In the child with monarthritis, other possible causes of inflammation in a single joint should be excluded. Evaluation by a physical therapist and occupational therapist to assess joint range, muscle strength, and function should be obtained. A slit-lamp examination by an experienced ophthalmologist is essential to exclude the possibility of uveitis, as soon as possible after the diagnosis of oligoarthritis.

Initial pharmacotherapy usually consists of a non-steroidal antiinflammatory drug (NSAID). Naproxen in a dosage of 15 to 20 mg/kg/day is often the drug of choice because of its twice-daily dosing and the availability of a suspension. The parents and patient should be cautioned to take the medication with food to minimize the risk of gastric upset and be reminded of the risk of naproxen-induced pseudoporphyria. A trial of at least 6 weeks is recommended. During this time, the physical therapist may recommend passive and active stretching for joints with limited motion. Consideration should be given to administration of intraarticular steroids, preferably triamcinolone hexacetonide (1 mg/kg with a maximum of 40 mg in large joints such as the knee, hip, and shoulder; 0.5 mg/kg in elbow and ankle with a maximum of 20 mg; and a maximum of 10 mg/joint in the wrist), either at diagnosis, or if NSAIDs fail to completely control the joint inflammation after 6 weeks of therapy. It may be necessary to serially cast joints with restricted range of motion. This can be done at the same time as joint injection using conscious sedation with a drug such as midazolam. Beukelman and colleagues used decision analysis to evaluate optimal initial therapy for monarthritis of the knee in JIA.[130] They compared the three most common approaches to initial management: NSAIDs alone, NSAIDs for 2 months followed by intraarticular corticosteroids, and intraarticular steroids alone. They concluded that the use of intraarticular steroids alone as initial therapy was the optimal strategy.

The response to NSAIDs and intraarticular glucosteroids is usually very good, and most patients with oligoarthritis respond to this approach. Joint injections can be repeated two or more times, but children who are resistant to such therapy require the addition of a second-line agent. A different NSAID may also be of benefit. The child who has an extended oligoarticular course is known to have a guarded outcome, and such children should be given the benefit of methotrexate earlier rather than later in the disease course. After a course of at least 6 months of NSAIDs and intraarticular steroids on one or two occasions, oral methotrexate (0.30 to 0.5 mg/kg/week; 10 to 15 mg/m^2) should be started with the dose increased as tolerated to 0.65 mg/kg/week (see Chapter 6).

The possible development of a leg-length inequality (in the child with a single affected knee) or contractures of affected joints requires ongoing assessment and physical therapy. Major leg-length inequalities are unusual in the child who is treated early and effectively. Sherry and colleagues[131] demonstrated the effectiveness of intraarticular steroids in preventing this complication. Should a leg-length inequality of greater than 1 cm develop, a lift to partially compensate for the difference should be applied to the sole of the shoe of the shorter leg. Flexion contractures around the knee or ankle are usually much more

FIGURE 16–3 These radiographs illustrate the 5-year progression of osteoporosis, joint space narrowing, and degenerative changes in the knees of a girl with oligoarticular juvenile rheumatoid arthritis. **A** In this radiograph, taken 2 years after onset of disease, there are only minimal epiphyseal advancement and osteoporosis. **B,** After 4 years of disease, there are increased prominence of the trabecular pattern secondary to osteoporosis, narrowing of the joint spaces, and remodeling of the normal contours of the articular surfaces. **C,** After 5 years of disease, there are marked narrowing of joint spaces and flattening of the tibial plateaus. Degenerative changes include squaring of the femoral condyles, development of osteophytes at the medial margin of the tibial plateaus, and development of subchondral cysts in the femoral epiphyses.

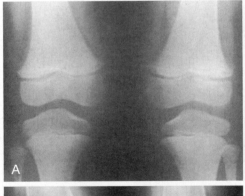
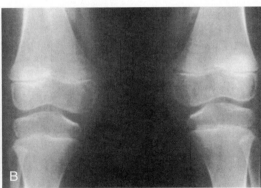
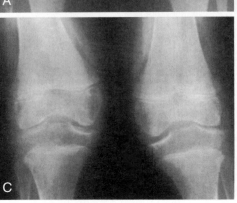

responsive to physical therapy after steroid injection of the affected joint. Serial casting may be initiated at the time of joint injection and is an effective way of regaining lost range of motion in the knee in particular. An active physical therapy program should be undertaken under the guidance of the therapist (see Chapter 12).

Surgical management of oligoarthritis is rarely necessary. Occasionally, soft tissue releases are required in the child who has not received early treatment and has developed a flexion contracture that is unresponsive to intraarticular corticosteroids and physical therapy.

DISEASE COURSE AND PROGNOSIS

The disease course and prognosis in children with oligoarthritis have improved considerably in the last 10 to 15 years. In particular, the frequency of significant joint contractures or leg-length inequalities has diminished, probably as the result of prompt institution of pharmacological and physical therapy, in particular the use of intraarticular steroids. Bowyer and colleagues[132] reported on the health status of 232 children with pauciarticular JRA who were monitored for 1 to 5 years. By 1 year after disease onset, one half no longer required medications, and 98% were in Steinbrocker functional class I or II. No patient with pauciarticular JRA was in Steinbrocker class III – IV 5 years after diagnosis. Childhood Health Assessment Questionnaire scores were 0 in the majority of patients, but approximately 25% had scores of between 0 and 0.5, and 12% had higher scores. Measures of psychosocial outcome were also evaluated in this study. Educational achievement and employment were comparable to the national norms. Bowyer and colleagues also found little negative impact of pauciarthritis on school participation: only 6% of the children were unable to participate in a full school program 5 years after diagnosis.

Sequelae from uveitis remain an important issue, although here, too, some centers report decreased frequency and severity of this complication (see Chapter 20).

Oen and associates[133] studied the outcomes of children with pauciarticular JRA who had been monitored for at least 5 years from disease onset and who were at least 8 years of age. Using stringent criteria for remission (absence of active arthritis, off medications for at least 2 years), these authors found that 47% of children with pauciarticular JRA were in remission 10 years after disease onset. Ninety-four percent of the remissions occurred before the age of 16 years. Although some patients had a monocyclical course, 25% relapsed approximately 5 years after the end of the first episode. An extended pauciarticular course was observed in 20% of children with pauciarticular onset, at a median of 3.9 years after disease onset. Children with pauciarticular JRA were mostly (85%) in Steinbrocker functional class I; 14.5% were in class II, and 0.5% in class III or IV.

Radiographic outcome was evaluated in the same population group.[127] Although joint erosion is unusual, it was demonstrable by plain radiographs in 10% of patients early in the disease course and in 25% of patients at some time during the disease course, most commonly

in knees, elbows, and shoulders. Joint space narrowing was even less frequent, but growth abnormalities occurred in approximately one quarter of the patients, most commonly in the knees and elbows. These results were confirmed by Bowyer and coworkers.[132] Al-Matar and colleagues[134] studied the patterns of joint involvement that would predict progression of disease in 205 children with oligoarthritis (ACR) who were monitored for 5 to 26 years. They concluded that the early presence of ankle or wrist disease, symmetrical joint involvement, and an elevated ESR predicted the progression of disease to affect more than four joints. ANA test positivity (titer of 1:40 or greater on HEp-2 cell substrate or 1:20 or greater on mouse liver substrate) and younger age at onset of disease correlated with longer active disease duration in a study by Oen and colleagues.[135] ANA positivity also correlated with worse outcome in this group of patients.

Fantini and colleagues[136] reported the follow up of 420 children with pauciarticular-onset JCA. Mean follow-up for these patients was 8.1 years, with a range from less than 1 year to more than 30 years. At last follow-up, 36% of these patients were in remission, which was defined as absence of clinical or laboratory evidence of active arthritis for a period of at least 6 months in the absence of antirheumatic therapy. Fifty-three percent of children with oligoarticular JCA had never gone into remission, and 13% had remitted but relapsed. Twenty-four percent of these patients had a polyarticular course.

Flato and associates[137] compared physical and psychosocial status in patients with pauciarticular JRA, who were monitored for a median of 14.9 years, with those of the healthy population. They found that early age at onset and an elevated ESR on first admission to hospital predicted persistent disease. In addition to these factors, DRB1*01 was found to predict joint erosions in these patients. Elevated ESR at onset, early age at onset, and the presence of hip disease in the first 6 months were predictors of disability. Early age at onset has not always been found to be a predictor of bad outcome, however.[138,139] Patients with persistent pauciarticular disease fared better than those with extended pauciarticular disease with respect to development of erosions, Health Assessment Questionnaire scores, and remission rates.[138,139]

The course of oligoarthritis is variable. Some children pursue an oligoarticular course and never have more than four affected joints (persistent oligoarthritis). In such children, the disease often goes into remission, although flares of the disease may occur many years later. In a second group, there is a progressive increase in the number of affected joints after the first 6 months of disease (extended oligoarthritis), so that by 1 or 2 years after onset, they have polyarthritis, although the number of affected joints is often much lower than in children with polyarthritis at onset. In this group, the prognosis is somewhat guarded, and fewer children enter remission. Because of the limited extent of the joint involvement, serious functional disability is uncommon. Fixed flexion contractures may persist, however, or osteoarthritis of a weight-bearing joint may eventually develop late in the course of the disease after clinical remission. Mortality is extremely rare.

PERSPECTIVE

Oligoarthritis is complex. Current understanding recognizes two subcategories (persistent and extended), and further studies may reveal other groups within this disease category. Its early recognition is essential to optimal management, which usually leads to a good functional outcome. Nonetheless, the disease is chronic and is complicated by chronic anterior uveitis, which may further compromise function.

REFERENCES

1. R.E. Petty, T.R. Southwood, P. Manners, et al., International League of Associations for Rheumatology classification of juvenile idiopathic arthritis, Second Revision J. Rheumatol. 31. Edmonton 2001, 31 (2004) 90–392.
2. European League Against Rheumatism, EULAR bulletin no. 4: nomenclature and classification of arthritis in children, National Zeitung AG, Basel, 1977.
3. E.J. Brewer, J. Bass, J. Baum, et al., Current proposed revision of JRA criteria, Arthritis Rheum. 20 (suppl) (1977) 195–199.
4. K.G. Oen, M. Cheang, Epidemiology of chronic arthritis in childhood, Semin. Arthritis Rheum. 26 (1996) 575–591.
5. R.K. Saurenmann, J.B. Rose, P. Tyre, et al., Epidemiology of juvenile idiopathic arthritis in a multiethnic cohort, Arthritis Rheum. 56 (2007) 1974–1984.
6. B. Andersson-Gare, Juvenile arthritis—who gets it, where and when? A review of current data on incidence and prevalence, Clin. Exp. Rheumatol. 17 (1999) 367–374.
7. P.J. Manners, C. Bower, Worldwide prevalence of juvenile arthritis—why does it vary so much? J. Rheumatol. 29 (2002) 520–530.
8. K. Oen, Comparative epidemiology of the rheumatic diseases in children, Curr. Opin. Rheumatol. 12 (2000) 410–414.
13. P.J. Manners, D.A. Diepeveen, Prevalence of juvenile chronic arthritis in a population of 12-year-old children in urban Australia, Pediatrics 98 (1996) 84–90.
15. J.T. Cassidy, D.B. Sullivan, R.E. Petty, Clinical patterns of chronic iridocyclitis in children with juvenile rheumatoid arthritis, Arthritis Rheum. 20 (suppl) (1977) 224–227.
17. J. Schaller, C. Kupfer, R.J. Wedgwood, Iridocyclitis in juvenile rheumatoid arthritis, Pediatrics 44 (1969) 92–100.
19. M.B. Moroldo, M. Chaudhari, E. Shear, et al., Juvenile rheumatoid arthritis affected sibpairs: Extent of clinical phenotype concordance, Arthritis Rheum. 50 (2004) 1928–1934.
20. K. Oen, R.E. Petty, M.L. Schroeder, An association between HLA-A2 and juvenile rheumatoid arthritis in girls, J. Rheumatol. 9 (1982) 916–920.
21. K.J. Murray, M.B. Moroldo, P. Donnelly, et al., Age-specific effects of juvenile rheumatoid arthritis-associated HLA genes, Arthritis Rheum. 42 (1999) 1843–1853.
22. E. Zeggini, R.P. Donn, W.E.R. Ollier, W. Thomson, the British Paediatric Rheumatology Study Group: Evidence of linkage of HLA loci in juvenile idiopathic oligoarthritis: independent effects of HLA-A and HLA-DRB1, Arthritis Rheum. 46 (2002) 2716–2720.
23. M.B. Moroldo, P. Donnelly, J. Saunders, et al., Transmission disequilibrium as a test of linkage and association between HLA alleles and pauciarticular-onset juvenile rheumatoid arthritis, Arthritis Rheum. 41 (1998) 1620–1624.
25. A. Smerdel, R. Ploski, B. Flato, et al., Juvenile idiopathic arthritis (JIA) is primarily associated with HLA-DR8, but not DQ4 on the DR8-DQ4 haplotypes, Ann. Rheum. Dis. 61 (2002) 354–357.
29. D. Glass, D. Litvin, K. Wallace, et al., Early onset pauciarticular juvenile rheumatoid arthritis associated with human leukocyte antigen-DRw5, iritis and antinuclear antibody, J. Clin. Invest. 66 (1980) 426–429.
34. S. Prahalad, M.H. Ryan, E.S. Shear, et al., Juvenile rheumatoid arthritis: linkage to HLA demonstrated by allele sharing in affected sibpairs, Arthritis Rheum. 43 (2004) 2335–2338.
39. D.N. Glass, E.H. Giannini, JRA as a complex genetic trait, Arthritis Rheum. 42 (1999) 2261–2268.
40. C. Van Kerckhove, L. Luyrink, J. Taylor, et al., HLA-DQA1*0101 haplotypes and disease outcome in early onset pauciarticular juvenile rheumatoid arthritis, J. Rheumatol. 18 (1991) 874–879.
44. I.S. Szer, H. Sierakowska, W. Szer, A novel autoantibody to the putative oncoprotein DEK in pauciarticular onset juvenile rheumatoid arthritis, J. Rheumatol. 21 (1994) 2136–2142.
45. X. Dong, J. Wang, F.N. Kabir, et al., Autoantibodies to DEK oncoprotein in human inflammatory disease, Arthritis Rheum. 43 (2000) 85–93.
46. R.P. Donn, W. Thomson, L. Pepper, et al., Antinuclear antibodies in early onset pauciarticular juvenile chronic arthritis (JCA) are associated with HLA-DQB1*0603: a possible JCA-associated human leucocyte antigen haplotype, Br. J. Rheumatol. 34 (1995) 461–465.
52. S.D. Thompson, M.B. Moroldo, L. Guyer, et al., A genome-wide scan for juvenile rheumatoid arthritis in affected sibpair families provides evidence of linkage, Arthritis Rheum. 50 (2004) 2920–2930.
61. J. Vencovsky, K. Jarosová, S. Ruzicková, et al., Higher frequency of allele 2 of the interleukin-1 receptor antagonist gene in patients with juvenile idiopathic arthritis, Arthritis Rheum. 44 (2001) 2387–2391.
63. E. Crawley, R. Kay, J. Sillibourne, et al., Polymorphic haplotypes of the interleukin-10 5¢ flanking region determine variable interleukin-10 transcription and are associated with particular phenotypes of juvenile rheumatoid arthritis, Arthritis Rheum. 42 (1999) 1101–1108.
66. E. Zeggini, W. Thompson, D. Kwiatkowski, et al., Linkage and association studies of single-nucleotide polymorphism-tagged tumor necrosis factor haplotypes in juvenile oligoarthritis, Arthritis Rheum. 46 (2002) 3304–3311.
67. S. Prahalad, D.N. Glass, A comprehensive review of the genetics of juvenile idiopathic arthritis, Pediatric. rheum. 6 (2008) 11.
76. K.J. Murray, L. Luyrink, A.A. Grom, et al., Immunohistological characteristics of T cell infiltrates in different forms of childhood onset chronic arthritis, J. Rheumatol. 23 (1996) 2116–2124.
77. K.J. Murray, A.A. Grom, S.D. Thompson, et al., Contrasting cytokine profiles in the synovium of different forms of juvenile rheumatoid arthritis and juvenile spondyloarthropathy: prominence of interleukin 4 in restricted disease, J. Rheumatol. 25 (1998) 1388–1398.
79. A.M. Rosenberg, D.M. Cordeiro, Relationship between sex and antibodies to high mobility group proteins 1 and 2 in juvenile idiopathic arthritis, J. Rheumatol. 27 (2000) 2489–2493.
80. R.W. McMurray, S.H. Allen, P.H. Pepmueller, et al., Elevated serum prolactin levels in children with juvenile rheumatoid arthritis and antinuclear antibody seropositivity, J. Rheumatol. 22 (1995) 1577–1580.
81. P. Picco, M. Gattorno, A. Buoncompagni, et al., Prolactin and interleukin 6 in prepubertal girls with juvenile chronic arthritis, J. Rheumatol. 25 (1998) 347–351.
89. A.B. Prakken, M.J. van Hoeij, W. Kuis, et al., T-cell reactivity to human HSP60 in oligo-articular juvenile chronic arthritis is associated with a favorable prognosis and the generation of regulatory cytokines in the inflamed joint, Immunol. Lett. 57 (1997) 139–142.
90. A.B. Prakken, W. van Eden, G.T. Rijkers, et al., Autoreactivity to human heat-shock protein 60 predicts disease remission in oligoarticular juvenile rheumatoid arthritis, Arthritis Rheum. 39 (1996) 1826–1832.
96. B. Prakken, M. Wauben, P. van Kooten, et al., Nasal administration of arthritis-related T cell epitopes of heat shock protein 60 as a promising way for immunotherapy in chronic arthritis, Biotherapy. 10 (1998) 205–211.
97. K. Nistala, H. Moncrieffe, K.R. Newton, et al., Interleukin-17-producing T cells are enriched in the joints of children with arthritis, but have a reciprocal relationship to regulatory T cell numbers, Arthritis Rheum. 58 (2008) 875–887.
98. C. Huemer, P.N. Malleson, D.A. Cabral, et al., Patterns of joint involvement at onset differentiate oligoarticular juvenile psoriatic arthritis from pauciarticular juvenile rheumatoid arthritis, J. Rheumatol. 29 (2002) 1531–1535.
99. S. Sharma, D.D. Sherry, Joint distribution at presentation in children with pauciarticular arthritis, J. Pediatr. 134 (1999) 642–643.
115. R.C. Allen, P. Dewez, L. Stuart, et al., Antinuclear antibodies using HEp-2 cells in normal children and in children with common infections, J. Paediatr. Child Health 27 (1991) 39–42.

116. D.A. Cabral, R.E. Petty, M. Fung, et al., Persistent antinuclear antibodies in children without identifiable inflammatory rheumatic or autoimmune disease, Pediatrics 89 (1992) 441–444.

119. R.E. Petty, J.T. Cassidy, D.B. Sullivan, Clinical correlates of antinuclear antibodies in juvenile rheumatoid arthritis, J. Pediatr. 83 (1973) 386–389.

120. J.G. Schaller, G.D. Johnson, E.J. Holborow, et al., The association of antinuclear antibodies with the chronic iridocyclitis of juvenile rheumatoid arthritis (Still's disease), Arthritis Rheum. 17 (1974) 409–416.

122. W. Hassfeld, O. Vinje, B. Flato, et al., Anti-citrulline autoantibodies in juvenile rheumatoid arthritis (JRA), Arthritis Rheum. 48 (2003) S100.

124. M. Van Rossum, R. Van Soesbergen, S. De Kort, et al., Anti-cyclic citrullinated peptide (anti-CCP) antibodies in children with juvenile idiopathic arthritis, J. Rheumatol. 30 (2003) 825–828.

127. K. Oen, M. Reed, P.N. Malleson, et al., Radiologic outcome and its relationship to functional disability in juvenile rheumatoid arthritis, J. Rheumatol. 30 (2003) 832–840.

128. S.E. Ramsey, R.A. Cairns, D.A. Cabral, et al., Knee magnetic resonance imaging in childhood chronic monarthritis, J. Rheumatol. 26 (1999) 2238–2243.

129. S. Magni-Manzoni, O. Epis, A. Ravelli, et al., Comparison of clinical versus ultrasound-determined synovitis in juvenile idiopathic arthritis, Arthritis Rheum. 61 (2009) 1497–1504.

130. T. Beukelman, J.P. Guevara, D.A. Albert, et al., Optimal treatment of knee monarthritis in juvenile idiopathic arthritis: a decision analysis, Arthritis Rheum. 59 (2008) 1580–1588.

131. D.D. Sherry, L.D. Stein, A.M. Reed, et al., Prevention of leg length discrepancy in young children with pauciarticular juvenile rheumatoid arthritis by treatment with intraarticular steroids, Arthritis Rheum. 42 (1999) 2330–2334.

132. S.L. Bowyer, P.A. Roettcher, G.C. Higgins, et al., Health status of patients with juvenile rheumatoid arthritis at 1 and 5 years after diagnosis, J. Rheumatol. 30 (2003) 394–400.

133. K. Oen, P.N. Malleson, D.A. Cabral, et al., Disease course and outcome of JRA in a multicenter cohort, J. Rheumatol. 29 (2002) 1989–1999.

134. M.J. Al-Matar, R.E. Petty, L.B. Tucker, et al., The early pattern of joint involvement predicts disease progression in children with oligoarticular (pauciarticular) juvenile rheumatoid arthritis, Arthritis Rheum. 46 (2002) 2708–2715.

135. K. Oen, P.N. Malleson, D.A. Cabral, et al., Early predictors of longterm outcome in patients with juvenile rheumatoid arthritis: subset-specific correlations, J. Rheumatol. 30 (2003) 585–593.

136. F. Fantini, V. Gerloni, M. Gattinara, et al., Remission in juvenile chronic arthritis: a cohort study of 683 consecutive cases with a mean 10 year followup, J. Rheumatol. 30 (2003) 579–584.

137. B. Flato, G. Lien, A. Smerdel, et al., Prognostic factors in juvenile rheumatoid arthritis: a case-control study revealing early predictors and outcome after 14.9 years, J. Rheumatol. 30 (2003) 386–393.

138. N. Ruperto, A. Ravelli, J.E. Levinson, et al., Longterm health outcomes and quality of life in American and Italian inception cohorts of patients with juvenile rheumatoid arthritis. II: Early predictors of outcome, J. Rheumatol. 24 (1997) 952–958.

139. K. Minden, U. Kiessling, J. Listing, et al., Prognosis of patients with juvenile chronic arthritis and juvenile spondyloarthropathy, J. Rheumatol. 27 (2000) 2256–2263.

Entire reference list is available online at www.expertconsult.com.

Chapter 17

ENTHESITIS-RELATED ARTHRITIS (JUVENILE ANKYLOSING SPONDYLITIS)

Ross E. Petty and James T. Cassidy

DEFINITION AND CLASSIFICATION

Enthesitis-related arthritis (ERA), a term introduced in the International League of Associations for Rheumatology (ILAR) classification of juvenile idiopathic arthritis (JIA),[1] is defined according to the inclusion and exclusion criteria shown in Table 17–1. It is predominantly a disease affecting joints of the lower extremities and, eventually, the axial skeleton, and it is characterized by the absence of autoantibodies such as rheumatoid factor (RF) and antinuclear antibodies (ANA) and by a strong association with the human leukocyte antigen–B27 (HLA-B27). In many instances, the disease evolves to closely resemble ankylosing spondylitis (AS), although the characteristic features of AS are seldom present in childhood or adolescence. Its relationship to subtypes of JIA, such as psoriatic arthritis, is not entirely clear.

Like ERA, juvenile ankylosing spondylitis (JAS) is a chronic inflammatory arthritis of the axial and peripheral skeletons, frequently accompanied by enthesitis, characterized by RF and ANA seronegativity, and having a firm genetic basis. Unlike ERA, radiological evidence of bilateral inflammation of the sacroiliac joints is required for a definitive diagnosis. AS in adults is defined by sets of criteria that are based on clinical, laboratory, and radiographic abnormalities. Only a few children or adolescents meet these criteria, principally because of the low frequency of spinal or sacroiliac signs or symptoms in the young patient. In addition, criteria for the diagnosis of AS in adults (Tables 17–2 through 17–4)[2-4] are not applicable to the younger age group for a number of reasons: Normal values for some of the required physical measurements have not been published for children, or, if reported (back range),[5] they have not yet been validated. In addition, limitations of spine and chest motion may reflect disease duration and are therefore of little aid in facilitating early diagnosis.[2,6] The fact that peripheral joint disease precedes clinical axial involvement by years in many children precludes an early diagnosis by criteria in which abnormalities of

spinal mobility or radiological changes are essential diagnostic features. Reasons for these differences between adults and children, whether they have an immunological, genetic, biochemical, or structural basis, are not understood.[7,8]

Historical Review of the Spondyloarthropathy Concept

In order to understand the relationship of ERA and JAS to psoriatic arthritis (Chapter 18) and the arthritides of inflammatory bowel disease (Chapter 19), it is useful to review the evolution of terminology in this group of diseases. Wright and Moll[9] introduced the term *spondarthritis* to include AS, psoriatic arthritis, ulcerative colitis, Crohn disease, juvenile chronic arthritis, Whipple disease, Behçet syndrome, reactive arthritis, and acute anterior uveitis. They observed that these patients were RF seronegative, lacked subcutaneous nodules, and had inflammatory peripheral arthritis; many had radiological evidence of sacroiliac arthritis. They also observed a tendency toward familial aggregation. It is the familiality of these disorders, based principally on transmission of the histocompatibility antigen HLA-B27, that currently unites the somewhat smaller group included under the title *seronegative spondyloarthritides*: AS, the arthritides of inflammatory bowel disease (IBD), reactive arthritis, and psoriatic arthritis.

There are several reasons for grouping these disorders together under the heading of spondyloarthropathy:

1. Inflammation of the joints of the axial skeleton and of entheses is the most important clinical feature exhibited by members of this group of diseases, a symptom that is less often observed in the other chronic arthritides.
2. Relatives of children with JAS or ERA commonly have AS, psoriatic arthritis, IBD, or, less commonly, reactive arthritis, related in part to the high frequency of B27 in these families.

3. Several diseases in this group share a number of extraarticular features. Uveitis, usually acute, occurs in all members of the group. The cutaneous manifestations of psoriasis and reactive arthritis may be indistinguishable.
4. RFs are absent, and other autoantibodies are infrequent.

Thus, although individual members of the spondyloarthropathy group differ from each other, they share some important characteristics that distinguish them from the other categories of JIA and the connective tissue diseases (Table 17–5). Nonetheless, this grouping has important limitations when applied to children. It does not recognize the heterogeneity within psoriatic arthritis in general and within the arthritis of IBD in particular. Only

---

Table 17–1

Enthesitis-related arthritis (ILAR classification) definition

Arthritis and enthesitis
or
Arthritis or enthesitis with at least two of the following:
  Sacroiliac joint tenderness and/or inflammatory spinal pain
  Presence of HLA-B27
  Family history in at least one first- or second-degree relative with medically confirmed HLA-B27-associated disease
  Anterior uveitis that is usually associated with pain, redness, or photophobia
  Onset of arthritis in a boy after 8 yr of age
Exclusions
  Psoriasis confirmed by a dermatologist in at least one first- or second-degree relative
  Presence of systemic arthritis

ILAR, International League of Associations for Rheumatology.
From Petty RE, Southwood TR, Baum J, et al: Revision of the proposed classification criteria for juvenile idiopathic arthritis: Durban, 1997, *J Rheumatol* 25:1991-1994, 1998.

Table 17–2

New York criteria for a diagnosis of ankylosing spondylitis (AS)

Clinical Criteria
1. Limitation of lumbar spine motion in all three planes
2. Pain or history of pain at the dorsolumbar junction or lumbar spine
3. Limitation of chest expansion to 2.5 cm or less at the level of the fourth intercostal space

Definite AS

Grade 3-4 bilateral sacroiliac arthritis on radiography with at least one clinical criterion,
or
Grade 3-4 unilateral or grade 2 bilateral sacroiliac arthritis on radiography with clinical criterion 1 or clinical criteria 2 and 3

Probable AS

Grade 3-4 bilateral sacroiliac arthritis on radiography without clinical criteria

From Bennett PH, Wood PHN: Population studies of the Rheumatic disease New York, Excerpta Medica 1968, P 456.

Table 17–3

Amor criteria for the classification of spondyloarthropathies

	Criteria	Points
Clinical		
	Lumbar or thoracic night pain or stiffness	1
	Asymmetrical oligoarthritis	2
	Buttock pain alternating in site	1
	Buttock pain triggered by pelvic movement	2
	Sausage digit	2
	Enthesopathy	2
	Uveitis	2
	Nonspecific urethritis or cervicitis within 1 mo before onset	1
	Diarrhea within 1 mo before onset	1
	Psoriasis, balanitis, or chronic enterocolitis	2
Radiological		
	Sacroiliitis (= stage 2 if bilateral; = stage 3 if unilateral)	3
Genetic		
	Presence of HLA-B27, family history of pelvospondylitis, reactive arthritis, psoriasis, uveitis, or chronic enterocolitis	2
Therapeutic		
	Amelioration of pain within 48 hr of treatment with nonsteroidal antiinflammatory drug	2

A definite diagnosis of spondyloarthropathy is confirmed if six or more points are present (sensitivity, 91.9%; specificity, 97.9%).

From Amor B, Dougados M, Mijiyawa M: Critères de classification des spondylarthropathies, *Rev Rhum Mal Osteoartic* 57:85-89, 1990.

Table 17–4

Classification criteria of the European Spondyloarthropathy Study Group (ESSG)

Inflammatory spinal pain
or
Synovitis (asymmetrical or predominantly in lower limbs)
plus
One of the following:
Positive family history
Psoriasis
Inflammatory bowel disease
Urethritis, cervicitis, or diarrhea within 1 mo before arthritis
Buttock pain alternating between right and left gluteal areas
Enthesopathy
Sacroiliac arthritis

Modified from Dougados M, van der Linden S, Juhlin R et al: The European Spondyloarthropathy Study Group preliminary criteria for the classification of spondyloarthropathy, *Arthritis Rheum* 34:1218-1227, 1991. Copyright © 1991 John Wiley & Sons, Inc. Reprinted with permission of Wiley-Liss, Inc., a subsidiary of John Wiley & Sons, Inc

Table 17–5

Overlapping characteristics of the spondyloarthropathies

Characteristic	Juvenile Ankylosing Spondylitis	Reactive Arthritis	Bowel Disease	Juvenile Psoriatic Arthritis
Enthesitis	+++	+	+	++
Axial arthritis	+++	++	++	+
Peripheral arthritis	+++	+++	+++	+++
HLA-B27 positive	+++	+	+++	+++
ANA positive	–	++	–	–
RF positive	–	–	–	–
Systemic disease				
Eyes	+	+	+	+
Skin	–	+++	+	+
Mucous membranes	–	–	+	+
Gastrointestinal tract	–	–	++++	+++

ANA, antinuclear antibodies; RF, rheumatoid factor.
Frequency of characteristics: –, absent; +, <25%; ++, 25-50%; +++, 50-75%; ++++, 75% or more.

a minority of the patients with psoriasis have involvement of axial joints, and most have chronic asymptomatic uveitis rather than acute symptomatic uveitis; most children with arthritis related to IBD have peripheral arthritis rather than spinal involvement.

Arthritis that is predominantly accompanied by inflammation of the entheses is recognized to be different from other types of inflammatory arthritis (although enthesitis occurs in a number of the chronic arthropathies of children). Although in some ways it resembles adult AS, it rarely exhibits early spinal involvement, making its early identification difficult. As a consequence, other approaches to the definition of these types of arthropathy have emerged. Recognition of the seronegative enthesitis and arthritis (SEA) syndrome[10] permitted the identification of children who were different from other children with chronic inflammatory joint disease: although they did not satisfy the criteria for adult AS, in addition to peripheral arthritis, they had inflammation of entheses. The absence or rarity of axial spinal involvement in childhood led, also, to the definition of ERA in the ILAR classification.[1,11,12] The suggested relationship among these three definitions is illustrated in Figure 17–1.

Children with the SEA syndrome have some of the characteristics of JAS but, at least at onset, lack the sacroiliac joint involvement needed to confirm that diagnosis.[10] These children are seronegative (lack RF and ANA), have enthesitis (usually around the heel or knee), and have arthritis of a few joints, particularly the large and small joints of the lower extremities. The SEA syndrome probably represents, for the most part, children with very early JAS or ERA, rather than a separate disease. It will take decades of observation and evaluation to determine whether JAS, ERA, and the SEA syndrome are simply earlier or later, milder or more severe versions of the same disease, although it seems highly likely that this will be the case. Of the 39 children in the original report of SEA syndrome, 8 had bilateral sacroiliac arthritis consistent with a diagnosis of JAS; 2 each had IBD and reactive arthritis; and 1 had psoriatic arthritis.[10] The remaining

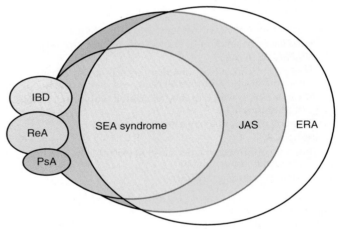

FIGURE 17–1 Representation of relationship between enthesitis related arthritis (ERA), juvenile ankylosing spondylitis (JAS), seronegative enthesitis and arthritis syndrome (SEA), arthritis with inflammatory bowel disease (IBD), reactive arthritis (ReA) and psoriatic arthritis (PsA).

26 children had no rheumatic disease that could be identified. A follow-up study of 23 of the 26 children with idiopathic SEA syndrome at a mean of 11 years after onset[13] indicated that 12 (52%) of 23 who did not have a definite spondyloarthropathy at the time of the original report now had definite or possible spondyloarthropathy. The presence of HLA-B27 (62%, p < .004) and arthritis (as opposed to arthralgia, p < .05) and onset of disease after the age of 5 years (p < .01) correlated with the evolution of the SEA syndrome to an identifiable spondyloarthropathy. Overall, 64% had definite or possible spondyloarthropathy, 10% JRA (American College of Rheumatology [ACR] criteria), 13% noninflammatory diseases, and 5% had continuing idiopathic SEA syndrome.

Burgos-Vargas and Clark[14] described a group of Mexican children with the SEA syndrome who developed an inexorable course of progressive axial disease and sacroiliac arthritis. Within 5 years after onset, 75%

had definite JAS. This was in contrast with the aforementioned report,[13] in which clinical progression was varied and remissions more frequent. A definite diagnosis in these latter children was often achieved only after a follow-up of approximately 10 years.

Jacobs and associates[15] studied 58 children with chronic arthritis selected on the basis of the presence of HLA-B27 who had been monitored for a mean of 5 years. Two-thirds were boys, and most had onset of symptoms after 9 years of age; none had RF, and only 7 had ANA (8.6%). Altogether, 51 of 58 had disease that satisfied the ACR criteria for a diagnosis of JRA,[16] 1 had reactive arthritis, and 6 had episodic arthritis and enthesitis. In all, 75% of the children with HLA-B27 had enthesitis, and many had other features of one of the spondyloarthropathies, although definitive diagnostic outcomes were not presented.

Sheerin and associates[17] monitored 36 of 85 children with arthropathy and HLA-B27 positivity for a mean of approximately 9 years. Only 2 of these children met New York criteria for AS. Five patients (24%) had enthesitis at onset, and at follow-up 22 patients (61%) had enthesitis or a history compatible with enthesitis. A group of 26 children who fulfilled the diagnostic criteria for the SEA syndrome or one of the other HLA-B27–associated syndromes were monitored by Hussein and colleagues[18] in an effort to define common characteristics among these various diseases. No diagnostic outcomes at follow-up were described in this study, although the proposed criteria tested favorably.

In the ILAR classification of juvenile idiopathic arthritides,[1] the dilemma of categorization of these diseases is dealt with by recognizing ERA, juvenile psoriatic arthritis, and arthritis related to IBD as separate categories. In this classification, the category ERA best describes what had been called JAS. The unifying, if not entirely unique, feature of these disorders is the presence of inflammation of the enthesis: enthesitis. ERA can be viewed as an umbrella term that includes children with JAS (who fulfill the New York criteria for AS) and most patients with SEA syndrome (especially those who are HLA-B27 positive).

There remains a clear need for development and standardization of diagnostic criteria for JAS and ERA. In one study,[19] 2958 consecutive children with various forms of childhood arthritis (including 324 definite spondyloarthropathies and 334 possible spondyloarthropathies) and 2300 control subjects were evaluated with the adult AS criteria of Amor and coworkers[3] and those of the European Spondylarthropathy Study Group (ESSG)[4] (Tables 17–3 and 17–4). Children with JAS were identified by the Amor criteria with a sensitivity of 73.5% and specificity of 97.6% and by the ESSG criteria with a sensitivity of 78.7% and specificity of 92.2%.

Inflexible application of any system of classification risks putting patients into categories in which they do not belong. This was a major problem with the spondyloarthropathy concept, but it could equally be problematic with the ILAR classification. Using the spondyloarthropathy concept, many patients with psoriatic arthritis did not have enthesitis or disease of the axial skeleton, although they were categorized as having a "spondyloarthropathy." On the other hand, the occasional child with

psoriatic arthritis and sacroiliac arthritis would probably best be categorized as having ERA but is excluded from that category because of the presence of psoriasis. Thus many classification problems still await clinical and laboratory evidence for their scientific resolution.

EPIDEMIOLOGY

The data examining the epidemiology of ERA are sparse. For this reason, the discussion that follows relies heavily on the study of patients who fulfilled traditional criteria for ankylosing spondylitis. Where there is sufficient evidence, ERA-specific information is included.

Incidence and Prevalence

Children with JAS accounted for 1% to 7% of children in national pediatric rheumatic disease registries of the United States,[20] Canada,[21] and the United Kingdom[22] and from studies in Sweden[23] and Finland.[24] A recent study noted that 10.6% of 1082 children with juvenile idiopathic arthritis had ERA.[25] Increasing awareness of the possibility of the occurrence of ERA in childhood and its clinical and laboratory differentiation from other chronic arthritides of childhood will probably result in an increase in the proportion of children with inflammatory arthritis in this category.

The proportion of adults with AS who had onset of the disease in childhood ranges from 8.6%[4] to 11%.[26] It is estimated that the prevalence of AS in adults is from 0.5% to 1.9%.[27,28] Among ethnic and racial groups, however, estimates of the frequency of AS range widely. Using modified New York criteria,[29] including radiographic evidence of sacroiliac arthritis, Carter and coworkers[30] determined a prevalence of 129/100,000 (0.13%) in an American population of Northern European extraction. A follow-up study of the same population confirmed that the incidence of AS was not changing over time.[31] On the basis of the prevalence of B27 antigen and the frequency of sacroiliac arthritis in the B27-positive population, the prevalence of AS was estimated to be 0.86% to 1%[27,32] and was highest in B27-positive persons.[32] Although this estimate includes asymptomatic persons, it also excludes the 8% to 10% of the AS population who do not have B27, and it may be a more accurate reflection of the prevalence of the entire spectrum of AS, whereas the estimate of Carter and colleagues[30] more accurately represents patients with clinically and radiologically evident disease.

Age at Onset

JAS usually has its onset in late childhood or adolescence, although instances of onset in younger children have been reported. The mean age at diagnosis in 115 children with ERA was 11.7 years (range: 2.8 to 17.6 years).[25] The age distribution appears to be homogeneous and presumably is continuous with that described in adult populations, suggesting that, at least on this basis, the disease as seen in adults is the same or very similar to that in children.

Sex Ratio

JAS has a much higher frequency in boys than in girls: of 247 children with this disorder, 216 were boys, for a male/female ratio of 7:1.[33-39] A ratio of 3.4 males to 1 female was observed in children with ERA.[25] This disproportionate representation of boys may not accurately represent the actual occurrence of the disease in girls. The strong correlation of JAS and ERA with HLA-B27 and the equal distribution of this antigen in males and females suggest that JAS and ERA could be as common in girls as in boys. Furthermore, in radiographic surveys of B27-positive adult blood donors, sacroiliac arthritis was as common in women as in men.[40] In a questionnaire survey of members of the National Ankylosing Spondylitis Society in the United Kingdom, the male/female ratio was 2.7:1.[26] However, in women, manifestations of the disease may occur later[26] and be less severe,[41] and they may have more peripheral and less axial disease.[42] It is possible that these observations contribute to the relative infrequency of the diagnosis in women.

Geographic and Racial Distribution

Few data are specifically related to geographic and racial differences in the frequency of JAS.[43] The low incidence of AS in African Americans[44] and in Japanese[45] and the high frequency in the Haida Indians of Pacific Canada[46] reflect, in part, the frequency of B27 in these populations. Other factors may be significant, however, because this antigen occurs in only 50% of African Americans with AS[47] and in 65% to 90% of Japanese with the disease.[45] In a multiethnic Canadian population, ERA was twice as common in children of European ancestry as in those of non-European origin.[25]

ETIOLOGY AND PATHOGENESIS

The cause of JAS or ERA is unknown. The clinical, genetic, and epidemiological similarities of these disorders and diseases such as reactive arthritis, in which enteric or genitourinary tract infections play a triggering role, suggest the possibility of an infectious etiology, although none has been proven. Although no organisms can be isolated from the joints, evidence of a local inflammatory response to antigen is supported by antibody and cellular immune studies.[48,49]

The strong association with HLA-B27 suggests that a genetically determined mechanism is central to pathogenesis.[50-54] The relationships between gastrointestinal infection and B27 are complex. The B27 transgenic rat develops a disease that is remarkably like ankylosing spondylitis[55-57] in the presence of intestinal bacteria. In humans there is a strong association of inflammatory bowel disease, HLA-B27, and sacroiliitis. Reports of an association between B27 and gastrointestinal (GI) isolation of *Klebsiella* species in adults with AS[48,49] remain largely unconfirmed.[58,59] Mielants and associates[60,61] described the presence of inflammatory gut changes in adolescents with spondyloarthropathies, supporting a pathogenic relationship between spondylitis and inflammation of the GI tract. Clinical or occult GI inflammation may be related in AS to the association with HLA antigens[62] as well as to cellular immunity to cartilage proteoglycans.[63]

There are at least 31 different HLA-B27 subtypes.[51] The most common subtype, B27*05, is most strongly associated with AS, at least in Caucasians. Two subtypes, B*2706 and B*2709, are rarely associated, and the others have not been sufficiently studied to establish an association.[51,54]

The mechanisms whereby B27 is involved in disease pathogenesis have been the subject of much debate. As a Class I MHC molecule, the role of HLA-B27 is to present endogenous peptides to the T-cell receptor on CD8+ lymphocytes. It has been proposed that the B27 molecule or peptides it presents share amino acid sequences with a microbial antigen (molecular mimicry) and thereby becomes a target for CD8+ T cells or crossreacting antibody, resulting in an inflammatory response.[64,65] Misfolding of the HLA-B27 heavy chain in the endoplasmic reticulum may invoke an inflammatory response. Folding of the heavy chains of HLA-B27 is much slower than for other HLA antigens. The result is that these molecules are degraded in the endoplasmic reticulum.[66-68] A modulatory effect of the surface expression of the B27 molecule on the invasive capability of arthritogenic bacteria, such as *Yersinia enterocolitica* and *Salmonella enteritidis*, has been demonstrated in murine cells [69,70] but not in human fibroblasts or lymphocytes.[71,72] Some investigators have found that, although bacterial invasion of B27-expressing cells is normal, killing of the organisms in such cells is impaired, with the result that infective organisms persist within the host.[73]

The pathogenesis of enthesitis, the characteristic abnormality of ERA and JAS, has been extensively studied by Benjamin and McGonagle.[74] An inflammatory infiltrate that includes CD8+ and CD14+ cells develops at sites of enthesitis in subchondral bone with bone absorption and new bone formation.[64] Tumor necrosis factor-α (TNF-α) messenger RNA is increased in affected bone.[75] CD2R, a T-cell activation marker, is expressed at high level in patients with JAS and JRA.[76] A type 1 helper T-cell (Th1) response has been suggested, with lymphocytic and mononuclear cellular infiltrates. Cells of the synovial membrane express TNF-α, TNF-β, and TNF receptors similar to those of children with other types of JIA.[77]

GENETIC BACKGROUND

There is often a striking familial occurrence of spondylitis and related diseases in adults and children.[78] Ansell and colleagues[79] noted that 6 of 12 monozygotic twin pairs concordant for arthritis were B27 positive, which made the diagnosis of JAS likely (if not certain) in these children. Family studies have indicated that AS is inherited as an autosomal dominant trait with penetrance of about 20%.[80] Although the risk of development of AS in a B27-positive person is not precisely known (approximately 1% to 3%), epidemiological studies suggest that AS occurs 10 to 20 times more frequently in relatives of patients with AS (20%) and 50 to 80 times more frequently in their siblings.[81,82] Thus, B27-positive persons with a family history of AS have a tenfold greater risk of AS than that of B27-positive persons with no family history of AS.[82] The general risk that a B27-heterozygous parent with AS will have a male child with the disease is approximately 5% to 10% (20% if the child is also B27 positive; close to zero if the child is B27 negative).[82] The risk of having a female child with JAS is lower. Risk may or may not be increased in first-born children.[83] Familial disease may not be concordant for phenotypes in each member.

The association between JAS and the B27 antigen is as strong in children as in adults. Of 247 children with JAS, B27 was present in 91%.[33-39] The possibility that homozygosity for B27 was responsible for the juvenile onset of AS was not supported by data in one small study,[84] and the idea that disease severity is genetically determined is unresolved.[85,86]

Although B27 has the strongest genetic association with AS and contributes the greatest share (15% to 60%) of the attributable genetic risk,[82,87] other genetic factors undoubtedly play a role. Van der Linden and colleagues found that only about 5% of the HLA-B27–positive population develops AS.[81] In contrast ~20% of the HLA-B27–positive relatives of patients with AS develop a similar disease, indicating that there are additional genetic factors that contribute to the predisposition to these diseases. There is also an increase in HLA-A2, an association that is shared with other chronic arthritides of childhood.[88] Woodrow[89] used meta-analysis to calculate a relative risk of spondylitis of 1.72 in A2-positive patients. Reports of an increased frequency of HLA-A28 in B27-positive patients with AS suggest that this antigen also may contribute to disease susceptibility.[90,91] HLA-B60 is increased in adults with AS, independent of the presence of B27.[92,93] The reported increased frequency of Cw1 and Cw2 [94,95] probably reflects a linkage disequilibrium with B27. One study alleged that a −308.1 polymorphism in the promoter region of the TNF gene was associated with AS and independent of B27.[96] A polymorphism in the interleukin-1 receptor antagonist (IL-1 Ra) gene has also been associated with ankylosing spondylitis.[97]

There are few known class II associations with JAS. A higher frequency of HLA-DRB1*08 (44.9%) was reported in a Mexican population with JAS than in a control population (25.4%).[98] Maksymowych and colleagues[99] reported that the LMP2A allele frequency in patients with adult- and juvenile-onset AS with uveitis was twice that in those without this complication (odds ratio, 2.51). Ploski and colleagues[100] reported an increase of B*4001, DRB1*08, and DPB1*0301 and the LMP2 b/b phenotype in patients with JAS compared with B27-positive controls or adults with AS. It is very likely that JAS and ERA are polygenic disorders. These and other associations are reviewed by Reveille[53,101] and Brown.[54,102,103]

CLINICAL MANIFESTATIONS

The onset of JAS or ERA may be insidious and characterized by intermittent musculoskeletal pain and stiffness or objective inflammation of peripheral joints, particularly those of the lower extremities, together with enthesitis at one or more sites around the knee or foot. Occasionally,

the disease may have an abrupt onset. Systemic signs are often minimal, but fatigue, sleep disturbances, and low-grade fever may be present. Symptoms related to the back are usually absent at onset but become increasingly evident during the disease course in adolescents. Differing modes of presentation and course may characterize specific population groups.[104,105]

Enthesitis

Entheses—the sites of attachment of ligament, tendon, fascia, or capsule to bone—are characteristic sites of inflammation in the spondyloarthropathies. Although the presence of exquisite, well-localized tenderness at characteristic entheses strongly suggests ERA, it must be noted that enthesitis occurs occasionally in other types of JIA and occasionally in normal children.[106] The presence of enthesitis is, however, the most helpful feature in differentiating ERA from other types of JIA. Enthesitis[107] is a characteristic early manifestation of JAS and occurs with greater frequency in JAS than in adult-onset AS. It frequently produces severe pain and resultant disability, which may be the child's most important complaints.[108] Deposits of acid mucopolysaccharides in the extensor tendons of the adult foot, resembling tendonitis, have been described as "tamale foot."[109]

Arthritis

The presenting joint symptoms recorded in the largest reported series of patients with JAS are summarized in Table 17-6. Initial musculoskeletal symptoms are often difficult for the child to localize and include pain in the buttocks, groin, thighs, heels, or around the shoulders. The vague quality and localization of this pain and its frequent spontaneous disappearance early in the disease are recurring sources of delay and confusion in the diagnosis.

In distinction to AS in adults, children seldom have symptoms of involvement of the axial skeleton at onset; only 24% of children with JAS are reported to have pain, stiffness, or limitation of motion of the lumbosacral spine or sacroiliac joints at presentation. In contrast, peripheral joint symptoms occur at onset in 82%, whereas only 16% have involvement of the upper extremities (see Table 17-6). With the exception of one report in which hip disease was frequent at onset,[110] distal joints are affected more commonly than proximal joints.

In most instances, the number of joints involved is limited (four or fewer), although approximately 25% of children have a polyarticular onset. Shoulders are not uncommonly affected, and even the temporomandibular joint may be involved. The least commonly affected joints are the small joints of the hands. Pain at the costosternal and sternoclavicular joints and the sternomanubrium, often in conjunction with tenderness over the proximal clavicle, may be associated with significant impairment of chest expansion. In the series of Schaller and associates,[34] five of seven patients had decreased chest expansion. Aside from the number and distribution of the affected joints, there is nothing clinically to distinguish the peripheral joint disease of ERA from that of other types of JIA. Burgos-Vargas and colleagues[111] have identified a

Table 17–6

Musculoskeletal signs and symptoms in juvenile ankylosing spondylitis (JAS)*

Clinical Evidence of Joint Involvement at Onset	Percentage
Arthritis, Painful Limitation of Range of Motion	
Proximal limb joints	35
Distal limb joints	44
Upper limb joints	16
Lower limb joints	82
Axial skeleton joints	24
Joint Involvement During Course	
No peripheral joints affected	3
1 to 4 peripheral joints affected	43
More than 4 peripheral joints affected	54
Sacroiliac involvement†	95
Lumbosacral spine affected†	90
Cervical spine involvement	-
Enthesitis	
Around the knee†	80
Around the ankle and foot†	90
Myopathy	
Pain/Wasting†	50

*Clinical or radiographic evidence of involvement of the sacroiliac joints, and particularly the lumbosacral spine, may not be evident until adulthood. Data are from published studies.
†Estimate.

subgroup of children with typical adult-type onset of disease. Whether this presentation represents a distinct entity or merely an extreme end of the clinical spectrum is not certain.[112]

Uveitis

The uveitis seen in JAS or ERA is characterized by an acutely red, painful, photophobic eye. It is usually unilateral, is frequently recurrent, and usually, but not always, leaves no ocular residua. It rarely precedes the onset of musculoskeletal complaints.[113] Acute uveitis occurs in 20% of adults with AS, particularly in those with HLA-B27, but may be less common in children.[114] In the series of Ladd and colleagues,[33] only 1 of 15 patients developed an acute uveitis; in the series of Schaller and associates,[34] 2 of 20 patients had this complication. However, Hafner[39] indicated that 14% of 71 patients had a history of an acute uveitis, and Ansell[115] observed this complication in 21 of 77 patients with JAS. These higher figures may reflect a longer follow-up time in the latter two studies or other confounding factors.

Cardiopulmonary Disease

Although cardiovascular disease is uncommon, it can occasionally be severe,[116] and marked aortic insufficiency has been reported in at least 7 patients with JAS.[117-123] The apparently low frequency of such complications in children may reflect the fact that follow-up is generally of shorter duration than in adults in whom cardiac disease

(aortic insufficiency, heart block) develops in approximately 5% of patients an average of 15 years after onset.[124] Rarely, cardiac involvement precedes development of sacroiliac disease.[125]

None of 36 consecutive patients with JAS who were monitored for a mean of 4.3 years had symptoms related to the cardiovascular system, and only one developed the murmur of aortic regurgitation.[126] Echocardiographs documented no structural cardiac abnormalities and electrocardiography no conduction defects, but color Doppler assessment confirmed mild mitral regurgitation in two patients and mild aortic regurgitation in three; systolic ventricular function was impaired in one. Transesophageal echocardiography demonstrated aortic root abnormalities and valvular disease in 82% of adults as compared with 27% of controls.[127] Valve thickening was demonstrable as nodularity of the aortic cusps and basal thickening of the anterior mitral valve leaflet, creating the characteristic subaortic bump. Aortic valve regurgitation was present in almost one half of the patients.

Few data relating to pleuropulmonary disease are available. In a study of 18 children aged 8 to 17 years who fulfilled the Amor criteria,[3] abnormalities of pulmonary function were present in 33%.[128] All patients had normal chest radiographs at baseline and on follow-up at 2 years. No patient had symptoms attributable to the respiratory system, and all had normal chest expansion. Nonetheless, 6 patients (33%) had abnormal pulmonary function tests. The most common abnormality was reduction in the forced vital capacity (22%); occasionally, increased functional residual capacity (11%) and residual volume (5%) were observed. Restrictive patterns were more common than diffusion defects, and diffusing capacity of the lungs for carbon monoxide was reduced in only 11%. Small airways disease was not present.

In adults, although diminished chest expansion and resultant decreased vital capacity are not infrequent, clinical parenchymal pulmonary disease is rare. In the review by Rosenow and associates,[129] 1.3% of 2080 adults with AS had radiographic evidence of pleuropulmonary disease (apical pleural thickening). High-resolution computed tomography (CT) in 26 adults with AS demonstrated a much higher frequency of pulmonary parenchymal abnormalities (69%) than was evident on plain radiography (15%).[127] These findings included interstitial lung disease in four patients, bronchiectasis in six, paraseptal emphysema in three, and tracheal dilatation and apical fibrosis in two each. Cor pulmonale can develop secondary to kyphoscoliosis and decreased chest wall movement, characteristic of advanced spondylitis, but it has not been reported in children or adolescents.

Nervous System Disease

Central nervous system disease is rare. Atlantoaxial subluxation leading to severe cervico-occipital pain was reported in one boy with JAS[131] and in two boys with the SEA syndrome.[132] The cauda equina syndrome, caused by bony impingement on the cauda equina and characterized by weakness of bowel and bladder sphincters, saddle anesthesia, and leg weakness, occurs in adults[133] but has not been reported in children.

Renal Disease

Renal abnormalities are rare. Papillary necrosis, perhaps secondary to nonsteroidal antiinflammatory drugs (NSAIDs), has been reported.[134] Immunoglobulin A (IgA) nephropathy, occasionally with uveitis,[135] was observed in 115 adults with spondyloarthropathies.[136] Most of these patients had elevated serum IgA concentrations; some had impaired renal function and hypertension. Ansell[115] documented amyloidosis in 3.8% of 77 patients with JAS seen before 1980; she noted its association with severe peripheral arthropathy and a persistently elevated erythrocyte sedimentation rate (ESR).

Cardiopulmonary, central nervous system, and renal disease appear to be very rare in children with ERA. Most of these complications occur after many years of disease in patients with JAS or AS. The diagnosis of ERA is usually made much earlier in the disease course, and it is likely that with very long-term follow-up these rare, but important, complications will be recognized in children with ERA.

PATHOLOGY

The pathology of JAS or ERA has not been studied, but it is probable that abnormalities are similar to those of AS. However, the synovitis is in general much milder, and the degree of cartilage erosion in peripheral joints much less, in AS compared with adult rheumatoid arthritis (RA).[137] The synovitis itself is otherwise virtually indistinguishable from that of RA, although there may be relatively more polymorphonuclear leukocytes present.

The characteristic pathological changes in the apophyseal and sacroiliac joints are enchondral and capsular ossification. The earliest lesion in the sacroiliac joints is subchondral inflammation, rather than synovitis, with formation of granulation tissue with few inflammatory cells. The surfaces of the sacroiliac joints are little affected and pannus is not present.[138] Enchondral ossification on the iliac side of the joint accounts for the radiographic appearance of erosions. Ball commented,[139] "As a rule, it seems that in any synovial joint in ankylosing spondylitis the outcome represents a balance of erosive synovitis and capsular and/or ligamentous ossification. In joints of low mobility the ossific process tends to be the dominant feature."

Enthesitis is characterized by nonspecific inflammation.[140] Granulation tissue, infiltrated with lymphocytes and plasma cells and causing a localized osteitis, undermines the bony and cartilaginous attachment of the ligament or tendon. Healing of this lesion gives rise to a bony spur, such as a calcaneal spur at the insertion of the plantar fascia into the calcaneus or a syndesmophyte at the attachment of the outer fibers of the annulus fibrosus to the anterolateral aspects of the rim of the vertebral body.

DIFFERENTIAL DIAGNOSIS

At onset, ERA most closely resembles oligoarticular JIA (OJIA). However, whereas OJIA is characteristically a disease of young girls, ERA typically occurs in older boys and adolescents. The presence of enthesitis is the distinguishing clinical feature in children with ERA. ERA may mimic other inflammatory arthropathies, mechanical causes of back or lower extremity pain, or, very occasionally, infection or malignancy. A history of cramping abdominal pain, diarrhea, weight loss, and fever suggests an accompanying inflammatory bowel disease in a child who otherwise has typical ERA. A few children with ERA also have psoriasis and would fulfill criteria for psoriatic arthritis. In most instances, however, children with ERA lack sacroiliac and back symptoms at onset, but, unlike children with OJIA, may have hip joint involvement.

In older children with established ERA, signs and symptoms of spine and sacroiliac inflammation clearly differentiate the child from one with OJIA. The disease then resembles JAS or AS. Arthritis of the cervical spine is infrequent and, when present, mimics that in children with polyarticular JIA. Thoracolumbar pain may reflect Scheuermann disease. Lumbar and lumbosacral pain has a myriad of causes, including spondylolysis, spondylolisthesis, osteoid osteoma, osteomyelitis, diskitis, and (rarely) lumbar disk herniation. Trauma may cause chronic pain in the sacrum and coccyx. Sacroiliac tenderness and pain occurs in many patients with JAS, but septic sacroiliac disease, osteomyelitis, Ewing sarcoma of the ilium, and familial Mediterranean fever[141] also produce pain in and around these joints.

Pain that mimics enthesitis may result from a number of causes, including excessive running or jogging. Usually, the pain of traumatic enthesopathy is less severe and more diffuse than that caused by inflammation. Osteochondrosis of the tibial tuberosity (Osgood-Schlatter disease), of the inferior pole of the patella (Sinding-Larsen-Johansson syndrome), or of the apophysis of the calcaneus (Sever disease) may mimic inflammatory enthesitis at those sites. The coexistence of enthesitis at multiple sites usually eliminates these disorders from consideration. The absence of B27 positivity also assists in differentiating these disorders from the inflammatory enthesitis of JAS.[142] Pressure over bony prominences, including entheses, may produce pain in children with leukemia or bone tumors. In most instances, however, the pain resulting from such infiltrative diseases is less discrete and more severe than that of inflammatory enthesitis and frequently awakens the child from sleep.

MUSCULOSKELETAL EXAMINATION

The musculoskeletal examination can be divided into three parts: (1) the entheses, (2) the peripheral joints, and (3) the axial skeleton including joints of the pelvis, spine, and chest.

Entheses

A careful history and a thorough but gentle palpation of entheses may document evidence of past or present inflammation. A diagnosis of ERA is strongly supported by the presence of marked localized tenderness on the patella at the 2-, 6-, and 10-o'clock positions, at the tibial tuberosity, at the attachment of the Achilles tendon or plantar fascia to the calcaneus, at the attachment of the plantar fascia to the base of the fifth metatarsal, and at the heads of the metatarsals (Fig. 17–2). Tenderness is less commonly demonstrable at the greater trochanters of the femurs, superior anterior iliac spines and iliac crests, pubic symphysis, and ischial tuberosities, and seldom at entheses of the upper extremities. Symptoms of pain or tenderness at the origin of the adductor longus near the symphysis pubis,[143] at the costochondral junctions, and over spinous processes, although infrequent, support a diagnosis. Observation of stance and gait (including walking on the toes and heels), may reveal altered weight-bearing as the child avoids pressure on inflamed entheses.

Peripheral Joints

The peripheral arthropathy of ERA is often asymmetrical and predominantly involves the lower extremities. Isolated hip disease may be the presenting feature,[144] but this would be highly unlikely in a child with other types of JIA. Although involvement of one or both knees is characteristic of both oligoarticular JIA and ERA, the child's age at onset, especially if a boy, is a useful distinguishing feature. Small joints of the foot and toes are commonly involved. In contrast, symmetrical disease of the small joints of the hands or polyarticular disease, particularly in a girl, is more likely to be another type of JIA.

A highly characteristic intertarsal joint inflammation occurs in many children with ERA or JAS. This tarsitis is accompanied by pain, tenderness, and restriction of movement in the midfoot that, in the presence of disease of the first metatarsophalangeal joint, results in a characteristic deformity of the foot. Burgos-Vargas and associates[145] concluded that a diagnosis of JAS could be confirmed or strongly suspected shortly after onset of disease in children who displayed enthesopathy, midtarsal foot involvement, sparing of the hands, and progressive onset of lumbosacral disease.

Axial Skeleton

Involvement of the joints of the axial skeleton is characteristic. In children with sacroiliac inflammation, pain may be elicited by direct pressure over one or both sacroiliac joints, compression of the pelvis, or distraction of the sacroiliac joints by Patrick test (Faber test). Examination of the back may demonstrate abnormalities in contour, such as loss of the normal lumbar lordosis, exaggeration of the thoracic kyphosis, or increased occiput-to-wall distance. The contour of the back on full forward flexion may demonstrate loss of the normal smooth curve in the lower part of the thoracolumbar spine (Fig. 17–3), or there may be restriction of hyperextension, signifying early axial disease. The rigid spine of long-standing AS is rare in children. Cervical spine involvement is also a late development.[146] Although observations of abnormalities of the contour of the back are often more informative than actual numerical measurements, sequential measurement of thoracolumbar mobility is useful in documenting progression of the disease.

The modified Schober test[147,148] provides one index of abnormality (Fig. 17–4). With the child standing with the feet together, a line joining the dimples of Venus is used as a landmark for the lumbosacral junction. A mark is made 5 cm below (point A) and 10 cm above (point B) the lumbosacral junction. With the patient in maximum forward flexion with the knees straight, the increase in distance between points A and B is used as an indicator of lumbosacral spine mobility. Normal values plus or minus 1 standard deviation are indicated in Figure 17–5. In general, a modified Schober measurement of less than 6 cm (e.g., an increase from 15 cm to less than 21 cm) should be regarded as abnormal. However, care should be exercised in interpreting this measurement, because there are large normal variations at each age and the data have not been adequately validated in children with musculoskeletal

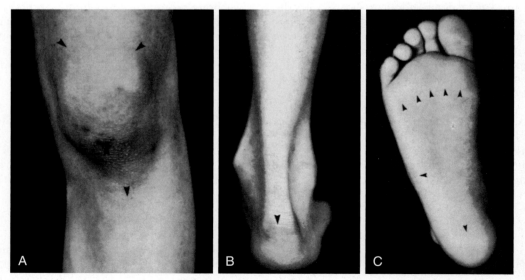

FIGURE 17–2 **A,** *Arrows* indicate the most common sites of tenderness associated with enthesitis at the insertions of the quadriceps muscles into the patella and the attachments of the patellar ligament to the patella and tibial tuberosity. **B,** *Arrow* indicates the site of tenderness at the insertion of the Achilles tendon into the calcaneus. **C,** *Arrows* indicate the most common sites of tenderness associated with enthesitis at the insertion of the plantar fascia into the calcaneus, base of the fifth metatarsal, and heads of the first through fifth metatarsals. Swelling in this area is best visualized by having the child lie prone on the examining table with the feet over the edge. (*B* and *C,* From Petty RE, Malleson P: Spondyloarthropathies of childhood, *Pediatr Clin North Am* 33:1079-1096, 1986.)

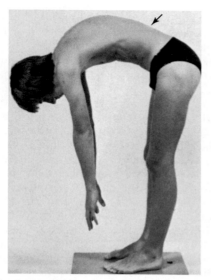

FIGURE 17–3 A 15-year-old boy shown in the position of maximal forward flexion. Note the flattened back *(arrow)*. Radiographs demonstrated bilateral sacroiliac arthritis but no abnormality of the lumbosacral spine.

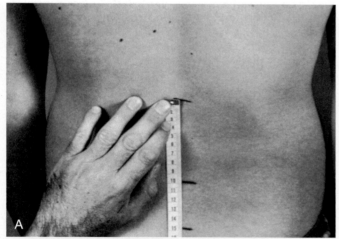

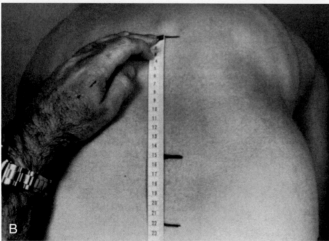

FIGURE 17–4 Schober test. **A,** Measurement 10 cm above and 5 cm below the lumbosacral junction (the dimples of Venus) in the upright position. **B,** Measurement of the distance between the upper and the lower marks when the child is bending forward.

disease. Measurement of the distance from the fingertips to the floor on maximum forward flexion is often used to quantitate spinal motion but is poorly reproducible and does not correlate with the Schober measurement. Furthermore, finger-to-floor distance reflects hip as well as back flexion.

Thoracic disease may be reflected in limitation of chest expansion. Normal thoracic excursion varies a great deal, and normal age- and sex-adjusted ranges have not been established. However, in a specific child, sequential measurement of thoracic motion may be useful in documenting progressive loss of range. In the adolescent, any thoracic excursion of less than 5 cm (maximum expiration to maximum inspiration, measured at the fourth intercostal space) should be regarded as probably abnormal. Even in the absence of symptoms, chest expansion in children with JAS may be restricted to 1 or 2 cm. Pain and tenderness at the costosternal and costovertebral joints may be elicited by firm palpation. Sternomanubrial tenderness sometimes occurs, but sternoclavicular pain is more common.

LABORATORY EXAMINATION

There are few distinguishing laboratory features. Anemia is usually mild and characteristic of the anemia of chronic disease. White blood cell counts are usually normal or moderately elevated with normal differential counts. Indices of inflammation are frequently abnormal. The platelet count and the ESR are often elevated and may remain so for years. Very high values for the ESR (>100 mm) occasionally occur but should also suggest the possibility of occult IBD. Conversely, a normal ESR may accompany clinically active disease.

Elevated immunoglobulin levels reflect inflammation, and selective IgA deficiency has been reported.[149,150] High levels of IgA and C4[151,152] and of circulating immune complexes[153] in adults with AS suggest an immunoreactive state. Characteristically, RFs are absent. ANAs do not occur in children with ERA more commonly than in

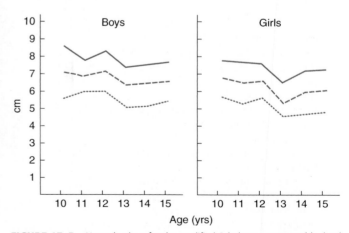

FIGURE 17–5 Normal values for the modified Schober test: mean *(dashed line)* ± 1 standard deviation *(solid lines)*. (Adapted from Moran HM, Hall MA, Barr A et al: Spinal mobility in the adolescent, *Br J Rheumatol Rehab* 18: 181-185, 1979.)

a healthy population. Antiphospholipid antibodies have been demonstrated in 29% of adults with AS,[154] but children with ERA have not been studied. Although there are no reports of systematic studies of other autoantibodies in ERA or JAS, experience suggests that they are not common.

HLA-B27 is present in 90% of children with JAS or ERA and in approximately 8% of the overall white population; it does not constitute a diagnostic test but rather an indicator of risk. The diagnosis of ERA rests on clinical characteristics, and the use of HLA typing for diagnosis may lead to misdiagnosis, although typing is important as a criterion to classify patients for study.

There are no specific studies of synovial fluid, but the changes are probably similar to those in adults with AS, in which the differential white blood cell count includes more neutrophils and fewer lymphocytes than in RA.[155] It has been reported that the predominant large mononuclear cell in synovial fluid in RA is lymphocyte derived, whereas that in AS is of macrophage origin.[156] Macrophages containing degenerated neutrophils are more common in the synovial fluid of patients with AS and related diseases such as reactive arthritis than in those with RA.[157] Descriptions of the synovial fluid are otherwise similar to those for RA, except that the complement level is usually normal[158] or increased.[115]

RADIOLOGICAL EXAMINATION

Sacroiliac Joints

The sacroiliac joint has some unique anatomical characteristics, an understanding of which assists in the interpretation of certain radiological features. The sacral side of the joint is covered by hyaline cartilage, whereas the iliac side is protected by a thin layer of fibrocartilage. These differences may account for the higher frequency of abnormalities on the iliac side. Only the lower one third to one half of each joint is diarthrodial and enclosed in a synovial membrane; the upper portion is a fibrous synostosis.[159]

Early radiographic changes in peripheral joints in ERA are like those of any type of JIA (Table 17–7). (see Chapter 10.) Evidence of enthesitis is most commonly seen at the plantar fascia insertion to the calcaneus (Fig. 17–6) or the insertion of the Achilles tendon to the calcaneus. Radiographic demonstration of sacroiliac arthritis often follows the onset of peripheral arthritis by years but is the first radiological evidence of inflammation affecting the axial skeleton. Radiological evidence of bilateral sacroiliac arthritis is necessary to establish an unequivocal diagnosis of AS, although the classic radiographic changes may not be seen for many years after the onset of ERA.

Radiological evaluation of the sacroiliac joints is difficult, and the preferred techniques used vary from one radiologist to another. It is the authors' practice to obtain a standard anteroposterior view of the pelvis, looking for apparent widening of the joint as a result of erosions of the subchondral bone, particularly in the inferior synovial portion of the joint, together with sclerosis of the iliac or sacral sides of the joint (Fig. 17–7). The lesion may appear initially as haziness of the cortical margins, followed by dissolution of the subchondral plate, which results in a punched-out appearance. Although these changes may be unilateral initially, they eventually become bilateral and symmetrical. An osteoblastic reaction occurring on both sides of the joint results in increased density or reactive sclerosis. Late changes may include fusion of the sacroiliac joints and regional osteoporosis. A normal or equivocal plain radiograph does not exclude the diagnosis of sacroiliitis, however, and in that circumstance magnetic resonance imaging (MRI) is helpful.

MRI identifies early changes in both the sacroiliac joints and the spine and may be the most sensitive

Table 17–7
Radiological characteristics of juvenile ankylosing spondylitis

Sacroiliac disease (bilateral)
  Diffuse osteoporosis of the pelvis
  Blurring of subchondral margins
  Erosions (iliac side first)
  Reactive sclerosis
  Joint-space narrowing
  Fusion (late)
Vertebral column
  Vertebral epiphysitis with anterior vertebral squaring
  Anterior ligament calcification
  "Bamboo spine"
Enthesitis (e.g., at calcaneus, tibial tuberosity)
  Soft tissue swelling
  Erosions or spur formation at insertions
Peripheral joints
  Soft tissue swelling
  Accelerated ossification and epiphyseal overgrowth
  Periostitis
  Joint-space narrowing, erosions
  Ankylosis

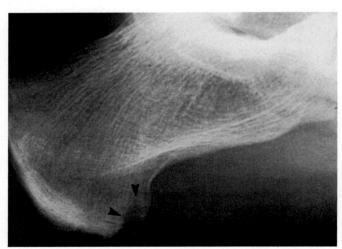

FIGURE 17–6   Lateral radiographs of the calcaneus with erosions at the site of insertion of the plantar fascia into the calcaneus (*arrowheads*). (From Petty RE, Malleson P: Spondyloarthropathies of childhood, *Pediatr Clin North Am* 33:1079-1096, 1986.)

indicator of inflammation.[160] It is critical in establishing an early diagnosis in specific patients and in determining therapy. Studies in adults show that evidence of bone marrow edema and osteitis was believed to be the MRI abnormality most indicative of active sacroiliitis, although synovitis, enthesitis, and capsulitis can also be demonstrated.[161] In one large study[162] dynamic MRI was used to evaluate 100 children younger than 6 years of age with probable spondyloarthropathies (ESSG criteria) and 30 control children. Early sacroiliac joint inflammation was confirmed in many patients for whom other studies were unrevealing, particularly in children with acute onset of disease. The investigators pointed out that this technique should not be used in every child with back pain because of cost; nevertheless, demonstration of involvement of the sacroiliac joints could influence the choice of antiinflammatory therapy.

Although computed tomography gives excellent images of the sacroiliac joints, its use requires a high radiation dose, and for this reason it is less often used. Scintigraphic study of the sacroiliac joint is of limited value in the growing child or adolescent unless there are distinct unilateral abnormalities. Sufficient experience in the interpretation of radionuclide scans in this age group is required before interpretation of bone scans can be relied on, and even then the yield is limited. Increased uptake in one sacroiliac joint can result not only from inflammation or infection but from asymmetrical weight-bearing caused by arthritis in a lower extremity joint or from enthesitis around the foot.

Spine

Radiological changes in the lumbosacral spine are less frequent and occur much later than abnormalities in the sacroiliac joints.[163] Periostitis with deposition of new bone along the anterior margin of the vertebral border results first in the shining corner and then in flattening of the normally concave anterior margin of the vertebral body. Syndesmophyte formation, the hallmark of advanced disease in adults, is rare in children and adolescents but develops during the adult years in some patients with juvenile-onset disease. Periostitis at the iliac crests or the inferior pubic rami and erosion at the symphysis pubis are uncommon. Arthritis affecting the cervical spine is

less commonly symptomatic than that of the lumbosacral spine but can cause severe damage.[164] This is documented by the study shown in Figure 17–8 A-C.

Entheses

Radiographic evaluation of entheses around the calcaneus, and rarely the patella, may demonstrate subtle changes in soft tissue density. Loss of the distinct margins at the insertion of the Achilles tendon, together with effacement of the triangular fat shadow, may be an early sign of inflammation. Erosion of bone at the insertion of the Achilles tendon or spur formation at that site is readily evaluated by a lateral radiograph of the calcaneus (see Fig. 17–6 and Chapter 10). Azouz and Duffy[165] have described changes in the bone marrow subjacent to an inflamed enthesis in children with JAS. A comparison of adult-onset and juvenile-onset ankylosing spondylitis documented exclusively peripheral joint disease in 26% of those with juvenile-onset AS, compared with 4.6% in adult-onset AS.[166]

TREATMENT

General Management

Children with ERA have frequently had undiagnosed symptoms for months or years. Explanation of the correct diagnosis, its chronicity, possible complications, and the need for long-term medical treatment, physical therapy, and follow-up facilitates compliance with the therapeutic recommendations. A team of health professionals helps to provide necessary education and care. In the older adolescent, realistic career goals must be discussed along with current means of minimizing work-related stress to the low back and joints of the lower extremities. The patient should be encouraged to participate as fully as possible in age-appropriate social and recreational activities. The relatively good long-term prognosis should be emphasized, particularly in the adolescent, who may regard the diagnosis as marking the end of recreational, social, educational, and career goals.

Management should be individualized according to the patient's specific problems. Current treatments are most successful in controlling the signs and symptoms

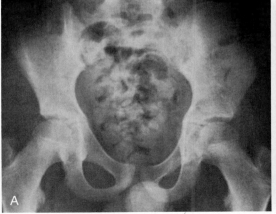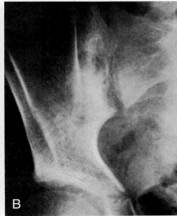

FIGURE 17–7 Juvenile ankylosing spondylitis. Moderately advanced radiographic changes. **A,** The widening, erosions, and reactive sclerosis are marked on this anteroposterior view of the pelvis. **B,** Oblique view of right sacroiliac joint demonstrates the same changes in more detail.

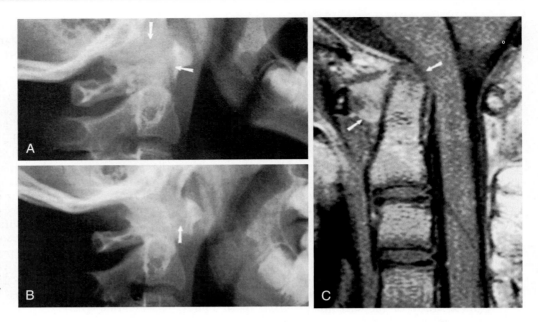

FIGURE 17–8 Radiographs of the upper cervical spine in a child with juvenile ankylosing spondylitis. **A,** Extension view identifies the upper limit of the odontoid process of C2 *(upper arrow)* and the posteroinferior margin of the anterior arch of C1 *(lower arrow)*. **B,** Flexion view documents a widened atlantoaxial space *(arrow),* confirming the presence of subluxation. **C,** T2-weighted magnetic resonance image delineates an inflammatory mass in the space between the C1 anterior arch and the odontoid process *(lower arrow),* as well as indentation of the odontoid on the lower medulla/upper cervical cord *(upper arrow).*

of the disease; none has been demonstrated to alter the progression of ankylosis. If widespread, severe joint inflammation is the overwhelming problem, systemic antiinflammatory medications (NSAIDs, sulfasalazine, glucocorticoids) are appropriate. If the joint disease is localized, it may be more useful to use NSAIDs and intraarticular glucocorticoid in joints that are particularly problematic. Enthesitis, particularly around the foot, is unlikely to respond to systemic anti-inflammatory drugs alone; the use of custom-made orthotics often provides relief. In all patients, exercise and maintenance of good posture to minimize loss of range of motion (ROM) in the spine and its articulations are recommended. A firm mattress and thin pillow are important adjuncts to the program. Smoking should be discouraged because of its demonstrated adverse effects on pulmonary function.[167]

Antiinflammatory Medications

NSAIDs are the initial pharmacological management. Although there are no reported trials of NSAIDs in JAS, it is probable that these children respond best to naproxen or indomethacin. Because of lower toxicity, the use of naproxen (15 to 20 mg/kg/day) is recommended before indomethacin (1 to 2 mg/kg/day). Although indomethacin is often effective, toxicity is common, and the drug must be monitored carefully, beginning with low doses. Headache, epigastric pain, and inability to pay attention in school occur in 20% to 30% of children taking this drug and frequently necessitate cessation of its use (see Chapter 6 for a warning on a potential risk of cardiovascular events).

Sulfasalazine (40 to 50 mg/kg/day: upper limit 2000 mg) has widespread currency in treatment,[168] based largely on experience in adults,[169-174] although no prospective, randomized, placebo-controlled trials have been reported. In an open-label, multicenter study, children with B27-positive late-onset oligoarthritis responded well to sulfasalazine.[175] This group of patients were those whose peripheral disease responded best in other small

trials as well.[175-178] Beneficial effects are usually not evident for several weeks after initiation of treatment. Toxicity to bone marrow and liver must be monitored closely.

Glucocorticoids have a role only in short-term therapy in the severely ill patient,[179] as topical agents in the management of acute uveitis, and for intraarticular administration in children with limited joint disease.[180,181] Triamcinolone hexacetonide is the preferred intraarticular steroid and can be given in a dose of 1 mg/kg to a maximum of 40 mg in large joints (hip, knee, ankle), or a maximum of 20 mg in wrist or elbow (see Chapter 6). The use of CT to guide injection of 40 mg of triamcinolone into the sacroiliac joints was reported in 30 adults with AS.[182] The injections were considered effective as judged both clinically and by dynamic MRI. Local injections of glucocorticoids at sites of enthesitis may occasionally be useful.

Hydroxychloroquine and methotrexate are sometimes used, but there are no reports of their efficacy in children. In a study of adults who had not responded to NSAIDs and sulfasalazine, modest benefit was demonstrated with the use of methotrexate in a dose of 7.5 to 15 mg/week.[183,184] By anecdotal report, methotrexate appears to be less effective in treating ERA than other types of JIA.

Etanercept has been advocated for refractory disease.[185,186] In a controlled trial in AS, it significantly improved signs and symptoms of the disease.[187] Infliximab in another trial produced a 50% improvement in 53% of the patients at week 12.[188]

In a group of 10 children with longstanding treatment-resistant HLA-B27–positive ERA treated with etanercept (n-2) or infliximab (n-8), Tse and colleagues noted almost total remission in tender enthesitic count and active joint count by 6 months.[189] This response was sustained during the 1-year follow-up period. Anti-TNF agents have an important and growing role in the management of children with ERA that is resistant to sulfasalazine. Pamidronate (60 mg IV/mo in adults) impressively reduced bone turnover but did not alter inflammatory indices.[190]

Physical and Occupational Therapy

Physical therapy should be directed at preventing loss of range of motion (ROM) and poor functional positioning in the spine and chest, as well as stabilizing or regaining lost ROM in peripheral joints. Attention to posture and daily active ROM exercises for the back and deep-breathing exercises for the chest help to preserve range. Some young patients with JAS breathe predominantly with the diaphragm and have to relearn to use the intercostal muscles. Strengthening of abdominal and back muscles should be undertaken cautiously. Swimming is an ideal form of physical activity that can be encouraged to augment these specific exercises. (See Chapter 12.)

Painful enthesitis in the feet may be relieved by the use of custom-made orthotics, fitted to support the fat cushion under the heel and to take pressure off the plantar aspects of the heel and metatarsophalangeal joints. If the Achilles enthesis alone is involved, the use of a slightly higher heel may help to reduce stress at this site. Therapeutic ultrasound and transcutaneous nerve stimulation are sometimes useful in the management of pain caused by enthesitis around the foot. Enthesitis can be quite resistant to therapy and may be the most functionally limiting aspect of the disease.

Surgery

Orthopaedic surgery has a very limited role in management of ERA in childhood or adolescence. Later in life, joint reconstruction and replacement are invaluable contributions to function and quality of life in the patient with severely damaged joints. The outcome of total hip replacement in young adults who were monitored for up to 30 years indicates that the probability that both components of low-friction arthroplasty will survive 10 years is 91%; this figure was 70% at 20 years.[191,192] Advances in total joint replacement will undoubtedly continue to improve long-term outcome. Bony ankylosis as a result of exuberant overgrowth of bone around the prosthesis has been reported after hip joint replacement as an almost unique complication related to AS. This complication may be amenable to the prophylactic use of medication.[115]

COURSE OF THE DISEASE AND PROGNOSIS

The early course of ERA is often remitting and may be mild. Often, it is only in retrospect that the initial musculoskeletal complaints are recognized as harbingers of this disorder. Almost one-half of these children have four or fewer joints affected during the entire course of the disease; even in those in whom this number is exceeded, it is uncommon cumulatively to have more than six or seven inflamed joints. Most children eventually develop arthritis affecting joints of the axial skeleton. Lower extremity predominance remains the rule throughout the course, with hips, knees, ankles, and feet more commonly affected than upper extremity joints.

Subtle losses in ROM of the thorax or back should be documented as early as possible. Ansell[115] noted that limitation of ROM of the spine was not detected until 11 to 33 years after onset of symptoms in patients who had JAS. However, from more recent experience, it is an impression that limitation of range of back motion may occur much earlier. In the study of Burgos-Vargas and colleagues,[14] all patients had decreased back mobility by 5 years.

Life expectancy in AS is reduced compared with the U.S. population as a whole. Cardiopulmonary and cerebrovascular diseases are the leading causes of death. At least during the years of childhood and adolescence, functional outcome probably remains good.[193] In one study,[194] however, outcome in JAS was worse than in AS. Peripheral joint disease may be more common in children than in adults, and persistent hip disease, in particular, is associated with a poor functional outcome.[195,196] Acute uveitis seldom leaves significant residua, even if recurrent, but uncommonly can be severe. Aortitis is rare but, if present, contributes to late morbidity and mortality. Although amyloidosis may develop in adults with AS, little information is available in children.[37]

REFERENCES

1. R.E. Petty, T.R. Southwood, P. Manners, et al., International League of Associations for Rheumatology classification of juvenile idiopathic arthritis: second revision, Edmonton 2001, J. Rheumatol. 31 (2004) 390–392.
2. P.H. Bennett, P.H.N. Wood, Population studies of the Rheumatic Diseases, Excerpta Medica, New York, 1968.
3. B. Amor, M. Dougados, M. Mijiyawa, Criteria of the classification of spondylarthropathies, Rev. Rhum. Mal. Osteoartic. 57 (1990) 85–89.
4. M. Dougados, L.S. van der Linden, R. Juhlin, et al., The European Spondylarthropathy Study Group preliminary criteria for the classification of spondylarthropathy, Arthritis Rheum. 34 (1991) 1218–1227.
9. V. Wright, J.M. Moll, Seronegative polyarthritis, North Holland, Amsterdam, The Netherlands, 1976.
10. A.M. Rosenberg, R.E. Petty, A syndrome of seronegative enthesopathy and arthropathy in children, Arthritis Rheum. 25 (1982) 1041–1047.
11. C.W. Fink, Proposal for the development of classification criteria for idiopathic arthritides of childhood, J. Rheumatol. 22 (1995) 1566–1569.
12. R.E. Petty, T.R. Southwood, J. Baum, et al., Revision of the proposed classification criteria for juvenile idiopathic arthritis: Durban, J. Rheumatol. 25 (1997) 1991–1994. 1998.
13. D.A. Cabral, K.G. Oen, R.E. Petty, SEA syndrome revisited: a longterm followup of children with a syndrome of seronegative enthesopathy and arthropathy, J. Rheumatol. 19 (1992) 1282–1285.
14. R. Burgos-Vargas, P. Clark, Axial involvement in the seronegative enthesopathy and arthropathy syndrome and its progression to ankylosing spondylitis, J. Rheumatol. 16 (1989) 192–197.
19. A.M. Prieur, V. Listrat, M. Dougados, et al., Criteria for classification of spondylarthropathies in children, Arch. Fr. Pediatr. 50 (1993) 379–385.
20. S. Bowyer, P. Roettcher, Pediatric rheumatology clinic populations in the United States: results of a 3 year survey. Pediatric Rheumatology Database Research Group, J. Rheumatol. 23 (1996) 1968–1974.
21. P.N. Malleson, M.Y. Fung, A.M. Rosenberg, The incidence of pediatric rheumatic diseases: results from the Canadian Pediatric Rheumatology Association Disease Registry, J. Rheumatol. 23 (1996) 1981–1987.
22. D.P. Symmons, M. Jones, J. Osborne, et al., Pediatric rheumatology in the United Kingdom: data from the British Pediatric Rheumatology Group National Diagnostic Register, J. Rheumatol. 23 (1996) 1975–1980.

25. R.K. Sauernmann, J.B. Rose, P. Tyrell, et al., Epidemiology of juvenile idiopathic arthritis in a multiethnic cohort, Arthritis Rheum. 56 (2007) 974–1984.

33. J.R. Ladd, J.T. Cassidy, W. Martel, Juvenile ankylosing spondylitis, Arthritis Rheum. 14 (1971) 579–590.

34. J. Schaller, S. Bitnum, R.J. Wedgwood, Ankylosing spondylitis with childhood onset, J. Pediatr. 74 (1969) 505–516.

39. R. Hafner, Juvenile spondarthritis: retrospective study of 71 patients, Monatsschr. Kinderheilkd. 135 (1987) 41–46.

50. T.-H. Kim, W.-S. Uhm, R.D. Inman, Pathogenesis of ankylosing spondylitis and reactive arthritis, Curr. Opin. Rheumatol. 17 (2005) 400–405.

51. T. Pham, Pathophysiology of ankylosing spondylitis: what's new? Joint. Bone Spine 75 (2008) 656–660.

52. J. Sieper, Developments in the scientific and clinical understanding of the spondyloarthritides, Arthritis Res. Therapy 11 (2009) 208.

53. J.D. Reveille, The genetic basis of ankylosing spondylitis, Curr. Opin. Rheumatol. 18 (2006) 332–341.

54. Brown MA: Genetics and the pathogenesis of ankylosing spondylitis, Curr. Opin. Rheumatol. 21 (2009) 318-323.

57. M. Breban, R.E. Hammer, J.A. Richardson, et al., Transfer of the inflammatory disease of HLA-B27 transgenic rats by bone marrow engraftment, J. Exp. Med. 178 (1993) 1607–1616.

60. H. Mielants, E.M. Veys, S. Goemaere, et al., A prospective study of patients with spondyloarthropathy with special reference to HLA-B27 and to gut histology, J. Rheumatol. 20 (1993) 1353–1358.

61. H. Mielants, E.M. Veys, C. Cuvelier, et al., The evolution of spondyloarthropathies in relation to gut histology. III. Relation between gut and joint, J. Rheumatol. 22 (1995) 2279–2284.

65. R.A. Colbert, The immunobiology of HLA-B27: variations on a theme, Curr. Mol. Med. 4 (2004) 1–30.

66. J.P. Mear, K.L. Schreiber, C. Munz, et al., Misfolding of HLA-B27 as a result of its B pocket suggests a novel mechanism for its role in susceptibility to spondyloarthropathies, J. Immunol. 163 (1999) 6665–6670.

67. M.J. Turner, M.L. Delay, S. Bai, et al., HLA-B27 upregulation causes accumulation of misfolded heavy chains and correlates with the magnitude of the unfolded protein response in transgenic rats: implications for the pathogenesis of spondarthritis-like disease, Arthritis Rheum. 56 (2007) 215–223.

68. K. Kapasi, R.D. Inman, HLA-B27 expression modulates gram-negative bacterial invasion into transfected L cells, J. Immunol. 148 (1992) 3554–3559.

71. O. Ortiz-Alvarez, D.T. Yu, R.E. Petty, et al., HLA-B27 does not affect invasion of arthritogenic bacteria into human cells, J. Rheumatol. 25 (1998) 1765–1771.

72. H.I. Huppertz, J. Heesemann, Invasion and persistence of Salmonella in human fibroblasts positive or negative for endogenous HLA B27, Ann. Rheum. Dis. 56 (1997) 671–676.

73. K. Granfors, Host-microbe interaction in HLA-B27-associated diseases, Ann. Med. 29 (1997) 153–157.

74. M. Benjamin, D. McGonagle, The enthesis organ concept and its relevance to the spondyloarthropathies, Adv. Exp. Med. Biol. 649 (2009) 57–70.

75. M. Benjamin, H. Toumi, D. Suzuki, et al., Microdamage and microvascularity at the enthesis-bone interface provides an anatomic explanation for bone involvement in the HLA-B27 associated spondyloarthritides and related disorders, Arthritis Rheum. 56 (2007) 224–233.

78. S. Brophy, A. Calin, Ankylosing spondylitis: interaction between genes, joints, age at onset, and disease expression, J. Rheumatol. 28 (2001) 2283–2288.

81. S.M. van der Linden, H.A. Valkenburg, B.M. de Jongh, et al., The risk of developing ankylosing spondylitis in HLA-B27 positive individuals. A comparison of relatives of spondylitis patients with the general population, Arthritis Rheum. 27 (1984) 241–249.

101. J.D. Reveille, Recent studies on the genetic basis of ankylosing spondylitis, Cur. Rheum. Rep. 11 (2009) 340–348.

102. M.A. Brown, Progress in spondylarthritis: progress in studies of the genetics of ankylosing spondylitis, Arth. Res. 11 (2009) 340–348.

103. M.A. Brown, Genome-wide screening in ankylosing spondylitis, Adv. Exp. Med. Biol. 649 (2009) 148–158.

107. G.A. Niepel, S. Sit'aj, Enthesopathy, Clin. Rheum. Dis. 5 (1979) 857.

111. R. Burgos-Vargas, J. Vazquez-Mellado, N. Cassis, et al., Genuine ankylosing spondylitis in children: a case-control study of patients with early definite disease according to adult onset criteria, J. Rheumatol. 23 (1996) 2140–2147.

113. D. Monnet, M. Breban, C. Hudry, et al., Ophthalmic findings and frequency of extraocular manifestations in patients with HLA-B27 uveitis: a study of 175 cases, Ophthalmology 111 (2004) 802–809.

116. H. Huppertz, I. Voigt, J. Muller-Scholden, et al., Cardiac manifestations in patients with HLA B27-associated juvenile arthritis, Pediatr. Cardiol. 21 (2000) 141–147.

126. T. Stamato, R.M. Laxer, C. de Freitas, et al., Prevalence of cardiac manifestations of juvenile ankylosing spondylitis, Am. J. Cardiol. 75 (1995) 744–746.

128. G. Camiciottoli, S. Trapani, M. Ermini, et al., Pulmonary function in children affected by juvenile spondyloarthropathy, J. Rheumatol. 26 (1999) 1382–1386.

132. H.E. Foster, R.A. Cairns, R.H. Burnell, et al., Atlantoaxial subluxation in children with seronegative enthesopathy and arthropathy syndrome: 2 case reports and a review of the literature, J. Rheumatol. 22 (1995) 548–551.

139. J. Ball, Pathology and pathogenesis, in: J.M.H. Moll (Ed.), Ankylosing spondylitis, Churchill Livingstone, Edinburgh, 1980.

140. J. Ball, Enthesopathy of rheumatoid and ankylosing spondylitis, Ann. Rheum. Dis. 30 (1971) 213–223.

147. I.F. Macrae, V. Wright, Measurement of back movement, Ann. Rheum. Dis. 28 (1969) 584–589.

159. N. Bellamy, W. Park, P.J. Rooney, What do we know about the sacroiliac joint? Semin. Arthritis Rheum. 12 (1983) 282–313.

165. E.M. Azouz, C.M. Duffy, Juvenile spondyloarthropathies: clinical manifestations and medical imaging, Skeletal Radiol. 24 (1995) 399–408.

168. R. Burgos-Vargas, J. Vazquez-Mellado, C. Pacheco-Tena, et al., A 26 week randomised, double blind, placebo controlled exploratory study of sulfasalazine in juvenile onset spondyloarthropathies, Ann. Rheum. Dis. 61 (2002) 941–942.

180. R.C. Allen, K.R. Gross, R.M. Laxer, et al., Intraarticular triamcinolone hexacetonide in the management of chronic arthritis in children, Arthritis Rheum. 29 (1986) 997–1001.

181. H.I. Huppertz, A. Tschammler, A.E. Horwitz, et al., Intraarticular corticosteroids for chronic arthritis in children: efficacy and effects on cartilage and growth, J. Pediatr. 127 (1995) 317–321.

184. B. Roychowdhury, S. Bintley-Bagot, D.Y. Bulgen, et al., Is methotrexate effective in ankylosing spondylitis? Rheumatology (Oxf.) 41 (2002) 1330–1332.

185. G. Homeff, R. Burgos-Vargas, TNF-alpha antagonists for the treatment of juvenile-onset spondyloarthritides, Clin. Exp. Rheumatol. 20 (2002) S137–S142.

189. S.M.L. Tse, R. Burgos-Vargas, R.M. Laxer, Anti-tumor necrosis factor alpha blockade in the treatment of juvenile spondylarthropathy, Arthriris Rheum. 52 (2005) 2103–2108.

193. A. Calin, J. Elswood, The natural history of juvenile-onset ankylosing spondylitis: a 24-year retrospective case-control study, Br. J. Rheumatol. 1 (27) (1998) 91–93.

Entire reference list is available online at www.expertconsult.com.

Chapter 18

JUVENILE PSORIATIC ARTHRITIS

Peter A. Nigrovic, Robert P. Sundel, and Ross E. Petty

An association between psoriasis and arthritis in the adult patient was described almost 200 years ago, but has been recognized in children only since the 1950s.[1-4] Juvenile psoriatic arthritis (JPsA) encompasses a heterogeneous set of arthritic phenotypes characterized by certain hallmark clinical features as well as considerable overlap with other subtypes of juvenile idiopathic arthritis (JIA). It is recognized both in children with frank cutaneous psoriasis as well as those in whom a psoriatic diathesis is suspected on other grounds.

DEFINITION AND CLASSIFICATION

As classified by the criteria of the International League of Associations for Rheumatology (ILAR), JPsA is arthritis that has its onset before the 16th birthday, lasts for at least 6 weeks, and is associated either with psoriasis or with two of the following: dactylitis, nail pitting or onycholysis, or psoriasis in a first-degree relative.[5] This definition resembles that of the "Vancouver criteria" (Table 18–1).[6] However, under ILAR criteria the diagnosis of JPsA cannot be made if the patient has a positive test for rheumatoid factor, a first-degree family history of an human leukocyte antigen B-27 (HLA-B27)–associated disease, or if the arthritis began in a boy over the age of 6 years who is HLA-B27 positive.

The diagnosis of JPsA is complicated by the presentation of psoriasis in children. Psoriasis in the young child may be subtle, atypical, and transient; initial misdiagnosis as eczema is common.[7-9] Psoriasis occurs in about 0.5% to 1% of children, with a prevalence rising to 2% to 3% in adulthood.[10-12] Since skin disease lags behind arthritis in about half of children with JPsA, sometimes by a decade or more (Table 18–2), the diagnosis may often rest on the presence of dactylitis or family history.[6-8,13-24] Not every patient with arthritis and psoriasis has psoriatic arthritis. Typical seropositive rheumatoid arthritis (RA) with coincidental psoriasis is well recognized.[25] Finally, agents such as methotrexate and tumor necrosis factor (TNF) blockers are effective treatments for cutaneous psoriasis and could potentially forestall its appearance in a child treated for joint inflammation. Confirming that a particular child does or does not have JPsA is therefore challenging, and diagnostic uncertainty is common.

These challenges have been reflected in the evolution of diagnostic criteria for JPsA. Initially, JPsA was limited to children with chronic arthritis who developed classic psoriasis.[3,7,13-16,26] Recognizing that the psoriatic diathesis may be suggested by features beyond the classic eruption, including dactylitis, nail pits, and a family history of psoriasis, Southwood and colleagues extended the diagnosis of JPsA to patients with such features even in the absence of the typical rash, yielding the "Vancouver criteria" for JPsA (see Table 18–1).[6] These criteria have been validated.[19,23,24] With the development of the ILAR nomenclature, the definition of JPsA was restricted to make it and other subtypes of JIA mutually exclusive. These definitions remain a work in progress.[5,23,24,27-29] Both the Vancouver and ILAR criteria were designed for research, and in practice the diagnosis of JPsA is often used more flexibly.

EPIDEMIOLOGY

Incidence and Prevalence

The incidence and prevalence of JPsA are unknown. Population data, enumerating largely patients with adult-onset psoriatic arthritis (PsA), suggest a prevalence of 0.10% to 0.25% in the United States.[30,31] It occurs in all ethnic groups.[32] The proportion of JIA patients with JPsA varies widely depending on the population studied and the diagnostic criteria employed. Series that recognize patients on the basis of frank psoriasis, or using ILAR criteria, find that JPsA represents approximately 7% (range: 0% to 11.3%) of patients with JIA.[6,8,18,21,24,33-40] Series employing the more inclusive Vancouver criteria identify JPsA in 8% to 20% of patients with JIA.[6,21,24,41]

Age at onset and Sex Ratio

The age at onset of JPsA is biphasic (Figure 18–1).[6,21] A first peak occurs during the preschool years, and a second is seen during middle to late childhood. JPsA is uncommon before the age of 1 year. It is somewhat more frequent in girls than in boys (see Table 18–2), with girls accounting for 60% of cases in larger series.[21,42]

ETIOLOGY, PATHOLOGY, AND PATHOGENESIS

The cause of JPsA and the reasons for the link between psoriasis and arthritis are unknown.

PATHOLOGY

Synovial Pathology

Data concerning the pathology of psoriatic synovium are available largely from adult-onset disease, with rare exception.[43] Gross examination, as performed by arthroscopy, reveals a synovial lining that is less villous than in adult RA but with distinctive tortuous, bushy superficial blood vessels.[44,45] This microvascular pattern resembles that of the psoriatic plaque and is observed also

---

Table 18–1

Vancouver and ILAR criteria for Juvenile Psoriatic Arthritis

	Vancouver	ILAR (Edmonton revision)

Inclusion	Arthritis plus psoriasis or arthritis plus at least two of
	  Dactylitis
	  Nail pits
	  Psoriasis in a first- or second-degree relative
	  Psoriasis-like rash
		Arthritis plus psoriasis, or arthritis plus at least two of
		  Dactylitis
		  Nail pits or onycholysis
		  Psoriasis in a first-degree relative

Exclusion	None	1. Arthritis in an HLA-B27–positive male beginning after the sixth birthday 2. AS, ERA, sacroiliitis with IBD, reactive arthritis, or acute anterior uveitis, or a history of one of these disorders in a first-degree relative 3. The presence of IgM RF on at least 2 occasions at least 3 months apart 4. The presence of systemic JIA 5. Arthritis fulfilling two JIA categories

For both criteria sets, arthritis must be of unknown etiology, begin before the sixteenth birthday, and persist for at least 6 weeks. Under the Vancouver criteria, "definite JPsA" is arthritis plus psoriasis or arthritis plus three minor criteria, while "probable JPsA" is arthritis plus two minor criteria.

AS, ankylosing spondylitis; ERA, enthesitis-related arthritis; IBD, inflammatory bowel disease; RF, rheumatoid factor.

Table 18–2

Clinical series of patients with Juvenile Psoriatic Arthritis

Year	First author	N	F (%)	Definition of JPsA	Follow-up (yr, mean)	Psoriasis (%)	Arthritis Before Rash (%)	FHx of Psoriasis (%)	Dac-tylitis (%)	Nail Changes (%)	Uveitis (%)
1976	Lambert	43	74	Lambert	11	100	53	40		71	9.3
1977	Calabro	12	58	Arthritis+Psoriasis		100	33		58	92	0
1980	Sills	24	71	Lambert*		71*	58			83	8.3
1982	Shore	60†	58	Lambert	10.8	100	43	42	23	77	8.3
1985	Wesolowska	21	38		4.2		56			86	14.3
1989	Southwood	35	69	Vancouver	4.4	60	48	88	49		17.1
1990	Truckenbrodt	48	44	Arthritis+Psoriasis	5	100	50	42	17	67	10.4
1990	Hamilton	28	57	Arthritis+Psoriasis	8.8	100	21	73	39	71	0
1991	Koo	11	55	Arthritis+Psoriasis		65	36	18		45	18
1996	Roberton	63	70	Vancouver	7		56	85	35		14.3
2006	Stoll	139	59	Vancouver	2	25	29	53†	37	47‡	7.9
2009	Flato	31	77	ILAR	>15	39	50	75	42	30.4	19.4

Blank = not specified
F = Female
*Nail disease counted as cutaneous psoriasis
†Includes 32 from Lambert 1976.
‡M. Stoll, P.A. Nigrovic, unpublished data.
Lambert criteria: inflammatory arthritis beginning before 16 years of age, psoriasis preceding or within 15 years of onset, usually negative for rheumatoid factor.
FHx, family history.

in synovial tissue from the spondyloarthropathies.[44,46] There are histological changes throughout the psoriatic synovium (Figure 18–2). The lining becomes hypertrophic with expansion of both type A (macrophage-like) and type B (fibroblast-like) synoviocytes.[47] The infiltrate in the loose connective tissue beneath the synovial lining is composed principally of lymphocytes and monocyte/macrophage lineage cells, with occasional neutrophils, plasma cells, and mast cells.[48-51] Lymphoid follicles may be observed. Compared with RA, lining hypertrophy and sublining infiltrates are typically less extensive. Infiltrating neutrophils are more prevalent in PsA, but they are not invariably present.[48,49,51] In general, given the variability between patients and within different parts of the same synovium, pathological findings generally are inadequate to define the diagnosis in an individual patient.

Characterization of the psoriatic synovial infiltrate by immunohistochemistry shows that the majority of infiltrating lymphocytes are T cells that express the memory CD45RO phenotype, with CD4 helper cells predominating over CD8 cytotoxic cells.[48,49,52-54] These cells are present at frequencies similar to that in RA, as are CD20+ B cells, plasma cells, and CD68+ macrophages. T cell oligoclonality suggests local antigen-driven expansion.[55] CD83+ dendritic cells are less common than in RA.

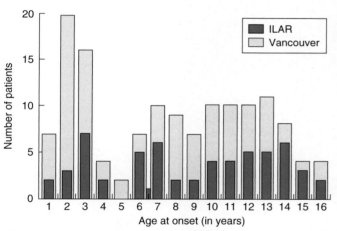

FIGURE 18–1 Age at onset of patients with juvenile psoriatic arthritis. (Data from Stoll, Lio P, Sundel RP, Nigrovic PA: Comparison of Vancouver and International League of Associations for rheumatology classification criteria for juvenile psoriatic arthritis, *Arthritis Rheum* 59:51-58, 2008.)

By contrast, increased numbers of macrophages expressing CD163 are identified in PsA and the adult spondyloarthropathies,[49,56] although not as clearly in juvenile-onset disease.[43] CD163 is a scavenger receptor, typically expressed on mature resident tissue macrophages that may help to limit rather than promote inflammation. However, the activity of these cells in the psoriatic synovium is unknown.[56,57]

Complement-fixing immune complexes are not typically found in the psoriatic synovium, and synovial fluid complement levels are usually normal.[58-60] Similarly, citrullinated peptides are observed commonly in the rheumatoid synovium but rarely in PsA.[49]

Entheseal Pathology

Entheseal sites are not readily accessible to biopsy, but small series in adult patients provide a degree of histological insight.[61-63] A low-grade inflammatory infiltrate is observed, often in association with underlying erosion of bone. This infiltrate is not limited to the surface of the bone and is often more extensive in the bone marrow underlying the enthesis. Such osteitis can be visualized as bone marrow edema by magnetic resonance imagining (MRI).[63-65] Cells observed at the interface include macrophages, lymphocytes (particularly CD8+ T cells), and occasional neutrophils. Bone healing is commonly evident, with woven bone filling in the defect left by erosions. This new bone often extends beyond the previous bony surface to interface with the ligament.[61] These observations have given rise to the hypothesis that the new bone formation characteristic of the spondyloarthropathies results from recurrent cycles of injury and healing, perhaps enabled by fluctuations in the degree of inflammation.[61,66] Whether such a mechanism underlies the hypertrophic periostitis observed in some patients with JPsA (Figure 18–3C) is unknown.

PATHOGENESIS

Environmental Contribution

Both psoriasis and psoriatic arthritis exhibit only limited concordance in monozygotic twins, suggesting that environmental contributions play a pivotal role in the

FIGURE 18–2 Synovial pathology in juvenile psoriatic arthritis. **A,** normal synovium with gracile synovial lining layer supported by a loose connective tissue sublining containing small blood vessels. **B,** synovium from 35-year old patient with juvenile-onset psoriatic arthritis, demonstrating lining hyperplasia, mononuclear infiltration of the subsynovium, and striking vascular hyperplasia. (Panel B courtesy of D.L. Baeten, University of Amsterdam, The Netherlands.)

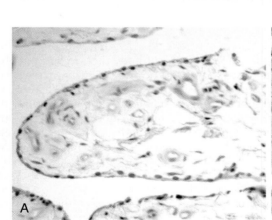
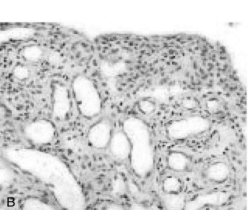

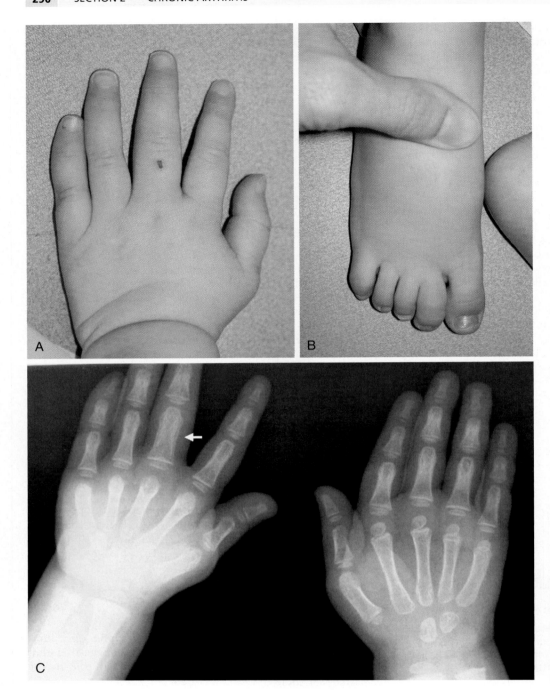

FIGURE 18–3 Dactylitis in juvenile psoriatic arthritis. **A,** dactylitis of the third finger (with incidental abrasion). **B,** dactylitis of the second and fifth toes. **C,** radiograph of the hands from the patient in **A,** demonstrating periosteal reaction in the affected digit *(arrow).*

development of disease.[67-69] The Koebner phenomenon, in which physical trauma precipitates skin disease, is evident in at least one-third of patients with psoriasis.[70,71] There have been reports of psoriatic arthritis being precipitated by physical trauma.[72] Because the entheses are points of mechanical stress, an exaggerated reaction to injury ("deep Koebner phenomenon") could contribute to clinical enthesitis in JPsA, with potential spread to adjacent structures. Streptococcal infection is a known precipitant for guttate psoriasis, raising the possibility that infection with streptococci or other agents could trigger joint inflammation.[73,74] Indeed, elevated antistreptococcal antibody titers have been observed in patients with psoriatic arthritis compared with other arthritides.[75] In support of such a role for bacteria, many rodent arthritis models fail to develop joint disease if deprived of normal bacterial flora. Among these is the rat transgenic for human HLA-B27, which develops features reminiscent of PsA including synovitis, spondylitis, and nail dystrophy.[76,77] Varicella infection has been reported to precipitate JPsA,[15] but a survey of childhood arthritis found no correlation between the onset of JPsA and coincident infections with *Mycoplasma,* respiratory syncytial virus, adenovirus, influenza A or B, parainfluenza, rubella, or herpes simplex.[41]

Exacerbation of psoriatic arthritis by emotional stress has also been observed in adults[67] and may potentially be modeled by the male DBA/1 mouse, which develops arthritis, dactylitis, and nail dystrophy with aging, but only if caged with other mice not originally from the same litter.[78]

Genetic Contribution

There is convincing clinical evidence for a genetic contribution to psoriasis and PsA. More than 50% of patients with childhood-onset psoriasis, with or without JPsA, have a family history of psoriasis (see Table 18–2).[9,70,79] The risk for both psoriasis and psoriatic arthritis appears to be transmitted more effectively via the paternal line (genetic imprinting).[80,81] A fifty-fold increased risk for PsA was observed in family members of the adults with PsA, suggesting that a propensity for arthritis is inherited over and above the propensity for psoriasis.[67] Similar results were noted in other studies.[82,83]

Association studies have begun to shed light on the genes that explain these strong familial associations.[68,84] In adults, psoriasis with onset age ≤ 40 years (Type I psoriasis) is more strongly familial than older-onset (Type II) disease.[85,86] Type I psoriasis is strongly associated with the MHC class I allele HLA-Cw6. This allele is also associated with adult PsA, and possibly with older-onset JPsA in children, but the link appears secondary to risk for psoriasis.[86,87] The results of studies of HLA associations in JPsA have been inconsistent, likely because of differences in definitions employed and variability within JPsA across the pediatric age spectrum.[6,7,17,19,87,88]

Beyond the MHC, JPsA has been linked with single nucleotide polymorphisms (SNPs) near genes involved in the autoinflammatory diseases (MEFV, NLRP3, NOD2, and PSTPIP1).[89] These associations have not emerged in adult genomewide association scans and have yet to be replicated. In adult studies, psoriasis and psoriatic arthritis have been associated with SNPs in a range of genes, including HCP5 (involved with control of viral replication) and genes related to the cytokines TNF, IL-13, and IL-23.[90-92] The functional consequences of these SNPs remain to be determined, but the cytokine findings are of particular interest. TNF blockade is markedly beneficial in psoriasis and psoriatic arthritis. IL-23 is involved in the differentiation of pro-inflammatory Th17 cells, which are increased in frequency in the circulation of patients with PsA and are present in psoriatic plaques.[93-95] Genetic studies have linked both psoriasis and PsA to IL12B, encoding the common p40 subunit of both IL-12 and IL-23, as well as to the IL-23 receptor IL23R. IL-13 suppresses the Th17 axis in favor of differentiation along a Th2 pathway, and the "risk" allele linked to psoriasis is associated with decreased cytokine production. Although no data from psoriatic synovium have been reported to date, murine models suggest that Th17 cells may contribute importantly to arthritis.[96] The implication of these findings is that the Th17 axis may be important in both psoriasis and its associated arthritis. Indeed, the anti–IL-12/IL-23 agent ustekinumab is highly effective for cutaneous psoriasis, although its efficacy for PsA is more modest.[97,98]

Cytokines and Other Mediators

Data on cytokine expression in psoriatic synovium and synovial fluid exhibit considerable variability. The range of mediators expressed is broadly similar to that in other inflammatory arthritides and includes the classical pro-inflammatory cytokines TNF, IL-1β and IL-6 as well as IL-1α, the neutrophil chemoattractant IL-8, the IL-2–like cytokine IL-15, IFN-γ, and others.[51-53,57,99-102] Pro-angiogenic factors such as VEGF are also elevated,[53,103,104] as are matrix metalloproteinases and their inhibitors.[53,57,105] No pattern of mediators has yet emerged as being specific for PsA, although compared with RA there are typically higher levels of pro-angiogenic factors and lower levels of pro-inflammatory mediators.

Synthesis: Pathogenesis of Juvenile Psoriatic Arthritis

Despite substantial advances in understanding, much remains to be learned about the pathogenesis of psoriatic arthritis. In the proper genetic context, an environmental trigger such as infection or trauma appears to unleash an inflammatory process involving infiltration of lymphocytes as well as neutrophils and other effectors of innate immunity into entheses and synovium. The target of this immune response remains unknown. Lymphocytes likely play a key role, as suggested by clonal expansion of these cells within the synovium and the requirement for lymphocytes in a murine model of psoriatic arthritis.[55,106] Joint inflammation is accompanied by an exuberant vascular expansion reminiscent of cutaneous psoriasis, with a tendency to promote bone formation as well as injury to cartilage and bone. Whether these principles apply equally to patients with JPsA, including those with early-onset disease, is unknown.

CLINICAL MANIFESTATIONS

Subgroups Within JPsA

JPsA is clinically heterogeneous. Age of onset data suggest a biphasic distribution, particularly in JPsA defined under the Vancouver criteria (see Figure 18–1).[6-8,21,23] This distribution is similar to that of JIA as a whole, with a peak around age 2 to 3 years and a second, less prominent peak in adolescence.[22,38,107] Younger children, presenting before the age of 5 years, tend to be female, ANA positive, and affected by dactylitis, the sausage-like swelling of individual digits.[15,21] This subgroup bears marked clinical and demographic similarity to early-onset oligoarticular JIA, although clinical differences include the tendency to develop dactylitis, to involve the wrists and small joints of the hands and feet, and to progress to polyarticular disease in the absence of effective therapy.[20,24,108] The merit of distinguishing these younger patients from oligoarticular JIA is controversial (Box 18–1). By contrast, older children exhibit a gender ratio closer to 1:1, with a tendency to enthesitis and axial disease, more closely resembling adult psoriatic arthritis.[8,15,17,21]

BOX 18–1

Psoriatic Arthritis, or Arthritis with Psoriasis?

The recognition of psoriatic arthritis in adults as an entity in its own right emerged gradually out of a number of observations. Inflammatory joint disease is encountered at a rate far higher than expected (10% to 20%) among patients with psoriasis.[31,148,149] This arthritis was often clinically distinctive. RF was usually absent or present in low titer, DIP and sacroiliac joints were commonly involved, and radiographs demonstrated new bone formation as well as erosions.[1] Even where arthritis was clinically indistinguishable from RA, it appeared at a younger age and in males and females equally, often clustered within certain psoriatic families.[25,67] Finally, PsA and RA synovial tissue could be differentiated, to some degree, on the basis of distinctive gross and microscopic features (see Pathology). Taken together, these data have provided strong support for the existence of psoriatic arthritis as a distinctive syndrome rather than simply the coincident occurrence of two common diseases.

By contrast, in children the case for JPsA remains controversial.[108,124,150] In most respects patients with JPsA fit somewhere in the spectrum of JIA. The hallmark psoriatic rash may take years to emerge. Absence of rheumatoid factor does not separate JPsA from most other JIA subtypes. Histopathological data are limited, and interpretation of genetic studies is complicated by issues of definition.[21,23,150,151] Finally, patients with JPsA respond to the therapies used in other JIA patients, and generally appear to do equally well.

Nevertheless, there are reasons to suspect that the association between psoriasis and arthritis spans both adults and children.[125] The prevalence of psoriasis in children is 0.5% to 1%; most present in adolescence.[10,11,70] Thus, the identification of a psoriatic diathesis in 7% or more of patients with JIA (of whom 40% to 60% have the classic rash) is not likely to reflect a chance association. Further, the pattern of arthritis in these children is distinctive in aggregate, if not always in an individual patient. Among younger patients, this includes dactylitis and involvement of small joints in the setting of oligoarthritis; in older patients, it includes an even gender ratio and an appreciable incidence of enthesitis and sacroiliitis.[20,21] Disease outcome may also differ.[24]

Although older-onset JPsA patients rather clearly resemble their adult counterparts, questions remain about arthritis that begins before the age of 5 or 6 years.[22,150] Like patients with early-onset oligoarticular JIA, these children tend to be female, are commonly ANA positive, and are prone to chronic asymptomatic uveitis.[21] Some share expression of the MHC II antigen HLA-DRB1*0801 (DRw8), associated with early-onset oligoarticular and polyarticular arthritis.[7,152,153] It seems very likely that shared pathophysiological mechanisms underlie these similarities,[22] and it has been proposed that JPsA in this age group is simply a variant of early-onset oligoarticular or polyarticular JIA.[150] However, at least under the Vancouver criteria, the proportion of these patients with a recognizable psoriatic diathesis greatly exceeds the 0.5 to 1.0% prevalence of psoriasis in this age group.[11] Further, young patients with JPsA manifest changes such as nail pits and dactylitis that are highly specific for adult psoriatic arthritis, an association noted even before these features were incorporated into the diagnostic criteria.[7,15,154] Therefore, even among younger children, the psoriatic diathesis seems to carry an elevated risk of an arthritis that is phenotypically distinct from other types of JIA. Clarification of the relationship between JPsA and other types of JIA awaits an improved understanding of the biology of these diseases.

Table 18–3

Joint involvement in Juvenile Psoriatic Arthritis

Series	Sills	Shore	Southwood	Truckenbrodt	Roberton	Stoll	Flato
Year	1980	1982	1989	1990	1996	2006	2009
Oligoarticular onset		73	94	85	73	84	68
Cervical spine		32	17		25		
TMJ			34		40	7	
Shoulder		23	9	8		3	
Elbow		43	20	15	30	13	33
Wrist	33	62	43	31	43	25	42
Small hand joints	88		60	31	62		61
MCP		53			43		
PIP		40			51		
DIP	63	42			27		
Sacroiliac joint	29		11	17	5	1	0
Hip	33	38	23	21	32	11	23
Knee	67	77	89	67	84	60	87
Ankle		63	63	50	60	51	71
Small foot joints	67		46	25	56		42
Any peripheral small joint	>88	>53	69	>31	>62	57	65

All numbers indicate percentage of patients

The presence of these clinical subgroups helps to explain the longstanding observation that girls with JPsA present at an earlier age than do boys[7,8,15,19] and corroborates data that HLA associations within JPsA depend on the age at onset of disease, as is also true in other subtypes of juvenile arthritis.[87,107]

Peripheral Arthritis

Arthritis in JPsA begins as an oligoarthritis in approximately 80% of children (Table 18–3). Initial presentation as monoarthritis is relatively common, and in some patients the disease begins with dactylitis in the absence of other joint involvement.[15] The knee is affected most

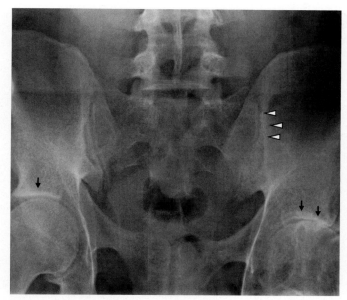

FIGURE 18–4 Sacroiliitis and hip arthritis in juvenile psoriatic arthritis. This radiograph depicts the pelvis and hip joints of a 23-year-old man with psoriasis who developed psoriatic arthritis at age 15. Note sclerosis at the left sacroiliac joint *(arrowheads)* and loss of joint space with reactive sclerosis at the hips, left greater than right *(arrows)*.

frequently, followed by the ankle; hip arthritis occurs in 20% to 30% (see Table 18–3). Even in children in whom arthritis remains oligoarticular, wrists, ankles, and small joints of the hands are more frequently affected than in other subtypes of oligoarthritis.[20,24] Without effective therapy, progression from oligoarticular to polyarticular involvement occurs in 60% to 80% of patients.[6,15,19] Polyarticular onset is observed in 20% of cases, although the number of joints involved is often lower than in other forms of childhood-onset polyarthritis, especially seropositive disease. As a result, joints affected by JPsA are often asymmetrically distributed.[6,109] Distal interphalangeal (DIP) involvement was identified in 30% to 50% of patients in early JPsA series[16-18] but is less common (10% to 30%) in patients diagnosed according to more inclusive criteria.[6,19,21] Fortunately, the highly destructive form of adult PsA known as arthritis mutilans is rare in children.

Axial Arthritis

Unlike most forms of JIA, JPsA is accompanied by an appreciable incidence of sacroiliitis, affecting from 10% to 30% of patients in some studies (see Table 18–3). Sacroiliitis affects principally patients with older age at onset.[21] These patients exhibit other features reminiscent of the adult spondyloarthropathies, including a balanced gender ratio, a tendency to manifest enthesitis, and an elevated frequency of the HLA-B27 antigen.[21,87] Patients in this older subgroup resemble adults with psoriatic arthritis, in whom definite radiographic sacroiliitis is detected in 30% to 70%.[110-112] Inflammatory disease of the lumbar spine occurs in less than 5% of children with JPsA.[6,19,21] Axial disease in JPsA is generally milder than in ankylosing spondylitis, with a tendency for asymmetric SI joint involvement and a failure to progress to spinal ankylosis (Figure 18–4).[113]

Enthesitis

Enthesitis denotes inflammation localized to the insertion of a tendon, ligament, fascia, or joint capsule into bone. Clinically, enthesitis is diagnosed in children with specific tenderness and occasionally swelling at characteristic sites, in the absence of an alternative, explanation (e.g. trauma). Using this standard, enthesitis is prevalent in patients within the older onset subgroup of JPsA, where it was observed in 57%, compared to 22% in younger patients.[21] This finding is in line with adult PsA, where enthesitis is considered a hallmark feature of the disease and can be documented radiographically in at least one site in almost all patients[114-116] (see Box 18–2). Typical sites of symptomatic enthesitis include the insertion of the Achilles tendon into the calcaneus and the insertions of the plantar fascia; other sites accessible to examination include the poles of the patellae, the iliac crests, the medial femoral condyles, and lateral epicondyles of the elbow.[115,117] Suspected enthesitis can be confirmed by ultrasound or by MRI.[118] Using the ILAR criteria, most children with arthritis and enthesitis are classified as having enthesitis-related arthritis (See Chapter 17), although patients with enthesitis may still be diagnosed with JPsA if they fulfill appropriate criteria.[5,23]

Dactylitis

Dactylitis refers to swelling within a digit that extends beyond the borders of the joints. Such swelling is typically uniform, giving the appearance of a "sausage digit," but can also be fusiform with accentuation around the PIP joint (Fig. 18–3A and B). Radiographically, tenosynovitis is often the dominant finding, with or without accompanying synovitis in the nearby joints; edema beyond the tendon sheath is common, suggesting the importance of enthesitis in the full phenotype (Box 18–2).[119-122] Subperiosteal new bone growth can also contribute to the thickness of the digit (Figure 18–3C). In children with JPsA, dactylitis is observed in 20% to 40% of patients (see Table 18–2). Commonly, only one or a few digits are affected, most commonly the second toe and index finger.[19] Dactylitis may be symptomatic or asymptomatic, and in one series it was the only musculoskeletal finding at presentation in 12% of children with JPsA.[15] Onset after trauma has been reported, and may explain the predilection for particular digits.[123] The specificity of dactylitis for psoriatic arthritis is incompletely defined. It has been reported in up to 18% of children with non-psoriatic JIA, although some of these children might actually have had JPsA.[6,124,125] Digital swelling also occurs in children with sickle cell disease, tuberculous osteomyelitis, and sarcoid arthropathy, but these are rarely confused with JPsA.

Extraarticular Manifestations

SKIN AND NAIL DISEASE

Overt psoriasis occurs in 40% to 60% of patients with JPsA.[6,24] In the large majority of patients, psoriasis presents as the classic vulgaris form, although guttate psoriasis is also observed.[7,8,14,15,17] Pustular and erythrodermic variants are rare.[8] This pattern approximates the presentation of psoriasis in childhood in general.[9] Psoriasis in children

---

BOX 18–2

Enthesitis: A Unifying Characteristic of Juvenile Psoriatic Arthritis?

Entheses are subject to substantial mechanical stresses. To dissipate these forces, a number of adaptations have emerged. For example, tendons often become infiltrated with fibrocartilage as they approach the site of insertion into bone, increasing in stiffness in order to limit the concentration of shear stress at the bone/tendon interface. Since the insertion of the joint capsule into bone is itself an enthesis, and tendons and ligaments frequently insert near joints, the synovial lining is usually in intimate contact with entheses.[156]

MRI studies of adults with psoriatic synovitis have identified edema at periarticular entheses.[64] McGonagle and colleagues have proposed that psoriatic arthritis begins at the enthesis and subsequently extends into the joint.[116] Since entheses are frequent sites of microtrauma, this process may be initiated by mechanical injury.[156]

Entheses in the lower extremity are more prone to inflammation, presumably related to mechanical loading, and this may explain the predilection of PsA for joints of the lower extremity (knee, ankle).[115]

Enthesitis also unifies hallmark features of the psoriatic hand. The finger contains a large number of entheses at sites where intrinsic and extrinsic muscles of the hand insert, as well as all along the shaft of the finger where the fibrous tendon sheath is anchored to prevent "bowstringing" with flexion.[155] Ultrasound and MRI have identified inflammation at these entheses in some, but not all, studies.[119-122] Such enthesitis may explain why the "sausage digit" is rarely observed in RA despite the occurrence of hand tenosynovitis at least as frequently in RA as in PsA.[157] The DIP joint may be particularly susceptible to inflammation originating at entheses, because the joint capsule is largely replaced by ligaments and tendons, residing therefore in unusually close proximity to the synovium.[155] These structures become inflamed in PsA of the DIP.[158] Interestingly, the extensor tendon enthesis extends distally along the DIP to interact with the nail bed. By MRI, thickening of the nailbed is present in almost all adults with PsA; more severe thickening is associated with visible changes in the nails, and these patients are prone to DIP synovitis.[128,159] Indeed, flares at the DIP often coincide with worsening psoriatic nail disease, while psoriasis and arthritis elsewhere are largely uncorrelated.[25] These results suggest that the primary lesion affecting the distal finger is enthesitis, with "spillover" into DIP synovitis when severe. The connection between finger entheses and the nailbed also explains the otherwise puzzling observation that nail changes are much more common in patients with psoriatic arthritis than in those with isolated skin disease (~50% to 80% versus ~10% to 30% in both adults and children)[1,160,161] (see Table 18–2). Taken together, these insights suggest that enthesitis is a distinguishing feature of JPsA not just among older patients, but also among younger children in whom dactylitis and nail changes are common presenting features.[21]

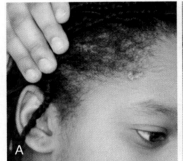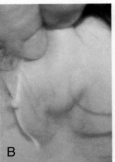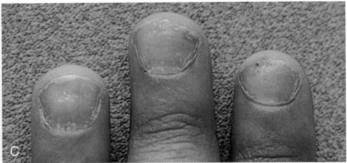

FIGURE 18–5 Cutaneous manifestations in juvenile psoriatic arthritis. **A,** psoriasis vulgaris on the scalp of a child with polyarticular JPsA. **B,** scaling behind the retracted ear of a 2–year-old girl with knee monoarthritis and a first-degree family history of psoriasis. This rash is suggestive of psoriasis but not diagnostic. **C,** nail dystrophy in JPsA. Findings include multiple nail pits, discoloration, and early onycholysis. This example shows florid changes, but more commonly nail findings are subtle and easily missed.

---

tends to be subtle, with thin, soft plaques that may come and go.[9,70] Lesions may be isolated to the hairline, umbilicus, behind the ears, or in the intergluteal crease, and thereby escape ready notice (Figures 18–5A and B). Misidentification as eczema is common, and some lesions are in fact ambiguous even to expert examination.[9] There are insufficient data to determine whether psoriasis associated with JPsA differs in age of onset or clinical course from the rest of childhood-onset psoriasis.

One substantial difference between children with JPsA and those with non-arthritic psoriasis is the prevalence of nail changes. Psoriatic changes in the nail surface include pits, onycholysis, horizontal ridging, and discoloration (Figure 18–5C). Nail changes accompany childhood psoriasis in up to 30% of cases.[126,127] By contrast, the prevalence of nail changes in JPsA is approximately 50% to 80%.[8,14,15,21] Nail changes are almost uniformly present in patients with DIP involvement in both adults and children, although nail pits are commonly found in the absence of overt DIP arthritis.[128] In adults, the presence of nail pits correlates with a more severe arthritis course, but this association is not obvious in children.[129]

UVEITIS

Chronic uveitis, indistinguishable from that in oligoarticular and polyarticular JIA, occurs in 10% to 15% of children with JPsA (see Table 18–2).[38,130] As in other JIA subsets, young patients with ANA are at highest risk, and standard uveitis screening guidelines apply (see Chapter 20). Acute anterior uveitis can occur in older children, although chronic uveitis is also observed in this subgroup.[8,18,21,23,131] Acute uveitis is associated with the presence of HLA-B27.[132] In one study, the rate of complications of uveitis was higher in JPsA than in other subtypes of juvenile arthritis.[133]

Other Systemic Manifestations

Children with significant polyarticular JPsA may have the constitutional features of chronic inflammatory disease, including anorexia, anemia, and poor growth.

Histological enteritis and occasionally symptomatic colitis are reported.[134] Fever may rarely occur in very severe cases but should not be ascribed to JPsA without a careful search for alternate causes.[7,25]Amyloidosis is a rare complication of longstanding active disease.[7,16] The SAPHO syndrome (synovitis, acne, pustulosis, hyperostosis, and osteitis) and CRMO (chronic recurrent multifocal osteomyelitis) have been associated with psoriasis and may be related to JPsA.[135] Other rare complications include lymphedema, aortic incompetence, and mitral valve prolapse.[136-138]

LABORATORY EXAMINATION

Laboratory tests are of limited diagnostic value in JPsA. Inflammatory markers, including ESR and CRP, may exhibit mild to moderate elevation, but are frequently normal.[15,21] Elevation of the platelet count has been noted in younger patients.[21] ANA is found in low or moderate titer in 60% of younger patients and 30% of older patients and is helpful primarily to define uveitis risk for the purpose of ophthalmologic screening.[21] Antibodies against extractable nuclear antigens are usually absent. Rheumatoid factor (RF) is typically absent, and indeed its presence excludes a diagnosis of JPsA under ILAR criteria (see Table 18–1). The presence of psoriasis may be considered incidental in patients with symmetrical polyarthritis who are positive for RF or anticyclical citrullinated peptide antibodies.[25]

RADIOLOGICAL EXAMINATION

Plain radiographic features of JPsA generally follow a sequence of changes similar to those in other forms of childhood arthritis. In early arthritis, soft tissue swelling around the joint (with or without joint effusion) is the only abnormality. Periarticular osteoporosis may occur within a few months after the onset of joint swelling, and periosteal new bone formation is common in digits affected by dactylitis (see Figure 18–3C). Joint-space narrowing, indicating significant cartilage loss, and erosive disease of bone are usually late features of JPsA (Figure 18–6). Bone remodeling may eventually occur, secondary to persistent periostitis and altered epiphyseal growth, though proliferative new bone formation is less often evident in children than in adults.[65] Sacroiliitis is commonly asymmetric (Figure 18–4).[113] MRI findings in JPsA include synovitis, tendinitis, and bone marrow edema at both articular and nonarticular sites, though the specificity of individual findings for JPsA has not been determined.[65] Both ultrasound and MRI can be used to assess entheseal involvement. In experienced hands ultrasound may be superior.[118]

TREATMENT

No randomized controlled trials (RCTs) have been conducted in JPsA. Recommendations are therefore extrapolated from trials of therapy in children with polyarticular course JIA,[139-141] from RCTs and clinical practice in adult

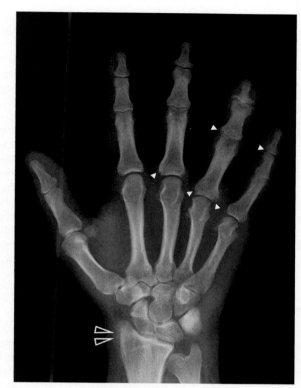

FIGURE 18–6 Radiographic changes in juvenile psoriatic arthritis include soft tissue swelling (dactylitis) of the 4th digit, arthritic and secondary degenerative changes of the 4th DIP joint, joint space loss at 4th and 5th PIP joints, multiple erosions of MCP, PIP and DIP joints (solid arrowheads) in the absence of periarticular osteopenia, and fluffy periostitis (open arrowheads).

PsA, and from experience in the treatment of JPsA and other types of JIA.[142] Roles for newer agents, including those that block IL-1, IL-6, and IL-12/23, remain to be defined.

Peripheral Arthritis

Psoriatic synovitis is potentially destructive of cartilage and bone, and like other types of synovitis may compromise bone growth in the immature skeleton. The goal of therapy is therefore remission, with normalization of physical findings and laboratory markers of inflammation. Efficacy has been demonstrated for nonsteroidal anti-inflammatory drugs (NSAIDs), sulfasalazine, methotrexate, leflunomide, cyclosporine, and the anti-TNF agents.[143] The basic treatment algorithm is similar to that employed in other subtypes of JIA. NSAIDs are often employed initially but typically do not induce remission. Individual large joints can be treated effectively with glucocorticoid injection. In patients with involvement of multiple joints, disease-modifying antirheumatic drugs (DMARDs) such as sulfasalazine or methotrexate are indicated. An inadequate response is addressed by addition of a second DMARD or, increasingly, the addition/substitution of anti-TNF therapy with any of the available agents. TNF blockade is particularly useful when there is axial disease, since no other treatment is effective for inflammation of the spine and sacroiliac joints (see Chapter 17). Anti-TNF agents are also the only medications with demonstrated activity against dactylitis and enthesitis. Abatacept has not been tested specifically in PsA or JPsA but has been shown to be effective and well tolerated in polyarticular-course JIA.[140]

Several specific considerations apply in the choice of agents for psoriatic disease. Based on anecdote and experience, PsA has been thought to be less responsive to systemic or intraarticular corticosteroids than other types of arthritis. This observation has not been examined rigorously, and both modes of administration are in common use. Substantial doses of systemic corticosteroids can provoke a flare of cutaneous psoriasis when tapered and should be avoided when possible. Similarly, antimalarials can worsen cutaneous psoriasis, although the magnitude of this risk is uncertain.[144,145] In any case, evidence for the efficacy of these agents is limited. Methotrexate has been associated with a higher risk of hepatotoxicity in adults with PsA than in RA.[143] It is not clear that this experience is relevant in JPsA, where methotrexate is typically well tolerated.

Spondylitis

Treatment of psoriatic spondylitis is based primarily on experience with ankylosing spondylitis.[144] Although axial disease is relatively common in older children and adults with JPsA, it tends to run a milder course. Treatment should be considered in patients who experience axial symptoms or show substantial or progressive limitation of spinal mobility. Continuous treatment with NSAIDs results in measurable radiographic improvement, but the effect is small.[146] Standard DMARDs, including sulfasalazine, methotrexate and leflunomide, are of minimal benefit. Anti-TNF therapy is highly effective for axial disease as assessed both by symptoms and by MRI evidence of inflammation.[144] However, studies in adults have so far failed to show a corresponding reduction in radiographic progression.[66,147]

COURSE AND PROGNOSIS

The long-term outcome of children with JPsA is incompletely defined. Patients followed at least 15 years demonstrated worse functional outcome than patients with oligoarticular or polyarticular JIA, and 33% still required DMARD therapy.[24] Another study of patients with JPsA followed for at least 5 years demonstrated persistently active disease in 70% and limitations of physical activity in one-third.[19] A more recent study with shorter follow-up documented achievement of clinical remission (on medication) in approximately 60% in both younger and older children, although younger patients required longer to achieve this endpoint.[21] Impaired visual function may also occur, especially if uveitis is not discovered promptly.

REFERENCES

1. J.M. Moll, V. Wright, Psoriatic arthritis, Sem. Arthritis Rheum. 3 (1973) 55–78.
5. R.E. Petty, T.R. Southwood, P. Manners, et al., International League of Associations for Rheumatology classification of juvenile idiopathic arthritis: second revision, Edmonton, 2001, J. Rheumatol. 31 (2004) 390–392.
6. T.R. Southwood, R.E. Petty, P.N. Malleson, et al., Psoriatic arthritis in children, Arthritis Rheum. 32 (1989) 1007–1013.
7. J.R. Lambert, B.M. Ansell, E. Stephenson, et al., Psoriatic arthritis in childhood, Clin. Rheum. Dis. 2 (1976) 339–352.
15. A. Shore, B.M. Ansell, Juvenile psoriatic arthritis—an analysis of 60 cases, J. Pediatr. 100 (1982) 529–535.
17. M.L. Hamilton, D.D. Gladman, A. Shore, et al., Juvenile psoriatic arthritis and HLA antigens, Ann. Rheum. Dis. 49 (1990) 694–697.
19. D.M. Roberton, D.A. Cabral, P.N. Malleson, et al., Juvenile psoriatic arthritis: followup and evaluation of diagnostic criteria, J. Rheumatol. 23 (1996) 166–170.
20. C. Huemer, P.N. Malleson, D.A. Cabral, et al., Patterns of joint involvement at onset differentiate oligoarticular juvenile psoriatic arthritis from pauciarticular juvenile rheumatoid arthritis, J. Rheumatol. 29 (2002) 1531–1535.
21. M.L. Stoll, D. Zurakowski, L.E. Nigrovic, et al., Patients with juvenile psoriatic arthritis comprise two distinct populations, Arthritis Rheum. 54 (2006) 3564–3572.
23. M.L. Stoll, P. Lio, R.P. Sundel, et al., Comparison of Vancouver and International League of Associations for Rheumatology classification criteria for juvenile psoriatic arthritis, Arthritis Rheum. 59 (2008) 51–58.
24. B. Flato, G. Lien, A. Smerdel-Ramoya, et al., Juvenile psoriatic arthritis: longterm outcome and differentiation from other subtypes of juvenile idiopathic arthritis, J. Rheumatol. 36 (2009) 642–650.
25. V. Wright, Rheumatism and psoriasis: a re-evaluation, Amer. J. Med. 27 (1959) 454–462.
38. R.K. Saurenmann, A.V. Levin, B.M. Feldman, et al., Prevalence, risk factors, and outcome of uveitis in juvenile idiopathic arthritis: a long-term followup study, Arthritis Rheum. 56 (2007) 647–657.
43. E. Kruithof, V. Van den Bossche, L. De Rycke, et al., Distinct synovial immunopathologic characteristics of juvenile-onset spondylarthritis and other forms of juvenile idiopathic arthritis, Arthritis Rheum. 54 (2006) 2594–2604.
44. R.J. Reece, J.D. Canete, W.J. Parsons, et al., Distinct vascular patterns of early synovitis in psoriatic, reactive, and rheumatoid arthritis, Arthritis Rheum. 42 (1999) 1481–1484.
45. J.D. Canete, J.R. Rodriguez, G. Salvador, et al., Diagnostic usefulness of synovial vascular morphology in chronic arthritis: a systematic survey of 100 cases, Sem. Arthritis Rheum. 32 (2003) 378–387.
48. D. Veale, G. Yanni, S. Rogers, et al., Reduced synovial membrane macrophage numbers, ELAM-1 expression, and lining layer hyperplasia in psoriatic arthritis as compared with rheumatoid arthritis, Arthritis Rheum. 36 (1993) 893–900.
49. E. Kruithof, D. Baeten, L. De Rycke, et al., Synovial histopathology of psoriatic arthritis, both oligo- and polyarticular, resembles spondyloarthropathy more than it does rheumatoid arthritis, Arthritis Res. Therapy 7 (2005) R569–580.
53. A.W. van Kuijk, P. Reinders-Blankert, T.J. Smeets, et al., Detailed analysis of the cell infiltrate and the expression of mediators of synovial inflammation and joint destruction in the synovium of patients with psoriatic arthritis: implications for treatment, Ann. Rheum. Dis. 65 (2006) 1551–1557.
55. P.J. Costello, R.J. Winchester, S.A. Curran, et al., Psoriatic arthritis joint fluids are characterized by CD8 and CD4 T cell clonal expansions that appear antigen driven, J. Immunol. 166 (4) (2001) 2878–2886.
56. D. Baeten, P. Demetter, C.A. Cuvelier, et al., Macrophages expressing the scavenger receptor CD163: a link between immune alterations of the gut and synovial inflammation in spondyloarthropathy, J. Pathol. 196 (2002) 343–350.
57. B. Vandooren, T. Noordenbos, C. Ambarus, et al., Absence of a classically activated macrophage cytokine signature in peripheral spondylarthritis, including psoriatic arthritis, Arthritis Rheum. 60 (2009) 966–975.
58. T.J. Pekin Jr., N.J. Zvaifler, Hemolytic complement in synovial fluid, J. Clin. Invest. 43 (1964) 1372–1382.
59. O. Fyrand, O.J. Mellbye, J.B. Natvig, Immunofluorescence studies for immunoglobulins and complement C3 in synovial joint membranes in psoriatic arthritis, Clin. Exp. Immunol. 29 (1977) 422–427.

61. J. Ball, Enthesopathy of rheumatoid and ankylosing spondylitis, Ann. Rheum. Dis. 30 (1971) 213–223.
63. D. McGonagle, H. Marzo-Ortega, P. O'Connor, et al., Histological assessment of the early enthesitis lesion in spondyloarthropathy, Ann. Rheum. Dis. 61 (2002) 534–537.
64. D. McGonagle, W. Gibbon, P. O'Connor, et al., Characteristic magnetic resonance imaging entheseal changes of knee synovitis in spondylarthropathy, Arthritis Rheum. 41 (1998) 694–700.
65. E.Y. Lee, R.P. Sundel, S. Kim, et al., MRI findings of juvenile psoriatic arthritis, Skeletal. Radiol. 37 (2008) 987–996.
67. J.M. Moll, V. Wright, Familial occurrence of psoriatic arthritis, Ann. Rheum. Dis. 32 (1973) 181–201.
68. P. Rahman, J.T. Elder, Genetic epidemiology of psoriasis and psoriatic arthritis, Ann. Rheum. Dis. 64 (Suppl. 2) (2005) ii37–ii39. discussion ii40-41.
69. O.B. Pedersen, A.J. Svendsen, L. Ejstrup, et al., On the heritability of psoriatic arthritis: disease concordance among monozygotic and dizygotic twins, Ann. Rheum. Dis. 67 (2008) 1417–1421.
72. I. Olivieri, A. Padula, S. D'Angelo, et al., Role of trauma in psoriatic arthritis, J. Rheumatol. 35 (2008) 2085–2087.
79. R. Church, The prospect of psoriasis, Br. J. Dermatol. 70 (1958) 139–145.
81. P. Rahman, D.D. Gladman, C.T. Schentag, A. Petronis, Excessive paternal transmission in psoriatic arthritis, Arthritis Rheum. 42 (1999) 1228–1231.
82. A. Myers, L.J. Kay, S.A. Lynch, et al., Recurrence risk for psoriasis and psoriatic arthritis within sibships, Rheumatology (Oxford) 44 (2005) 773–776.
83. V. Chandran, C.T. Schentag, J.E. Brockbank, et al., Familial aggregation of psoriatic arthritis, Ann. Rheum. Dis. 68 (2009) 664–667.
86. P.Y. Ho, A. Barton, J. Worthington, et al., Investigating the role of the HLA-Cw06 and HLA-DRB1 genes in susceptibility to psoriatic arthritis: comparison with psoriasis and undifferentiated inflammatory arthritis, Ann. Rheum. Dis. 67 (2008) 677–682.
87. B. Ansell, M. Beeson, P. Hall, et al., HLA and juvenile psoriatic arthritis, Br. J. Rheumatol. 32 (1993) 836–837.
99. G. Partsch, G. Steiner, B.F. Leeb, et al., Highly increased levels of tumor necrosis factor-alpha and other proinflammatory cytokines in psoriatic arthritis synovial fluid, J. Rheumatol. 24 (1997) 518–523.
100. C. Ritchlin, S.A. Haas-Smith, D. Hicks, et al., Patterns of cytokine production in psoriatic synovium, J. Rheumatol. 25 (1998) 1544–1552.
102. A.J. Hueber, I.B. McInnes, Immune regulation in psoriasis and psoriatic arthritis–recent developments, Immunol. Let. 114 (2007) 59–65.
110. D.D. Gladman, R. Shuckett, M.L. Russell, et al., Psoriatic arthritis (PSA)—an analysis of 220 patients, Q. J. Med. 62 (1987) 127–141.
114. P.V. Balint, D. Kane, H. Wilson, et al., Ultrasonography of entheseal insertions in the lower limb in spondyloarthropathy, Ann. Rheum. Dis. 61 (2002) 905–910.
115. M.A. D'Agostino, R. Said-Nahal, C. Hacquard-Bouder, et al., Assessment of peripheral enthesitis in the spondylarthropathies by ultrasonography combined with power Doppler: a cross-sectional study, Arthritis Rheum. 48 (2003) 23–33.
116. D. McGonagle, R.J. Lories, A.L. Tan, et al., The concept of a "synovio-entheseal complex" and its implications for understanding joint inflammation and damage in psoriatic arthritis and beyond, Arthritis Rheum. 56 (2007) 2482–2491.
120. I. Olivieri, C. Salvarani, F. Cantini, et al., Fast spin echo-T2-weighted sequences with fat saturation in dactylitis of spondylarthritis: no evidence of entheseal involvement of the flexor digitorum tendons, Arthritis Rheum. 46 (2002) 2964–2967.
122. P.J. Healy, C. Groves, M. Chandramohan, P.S. Helliwell, MRI changes in psoriatic dactylitis–extent of pathology, relationship to tenderness and correlation with clinical indices, Rheumatology (Oxford) 47 (2008) 92–95.
124. Y. Butbul, P. Tyrrell, R. Schneider, et al., Comparison of patients with juvenile psoriatic arthritis (JPsA) and non-psoriatic juvenile idiopathic arthritis (JIA): are they distinct diseases? J. Rheumatol. 36 (2009) 2033–2041.
125. P.A. Nigrovic, Juvenile psoriatic arthritis: baby or bathwater? J. Rheumatol. 36 (2009) 1861–1863. (editorial).
128. R. Scarpa, E. Soscia, R. Peluso, et al., Nail and distal interphalangeal joint in psoriatic arthritis, J. Rheumatol. 33 (2006) 1315–1319.
130. A. Heiligenhaus, M. Niewerth, G. Ganser, et al., Prevalence and complications of uveitis in juvenile idiopathic arthritis in a population-based nation-wide study in Germany: suggested modification of the current screening guidelines, Rheumatology (Oxford) 46 (2007) 1015–1019.
150. A. Martini, Are the number of joints involved or the presence of psoriasis still useful tools to identify homogeneous disease entities in juvenile idiopathic arthritis? J. Rheumatol. 30 (2003) 1900–1903.
151. A. Ravelli, E. Felici, S. Magni-Manzoni, et al., Patients with antinuclear antibody-positive juvenile idiopathic arthritis constitute a homogeneous subgroup irrespective of the course of joint disease, Arthritis Rheum. 52 (2005) 826–832.
154. W. Taylor, D. Gladman, P. Helliwell, et al., Classification criteria for psoriatic arthritis: development of new criteria from a large international study, Arthritis Rheum. 54 (2006) 2665–2673.
155. M. Benjamin, D. McGonagle, The anatomical basis for disease localisation in seronegative spondyloarthropathy at entheses and related sites,, J. Anatomy 199 (Pt 5) (2001) 503–526.
156. M. Benjamin, H. Toumi, D. Suzuki, et al., Microdamage and altered vascularity at the enthesis-bone interface provides an anatomic explanation for bone involvement in the HLA-B27-associated spondylarthritides and allied disorders, Arthritis Rheum. 56 (2007) 224–233.
157. H. Marzo-Ortega, S.F. Tanner, L.A. Rhodes, et al., Magnetic resonance imaging in the assessment of metacarpophalangeal joint disease in early psoriatic and rheumatoid arthritis, Scand. J. Rheumatol. 38 (2009) 79–83.
158. A.L. Tan, A.J. Grainger, S.F. Tanner, et al., A high-resolution magnetic resonance imaging study of distal interphalangeal joint arthropathy in psoriatic arthritis and osteoarthritis: are they the same? Arthritis Rheum. 54 (2006) 1328–1333.
159. A.L. Tan, M. Benjamin, H. Toumi, et al., The relationship between the extensor tendon enthesis and the nail in distal interphalangeal joint disease in psoriatic arthritis—a high-resolution MRI and histological study, Rheumatology (Oxford) 46 (2007) 253–256.
160. V. Wright, M.C. Roberts, A.G. Hill, Dermatological manifestations in psoriatic arthritis: a follow-up study, Acta. Dermato-Venereologica. 59 (3) (1979) 235–240.

Entire reference list is available online at www.expertconsult.com.

Chapter 19

ARTHROPATHIES OF INFLAMMATORY BOWEL DISEASE

Carol B. Lindsley and Ronald M. Laxer

DEFINITION AND CLASSIFICATION

The arthropathies of inflammatory bowel disease (IBD) may be defined as any noninfectious arthritis occurring before or during the course of Crohn's Disease (CD), indeterminate colitis (IC), or ulcerative colitis (UC). Arthritis is the most common extraintestinal complication of these disorders.[1] There are two patterns of joint inflammation: peripheral polyarthritis and, less commonly, involvement of the sacroiliac (SI) joints and axial skeleton. Arthritis associated with IBD is not included in the American College of Rheumatology classification of childhood arthritis but is included in both the European League Against Rheumatism and International League of Associations for Rheumatology criteria (see Chapter 13).

EPIDEMIOLOGY

Incidence and Prevalence

Arthropathy has been reported in 7% to 21% of children with IBD[2-6] (Table 19–1). Passo and colleagues[6] found arthritis in 9% of 44 children with UC and in 15.5% of 58 children with CD. Arthralgia was much more common, occurring in 32% of those with UC and 22% of those with CD.[6] Differentiation of UC from CD is not always easy, and differences in the reported frequencies of arthritis in each may reflect the accuracy of diagnosis in these types of IBD.[3,4] A recent study showed much lower frequencies of 1% in CD and 2% in UC. These lower frequencies may reflect the current therapies for the IBD.[7] Other children have myalgia, skeletal pain associated with glucocorticoid-induced osteopenia, or secondary hypertrophic osteoarthropathy without objective arthritis. Although there has been concern about an increasing incidence of IBD worldwide, a recent Swedish study reported a stable and unchanged rate of UC and CD during the past 30 years.[8]

Age at Onset and Sex Ratio

In a study of 136 patients with onset of IBD before the age of 20 years,[5] age at onset did not differ in patients with and without arthritis. The ratios of boys to girls in those with and without peripheral arthritis were almost identical, although the five children who developed spondylitis were boys.

ETIOLOGY AND PATHOGENESIS

The causes of both IBD and the accompanying arthritis are obscure. The possible roles of gastrointestinal (GI) infections or allergic reactions to foods absorbed across an inflamed mucosa remain speculative. The SI arthritis probably shares its etiology with that of ankylosing spondylitis (AS), and studies of associated enteric species and immunity to them may be relevant.[9] Peripheral arthropathy may involve entirely different immunoinflammatory mechanisms (immune complexes), however, and it is clinically more closely related to the activity of the intestinal disease. Picco and colleagues[10] found increased gut permeability in all subtypes of juvenile arthritis using the lactulose/mannitol test, but IBD patients with spondyloarthropathy had the highest levels. Reciprocally, subclinical gut inflammation in the majority of patients with seronegative spondyloarthropathy has been described.[11]

GENETIC BACKGROUND

There is a pronounced tendency for familial, racial, and ethnic clustering of UC and CD. Hamilton and associates[3] reported that approximately 15% of children with UC and 8% of those with CD had first-degree relatives with IBD. Both diseases are more common in children of Jewish descent, who composed 21% of the IBD population but only 2% of the general population in one study.[3] Published reports support the view that genes

Table 19–1

Arthritis in inflammatory bowel disease in children

Author and Year (ref. no.)	Disease	No. Patients	No. with Arthritis	% with Arthritis
Farmer & Michener, 1979 (2)	CD	522	39	7
Hamilton et al, 1979 (3)	CD	58	11	19
Burbige et al, 1975 (4)	CD	58	6	10
Lindsley & Schaller, 1974 (5)	CD	50	5	10
Passo et al, 1986 (6)	CD	58	9	15
Lindsley & Schaller, 1974 (5)	UC	86	18	21
Hamilton et al, 1979 (3)	UC	87	8	9
Passo et al, 1986 (6)	UC	44	4	9

CD, Crohn's Disease (regional enteritis); UC, ulcerative colitis.

of the major histocompatibility complex are important in determining susceptibility to UC in particular,[12] but inherited predispositions are undoubtedly polygenic. In Japanese[13] and Jewish patients,[14] but not in other ethnic groups, the human leukocyte antigen (HLA) DRB1*1502 (DR2) allele is increased in frequency. It is estimated that SI arthritis is at least 30 times more common in patients with IBD than in the general population,[15] a fact that reflects the high frequency of HLA-B27 in such patients. The peripheral polyarthritis accompanying IBD has no known HLA association.

Studies have identified NOD2/Card 15 variants that are associated with CD in both children and adults, particularly in those with ileal disease and lower weight at time of diagnosis.[16] However, no association has been reported with articular involvement or AS.[17] Recently, genome-wide associations between the IL-23 R gene and CD have been shown in the pediatric age group.[18] In a separate study, Leshinsky and colleagues showed that haplotypes without the common disease-associated mutations in the NOD2/Card 15 and TLR genes are associated with age at onset of the IBD.[19]

CLINICAL MANIFESTATIONS

Arthritis and Enthesitis

Two distinct patterns of joint disease occur. The more common one in patients with IBD is inflammation affecting peripheral joints. Lower extremity joints, especially ankles and knees, are most frequently affected,[4-6] although upper extremity joints, occasionally also including small joints of the hand and the temporomandibular joints, may be involved. Lindsley and Schaller[5] reported that 4 or fewer joints were affected at onset or during the

course of the illness in 11 of 18 children; in 5 children, 5 to 9 joints were affected; in only 2 children were more than 10 joints affected, including small joints of the hand. Episodes of acute peripheral arthritis are usually brief, lasting 1 or 2 weeks (occasionally longer), and tend to recur.[6] In some children, arthritis may last for several months, particularly if the GI disease is active. Rarely, joint inflammation persists for months, although permanent functional loss or joint damage is unusual. However, erosive disease has been described in young adults with juvenile-onset disease.[20,21] Whereas the SI arthritis bears little relation to the activity of the gut disease, the peripheral arthritis reflects the activity and course of the GI inflammation. A clinical flare-up in a child's arthritis is suggestive of poor control of the underlying IBD.

In adult patients, additional clinical phenotypes have been described in the peripheral arthropathy group (non–HLA-B27 associated): type I, which is similar to the previously described disease and is frequently associated with uveitis and erythema nodosum (EN), and type II, which is a symmetrical polyarthritis that is independent of IBD activity, of longer duration, and rarely associated with EN.[22]

SI arthritis, which may be asymptomatic but often is characterized by pain and stiffness in the lower back, buttocks, or thighs, is a much less common complication of IBD than is polyarthritis. It is sometimes accompanied by enthesitis identical to that occurring in other forms of spondyloarthritis. SI arthritis may also be associated with chronic symmetrical oligoarthritis predominantly affecting the joints of the lower limbs: 5% to 10% of established cases of AS in adults are associated with chronic IBD.[23] Also, an additional category of asymptomatic SI disease (18%) occurs in patients with IBD, most often in those with greater disease duration.[24]

Hypertrophic osteoarthropathy is a relatively rare, very painful musculoskeletal complication of IBD.[25] The pain occurs symmetrically in the limbs (rather than the joints) and may be accompanied by increased sweating and purple discoloration of the affected limbs.

Osteoporosis can be a significant component of articular disease or, rarely, a presenting manifestation when associated with fractures.[26] Patients treated with steroids are especially at high risk, and in addition they may develop avascular necrosis, most commonly involving the femoral head. However, non–steroid-treated patients have about a 12% risk to develop osteoporosis as well.[27] Chronic recurrent multifocal osteomyelitis has been associated with IBD in some patients.[28]

Gastrointestinal Disease and Extraarticular Manifestations

Gastrointestinal Disease

Cramping abdominal pain, often with localized or generalized tenderness, anorexia, and diarrhea, sometimes occurring at night, is characteristic of IBD. Differentiation of UC and CD on the basis of GI symptoms alone is unreliable, although bloody diarrhea is highly suggestive of UC, whereas perianal skin tags and fistulae are typical of CD (Table 19–2). More recent terminology adds the

Table 19–2

Gastrointestinal and other systemic diseases in children with inflammatory bowel diseases

Symptom or Sign	Ulcerative Colitis	Crohn's Disease
Diarrhea	++++	++
Hematochezia	++	+
Abdominal pain	++	+++
Weight loss	++	++++
Fever	+	+++
Vomiting	+	++
Perianal disease	+	+++
Finger clubbing	+	++
Erythema nodosum	+	+
Oral lesions	+	+
Uveitis	(+)	(+)
Pyoderma gangrenosum	(+)	(+)

Frequency: (+), rare; +, <25%; ++, 25-50%; +++, 50-75%; ++++, ≥75%.

category of IC.[7] Many of these patients will meet criteria for a revised diagnosis, usually UC, within 2 years.[7]

GI symptoms usually precede joint disease by months or years, although occasionally both systems are affected simultaneously or joint symptoms precede intestinal disease. In the latter case, the arthritis resembles that of juvenile idiopathic arthritis, juvenile AS, or the seronegative enthesopathy and arthropathy syndrome, with a course punctuated by intermittent abdominal pain that may be incorrectly ascribed to the effects of antiinflammatory drugs. Low-grade diarrhea, anemia, unexplained fever, weight loss, growth retardation out of proportion to the extent and activity of the joint disease, or a family history of IBD should alert the physician to the possibility of occult IBD. Mucocutaneous lesions (EN, aphthous stomatitis, pyoderma gangrenosum) seem to be more common in children who have arthritis (especially peripheral arthritis) as a complication of IBD, although this association is not supported by some clinical studies.[6]

Although there are no clear cut correlations between the extent of GI inflammation and arthritis, most reports support the view that there is a higher frequency of arthritis in children with extensive, as opposed to segmental, bowel disease.[2,3,6] Patients with arthritis usually have active gut disease, although the onset of arthritis is not necessarily related to obvious flare-ups in GI tract inflammation. The occurrence of first-time joint symptoms after proctocolectomy for UC has been associated with the development of "pouchitis."[29]

Erythema Nodosum

The lesions of EN (nodular panniculitis) occur most commonly in the subcutaneous fat of the pretibial region (Fig. 19–1) as erythematous, painful, slightly elevated lesions, 1 to 2 cm in diameter, that erupt in groups and reappear sequentially in new areas after several days. The nodules tend to persist for several weeks and recur in crops for several months. As they heal, they frequently leave pigmented areas that persist for many months. Articular pain and synovitis accompany each exacerbation in

approximately two-thirds of instances. Erythema nodosum is more likely associated with peripheral arthritis that is of short duration and involving few joints.[22]

Although EN may also occur as a distinct, isolated clinical syndrome, it is commonly associated with systemic illness of diverse causes, including IBD.[30,31]

Pyoderma Gangrenosum

The lesions of pyoderma gangrenosum may occur alone or in concert with IBD (Fig. 19–2). They often arise after minor trauma, may be single or multiple, and usually begin as a pustule that breaks down and rapidly enlarges to form a chronic, painful, deep, undermined ulcer with a red, raised border. They have rarely been reported in children but may in fact be the initial clinical manifestation. In adults, the lesions occur with IBD, rheumatoid arthritis, or other systemic diseases.[32] A single report, not confirmed, of pyoderma gangrenosum in a 2-year-old boy with joint effusions but without IBD was associated with enhanced leukocyte mobility.[33] This may have been an early description of the pyogenic arthritis, pyoderma gangrenosum and acne syndrome (see chapter 43).

Oral Lesions

Occasionally, painful oral ulcerations are seen, particularly in CD (Fig. 19–3). These may precede the onset of prominent GI symptoms. If recurrent, the patient may be misdiagnosed as having Behçet disease.

Vasculitis

Vasculitis of several types has been reported in patients with IBD and arthritis. Involvement of large vessels was found in at least two studies.[34,35] Takayasu arteritis in patients with CD was first described in 1970[36] and has been reported in several other adults and in a 15-year-old boy,[37] as well as in a young adult with UC and juvenile AS.[38] It seems unlikely that coincidence could account for the simultaneous occurrence of these rare diseases, but the data are insufficient to allow for certainty. A syndrome of cutaneous vasculitis, glomerulonephritis, and circulating immune complexes was reported in two adults with IBD and spondyloarthritis (one with juvenile-onset colitis).[39] Immunoglobulin A nephropathy has been described in AS and in at least three patients with IBD.[40,41] Cutaneous vasculitis was reported as the presenting feature in a 14-year-old girl with CD.[42]

Uveitis

Lyons and Rosenbaum[43] compared the characteristics of uveitis in 17 adults with IBD and 89 patients with spondyloarthritis. Twelve of the 15 patients with uveitis and IBD had CD, and 82% were female. Uveitis accompanying IBD was usually bilateral, posterior, and of insidious onset and chronic duration. The frequency of HLA-B27 was one half that in the spondyloarthritis group. Episcleritis, scleritis, and glaucoma were more common among patients with IBD. At least in adults, the uveitis associated with IBD was frequently complicated by cataract (35%), glaucoma (24%), cystoid macular edema (24%), or posterior synechiae (29%).[43] There are no reported studies of uveitis in children with IBD and arthritis. However, it is known that children with IBD may develop asymptomatic uveitis.[44]

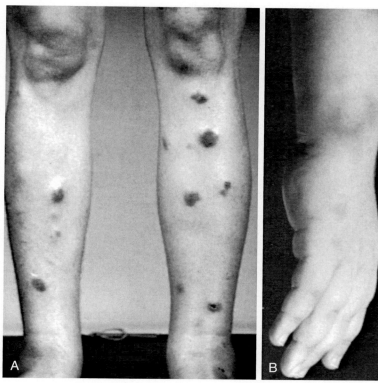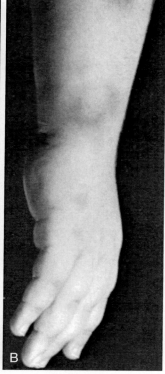

FIGURE 19–1   Erythema nodosum. **A,** This young girl had tender, circumscribed purple-red nodules on the shins. **B,** Lesions on the forearm of a child.

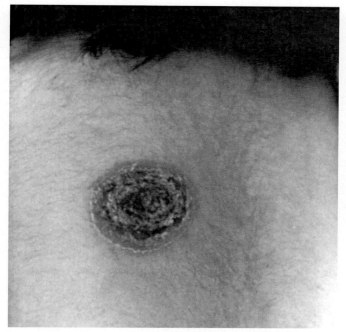

FIGURE 19–2   Pyoderma gangrenosum on the upper back of a child. These lesions begin as nodules but progress to ulcers with considerable loss of subcutaneous tissue.

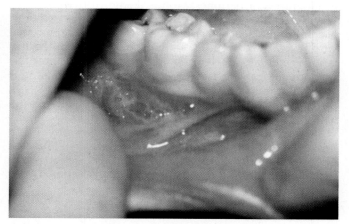

FIGURE 19–3   Oral ulcer in a child with ulcerative colitis

histiocytes.[45] Granulomatous synovitis occasionally occurs.[46] For a discussion on the full spectrum of the histopathology of IBD, the reader is referred to current textbooks of gastroenterology.

DIAGNOSIS AND LABORATORY EXAMINATION

Making the diagnosis of arthritis associated with IBD rests on recognition of the significance of this association and on a high level of clinical suspicion. A diagnosis of IBD should be suspected in any child with arthritis accompanied by lower abdominal pain, hematochezia, unexplained weight loss, anemia, fever, or poor growth.

PATHOLOGY

The histopathology of the synovitis of IBD is nonspecific with proliferation of lining cells and infiltration of the synovium with lymphocytes, plasma cells, and

Occult GI blood loss can be verified by repeated stool guaiac examinations.

This suspicion would be supported by laboratory evidence of inflammation (high erythrocyte sedimentation rate and other acute phase reactants, low serum albumin), and negative results for rheumatoid factor and antinuclear antibody tests. Antibodies to neutrophil cytoplasmic antigens (pANCA—a perinuclear pattern on immunofluorescence) and anti–Saccharomyces cerevisiae antibody (ASCA) are frequently present in the sera of children with IBD.[47] Tests for antineutrophil cytoplasmic antibody (ANCA) were positive in 73% of children with UC and 14% of those with CD.[48] In spite of the known association of this autoantibody with systemic vasculitis, vasculitis does not appear to be more frequent in ANCA-positive patients with IBD.[49] A potential new marker for intestinal inflammation in IBD is the fecal pyruvate kinase test.[50]

Synovial fluid analyses of children with IBD have not been reported, although in adults counts of synovial fluid white blood cells have ranged from 5000 to 15,000/mm³ (5 to 15 × 10⁹/L), with a predominance of neutrophils. Synovial fluid protein, glucose, and hemolytic complement levels have been normal.[51]

RADIOLOGICAL EXAMINATION

Radiographs of peripheral joints document only soft tissue thickening and joint effusions. SI arthritis, when it occurs, is not clearly distinguishable from that associated with juvenile AS. Spur formation, the result of enthesitis, is sometimes identified at the insertion of the plantar fascia into the calcaneus. Periostitis may be demonstrable by radiography or by radionuclide scanning (Fig. 19–4). Burbige and coworkers[4] noted erosive lesions secondary to granulomatous synovitis in one child. Although radionucleotide scanning or magnetic resonance imaging is optimal for documenting early changes in SI joints, high-resolution computed tomography is more reliable in detecting erosions and documenting calcifications.[52]

TREATMENT

Successful management of the peripheral arthritis generally depends on effective treatment of the GI disease: Control of the primary disease usually results in remission of the peripheral arthritis. Colectomy in UC may be followed by a striking remission in peripheral joint symptoms, although colectomy for the control of peripheral joint arthritis alone is certainly not indicated. Peripheral arthritis may be managed with nonsteroidal antiinflammatory agents, but there is increasing evidence that these drugs can exacerbate IBD.[53] Selective cyclooxygenase-2 inhibitors may be preferred in this situation. Early use of sulfasalazine or glucocorticoids may provide the best management of the arthropathy of IBD directly by way of a beneficial effect on the GI inflammation, although no therapeutic trials have been published. For persistent arthritis in one or two joints, intra-articular glucocorticoid should be considered. In CD, the use of oral budesonide,

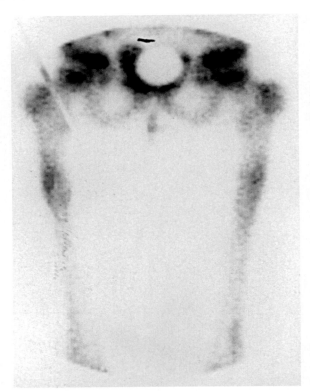

FIGURE 19–4   Bone scan documents increased uptake in the sacroiliac joints and along the femoral shafts, representing sacroiliac joint arthritis and periostitis in a 14-year-old girl with ulcerative colitis.

predominantly a topically acting steroid, resulted in the remission of joint symptoms in 74% of affected patients.[54]

Methotrexate results in improvement of both GI symptoms and arthritis in CD.[55] Anti-TNF therapy, particularly infliximab, produced prompt, substantial improvement in CD of GI symptoms as well as arthritis.[56] Adalimumab may be useful as well, and there is reported improvement in bowel manifestations in patients who failed infliximab and subsequently were treated with adalimumab.[57] However, etanercept has not been reported to be effective in IBD. As these potent antiinflammatory drugs are used earlier and more aggressively in the treatment of IBD, it is possible that the associated arthropathies will decrease in frequency or severity. However, patients with JIA have developed CD while on therapy with etanercept.[58]

The HLA-B27–associated spondylitis of IBD is much more likely than the peripheral arthritis to persist and progress without remission, independent of the activity of the GI disease and unaffected by procedures such as colectomy. It is therefore much more difficult to manage in the long term. Sulfasalazine is the initial drug choice, in a dose of 30 to 50 mg/kg/day to a maximum of 2.5 g/day. Methotrexate and anti-TNF agents may also be helpful in patients who have no response to initial therapy. A physical therapy program with range-of-motion exercises to maintain back and chest motion (as for juvenile AS) may help to prevent or slow the effects of the disease. Custom-made orthotics may be useful to minimize pain secondary to enthesitis around the foot. Vasculitis accompanying IBD should be treated with systemic glucocorticoids. Topical glucocorticoids are used to treat uveitis.

COURSE OF THE DISEASE AND PROGNOSIS

The outcome of GI disease is the most important determinant of overall prognosis in the child with IBD and arthritis.[2] Prognosis of the peripheral joint disease is usually excellent, although axial disease may progress independent of the course of the GI inflammation. Permanent changes in the spine and hips are frequent in this group of children. Poor nutrition and accompanying growth retardation may be major problems in poorly controlled disease. Advances in therapeutics will no doubt result in improved short- and long-term outcomes for patients with IBD.

REFERENCES

1. F.A. Jose, E.A. Garnett, E. Vittinghoff, et al., Development of extraintestinal manifestations in pediatric patients with inflammatory bowel disease, Inflamm. Bowel Dis. 15 (2009) 63–83.
2. R.G. Farmer, W.M. Michener, Prognosis of Crohn's Disease with onset in childhood or adolescence, Dig. Dis. Sci. 24 (1979) 752.
3. J.R. Hamilton, M.D. Bruce, M. Abdourhaman, et al., Inflammatory bowel disease in children and adolescents, Adv. Pediatr. 26 (1979) 311–341.
4. E.J. Burbige, H. Shi-Shung, T.M. Bayless, Clinical manifestations of Crohn's Disease in children and adolescents, Pediatrics 55 (1975) 866–871.
5. C. Lindsley, J.G. Schaller, Arthritis associated with inflammatory bowel disease in children, J. Pediatr. 84 (1974) 16–20.
6. M.H. Passo, J.F. Fitzgerald, K.D. Brandt, Arthritis associated with inflammatory bowel disease in children: relationship of joint disease to activity and severity of bowel lesion, Dig. Dis. Sci. 31 (1986) 492–497.
7. E.A. Newby, N.M. Croft, M. Green, et al., Natural history of paediatric inflammatory bowel diseases over a two-year follow-up: a retrospective review of data from the register of paediatric inflammatory bowel diseases, J. Pediatr. Gastroenterol. Nutr. 46 (2008) 539–545.
8. B.S. Bensen, B. Moum, A. Ekbom, Incidence of inflammatory bowel disease in children in southeastern Norway, Scand. J. Gastroenterol. 37 (2002) 540–545.
9. A. Keat, Infections and the immunopathogenesis of seronegative spondyloarthropathies, Curr. Opin. Rheumatol. 4 (1992) 494–499.
10. P. Picco, M. Gattorno, N. Marchese, et al., Increased gut permeability in juvenile chronic arthritides: a multivariate analysis of the diagnostic parameters, Clin. Exp. Rheumatol. 18 (2000) 773–778.
11. M. Devos, C. Cuvelier, H. Mielants, et al., Ileocolonoscopy in seronegative spondyloarthropathy, Gastroenterology 96 (1989) 339–344.
12. J. Satsangi, D.P. Jewell, J.I. Bell, The genetics of inflammatory bowel disease, Gut 40 (1997) 572–574.
13. S. Futami, N. Aoyama, Y. Honsako, et al., HLA-DRB1*1502 alleles, subtype of DR15 is associated with susceptibility to ulcerative colitis and its progression, Dig. Dis. Sci. 40 (1995) 814–818.
14. H. Toyoda, S-J. Wang, H. Yang, et al., Distinct association of HLA class II genes with inflammatory bowel disease, Gastroenterology 104 (1993) 741–748.
15. D.A. Brewerton, D.C.O. James, The histocompatibility antigen HLA-27 and disease, Semin. Arthritis Rheum. 4 (1975) 191–207.
16. G. Tomer, C. Ceballos, E. Concepcion, et al., NOD2/CARD15 variants are associated with lower weight at diagnosis in children with Crohn's Disease, Am. J. Gastroenterol. 98 (2003) 2479–2484.
17. I. Ferreiros-Vidal, J. Amarelo, F. Barros, et al., Lack of association of ankylosing spondylitis with the most common NOD2 susceptibility alleles in Crohn's Disease, J. Rheumatol. 30 (2003) 102–104.
18. D.K. Amre, D. Mack, D. Israel, et al., Association between genetic variants in the IL-23R gene and early-onset Crohn's disease: Results from a case-control and family-based study among Canadian children, Am. J. Gastroenterol. 103 (2008) 615–620.
19. E. Leshinsky-Silver, A. Karban, E. Buzhakor, et al., Is age of onset of Crohn's Disease governed by mutations in NOD2/caspase recruitment domains 15 and Toll-like receptor 4? Evaluation of a pediatric cohort, Pediatr. Res. 58 (2005) 499–504.
20. A. el Maghraoui, A. Aouragh, M. Hachim, et al., Erosive arthritis in juvenile onset Crohn's Disease, Clin. Exp. Rheumatol. 18 (2000) 541.
21. K. Benbouazza, R. Bahiri, H.E. Krami, et al., Erosive polyarthritis in Crohn's Disease: report of a case, Rev. Rhum. 66 (1999) 743–746.
22. T.R. Orchard, B.P. Wordsworth, D.P. Jewell, Peripheral arthropathies in inflammatory bowel disease: their articular distribution and natural history, Gut 42 (1998) 387–391.
23. P. Wordsworth, Arthritis and inflammatory bowel disease, Curr. Rheumatol. Rep. 2 (2000) 87–88.
24. K. de Vlam, H. Mielants, C. Cuvelier, et al., Spondyloarthropathy is underestimated in inflammatory bowel disease: prevalence and HLA association, J. Rheum. 27 (2000) 2860–2865.
25. G. Neale, A.R. Kelsall, F.H. Doyte, Crohn's Disease and diffuse symmetrical periostitis, Gut 9 (1968) 383–387.
26. M. Thearle, M. Horlick, J.P. Bilezikian, et al., Osteoporosis: an unusual presentation of childhood Crohn's Disease, Endocrinol. Metab. 85 (2000) 2122–2126.
27. F. Walther, C. Fusch, M. Radke, et al., Osteoporosis in pediatric patients suffering from chronic inflammatory bowel disease with and without steroid treatment, J. Pediatr. Gastroenterol. Nutr. 43 (2006) 42–51.
28. A.M. Huber, P.Y. Lam, C.M. Duffy, et al., Chronic recurrent multifocal osteomyelitis: clinical outcomes after more than five years of follow-up, J. Pediatr. 141 (2002) 198–203.
29. A. Balbir-Gurman, D. Schapira, M. Nahir, Arthritis related to ileal pouchitis following total proctocolectomy for ulcerative colitis, Semin. Arthritis Rheum. 30 (2001) 242–248.
30. J. Lorber, The changing etiology of erythema nodosum in children, Arch. Dis. Child 33 (1958) 137–141.
31. R.K. Winkelmann, L. Forstrom, New observations in the histopathology of erythema nodosum, J. Invest. Dermatol. 65 (1975) 441–446.
32. S. Hurwitz, Clinical Pediatric Dermatology, second ed., WB Saunders, Philadelphia, 1993.
33. J.C. Jacobs, E.J. Goetzl, "Streaking leukocyte factor," arthritis and pyoderma gangrenosum, Pediatrics 56 (1975) 570–578.
34. S. Yassinger, R. Adelman, D. Cantor, Association of inflammatory bowel disease and large vascular lesions, Gastroenterology 71 (1976) 844–846.
35. S. Gormally, W. Bourke, B. Kierse, et al., Isolated cerebral thrombo-embolism and Crohn's Disease, Eur. J. Pediatr. 154 (1995) 815–818.
36. M. Soloway, T.W. Moir, D.W. Linton, Takayasu's arteritis: report of a case with unusual findings, Am. J. Cardiol. 25 (1970) 258–263.
37. M.O. Hilário, M.T. Terreri, G. Prismich, et al., Association of ankylosing spondylitis, Crohn's Disease and Takayasu's arteritis in a child, Clin. Exp. Rheumatol. 16 (1998) 92–94.
38. S. Aoyagi, H. Akashi, T. Kawara, et al., Aortic root replacement for Takayasu arteritis associated with ulcerative colitis and ankylosing spondylitis-report of a case, Jpn. Circ. J. 62 (1998) 64–68.
39. A.J. Peeters, B.A.W. van den Wall, M.R. Daha, et al., Inflammatory bowel disease and ankylosing spondylitis was associated with cutaneous vasculitis, glomerulonephritis and circulating IgA immune complexes, Ann. Rheum. Dis. 49 (1990) 638–640.
40. S. Dard, S. Kenouch, J.P. Mery, et al., A new association: ankylosing spondylitis (AS) and Berger disease (BD), Kidney Int. 24 (1983) 129.
41. D. McCallum, L. Smith, F. Harley, et al., IgA nephropathy and thin basement membrane disease in association with Crohn's Disease, Pediatr. Nephrol. 11 (1997) 637–640.
42. M.H. Kay, R. Wyllie, Cutaneous vasculitis as the initial manifestation of Crohn's Disease in a pediatric patient, Am. J. Gastroenterol. 93 (1998) 1014.
43. J.L. Lyons, J.T. Rosenbaum, Uveitis associated with inflammatory bowel disease compared with uveitis associated with spondyloarthropathy, Arch. Ophthalmol. 115 (1997) 61–64.
44. P. Hofley, J. Roarty, G. McGinnity, et al., Asymptomatic uveitis in children with chronic inflammatory bowel disease, J. Pediatric Gastroenterol. Nutr. 17 (1993) 397–400.
45. B.M. Ansell, R.A.D. Wigley, Arthritis manifestations in regional enteritis, Ann. Rheum. Dis. 23 (1964) 64–72.

46. H. Lindstrom, H. Wramsby, G. Ostberg, Granulomatous arthritis in Crohn's Disease, Gut 13 (1972) 257–259.
47. K. Khan, S.J. Schwarzenberg, H. Sharp, et al., Role of serology and routine laboratory tests in childhood inflammatory bowel disease, Inflamm. Bowel Dis. 8 (2002) 325–329.
48. J.P. Olives, A. Breton, J.P. Hugot, et al., Antineutrophil cytoplasmic antibodies in children with inflammatory bowel disease: prevalence and diagnostic value, J. Pediatr. Gastrol. Nutr. 25 (1997) 142–148.
49. C. Rosa, C. Esposito, A. Caglioti, et al., Does the presence of ANCA in patients with ulcerative colitis necessarily imply renal involvement? Nephrol. Dial. Transplant. 11 (1996) 2426–2429.
50. E. Czub, K.H. Herzig, A. Szaflarska-Popawska, et al., Fecal pyruvate kinase: a potential new marker for intestinal inflammation in children with inflammatory bowel disease, Scand. J. Gastroenterol. 42 (2007) 1147–1150.
51. T.W. Bunch, G.G. Hunder, F.C. McDuffie, et al., Synovial fluid complement determination as a diagnostic aid in inflammatory joint disease, Mayo. Clin. Proc. 49 (1974) 715–720.
52. A.R. Mester, E.K. Makò, K. Karlinger, et al., Enteropathic arthritis in the sacroiliac joint: imaging and different diagnosis, Eur. J. Radiol. 35 (2000) 199–208.
53. J.M. Evans, A.D. McMahon, F.E. Murray, et al., Non-steroidal anti-inflammatory drugs are associated with emergency admission to hospital for colitis due to inflammatory bowel disease, Gut 40 (1997) 619–622.
54. T.H.J. Florin, H. Graffner, L.G. Nilsson, et al., Treatment of joint pain in Crohn's patients with budesonide controlled ileal release, Clin. Exp. Pharmacol. Physiol. 27 (2000) 295–298.
55. D.R. Mack, R. Young, S.S. Kaufmann, et al., Methotrexate in patients with Crohn's Disease after 6-mercaptopurine, J. Rheumatol. 132 (1998) 830–835.
56. F. Van den Bosch, E. Kruithof, M. De Vos, et al., Crohn's Disease associated with spondyloarthropathy: effect of TNF-alpha blockade with infliximab on articular symptoms, Lancet 356 (2000) 1821–1822.
57. J.D. Noe, M. Pfefferkorn, Short-term response to adalimumab in childhood inflammatory bowel disease, Inflamm. Bowel Dis. 14 (2008) 1683–1687.
58. F.M. Ruemmle, A.M. Prieur, C. Talbotec, et al., Development of Crohn's disease during anti-TNF alpha therapy in a child with juvenile idiopathic arthritis, J. Pediatr. Gastroenterology Nutr. 39 (2004) 203–206.

Chapter 20

UVEITIS IN JUVENILE IDIOPATHIC ARTHRITIS

Ross E. Petty and James T. Rosenbaum

Inflammatory eye diseases comprise some of the most devastating complications of childhood rheumatic diseases, especially juvenile idiopathic arthritis (JIA). Chronic (initially asymptomatic) uveitis is the most common ocular complication of oligoarticular JIA. It is predominantly an insidious onset, anterior, nongranulomatous inflammation affecting the iris and ciliary body—an iridocyclitis (Fig. 20–1). Acute (symptomatic) anterior uveitis is characteristic of human leukocyte antigen-B27 (HLA-B27)–associated diseases such as enthesitis-related arthritis. The posterior uveal tract, the choroid, is rarely affected clinically.

CLASSIFICATION OF UVEITIS

It has been customary to classify anterior uveitis as *acute* or *chronic*, terms that are used imprecisely, and often synonymously, with *symptomatic* and *asymptomatic* respectively. The Standardization of Uveitis Nomenclature (SUN) Working Group has proposed a framework for the classification of uveitis, a standardized grading system and definitions of other terminology used to describe uveitis[1] (Table 20–1). The SUN working group suggests the use of the terms *insidious* or *sudden* to describe the onset of uveitis, and *limited* (if the duration is 3 months or less), or *persistent* (if the duration exceeds 3 months). It recommended that the term *acute* be applied to those instances in which the onset was sudden and the duration limited (as seen in HLA-B27–associated acute anterior uveitis), and that the term *chronic* be used to describe persistent disease with prompt (within 3 months) relapses after discontinuation of therapy (Table 20–2). Pars planitis, a form of intermediate uveitis, is occasionally described in JIA. For orientation, a schematic view of a sagittal section of the eye is shown in Figure 20–1.

UVEITIS IN JUVENILE IDIOPATHIC ARTHRITIS

The uveitis associated with JIA is the most common form of childhood anterior uveitis, accounting for up to 40% of cases in some large series.[2] Interpretation of data on this subject is hindered by the use of different classifications to describe chronic arthritis in children (see Chapter 13), different types of uveitis, different definitions of response and remission of uveitis, and different types of study populations. For these reasons, care must be taken in interpreting and generalizing conclusions from published information.

History: The Association of Arthritis and Uveitis

Ohm[3] first described chronic uveitis and band keratopathy in a child with arthritis in 1910. The association of ocular disease and juvenile arthritis was confirmed by several authors.[4-6] In Sury's large series of children with chronic arthritis,[7] chronic uveitis was found in 15% of the total, and two-thirds of these patients had band keratopathy. The majority of his patients had an insidious onset of uveitis with little or no early disturbance of vision; diagnosis was often delayed until slit-lamp examination was performed. The occurrence of "chronic, asymptomatic, non-granulomatous anterior uveitis" became recognized as an important complication of juvenile rheumatoid arthritis, particularly the limited joint disease referred to as oligoarthritis, a subset of juvenile idiopathic arthritis in the International League of Associations for Rheumatology (ILAR) classification, but also rheumatoid factor (RF)–negative polyarthritis and psoriatic arthritis. The term *acute symptomatic anterior uveitis* is usually applied to the disease complicating HLA-B27–associated diseases especially enthesitis-related arthritis (ERA).

Epidemiology

Chronic uveitis is especially likely in young girls who have oligoarthritis with an early age at onset and who are antinuclear antibody (ANA) seropositive (Table 20–3).[8-19] The frequency of chronic uveitis has varied considerably in reported series of children with chronic arthritis, from 2% in Costa Rica[20] to 10% in the United States,[19] 13% in Canada,[21] and 16% in the Nordic countries.[22,23] It appears to be particularly uncommon in Asian and African populations but has been reported worldwide.

The frequency of chronic uveitis is highly dependent on the subtype of JIA: it occurred in 15% to 20% of children with oligoarthritis (in up to 30% of those with extended oligoarthritis), 10% of those with psoriatic arthritis, and 14% of those with polyarthritis (RF negative). It is very uncommon in children with systemic JIA or RF-positive polyarthritis.[21] Acute (rather than chronic) anterior uveitis is characteristic of ERA.

Sudharshan and colleagues[24] described uveitis in 40 Indian children (64 eyes) with JIA who were referred for ophthalmological evaluation between 1988 and 1994 because of eye symptoms. These patients differed considerably from study cohorts in Europe and North America in that most were boys, (sex ratio 1.3 M to 1 F), the mean age at evaluation was 9 years, and complications were very common (cataract in 63% of eyes and band keratopathy in 62% of eyes). Only two patients were ANA positive. Whether these findings reflect differences in the disease (i.e., HLA-B27–associated arthritis) or in the pattern of referral (they were all symptomatic) is not entirely certain.

Etiology and Pathogenesis

The pathogenesis of chronic uveitis and the basis of its association with JIA are not known, although it is evident that T lymphocytes and their products are vital participants in the process. Involvement of the immune response and perturbation of inflammatory cytokines is documented in animal and human studies, although there is limited direct evidence from studies of uveitis in JIA. Ooi and colleagues[25] have reviewed the evidence that interleukin (IL)-1ß, IL-2, IL-6, interferon-γ, and tumor necrosis factor (TNF)-α are present in ocular fluids and tissues and that higher levels of these cytokines are associated with more severe uveitis. Levels of TNF-α were especially elevated in the aqueous of patients with ankylosing spondylitis–associated uveitis. The clinical responsiveness of uveitis to the administration of some, but not all, anti–TNF-α agents provides strong support for the premise that TNF-α is at least in part responsible for the inflammation. Serum levels of IL-6 and IL-8 are higher when uveitis is active in adults with posterior uveitis, anterior uveitis, or panuveitis.[26] IL-6 influences the maturation

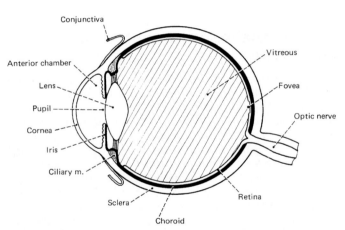

FIGURE 20–1   Schematic view of a sagittal section of the eye. Chronic anterior uveitis (iridocyclitis) involves the iris and ciliary body primarily, but secondary effects occur in the cornea, anterior chamber, lens, vitreous, and (rarely) retina.

Table 20–2

The SUN[1] working group descriptors of uveitis

Category	Descriptor	Comment
Onset	Sudden	
	Insidious	
Duration	Limited	≥3 months duration
	Persistent	>3 months duration
Course	Acute	Episode of sudden onset and limited duration
	Recurrent	Repeated episodes separated by periods of inactivity without treatment > 3 months in duration
	Chronic	Persistent uveitis with relapses in < 3 months after discontinuing treatment

Table 20–1

The SUN[1] working group classification of uveitis

Type	Primary Site of Inflammation	Includes
Anterior uveitis	Anterior chamber	Iritis
		Iridocyclitis
		Anterior cyclitis
Intermediate uveitis	Vitreous	Pars planitis
		Posterior cyclitis
		Hyalitis
Posterior uveitis	Retina or choroid	Focal, multifocal, or diffuse choroiditis
		Chorioretinitis
		Retinochoroiditis
		Retinitis
		Neuroretinitis

Table 20–3

Characteristics of children with chronic uveitis and arthritis

Characteristic	Overall Average
Female/male ratio	4.4:1
Mean age at onset of arthritis (yr)	4
Arthritis subtype (% with uveitis)	
Oligoarthritis	30
Polyarthritis (RF negative)	15
Psoriatic arthritis	10
Polyarthritis (RF positive)	<1
Systemic arthritis	<1
Enthesitis-related arthritis	<1*
Serology (%)	
RF positive	<1
Antinuclear antibody positive	80

RF, rheumatoid factor.
*Acute uveitis ~7%.

of Th17 CD4+ T cells, which participate in autoimmune diseases. Yoshimura and colleagues[27] demonstrated in a murine model, primarily of posterior uveitis or retinitis, that absence of both IL-6 and IL-23 prevented the production of Th17 cells and reduced the ocular inflammation. Keino and colleagues[28] demonstrated that the oral administration of an inhibitor of IL-12/IL-23 prevented autoimmune uveoretinitis in animals by reducing production of IL-17–producing cells. Other animal studies have shown that anti-Th17 can block the development of uveitis in uveitis-susceptible mice, but that administration of the cytokine itself into uveitis-susceptible rats has a mitigating effect on disease development.[29] Despite the implication of IL-17 in uveitis, some models involve either Th1[30] or Th2[31] cells exclusively. Sijssens and colleagues have demonstrated age-related differences in aqueous humor cytokines in patients, including some with JIA.[32]

Parikh and colleagues[33] have suggested, on the basis of the characteristics of the cellular infiltrate seen in histological studies of enucleated eyes, that the pathogenesis probably involved B lymphocytes as well. In addition to the high frequency of antinuclear antibodies of undetermined specificity, autoantibodies to ocular antigens have been described in children with arthritis and uveitis. There have been unconfirmed reports that children with uveitis and JRA have a higher frequency of immunity to soluble retinal antigen (S antigen)[34-36] and to a low-molecular-weight iris antigen[37,38] than do children with arthritis alone. It is not clear whether immunity to these ocular antigens is pathogenic or merely reflects the inflammatory process.

The basis of the association between inflammatory joint disease and inflammatory ocular disease is unexplained.

Genetic Background

Genetic susceptibility to uveitis in JIA is complex. Although there is limited evidence for the familial occurrence of this disorder, a few case reports have documented the occurrence of oligoarthritis and chronic anterior uveitis in siblings.[39,40]

A number of sometimes contradictory studies have reported an array of HLA alleles associated with chronic anterior uveitis in JIA. The strongest associations appear to be with genes in the Class II region. Studies from the United States have documented a strong association with DRB1*1104 (formerly called DR5).[41,42] These studies also showed an association with DQA1*0501 and DQB1*0301, which are in linkage disequilibrium with DRB1*1104. An additive risk was noted if both DRB1*1104 and DPB1*0201 were present.[42] A protective effect of DR1 was noted.[41] The association of uveitis in JIA with DRB1*11 noted in American children was confirmed in a study of Italian children, 83.7% of whom had this gene.[43]

Another study of Italian children failed to show an association with DRB1*11, however, but noted an increased frequency of HLA-A19 (odds ratio [OR] 2.87), HLA-B22 (OR 4.52), and DR9 (DRB1*09) (OR 2.33).[44] Zeggini and colleagues[45] noted an association only between HLA DRB1*13 and chronic anterior uveitis in JIA in British Caucasians. Another study followed 130 patients with

oligoarthritis (ILAR criteria), 31 of whom had uveitis, and their families, and a second group of 228 patients with JIA. Twenty-seven markers in the MHC region and single nucleotide polymorphisms in the TNF-α, HLA-E and DIF-2 genes were evaluated. DRB1*13 was found to confer a threefold increased risk of developing uveitis. Pratsidou-Gertsi and colleagues[46] also noted an increased frequency of DRB1*13 in Greek children with JIA and uveitis. This study additionally identified an increased incidence of DPB1*0201.

Associations with genes in the Class I region appear to be less specific. Increased frequencies of A*30, and B*54 or 55 (previously B22) have been noted, however.[44] HLA-B27 is strongly linked to the presence of acute anterior uveitis, irrespective of the presence of joint disease.[40]

Clinical Manifestations

Insidious Onset, Chronic Uveitis

Insidious chronic uveitis is characteristic of oligoarthritis (persistent or extended), and most children with psoriatic arthritis or RF-negative polyarthritis who develop uveitis. (see Table 20–3) The onset of chronic uveitis is usually insidious and often entirely asymptomatic, although up to one-half of the children have some symptoms attributable to the uveitis (pain, redness, headache, photophobia, change in vision) later in the course of their disease (Table 20–4). Uveitis is detected in fewer than 10% of patients before the onset of arthritis,[47] usually in the course of a routine ophthalmic examination. In almost one-half of all patients with uveitis, it occurs just before arthritis is diagnosed, at the time of diagnosis, or shortly thereafter.[8,19,41] Most children develop uveitis within 5 to 7 years after onset of arthritis, although the risk is never entirely absent[8,48] (Fig. 20–2). The disease is bilateral in 70% to 80% of children.[8,18,49,50] Patients with unilateral disease are unlikely to develop bilateral involvement after the first year of disease; however, there are exceptions, and unilateral uveitis may persist for many years in a few children before the other eye is involved.

The early detection of chronic uveitis requires slit-lamp biomicroscopy, which should be performed at the time of diagnosis in every child with JIA and repeated at prescribed intervals during the first few years of the disease. The frequency of ophthalmological examinations

Table 20–4

Ocular signs and symptoms in children with chronic uveitis and arthritis

Characteristic	Percentage Affected	
	Mean	Range
Bilateral uveitis	64	25-89
Symptoms		
Ocular pain and or redness		0-25
Change in vision		0-20
Photophobia		0-8
Headache		0-6
None	65	51-97

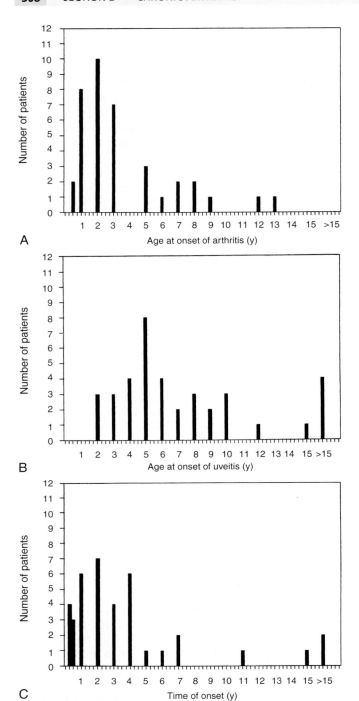

A

B

C

FIGURE 20–2   Graphs showing the temporal relationships between arthritis and uveitis in children with juvenile idiopathic arthritis. **A,** The distribution of age at onset of arthritis in a series of 38 children who developed uveitis. **B,** The distribution of age at onset of uveitis in the same children. Note that in four patients, uveitis began after their 15th birthday: at 15½, 18, 31, and 39 years of age. **C,** Interval between onset of arthritis and diagnosis of uveitis in these patients. Note that for one patient the interval was 29 years, and for another, 34 years.

is influenced by the level of risk of uveitis (Table 20–5). It is recommended that slit-lamp examinations be performed every 3 months for the first 2 years in children in the high-risk group (early age at onset, oligoarthritis or polyarthritis, female sex, ANA seropositivity) and every 4 to 6 months thereafter for a period of 7 years

at a minimum. In children with ANA-negative disease, slit-lamp examinations should be done initially at 4- to 6-month intervals. Children with psoriatic arthritis are also at considerable risk for the development of uveitis and should be followed at the same frequencies as children with oligoarthritis or polyarthritis. In children with a systemic onset, examinations once a year after the first year are probably sufficient. Any child who has had uveitis should be considered to be at high risk, even if it has remitted, and continued surveillance is essential.

The diagnostic signs of anterior uveitis on slit-lamp examination are the presence of inflammatory cells and increased protein concentration ("flare") in the aqueous humor of the anterior chamber of the eye (Figure 20–3). Deposition of inflammatory cells on the inner surface of the cornea (keratic precipitates) may be detected at presentation or develop later.

Complications of chronic anterior uveitis are frequent and increase with increasing duration of active disease. In recent series, the frequency is somewhat lower than in earlier reports, presumably due to earlier treatment. Posterior synechiae, inflammatory adhesions between the iris and the anterior surface of the lens, result in an irregular or poorly reactive pupil (Table 20–6; Fig. 20–4). This abnormality may be the first obvious clue to the presence of uveitis on ophthalmoscopic examination, but it is often a sign of disease of considerable duration or severity. Synechiae that are circumferential prevent the free flow of aqueous humor between the posterior and anterior chambers, resulting in bulging of the iris (iris bombé) and increased intraocular pressure. Synechiae are reported in from 22% to 51% of patients in recent series.[23,49,50]

Band keratopathy, occurring in 14% to 34% of children with uveitis, is caused by deposition of calcium in the corneal epithelium and tends to occur late (Figure 20–5). Initially crescentic grey-to-brown depositions are seen at the corneal limbus. With time the band progresses centrally at the equator of the eye to impair light entry through the pupil. Band keratopathy occurs in from 22% to 42% of affected children.[23,49,50] Cataracts result either from the inflammatory disease or the use of corticosteroids and are seen in approximately one-fifth of children with JIA and uveitis;[23,49] the prevalence is higher (42%) in children followed for a longer period of time (7 years).[50] The frequency of glaucoma ranges from 5% to 17%; hypotony is found in 5% to 10% and phthisis bulbi is rare and occurs late in the disease course.[23,49,50] Cystoid macular edema, which affects central vision,[51] is reported in 3.5% to 5.6% of children in some series[23,50] (Figure 20–6).These complications are still occasionally encountered in some children with chronic uveitis in spite of vigorous and carefully monitored ophthalmic treatment, although their frequency may be diminishing.

Keenan and colleagues[52] suggest that granulomatous uveitis may be more common than has been believed. Using a definition of granulomatous uveitis as the presence of Busacca or angle nodules, mutton-fat keratic precipitates (KP), or hyalinised ghost KPs, they observed granulomatous uveitis in 28% of 71 children with JIA. Granulomatous uveitis may be more common in black patients (67%) than white patients (25%). Many of these patients had only ghost KP as evidence of disease; this

Table 20–5

Guidelines for the ophthalmological screening of children with JIA

JIA Onset Type	ANA	Screening Schedule	
		Onset < 7 yr*	Onset ≥ 7 yr†
Oligoarticular	Positive	Every 3-4 mo‡	Every 4-6 mo
Oligoarthritis	Negative	Every 4-6 mo	Every 4-6 mo
Polyarthritis	Positive	Every 3-4 mo‡	Every 4-6 mo
Polyarthritis	Negative	Every 4-6 mo	Every 4-6 mo
Systemic	Neg. or Pos.	Every 12 mo	Every 12 mo
High risk: Screen every 3 months			
Moderate risk: Screen every 4-6 months			
Low risk: Screen every 12 months			

*All patients considered to be at low risk 7 yr after onset of arthritis; should have yearly ophthalmological examinations indefinitely.
†All patients are considered to be at low risk 4 yr after onset of arthritis; should have yearly ophthalmological examinations indefinitely.
‡All high-risk patients are considered to be at medium risk 4 years after onset of arthritis.
Modified from Yancey C et al: The Guidelines of the Rheumatology and Ophthalmology sections of the American Academy of Pediatrics, *Pediatrics* 92:295-296, 1993.

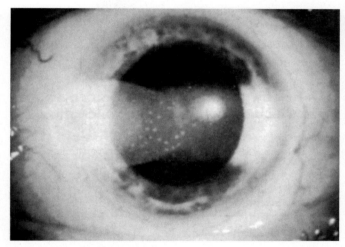

FIGURE 20–3 A slit-lamp examination shows "flare" in the fluid of the anterior chamber (caused by increased protein content) and keratic precipitates on the posterior surface of the cornea, representing small collections of inflammatory cells. (Courtesy of Dr. H. J. Kaplan.)

may account for the higher incidence of granulomatous uveitis than in other studies of juvenile arthritis.

Sudden Onset, (Acute) Uveitis

Sudden-onset (acute) uveitis differs in several ways from the more common insidious-onset, chronic uveitis and is strongly associated with HLA-B27 and ERA. In a large series reported by Saurenmann and colleagues,[21] 7.8% of children with ERA had uveitis. It is much more common in boys, is more often unilateral, and is characterized by a painful, red, photophobic eye. Until the patient is evaluated by an ophthalmologist, the symptoms are often mistakenly attributed to a foreign body, infection, or an allergy. Slit-lamp examination reveals the presence of cells and flare in the anterior chamber. Because of the symptomatic nature of this type of anterior uveitis, the process is usually identified and appropriately treated soon after onset; as a result, long-term sequelae are uncommon and visual prognosis is excellent. The reasons for the differences in

Table 20–6

Frequency of complications of chronic uveitis in reported cases

Complication	Approximate Frequency (%)	Reported Range (%)
Synechiae	62	37-75
Band keratopathy	37	11-56
Cataract	40	6-75
Glaucoma	10	8-25
Hypotony	5	
Phthisis bulbi	9	0-14
Cystoid macular edema	4	3-6

clinical appearance between sudden-onset acute uveitis and insidious-onset chronic uveitis are unknown. The strong association with HLA-B27 may reflect its association with ERA, rather than an independent association.

Differential Diagnosis

Uveitis is associated with a myriad of disorders.[53] Anterior uveitis may occur in children without evidence of joint or systemic involvement as an isolated disorder. This type of uveitis is probably the most common.[53] Such children should be evaluated for the presence of occult inflammatory joint disease and monitored for the possible development of arthritis or other systemic disease over time.

Uveitis and arthritis occur together with high frequency in a number of diseases other than JIA. Inflammation of the anterior uveal tract may complicate the arthropathy of inflammatory bowel disease and reactive arthritis. Uveitis also occurs in chronic infantile neurological cutaneous and articular syndrome, sarcoidosis, Blau syndrome, Behçet disease, and Kawasaki disease. Uveitis that occurs in these disorders is discussed in relevant chapters. Uveitis rarely occurs in systemic lupus erythematosus or Henoch Schonlein purpura. Rheumatoid arthritis in adults generally does not cause uveitis unless it induces scleritis

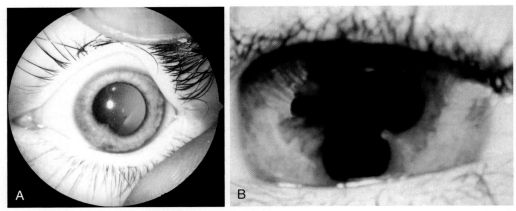

FIGURE 20–4 Posterior synechiae. **A,** Iris is tethered to the lens at a single point revealed only after mydriatics were given in this 4-year-old girl with oligoarthritis. **B,** The eye of a 7-year-old boy shows an irregular pupil that resulted from multiple adhesions of the iris to the anterior surface of the lens.

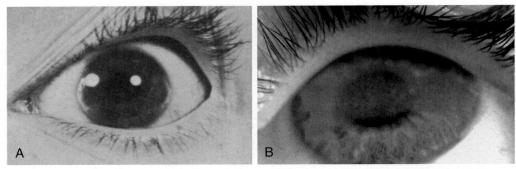

FIGURE 20–5 A, Early band keratopathy is noted as a semilunar band just inside the limbus medially and laterally. It does not extend across the pupil. **B,** the semiopaque band extends across the midplane of the cornea in this example of more advanced band keratopathy. It is fenestrated and does not extend to the limbus.

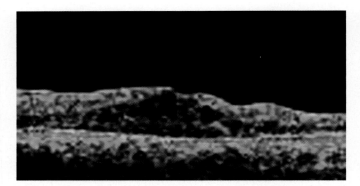

FIGURE 20–6 Cystoid macular edema. Ocular coherence tomography (OCT) images the retina and its layers by reflectance. The normal macula is concave. The convex appearance of the macula in this example is due to cystoid edema.

with secondary uveal involvement. Syndromes associated with uveitis are listed in Table 20–7.

Uveitis in Other Diseases

Tubulointerstitial Nephritis and Uveitis

Tubulointerstitial nephritis and uveitis (TINU) is the second most common type of childhood uveitis in Japan;[54] in an American series[55] one-third of patients under the age of 20 years with sudden-onset bilateral anterior uveitis had

Table 20–7
Diseases associated with anterior uveitis in children
Rheumatic Diseases
Juvenile Idiopathic Arthritis
Oligoarthritis
Psoriatic arthritis
Polyarthritis (rheumatoid factor negative)
Enthesitis-related arthritis (acute uveitis)
Reactive arthritis, urethritis, conjunctivitis syndrome
Lyme disease
Vasculitis
Kawasaki disease
Behçet disease
Henoch Schonlein purpura (very rare)
Wegener granulomatosis
Other
Vogt Koyangi Harada syndrome
Tubular interstitial nephritis and uveitis
Pars planitis
Masquerade syndromes
Human immunodeficiency virus infection, Epstein-Barr virus
Cat scratch disease
Herpes

TINU. This diagnosis is frequently missed and its prevalence may be underestimated.[56] TINU usually manifests as a bilateral sudden-onset anterior uveitis with eye redness and photophobia before or after the presentation of renal disease.[57] The child with TINU is usually systemically ill with fever, arthralgias, fatigue, and abdominal pain. The renal disease, manifested by sterile pyuria, may be transient. There may be elevation of liver enzyme levels, an elevated erythrocyte sedimentation rate, and mild anemia. Association with HLA DRB1*0102 and HLA DQA*01 is quite marked.[58] Treatment with moderate doses of corticosteroids for 8 to 12 weeks is usually effective treatment for all aspects of this syndrome, although some children go on to develop chronic uveitis.[57] The cause of TINU is unknown.

Infectious Causes of Uveitis

Uveitis was identified in seven South African boys who had human immunodeficiency virus–associated arthritis.[59] Intermediate uveitis was present in four children, and nongranulomatous anterior uveitis was present in three patients. The range of complications was similar to that seen in children with JIA.

Infection with *Bartonella henselae*, the most commonly identified cause of cat-scratch fever, may result in arthritis[60,61] and a neuroretinitis characterized by exudates in the retina (macular star).[62] Cells in the vitreous indicate the presence of uveitis. Diagnosis is confirmed serologically. Treatment with antibiotics is usually effective. Lyme disease is associated with a variety of ocular manifestations, including anterior and intermediate uveitis.[63] Rare causes of anterior uveitis include Epstein-Barr infection and infection with *Toxoplasma gondii*.

Other Syndromes Associated with Uveitis

Vogt-Koyanagi-Harada syndrome is a rare autoimmune disease possibly induced by immunity to an enzyme, tyrosinase, leading to changes in the retinal pigment epithelium, vitiligo, aseptic meningitis, uveitis, and hearing loss.[64] Poliosis (patchy loss of pigment of eyelashes, eyebrows, or hair) is a characteristic finding. The disease is usually responsive to corticosteroid given over a period of months. Some authorities recommend using pulse intravenous methylprednisolone for this disease when it presents in childhood.

Pars planitis is a form of uveitis characterized by inflammatory cells accumulating over the inferior pars plana, the portion of the eye just posterior to the ciliary body. Patients with this form of uveitis usually complain of visual floaters. The disease is generally bilateral with an insidious onset. This disease commonly begins in children or young adults and may last for decades. Visual acuity is often only moderately impaired by pars planitis, but macular edema is an especially common complication.

So-called masquerade syndromes, caused by juvenile xanthogranuloma or infiltration of the uveal tract with retinoblastoma or leukemic cells, may mimic the presence of uveitis.[65] Children with leukemia frequently have bone pain and occasionally frank joint effusions (see Chapter 46), suggesting the possible diagnosis of JIA and adding to the risk of misinterpretation of uveitis. Uveitis has been described in adults experiencing graft-versus-host disease after stem cell transplantation for malignancies.[66,67]

PATHOLOGY

Reports of the histopathology of uveitis in JIA are few. Descriptions of the pathology in patients with extremely severe, longstanding disease that led to blindness do not necessarily illuminate the pathogenic process. Such studies report an intense immunoinflammatory response in the iris, ciliary body, and pars plana, as well as increased iris vascularity.[68] Evidence of B lymphocyte involvement is suggested by the presence of scanty lymphocyte and plasma-cell infiltrates;[33,69-71] increased immunoglobulin (Ig) levels in the aqueous humor;[71-73] and high IgG concentration, activated complement, and C1q binding in the vitreous.[74] Kaplan and associates[75] found that 90% of vitreous lymphocytes in one adult with uveitis and "juvenile" RA were B lymphocytes. Evidence of T cell infiltrations is limited.[71] The keratic precipitates on the endothelial surface of the cornea consist of mononuclear phagocytes, with plasma cells and lymphocytes.[76]

LABORATORY EXAMINATION

The most characteristic laboratory abnormality found in children with arthritis and insidious chronic uveitis is the presence of ANAs, usually in low titer (less than 1:640). The specificities of these antibodies are usually unknown, although reactivity to histones has been reported to occur more commonly in children with JIA and uveitis than those with JIA alone.[77] ANAs and RFs are uncommon in children with sudden onset uveitis, as they are in the JIA subtype (ERA) with which this type of uveitis is usually seen. In children with acute anterior uveitis, HLA-B27 is often present. Abnormalities of the acute phase response reflect the extent and activity of arthritis, rather than uveitis.

MANAGEMENT

Medical Management

The treatment of chronic uveitis should be supervised by an ophthalmologist who is experienced in management of this disease.[78] The initial approach consists of glucocorticoid eye drops (such as dexamethasone or methylprednisolone), with or without a mydriatic agent to dilate the pupil and help prevent the development of posterior synechiae. A short-acting mydriatic drug is preferred, given if possible once a day in the evening, so that pupillary dilatation does not interfere with school work and reading. Some data suggest that oral nonsteroidal antiinflammatory drugs (NSAIDs) may be of some benefit.[79,80] Although this effect is not a major one, it should be considered when NSAID treatment of arthritis is altered.

In unresponsive disease, glucocorticoid drops may be given hourly during waking hours, with glucocorticoid ointment placed in the conjunctival sac at bedtime. The approach to management of uveitis that does not respond completely to the use of topical corticosteroids is changing rapidly. Systemic corticosteroids (prednisone 1 to 2 mg/kg/d orally), or methylprednisolone, 30 mg/kg intravenously on 1 to 3 consecutive days) are occasionally used to achieve rapid control of inflammation prior to surgery or to help manage hypotony (dangerously low intraocular pressure). In a few instances, subtenon injections of glucocorticoid may be required. Although the results of slit-lamp examination may quickly return to normal soon after treatment is initiated, relapses are common. Long-term ophthalmic or systemic administration of corticosteroids may lead to the development of Cushing syndrome, cataracts, and increased intraocular pressure, and should be avoided if possible. Limited response to corticosteroids requires initiation of second-line therapy, most commonly methotrexate. Foeldvari and Wierk[81] reviewed the treatment of 38 children with uveitis (31 associated with oligoarticular JIA and 7 with psoriatic JIA). Twenty-five patients were treated with methotrexate. Remission (no active uveitis without topical or systemic corticosteroids) occurred in 21 of 25 patients. Heiligenhaus and colleagues[82] reported that methotrexate allowed control of uveitis with (n = 21) or without (n = 4) topical corticosteroids in 25 of 35 patients. Both of these studies concluded that methotrexate was very effective in managing uveitis in children with JIA, but that topical corticosteroids were often required in addition. It is not entirely clear how rigorous the definition of remission was in these studies. Charuvanij and colleagues[83] reviewed the medication history in 43 children with JIA and anterior uveitis. Only 16% achieved satisfactory control with topical corticosteroids alone. The addition of methotrexate controlled the uveitis in three-quarters of the children, but 6 required the addition of infliximab, with disease control in 4 patients.

Cyclosporine has been used to treat uveitis of JIA. Cyclosporine was given to 14 children with chronic uveitis refractory to glucocorticoids for a mean duration of 21 months.[84] Visual acuity was improved or did not deteriorate further in 92% of eyes, and results of the ophthalmic examination were improved in 76%. In a review of 82 children with JIA who received cyclosporine for treatment of uveitis, Tappeiner[85] concluded that the drug had a limited role in treating uveitis that was resistant to topical or systemic corticosteroid. In addition, 55% had received methotrexate and 18% azathioprine prior to initiation of cyclosporine therapy. Remission (≤1 cell in the anterior chamber) occurred in 6 of 25 patients receiving cyclosporine as monotherapy. When cyclosporine was added to methotrexate, uveitis became inactive in approximately one-half of patients, with reduction in requirements for topical or systemic corticosteroids in many.[85] However, over the 2.9 year follow-up period, 45% developed new complications of uveitis.

Mycophenolate mofetil (MMF) has recently received attention as an effective agent in patients resistant to other therapy.[86,87] Doycheva and colleagues[86] noted a considerable steroid sparing effect, improvement in inflammation, and reduction in relapse rate in 17 children with uveitis (only one with JIA) treated with MMF (600 mg/m^2/day) during the average of 3 years follow-up. However, additional immunosuppression was required in some patients. Sobrin and colleagues[87] reported that MMF was effective in treating uveitis in children but was less effective in those with JIA.

The anti-TNF-α agents etanercept, infliximab, and adalimumab have advanced the therapy of methotrexate-resistant uveitis, including that associated with JIA. Reiff[88] reported effectiveness of etanercept in an uncontrolled study of seven children with active uveitis and JRA who had not responded satisfactorily to corticosteroids and methotrexate or cyclosporine. Follow up of these patients indicated that at least four had a sustained response.[89] Smith and coworkers[90] conducted a randomized, blinded, placebo-controlled trial in 12 children with JRA and uveitis in whom the methotrexate response was insufficient and found no difference between etanercept and placebo at 6 months. Saurenmann and colleagues[91] reported results of treatment with etanercept (n = 6) or infliximab (n = 8) in 12 patients with JIA and concluded that infliximab was superior to etanercept in both clinical response and frequency of complications. Tynjala and colleagues[92] reported similar results. In most studies, the response was partial, with approximately one-third of patients achieving complete remission of uveitis. Simonini[93] reported complete remission in eight children with JIA and uveitis receiving infliximab but noted that the beneficial effect waned over time. Similar results were noted by Tugal-Tutkun.[94] There are also reports of new onset or worsening of uveitis during treatment with anti-TNF agents, particularly etanercept.[95]

Vazquez-Cobian and colleagues[96] treated 14 children with JIA and chronic uveitis with adalimumab and noted improvement in anterior chamber cells and flare in 65% and in visual acuity in 38% of affected eyes. In many children, concomitant medications (NSAIDs, topical corticosteroids, methotrexate, cyclosporine) could be decreased or discontinued. Beister and colleagues reported similar results in the same patient group.[97] There is probably no longer a role for chlorambucil in the management of uveitis in children with JIA.

Case reports record the benefit of abatacept (anti-CTLA4)[98] and rituximab (anti-CD20).[99] Refractory uveitis has also been treated with intravenous immunoglobulin.[100]

Surgical Management

Band keratopathy has been treated with topical chelation and by lasers. Cataracts seldom interfere significantly with vision in childhood, but they may require surgical removal. The management of complicated uveitis and glaucoma remains unsatisfactory, but results of lensectomy or vitrectomy for complicated cataract are improved.[82] It is recommended that cataract surgery be performed only in the absence of vitreous opacities, hypotony, or cyclitic membrane formation and that the anterior chamber be free of inflammatory cells. Perioperative glucocorticoids are recommended. The timing of cataract extraction challenges the judgment of the ophthalmologist in weighing the danger of operation on an inflamed eye against the risk of amblyopia. An unresolved controversy is whether to replace the lens with an intraocular lens or require that the child use a contact lens or a thick corrective lens. Operative complications are minimized with microsurgery and cryoextraction.

DISEASE COURSE AND PROGNOSIS

The course of chronic anterior uveitis in patients with JIA is variable; it may last for months to a decade or longer, although new approaches to therapy suggest that the course may be much shorter if it is treated aggressively. It has been suggested that the frequency and severity of uveitis may actually be decreasing.[101] In some children, the course is intermittent; in others it is persistent. The activity of the uveitis does not appear to parallel that of the arthritis,[102] and it may occur for the first time after the arthritis is in remission. Visual loss may occur because of complications of the uveitis or as a result of amblyopia related to suppression of visual images from a cataract in a young child.

In early studies, the frequency of blindness (less than 20/400 OU) in both eyes was as high as 15% to 30%. In more recent reports,[18] visual outcome is much improved. Cabral and colleagues,[17] in a 1994 study of 49 patients (82 affected eyes), reported that only 15 affected eyes had corrected visual acuity of 20/40 or worse, at an average of 9.4 years after onset of uveitis, and 8 had corrected visual acuity of 20/200 or worse. In a large series of patients reported by Sabri and colleagues[49] followed for a mean of 6.3 years, visual acuity of 20/40 or better was present in 91% of affected eyes; 3.4% had visual impairment, and 5.7% were blind. It seems likely that earlier identification of the disease and more aggressive therapy is responsible for this improvement in outcome in the last decade.

The prognosis for uveitis is worse in children in whom the onset of uveitis occurs before diagnosis of arthritis or shortly thereafter.[16,19] It is also worse in those with an initial severe inflammatory response,[19] chronicity of inflammation,[9] or ANA seronegativity.[19]

In a long-term follow-up study of 123 patients with onset of JIA between 1976 and 1995,[103] active uveitis was defined as the presence of ≥ 3 cells in the anterior chamber or the requirement of topical corticosteroids. At the time of clinic re-evaluation (a mean of 16 years after diagnosis), uveitis was still active in 8 of 19 patients with insidious-onset chronic disease. Oligoarthritis tended to become extended and to be active in those with active uveitis. Acute symptomatic anterior uveitis was seen in 6 patients, between the ages of 14.5 and 22 years, all of whom were HLA-B27 positive. Visual outcome was good. These observations are similar to those reported by Skarin and colleagues.[23]

Complications of uveitis were frequent in the recent series reported by Paroli and associates.[43] Of 42 children with JRA-associated uveitis who were observed for at least 1 year, cataract was present in 64%, band keratopathy occurred in 59%, and glaucoma occurred in 25%. Nonetheless, visual acuity was normal or good in almost two thirds of these children. Rare ocular complications include papillitis, scleritis, episcleritis, and keratoconjunctivitis sicca.

REFERENCES

3. J. Ohm, Bandformige Hornhauttrubung bei einem neunjhrigen Madchen und ihre Behandlung mit subkonjunktivalen Jodkaliumeinspritzungen, Klin. Monatsbl. Augenheilkd. 48 (1910) 243.
4. A. Friedlander, 2 Tilfaelde af kronisk septisk Polyartritis i Barnealderen med Ojenkomplikationer, Ugeskr. Laeger. 95 (1933) 1190.
5. E. Holm, Iridocyclitis and ribbon-like keratitis in cases of infantile polyarthritis (Still's disease), Trans. Ophthalmol. Soc. U.K.55 (1935) 478.
6. O. Blegvad, Iridocyclitis and disease of the joints in children, Acta. Ophthalmol. (Copenh) 19 (1941) 219.
7. B. Sury, Rheumatoid arthritis in children: a clinical study, Munksgaard, Copenhagen, 1952.
10. L.T. Chylack, Jr., The ocular manifestations of juvenile rheumatoid arthritis, Arthritis Rheum. 20 (suppl.) (1977) 217–223.
12. L.T. Chylack Jr., D.C. Bienfang, A.R. Bellows, et al., Ocular manifestations of juvenile rheumatoid arthritis, Am. J. Ophthalmol. 79 (1975) 1026–1033.
13. W.K. Smiley, The eye in juvenile chronic polyarthritis, Clin. Rheum. Dis. 2 (1976) 413.
14. J.G. Schaller, Iridocyclitis, Arthritis Rheum. 20 (suppl.) (1977) 227.
19. E.C. Chalom, D.P. Goldsmith, M.A. Koehler, et al., Prevalence and outcome of uveitis in a regional cohort of patients with juvenile rheumatoid arthritis, J. Rheumatol. 24 (1997) 2031–2034.
20. P. Arguedas, A. Fasth, B. Andersson-Gäre, a prospective population based study of outcomes of juvenile chronic arthritis in Costa Rica, J. Rheumatol. 29 (2002) 174–183.
22. I. Kunnamo, P. Kallio, P. Pelkonen, Incidence of arthritis in urban Finnish children: a prospective study, Arthritis Rheum. 29 (1986) 232–1238.
24. S. Sudharshan, J. Biswas, S.K. Ganesh, Analysis of juvenile idiopathic arthritis associated uveitis in India over the last 16 years, Indian J. Ophthalmol. 55 (2007) 199–202.
31. S.J. Kim, M. Zhang, B.P. Vistica, et al., Induction of ocular inflammation by T helper lymphocytes type 2, Invest. Ophthalmol. Vis. Sci. 43 (2002) 758–765.
34. R.E. Petty, D.W. Hunt, D.F. Rollins, et al., Immunity to soluble retinal antigen in patients with uveitis accompanying juvenile rheumatoid arthritis, Arthritis Rheum. 30 (1987) 287–293.
35 R.E. Petty, D.W. Hunt, Immunity to ocular and collagen antigens in childhood arthritis and uveitis, Int. Arch. Allergy Appl. Immunol. 89 (1989) 31–37.
36. D. Gupta, V.K. Singh, J. Rajasingh, et al., Cellular immune responses of patients with juvenile chronic arthritis to retinal antigens and their synthetic peptides, Immunol. Res. 15 (1996) 74–83.
37. R.C. Uchiyama, T.G. Osborn, T.L. Moore, Antibodies to iris and retina detected in sera from patients with juvenile rheumatoid arthritis with iridocyclitis by indirect immunofluorescence studies on human eye tissue, J. Rheumatol. 16 (1989) 1074–1078.

Table 20–8

Suggested guidelines for the treatment of uveitis in juvenile idiopathic arthritis

Initial Therapy

Topical corticosteroids +/- mydriatics

Continue for up to 3 months provided inflammation is controlled before gradually tapering frequency of eye drops.

If disease activity increases or does not respond, add second line agent.

Second Line Therapy

Add methotrexate (0.35-0.65 mg/kg) by mouth or by subcutaneous injection once a week for up to 3 months. If inflammation is controlled, continue using methotrexate and taper topical corticosteroids. Monitor methotrexate toxicity (liver enzymes, albumin, complete blood count every 2 months) If disease control is unsatisfactory or disease worsens, add third-line therapy.

Third-Line Therapy

Add anti TNF-α agent—preferably intravenous infliximab (4-10 mg/kg every 6-8 weeks), or adalimumab (20-40 mg subcutaneously every 1 to 2 weeks). If rapid control of inflammation is not achieved, consider substituting mycophenolate mofetil or cyclosporine; local corticosteroid injections.

38. D.W. Hunt, R.E. Petty, F. Millar, Iris protein antibodies in serum of patients with juvenile rheumatoid arthritis and uveitis, Int. Arch. Allergy Appl. Immunol. 100 (1993) 314–318.

46. P. Pratsidou-Gertsi, F. Kanakoudi-Tsakalidou, M. Spyropoulou, et al., Nationwide collaborative study of HLA class II associations with distinct types of juvenile chronic arthritis (JCA) in Greece, Eur. J. Immunogenet. 26 (1999) 299–310.

47. J.J. Kanski, Anterior uveitis in juvenile rheumatoid arthritis, Arch. Ophthalmol. 95 (1977) 1794–1797.

52. J.D. Keenan, H.H. Tessler, D.A. Goldstein, Granulomatous inflammation in juvenile idiopathic arthritis-associated uveitis, J. AAPOS 12 (2008) 546–550.

55. F. Mackensen, J.R. Smith, J.T. Rosenbaum, Enhanced recognition, treatment, and prognosis of tubulointerstitial nephritis and uveitis syndrome, Ophthalmology 114 (2007) 995–999.

56. R.D. Levinson, J.T.H. Mandeville, G.N. Holland, et al., Tubulointerstitial nephritis and uveitis syndrome: Recognizing the importance of an uncommon disease, Am. J. Ophthalmol. 629 (2000) 798–799.

57 J.T. Mandeville, R.D. Levinson, G.N. Holland, The tubulointerstitial nephritis and uveitis syndrome, Surv. Ophthalmol. 46 (2001) 195–208.

60. M. Giladi, E. Maman, D. Paran, et al., Cat scratch disease–associated arthropathy, Arthritis Rheum. 52 (2005) 3611–3617.

61. M.J. Al-Matar, R.E. Petty, D.A. Cabral, et al., Rheumatic manifestations of Bartonella infection in two children, J. Rheumatol. 29 (2002) 184–186.

65. S.V. Patel, D.C. Herman, P.M. Anderson, et al., Iris and anterior chamber involvement in acute lymphoblastic leukemia, J. Pediatr. Hematol. Oncol. 25 (2003) 653–656.

66. M. Wertheim, J.T. Rosenbaum, Bilateral uveitis manifesting as a complication of chronic graft-versus-host disease after allogeneic bone marrow transplantation, Ocular. Immunol. Inflamm. 13 (2005) 403–404.

67. Y.M. Hettinga, L.F. Verdonck, R. Fijnheer, et al., Anterior uveitis: a manifestation of graft-versus- host disease, Ophthalmology 114 (2007) 794–797.

68. L.T. Chylack Jr., D.K. Dueker, D.J. Pihlaja, Ocular manifestations of juvenile rheumatoid arthritis: pathology, fluorescein iris angiography, and patient care patterns, in: J.J. Miller III (Ed.), Juvenile Rheumatoid Arthritis, PSG, Littleton, MA, 1978.

69. R. Sabates, T. Smith, D. Apple, Ocular histopathology in juvenile rheumatoid arthritis, Ann. Ophthalmol. 11 (1979) 733–737.

70. J.C. Merriam, L.T. Chylack Jr., D.M. Albert, Early-onset pauciarticular juvenile rheumatoid arthritis: a histopathologic study, Arch. Ophthalmol. 101 (1983) 1085–1092.

71. W.A. Godfrey, C.B. Lindsley, F.E. Cuppage, Localization of IgM in plasma cells in the iris of a patient with iridocyclitis and juvenile rheumatoid arthritis, Arthritis Rheum. 24 (1981) 1195–1198.

72. A.H. Rahi, J.J. Kanski, A. Fielder, Immunoglobulins and antinuclear antibodies in aqueous humour from patients with juvenile "rheumatoid" arthritis (Still's disease), Trans. Ophthalmol. Soc. U.K. 97 (1997) 217–222.

73. J.J. Kanski, Clinical and immunological study of anterior uveitis in juvenile chronic polyarthritis, Trans. Ophthalmol. Soc. U.K. 96 (1976) 123–130.

74. D.A. Person, C.M. Leatherwood, E.J. Brewer, et al., Immunology of the vitreous in juvenile rheumatoid arthritis, Arthritis Rheum. 24 (1981) 591.

75. H.J. Kaplan, T.M. Aaberg, R.H. Keller, Recurrent clinical uveitis: cell surface markers on vitreous lymphocytes, Arch. Ophthalmol. 100 (1982) 585–587.

76. M. Hogan, S.J. Kimura, P. Thygeson, Signs and symptoms of uveitis. I. Anterior uveitis, Am. J. Ophthalmol. 47 (1959) 155–170.

79. N.Y. Olson, C.B. Lindsley, W.A. Godfrey, Treatment of chronic childhood iridocyclitis with nonsteroidal anti-inflammatory drugs, J. Allerg. Clin. Immunol. 79 (1981) 220.

80. W.F. March, T.C. Coniglione, Ibuprofen in the treatment of uveitis, Ann. Ophthalmol. 17 (1985) 103–104.

Entire reference list is available online at www.expertconsult.com.

Chapter 21

SYSTEMIC LUPUS ERYTHEMATOSUS

Earl Silverman and Allison Eddy

Systemic lupus erythematosus (SLE) is a systemic multi-system autoimmune disease characterized by the presence of autoantibodies and multiorgan system involvement. It should be considered as a potential diagnosis in all patients who present with multiorgan system disease. Antinuclear antibodies (ANAs) are present in >90% of patients with SLE, most of whom have specific autoantibodies. The clinical presentation is very diverse, ranging from a mild disease characterized by rash and arthritis to a severe life-threatening disease involving one or multiple organs. SLE is characterized by flares and remission and the flares tend to be mimetic. In many patients intermittent symptoms may precede the diagnosis by months to years and may initially spontaneously remit without treatment. Even following diagnosis spontaneous remissions of disease have been reported. The goal of treatment is to reset the immune system to a state of remission.

HISTORICAL REVIEW

Medical literature described the dermatitis of SLE as early as the 13th century. The butterfly rash was recognized in 1845, and in 1852 the term *lupus erythemateux* was coined. Osler described the clinical features, and in 1924 Libman and Sacks reported the characteristic endocarditis. In 1948 Hargroves and colleagues described the lupus erythematosus (LE) cell and one year later cortisone was first used. In 1957 the association of a positive ANA and SLE was made.

CLASSIFICATION CRITERIA

Because SLE is manifested by multiple different organ involvement, in 1971 the American Rheumatism Association, now the American College of Rheumatology (ACR)

devised a classification system for the disease, modified in 1982 and again in 1997 (Table 21–1).[1-2] The system was designed to allow comparison between different populations and enable research. According to the ACR system 4 of 11 ACR criteria must be found in a patient to fulfill the classification of SLE. However, it is important to emphasize that these are classification, not diagnostic criteria. The criteria are useful for diagnosis, but patients are not required to meet more than 4 of the criteria to have definite SLE. However, in most studies 90% to 95% of patients do, in fact, meet more than 4 of the criteria. The ACR criteria were developed and validated in adults rather than pediatric patients, and certain features such as a discoid lupus rash are rarely seen in children. However, the ACR criteria appear to be very useful in pediatric SLE (pSLE).[3]

ETIOLOGY AND PATHOGENESIS

Environmental Factors

It is likely that lupus is a combination of genetic susceptibility and environmental factors, including exposure to sunlight, infections, drugs, and chemicals (Table 21–2 [online only]).[4-10] Although almost all of the environmental studies were performed in adults, it is likely that these data can be extrapolated to pSLE. Patients with SLE have a high incidence of drug allergies.

Ultraviolet Radiation

It is well recognized that in some patients exposure to ultraviolet radiation, and in particular ultraviolet (UV)-B rays, may exacerbate either skin or systemic disease.[11-13] In vitro studies have shown that exposure of cells, and particularly keratinocytes, to UV radiation leads to

Table 21–1

The 1982 revised criteria for classification of systemic lupus erythematosus with 1997 revision

Criterion	Definition
Malar rash	Fixed erythema, flat or raised, over the malar eminences, tending to spare the nasolabial folds
Discoid rash	Erythematosus raised patches with adherent keratotic scaling and follicular plugging: atrophic scarring may occur in older lesions
Photosensitivity	Skin rash as a result of unusual reaction to sunlight, by patient history or physician observation
Oral ulcers	Oral or nasopharyngeal ulceration, usually painless, observed by physician
Arthritis	Nonerosive arthritis involving two or more peripheral joints, characterized by tenderness, swelling, or effusion
Serositis	Pleuritis—convincing history of pleuritic pain or rubbing heard by a physician or evidence of pleural effusion or pericarditis— documented by ECG or rub or evidence of pericardial effusion
Renal disorder	Persistent proteinuria greater than 0.5 g/d (or >3 + if quantitation nor performed) or cellular casts—may be red cell, hemoglobin, granular, tubular, or mixed
Neurological disorder	Seizures in the absence of offending drugs or known metabolic derangements (e.g., uremia, ketoacidosis, or electrolyte imbalance) or psychosis in the absence of offending drugs or known metabolic derangements (e.g., uremia, ketoacidosis, or electrolyte imbalance)
Hematological disorder	Hemolytic anemia with reticulocytosis or leukopenia less than 4000/mm^3 total on two or more occasions, or lymphopenia less than 1500/mm^3 on two or more occasions, or thrombocytopenia less than 100,000/mm^3 in the absence of offending drugs
Immunological disorder	a) Positive anti-DNA antibody to native DNA in abnormal titer, or b) Presence of anti-Sm nuclear antigen, or c) Positive finding of antiphospholipid antibodies based on 1) an abnormal serum level of IgG or IgM anticardiolipin antibodies, 2) a positive test result for lupus anticoagulant using a standard method, or 3) a false-positive serological test and confirmed by *Treponema pallidum* immobilization or fluorescent treponemal antibody absorption test.
Antinuclear antibody	An abnormal titer of antinuclear antibody by immunofluorescence or an equivalent assay at any point in time and in the absence of drugs known to be associated with drug-induced lupus syndrome

The proposed classification is based on 11 criteria. For the purpose of identifying patients in clinical studies, a person is defined as having SLE if any 4 or more of the 11 criteria are present, serially or simultaneously, during any interval of observation.

Data from Tan EM, Cohen AS, Fries JF et al: The 1982 revised criteria for the classification of systemic lupus erythematosus, *Arthritis Rheum* 25:1271-1277, 1982; Hochberg MC: Updating the American College of Rheumatology revised criteria for the classification of systemic lupus erythematosus, *Arthritis Rheum* 40:1725, 1997.

ECG, electrocardiogram; IgG, immunoglobulin G; IgM, immunoglobulin M.

apoptosis, allowing blebs containing autoantigens to appear on the cell surface, which can then be processed and lead to an autoimmune response.[11,14-19]

Viral Infection

For many years it has been proposed that exposure to viruses, in particular herpes families of viruses, can lead to polyclonal immune activation of the immune system, molecular mimicry, and then to the development of SLE.[5-6,20-27] Studies of adults with SLE have demonstrated that a significantly higher percentage of patients had exposure to Epstein-Barr virus (EBV) than did those in a control group.[28-29] Although parvovirus B19 infection can appear to mimic the clinical features of SLE, there is no evidence that it leads or predisposes to SLE.[30-36]

Drugs and Chemicals

Drug-induced lupus is a well-recognized form of SLE (see below). Exposure to many chemicals, including hair dye, tobacco, L-canavanine, and other environmental factors have been associated with SLE (see Table 21–2 [online only]).[6]

Immunological Abnormalities

SLE is characterized by immune dysregulation involving both the innate and adaptive immune systems and all effector mechanisms have been shown to be defective (Table 21–3 [online only]). Much of our knowledge about immune dysregulation has been adapted from animal models because immune dysregulation in human SLE is much more difficult to study.[37-42] Current hypotheses regarding loss of tolerance in SLE suggests that one or more of the following factors play a role: the generation of self-antigens on cell surfaces following apoptosis[14,43-47]; abnormalities of innate immunity including Toll-like receptors[48-51]; abnormalities of all arms of the adaptive immune system including antigen-presenting cells, T cells, and B cells[52-63]; epigenetics[64-68]; and, most recently, abnormal regulation of interferon-α.[54,69-71,72]

Apoptosis and Abnormal Cell Death

During normal apoptosis nuclear and cytoplasmic antigens appear on the surface of the dying cells within blebs surrounded by the cell membrane. Abnormal clearance and/or regulation of clearance or abnormal presentation of blebs (containing autoantigens) to autoreactive cells may drive the autoimmune process. Abnormal clearance may be secondary to defects in complement components and/or abnormal complement receptors. In human SLE there is evidence of abnormal apoptosis of lymphocytes, macrophages and neutrophils, and sera from SLE patients is pro-apoptotic.[43,73-75] It has been shown that SLE patients may have abnormal production of anti-apoptotic molecules (such as the Bcl-2 family of proteins), programmed cell death 1 (PD1), and/or Fas, any of which can lead to a prolonged lifespan of autoreactive cells.[76-82]

CLINICAL DISEASE

The true incidence and prevalence of pSLE is difficult to estimate because there have been very few studies focusing on the pediatric population. Most data have been extrapolated from adult studies. Approximately 15% to 20% of SLE cases begin before age 19. Incidence and prevalence rates vary by ethnicity and are higher in Hispanic, Black, North American First Nations, and South-East and South Asian populations.[7,87-100] Data suggest a prevalence of SLE beginning before age 19 of from 6 to18.9 cases/100,000 white females, with higher rates among Blacks and Puerto Ricans.[83-86] Although it has been estimated that 5% to 10% of patients followed in pediatric rheumatology clinics in North America and England have pSLE,[85,101-103] in Asia and South Asia and in patients of African or Afro-Caribbean origin in North America, it has been estimated that SLE in adolescents has a prevalence similar to that of juvenile idiopathic arthritis (JIA).[84,104-107]

Some early small studies had suggested that the male/female ratio was similar to that seen in adults; however, most large reviews of pediatric populations show a male/female ratio of 1:2 to 1:5. This large variation in the male/female ratio appears to be secondary to racial/ethnic differences in the percentage of males.[87,89,108-115]

The mean age at pSLE diagnosis is approximately 12 to 13 years; however, in some countries the mean age is affected by the upper limit of the "pediatric age" of the population being studied. In clinics who only follow patients up to age 14 to 16 years, the mean age of diagnosis is lower.[109] The time to diagnosis of SLE from onset of symptoms is variable and can range from 1 month to 5 years (median 4 to 8 months), varying by country of origin.

The overall 10-year survival rate for adult patients with SLE is between 85% to 92% with 5-year survival rates 3% to 5% higher.[116-117] Thirty years ago the reported survival of pSLE patients at 5 years was 82.6% and at 10 years 76.1%.[118] Recent pSLE studies have shown 5-year survival rates of > 95%, with 10-year survival rates reported to be as high as 86%.[88] Mortality rates have been shown to be associated with socioeconomic status and individual access to health care, educational background, racial/ethnic background, endemic infection rates, disease activity, and renal or central nervous system (CNS) involvement.[88,114,119-125] Table 21–4 shows trends in mortality rates by decade and reported causes of death. Common causes of death within the first 2 years are pancreatitis, pulmonary hemorrhage, infection, thromboembolic disease, and active neuropsychiatric disease. The causes of late death (>5 years) are complications of end-stage renal disease (ESRD), atherosclerosis, suicide, and less commonly active SLE or infection.[120,126-138]

Clinical Patterns

Children and adolescents with SLE frequently present with systemic, constitutional symptoms such as fever, diffuse hair loss, fatigue, weight loss, and diffuse generalized inflammation as demonstrated by lymphadenopathy and hepatosplenomegaly—in addition to specific organ

Table 21–4

Rates and causes of death in pSLE covering multiple decades

Author (Ref no.)	Publication Date	Total Number of Patients	Death (Percentage)	Infection	Active CNS	Renal Failure	Cardiac/ Pulmonary	Other
Meislin & Rothfield (130)	1968	42	43%	39%	11%	33%	0%	11%
Walraven & Chase(128)	1976	50	24%	8%	0%	33%	42%	25%
Garin et al* (129)	1976	49	12%	33%	33%	33%	0%	0%
King et al (126)	1977	108	26%	29%	0%	43%	0%	0%
Cassidy et al* (127)	1977	58	19%	73%	9%	64%	27%	9%
Abeles et al (132)	1980	67	15%	10%	0%	30%	0%	60%
Platt et a l(132)	1982	70	16%	82%	0%	18%	9%	18%
Glidden et al (133)	1983	55	16%	33%	33%	33%	0%	11%
Wang et al (120)	2003[1980-1990†]	52	63%	78%	13%	35%	25%	64%
Wang et al (120)	2003[1991-2000†]	101	18%	72%	28%	0%	22%	55%
Yu et al (NP patients) (134)	2006[1985-1994†]	46	52%	71%	29%	63%	29%	12%
Yu et al (NP patients) (134)	2006[1995-2005]	18	28%	28%	60%	20%	20%	20%
Yu et al (134) (non-NP patients)	2006[1985-1994†]	55	34%	No details	No details	No details	No details	No details
Yu et al (non-NP patients) (134)	2006[1995-2005†]	66	3%	No details	No details	No details	No details	No details
Descloux et al (135)	2009	56	6%	No details	No details	No details	No details	No details
Hari* (136)	2009	54	16%	45%	0%	33%	11%	11%

*Cohorts were divided into 2 different decades.
†Only renal patients were studied.

Table 21–6

Frequencies of clinical features of children and adolescents: Within 1 year of diagnosis and any time during their disease

Clinical Features*	Within First Year of Diagnosis	Any Time
Constitutional and generalized symptoms		
Fever	35-90%	37-100%
Lymphadenopathy	11-45%	13-45%
Hepatosplenomegaly	16-42%	19-43%
Weight loss	20-30%	21-32%
Organ Involvement		
Musculoskeletal		
Arthritis	60-88%	60-90%
Myositis	<5%	<5%
Any skin involvement	60-80%	60-90%
Malar rash	22-68%	30-80%
Discoid rash	<5%	<5%
Photosensitivity	12-45%	17-58%
Mucosal ulceration	25-32%	30-40%
Alopecia	10-30%	15-35%
Other rashes	40-52%	42-55%
Nephritis	20-80%	48-100%
Neuropsychiatric disease	5-30%†	15-95%‡
Psychosis	5-12%	8-18%
Seizures	5-15%	5-47%
Headache	5-22%	10-95%
Cognitive dysfunction	6-15%	12-55%
Acute confusional state	5-15%	8-35%
Peripheral nerve involvement	<5%	<5%
Cardiovascular disease	5-30%	25-60%
Pericarditis	12-20%	20-30%
Myocarditis	<5%	<5%
Pulmonary disease	18-40%	18-81%
Pleuritis	12-20%	20-30%
Pulmonary hemorrhage	<5%	<5%
pneumonitis	<5%	<5%
Gastrointestinal disease	14-30%	24-40%
Peritonitis (sterile)	10-15%	12-18%
Abnormal Liver Function Tests	20-40%	25-45%
Pancreatitis	<5%	<5%

*Not all reports commented on all features or incidence in first year.
†Had highest prevalence of CNS disease but did not describe incidence in first year.[245]
‡Headache reported in 95% of patients.[245]
Data from references 88, 89, 110-115, 118, 120, 123, 125, 135, 242, 245, 268, 613-618.

involvement (Table 21–5 [online only]). This is true both at diagnosis and throughout the disease course at times of disease flare. Mucocutaneous, musculoskeletal and kidney disease are the most common manifestations of pSLE.

Musculoskeletal Disease

Musculoskeletal disease (MSK) is common both at presentation and during the course of pSLE (see Table 21–5 [online only] and Table 21–6). The main features are arthritis, arthralgia, and/or tenosynovitis. The arthritis may be a painful, symmetric polyarthritis affecting both large and small joints, although a relatively asymptomatic arthritis similar to that seen in JIA is common. Morning stiffness is also common. Because more than 90% of patients who will develop arthritis have developed the arthritis within the first year of diagnosis (frequently at diagnosis), it is important to look for other causes of new-onset joint inflammation (such as infection, avascular necrosis, and injury) in patients who present with "SLE arthritis" after more than 1 year following diagnosis. Radiographic changes are rarely seen. An ultrasound study of pSLE patients showed that arthritis of fingers and wrists was accompanied by flexor and extensor tenosynovitis that led to thinning of the tendons but not to rupture without bony erosions.[139]

The deforming arthritis associated with ligament and tendon laxity (Jaccoud arthritis) is rarely seen in pSLE, nor is the destructive arthritis associated with a positive rheumatoid factor (rhupus).[140-146] More commonly seen is the development of pSLE in patients with longstanding definite polyarticular or systemic JIA.[147-149]

Although myalgia is seen in 20% to 30% of patients, true myositis occurs much less frequently, but when present, it is difficult to differentiate from juvenile dermatomyositis (JDM). Noninflammatory musculoskeletal pain frequently occurs following treatment and may be the result of a pain amplification syndrome secondary to glucocorticoid therapy.

Treatment-induced MSK Disease

Treatment-induced MSK complications include avascular necrosis (AVN), osteoporosis with or without fracture or vertebral body collapse (see Morbidities), and growth failure. A steroid-induced myopathy is rarely seen in pSLE. However, a statin-associated myopathy will likely be seen more commonly as these drugs are increasingly used to treat pSLE.[150-153] Approximately 5% to 10% of pSLE patients develop AVN.[154] When the diagnosis is based on MRI only, AVN is seen in up to 40% of patients, but most will not progress to x-ray changes.[155-156] Typically AVN occurs in the juxtaarticular regions of the large weight-bearing bones (femur and tibia being the most commonly involved). In general, AVN is associated with long-term, high-dose steroid therapy; however, it may occur with standard therapy, within weeks of initiation of steroids, and may be associated with high disease activity.[154,155,157-159] Although suggested in early studies, there is no consistent association with antiphospholipid antibodies (aPLs).[154,157,160-162] In the past, core decompression and avoidance of weight bearing were suggested for patients with AVN, but these therapies have not been shown to be beneficial.[163] In contrast, vascularized fibular grafting has been shown to be of benefit.[164,165] Arthroplasty and joint replacement are reserved for patients with severe, intractable pain and/or disability and tend to be deferred until fusion of the growth plate.

Treatment of MSK Disease

In many pediatric patients arthritis occurs, or flares, at the times of high disease activity in other organs and will respond to treatment related to specific organ involvement. Arthritis may herald a systemic flare. In patients

Table 21–7

Medications commonly used in pediatric SLE (excluding corticosteroids)

Medication	Major Indications	Usual Dose	Major Side Effects	Precautions
Hydroxychloroquine	Most patients	5-6 mg/kg/day maximum 400 mg	Ophthalmological Cardiac muscle	Reduce dose in renal insufficiency Ophthalmological exam q 6 months
Nonsteroidal antiinflammatory drugs (NSAIDs)	Systemic features Musculoskeletal	Varies by drug	Gastrointestinal Aseptic meningitis	Give with caution with decreased renal function
Methotrexate	Steroid sparing	Up to 15 mg/m^2/wk: orally or subcutaneously maximum 25 mg	Hepatitis Bone marrow suppression	Monitor CBC and LFTs Alter dose in renal insufficiency
Azathioprine	Proliferative nephritis Steroid sparing	3 mg/kg/day maximum 150 mg	Bone marrow suppression Hepatitis infection	Monitor CBC and LFTs
Cyclophosphamide	NP disease Proliferative nephritis	1 g/m^2/mo intravenously	Bone marrow suppression Infection Infertility Malignancy	Alter dose with renal insufficiency Give PCP prophylaxis Give mesna Monitor CBC and urine
Mycophenolate mofetil	Proliferative and membranous lupus nephritis NP disease Steroid-sparing when other drugs fail	1 g/m^2/day (can measure levels)	Bone marrow suppression Hepatitis infection	Monitor CBC and LFTs May need to alter dose with renal insufficiency

CBC, complete blood count; LFT, liver function test; NP, neuropsychiatric; PCP, *Pneumocystis jiroveci* pneumonia.

with relatively mild systemic disease, treatment with nonsteroidal antiinflammatory drugs (NSAIDs) combined with an antimalarial drug usually suffices. However, steroids are frequently required, although an immunosuppressive agent (methotrexate, azathioprine, and occasionally mycophenolate mofetil) may be used to decrease corticosteroid dosage (Tables 21–7 and 21–8).

Mucocutaneous Involvement

The reported incidence of cutaneous involvement at presentation of pSLE varies from to 60% to 80% of patients, with up to 85% of patients having skin involvement during the course of the disease (see Tables 21–5 and 21–6). A list of mucocutaneous features seen in pSLE is shown in Table 21–9. The characteristic rash of SLE maculopapular in a malar distribution, the so-called "butterfly" rash. It extends over the bridge of the nose. It may not involve the whole malar area, and the extension from the malar area to the bridge of the nose does not need to be contiguous. Specific features that help to distinguish it from sunburn include the sparing of the nasolabial folds, extension onto the nose, and the frequent occurrence of the rash on the chin (Figures 21–1, 21–2). It usually has distinctive borders, and it is may be raised. The rash tends to be photosensitive (nonmandatory) and heals without scarring (Figures 21–3, 21–4). The only other disease that can give an identical rash, both clinically and histologically, is JDM. There are other rare syndromes that may cause a photosensitive rash in the malar area, but generally they have different distinguishing features (Table 21–10 [online only]).

Sun exposure may precipitate a rash over the neck or arms and legs. This rash, annular erythema, tends to be circular or "discoid-shaped." It is seen in 10% to 20% of patients and should not be confused with a true discoid lupus rash (Figures 21–5, 21–6). A true discoid lesion, as described in the classification criteria, is uncommonly seen in pSLE, as is isolated discoid lupus erythematosus (DLE).[166,167] Discoid lesions may be photosensitive, frequently occur on the forehead and in the scalp, are rarely bilateral, tend to be more orange-red as (as opposed to the more pink lesions of annular erythema), and tend to have more of a scale. The importance of this lesion is that it heals with atrophy, scarring, and possible pigmentary changes. Discoid lesions may have a distinct histology but also may resemble the skin lesions of SLE.[167,168]

Annular erythema is also the characteristic lesion seen in subacute cutaneous lupus (SCLE), which is associated with anti-Ro and anti-La antibodies (Figure 21–7).[169-171] Isolated SCLE is more common in adult SLE than in pSLE.

Hyperemia of the oral and nasal mucosa is common but nonspecific. Oral mucosal lesions tend occur on the hard palate, although involvement of the buccal mucosa may occur. Hard palate lesions range from hyperemia, to petechial rashes, to true ulceration. The ulcers are usually painless unless they come in contact with an irritant (Figure 21–8). Although more usually associated with Wegener granulomatosis, nasal septal involvement with perforation occurs in pSLE[172]; however, shallow ulcerations or mucosal hyperemia are more common.

Table 21–8

Approach to Management of pSLE

General
Counseling, education, team approach
Adequate rest, appropriate nutrition
Appropriate exercise
Vitamin D supplementations and ensure adequate calcium intake
Use of sunscreen
Immunizations, especially antipneumococcal vaccine
Prompt management of infection

Indications for Nonsteroidal antiinflammatory drug use
Mild constitutional symptoms
Musculoskeletal signs and symptoms
Mild pleuritis and pericarditis

Indications for Hydroxychloroquine Use
Mild systemic disease
Cutaneous disease
Alopecia
Arthritis
Adjunctive therapy for most patients
    May delay development of overt autoimmune disease in "preautoimmune" patient

Indications and Use of Glucocorticoids

General systemic disease, cutaneous disease, serositis, or musculoskeletal disease
Oral prednisone 0.25-0.75 mg/kg/day as single dose is usually adequate for most patients. Occasionally split doses may be possible
For serositis 0.5-1.0 mg/kg/day (maximum 60 mg/day) and frequently BID dosing may be required. Always use minimal dose possible

Major organ involvement—Renal (Class III or IV) or significant NP involvement
Oral prednisone
- Initial 6 weeks: 2 mg/kg/day (maximum 60-80 mg/day) divided TID for 4 weeks then OD
- Subsequent 3 months: taper by 10 mg monthly
- When dosage reaches 30 mg/day: taper 5 mg q 4-8 depending on response (flares frequently occur between 20-25 mg/day)
- When dosage reaches 20 mg/day: Slow taper to 2.5 mg q6-8 weeks depending on response (flares frequently occur between 10-15 mg/day)
- When dosage reaches 10-15 mg/day consider alternate prednisone and when reach 15 mg alternate day then slow taper to 2.5-5.0 mg/day alternate q 3-6 months
Intravenous pulse methylprednisolone (10-30 mg/kg/day; maximum 1 g/day). May be considered early in patients with severe disease but is rarely required for >3 doses. There is no evidence monthly maintenance therapy is of benefit when oral prednisone is used.

Indications and Use of Immunosuppressive Agents
Methotrexate
- Indications: musculoskeletal or skin disease, Steroid-sparing agent
- Dosage: 10-15mg/m^2/week either orally or subcutaneously
- Folate supplementation strongly recommended

Azathioprine
- Indications: Class III or IV lupus nephritis, NP disease when mild, Steroid-sparing agent
- Dosage: 3 mg/kg/day (maximum 150 mg/day)

MMF or MPA
- Indications: Class III or IV lupus nephritis, NP diseases, Steroid-sparing agent when methotrexate and azathioprine fail or patient is intolerant
- Dosage: 1 g/m^2/day divided twice daily for MMF and 720 mg/m^2/day for MPA
- Can increase if tolerate
- Able to measure serum levels

Cyclophosphamide
- Indications: Severe NP disease
  Consider for Class III or IV nephritis if azathioprine or MMF is not effective or patient is intolerant. There is no evidence that cyclophosphamide is superior to the other two agents in patients with severe renal disease or patients at high risk for poor long-term outcome
- Dosage: Standard: begin at 500 mg/m^2; can increase to 1000 mg/m^2 (intravenous)
  Alternatively, Eurolupus protocol
- Use mesna
- Ensure high urine flow
- Metabolism of drug is under control of cytochrome p450 enzyme genetic polymorphisms

Cyclosporine
- Indications:
  Class V lupus nephritis
  Macrophage activation syndrome
- Dosage: 2-5 mg/kg/day divided BID
  Use levels to help in dosing
  Minimum dose to control disease should be used and monitor for toxicities

MMF, mycophenolate mofetil; MPA, mycophenolic acid; NP, neuropsychiatric.

Raynaud phenomenon is seen in 15% to 20% of patients with pSLE (see Chapter 29). Patients may have the classic triphasic changes or only two color changes. However, if there are only two color changes, one of them must be the reflex hyperemia. Many patients will respond to non-medical interventions that include cold avoidance, the use of insulated mittens rather than gloves, multiple layers of light clothing rather than a single heavy piece of clothing, hats, and/or hand/feet warmers. If these measures are not adequate, calcium-channel blocking agents may be used, preferably long acting or sustained release. Nailfold abnormalities are frequently seen but are not specific for SLE. They include abnormal capillary loops with sludging, drop-out of capillaries, and loop length variability.[173]

Although the pathology of SLE is generally not a vasculitis, true vasculitic rashes do occur and these include: 1) frank ulceration (Figure 21–9); 2) nodules;

Table 21–9

Spectrum of skin involvement

Malar "butterfly" rash
Photosensitivity
Annular rash*
Alopecia
Raynaud phenomenon
Vasculitis
  petechiae
  palpable purpura (leukocytoclastic vasculitis)
  urticarial vasculitis
  digital ulcers
  periungual gangrene
Livedo reticularis
Periungual erythema
Subacute lupus erythematosus*
Linear
Discoid lupus erythematosus
Panniculitis
Chilblains
Bullous lupus erythematosus

*Frequently associated with anti-Ro/La antibodies

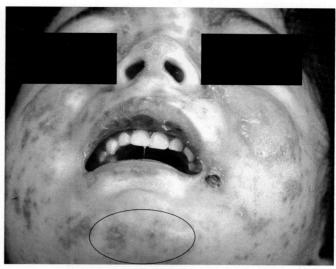

FIGURE 21–2 **Malar rash.** Butterfly rash extending over bridge of nose. There is sparing below the lip chin involvement.

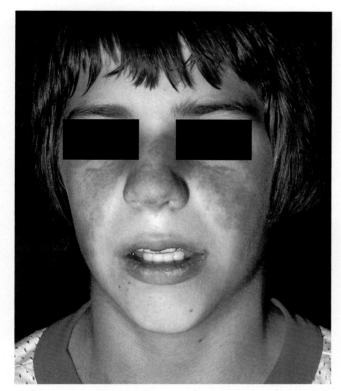

FIGURE 21–1 Malar erythema of acute systemic lupus erythematosus. The classic butterfly rash has erupted over both cheeks and spread over the bridge of the nose. It may be punctate and follicular or an erythematous blush. The rash does not leave a scar.

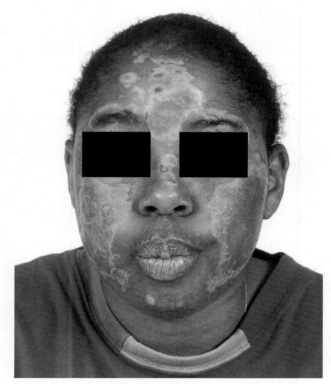

FIGURE 21–3 **Photosensitive rash.** Rash appeared after significant sun exposure.

3) punctate erythema (Figure 21–10); and 4) palpable purpura (Figure 21–11) which may be confused with Henoch Schonlein Purpura (HSP). Ulcerative skin lesions tend to be painful and are most frequently found on fingers or toes.

A nodular skin lesion resembling chilblains, both clinically and histologically may be seen.[174-176] Resistant ulcerative skin lesions have been associated with congenital complement deficiencies (Figure 21–12).[177-181]

Alopecia is common but scarring alopecia is rare. When the latter is present, it is frequently associated with discoid lesions in the scalp.[182,183] Alopecia tends to mild, but it can be severe and may be the presenting feature.

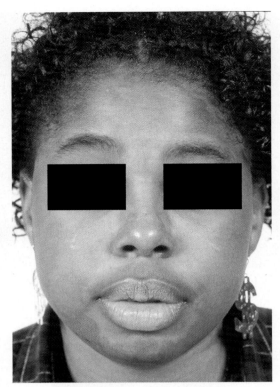

FIGURE 21–4 Healed malar rash. Same patient as seen in Figure 21–3, now 4 months later with healing without a scar.

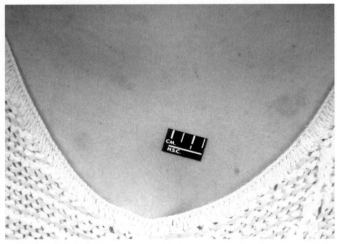

FIGURE 21–5 Photosensitive annular (discoid shaped) rash associated with anti-Ro antibodies.

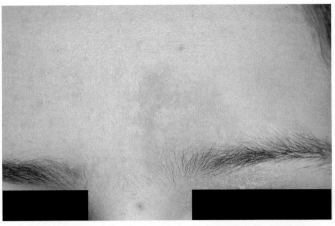

FIGURE 21–6 Discoid rash. Discoid over the eye with evidence of scaly rash and induration

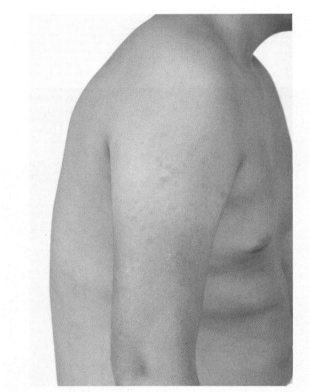

FIGURE 21–7 Subacute cutaneous lupus. Isolated rash of subacute cutaneous lupus is less commonly seen in pediatric patients in association with SLE.

Treatment of Mucocutaneous Disease

Avoidance of sunbathing and the use of sun-blocking agents (with high sun-protecting factor) and protective clothing (including long-sleeved shirts and hats) are recommended. Skin flares frequently accompany systemic flares, and treatment of the systemic flare usually improves skin disease. However, topical treatment may be required and, when severe, corticosteroids and rarely other immunosuppressive agents may be required (Tables 21–7, 21–8, and Table 21–11 [online only]). All patients with skin disease should be on antimalarials.

Renal Involvement

Involvement of the kidneys is a significant cause of morbidity and mortality in patients with pSLE and thus has a major impact on the choice of immunosuppressive therapy—in both the induction and maintenance (of remission) phases.[184] In the Euro-Lupus project of 1000 adult patients with SLE, the 10-year patient survival was 94% without and 88% with nephritis.[117] Approximately 50% of pSLE patients have evidence of renal involvement, 80% to 90% within first year of diagnosis

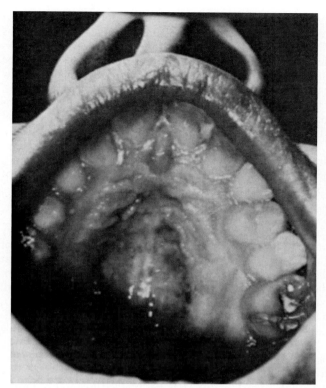

FIGURE 21–8   Mucocutaneous ulcerations of acute systemic lupus erythematosus. A shallow, painless, erythematous ulceration with an irregular margin is seen on the hard palate.

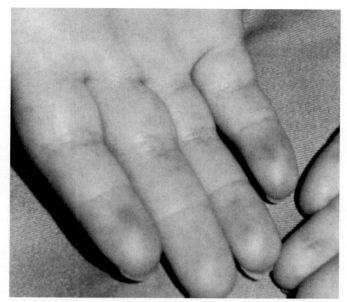

FIGURE 21–10   Vasculitis seen as punctate erythema of the fingertips of a child with systemic lupus erythematosus.

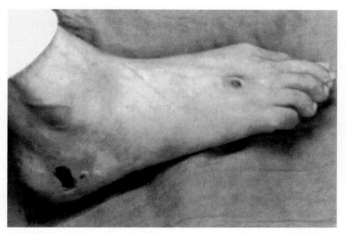

FIGURE 21–9   Chronic and well-demarcated ulcers of the skin in a child with systemic lupus erythematosus.

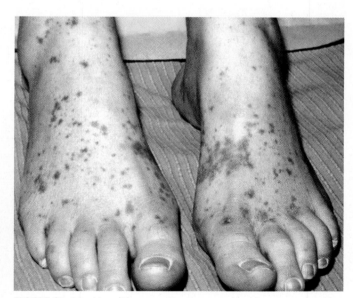

FIGURE 21–11   Vasculitic purpura in a teenage girl with an acute exacerbation of systemic lupus erythematosus.

(see Table 21–6). In 10% to 20% of patients, the nephritis usually occurs between year 1 and year 2 after diagnosis, but late development beyond 5 years can occur.[89,185,186] In 1974 the World Health Organization (WHO) introduced a classification for lupus glomerular disease that most recently was revised by the International Society of Nephrology/Renal Pathology Society in 2004 (Table 21–12 and Table 21–13 [online only]).[187,188] This almost universally accepted classification system attempts to integrate acute and chronic disease and to take interstitial and vascular complications into consideration.

A particularly helpful feature is the separate reporting of membranous and proliferative lesions when both occur together in a single patient. The relative frequency of each subclass in pediatric SLE patients is summarized in Table 21–12.[89,109,136,189-194] In most studies, the distribution of the various forms of lupus nephritis is similar in childhood- and adult-onset SLE, although the incidence of nephritis may be higher in children.[195]

Lupus Glomerulonephritis

The most common patterns of lupus glomerulonephritis seen in pSLE are (in order): 1) proliferative glomerulonephritis (Classes III and IV); 2) mesangial proliferative glomerulonephritis (Class II); and 3) membranous

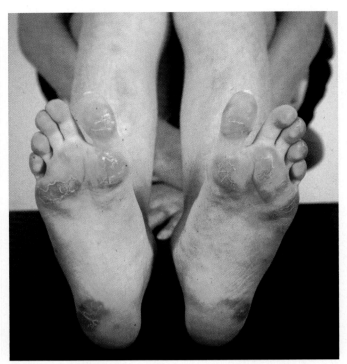

FIGURE 21–12 Significant persistent ulceration of feet in a patient with C4 deficiency.

nephropathy (Class V) (Figure 21–13; see Table 21–12). Other lesions that are less common and may occur either as isolated findings or in association with the other common patterns are: 1) thrombotic microangiopathy—similar to hemolytic uremic syndrome (HUS), which is frequently associated with aPLs; and 2) focal necrotizing lesions, similar to ANCA-positive vasculitis (seen with Class III or IV lesions only). No matter what the primary lesion, renal outcomes most closely parallel the degree of fibrosis. Even today chronic and end-stage kidney disease remains a significant cause of morbidity and mortality. Advanced renal scarring with significant loss of functional nephrons cannot be reversed with immunosuppressive therapy. Presentation with advanced renal scarring or crescents and focal necrotizing lesions is associated with a poor prognosis.[196]

PATHOGENESIS

Lupus glomerulonephritis is an immune complex–mediated glomerular disease.[197-199] It is generally accepted that the immune complexes form locally within the glomerulus as lupus autoantibodies react with intraglomerular antigens (Figure 21–14). Most investigators now believe that there is in situ deposition of immune complexes rather than deposition of circulating preformed complexes. The target antigen(s) is still not clear and candidate antigens include any or all of: 1) cell membrane components (mesangial cells, endothelial cells, podocytes); 2) basement membrane proteins; 3) intracellular proteins (nucleosome-derived peptides, α-actinin); and 4) other unknown antigens. Immune deposits are almost universally found within the mesangial regions of glomeruli. Deposits along the endothelial aspect of the glomerular capillary wall (wire

loop lesions develop when numerous deposits are present) are characteristic of diffuse proliferative lupus nephritis (DPLN), while membranous lupus nephropathy (MLN) is defined by the presence of immune complexes along the subepithelial aspect (urinary space side) of the glomerular basement membrane beneath the podocyte foot processes. The coexistence of subendothelial deposits and/or mesangial hypercellularity is more suggestive of MLN than of idiopathic membranous nephropathy.

Glomerular immune deposits contain immunoglobulin G (IgG), IgM, IgA, and complement. (The presence of complement deposition illustrates the importance of complement activation.)

CLINICAL SYNDROMES

Patients may present with identical clinical and laboratory manifestations but have a different histological pattern of glomerular involvement. Given this fact and evidence that different forms of kidney involvement require different therapy, a kidney biopsy is strongly recommended in all patients with evidence of renal involvement. In particular, it is well recognized that relatively mild clinical manifestations may be present in biopsy-confirmed DPLN (see Table 21–12). However, initial treatment does not necessarily need to be delayed because the short-term use of corticosteroids will not change the glomerular histology. However, it is that important NSAIDs be avoided in the pre-biopsy period.

There are 5 major clinical syndromes of lupus nephritis (see Table 21–12):

1) Isolated asymptomatic hematuria and proteinuria. (Microscopic hematuria alone may also occasionally occur, usually, but not always, as a result of mesangial lupus.)
2) Acute nephritic syndrome. Hypertension at diagnosis suggests more serious disease—DPLN, thrombotic microangiopathy, or advanced disease (or, rarely, renal infarction associated with aPLs).
3) Nephrotic syndrome. This may occur in isolation or associated with nephritic features. DPLN and MLN are the most common causes of nephrotic syndrome. Rarely a unique variant of mesangial lupus nephritis may present as nephrotic syndrome. This appears to be a cytokine-mediated (nonproliferative/noninflammatory) disease that (like isolated idiopathic steroid-responsive nephrotic syndrome) responds rapidly to corticosteroids.[200]
4) Gross hematuria may be a manifestation of the acute nephritic syndrome, but it is not commonly seen in patients with SLE. When gross hematuria is present in a patient with SLE, it should raise suspicion for other causes such as renal vein thrombosis (as a complication of nephrotic syndrome or antiphospholipid antibodies) and a clotting factor deficiency (such as prothrombin deficiency).[201,202]
5) Chronic kidney disease (CKD).

Treatment of Renal Disease

Although lupus nephritis can be controlled with medical therapy, there is no known cure. The class and severity of the renal disease guides the approach to immunosuppression (Tables 21–14, 21–7, and 21–8). Severe lupus

Table 21-12

Pathological and clinical features of lupus nephritis

Class	Name	Histology			Frequency		Clinical		
		Light	IF	EM	Biopsy data	No symptoms	Nephritic syndrome	Nephrotic Syndrome	BP↑
I	Minimal Mesangial	Deposits, normal cellularity	Immune deposits positive for complement and immunoglobulins (IgG>IgM>IgA)	Electron dense deposits in the location suggested by immunofluorescence microscopy	<5%	√			
II	Mesangial Proliferative	Mild increase in mesangial matrix and cells	mesangial deposits, rare GBM deposits		19-27%	√		Rare	
III	Focal Proliferative	<50% glomeruli hypercellular with increased matrix	mesangial deposits> subendothelial GBM deposits		15-24%	√		Rare	
IV	Diffuse Proliferative	>50% glomeruli have increased cells and matrix, may be thickened GBM segments ("wire-loops")	Mesangial and diffuse subendothelial deposits		40-50%	√	√	√	√
V	Membranous	Thickened GBM, cellularity normal or mildly increased	Subepithelial deposits > mesangial deposits		10-20%	√		√	Rare
VI	Advanced Sclerosing	Irreversible advanced disease, >90% glomerulosclerosis	Staining may be positive in sclerotic areas		<5%		√	√	√
Other Lesions									
	Thrombotic microangiopathy	Glomerular capillaries thickened and congested with RBCs, arteriolar thrombi	Fibrin deposits	Endothelial cells swollen, subendothelial space filled with fluffy material	Low		√	Rare	
	Interstitial nephritis (isolated)	Interstitial inflammation, tubular damage	Tubular immune deposits may be present, but not a universal finding		Low	√ (or tubular dysfunction)			√

BP, blood pressure; EM, electron microscopy; GBM, glomerular basement membrane; IF, immunofluorescence; RBCs, red blood cells

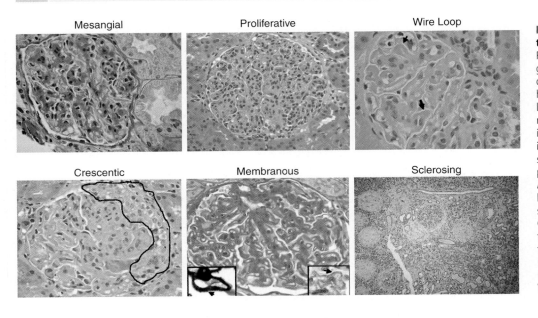

FIGURE 21–13 Histological patterns of lupus glomerulonephritis. Representative kidney photomicrographs illustrate the primary patterns of lupus glomerulonephritis. *Arrows* highlight two of the several wire loop lesions in the upper right image that represent coalescent subendothelial immune deposits. The small inserts in the membranous photomicrograph show subepithelial immune deposits present between the "spikes" *(arrowhead)* of glomerular basement membrane (GBM) on Jone's methenamine silver staining (left) and as red-stained GBM deposits *(arrow)* on Masson's trichrome staining (right insert). (Photomicrographs provided by Dr. Laura Finn, Department of Pathology, Seattle Children's Hospital and the University of Washington.)

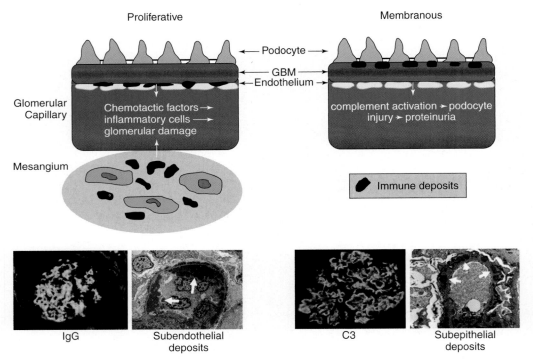

FIGURE 21–14 Pathogenesis of lupus nephritis. The diagram schematically summarizes two distinct patterns of glomerular injury that may develop in SLE patients. Shown below are representative histological photomicrographs illustrating subendothelial immune deposits *(arrows)*. Small subepithelial deposits are also present in a patient with diffuse proliferative lupus nephritis (left) and subepithelial immune deposits *(arrows)* in a patients with membranous lupus glomerulonephritis. (Photomicrographs provided by Dr. Laura Finn, Department of Pathology, Seattle Children's Hospital and the University of Washington.)

nephritis typically takes many months to years to completely respond once induction therapy is initiated. It is important to note that the degree of proteinuria will almost universally increase before it decreases. In fact when the renal lesion is severe, the proteinuria frequently increases for 3 to 4 months. The increase in proteinuria is thought to represent improved perfusion of damaged glomerular capillaries as the inflammation begins to subside; the lesions must begin to heal before the proteinuria can decrease. Therefore, patience and meticulous supportive medical care (not additions or alterations to the induction treatment protocol) are required during the initial phase of management: most patients generally

achieve remission, although it usually takes many months to years if the lesion is severe. For refractory patients, the possibility of medication non-compliance and the presence of irreversible glomerular scarring (which may cause proteinuria but not an active urine sediment) need to be considered. When there is a sudden deterioration of renal function, a secondary cause such as renal vein or artery thrombosis, poor renal perfusion secondary to medication (ACE-inhibitors in particular), infection, or contracted intravascular volume or drug-induced interstitial nephritis should be considered. Optimal therapy for true refractory patients with aggressive uncontrolled nephritis is unclear,[203-205] but plasmapheresis has been shown

Table 21-14

General guidelines for immunosuppressive therapy in lupus nephritis

Class	Name	Treatment
I	Minimal mesangial	Determined by extrarenal manifestations
II	Mesangial proliferative	Determined by extrarenal manifestations. Antiproteinuric antihypertensives may be considered.
III	Focal proliferative	Corticosteroids plus immunosuppressive agents (especially if crescents or focal necrotizing lesions)
IV	Diffuse proliferative	Corticosteroids plus immunosuppressive agents induce response in >80%
V	Membranous	When associated with proliferative lesions, treatment guided by the latter. Evidence-based guidelines for pure membranous lacking: steroids plus calcineurin inhibitors (MMF and cyclophosphamide are alternatives). Proteinuria levels usually guide therapy. Antiproteinuric antihypertensives should be considered.
VI	Advanced sclerosing	Determined by extrarenal manifestations.
	Interstitial nephritis	Isolated disease is rare; treated with steroids ± immunosuppressive agents.
	Thrombotic microangiopathy	Isolated disease is rare; may be role for apheresis and anticoagulation for antiphospholipid antibody–associated disease in addition to immunosuppression.

not to improve renal outcomes.[206] Hydroxychloroquine has been shown to have reno-protective effects in lupus nephritis but should not be added until the renal function has stabilized (see Table 21–7).[207]

Lupus nephritis can recur after variable periods of remission with relapse rates of 40% to 50% for DPLN.[208-212] Maintenance immunosuppressive therapy with either mycophenolate mofetil or azathioprine is the standard of care for proliferative nephritis.[213-217] The calcineurin-inhibiting drugs are an acceptable alternative for membranous nephropathy.[218-221]

There is considerable interest in identifying urinary biomarkers as sensitive and early predictors of a nephritic flare with some recent promising studies, but these markers should be considered experimental and have not demonstrated clinical utility.[222-224] Careful examination of the urine sediment should be routinely performed at each clinic visit for evidence for new hematuria, pyuria, and/or cellular casts because these biomarkers may be an equally sensitive early indicator of renal disease reactivation. First-morning urine protein:creatinine ratios are a reliable way to monitor protein excretion rates in SLE patients on maintenance therapy, although they may not be as accurate as 24-hour urine collections.[225-227]

A feature of lupus nephritis is its potential to transform from one class to another over time. Proliferative lesions occasionally transform to non-proliferative MLN or class II LN, and a class II lesion can transform to proliferative LN. Repeat renal biopsies may be indicated when such transformations are clinically suspected and will influence therapeutic choices.

Interstitial Nephritis

Interstitial inflammation is typically present in association with proliferative lupus nephritis and at times may be severe. Several pathogenic mechanisms have been suggested, including leakage of inflammatory cytokines from damaged glomeruli directly into the interstitium (via breaks in the Bowman capsule or disruption of glomerular-tubular junctions) or interaction of inflammatory cytokines or other urinary proteins (including modified albumin) with the apical membrane of proximal tubules to trigger interstitial inflammation.[228,229]

On rare occasions, interstitial nephritis may develop as the predominant renal lesion in SLE (Figure 21–15)[230] and may be associated with clinical and/or laboratory abnormalities resulting from tubular injury and dysfunction of the proximal tubular (acidosis, phosphaturia, glycosuria, low–molecular weight proteinuria), distal tubular (acidosis, hyperkalemia), and collecting duct (polyuria).[231]

Important alternative causes of interstitial nephritis that should be considered include a variety of infections (including several viral infections) and drugs (antibiotics, NSAIDs, thiazide diuretics, and proton pump inhibitors).[231]

Renal disease secondary to blood vessel involvement is covered in APLA section.

Renal Outcomes

Renal outcomes have significantly improved with current induction and maintenance protocols, together with better prevention, early diagnosis, and treatment of infectious and thrombotic complications. The incidence of ESRD secondary to lupus nephritis has declined in the last decade (Figure 21–16).[232] Ethnicity influences prognosis—outcomes are worse in people of African descent and Hispanics than in people of other ethnicities.[192,233-235]

An integral component of treating patients with lupus nephritis is achieving optimal hypertension control. In patients with proteinuria, antihypertensive drugs that inhibit the renin-angiotensin system (angiotensin-converting enzyme inhibitors and angiotensin receptor blockers) and also reduce urinary protein excretion are the preferred chronic agents because proteinuria is an independent risk factor for faster rates of CKD progression and for cardiovascular morbidity and mortality.[236]

When lupus nephritis leads to ESRD, kidney transplantation is an option. If the systemic disease is quiescent at the time of transplantation, the risk of recurrence of lupus nephritis is low; however, with improved allograft survival

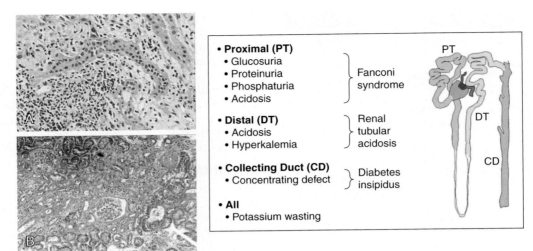

- **Proximal (PT)**
  - Glucosuria
  - Proteinuria
  - Phosphaturia
  - Acidosis
  } Fanconi syndrome

- **Distal (DT)**
  - Acidosis
  - Hyperkalemia
  } Renal tubular acidosis

- **Collecting Duct (CD)**
  - Concentrating defect
  } Diabetes insipidus

- **All**
  - Potassium wasting

FIGURE 21–15   Interstitial disease in lupus nephritis. Histological photomicrographs illustrate acute interstitial nephritis (**A**) that occasionally occurs as a manifestation of lupus nephritis in the absence of significant glomerular disease, and interstitial fibrosis identified by the blue interstitial staining with Masson's tri-chrome (**B**). The degree of interstitial fibrosis is an important predictor of renal functional impairment and long-term prognosis. The *nephron* on the right illustrates the pattern of renal tubular dysfunction that may develop in patients with significant tubulointerstitial disease. (Reproduced with permission from Verghese P Luckritz K, Eddy A: Interstitial nephritis. In Geary D, Schaefer F, editors: *Clinical pediatric nephrology*, Philadelphia, 2008, Mosby.)

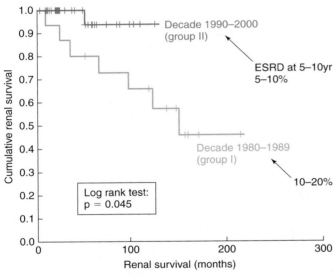

FIGURE 21–16   Renal survival in SLE. Comparison of incidence of terminal renal failure between two eras illustrates improved outcomes with newer treatment protocols. n = 15 group I patients and 41 group II patients. (Reproduced with permission from Fiehn C, Hajjar Y, Mueller K et al: Improved clinical outcome of lupus nephritis during the past decade: importance of early diagnosis and treatment, *Ann Rheum Dis* 62:435-439, 2003).

times, the rate of recurrence of lupus nephritis appears to be increasing.[237] Despite excellent allograft outcomes, there is some evidence that patient survival is lower in transplant patients with SLE than in patients with ESRD.[238] Cardiovascular disease, infections, and malignancy are important causes of death.[239] This fact deserves consideration when weighing the risks and benefits of aggressive immunosuppression with agents such as cyclophosphamide in patients with advanced chronic (and irreversible) kidney damage.

Neuropsychiatric Disease

Involvement of peripheral nervous system (PNS) and the CNS has been reported to occur in 20% to 95% of patients with pSLE (see Table 21–6).[110,131,240-245] This large variation in incidence and prevalence of nervous system involvement is the result of differing definitions (particularly for headaches) used in different studies, the small sample size of many studies, and referral bias. Because SLE can involve both the CNS and PNS, the term *neuropsychiatric systemic lupus erythematosus* (NP-SLE) has gained currency to describe this aspect of SLE. In 1999 the ACR developed a new classification system for NP-SLE that separated NP disease into 19 entities (see Table 21–15 [online only]).[246,247] (Table 21–16 reviews the frequency of the individual NP manifestations in pSLE). Although this classification system was defined in adult cohorts, it is generally useful in pSLE. The majority of patients with NP-SLE have the initial signs and symptoms within the first year of diagnosis of SLE; approximately 25% initially develop NP-SLE more than 2 years after disease onset.[240]

NP Disease Manifestations

HEADACHES

Headache is the most common NP manifestation. However, despite the use of 1999 case definitions, it can be difficult to differentiate a headache due to active SLE from other causes. A large study reported that "significant" headache occurred in approximately 50% of pSLE patients.[248] The term *lupus headache* is defined as a severe, unremitting headache requiring narcotic analgesic treatment.[249] This severe, unremitting headache is important to recognize because it usually reflects significant NP disease. It includes active CNS vasculitis, cerebral vein thrombosis, and raised intracranial

Table 21–16

Frequency of NP manifestations in pSLE

Central nervous system*	
Headache (any)	4-55% (95%)
Recurrent	10-50%
Migraine	3-10%
Benign Intracranial hypertension	2-4%
Cognitive dysfunction	
Acute confusional state	3-9%
Mood disorder	5-9%
Depression	5-9%
Maniac	0-3%
Mixed Features	0-1%
Seizure disorder (any)	4-20%
Single episode	4-20%
Epilepsy	0-2%
Anxiety disorder	1-10%
Cerebrovascular disease (any)	4-14%
Transient ischemic attack	0-2%
Cerebral Infarction (stroke)	2-9%
Venous thrombosis (sinus vein)	1-4%
Vasculitis	1-2%
Hemorrhage	1-3%
"Chronic multifocal disease"	1-2%
Psychosis	3-24%
Movement disorder (any)	0-6%
Chorea	0-5%
Parkinsonian	Case reports
Demyelinating syndrome	2-3%
Aseptic meningitis—may be idio-pathic (acute or chronic) or secondary to drugs[†]	0-2%
Myelopathy	1-2%
Peripheral nervous system	3-5%
Acute inflammatory demyelinating polyradiculoneuropathy (Guillain-Barré syndrome and its variants)	Case reports only
Chronic inflammatory demyelinating polyradiculoneuropathy	Case reports only
Autonomic disorder	Case reports only [‡]
Mononeuropathy, single/multiplex	1-2%
Myasthenia gravis	Case reports only
Neuropathy, cranial	1-4%
Plexopathy	No reported pediatric case
Polyneuropathy	0-2%

Sources: references 134, 240, 241, 244, 245, 250, 263, 268, 285, 632-635.
*Many patients have more than one manifestation
[†]Drugs associated with aseptic meningitis: NSAIDs (ibuprofen, tolmetin, sulindac, naproxen, diclofenac) lamotrigine, trimethoprim-sulfamethoxasole, influenza vaccination, azathioprine
[‡]One report suggested a 42% rate of subclinical autonomic nervous system involvement.[285]

pressure. Although a headache may occur in isolation, it is frequently seen in association with more significant NP involvement. It is important to determine the cause of migraine-like headaches because a migraine headache is a vascular headache and may represent significant pathology.

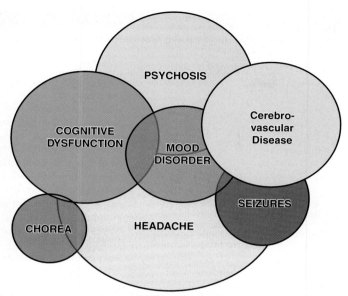

FIGURE 21–17   Overlapping NP symptoms in pSLE. Patients with pSLE most commonly have more than one NP symptom—in particular for seizures.

PSYCHOSIS

The diagnosis of psychosis is made in 30% to 50% of pediatric patients with NP involvement, or approximately 10% to 13% of all patients with pSLE (see Table 21–16). The hallucinations seen in pSLE resemble those seen in other organic psychoses, but with some unique features. They tend to be visual, although auditory (but rarely tactile) hallucinations occur and pSLE patients tend to have preserved insight.[240,250,251] Psychosis is frequently accompanied by cognitive dysfunction, confusion, and headaches (Figure 21–17). Both laboratory measurements and brain parenchymal imaging are frequently normal (Table 21–17); however, CNS imaging may be helpful in differentiating NP-SLE–associated psychosis from other forms of psychosis.[252] Antiribosomal P antibodies have been associated with depression and psychosis in SLE, but these antibodies are not specific for depression (Table 21–18). Steroid-induced psychosis is an infrequent complication of pSLE, and patients usually have different clinical features.[253-259]

COGNITIVE DYSFUNCTION AND ACUTE CONFUSIONAL STATE

Cognitive impairment ranges from concentration difficulties, a decrease in school performance, to frank confusion and coma. As seen in patients with psychosis, inflammatory markers and imaging are frequently normal in patients with cognitive dysfunction or acute confusional state. Although the diagnosis of overt organic brain syndrome is rarely in doubt, it is difficult to determine if subtle involvement and, in particular, new-onset learning difficulties are SLE-related. Neuropsychological testing reveals patterns of abnormalities similar to those seen in adults with SLE.[260] Although there have been efforts to develop a standardized battery of tests, currently there is no standardized testing for cognitive impairment in pSLE.[260-262] In adult SLE neurocognitive testing, abnormalities have been associated with presence

Table 21–17

Possible investigations for patients with NP involvement

Examination	Indication	Common findings
Cerebrospinal fluid	Possible infection (most important indication)	Increased WBC, protein, and/or opening pressure
	Subarachnoid hemorrhage	Increased RBC
	Demonstrate active inflammation	Increased WBC, protein and/or opening pressure[240, 244]
Neurocognitive testing	Detection of subtle changes in cognition	Executive function and spatial abnormalities
	Assessment to aid in schooling	
Computed tomography (usually unnecessary if magnetic resonance imaging available, although venogram can be helpful)	Demonstrate focal lesion secondary to large vessel disease	Bleed or infarction
	Detect raised intracranial pressure	Enlarged ventricles
	Venogram for sinus vein thrombosis	Absence of flow
Magnetic resonance imaging (MRI) (neuroimaging modality of choice)	Demonstrate focal lesion secondary to large vessel disease	Infarction
	Demonstrate small vessel disease (vasculitis)	Single or multiple areas of abnormal signal
	Severe Headache	Depends on cause (see Headache)
Magnetic resonance angiography or venogram (conventional angiogram usually not needed)	Suspected vasculitis or sinus vein thrombosis (venogram)	Demonstrates presence and degree of vessel involvement-may miss small vessel disease
MRI Spectroscopy	Limited to investigational	Abnormal metabolites
fluoro-2-deoxy-D-glucose positron emission tomography (FDG-PET)	Investigational	Abnormal perfusion (metabolism) but may be abnormal without NP involvement
Single photon emission computed tomography (SPECT)	Good if diagnosis of SLE in doubt in patient with psychosis or confusional state	Abnormal perfusion (metabolism) but may be abnormal without NP involvement

NP, neuropsychiatric; RBC, red blood cell count; WBC, white blood cell count.

of multiple antibodies, but the associations have not been validated in independent cohorts.

DEPRESSION

Depression is commonly seen in pSLE and may be reactive (most common form), a corticosteroid effect, or rarely the result of direct involvement of active SLE.[242] Other mood disorders are unusual manifestations in pSLE.[240,263]

CEREBROVASCULAR DISEASE

Cerebrovascular disease (CVD) occurs in 12% to 30% of cases with NP involvement. It can be a small vessel vasculitis involving the microcirculation with normal angiography; in the presence of a stroke it can involve a larger vessel with an abnormal angiogram.[264-265] Headaches and seizures are the most common clinical signs and symptoms of CNS vasculitis. Inflammatory markers are often elevated.

Cerebral vein thrombosis is an important manifestation to recognize and may present in the absence of other CNS manifestations. It occurs in 10% to 20% of pSLE patients with NP involvement and it is almost universally associated with the presence of aPLs, usually the lupus anticoagulant (LAC).[201,266,267] If neuroimaging studies demonstrate an absence of flow in the affected vein (Figure 21–18), anticoagulation is required on an urgent basis.

SEIZURES

Seizures are most frequently associated with other NP features, which include headaches, CVD, and cognitive dysfunction; more rarely they are found in isolation (see Table 21–15 [online only]). Generalized seizures are more

common than focal seizures. In patients with isolated seizures, inflammatory markers are commonly elevated and frequently MRI scans are abnormal.[240] Unlike studies in adult SLE, pSLE studies have only rarely found an association of aPLs and seizures.[268-272] Seizures in pSLE may also develop secondary to uremia, hypertension, or CNS infections in addition to active SLE.

MOVEMENT DISORDERS

A variety of movement disorders are seen, but chorea is the most common (see Table 21–16).[271,273] aPLs (especially LAC) are almost universally present in patients with chorea.[243-244,274-279] With the decline in rheumatic fever in developed countries, the diagnosis of SLE or isolated anti-phospholipid antibody syndrome should be considered in pediatric patients with chorea.[280]

PERIPHERAL NERVOUS SYSTEM

Involvement of either cranial or peripheral nerves has been infrequently described in pSLE, usually as case reports only.[281-283] Cranial nerve involvement is more frequently seen than peripheral nerve involvement (see Table 21–16). Transverse myelitis, almost universally associated with aPLs, usually presents with acute paraplegia or quadriplegia and may be the presenting sign of SLE.[244,274,284] Autonomic nerve dysfunction has been reported to occur frequently in adults with SLE and recently in pSLE (asymptomatic).[285-287]

NP Disease Investigations

Investigation of patients with psychosis and significant neurocognitive dysfunction are frequently normal, as described above, but it is important to exclude other

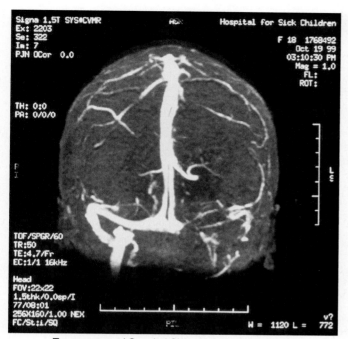

Transverse and Saggital Sinus Venous Thrombosis

FIGURE 21–18 **MRI venogram of cerebral vein thrombosis.** Patient presenting with severe, unremitting headache should be investigated for a cerebral vein thrombosis. MR venogram demonstrates occlusion of the transverse sinus.

non-SLE causes—infection, in particular—of NP signs and symptoms. Research studies have shown a variety of cerebrospinal fluid (CSF) abnormalities, including elevated cytokine and chemokine levels. Measurement of these important mediators of inflammation may help us to understand the pathophysiology of NP-SLE but currently have no clinical utility.[288-290] Although routine measurement of autoantibody levels either in the peripheral blood or CSF is not helpful, specific mention of antiribosomal P antibodies is required. The presence of antiribosomal P antibodies was initially heralded as a sensitive and specific test for depression and psychosis in SLE. However, they are frequently present in patients without any CNS disease and although it is appears to have good sensitivity for the presence of depression and psychosis, the lack of specificity makes the clinical utility of measuring anti-ribosomal P antibodies low. The results of investigations into the clinical utility of some "CNS-specific" autoantibodies are shown in Table 21–18.

Neuroimaging studies are best used to demonstrate arterial or venous occlusion and are important investigations in the presence of a stroke or seizures and to demonstrate cerebral vein thrombosis (see Table 21–17). NP-SLE–related CNS perfusion defects may be assessed by CNS SPECT or PET scans. However, they are best used to help differentiate SLE psychosis and non-SLE psychosis. In patients with SLE they are less useful to determine CNS involvement because abnormalities may be seen in patients without a history of NP involvement.[252,291-298]

Treatment of NP Disease

Treatment of NP-pSLE usually requires an interdisciplinary approach, with involvement of psychiatrists, psychologists, and/or neurologists in addition to rheumatologists. Patients with psychosis, acute confusional state, and/or organic brain syndrome have a potentially life-threatening illness. When the condition is severe, a combination therapy of high-dose steroids and an additional immunosuppressive agent such as azathioprine or cyclophosphamide (generally drug of choice) is frequently required (see Tables 21–7 and 21–8). Psychotropic drugs and supportive therapies are frequently needed. When depression is severe, antidepressants should be added. Because seizures are rarely seen in isolation, an associated underlying non-NP cause or NP cause should be pursued if seizures occur alone. Headaches resistant to analgesia are frequently caused by significant underlying CNS disease, including cerebral vein thrombosis, vasculitis, or infection; therefore, identification of the underlying cause is required. Of note, emotional ability is common with steroids.

Hematologic Involvement

Hematological involvement has been reported to occur in up to 100% of patients (Table 21–19 [online only]). There is a large variation in frequency of hematological involvement based on the racial/ethnic background of the patient group described. The most common anemia in pSLE is the anemia of chronic disease. It tends to be a mild normochromic, normocytic condition. When it is persistent, however, it can become hypochromic and microcytic, which may make it difficult to distinguish from iron deficiency anemia.[299,300] Serum iron levels tend to be low in both types of anemia, while the transferrin is helpful as a diagnostic marker only if it is high. Ferritin levels are rarely low even with true iron deficiency because ferritin is an acute phase reactant. More promising is measuring soluble transferrin receptor, which is elevated when iron deficiency anemia is present.[301] The Coombs test is positive in approximately 30% to 40% of patients but only 10% to 15% of patients have overt hemolysis.[112,113,115,302] When determining the cause of anemia in pSLE patients, hemoglobinopathies such as sickle cell anemia and thalassemia trait should be considered.[113,303-307] Hypersplenism, gastrointestinal (GI) and menstrual loss, aplastic anemia, and autoantibodies against erythrocytes or stem cells may also contribute to or cause anemia.[308-315]

Thrombocytopenia is present in 15% to 45% of patients and may be the initial presentation in up to 15% of pediatric cases (see Table 21–19 [online only]). Patients with chronic autoimmune "idiopathic" thrombocytopenic purpura (AITP) should be assessed for presence of antinuclear antibodies since they are at high risk to develop SLE.[316] Pediatric patients with AITP and a Coombs-positive hemolytic anemia (Evans syndrome) frequently have evidence of SLE at presentation of the cytopenias or will develop SLE.[316-319] Many patients with AITP secondary to SLE have a resistant thrombocytopenia, which usually requires prolonged use of steroids and/or multiple courses of intravenous immunoglobulin. When resistant, other agents, including anti–B cell

Table 21–18

Autoantibodies and NP-SLE

Antibody (Ref nos. in order of year of first study)	Proposed NP Association	Sensitivity for NP Disease Manifestation in SLE	Specificity for NP Disease Manifestation in SLE
Anti-neuronal (636,* 637,* 638,† 639-645)	General cognitive dysfunction	Fair-Good	Fair
	Psychosis, seizures	Poor-Good	Fair
		Poor	Poor
Antiganglioside (646-651)	Any NP involvement	Poor-Good	Poor-good
Antineurofilament (652, 653)	Any NP involvement	Fair	Fair
	Diffuse	Good	Fair
Brain synaptic terminals (639, 654)	Any NP involvement	Good	Fair
Antiglial fibrillary acid protein (298)	Any NP involvement	Fair	Good
Anti–microtubule-associated protein-2 (655)	Any NP involvement	Fair	Fair
Anti-mouse choriod plexus (656)	Any involvement	Good	Fair
NMDAR (657, 658)	Cognitive dysfunction or mood disorders	Fair	Poor
Anti-NR2 subunit of NMDAR (659, 660)	Cognitive dysfunction or mood disorders	Poor	Poor
Antiaquaporin 4 (661, 662)	Either transverse myelitis +/- optic neuritis	Unknown	Unknown
Antiribosomal P (663,* 664, 665-668, 683, 684)	Depression, psychosis	Excellent	Fair
	Cognitive dysfunction	Poor	Poor
	Diffuse vs. focal	Good	Poor
Lupus anticoagulant (660, 669)†	Cerebrovascular events	Excellent	
	Cognitive dysfunction	Fair	Poor
	Movement disorders	Excellent	Good
			Poor
Anticardiolipin antibodies‡ (645, 647, 650)	Cognitive impairment	Poor	Poor
	Any NP involvement	Poor	Poor
Lymphocytotoxic (645, 670-673)	Cognitive dysfunction	Fair-Good	Poor
	Any NP involvement	Good	Poor

*Pediatric studies.
†Some pediatric patients.
‡See NP-SLE for pediatric references.
NMDAR, anti–N-methyl-D-aspartate receptor; NP, neuropsychiatric.

therapy, may be used.[320-324] Although previously suggested to be of benefit in SLE, splenectomy should be avoided[320,322,325-330] because of the increased risk of infection and the efficacy of other therapies.[320,322,325-330] The etiologies of thrombocytopenia in pSLE include antiplatelet antibodies, impaired thrombopoiesis, microangiopathic thrombotic thrombocytopenic purpura (TTP) or HUS, APLA, hemophagocytic syndrome/macrophage activation syndrome (MAS), drug side effects, and rarely anti-CD40 ligand antibodies.[316,321,331-346]

Classic TTP presenting with a microangiopathic hemolytic anemia and neurological and renal disease is unusual in children. When it is present, an underlying diagnosis of SLE should be sought.[341] These patients may have widespread occlusion of arterioles and capillaries with fibrin deposit in the kidney and/or skin. Aggressive treatment with anticoagulation and plasmapheresis is usually required.

Leucopenia is seen in 20% to 40% of cases of pSLE (see Table 21–19 [online only]). Both lymphopenia and granulocytopenia can be found, although lymphopenia is more common and usually does not require specific therapy. When the lymphopenia is profound (an absolute count persistently < 500), an underlying infection with the herpes family of viruses or MAS should be sought. Granulocytopenia is usually secondary to a central

depression of granulopoiesis, splenic sequestration, or more rarely antigranulocyte antibodies or suppression of progenitor.[75,347-352] It is not clear whether patients with leucopenia or lymphopenia secondary to active SLE are at an increased risk of infection.[335,353-356]

When two to three lineages are depressed, then another cause, rather than just active SLE should be considered. These causes include: 1) secondary hemophagocytic syndrome/MAS[342,343,357-360]; 2) infection with herpes family viruses—in particular EBV and (cytomegalovirus) CMV and less commonly herpes simplex; and 3) bone marrow aplasia secondary to antibody- or cytokine-mediated suppression of bone marrow progenitor cells or myelofibrosis.[361-366]

Coagulation abnormalities are common. The LAC is positive in approximately 20% of patients with pSLE. Patients with the LAC do not bleed but rather develop thromboembolic events (TEs) and in particular venous rather than arterial occlusions. The most common areas for TEs are the legs, cerebral veins, and pulmonary vasculature.[201] Patients with the LAC have approximately a 25 to 30 time greater risk of thrombosis than do patients without the LAC. Patients with an arterial thrombosis tend to have a true vasculitis in addition to the LAC.[201] When patients with the LAC present with bleeding, a second coagulation abnormality should be considered such as an acquired prothrombin deficiency (seen in about 5% of pSLE patients with the LAC) or less commonly acquired Factor VIII and IX or Van Willebrand deficiencies. Elevated homocysteine levels or acquired protein S, protein C, or anti–thrombin III deficiency may also increase risk of thrombosis while congenital thrombophilia defects do not seem to be increased in SLE patients.[201,367-376]

Antiphospholipid Antibody Syndrome

The antiphospholipid antibody syndrome (APS) is characterized by the presence of antibodies directed against phospholipids (usually cardiolipin, phospholipids present in the LAC, and anti–β2-glycoprotein1) (see chapter 22). It is referred to as primary APS when there is no evidence of another autoimmune disease and secondary when it is associated with another autoimmune disease. In children secondary APS is more common than primary and SLE is the most common secondary cause. The international classification for APS has undergone multiple revisions, the most recent in 2006 (Table 22–1), but there are still concerns about standardization and validation of the laboratory tests used in different centers.[377-380] The characteristic clinical and laboratory features of APS are shown in Table 21–20. SLE may develop many years after the presentation of primary APS.[381-384] Venous events are more common than arterial events and occur in the following order (beginning with the most frequent): deep venous thrombosis of the lower extremities, pulmonary embolism, and cerebral events.[201, 267, 270, 334, 381, 383, 385-389]

Secondary APS can occur in other autoimmune diseases in addition to SLE including Wegener granulomatosis and a wide variety of neoplastic, infectious, and inflammatory diseases.[390]

Renal disease in APS may manifest as a small vessel microangiopathy or as large vessel involvement of the renal arteries (leading to hypertension from renal artery stenosis) or vascular occlusion leading to renal infarction (Figure 21–19). Radiological imaging is required to establish the diagnosis. More commonly thrombosis will involve the renal vein (which may present clinically as gross hematuria, often associated with flank pain). This is particularly true in patients with nephrotic syndrome. The presence of aPLs carries an increased risk of renal allograft thrombosis.

APS nephropathy is characterized as a small vessel vasculopathy that resembles the thrombotic microangiopathy seen in hemolytic uremic syndrome. Hypertension is common and is often associated with livedo reticularis.[391,392]

Catastrophic antiphospholipid syndrome (CAPS) is a term applied to an aPL-mediated disorder in which there are multiple thrombi of small vessels affecting viscera over a relatively short period. In approximately 50% of patients CAPS was the initial presentation of APS.[292,393] Thrombocytopenia and hemolytic anemia are frequent, and disseminated intravascular may be present. The sites of organ thrombosis include CNS, lung, liver, kidney, and heart. CAPS has a reported mortality of 40% to 50%.

Treatment of APS and CAPS is heparin followed by low–molecular weight heparin or coumadin (lifelong). Avoidance of estrogen-containing birth control pills is recommended.

Table 21–20

Clinical and laboratory measurements of antiphospholipid antibodies in pSLE

Clinical Presentations
Venous thrombosis—deep and superficial
Arterial thrombosis (less common than venous)
Dermatologic
   Livedo reticularis
   Sneddon syndrome
   Cutaneous ulcers
   Skin necrosis
Non-infective endocarditis
Pulmonary hypertension (recurrent thrombosis or emboli)
Renal dysfunction and/or hypertension secondary to recurrent thrombosis or emboli
Central nervous system involvement
   Stroke (thrombotic or embolic)
   Transient ischemic attacks
   Chorea
   Guillain-Barré
   Transverse myelitis
   Multiple sclerosis–like
   Migraine
   Seizure

Antibody	Frequency at Presentation	Frequency During Disease Course
Anti-β2glycoprotein 1	No reported data	53%
Anticardiolipin	26-50%	40-59%
Lupus Anticoagulant i. Antiprothrombin antibodies* ii. Directed against neutral lipid*	9%	13-23%
Antiannexin	No reported data	No reported data
Biological false-positive test for syphilis	No reported data	No reported data

Sources: see references 89, 398, 675, 676.
*May be measured directly but are part of lupus anticoagulant.

Cardiovascular Disease

Pericarditis with pericardial effusion is the most commonly described cardiovascular involvement while endocarditis, myocarditis, and valvular disease are less common. Rarely acute ischemic heart disease secondary to coronary artery vasculitis may be seen.[138,394,395] Premature atherosclerosis with cardiovascular events is likely to be increasingly important as a late complication (see premature antherosclerosis in this chapter). An association of pericarditis and myocarditis with specific autoantibodies is controversial.[396-398]

Pericarditis

Pericarditis may be relatively asymptomatic. Patients may present with only a resting tachycardia or precardial pain that is worse when lying down or with a deep breath. Heart sounds are usually normal but, when the pericardial effusion is large, there may be a pericardial friction rub or muffling of the heart sounds and/or the pericardial friction rub in the presence of a large pericardial effusion. The chest x-ray maybe normal or show cardiomegaly. The electrocardiogram may show S-T segment elevation or nonspecific changes while sinus tachycardia is frequent. The diagnosis is confirmed with echocardiogram. Symptomatic pericarditis occurs in 15% to 25% of patients and with echocardiographic abnormalities in up to 68% of patients.[399] Rarely pericarditis can lead to tamponade or a restrictive pericarditis.[396-397,400] SLE should be considered in patients with pericarditis of unknown etiology. When mild, NSAIDs may be initially tried but frequently corticosteroids, including pulse methylprednisolone, are required. Divided dosing appears to be better than single daily dosing of corticosteroids.

Myocarditis

Clinically significant myocarditis is rare, although echocardiogram changes have been reported in 5% to 15% of patients, and a study in adults with SLE suggested that up to 40% of patients had some evidence of myocarditis.[401-404] Patients may present with congestive heart failure, or when less severe isolated tachycardia (similar to the findings seen with pericarditis), cardiomegaly, and/or narrow pulse pressure. SLE should be considered in all pediatric patients who present with myocarditis because it may be the initial manifestation of pSLE.[405,406] Cardiac enzymes should be obtained if the diagnosis is suspected. The gold standard of diagnosis is endomyocardial biopsy, although it is rarely required.[407] Cardiac MRI scans have been abnormal in adults with SLE-associated myocarditis.

Endocarditis

Non-infective, or Libman-Sacks, endocarditis, associated with aPLs, may lead to either valvular stenosis or regurgitation.[408-413] Histologically noninfective endocarditis is a nodular lesion of the valve associated with fibrinoid necrosis.[402,413,414] The most commonly affected valves are the aortic, mitral and tricuspid.[408-413] These patients are at risk for secondary infective endocarditis. Unlike in adults, where transesophageal echocardiogram is frequently required to diagnose endocarditis, transthoracic echocardiograms are usually sufficient to diagnosis endocarditis in pSLE.[415,416] It is not clear what is the best treatment for non-infective endocarditis to prevent significant valvular disease.

Pleuropulmonary involvement

Pulmonary involvement is common in pSLE, occurring in 25% to 75% of cases (frequently asymptomatic pulmonary function test abnormalities [PFTs]).[417,418] There is a wide range of manifestations from asymptomatic to life-threatening (Table 21–21). Clinically significant pulmonary parenchymal involvement has been reported to occur in 5% of patients with pSLE.

Pleural Involvement

Pleuritis is the most common, clinically significant, pleuropulmonary manifestation of pSLE (frequently associated with pericarditis). Symptoms are chest pain, orthopnea, and dyspnea. Chest x-ray will show a pleural effusion (frequently unilateral), and autopsies have suggested at least some pleural involvement in >90% adults with SLE.[419] Bilateral pleural effusions may also be secondary to hypoalbuminemia from nephrotic syndrome or other causes and/or volume overload. Treatment is similar to that of pericarditis, but pulse methylprednisolone is rarely required.

Lupus Pneumonitis

Acute lupus pneumonitis presents with respiratory distress with or without fever and/or pleuritic chest pain. Acute lupus pneumonitis must be distinguished from

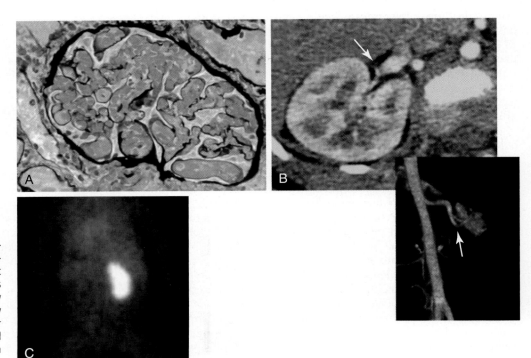

FIGURE 21–19 Renal manifestations of the antiphospholipid antibody syndrome. Kidney involvement may involve **(A)** glomerular capillaries to cause thrombotic microangiopathy **(B)** renal artery stenosis (identified by CT angiography) and hypertension, or **(C)** renal vein thrombosis (suggested by the nonfunctioning right kidney on a radionucleotide scintigraphic study).

infective pneumonia and pulmonary hemorrhage. A chronic, indolent interstitial lung disease is reported in 3% to 15% of adults but is rarely seen in pSLE. Chest radiographs usually show linear opacities and pleural thickening with or without effusions similar to findings in infection and pulmonary hemorrhage.[420] The characteristic finding on high-resolution CT scan is a ground glass appearance (vasculitic-type inflammation) with occasional nodules.[421]

Table 21–21

Presentation pulmonary manifestations of pSLE: Type of presentation and most common causes

Presentation*	Cause	Frequency
Subclinical	Abnormal pulmonary function tests†	Common
	Abnormal computerized tomography	
	Pleural effusions from volume overload	
Acute	Infection	Common
	Bacterial	
	Viral	
	Opportunistic	
	Pulmonary hemorrhage	Uncommon
	Acute lupus pneumonitis	Uncommon
	Pulmonary embolus	Uncommon
Subacute/chronic	Subacute interstitial lung disease	Uncommon
	Bronchiolitis obliterans organizing pneumonia	Uncommon
	Shrinking lung syndrome‡	Uncommon
	Pulmonary arterial hypertension (causes)	Uncommon
	Vasculitis	
	Pulmonary embolism (acute/chronic)	
	Valvular heart disease	
	Primary	
	Chronic	
	Chronic interstitial lung disease	Rare

*Presented in order of frequency
†Most common finding: restive lung disease and abnormal DLCO
‡Diaphragmatic or phrenic nerve dysfunction

Pulmonary Hemorrhage

Pulmonary hemorrhage, occurring in 5% to 10% of pSLE patients with lung involvement, can present as a chronic low-grade hemorrhage with few early symptoms, but more frequently it presents as acute respiratory distress. The clues are tachypnea and tachycardia even without overt hemoptysis. If acute, there is a sudden fall in the hemoglobin with accompany respiratory symptoms, and the chest x-ray shows a diffuse air space and interstitial disease (Figure 21–20). PFTs may show an increased diffusing capacity. SLE should be considered in the differential diagnosis of pulmonary hemorrhage in children.[422] Aggressive treatment is required.

Shrinking Lung Syndrome

Loss of lung volume resulting from diaphragmatic dysfunction and/or phrenic nerve dysfunction is uncommon.[423-426] Patients may present with restrictive lung disease with few if any changes on radiographic investigations (early), while with progression x-rays show decreased volumes and basilar atelectasis.

Infection

Patients with pSLE are at high risk for lung infection as a result of immunosuppression secondary to disease activity and treatment. If present, infection may complicate other acute lung presentations.[427] When patients present with acute respiratory failure and fever, treatment with broad-spectrum antibiotics and high-dose corticosteroids, including pulse therapy, may be required. Bronchoscopy with bronchial washings should be considered early,[420] but frequently patients require an open lung biopsy. SLE patients are at high risk for infection with opportunistic organisms (herpes viruses, *Pneumocystis jiroveci*, *Legionella*, and fungi).[427-436] These infections must be ruled out prior to the introduction of significant immunosuppressive therapy.

Pulmonary Hypertension

Pulmonary vascular disease leading to pulmonary hypertension is a rare but life-threatening complication.[437-440] It is likely the result of a combination of vasculitis, vaso-occlusion, and/or thrombosis and is frequently associated with Raynaud phenomenon.[441]

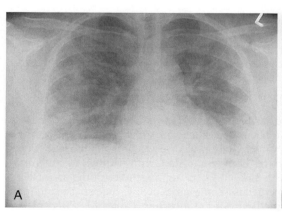
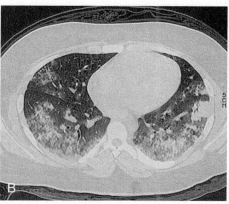

FIGURE 21–20 Radiograph (A) and thin-section computed tomogram (B) of the chest of a 14-year-old girl with acute onset of pulmonary hemorrhage and thrombocytopenia. There is evidence of widespread airspace and interstitial disease. The abnormalities completely resolved after therapy with high-dose prednisone.

Gastrointestinal Manifestations Including Liver Involvement

GI involvement occurs in approximately 20% of patients (see Table 21–7). The most common symptoms are abdominal pain and diarrhea, which have a large number of causes.[442-444] Lupus peritonitis occurs in <10% of patients and will lead to crampy abdominal pain with ascites. It must be distinguished from infective peritonitis. Lupus enteropathy, frequently associated with lupus cystitis, may present as crampy abdominal pain and diarrhea or as a protein-losing enteropathy.[442,443,445-447] Protein-losing enteropathy and pseudo-obstruction may occur with or without evidence of bowel wall inflammation.[447] Bowel wall inflammation on x-ray or ultrasound examination can reflect lupus enteritis or may be secondary to a mesenteric vasculitis and/or thrombosis. A CT scan may be required to determine the cause of abdominal symptoms.[448] When GI vasculitis is present, patients are at risk for perforation.[444] In patients on high doses of corticosteroids, signs and symptoms of perforation may be masked. Rare cases of the coexistence of SLE and inflammatory bowel disease have been described.[449,450] The only large study of the pathology of the GI tract in pSLE examined 26 autopsies (all causes of death) and commonly found chronic nonspecific inflammation of the mucosa and/or ascites, ischemic lesions, and peritoneal inflammation.[451]

Studies have shown an association between pSLE and celiac disease. Therefore, when abdominal pain is persistent and/or unexplained weight loss is present, celiac disease should be excluded.[452-455]

Pancreatitis

Pancreatitis, an uncommon but potentially life-threatening SLE manifestation (overall incidence of <5%), may present at SLE diagnosis. It usually presents with diffuse abdominal pain, nausea, and vomiting.[456-457] Laboratory investigations reveal an increased amylase and/or lipase level. Pancreatitis may reflect active SLE, be secondary to infection, or be drug related (in particular to corticosteroids or azathioprine).[456,458-466] SLE-associated pancreatitis usually requires corticosteroid treatment, and it may present at SLE diagnosis. Rarely pseudocyst formation and pancreatic insufficiency may be a sequelae.[462]

Splenomegaly

Splenomegaly, seen in 20% to 30% of patients, reflects the generalized inflammatory state. A more serious manifestation is functional asplenia, secondary to either splenic infarction or immune dysfunction. It is important to recognize this complication because it increases the risk of sepsis.

Hepatomegaly

Hepatomegaly occurs in 40% to 50% of patients, with abnormal liver function tests (LFTs) in up to 25%. Hepatomegaly with or without elevated LFTs may be secondary to multiple causes, which include drug side effect, active SLE, infection, fatty infiltration, hepatic vein or artery thrombosis, and congestion secondary to right heart failure. When liver involvement is the major manifestation or the LFTs are markedly elevated (so-called lupoid hepatitis), the differentiation of SLE involving the liver from autoimmune hepatitis may be difficult because both have similar laboratory and pathological features.[467] Budd-Chiari syndrome, acute hepatic vein thrombosis associated with aPLs, is important to diagnose because it requires rapid anticoagulation to preserve liver function.

Endocrine Involvement

The thyroid gland is the most common endocrine organ involved in pSLE. Up to 35% of pSLE patients have antithyroid antibodies, with 10% to 15% developing overt hypothyroidism.[468] As a result thyroid function should be checked annually. In contrast, there is not an increased incidence of Grave disease in pSLE. There have been case reports of hypo- and hyperparathyroidism, Addison disease, and type I diabetes mellitus (DM). Corticosteroid-induced DM requiring insulin treatment occurs in 5% to 10% of patients. Nonautoimmune adrenal insufficiency may develop secondary to thrombosis in patients with aPLs or prolonged corticosteroid use.

Growth failure is frequent and is usually attributable to a combination of chronic disease and corticosteroids. However, pSLE patients have an increased incidence of growth hormone deficiency. Delayed puberty and menstrual abnormalities are common. Ovarian failure is a potential complication of cyclophosphamide therapy and is dose dependant.[469,470]

Ocular Disease

Few studies have described the incidence of ocular involvement in pSLE. The most common ocular finding associated with pSLE is cotton-wool spots (cytoid bodies), indicative of retinal vasculitis (Figure 21–21; Table 21–22). Cotton-wool spots tend to have a para-arteriolar location in the posterior pole of the retina. Occlusion of the central retinal vein, usually associated with aPLs or CNS vasculitis, and severe diffuse retinal vasculitis may occur. Both of these entities are frequently associated with visual loss.[471-473] Both episcleritis and scleritis may be seen. Keratoconjunctivitis sicca is seen in patients with secondary Sjögren syndrome.

PHARMACOLOGIC THERAPY

Specific treatment should be individualized and based on the extent and severity of the disease.

Nonsteroidal Antiinflammatory Drugs

The primary role of NSAIDs in the management of pediatric SLE is to treat musculoskeletal complaints. Myalgia, arthralgia, or arthritis may respond well to antiinflammatory doses. NSAIDs have been associated with aseptic meningitis in patients with SLE.[474] There are no studies of the use of selective cyclooxygenase-2 inhibitors in SLE. Side effects and monitoring of medications are shown in Tables 21–7 and 21–8.

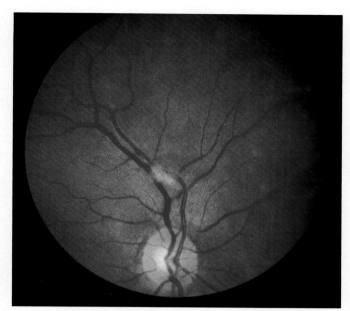

FIGURE 21–21   An oval white cotton-wool spot (CWS) in the posterior retinal pole. A CWS is invariably in a para-arteriolar position and often partially obliterates the adjacent arteriole. CWSs arise from segmental vasculitis within and adjacent to these vessels. The surrounding retina generally shows an edematous sheen. In systemic lupus erythematosus, usually only a few CWSs are present. Identical lesions may rarely be seen in other connective tissue diseases. In hypertension, diabetes, or septicemia, numerous CWSs may be present.

Table 21–22

Ocular manifestations

External eye disease: discoid rash over eyelids
Lacrimal system: keratoconjunctivitis sicca
Orbital disease: periorbital edema, orbital masses, myositis, panniculitis, ischemia/infarction
Anterior segment: corneal-dry eyes, erosions, punctuate epithelial loss, ulcerative keratitis, conjunctival inflammation (rare), uveitis (rare)
Episcleritis
Scleritis: either anterior or posterior
Posterior segment
   Retinopathy-cotton-wool spots, perivascular hard exudates, retinal hemorrhages and vascular tortuosity, vasoocclusive retinopathy (or "retinal vasculitis"), retinal infections
   Choroidal-uni/multifocal retinal detachments and choroidal effusions or ischemia
Infections
Optic nerve disease: optic neuritis and ischemic optic neuropathy (anterior or posterior).
Ocular motor abnormalities: diplopia, internuclear ophthalmoplegia, nystagmus and Miller Fisher syndrome
Drug-induced

Adapted from reference[77]

Hydroxychloroquine/Chloroquine

Hydroxychloroquine is given to most patients with SLE to maintain rather than induce remission.[475-479] However, in patients with mild disease, including systemic, skin, or MSK disease, hydroxychloroquine and NSAIDS may suffice without the need for corticosteroids.[480,481]

If hydroxychloroquine is not tolerated, chloroquine may be used. The use of both drugs is associated with an improved lipid profile.[482-485]

Glucocorticoids

Glucocorticoids are the mainstay of pharmacological therapy, and >90% of children with SLE receive them at some stage of the disease. The dosing and duration is based on the severity and response to treatment. No studies in children have been performed to determine optimal dose. One study reported a wide practice variation among North American pediatric rheumatologists.[486]

Immunosuppressive Agents

There are two major indications for the use of immunosuppressive agents in pSLE: 1) To improve outcome in patients with severe renal (Class III and IV) or NP involvement; and 2) As a steroid-sparing agent in patients with milder disease but who are corticosteroid dependent. The indication dictates the choice, dosage, and duration of corticosteroid therapy.

Azathioprine

Azathioprine has probably been used longer to treat childhood lupus than any other second-line agent and has safety, cost, and/or dosing frequency advantages over other agents (except methotrexate). A problem in the past has been that some investigators used a low (1-2 mg/kg/day) rather than an optimal (3mg/kg/day; maximum 150 mg/day) dosage.[211,242,244]

Cyclophosphamide

Cyclophosphamide is a commonly used drug for management of severe SLE but has significant toxicity. Controlled trials and metaanalyses have failed to demonstrate a superiority of cyclophosphamide over azathioprine or mycophenolate mofetil in proliferative lupus nephritis.[184,213,470,487-496,497,498] Despite these data, many pediatric (and adult) rheumatologists still use cyclophosphamide as the immunosuppressive agent of choice in proliferative lupus nephritis. Although no controlled trials have been performed, open label trials and case series suggest that cyclophosphamide should be used with corticosteroids in patients with severe NP involvement.[499]

Methotrexate

Methotrexate has a role in the management of resistant arthritis and skin disease as a steroid-sparing agent.[500-505]

Cyclosporine

Although early studies suggested that cyclosporine may be of benefit in SLE, currently its use should be reserved for patients with membranous nephritis or MAS, and possibly in severe treatment resistant skin disease.[221,506-511]

Mycophenolate Mofetil

Experience with the use of mycophenolate mofetil (MMF) in pSLE is limited. However, multiple studies, meta-analyses in adults, demonstrated that MMF is equivalent or superior to intravenous cyclophosphamide in inducing remission in patients with proliferative nephritis and is associated with a better safety profile.[184,488,490,493,495,497,512-514] However, currently there is very little data at 5- and 10 -year follow-up.

Biologic Therapies

Intravenous Immunoglobulin

Currently there is a limited role for intravenous immunoglobulin except in the treatment of autoimmune cytopenias and MAS.

Plasmapheresis

Plasmapheresis should be reserved for a severe acute complications such as TTP or pulmonary hemorrhage. It has not been shown to be of benefit in the long-term management of SLE.[206,424,515-519]

Monoclonal Antibodies

Anti-CD20 (rituximab) has been reported to be of benefit in multiple open label studies of hundreds of patients with all types of SLE, and these series suggest that it is particularly effective in patients with treatment-resistant SLE-associated cytopenias.[520-525] However, randomized controlled trials failed to show a benefit over placebo. Other monoclonal therapies currently in early trials include targeting B cells (anti–B-lymphocyte stimulator, anti–B7-related protein-1, anti-CD22, and other anti-CD20 monoclonal antibodies), T cells (anti-CTLA4), and cytokines (anti-TNF and antiinterferon agents).

TRANSPLANTATION

Autologous bone marrow transplantation (ABMT) has been performed in adult and pSLE patients, but the long-term safety and effectiveness of ABMT is not yet known.[526] Recent changes to ABMT protocols, such as T cell depletion and/or nonmyeloablative conditioning, have been advocated to enhance engraftment and to decrease morbidity and mortality associated with the procedure.[527-529] There have been reports of the successful use of allogenic bone marrow transplantation and allogenic bone marrow mesenchymal stem cells in adult SLE patients.[529,530]

MORBIDITIES

A list of morbidities seen in patients with pSLE is shown in Table 21–23. This part of the chapter will focus on two of the more common and significant morbidities not previously covered.

Premature Atherosclerosis

With increased survival of patients with SLE, premature atherosclerosis has come to be recognized as a leading cause of morbidity and mortality. Both traditional and nontraditional atherosclerotic risk factors are implicated in premature atherosclerosis in patients with adult SLE and pSLE. Preliminary studies have shown abnormalities of myocardial perfusion and early signs of atherosclerosis, including abnormal pulse wave velocity, vascular reactivity, and increased carotid intima-media thickness.[531-536] There are reports of early myocardial infarction and cerebral vascular events in pSLE in addition to late events.[138,240,537,538] Although lipid abnormalities, autoantibodies, vasculitis, hypertension, and possibly steroid use all contribute, it is likely that the chronic inflammation of SLE is the major risk factor for premature atherosclerosis (Table 21–24 [online only]).

Osteoporosis

Low bone mineral density (BMD), seen in to 20% of patients with pSLE, is likely the result of both chronic inflammation and steroid use.[539,540] The rate of vertebral fracture is <5%.[539,541-544] Hip fractures are rarely seen in patients with pSLE, even in the presence of significantly low BMD. Factors reported to be associated with low BMD include disease duration, dosage and duration of steroid use, high disease activity, low physical activity from chronic disease, sun avoidance, low vitamin D levels, and inadequate calcium intake. Low bone mass during adolescence may be a more significant long-term problem because peak bone mass is reached between 18 and 20 years of age. Therefore, the low bone mass seen in adolescents with SLE may lead to premature osteoporosis and increased fractures rates in midlife. Currently there have been no studies addressing this issue.

The current recommendations for patients on chronic corticosteroids and/or with low BMD are is physical activity and optimizing vitamin D and calcium intake. However, there are no guidelines for vitamin D doses or for a target vitamin D level. Currently, because of safety concerns, it is recommended that bisphosphonates should not be given prophylactically but reserved for patients with BMD in the osteoporotic range who experience fragility fractures.[545,546]

AUTOANTIBODIES

Autoantibodies directed against histone, nonhistone, RNA-binding, cytoplasmic, and nuclear proteins are the hallmark of SLE. Autoantibodies tend to appear in

Table 21–23	
Morbidities associated with pSLE	
System	**Morbidity**
Renal	Hypertension, dialysis, transplantation
Central nervous system	Organic brain syndrome, seizures, psychosis, neurocognitive disorder
Cardiovascular	Atherosclerosis, myocardial infarction, cardiomyopathy, valvular disease
Immune	Recurrent infection, functional asplenia, malignancy
Musculoskeletal	Osteoporosis, compression fractures, avascular necrosis
Ocular	Cataracts, glaucoma, retinal detachment, blindness
Endocrine	Diabetes, obesity, growth failure, infertility, fetal wastage

patterns: antibodies associated with chromatin (DNA and histones), those binding to proteins associated with the U series of human RNAs (Sm and RNP), those binding to proteins associated with Y series of human RNAs (Ro and La), and aPLs (aCl, B2GP1, and LAC).[547-555] A more complete list of autoantibodies, frequencies, and associated disease manifestations is shown in Table 21–25.

GENERAL LABORATORY EVALUATION

Routine laboratory investigations are of benefit in measuring overall disease activity. Serum complement levels may reflect disease activity in major organ systems (see Nephritis and NP-SLE); however, they tend to be normal in mild disease such as malar rash and/or arthritis.

Persistently low complement levels in an otherwise well-appearing patient may indicate subclinical major organ involvement that will be revealed over time or reflect partial or complete complement component deficiency. SLE is one of the few chronic diseases to be associated with hypocomplementemia. Erythrocyte sedimentation rate is a good measure of overall inflammation, while C-reactive protein (CRP) levels tend to be normal even in active nephritis or NP disease. Elevated CRP levels are commonly seen only in patients with serositis and in the presence of infection. Elevated Ig levels (in particular IgG) are common as are elevated ferritin and other acute phase reactants (except CRP). Low IgG levels are seen in patients with severe nephrotic syndrome and who have SLE associated with a primary immune deficiency. There is a higher prevalence of isolated IgA deficiency in SLE patients than in the normal population.

Table 21–25

Autoantibodies in pSLE*

Particle Recognized	Specificity of Particle	Common Name for Antibody	Specific Protein	Frequency at Presentation†	Frequency at Any Time	Disease Association(s)
Nucleosome (chromatin)	Epitopes on nucleosome (chromatin)	Anti–ds-DNA	Native, ds-DNA	65-95%	84-100%	Highly specific for SLE
						Active glomerulonephritis
	Histone proteins complexes	Antihistone	Histone proteins H1, H2A, H2B, H3, H4	No large studies in pSLE	~90% 30-40%	Drug-induced LE SLE
Ro RNP	Proteins complexed to small cytoplasmic RNAs known as hY-RNAs	Anti-Ro	52- and 60-kD proteins	27-33%	38-54%	Neonatal LE
						Secondary SS
						Subacute cutaneous LE
						Cardiac (one study only)
		Anti-La	48kD protein	13-19%	16-32%	Neonatal LE
						Secondary SS
						Subacute cutaneous LE
						Cardiac (one study only)
Small nuclear (Sn) RNP	Proteins complexed to Uridine -rich (u) RNAs (U1,U2,U4,U5 SnRNP)	Anti-Sm	B/B/,† D1,‡ D2,‡ D3,‡ E, F, G proteins	32-34%	23-48%	Specific SLE
	Proteins associated with U1 RNP	U1RNP	70 Kd, A, C proteins	27-35%	31-62%	SLE MCTD
Rheumatoid factors	Gamma(g) globulins	RF	IgM antibodies	11%	15-35%	SLE JIA, SS
Ribosomal P proteins	Phosphorylated ribosomal proteins	Anti-P	P0 (38Kd), P1 (19Kd) and P2 (17Kd) proteins§	No large studies in pSLE	21-42%	SLE-hepatitis, renal and psychosis
Chromosomal protein	Nonhistone basic chromosomal protein	Anti–SCl-70	topoisomerase 1 (70Kd protein)	No large studies in pSLE	15%	More common in progressive systemic sclerosis

Sources: see references 89, 111 ,115,120, 123, 396, 398, 613, 618, 663, 675, 678, 679.
*APLA described separately in Table 21–21.
†Vey few studies reported autoantibodies at presentation.
‡Major antigens.
§Most antibodies bind to all three.

ds-DNA, double-stranded DNA; IgM, immunoglobulin M; JIA, juvenile idiopathic arthritis; LE, lupus erythematosus; MCTD, mixed connective tissue disease; pSLE, pediatric systemic lupus erythematosus; RNP, ribonuclear protein; SLE, systemic lupus erythematosus; SS, Sjogren syndrome.

DRUG-INDUCED LUPUS

It was recognized in the 1960s that patients on specific medications developed the clinical syndrome of SLE. The most commonly described drug was hydralazine. Currently drug-induced lupus in childhood is more frequently related to the use of antiepileptic medications (specifically diphenylhydantoin, ethosuximide, and carbamazepine); other drugs are implicated as well (Table 21–26). Clinically patients tend to have cutaneous, hematological, and pleural/pericardial disease.[556-559] ANA is common; in the past approximately 80% of patients had antihistone antibodies, with anti-DNA antibodies being much less common. It has been suggested that measuring antihistone antibodies may be of benefit, but, in fact, 20% to 40% of idiopathic SLE patients have antihistone antibodies. Therefore, the presence of these antibodies may be suggestive but not diagnostic of DLE. The association of antihistone antibodies and drug-induced LE was described for the drugs initially found to be associated with DLE. It is not clear that this association holds with the newer medications, although patients with minocycline-induced DLE have antihistone antibodies.[560]

Discontinuation of the offending medication and substitution of another to treat the underlying condition is usually sufficient to treat DLE, although occasionally corticosteroids are required. The recommended treatment is the discontinuation of the offending medication; fortunately, there are alternative medications for each of medication associated with DLE. The signs and symptoms should resolve within 6 months, although the ANA may persist for many years. Of note, the development of DLE takes weeks to months or even years to occur; therefore, DLE, rather than SLE, should be suspected in patients on the associated medications even if they have been treated long term.

ANIMAL MODELS OF SLE

The initial mouse model used to study SLE was a crossbreeding of the New Zealand Black and the New Zealand White mouse strains with the offspring developing a lupuslike condition. The second strain, the BXSB, was later developed but currently is rarely used. The most commonly used strain of mice to study lupus is the MRL/lpr mouse. This mouse has been extensively used and has led to very important genetic breakthroughs.

More recently genetically engineered mice and transgenic mice have been studied. The types of models are summarized in Table 21–27 [online only].

GENES

Several observations—including the facts that monozygotic twins have a higher concordance rate of SLE (20% to 30%) than do dizygotic twins (2% to 3%), that children born to mothers with SLE have a tenfold increased risk of developing SLE themselves, and that SLE appears

Table 21–26

Drugs associated with the development of SLE drug-induced lupus (DLE)

Agent	Risk
Antihypertensives	
Hydralazine	High
Enalapril	Low
Captopril	Low
Atenolol	Low
Acebutolol	Low
Methyldopa	Low
Clonidine	Low
Anticonvulsants	
Carbamazepine	Low
Phenytoin	Low
Ethosuximide	Low
Primidone	Low
Trimethadione	Low
Antibiotics	
Isoniazid	Low
Minocycline	Low
Antithyroidals	
Propylthiouracil	Low
Antiinflammatories	
D-penicillamine	Low
Sulfasalazine	Low
Diuretics	
Chlorthalidone	Low
Hydrochlorothiazide	Low
Miscellaneous	
Anti–tumor necrosis factor	Low
Statins	Low
Interferon	Low
Timolol eye drops	Low

Adapted from Rubin RL: Drug-induced lupus, *Toxicology* 209:135-147, 2005.

in "autoimmune families"—have led to the investigation of the role of genetics in development of SLE.[561] Initial studies in the genetics of SLE focused on human leukocyte antigen Class I, II, and III genes (genes involved in the immune response). Class II and Class III, but not Class I, genes have been consistently associated with SLE susceptibility in both pediatric and adult studies.[562] Later studies used a candidate gene approach to examine genes that had previously been identified as important in the immune response, suspected to be abnormal in SLE patients, or defined in studies of murine models. These studies identified that the following genes were important in both adult and pSLE: 1) Fc receptors for IgG (FcγR), which mediate clearance of immune complexes; 2)intracellular protein tyrosine phosphatase type N22 (PTPN22), which is an inhibitor of T cell activation[563-565]; 3) PD1 gene, involved in immune cell death[566-567]; 4) interferon regulator factor 5, which is important in type-1 interferon signaling[568-569];

and 5) signal transducer and activator of transcription 4 (STAT4), which is an important signaling pathway in lymphocytes.[570] The association with STAT4 gene polymorphism and SLE was originally established by genome-wide association studies (GWAS).

Using a candidate gene approach, the most recent advances into the genetics of SLE using GWAS have identified other genes that may lead to SLE that may otherwise not have been suspected. This so-called "shotgun" approach had led some to question the value of GWAS in identifying clinically or biologically relevant associations. The genes most frequently associated with SLE have been associated with components of the immune system, including both innate and adaptive immunity pathways that may otherwise not have been suspected of association. Importantly when the studies in SLE are combined with the studies in other autoimmune diseases, the concept that there may be genes that predispose to immunity in general has been validated. Therefore, specific genes may predispose an individual to SLE rather than RA, multiple sclerosis, or diabetes.[571-574] These findings support the previously suggested concept of "autoimmune families." Genes identified in GWAS that subserve immunological function can be divided those associated with the innate immune systems and those associated with the adaptive immune systems—and then further divided within these major arms of the immune system.

BIOMARKERS

In addition to examining genetic susceptibility, recent research has explored the possibility of measuring circulating or urinary molecules to predict disease outcome, activity, and damage (biomarkers). To date the following biomarkers have been proposed for pSLE (but none yet validated in large studies): 1) serum-melanoma–associated antigen gene B2,[575] angiogenic vascular endothelial growth factor,[576] neutrophil gelatinase–associated lipocalin (NGAL),[224] and adipokines (leptin, adiponectin, and ghrelin)[577]; and 2) urinary-NGAL, transferrin, alpha1-acid-glycoprotein, and lipocalin-type prostaglandin-D synthetase.[223,578-579]

OUTCOME MEASURES

Disease Activity

A number of measurement systems have been developed to determine the influence of active disease on outcome measures of disease activity for patients with adult SLE. Initial measures included physician's global assessment and composite indices measuring organ involvement and laboratory measures of activity. These were superseded by four different indices, usually derived by consensus conferences: 1) the Systemic Lupus Erythematosus Disease Activity Index, which has been modified twice[580-582]; 2) the Systemic Lupus Activity Measure with revisions[583-584]; 3) the British Isles Lupus assessment Group Index, which was later modified[585-586]; and 4) the European Consensus Lupus Activity Measurement.[587-589] These indices,

without modification, have been validated in pSLE, and none appears superior.[590-592] It should be remembered that these indices were developed to measure disease activity over time in longitudinal cohort studies and not for interventional studies because sensitivity to change with therapy was not a requirement for validation. This may be a significant problem in future drug studies if these indices are used as the primary outcome variable.[593]

Health-Related Quality of Life

Unlike the above-mentioned measures, which could be adapted for pSLE from adult SLE, measurement of health-related quality of life could not be adapted from adult measures. However, similar to what had occurred in adult SLE, adaption of currently available quality of life measures were assessed and validated in pediatric rheumatology and pSLE. The measures validated were: 1) the Childhood Health Assessment Questionnaire, 2) the Rhuematology Module of the Pediatric Quality of Life Inventory Generic Core Scale, 3) the Peds QL Multidimensional Fatigue Scale, and 4) the Child Health Questionnaire.[594-597] The Simple Measure of the Impact of Lupus Erythematosus in Youngsters was developed as a pSLE-specific instrument.[598-600]

Disease Damage

A separate instrument, the Systemic Lupus International Collaborating Clinics/American College of Rheumatology Damage Index was developed and validated to measure damage in adult SLE.[583,601] It was subsequently validated in pSLE,[602-603] but since that initial validation it has been suggested that a pediatric version should include the pediatric-specific measures of abnormal growth and delayed puberty.[604] However, because both are reversible, they do not fulfill the definition of organ damage (i.e., that the damage is permanent) and perhaps should not be included.[605]

REFERENCES

2. M.C. Hochberg, Updating the American College of Rheumatology revised criteria for the classification of systemic lupus erythematosus, Arthritis Rheum. 40 (1997) 1725.

6. G.S. Cooper, K.M. Gilbert, E.L. Greidinger, et al., Recent advances and opportunities in research on lupus: environmental influences and mechanisms of disease, Environ. Health Perspect. 116 (2008) 695–702.

25. B.D. Poole, A.K. Templeton, J.M. Guthridge, et al., Aberrant Epstein-Barr viral infection in systemic lupus erythematosus, Autoimmun. Rev. 8 (2009) 337–842.

38. D.H. Kono, A.N. Theofilopoulos, Genetics of SLE in mice, Springer. Semin. Immunopathol. 28 (2006) 83–96.

85. P.N. Malleson, M.Y. Fung, A.M. Rosenberg, The incidence of pediatric rheumatic diseases: results from the Canadian Pediatric Rheumatology Association Disease Registry, J. Rheumatol. 23 (1996) 1981–1987.

88. P.M. Miettunen, O. Ortiz-Alvarez, R.E. Petty, et al., Gender and ethnic origin have no effect on longterm outcome of childhood-onset systemic lupus erythematosus, J. Rheumatol. 31 (2004) 1650–1654.

89. L.T. Hiraki, S.M. Benseler, P.N. Tyrrell, D. Hebert, E. Harvey, E.D. Silverman, Clinical and laboratory characteristics and long-term outcome of pediatric systemic lupus erythematosus: a longitudinal study, J. Pediatr. 152 (2008) 550–556.

100. C.A. Peschken, S.J. Katz, E. Silverman, et al., The 1000 Canadian faces of lupus: determinants of disease outcome in a large multi-ethnic cohort, J. Rheumatol. 36 (2009) 1200–1208.

107. D. Kurahara, A. Tokuda, A. Grandinetti, et al., Ethnic differences in risk for pediatric rheumatic illness in a culturally diverse population, J. Rheumatol. 29 (2002) 379–383.

108. J.T. Lo, M.J. Tsai, L.H. Wang, et al., Sex differences in pediatric systemic lupus erythematosus: a retrospective analysis of 135 cases, J. Microbiol. Immunol. Infect. 32 (1999) 173–178.

109. R. Bogdanovic, V. Nikolic, S. Pasic, et al., Lupus nephritis in childhood: a review of 53 patients followed at a single center, Pediatr. Nephrol. 19 (2004) 36–44.

111. S. Salah, H.M. Lotfy, S.M. Sabry, et al., Systemic lupus erythematosus in Egyptian children, Rheumatol. Int. 29 (2009) 1463–1468.

112. I.E. Hoffman, B.R. Lauwerys, F. De Keyser, et al., Juvenile-onset systemic lupus erythematosus: different clinical and serological pattern than adult-onset systemic lupus erythematosus, Ann. Rheum. Dis. 68 (2009) 412–415.

115. L.A. Ramirez Gomez, O. Uribe Uribe, O. Osio Uribe, et al., Childhood systemic lupus erythematosus in Latin America, The GLADEL experience in 230 children, Lupus 17 (2008) 596–604.

120. L.C. Wang, Y.H. Yang, M.Y. Lu, et al., Retrospective analysis of mortality and morbidity of pediatric systemic lupus erythematosus in the past two decades, J. Microbiol. Immunol. Infect. 36 (2003) 203–208.

122. S. Vyas, G. Hidalgo, N. Baqi, et al., Outcome in African-American children of neuropsychiatric lupus and lupus nephritis, Pediatr. Nephrol. 17 (2002) 45–49.

123. K. Alsaeid, H. Kamal, M.Z. Haider, et al., Systemic lupus erythematosus in Kuwaiti children: organ system involvement and serological findings, Lupus 13 (2004) 613–617.

134. H.H. Yu, J.H. Lee, L.C. Wang, et al., Neuropsychiatric manifestations in pediatric systemic lupus erythematosus: a 20-year study, Lupus 15 (2006) 651–657.

135. E. Descloux, I. Durieu, P. Cochat, et al., Influence of age at disease onset in the outcome of paediatric systemic lupus erythematosus, Rheumatology (Oxford) 48 (2009) 779–784.

136. P. Hari, A. Bagga, P. Mahajan, et al., Outcome of lupus nephritis in Indian children, Lupus 18 (2009) 348–354.

160. F.A. Houssiau, A. N'Zeusseu Toukap, G. Depresseux et al., Magnetic resonance imaging-detected avascular osteonecrosis in systemic lupus erythematosus: lack of correlation with antiphospholipid antibodies, Br. J. Rheumatol. 37 (1998) 448–453.

166. M.C. Sampaio, Z.N. de Oliveira, M.C. Machado, et al., Discoid lupus erythematosus in children–a retrospective study of 34 patients, Pediatr. Dermatol. 25 (2008) 163–167.

171. A. Siamopoulou-Mavridou, D. Stefanou, et al., Subacute cutaneous lupus-erythematosus in childhood, Clin. Rheumatol. 8 (1989) 533–537.

177. V.M. Holers, Complement deficiency states, disease susceptibility, and infection risk in systemic lupus erythematosus, Arthritis Rheum. 42 (1999) 2023–2025.

184. G.B. Appel, G. Contreras, M.A. Dooley, et al., Mycophenolate mofetil versus cyclophosphamide for induction treatment of lupus nephritis, J. Am. Soc. Nephrol. 20 (2009) 1103–1112.

187. J.J. Weening, V.D. D'Agati, M.M. Schwartz, et al., The classification of glomerulonephritis in systemic lupus erythematosus revisited, Kidney Int. 65 (2004) 521–530.

189. S.D. Marks, N.J. Sebire, C. Pilkington, et al., Clinicopathological correlations of paediatric lupus nephritis, Pediatr. Nephrol. 22 (2007) 77–83.

190. P. Vachvanichsanong, P. Dissaneewate, E. McNeil, Diffuse proliferative glomerulonephritis does not determine the worst outcome in childhood onset lupus nephritis: a 23-year experience in a single centre, Nephrol. Dial. Transplant. 24 (2009) 2729–2734.

191. S.N. Wong, K.C. Tse, T.L. Lee, et al., Lupus nephritis in Chinese children—a territory-wide cohort study in Hong Kong, Pediatr. Nephrol. 21 (2006) 1104–1112.

195. H.I. Brunner, D.D. Gladman, D. Ibanez, et al., Difference in disease features between childhood-onset and adult-onset systemic lupus erythematosus, Arthritis Rheum. 58 (2008) 556–562.

201. D.M. Levy, M.P. Massicotte, E. Harvey, et al., Thromboembolism in paediatric lupus patients, Lupus 12 (2003) 741–746.

211. S.M. Benseler, J.M. Bargman, B.M. Feldman, et al., Acute renal failure in paediatric systemic lupus erythematosus: treatment and outcome, Rheumatology (Oxford) 48 (2009) 176–182.

212. G.G. Illei, K. Takada, D. Parkin, et al., Renal flares are common in patients with severe proliferative lupus nephritis treated with pulse immunosuppressive therapy: long-term followup of a cohort of 145 patients participating in randomized controlled studies, Arthritis Rheum. 46 (2002) 995–1002.

231. P. Verghese, K. Luckritz, A.A. Eddy, Interstitial nephritis, D. Geary and F. Schaefer (Eds.), In: Clinical Pediatric Nephrology, Mosby Elsevier, Philadelphia, Chapter 34 (2008) 527–538.

246. American College of Rheumatology, Nomenclature and case definitions for neuropsychiatric lupus syndromes, Arthritis Rheum. 42 (1999) 599–608.

248. H.I. Brunner, O.Y. Jones, D.J. Lovell, et al., Lupus headaches in childhood-onset systemic lupus erythematosus: relationship to disease activity as measured by the systemic lupus erythematosus disease activity index (SLEDAI) and disease damage, Lupus 12 (2003) 600–606.

260. D.M. Levy, S.P. Ardoin, L.E. Schanberg, Neurocognitive impairment in children and adolescents with systemic lupus erythematosus, Nat. Clin. Pract. Rheumatol. 5 (2009) 106–114.

268. M.J. Spinosa, M. Bandeira, P.B. Liberalesso, et al., Clinical, laboratory and neuroimage findings in juvenile systemic lupus erythematosus presenting involvement of the nervous system, Arq. Neuropsiquiatr. 65 (2007) 433–439.

272. L. Harel, C. Sandborg, T. Lee, et al., Neuropsychiatric manifestations in pediatric systemic lupus erythematosus and association with antiphospholipid antibodies, J. Rheumatol. 33 (2006) 1873–1877.

275. G. Zandman-Goddard, J. Chapman, Y. Shoenfeld, Autoantibodies involved in neuropsychiatric SLE and antiphospholipid syndrome, Semin. Arthritis Rheum. 36 (2007) 297–315.

343. A. Parodi, S. Davi, A.B. Pringe, et al., Macrophage activation syndrome in juvenile systemic lupus erythematosus: A multinational multicenter study of thirty-eight patients, Arthritis Rheum. 60 (2009) 3388–3399.

378. S. Miyakis, M.D. Lockshin, T. Atsumi, et al., International consensus statement on an update of the classification criteria for definite antiphospholipid syndrome (APS), J. Thromb. Haemost. 4 (2006) 295–306.

381. T. Avcin, R. Cimaz, E.D. Silverman, et al., Pediatric antiphospholipid syndrome: clinical and immunologic features of 121 patients in an international registry, Pediatrics 122 (2008) e1100–e1107.

386. E. Descloux, I. Durieu, P. Cochat, et al., Paediatric systemic lupus erythematosus: prognostic impact of antiphospholipid antibodies, Rheumatology (Oxford) 47 (2008) 183–187.

398. R. Jurencak, M. Fritzler, P. Tyrrell, et al., Autoantibodies in pediatric systemic lupus erythematosus: ethnic grouping, cluster analysis, and clinical correlations, J. Rheumatol. 36 (2009) 416–421.

486. H.I. Brunner, M.S. Klein-Gitelman, J. Ying, et al., Corticosteroid use in childhood-onset systemic lupus erythematosus-practice patterns at four pediatric rheumatology centers, Clin. Exp. Rheumatol. 27 (2009) 155–162.

490. F. Falcini, S. Capannini, G. Martini, et al., Mycophenolate mofetil for the treatment of juvenile onset SLE: a multicenter study, Lupus 18 (2009) 139–143.

493. A. Mak, A.A. Cheak, J.Y. Tan, et al., Mycophenolate mofetil is as efficacious as, but safer than, cyclophosphamide in the treatment of proliferative lupus nephritis: a meta-analysis and meta-regression, Rheumatology (Oxford) 48 (2009) 944–952.

521. M. Ramos-Casals, M.J. Soto, M.J. Cuadrado, et al., Rituximab in systemic lupus erythematosus: A systematic review of off-label use in 188 cases, Lupus 18 (2009) 767–776.

536. A.K. Nascif, M.O. Hilario, M.T. Terreri, et al., Endothelial function analysis and atherosclerotic risk factors in adolescents with systemic lupus erythematosus, Int. J. Adolesc. Med. Health 19 (2007) 497–505.

540. S. Compeyrot-Lacassagne, P.N. Tyrrell, E. Atenafu, et al., Prevalence and etiology of low bone mineral density in juvenile systemic lupus erythematosus, Arthritis Rheum. 56 (2007) 1966–1973.

550. Y. Sherer, A. Gorstein, M.J. Fritzler, et al., Autoantibody explosion in systemic lupus erythematosus: more than 100 different antibodies found in SLE patients, Semin. Arthritis Rheum. 34 (2004) 501–537.

557. A.T. Borchers, C.L. Keen, M.E. Gershwin, Drug-induced lupus, Ann. N. Y. Acad. Sci. 1108 (2007) 166–182.

562. L.A. Criswell, The genetic contribution to systemic lupus erythematosus, Bull. NYU. Hosp. Jt. Dis. 66 (2008) 176–183.

590. H.I. Brunner, B.M. Feldman, C. Bombardier, et al., Sensitivity of the Systemic Lupus Erythematosus Disease Activity Index, British Isles Lupus Assessment Group Index, and Systemic Lupus Activity Measure in the evaluation of clinical change in childhood-onset systemic lupus erythematosus, Arthritis Rheum. 42 (1999) 1354–1360.

598. L. Moorthy, M. Peterson, A. Hassett, et al., Relationship between health-related quality of life and SLE activity and damage in children over time, Lupus 18 (2009) 622–629.

604. R. Gutierrez-Suarez, N. Ruperto, R. Gastaldi, et al., A proposal for a pediatric version of the Systemic Lupus International Collaborating Clinics/American College of Rheumatology Damage Index based on the analysis of 1,015 patients with juvenile-onset systemic lupus erythematosus, Arthritis Rheum. 54 (2006) 2989–2996.

615. L.B. Tucker, A.G. Uribe, M. Fernandez, et al., Adolescent onset of lupus results in more aggressive disease and worse outcomes: results of a nested matched case-control study within LUMINA, a multiethnic US cohort (LUMINA LVII), Lupus 17 (2008) 314–322.

618. B. Bader-Meunier, J.B. Armengaud, E. Haddad, et al., Initial presentation of childhood-onset systemic lupus erythematosus: a French multicenter study, J. Pediatr. 146 (2005) 648–653.

677. R.R. Sivaraj, O.M. Durrani, A.K. Denniston, et al., Ocular manifestations of systemic lupus erythematosus, Rheumatology (Oxford) 46 (2007) 1757–1762.

Entire reference list is available online at www.expertconsult.com.

Chapter 22

ANTIPHOSPHOLIPID SYNDROME

Tadej Avčin and Kathleen M. O'Neil

The antiphospholipid syndrome (APS) is an autoimmune multisystem disease characterized by thromboembolic events, pregnancy morbidity, hematological, dermatological, neurological, and other manifestations in the presence of elevated titers of antiphospholipid antibodies (aPLs). It may occur as an isolated clinical entity (primary APS) or in association with other diseases, mainly systemic lupus erythematosus (SLE). It occasionally occurs with other autoimmune conditions, infections, and malignancies.

DEFINITION AND CLASSIFICATION

Preliminary classification criteria for APS were developed by consensus at the Sapporo, Japan, antiphospholipid meeting in 1998.[1] It was proposed that the term APS should designate patients who suffered from vascular thrombosis or recurrent fetal losses associated with the presence of aPL, namely the lupus anticoagulant (LA) or the anticardiolipin antibodies (aCLs) of immunoglobulin G (IgG) and/or IgM isotype in medium or high titers detected on two or more occasions at least 6 weeks apart.[1] These criteria were revised in 2006 after the consensus workshop held in Sydney, Australia. The revised classification criteria for definite APS include the presence of antibodies against β_2 glycoprotein I (anti-β_2GPIs) of IgG and/or IgM isotype as part of the updated laboratory criteria and require aPLs to be positive on more than one occasion at least 12 weeks apart[2] (Table 22–1). The revised 2006 criteria were evaluated only in a few studies in adult populations and require further validation; however, it is generally assumed that they limit the risk of misclassification of patients with transient aPLs and provide a more selective and risk-stratified framework for evaluating patients with persistently positive aPLs.[3,4]

APS in children has been largely reported in patients with vascular thromboses and less frequently in association with isolated neurological or hematological manifestations.[5-7] Pregnancy morbidity, which represents one of the two clinical criteria for definite APS in adults, is not applicable to the pediatric population, and it is possible that current consensus criteria may fail to recognize a subgroup of pediatric patients who do not present with vascular thrombosis but demonstrate typical nonthrombotic clinical features and fulfill the laboratory criteria for APS.[8] A classification of *probable APS* has been given to patients with aPLs who have non-criteria clinical features associated with APS, such as heart valve disease, livedo reticularis, thrombocytopenia, nephropathy, and neurological manifestations.[2] The term *probable APS* was proposed also to classify rare cases of patients who fulfill the clinical criteria for APS but test positive for non-criteria aPLs, such as IgA isotype of aCL or anti-β_2GPI, antiphosphatidylserine, antiphosphatidylethanolamine antibodies, or antibodies against prothrombin alone or against the phosphatidylserine-prothrombin complex.[2]

Catastrophic antiphospholipid syndrome (CAPS) is another subset of APS that is characterized by acute microvascular occlusive disease with subsequent multiorgan failure and a high mortality rate. Preliminary classification criteria for CAPS were established in 2002 at the consensus workshop held in Taormina, Italy[9] (Table 22–2). This syndrome is defined as clinical involvement of at least three organ systems and/or tissues over a very short period of time with histopathological evidence of small vessel occlusion and laboratory confirmation of the presence of aPLs.[9,10]

EPIDEMIOLOGY

There are no reliable data on the incidence or prevalence of APS in the pediatric population, since there are no validated criteria and the diagnosis rests on extension of adult guidelines and clinical judgment. In a large cohort study of 1000 consecutive patients with APS from 13 European countries, 85% of patients were diagnosed between ages 15 and 50 years. Those with disease onset before 15 years of age accounted for 2.8% of patients with APS.[11]

APS is considered the most common acquired hypercoagulation state of autoimmune etiology, and aPLs were reported in 12% to 25% of unselected children with thrombosis.[12,13] Although the incidence of thrombosis in children is significantly lower than in adults, the proportion of thrombosis that is attributable to aPLs in children appears to be higher than in the adult population, which has other common prothrombotic risk factors such as atherosclerosis, cigarette smoking, hypertension, and use of oral contraceptives.[14]

Table 22-1

Revised classification criteria for the Antiphospholipid Syndrome[2]

Clinical Criteria:

1. Vascular thrombosis

One or more clinical episodes of arterial, venous, or small vessel thrombosis in any tissue or organ. Thrombosis must be confirmed by objective validated criteria (i.e., unequivocal findings of appropriate imaging studies or histopathology). For histopathological confirmation, thrombosis should be present without significant evidence of inflammation in the vessel wall.

2. Pregnancy morbidity

(a) One or more unexplained deaths of a morphologically normal fetus at or beyond the 10th week of gestation, with normal fetal morphology documented by ultrasound or by direct examination of the fetus.

(b) One or more premature births of a morphologically normal neonate before the 34th week of gestation because of: (1) eclampsia or severe preeclampsia defined according to standard definitions, or (2) recognized features of placental insufficiency.

(c) Three or more unexplained consecutive spontaneous abortions before the 10th week of gestation, with maternal anatomical or hormonal abnormalities and paternal and maternal chromosomal causes excluded.

Laboratory Criteria:

1. Lupus anticoagulant (LA) present in plasma on two or more occasions at least 12 weeks apart, detected according to the guidelines of the International Society on Thrombosis and Hemostasis.
2. Anticardiolipin antibody of IgG and/or IgM isotype in serum or plasma, present in medium or high titer (i.e. > 40 GPL or MPL, or > the 99th percentile), on two or more occasions, at least 12 weeks apart, measured by a standardized ELISA.
3. Anti-β_2 glycoprotein-I antibody of IgG and/or IgM isotype in serum or plasma (in titer > the 99th percentile), present on two or more occasions, at least 12 weeks apart, measured by a standardized ELISA.

Note: APS is present if at least one of the clinical criteria and one of the laboratory criteria are met.

Table 22-2

Preliminary criteria for the classification of Catastrophic Antiphospholipid Syndrome

1. Evidence of involvement of three or more organs, systems, and/or tissues.
2. Development of manifestations simultaneously or in less than a week.
3. Confirmation by histopathology of small vessel occlusion in at least one organ or tissue.
4. Laboratory confirmation of the presence of antiphospholipid antibodies.

Definite catastrophic APS
- All four criteria

Probable catastrophic APS
- All four criteria, except only two organs, systems, and/or tissues involved
- All four criteria, except the absence of laboratory confirmation at least 6 weeks apart because of the early death of a patient never tested for aPLs before the catastrophic APS
- 1, 2, and 4
- 1, 3, and 4 and the development of a third event in more than a week but less than a month, despite anticoagulation

Modified from Asherson RA, Cervera R, de Groot PG et al: Catastrophic antiphospholipid syndrome: international consensus statement on classification criteria and treatment guidelines. *Lupus* 12:530-534, 2003.

The demographic characteristics of 121 pediatric patients with aPL-related thrombosis, included in an international registry of pediatric APS, revealed a mean age at disease onset of 10.7 years (range, 1.0 to 17.9 years).[15] There was a slight female predominance in pediatric APS studies with a female-to-male ratio ranging from 1.2:1 to 1.5:1,[15,16] whereas in adult APS studies the female-to male ratio is over 5:1.[11,17] This difference may reflect, in part, a sampling bias, because the adult APS studies included patients with thrombosis as well as women with pregnancy morbidity. Very little is known about the geographic and racial distribution of pediatric APS.

Primary Antiphospholipid Syndrome

Primary, isolated APS without other underlying disease accounts for approximately 50% of pediatric patients with APS.[15] This percentage may be somewhat overestimated because a number of children initially present with primary APS and later during the follow-up develop overt SLE.[15,16,18] During the 6.1-year mean follow-up period, 21% of children who were initially diagnosed with primary APS progressed to have either clear-cut SLE or lupus-like disease.[15] Comparisons between pediatric patients with primary APS and those with APS associated with underlying autoimmune disease suggest that children with primary APS are significantly younger and have a higher frequency of arterial thrombotic events, especially cerebrovascular ischemic events.[15]

Autoimmune Diseases

From the pediatric APS registry, it is estimated that approximately 50% of all APS cases in pediatric populations are associated with underlying autoimmune disease.[15] There are only limited data addressing how autoimmune disease can modify the clinical expression of APS, and sometimes the clinical distinction between primary APS and APS associated with autoimmune disease can be difficult to make. This is especially true in SLE, which has many overlapping features with APS, including thrombocytopenia, hemolytic anemia, seizures, and proteinuria.[19] Recent evidence suggests that children with APS associated with underlying autoimmune disease are significantly older and have a higher frequency of venous thrombotic events associated with hematological and skin manifestations than do children with primary APS.[15]

SLE and lupus-like disease account for the majority (83%) of pediatric APS cases associated with underlying autoimmune disease.[15] SLE is the autoimmune disease in which aPLs can be found most often, with the reported aPL frequencies ranging from 19% to 87% for aCL, 31% to 48% for anti-β_2GPI, and 10% to 62% for LA, respectively.[20-34] A metaanalysis of the published studies that investigated the prevalence and clinical significance of aPLs in pediatric SLE showed a global prevalence of 44% for aCL, 40% for anti-β_2GPI, and 22% for LA.[35]

Isolated cases of APS were reported in a variety of other pediatric autoimmune diseases, including juvenile idiopathic arthritis (JIA),[36,37] Henoch-Schönlein purpura,[38,39] Behçet disease,[15] hemolytic-uremic syndrome,[40] juvenile dermatomyositis,[41] and rheumatic fever.[15,42,43] In most of these diseases persistently positive aPLs were observed in a high percentage,[29,44-49] but in contrast to patients with SLE, these patients very rarely develop aPL-related thrombotic events. It appears that aPLs observed in autoimmune diseases other than SLE may have limited pathogenic potential; alternatively, some disease-specific factors in SLE may act as a second trigger, exacerbating the prothrombotic effect of aPLs. In JIA, aCL has been reported in 7% to 53% of patients,[20,24,28,29,46,50-52] but anti-β_2GPI and LA, felt to be more specific for thrombosis risk than aCL, were detected in fewer than 5% of patients.[29,46]

Infections

Various infectious processes may act as a triggering factor for thrombosis in aPL-positive patients.[53-55] Preceding or concomitant infections were found in approximately 10% of children with primary APS or APS associated with autoimmune disease.[15] Pediatric APS was most frequently reported in association with parvovirus B19,[56] varicella-zoster virus,[57,58] HIV,[59] streptococcal and staphylococcal infections, gram-negative bacteria,[60] and *Mycoplasma pneumoniae*.[61-63]

Many viral and bacterial infections in childhood can also induce de novo production of aPLs in previously negative patients.[64-67] Infection-induced aPLs tend to be transient and are generally not associated with clinical manifestations of APS.[54,55] The majority of postinfectious aPLs differ immunochemically from those seen in patients with autoimmune diseases and do not require the presence of cofactor plasma proteins such as β_2GPI for binding.[68,69] Because most children suffer from common viral and bacterial infections, a high percentage of incidental aPL positivity might be expected in a pediatric population.[70] The association between infections and aPLs is supported also by some indirect evidence, such as seasonal distribution of aPLs.[71]

Malignancies

There have been isolated case reports of the association of aPL with thrombotic events in children with various malignancies, including solid tumors and lymphoproliferative and hematological malignancies.[72-74] Published data suggest that APS associated with malignancies accounts for fewer than 1% of all children with APS.[15] It appears that aPL-related thrombotic events associated with malignancies are more common in elderly patients, particularly in association with solid tumors.[74,75]

Healthy Children

Low levels of aPL can be found in up to 25% of apparently healthy children, which is higher than the rate seen in the normal adult population.[70,76-79] Such naturally occurring aPLs are usually transient and could be the result of previous infections or vaccinations.[64,65,67,80,81] In apparently healthy children, the estimated frequency of aCL ranges from 3% to 28%, and of anti-β_2GPI from 3% to 7%, respectively.[70,79] LA have also been described in apparently healthy children, usually as an incidental finding of prolonged activated partial thromboplastin time (aPTT) in pre-operative coagulation screening.[76,77] The risk of future thrombosis is exceedingly low in otherwise healthy children who were incidentally found to have positive aPL.[76]

ETIOLOGY AND PATHOGENESIS

Although aPLs are found in healthy children, it is clear that their presence is associated with thrombosis (see Clinical Manifestations), pregnancy morbidity, hematological, skin, and neurological conditions, and microangiopathy. aPL production appears to be triggered by infections of all sorts, and in some instances, can be familial/hereditary.[82] It is apparent that many people with aPLs do not experience disease related to these antibodies, but the presence of any one of several prothrombotic risk factors, including underlying autoimmune disease such as SLE, will dramatically increase the risk of thromboembolic disease.

Pathophysiology

aPLs cause disease through a variety of effects on endothelial cells, platelets, monocytes, and neutrophils. Many of these important effects are mediated through complement activation, as has been described in the last few years, promoting both inflammation at sites of antibody deposition and thrombus formation. Phospholipids are a component of all membranes; thus it is not surprising that these autoantibodies have broad-ranging biological effects, perturbing the interaction between cells and the plasma that bathes them and disrupting the orderly function of biological membranes. In addition, aPLs promote thrombin assembly while inhibiting thrombolysis. There is emerging evidence, moreover, that aPLs promote atherosclerosis.

Platelet effects

In vitro pretreatment of platelets with clonal anti-β_2GPI can activate the platelets, promoting their adherence to endothelium.[83] In vivo platelet activation in patients with APS has been demonstrated by the finding of high levels of urinary thromboxane metabolites, and in vitro aPLs induce release of thromboxane from platelets.[84] In vitro platelet aggregation requires partial preactivation of the platelets with thrombin, collagen, or ADP; aPL then completes that activation via p39 MAP-kinase phosphorylation, leading to release of thromboxane B2 and activation of

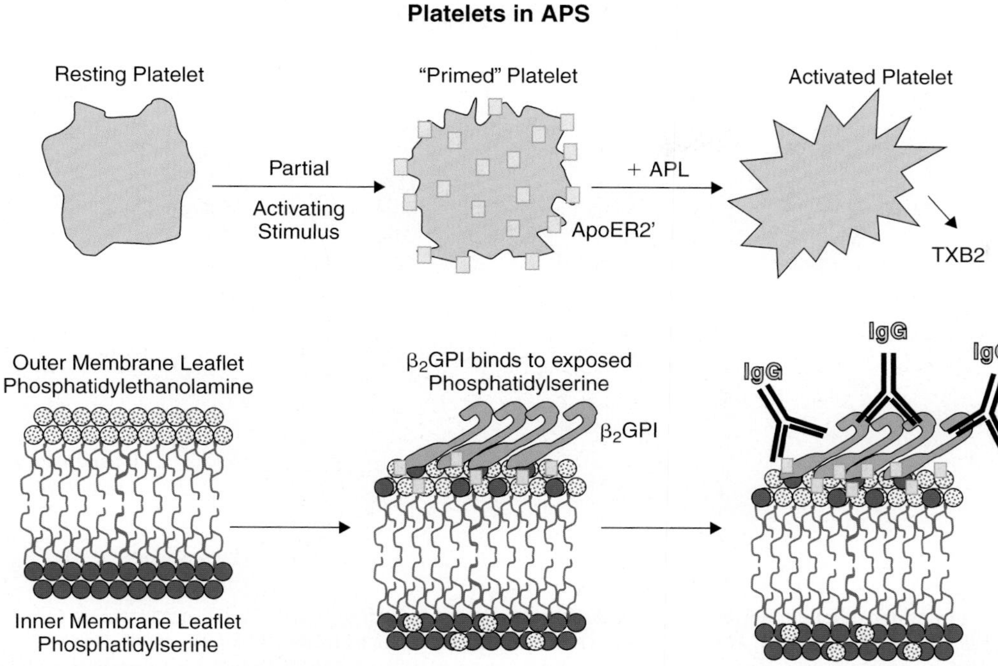

Platelets in APS

FIGURE 22–1   Effects of antiphospholipid antibodies on platelets. Upper images: Following a partial activating stimulus such as LPS or cytokine exposure, platelets increase expression of the apolipoprotein E2 receptor (ApoE2R), *yellow squares*, and bind β_2GPIs and aPLs, leading to platelet aggregation and release of thromboxane B2. The lower images show fine detail at the level of the platelet membrane. In the resting state, the neutral phospholipid, phosphatidylethanolamine, is maintained in the extracellular leaflet, and the negatively charged phosphatidylserine (PS) is on the intracellular membrane leaflet. With preactivation, this is perturbed, and PS is expressed on the platelet surface, exposing sites that can bind β_2GPI. This now produces binding sites for aPLs, and total activation of the platelet.

phospholipase A2.[85-89] For anti-β_2GPI to induce this effect, expression of the platelet type 2' receptor for apolipoprotein E (Apo E R2') and of platelet glycoprotein Ib alpha subunit is required.[90] The interaction of aPLs with platelets is illustrated in Figure 22–1. These platelet-activating effects of aPL can be blocked in vitro with pharmacological concentrations of hydroxychloroquine,[91] suggesting an important mechanism for the effect of this drug in APS.

Endothelial Cells in Antiphospholipid Syndrome

Antiphospholipid antibodies increase the adhesiveness of endothelial cells to leukocytes and platelets by increasing expression of ICAM-1, VCAM-1, and E selectin.[92,93] Mice genetically deficient in these adhesion molecules have impaired aPL-induced thrombus formation,[94,95] confirming the importance of this effect in the pathology of APS. Endothelial cells treated with aPL increase production of interleukin-6 and reactive oxygen species, promoting an inflammatory phenotype at the level of endothelium.[96,97] Tissue factor, an important initiator of coagulation via the extrinsic pathway, is highly expressed by endothelium of vessels from patients with APS.[98] Anti-β_2GPIs activate p38-MAP kinase in endothelium as well as platelets, and this results in increased expression of tissue factor by endothelium exposed to aPL.[89,99] This tissue factor overexpression contributes to the prothrombotic effects of aPL. Activation of NFκB is an essential step in the endothelial effects of aPL, and MG132, an inhibitor of

NFκB, blocks the tissue factor upregulation induced by aPL.[100,101] aPL treatment of mice in vivo increases VCAM and tissue factor expression in aortic and carotid artery endothelium, and this is dependent on activation of p38 MAPK and NFκB.[89,102] Pretreatment with fluvastatin blocks aPL endothelial cell effects on tissue factor and adhesion molecule expression.[103] β_2GPI blocks von Willebrand factor–dependent platelet aggregation, and aPLs interfere with this inhibition of platelet aggregation.[104] Plasma concentrations of von Willebrand protein are high in patients with primary APS,[105] further promoting platelet aggregation and the prothrombotic effects of aPL.

β_2GPI-aPL complexes bind tightly to endothelial cells, and that binding is mediated by annexin A2.[106,107] Antibodies to annexin A2 produce the same activation of endothelial cells as do anti-β_2GPIs, with the same kinetics. This effect is only present with cross-linking antibodies and not present with F(ab') monomers, suggesting that perturbation of annexin A2 in the membrane mediates the anti-β_2GPI–induced endothelial activation through effects on annexin A2.[107] β_2GPI promotes the activation of plasminogen by tissue plasminogen activator; this suggests that β_2GPI may be an endogenous regulator of fibrinolysis.[108] Consequently, impairment of β_2GPI-augmented fibrinolysis by anti-β_2GPI antibodies may contribute to thrombosis in patients with APS.

aPLs activate endothelial cells via the Toll-like receptor 4 (TLR4),[109] activating the adaptor protein MyD88 and downstream effects,[110] and TLR4 knock-out mice are resistant to aPL-induced thrombosis. In mouse fibroblasts a similar role for TLR2 has been demonstrated.[111]

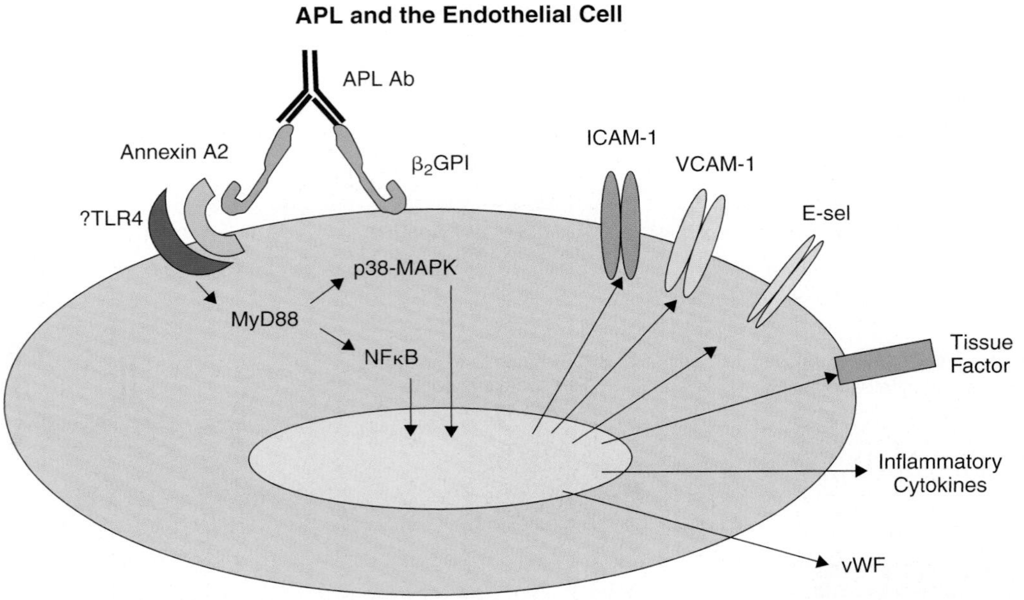

FIGURE 22–2   Effects of antiphospholipid antibodies on endothelial cells. β_2GPI binds to endothelial cell membranes via annexin A2, which does not contain a transmembrane domain. aPL binds to the β_2GPI, and through a signaling pathway involving MyD88, p38-MAPK, and NFκB activation (presumably mediated by TLR4), the endothelial cell becomes activated, increasing expression of the adhesion molecules ICAM-1, VCAM-1, E-selectin (E-sel) and the coagulation protein tissue factor. In addition, inflammatory cytokines and the von Willebrand factor (vWF, the factor VIII–associated antigen) are produced for local activity at the cell surface and are exported into the plasma.

This involvement of the innate immune system may be a critical link in comprehending the pathogenesis of this complex disease. The interaction of aPLs with endothelial cells is illustrated in Figure 22–2.

Monocyte and Neutrophil Activation by Antiphospholipid Antibodies

aPLs affect monocytes in ways similar to how they affect platelets. They upregulate tissue factor expression and adhesion molecule expression, the production of interleukins-1, -6 and -8 via phosphorylation of p38 MAPK, and the activation of NFκB and MEK/ERK kinases.[112] Dilazep, an inhibitor of platelet adenosine uptake, inhibits the increased tissue factor activity in monocytes induced by aPL.[113] These monocyte effects of aPL are likely important in preactivating endothelial cells to a prothrombotic phenotype. Neutrophils are required for fetal loss related to aPL, as neutrophil depletion in mice prevents the intrauterine growth retardation and fetal demise related to passive aPL antibody administration. Neutrophil accumulation in the decidual tissues is mediated by complement activation products, particularly C5a.[114] Tissue factor expression on neutrophils is increased by aPL, and blockade of tissue factor by monoclonal antibody treatment prevents fetal injury.[115,116]

aPLs' Effect on Placental Trophoblasts

In addition to promoting inflammation and coagulation at the level of endothelial cells and leukocytes within vessels, evidence is accumulating that aPLs have direct toxic effects on the function of a variety of other cells, most prominent among these are the effects on placental trophoblasts. This has best been demonstrated in a murine model of APS, where serum IgG antibody and monoclonal human aPL can induce fetal loss in pregnant mice.[117] In particular, aPLs can bind directly to trophoblast in the developing embryo,[118] and following binding, these antibodies inhibit the normal invasion of trophoblast into the decidual tissues, resulting in defective placentation. Trophoblast production of chorionic gonadotropin and placental lactogen is impaired following aPL treatment.[118,119] Because trophoblast expresses anionic phospholipids on the surfaces during differentiation, they bind β_2GPIs in vivo, making them a target for aPLs.[120] Matrix metalloproteinases, required for placental invasion, are underexpressed in APS, and heparin increases trophoblast invasiveness by increasing matrix metalloproteinases expression.[121]

Complement Activation in the Antiphospholipid Syndrome

Antigen-antibody complexes made of aPLs and the membrane phospholipids to which they are directed, like most immune complexes, can activate complement via the classical pathway. Complement activation generates a variety of biologically active cleavage fragments that have serine protease activity, anaphylatoxic effects, and promote neutrophil adhesion to activated endothelium, then influx into tissues. Early reports suggested that in very active thrombotic disease due to aPL, depletion of C3 and C4 could be found.[122,123] In an animal model of aPL-induced fetal loss, complement activation appears to be necessary for fetal demise and resorption[114,124,125] and

Table 22–3

Mechanisms of action of antiphospholipid antibodies

Platelet Activation
- Aggregation
- Thromboxane release

Monocyte Activation
- Inflammatory cytokine production
- Increased monocyte tissue factor expression

Endothelial Activation
- Tissue factor expression and secretion
- Increased vWF expression
- Expression of adhesion molecules

Impaired function of activated protein C

Decreased binding of C4 to C4BP
- Increased C4BP binding of protein S

Promote clot formation
Impair thrombolysis

vWF, von Willebrand factor.

aPL-induced thrombus formation.[125] This complement effect makes intuitive sense, as both complement and the thrombosis systems are cascades of interacting serine proteases. Serine protease inhibitors (serpins), several of which are common to both pathways, regulate both coagulation and thrombosis. Studies utilizing intravital microscopy following immunological "priming" with lipopolysaccharide then intraarterial injection of aPLs in rats demonstrated complement activation in the aPL-treated thrombotic vessels. In contrast, thrombus did not form as efficiently in complement-deficient C6-/- animals. In addition, an anti-C5 antibody that blocks C5 activation, C5a release, and C5b-9 assembly also had diminished thrombus formation.[126] Thus complement plays a crucial role in promoting the placental inflammation that leads to fetal demise in APS, and in promoting thrombus formation.

aPLs can have antifibrinolytic effects and have been shown to inhibit the activities of thrombin, activated protein C, plasminogen, and plasmin.[127-9] Anti-β_2GPIs inhibit the anticoagulant activity of activated protein C.[130] Some APS patients have demonstrable antibody to protein S and/or protein C. There is in vivo evidence that this inhibition of thrombolysis contributes to the pathogenicity of aPL.[131-133] In fact, measuring inhibition of activated protein C activity may be more sensitive for pathogenic aPLs than currently employed assays.[134]

In summary (see Table 22–3), aPLs have a variety of procoagulant effects, including the activation of platelets to aggregate and release thromboxane, activation of monocytes (inflammatory cytokine production and increased tissue factor expression), and activation of endothelium (increased tissue factor expression and secretion, increased von Willebrand factor, and expression of adhesion molecules). They also impede activated protein C. Furthermore, through aPL actions on complement, endothelium and neutrophils are activated to promote tissue accumulation of neutrophils, thus promoting local inflammation.

GENETIC BACKGROUND

The first suggestion that APS might cluster in families and therefore have a heritable basis was published over four decades ago, with the description of several family members with the biological false-positive serological test for syphilis, only some of whom were had a thrombotic diathesis.[135] Other similar reports in the 1980s[136,137] rekindled interest in a possible genetic component for this APS. The findings of a high incidence of aCL in first-degree relatives of people with APS or with SLE[138,139] suggested that the capacity to develop antibodies to charged phospholipids, at the least, may be influenced by genetics, probably with important environmental influences.[140] Family studies showed that APS and aPL can occur in family clusters,[138,141] but this is so only in a minority of patients. Inheritance in familial APS may be autosomal recessive,[138] or dominant/codominant.[142] In most cases, the disease does not appear to be familial, however, and in fact, the Thrombosis Interest Group of Canada website advises against testing for APS in the evaluation of familial hypercoagulability (http://www.tigc.org/pdf/antiphospholipid04.pdf).

In interpreting the studies of familial APS, it is important to remember several factors: although primary and secondary APS share a number of features, it is not clear that their genetic basis is similar. Most secondary APS occurs in SLE, but the majority of Lupus patients with aPLs do not have thromboembolic disease or APS. aPLs are common in SLE, seen in 25% to 40% of adult lupus patients, though one study reported a rate as high as 77%.[143] aPLs occur in people without apparent underlying autoimmunity or thromboembolic disease; and healthy children, in particular, may have a high rate of aCL positivity relative to adults.[70,78] Reports of aPL rates in pediatric family members of patients with APS must be interpreted in light a evidence of higher antibody positivity rates in healthy children than in adults.

There are several reports of familial Sneddon syndrome, which is often associated with aPLs and is inherited as an autosomal-dominant trait,[144,145] reminiscent of the thrombotic disease in the APS kindred reported by Ford and colleagues.[141] This may represent a variation of familial APS. Individual kindreds with the familial form of moyamoya disease, another cerebrovascular disease inherited in an autosomal dominant pattern,[146] have been assessed for the presence of aPLs, but these antibodies were rarely found. Rather, autosomal dominant moyamoya disease is due to mutations in tissue inhibitors of metalloproteinases.[147] Another form of autosomal dominant vascular neuropathology, Binswanger disease, that presents as early-onset familial dementia with multifocal abnormalities on MR imaging of the brain, has been associated with LA in one large kindred, but tests for aCLs were negative.[148] Whether this represents a linked genetic disorder or whether familial Binswanger disease might be caused by familial APS in more families is not known.

Most reports of familial APS are anecdotal and do not provide information on the genetic transmission of the disease.[145, 149-153] The number of reports and small

Table 22–4

HLA-alleles associated with Antiphospholipid Syndrome

Clinical Condition	HLA-Allele Association
Primary APS	DR4 (Asherson, 1992; Camps, 1995) DR5 (Vargas-Alarcon, 1995)
Secondary APS	DQB1*0301 (Arnett, 1991)
Lupus anticoagulant	DR5, DRw52b, DQB1*0301 (DQw7), or DQB1*0302 (DQw8) (Arnett, 1991)
Anticardiolipin antibody	DR7 (Camps, 1995; Savi, 1988; Granados, 1996) DR4 (McHugh, 1989)
Antiphosphatidylserine/ antiprothrombin antibodies	DQB1*0301/4; DQA1*0301/2;DRB1*04 (Bertolaccini, 2000)
Anti-β_2 glycoprotein-I antibody	DQB1*0604/5/6/7/9; DQA1*0102; DRB1*1302 and DQB1*0303 (Bertolaccini, 2000; Arnett, 1999)

series published provide evidence that familial occurrence and possibly genetic influence is important, at least in a subset of human APS. Other issues that cloud reports of familial APS are variations in whether, and how completely, patients were evaluated for other prothrombotic traits such as inherited heterozygous deficiency of protein C or protein S or resistance to activated protein C from such genetic disorders as factor V Leiden and methylenetetrahydrofolate reductase (MTHFR) deficiencies. Any of these defects can coexist with aPL[154-157] and increase the likelihood of thrombosis in the presence of aPL. The number of patients reported with aPLs who have genetic defects predisposing to pathological thrombosis raises the possibility that disordered coagulation itself might indeed predispose to the formation of aPLs. This question has not been directly addressed.

It is not known how often APS is familial. Estimates based on family history usually do not include complete laboratory evaluation[140,158] of family members. Consequently, such studies likely overestimate the rate of "affected" relatives. Prospective studies of families utilizing current definitions of APS and standardized testing technology are not yet available.

Genetic Studies

A variety of human leukocyte antigen (HLA) -DR and -DQ antigens have been associated with aPLs and both primary and secondary APS (summarized in Table 22–4). Many of these associations lose significance when corrected for the number of variables tested, however.[159] These studies are generally small series, and most do not include appropriate ethnic controls. One study of secondary APS looked for the "autoimmune" haplotype, HLA-B8, DR3, in lupus patients and found aCLs correlated with this haplotype.[160] Arnett and colleagues studied major histocompatibility complex (MHC) genotypes in 20 patients with LA, of whom 8 had primary APS and 12

had other rheumatic diseases (7 with significant thrombotic complications).[161] The strongest association with LA was seen for DQB1*0301 (DQw7), and all who were negative for this allele had DQB1*0302 (DQw8). These two antigens share an identical 7-amino acid sequence in the third hypervariable region of the DQ molecule, suggesting this epitope might be important in mediating an immune response to phospholipid. The large number of associations reported between various measures of aPL and its related thrombotic disease and alleles in the human MHC support the fact that these genes may play a significant role in facilitating formation of preceeding antibody to phospholipid antigens, but other factors are likely to be important in the familial APS.[140,142]

Genetic associations outside the HLA region have been sought in APS, but variants of β_2GPI[142,162] and the TNFa-238 promoter polymorphism[163] that lead to TNF overproduction did not correlate with APS. Other gene mutations that did not correlate with disease in a large study of seven extended families[142] included Fas and Fas ligand, T cell receptor β chain, Ig heavy chain, antithrombin III, factor V, complement factor H, and IgK. One study of 45 patients with APS found a possible association with the FcγRIIA-H131 allele (40% of affected patients were homozygous for that allele, compared to only 25% of disease-free controls),[164] suggesting that this allele might predispose to a greater risk of thrombosis in aCL-positive persons. As of now, however, single gene associations with APS are not confirmed, and remain an area of active investigation.

CLINICAL MANIFESTATIONS

Children with aPLs may present with any combination of vascular occlusive events or with a variety of nonthrombotic clinical manifestations. Most of the clinical features that occur in adults with aPLs have also been described in children. However, the clinical expression of aPLs in children is modified by several characteristics of the pediatric age group, such as the immaturity of the immune and other organ systems, the absence of common prothrombotic risk factors often present in adults, the lack of pregnancy morbidity, and the presence of routine immunizations and frequent exposure to viral and bacterial infections.[5-7] Data from the largest series of pediatric patients with APS (the international pediatric APS registry) have provided information on the spectrum of thrombotic and nonthrombotic clinical manifestations in children.[15] At the time of the initial thrombotic event in children with definite APS, the estimated frequencies of associated nonthrombotic manifestations were 38% for hematological manifestations, 18% for dermatological manifestations, and 16% for nonthrombotic neurological manifestations.[15]

A high percentage of children with persistently positive aPLs apparently do not present with overt thrombotic event. A retrospective study of 100 children with positive aPLs evaluated at the tertiary care pediatric hospital demonstrated that thromboses occurred only in 10% of patients, while the nonthrombotic aPL-related clinical manifestations alone were observed in 77% of patients.[165]

Thromboses

The classical clinical picture of APS in pediatric populations is characterized by venous, arterial, or small-vessel thrombosis. Vascular occlusion in APS may involve arteries and veins at any level of the vascular tree and in all organ systems, giving rise to a wide variety of clinical presentations (summarized in Table 22–5).[7,15] It is now well established that APS may develop as an initial manifestation of SLE, and all children presenting with aPL-related thrombosis require thorough assessment for evidence of underlying systemic disease.[15,31,166,167]

Venous thrombosis is the most common vascular occlusive event seen, occurring in up to 60% of pediatric APS patients.[15,16] The most frequently reported site of venous thrombotic event is deep vein thrombosis in the lower extremities, followed by cerebral sinus vein thrombosis, portal vein thrombosis, deep vein thrombosis in the upper extremities, and superficial vein thrombosis.[15] Venous thrombotic events are particularly common in APS associated with pediatric SLE. In a Canadian retrospective cohort study in pediatric SLE, 13 of the 149 patients (9%) had one or more thromboembolic events, and all 13 patients with thromboembolic events were LA positive.[31] In total, venous thrombosis occurred in 76% of episodes (cerebral venous thrombosis in nine, deep vein thrombosis in four, pulmonary embolism in two, and retinal vein occlusion in one) and arterial thrombosis in 24% (arterial stroke in three, retinal artery occlusion in one, and splenic infarct in one). The overall incidence of thromboembolic events in pediatric SLE patients with positive LA was 54% and with positive aCLs 22%.[31] LA was found to be the strongest predictor of thrombosis risk in another study in 58 children with SLE, and positivity for multiple aPL subtypes indicates stronger associations with thromboembolic events than for individual aCL, anti-β_2GPI or anti-prothrombin antibodies.[33] Overall, it has been estimated that pediatric SLE patients with persistent LA positivity have a twenty-eight fold increased risk of thrombotic events compared with patients who are negative for LA.[27]

Arterial thrombosis occurs in approximately 30% of pediatric APS patients. The most frequently reported site of arterial thrombotic event is ischemic stroke, followed by peripheral arterial thrombosis.[15] Arterial thrombotic events are significantly more common in primary APS patients than in APS associated with underlying autoimmune disease.[15] Several studies have demonstrated that the prevalence of aPL-related cerebral ischemia is particularly high in pediatric and young adult patients, ranging from 15% to 75 %.[168-173] In an Israeli study evaluating the importance of various thrombophilia markers in 58 pediatric patients with stroke, only factor V Leiden and aPL were found to be significant risk factors for ischemic stroke in children.[172] aPLs are also an independent risk factor for recurrent ischemic stroke in children, but this effect has not been confirmed for IgG aCLs.[174] Sneddon syndrome is a rare but potentially severe condition characterized by generalized livedo reticularis or racemosa and cerebrovascular ischemic arterial events, which is associated with aPL in approximately 50% of all patients.[175-178]

Table 22–5

Venous and arterial thrombosis manifestations of Pediatric Antiphospholipid Syndrome

Vessel Involved	Clinical Manifestations
Venous Sites	
Limbs	Deep vein thrombosis
Skin	Livedo reticularis, chronic leg ulcers, superficial thrombophlebitis
Large veins	Superior or inferior vena cava thrombosis
Lungs	Pulmonary thromboembolism, pulmonary hypertension
Brain	Cerebral venous sinus thrombosis
Eyes	Retinal vein thrombosis
Liver	Budd-Chiari syndrome, enzyme elevations
Adrenal glands	Hypoadrenalism, Addison disease
Arterial Sites	
Limbs	Ischemia, gangrene
Brain	Stroke, transient ischemic attack, acute ischemic encephalopathy
Eyes	Retinal artery thrombosis
Kidney	Renal artery thrombosis, renal thrombotic microangiopathy
Heart	Myocardial infarction
Liver	Hepatic infarction
Gut	Mesenteric artery thrombosis
Bone	Infarction

Small-vessel thrombosis occurs in fewer than 10% of pediatric APS patients and may present as an aggressive microvascular occlusive disease (catastrophic APS) or localized small vessel thrombosis. Localized small vessel thrombosis has been described primarily in children with isolated thrombosis of digital vessels or renal thrombotic microangiopathy.[15] Peripheral vascular disease leading to digital gangrene is a well-recognized complication of APS, particularly in patients with SLE, and it may be difficult to distinguish this from vasculitis, cryoglobulinemia, or disseminated intravascular coagulation.[179,180]

Hematological Manifestations

The most common hematological manifestations associated with APS in children are thrombocytopenia, autoimmune hemolytic anemia, and leucopenia. Thrombocytopenia was observed in 20% of children with APS, often in association with Coombs-positive hemolytic anemia (Evans syndrome).[15] Thrombocytopenia associated with APS is usually mild, with platelet counts greater than 50×10^9/l and is not associated with hemorrhagic phenomena. Occasionally, thrombocytopenia may be severe, causing major bleeding.[181] Thrombotic events are unusual with severe thrombocytopenia but may occur if the platelet counts increase during the disease course.

In a case control study of 42 children with immune thrombocytopenic purpura, IgG aCLs were found in 78% and anti-β_2GPIs in all chronic cases, while patients with acute immune thrombocytopenic purpura demonstrated IgG aCLs in just 27% and anti-β_2GPIs in 13%, respectively.[182] During a 4-year follow-up period, 17%

of children who were initially diagnosed with immune thrombocytopenic purpura developed overt SLE, and closer follow-up has been suggested for these children.[182] Several studies have reported an increased risk of aPL-positive patients who present with isolated hematological manifestations for the development of future thrombosis.[18,183]

The acquired LA-hypoprothrombinemia syndrome is a rare complication consisting of a severe bleeding diathesis associated with the presence of LA. It has been described in both primary APS and APS associated with SLE and is often preceded by a viral infection.[184-187] This complication has been attributed to the presence of antiprothrombin antibodies that cause rapid depletion of plasma prothrombin.

Dermatological Manifestations

A wide variety of dermatological manifestations have been reported in patients with APS, ranging from minor signs to life-threatening conditions such as widespread cutaneous necrosis.[11,188-190] In a single-center series of 200 consecutive pediatric and adult patients with APS, skin manifestations were observed in 49% of the patients and were the presenting symptom in 30%.[191] The most frequent manifestation was livedo reticularis (25%), followed by digital necrosis (7%), subungual splinter hemorrhages (5%), superficial venous thrombosis (5%), postphlebitic skin ulcers (4%), circumscribed cutaneous necrosis (3%), thrombocytopenic purpura (3%), and other (7%). Livedo reticularis and especially the coarser livedo racemosa variant are considered a major clinical feature of APS, strongly associated with arterial thrombotic events, primarily cerebral and ocular ischemic arterial events.[191,192] Livedo reticularis was observed less frequently in those who have only venous thrombosis.[191]

The most common dermatological manifestations present in children included in the pediatric APS registry were livedo reticularis (6%), Raynaud Phenomenon (6%), and skin ulcers (3%)[15] (Figure 22–3). Association of aPLs with Raynaud Phenomenon was noted also in a retrospective study of 123 children, where at least one aPL subtype was positive in up to 36% of patients with primary and 30% of patients with secondary Raynaud Phenomenon.[193]

Neurological Manifestations

Typical neurological manifestations of APS are ischemic stroke and cerebral sinus vein thrombosis, both caused by thrombotic occlusion of cerebral vessels.[15,172,194,195] Several other neurological manifestations have been associated with the presence of aPLs, including various movement disorders, epilepsy, migraine, transverse myelitis, multiple sclerosis–like disorders, sensorineural hearing loss, cognitive defects, psychiatric diseases, and Guillain-Barré syndrome.[196-199] These manifestations are not fully explained by the procoagulant effect of aPLs and may result from both thrombotic and nonthrombotic immune-mediated mechanisms such as direct interaction between aPLs and neuronal tissue or immune complex deposition in the cerebral blood vessels wall.[200-203]

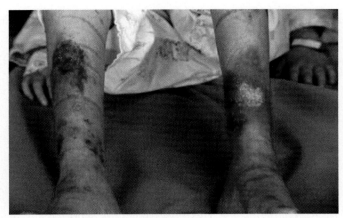

FIGURE 22–3 Chronic leg ulcers in a child with systemic lupus erythematosus and antiphospholipid antibodies.

The most common nonstroke neurological manifestations observed in children with APS were migraine headache (7%), chorea (4%), and seizures (3%).[15] Chorea has been strongly linked to the presence of aPLs as an isolated clinical finding or in children with SLE.[43,196,204-209] A large retrospective cohort study of 137 children with SLE demonstrated an association between LA and chorea over the disease course, but not between aPLs and other neuropsychiatric manifestations.[34] A significant association was found between aPLs and childhood seizure disorder in two prospective studies, but cerebrovascular disease should be excluded as a cause.[210,211] There has been controversy concerning a possible association of aPLs and migraine, which has not been confirmed in a prospective study in an unselected group of children with migraine.[212] Prospective studies of adult patients with SLE demonstrated an association between persistent aPLs and cognitive impairments, especially in areas of attention, concentration, and executive functioning.[213,214] In general, APS may constitute a potentially treatable cause of a variety of neurological diseases and it is recommended to routinely measure aPLs in children with otherwise unexplained neurological disorders.

Other Manifestations

Cardiac manifestations are frequent in adult patients with APS but have not been extensively investigated in childhood. The most prominent cardiac manifestations include valvular disease, occlusive coronary artery disease, cardiomyopathy, and intracardiac thrombosis.[11,215] Nonbacterial vegetations, known as Libman-Sacks endocarditis, were disclosed by echocardiographic studies in 11% of adult patients with APS,[11] but the frequency of this complication in pediatric APS is unknown. Several pediatric patients with aPL-related myocardial infarction have been reported, often in association with underlying SLE or congenital heart disease.[18,216-219] Multiple small vascular occlusions are responsible for APS cardiomyopathy, especially in catastrophic APS, where it is one of the most common causes of death.[220,221]

Pulmonary embolism and infarction constitute the most frequent pulmonary manifestation of APS.[31,57,63,222,223] Positive aPLs were reported in more than 40% of children with pulmonary embolism referred for hematology evaluation.[222] Rarely, recurrent pulmonary embolism may lead to pulmonary hypertension.[179,224]

The kidney is a major target organ of pediatric APS with manifestations that include renal vascular occlusion, thrombotic glomerular microangiopathy, and hypertension.[32,225-229] The term *aPL-associated nephropathy* was proposed to describe thrombotic microangiopathy involving both arterioles and glomerular capillaries causing hematuria and hypertension, often with minimal proteinuria.[2,230,231] This entity may be underrecognized in pediatric APS patients because of the rarity of clinical indications for percutaneous renal biopsy and its potential risks in thrombocytopenic patients. aPLs are also associated with hepatic, digestive, and adrenal manifestations resulting from occlusive vascular disease of intraabdominal vessels.[232-234]

Osteoarticular manifestations such as avascular necrosis of bone, nontraumatic fractures, and bone marrow necrosis are rarely seen in APS patients.[235,236] Adult patients with primary APS and no prior glucocorticoid treatment appear to have an increased risk of avascular necrosis.[237] Perthes disease has been linked with aPLs in two pediatric studies.[236,238]

Catastrophic Antiphospholipid Syndrome

Catastrophic APS is a rare, potentially life-threatening variant of APS, characterized by multiple small-vessel occlusions that can lead to multiorgan failure.[9,10] The most commonly affected organ systems include the kidney, lung, central nervous system, heart, and skin.[239] Catastrophic APS has been described in more than 20 pediatric case reports and commonly presents with microvascular thrombosis in renal, skin, and pulmonary vessels.[15,72,239-247] Thrombosis of large vessels is less frequent in catastrophic APS but may occur together with small vessel occlusion.[72] Catastrophic APS represents only a minor proportion of pediatric APS patients, and it is not known why this disorder behaves in such an aggressive fashion in some patients. Catastrophic APS in children most frequently appears to be triggered by preceding infections (especially acute gastroenteritis), SLE flares, or in the setting of a malignancy; it is rarely seen in primary APS.

In a cohort of 121 children included in the pediatric APS registry, six patients (5%) presented with life-threatening widespread thrombotic disease suggestive of catastrophic APS.[15] Three children had aggressive microvascular occlusive disease and three children developed mixed arterial and venous large-vessel thrombosis over a short period of time. Two of the six children with catastrophic APS died, resulting in a high mortality rate.[15] In the adult population, catastrophic APS occurs in fewer than 1% of patients with APS and has been associated with antecedent infections (22%), surgery (10%), oral anticoagulation withdrawal (8%), drugs (7%), obstetric complications (7%), malignancy (5%), or SLE flare (3%).[239] Among the 280 patients included in the international registry of catastrophic APS, 123 patients (44%) died at the time of the catastrophic APS event.[239]

Microangiopathic Antiphospholipid-Associated Syndrome

aPLs have been associated also with a variety of microangiopathic syndromes that cannot be attributed simply to the microvascular thrombotic process. The term *microangiopathic antiphospholipid-associated syndrome* was recently introduced to refer patients with aPLs and clinical features of thrombotic microangiopathy, such as thrombotic thrombocytopenic purpura, disseminated intravascular coagulation, and related syndromes.[240-248] There is usually accompanying hemolytic anemia, severe thrombocytopenia, and the presence of schistocytes. Hemolytic uremic syndrome (HUS) is a clinical entity characterized by endothelial damage associated with hemolytic anemia, thrombocytopenia, and microvascular thrombosis that resembles thrombotic thrombocytopenic purpura (TTP) in adults but has more frequent kidney involvement. Two pediatric series reported a high frequency of aCLs in children with diarrhea-associated HUS, but without clear clinical significance.[249,250] In adults, an association between TTP and APS has been suggested in a few case reports, implying that the underlying pathogenic mechanism may reflect the spectrum of a common autoimmune process.[251] The pathogenic role of aPLs in these clinical conditions remains controversial, and the presence of aPLs may merely reflect the induction of aPLs as an immune response to the endothelial cell perturbation and damage, or an immune response to the preceding infection. Recently, microangiopathic antiphospholipid-associated syndrome was reported in a 4-year-old child who presented with atypical HUS after acute tonsillitis and later developed rapidly progressive thrombotic microangiopathy associated with the presence of aPLs, decreased serum factor H, and positive anti–ADAMTS-13 antibodies[40] (Figure 22–4). It appears that aPLs may represent only one of the pathogenic factors in this condition, and various infectious and genetic causes such as deficiencies of factor H, membrane cofactor protein, von Willebrand factor–cleaving protease

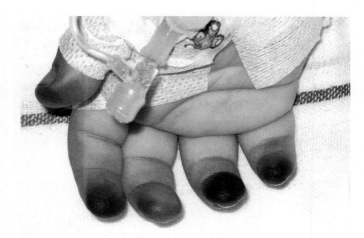

FIGURE 22–4   Necrotic changes on the fingertips in a child with microangiopathic antiphospholipid-associated syndrome (From Meglič A, Grosek S, Benedik-Dolničar M et al: Atypical haemolytic uremic syndrome complicated by microangiopathic antiphospholipid-associated syndrome, *Lupus* 17: 842-845, 2008.)

(ADAMTS 13), and inherited prothrombotic disorders must be taken into consideration, particularly in the pediatric population.

Perinatal Complications Associated with aPLs

The presence of maternal aPLs during pregnancy is associated with a number of serious obstetric and fetal complications, including preeclampsia, uteroplacental insufficiency, intrauterine growth restriction, fetal distress, and premature birth.[252,253] With recent therapeutic approaches including low–molecular weight heparin (LMWH) and aspirin, or aspirin alone, in pregnant women with aPL, the percentage of pregnancies ending in live births ranges from 75% to 80%.[254,255] The prematurity rate in babies born to mothers with APS is 10% to 15%, and the incidence of growth restriction is 15% to 20%.[256-259]

There is growing evidence that transplacentally transferred aPLs can contribute to the pathogenesis of perinatal thrombosis. However, aPLs alone are not usually sufficient for thrombosis, so other inherited and acquired thrombophilic risk factors should be systematically evaluated.[260-262] A recent metaanalysis reviewed clinical and immunological features of 16 infants with perinatal thrombosis born to mothers with aPLs.[263] Arterial thromboses were reported in 80% of the perinatal thrombotic events, and ischemic stroke occurred in half of the cases[264-269] (Figure 22–5). Thromboses occurred in other vessels including the aorta, peripheral arteries, mesenteric arteries, renal veins, and subclavian veins.[270-278] More than 60% of infants with aPL-related perinatal thrombosis had at least one additional thrombophilic risk factor identified, most commonly arterial or venous catheters, sepsis, asphyxia, and/or congenital thrombophilia.[263]

Perinatal thrombosis and other aPL-related clinical manifestations are rare complications of transplacental passage of aPLs.[263,279] Several cohort studies examining the outcome of infants born to mothers with APS have consistently shown that, except for prematurity and its potential associated complications, these neonates had no other clinical manifestations.[256-259] In contrast, preliminary results of a follow-up study of 31 infants born to mothers with APS beyond their second birthday revealed abnormal behavior in 3 children who were diagnosed with language delay, hyperactivity disorder, and autistic symptoms in 1 child.[259] Furthermore, a smaller Italian study of the neuropsychological development of children born to mothers with APS showed a high percentage of children with learning disabilities such as dyslexia and dyscalculia at school entry.[280] Regular neuropsychological assessments are recommended for long-term follow-up of these high-risk children.

It is well established that maternal aCLs and anti-β_2GPIs can cross the placenta and be detected in cord blood.[281-284] The estimated rate of transplacental passage of maternal aPL is 30% to 50%, significantly lower than that observed for antinuclear antibodies (~80%).[283,285] There is controversy regarding the persistence of transplacentally transferred aPLs after birth in infants. During the prospective follow-up of infants born to mothers with APS or aPL-positive autoimmune disease, it was observed that aCL titers in newborns' sera progressively decrease; at 6 and 12 months of age, all infants were negative for aCL.[281,283] In contrast, anti-β_2GPIs can be found at 12 months of age in up to 64% of infants born to aPL-positive mothers and in 33% of infants born to mothers with aPL-negative autoimmune disease.[283] This finding implies postnatal de novo synthesis of anti-β_2GPIs in infants, presumably associated with the exaggerated immune response to nutritional antigens, as originally described in healthy preschool children and infants with atopic dermatitis.[70,286] Current evidence suggests that anti-β_2GPIs detected in infants have low thrombosis risk and have different epitope specificity than do anti-β_2GPIs found in patients with APS.[286] For clinical practice it seems prudent to consider the detection of aCLs, but not

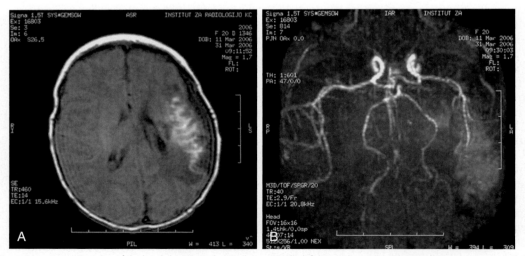

FIGURE 22–5　Magnetic resonance imaging of the head showing ischemic changes in the left hemisphere **(A)** and magnetic resonance angiography showing occlusion of the left middle cerebral artery **(B)** in a neonate with IgG anticardiolipin antibodies and heterozygous methylenetetrahydrofolate reductase C677T and prothrombin G20210A gene mutations (From Paro-Panjan D, Kitanovski L, Avčin T: Neonatal antiphospholipid syndrome associated with heterozygous methylenetetrahydrofolate reductase C677T and prothrombin G20210A gene mutations, *Rheumatology* 46:720-721, 2007.)

anti-β₂GPIs, to evaluate the disappearance of transplacentally acquired maternal aPLs and to assess the potential thrombosis risk associated with aPLs in infants.

PATHOLOGY

Histopathological changes in APS may be grouped under several categories, including thrombotic, microangiopathic, ischemic, or coincidental with underlying disease–related pathology.[287]

Classic vaso-occlusive lesions in APS are thrombotic, recent, or organized and can either be systemic or involve single organs.[288] Thrombotic lesions are characterized by predominant noninflammatory occlusive or mural thrombosis and its consequences. Acute thrombotic lesions may be seen as occlusive thrombi with or without features of thrombolysis and limited reactive changes. Microvascular thrombi can undergo rapid dissolution and disappear. Otherwise, thrombus organization starts early by proliferation of neighboring endothelial cells and is later dominated by intraluminal proliferation of myofibroblasts and recanalization. Occlusive vascular thrombosis causes secondary acute and chronic ischemic changes. True vasculitis may occur as a coincidental finding that is causally not related to APS but to the coexisting underlying disease, most commonly SLE.[288]

Microangiopathic lesions are characterized predominantly by endothelial cell injury—subendothelial plasma insudation often associated with thrombotic necrotizing lesions and its chronic consequences. This type of histopathological lesion has not been adequately recognized in the context of APS and appears to be significantly underestimated. Endothelial cells of the small blood vessels that are activated and injured by aPLs play a major role in the initiation and development of acute microangiopathic lesions. Acute phase is characterized by endothelial cell swelling, detachment, and necrosis as well as prominent insudation into the subendothelium of blood constituents through a leaky endothelium, which may be seen in an immunofluorescence micrography as intensely positive staining for IgM with a lumpy pattern along the small-vessel walls. Chronic microangiopathic glomerular lesions are characterized by a double-contoured basement membrane in the thickened glomerular capillary walls without thrombosis and unassociated with inflammatory cell proliferation and exudation. In addition, chronic microangiopathic vascular lesions with obliterating fibrous intimal hyperplasia of arterioles and interlobular arteries may become evident.[287,289]

DIAGNOSIS AND DIFFERENTIAL DIAGNOSIS

Children with APS present to a wide range of clinical specialists, including pediatric rheumatologists, hematologists, neurologists, and others. A multidisciplinary approach to investigation and management is often appropriate. The presence of aPLs should be investigated in every child presenting with thrombosis or clinical features that are suggestive of APS, such as unexplained thrombocytopenia,

hemolytic anemia, livedo reticularis, Raynaud Phenomenon, and chorea. Determination of aPLs may provide clinically relevant information in children with other clinical features associated with aPLs, including various neurological, dermatological, and renal manifestations.[7,290] In a child with SLE, it is recommended to perform aPL testing at the time of diagnosis and then at least once yearly as part of routine screening of the autoantibody profile.[35]

Given the spectrum of clinical manifestations, the differential diagnosis of APS is very broad and depends on target organ involvement. Characteristically, pathological thrombosis in children requires the presence of multiple risk factors to produce abnormal clotting[291]; therefore, clinical assessment of all children presenting with an aPL-related thrombotic event should include a search for additional congenital and acquired prothrombotic risk factors and thorough evaluation for evidence of underlying SLE or other systemic disease.

The main congenital prothrombotic states to be considered include factor V Leiden, prothrombin G20210A mutation, and deficiencies of antithrombin, protein C, and protein S. Factor V Leiden is the most common hereditary risk factor for venous thrombosis, and up to 5% of the Caucasian population carry this polymorphism.[292] The G20210A mutation of the prothrombin gene is a common polymorphism associated with venous thrombosis, and its prevalence in Caucasians is 2% to 4%.[293,294] Congenital deficiencies of antithrombin, protein C, and protein S are very uncommon, but acquired deficiency of protein S has been reported in children with APS, particularly in association with varicella infection.[295,296] The evaluation for congenital prothrombotic profile in children should also include testing of total cholesterol, triglycerides, lipoprotein (a), fasting homocysteine concentration and T677T polymorphism of the MTHFR gene.[297,298] The most common acquired factors that may contribute to the risk of thrombosis are infection, malignancy, congenital heart disease, nephrotic syndrome, systemic vasculitis, central venous lines, surgery, and immobilization.

The differential diagnosis of nonthrombotic aPL-related clinical manifestations encompasses a variety of hematological, dermatological, neurological, and other diseases. Differentiation of isolated aPL-related thrombocytopenia from classic idiopathic thrombocytopenic purpura is important to indicate closer follow-up regarding increased risk of future thrombosis or progression to SLE.[18,182] Neurological manifestations of aPL should be distinguished from idiopathic neurological conditions, neuropsychiatric involvement in systemic autoimmune diseases, Sydenham chorea, multiple sclerosis, infections, intoxications, and other causes.[299]

Catastrophic APS should be distinguished from severe SLE vasculitis, sepsis, thrombotic thrombocytopenic purpura, macrophage activation syndrome, and disseminated intravascular coagulation.[7,300]

LABORATORY EXAMINATION

Antiphospholipid antibodies is an umbrella term used to describe a heterogeneous group of autoantibodies directed against negatively charged phospholipids or phospholipid-binding plasma proteins. In clinical practice, the most relevant aPLs for identifying patients at risk for immune-mediated thrombosis are aCLs, anti-β_2GPIs, and LA. In a cohort of 121 children included in the pediatric APS registry, the presence of aCLs was detected in 81%, anti-β_2GPI in 67%, and LA in 72% of cases.[15]

Persistent positivity of aPLs is of major importance for diagnosing APS, and all abnormal aPL values should be verified on at least two occasions at least 12 weeks apart, preferably at a time when the child has not had a recent infection.[2]

aPLs can be detected by a variety of laboratory tests. The most sensitive test for aPLs is the aCL test, which uses enzyme-linked immunosorbent assay to determine antibody binding to solid plates coated either with cardiolipin or other phospholipids. The specificity of aCL for APS increases with titer and is higher for the IgG than for the IgM isotype. There have been numerous efforts to standardize the aCL test, but precise reproducible measurement of aCL levels is difficult; for clinical practice the use of semiquantitative measurements (low, medium, and high) is recommended.[301] aCLs must be persistently present in medium or high titer to meet the definition of APS. The observation that many aCLs are directed at an epitope on β_2GPIs led to the development of anti-β_2GPI immunoassays, which have improved specificities over the aCL test. Anti-β_2GPIs have been reported to be associated primarily with thrombosis in patients with APS, particularly in patients with underlying SLE.[302] The issue of the standardization of the anti-β_2GPI immunoassay has also been the subject of considerable debate, but despite these efforts, a considerable degree of interlaboratory variation has been reported.[303,304] The LA test is a functional assay measuring the ability of aPLs to prolong in vitro phospholipid-dependent clotting reactions such as the aPTT, the Russell viper venom time, or the kaolin clotting time. In vivo, however, the presence of LA is paradoxically associated with thrombotic events rather than with bleeding. According to the guidelines of the Scientific Standardization Committee of the International Society of Thrombosis and Haemostasis, the presence of LA should be confirmed with mixing tests with normal plasma and demonstration of the phospholipid-dependent nature of the inhibitor.[305,306] LA is less frequently positive in APS and is thus regarded as a less sensitive but more specific test for detection of aPLs. The LA assay has been shown to correlate much better with the occurrence of thromboembolic events than the aCL or the anti-β_2GPI assay and is considered to be the most important acquired risk factor for thrombosis.[31,33,307] Inadequate data exist as to the clinical utility of other aPL assays for antibodies to prothrombin, phosphatidylserine, phosphatidylethanolamine, and IgA isotype of aCL and anti-β_2GPI.[2]

Several assays may be required to confirm aPL in some patients, because they may be negative according to one test but positive according to another. Reliance on just one type of assay may lead to false negative aPL assessments. Recent evidence suggests that only 33% of pediatric APS patients are concurrently positive for all three aPL subtypes (aCL, anti-β_2GPI, and LA), while 67% of patients tests are negative for at least one of the aPL subtypes.

Measurement of the activation products of coagulation and fibrinolysis, such as D-Dimer, prothrombin fragment 1 and 2, soluble fibrin, and thrombin-antithrombin complexes provides additional information on the hypercoagulability state in patients with inherited and acquired prothrombotic disorders such as APS.[308] D-Dimer was most extensively studied, and there is substantial evidence that it is a sensitive but nonspecific indicator of deep-vein thrombosis. Because of its high negative predictive value, it is particularly useful for the exclusion of deep-vein thrombosis.[309,310] Persistently elevated concentrations of D-Dimer above 500 ng/mL and of coagulation factor VIII above 150 IU are associated with an increased risk of recurrent thromboembolism in children and adults.[311,312]

RADIOLOGICAL EXAMINATION

Thrombosis in patients with APS must be confirmed by objective validated criteria. The ability to detect thrombosis in target organs in infants and children was markedly improved by the development of noninvasive imaging techniques using color-flow and pulsed Doppler ultrasound (US), echocardiography, computerized tomography plus angiography (CT/CTA), and magnetic resonance imaging with or without angiography (MRI/MRA). The diagnosis of deep-vein thrombosis in the lower or upper extremity is usually established by compression and Doppler US, which can be easily performed in children (Figure 22–6). Echocardiography, CTA, or MRA can be used for thrombus imaging in the superior vena cava and proximal subclavian veins. CTA and ventilation-perfusion scan are used in children with suspected pulmonary embolism.[298] Except during interventional procedures, venography and angiography are rarely used in children because of technical difficulties (peripheral venous access or arterial catheterization), the requirement for iodinated contrast, and the possibility of extending thrombus. Brain MRI and positron emission tomography are utilized to assess structural brain lesions such as ischemic infarcts or hemorrhage but are poorly correlated with diffuse or global neurological dysfunction.

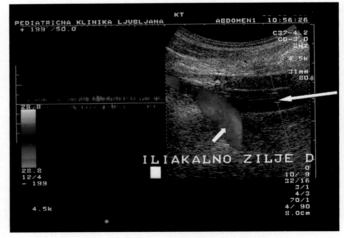

FIGURE 22–6 Color flow Doppler image showing occlusive thrombus in the right external iliac vein *(long arrow)* and normal blood flow in the internal iliac vein *(short arrow)*.

Cerebral ischemia in APS most often affects the territory of the middle cerebral artery. Cortical MRI findings of middle cerebral artery occlusion are similar to large-vessel strokes that result from other etiologies. Neuroimaging findings are often subtle or unremarkable in patients with small-vessel involvement. Magnetization transfer imaging (MTI) is a quantitative MRI technique that is sensitive to macroscopic as well as microscopic brain tissue changes. In SLE patients with neuropsychiatric manifestations and positive aCLs, MTI demonstrates brain damage in the absence of abnormalities on conventional MRI, suggesting that MTI may prove useful in detecting widespread microscopic damage associated with aPLs.[203,313]

TREATMENT

Treatment of pediatric patients with APS is challenging because of the clinical complexity of the syndrome, different pathogenic potential of aPL subtypes, and a lack of randomized controlled trials in children.[7,35,314,315] Management strategies for children with APS are based on a few pediatric observational cohort studies[15,16,18,31] and modified recommendations for adult patients with APS.[316-319] Several differences specific to children must be considered when using the adult recommendations— in particular, the different concentrations of plasma procoagulant and anticoagulant proteins, difficulty of maintaining the appropriate international normalization ratio (INR) levels in infants and children, anticoagulant side effects in growing children, variable metabolism of oral anticoagulants during infections, a higher risk of hemorrhage during play and sports activities, and important compliance issues.[298,320] The optimal management of children with positive aPLs, whether or not they have had a previous thrombosis, should include avoidance of additional risk factors for thrombosis such as smoking, hypertension, obesity, and hypercholesterolemia. Moreover, use of estrogen-containing oral contraceptives is contraindicated in adolescent girls with aPLs.

Primary Thromboprophylaxis

Given the severity of thrombotic complications associated with aPLs, the ideal therapeutic approach would be to avoid progression from asymptomatic aPL carriers to patients with definite APS. Primary thromboprophylaxis concerns asymptomatic children—in whom aPLs were incidentally found during laboratory testing performed for other reasons (e.g., LA discovered during routine preoperative coagulation screening)—and children with SLE found to have aPLs in routine serological screening.

The annual thrombosis risk in asymptomatic adult carriers of aPLs is estimated to be between 0% and 4%, and is higher in patients with positive LA and anti-β_2GPIs.[321-323] Based on retrospective studies,[324,325] an expert panel has recommended the use of low-dose aspirin (80 to 100 mg daily) for prevention of thrombosis in asymptomatic adult patients with persistently positive aPLs.[316] This recommendation was challenged by a placebo-controlled, randomized controlled trial (antiphospholipid antibody acetylsalicylic acid study) that failed to show a beneficial effect of aspirin for primary thrombosis prophylaxis in asymptomatic aPL-positive adults, but the study had important limitations, including the small sample size and the short follow-up period.[326] A recent Italian collaborative study evaluated the efficacy of prophylactic treatments including low-dose aspirin, long-term warfarin, or low-dose aspirin/heparin given during high-risk periods for prevention of a first thrombotic event in aPL carriers.[327] This study showed that long-term prophylaxis with aspirin does not have a protective role when considered alone; however, when analyzed together with a high-risk period prophylaxis in a multivariate regression model, such prophylaxis has been found to be an independent, protective factor against thrombosis.[327]

Future thrombotic events are very rare, if not exceptional, in apparently healthy children who were incidentally found to have positive aPLs,[76] and there is considerable controversy as to whether prophylactic treatment is indicated in this group of children. Because of the increased risk of bleeding during play and sports in children, which might outweigh the possible but unproven benefit of low-dose aspirin, it is generally recommended that asymptomatic children with aPLs do not need long-term prophylactic treatment. In clinical practice, the final decision on the use of specific prophylactic therapy should be individualized and based on the presence of additional congenital or acquired prothrombotic risk factors and the aPL profile (multiple aPL antibodies, high titers of aCLs and/or anti-β_2GPIs, presence of LA). Prophylaxis with LMWH administered subcutaneously should certainly be considered during high-risk situations, such as prolonged immobilization or surgery.

The coexistence of an underlying autoimmune disease, particularly SLE, represents a prothrombotic condition per se and significantly increases the thrombosis risk, primarily because of chronic systemic inflammation and nephrosis that depletes endogenous anticoagulants. Retrospective studies suggest that both pediatric and adult patients with SLE and aPLs have a 50% chance of suffering a thrombotic event within 10 years.[31,328] A Markov decision analysis demonstrated that in patients with SLE the benefit of primary prophylaxis with aspirin outweighs its risks and that aspirin should therefore be given to all patients with SLE to prevent both arterial and venous thrombotic events, especially in patients with aPLs.[329] In this sense, low-dose aspirin (3 to 5 mg/kg/ day) has been recommended as thromboprophylaxis in all pediatric SLE patients with persistently positive aPLs. Prophylactic oral anticoagulant therapy may provide further advantage in selected SLE patients with a low bleeding risk and a high thrombotic tendency, such as young SLE patients with positive LA, but there are insufficient data to support the latter recommendation at the present time.[329]

An additional protection for pediatric SLE patients with aPLs may be provided by hydroxychloroquine, which has modest anticoagulant properties and decreases endothelial and leukocyte expression of tissue factor.[91] There is well-established evidence about the protective role of this old drug against the development of both venous and arterial thrombosis in adult SLE patients.[330,331]

Antithrombotic Therapy and Prevention of Recurrent Thrombosis

Treatment of the acute thrombotic event in children with APS is no different from that of thrombosis arising from other causes and should be organized in consultation with a pediatric hematologist. Most children receive anticoagulation therapy with unfractionated heparin as a loading bolus injection followed by continuous infusion. Because LA prolongs the aPTT and alters the relationship of aPTT to heparin concentration, it is recommended to use anti-Xa activity for heparin monitoring. LMWHs are being used increasingly as initial therapy for acute thrombosis in children because of their subcutaneous administration, more predictable dose response, and reduced requirement for monitoring. The target therapeutic anti-Xa activity for children treated with LMWH ranges between 0.5 and 1.0 U/mL.[298] Systemic or local delivery of thrombolytic agents should be seriously considered in children with high-risk clots that present within 2 weeks of symptomatic onset. Successful outcome with the use of thrombolytic therapy has been reported in difficult pediatric APS patients.[332,333]

Children treated with unfractionated heparin or LMWH as an initial agent are often subsequently transitioned to warfarin for long-term oral anticoagulation. Among children included in the pediatric APS registry, all patients with venous thrombosis received long-term oral anticoagulation therapy, but only 40% of patients with arterial thrombosis received anticoagulation with or without concomitant antiaggregation therapy.[15] During the mean follow-up period of 6.1 years, 19% of pediatric patients with initial venous thrombosis and 21% of patients with initial arterial thrombosis developed recurrent thrombotic events.[15] Two previous studies in children with APS also reported a high thrombosis recurrence rate (29%),[16,18] which is significantly higher than recurrence rates reported in adult APS patients (3% to 11%).[334,335] Of note, 73% of recurrent thrombotic events in children evolved after cessation of anticoagulation therapy, which represents a situation with the highest risk for thrombosis.[16] Because of the ability of heparin to block complement activation, and in view of the important role of complement in APS pathophysiology, some physicians recommend long-term use of LMWH in children at very high risk of recurrent thrombosis.

Based on three randomized controlled trials in adult APS patients,[334-336] it has been recommended that patients with venous or noncerebral arterial thromboembolism be treated with oral anticoagulation at a target INR of 2.0 to 3.0, and patients with ischemic stroke should receive either low-dose aspirin or moderate-intensity warfarin with INR between 1.4 and 2.8.[317] This recommendation has been challenged by another systematic review that included observational cohort studies and advised life-long anticoagulation at a target INR of 2.0 to 3.0 in patients with first venous events and above 3.0 for those with recurrent and/or arterial events.[318] In the absence of controlled trials, the optimal intensity and duration of anticoagulation therapy in pediatric APS patients are still controversial. Given the higher recurrence rate of thrombosis, it seems reasonable to consider anticoagulation in all pediatric patients with definite APS, at least at a target INR suggested for the adult population. In a large retrospective study in pediatric SLE, none of the LA-positive patients who were maintained in the target INR range of 2.0 to 3.0 developed a second thrombotic event.[31] One of the problems of the high-intensity anticoagulation may be a higher risk of secondary bleeding, which should be assessed individually for each patient. Among adult patients with APS, the systematic review showed that repeated thromboses were more frequent and associated with a much higher mortality than hemorrhagic complications in patients taking warfarin.[318]

An improved understanding of the pathogenic mechanisms by which aPLs induce thrombosis has suggested some innovative treatments such as new anticoagulant and antiplatelet drugs, hydroxychloroquine, statins, complement inhibitors, rituximab, and other targeted therapies.[337] Rituximab, an anti-CD20 chimeric monoclonal antibody that selectively induces depletion of circulating B cells, has been shown to decrease aPL levels in individuals and small series and can be effective in aPL-related immune cytopenias and recurrent thrombosis.[338-340] A few pediatric case reports suggest that rituximab can also offer a therapeutic alternative in severe or resistant pediatric APS patients.[247,341]

Catastrophic Antiphospholipid Syndrome

If catastrophic APS is suspected, immediate aggressive treatment is required. Therapy must be multifaceted and include elimination of possible precipitating factors, treatment of the ongoing thrombotic events, and suppression of the excessive cytokine storm.[9,342] Analysis of 250 patients included in the catastrophic APS registry showed that the highest recovery rate was achieved by the combination therapy of anticoagulants, corticosteroids, and plasma exchange (78%), followed by the combination of anticoagulants, corticosteroids, plasma exchange and/or intravenous immunoglobulin (IVIG).[343] According to the results of this study, the use of a combined treatment of anticoagulants, corticosteroids, and plasma exchange has been recommended as first-line therapy for patients with catastrophic APS.[342] IVIG has multiple therapeutic actions and may improve outcome in catastrophic APS patients, but rapid infusion of high doses of IVIG may increase the risk of thrombosis. When IVIG and plasma exchange are used simultaneously in the same patient, IVIG is administered after the last day of the plasma exchange to prevent the removal of IVIG by plasma exchange. Concomitant treatment with cyclophosphamide did not demonstrate additional benefit in patients with primary catastrophic APS but improved survival in those with SLE-associated catastrophic APS.[344] Rituximab has been also successfully used in a limited number of catastrophic APS patients.[247,345] Treatment of known precipitating factors in catastrophic APS patients should include prompt use of antibiotics (if infection is suspected) and excision of necrotic tissues.

Perinatal Complications Associated with Antiphospholipid Antibodies

There are no uniform guidelines for the therapeutic approach in perinatal thrombosis associated with trans-placentally transferred aPLs.[263] Infants with stroke usually received only symptomatic treatment for the seizures, with or without antiaggregation, and infants with venous or disseminated thrombotic events received additional anticoagulation, thrombolytic therapy, and/or exchange transfusion. Children born to mothers with APS may exhibit a higher percentage of learning disabilities at school age, and it is recommended to include regular neuropsychological assessments during their long-term follow-up.[280]

COURSE OF THE DISEASE AND PROGNOSIS

An understanding of the course and prognosis of pediatric APS awaits prospective studies in large cohorts. Recent observations suggest that the risk of recurrent thrombosis in children with APS during the mean follow-up period of around 6 years is 20% to 30%.[15,16,18] In general, the risk of future thrombosis is very low in asymptomatic children who are incidentally found to have positive aPLs. However, it is high among those in whom thrombosis already occurred and extremely high in patients with catastrophic APS. A high titer of aPLs, and in particular the presence of LA, increases the risk of thrombosis, as do the concomitant presence of inherited prothrombotic disorders and/or other acquired thrombotic risk factors.[16,298,314,346] The time interval between recurrent thrombotic events varies considerably from weeks to months or even years.

APS is a serious and potentially life-threatening disease. In the cohort of 121 children included in the pediatric APS registry, the estimated mortality rate was 7%. In total, seven patients with APS associated with underlying SLE and two patients with primary APS died during the mean follow-up time of 6.1 years.[15] The most common cause of death was a thrombotic event (seven patients), followed by SLE complications (one patient) and hemophagocytic syndrome associated with splenic infarction (one patient).

Approximately 20% of children who initially present with the features of primary APS may progress over time to develop SLE or a lupus-like disease.[15,18] This percentage is almost three times higher than reported in adult patients with primary APS (7%)[347] and emphasizes the importance of careful follow-up of all children with primary APS for the subsequent appearance of manifestations of SLE. The presence of an underlying autoimmune disease influences the occurrence of clinical manifestations of APS. Hematological and skin manifestations have lower prevalence in patients with primary APS, whereas arterial occlusions are less frequent in APS secondary to SLE.[15]

Some pediatric studies noted a positive correlation of aCL titers with SLE disease activity indices.[20,23,25,34] The influence of SLE treatment on aPL titers may reflect the effect of therapy on SLE disease activity; however, there are some pediatric SLE patients who have persistently positive aPLs even when their disease is inactive, and these patients may develop thrombotic events even during SLE remission. Fluctuations of LA are less commonly seen than fluctuations in the level of aCL in SLE patients; this may also contribute to the more consistent relation of LA with thrombosis compared with aCL.[348]

The presence of aPLs may have a negative impact on the clinical outcome of both childhood-onset and adult-onset SLE.[349-351] Several studies of adult patients with SLE have reported that the presence of APS was an important predictor of irreversible organ damage and death in SLE.[352,353] A recent retrospective study of 56 children with SLE showed that the risk of irreversible organ damage (as scored by the Systemic Lupus International Collaborating Clinics/ACR Damage Index) in aPL-positive patients was three times higher than in aPL-negative patients.[351] Thus, the presence of aPLs in pediatric SLE patients could represent not only a risk factor for thrombosis but also a poor prognostic factor overall.

REFERENCES

2. S. Miyakis, M.D. Lockshin, T. Atsumi, et al., International consensus statement on an update of the classification criteria for definite antiphospholipid syndrome, J. Thromb. Haemost. 4 (2006) 295–306.
7. A. Ravelli, A. Martini, Antiphospholipid syndrome in pediatrics, Rheum. Dis. Clin. North Am. 33 (2007) 499–523.
9. R.A. Asherson, R. Cervera, P.G. de Groot, et al., Catastrophic antiphospholipid syndrome: international consensus statement on classification criteria and treatment guidelines, Lupus 12 (2003) 530–534.
11. R. Cervera, J.C. Piette, J. Font, et al., Antiphospholipid syndrome: clinical and immunologic manifestations and patterns of disease expression in a cohort of 1,000 patients, Arthritis Rheum. 46 (2002) 1019–1027.
14. J.S. Levine, D.W. Branch, J. Rauch, The antiphospholipid syndrome, N. Engl. J. Med. 346 (2002) 752–763.
15. T. Avčin, R. Cimaz, E.D. Silverman, et al., Pediatric antiphospholipid syndrome: clinical and immunologic features of 121 patients in an international registry, Pediatrics 122 (2008) e1100–1107.
16. Y. Berkun, S. Padeh, J. Barash, et al., Antiphospholipid syndrome and recurrent thrombosis in children, Arthritis Rheum. 55 (2006) 850–855.
18. M. Gattorno, F. Falcini, A. Ravelli, et al., Outcome of primary antiphospholipid syndrome in childhood, Lupus 12 (2003) 449–453.
27. C. Berube, L. Mitchell, E. Silverman, et al., The relationship of antiphospholipid antibodies to thromboembolic events in pediatric patients with systemic lupus erythematosus: a cross-sectional study, Pediatr. Res. 44 (1998) 351–356.
30. E. Von Scheven, D.V. Glidden, M.E. Elder, Anti-β2-glycoprotein I antibodies in pediatric systemic lupus erythematosus and antiphospholipid syndrome, Arthritis Rheum. 47 (2002) 414–420.
31. D.M. Levy, M.P. Massicotte, E. Harvey, et al., Thromboembolism in paediatric lupus patients, Lupus 12 (2003) 741–746.
33. C. Male, D. Foulon, H. Hoogendoorn, et al., Predictive value of persistent versus transient antiphospholipid antibody subtypes for the risk of thrombotic events in pediatric patients with systemic lupus erythematosus, Blood 106 (2005) 4152–4158.
53. R. Cervera, R.A. Asherson, M.L. Acevedo, et al., Antiphospholipid syndrome associated with infections: clinical and microbiological characteristics of 100 patients, Ann. Rheum. Dis. 63 (2004) 1312–1317.
70. T. Avčin, A. Ambrožič, M. Kuhar, et al., Anticardiolipin and anti-β2 glycoprotein I antibodies in sera of 61 apparently healthy children at regular preventive visits, Rheumatology 40 (2001) 565–573.
76. C. Male, K. Lechner, S. Eichinger, et al., Clinical significance of lupus anticoagulants in children, J. Pediatr. 134 (1999) 199–205.
77. H.J. Siemens, S. Gutsche, S. Brückner, et al., Antiphospholipid antibodies in children without and in adults with and without thrombophilia, Thromb. Res. 98 (2000) 241–247.
82. A.L. Sestak, K.M. O'Neil, Familial lupus and antiphospholipid syndrome, Lupus 16 (2007) 556–563.

87. S.S. Pierangeli, M. Vega-Ostertag, E.N. Harris, Intracellular signaling triggered by antiphospholipid antibodies in platelets and endothelial cells: a pathway to targeted therapies, Thromb. Res. 114 (2004) 467–476.

89. M.E. Vega-Ostertag, D.E. Ferrara, Z. Romay-Penabad, et al., Role of p38 mitogen-activated protein kinase in antiphospholipid antibody-mediated thrombosis and endothelial cell activation, J. Thromb. Haemost. 5 (2007) 1828–1834.

91. R.G. Espinola, S.S. Pierangeli, A.E. Gharavi, et al., Hydroxychloroquine reverses platelet activation induced by human IgG antiphospholipid antibodies, Thromb. Haemost. 87 (2002) 518–522.

96. N. Del Papa, L. Guidali, A. Sala, et al., Endothelial cells as target for antiphospholipid antibodies. Human polyclonal and monoclonal anti-beta 2-glycoprotein I antibodies react in vitro with endothelial cells through adherent beta 2-glycoprotein I and induce endothelial activation, Arthritis Rheum. 40 (1997) 551–561.

98. O. Amengual, T. Atsumi, M.A. Khamashta, Tissue factor in antiphospholipid syndrome: shifting the focus from coagulation to the endothelium, Rheumatology 42 (2003) 1029–1031.

102. G. Montiel-Manzano, Z. Romay-Penabad, Papalardo de Martinez, et al., In vivo effects of an inhibitor of nuclear factor-kappa B on thrombogenic properties of antiphospholipid antibodies, Ann. NY. Acad. Sci. 1108 (2007) 540–553.

104. J.J. Hulstein, P.J. Lenting, B. de Laat, et al., Beta2-Glycoprotein I inhibits von Willebrand factor dependent platelet adhesion and aggregation, Blood 110 (2007) 1483–1491.

109. S.S. Pierangeli, M.E. Vega-Ostertag, E. Raschi, et al., Toll-like receptor and antiphospholipid mediated thrombosis: in vivo studies, Ann. Rheum. Dis. 66 (2007) 1327–1333.

110. E. Raschi, C. Testoni, D. Bosisio, et al., Role of the MyD88 transduction signaling pathway in endothelial activation by antiphospholipid antibodies, Blood 101 (2003) 3495–3500.

112. C. Lopez-Pedrera, P. Buendia, M.J. Cuadrado, et al., Antiphospholipid antibodies from patients with the antiphospholipid syndrome induce monocyte tissue factor expression through the simultaneous activation of NF-kappaB/Rel proteins via the p38 mitogen-activated protein kinase pathway, and of the MEK-1/ERK pathway, Arthritis Rheum. 54 (2006) 301–311.

113. H. Zhou, A.S. Wolberg, R.A. Roubey, Characterization of monocyte tissue factor activity induced by IgG antiphospholipid antibodies and inhibition by dilazep, Blood 104 (2004) 2353–2358.

114. G. Girardi, J. Berman, P. Redecha, et al., Complement C5a receptors and neutrophils mediate fetal injury in the antiphospholipid syndrome, J. Clin. Invest. 112 (2003) 1644–1654.

115. P. Redecha, R. Tilley, M. Tencati, et al., Tissue factor: a link between C5a and neutrophil activation in antiphospholipid antibody mediated fetal injury, Blood 110 (2007) 2423–2431.

117. N. Di Simone, P.L. Meroni, D. Marco, et al., Pregnancies complicated with antiphospholipid syndrome: The pathogenic mechanism of antiphospholipid antibodies, a review of the literature, Ann. NY. Acad. Sci. 1108 (2007) 505–514.

119. H. Katsuragawa, H. Kanzaki, T. Inoue, et al., Monoclonal antibody against phosphatidylserine inhibits in vitro human trophoblastic hormone production and invasion, Biol. Reprod. 56 (1997) 50–58.

121. N. Di Simone, F. Di Nicuolo, M. Sanguinetti, et al., Low-molecular weight heparin induces in vitro trophoblast invasiveness: role of matrix metalloproteinases and tissue inhibitors, Placenta 28 (2007) 298–304.

124. V.M. Holers, G. Girardi, L. Mo, et al., Complement C3 activation is required for antiphospholipid antibody-induced fetal loss, J. Exp. Med. 195 (2002) 211–220.

125. J.E. Salmon, G. Girardi, V.M. Holers, Activation of complement mediates antiphospholipid antibody-induced pregnancy loss, Lupus 12 (2003) 535–538.

126. F. Fischetti, P. Durigutto, V. Pellis, et al., Thrombus formation induced by antibodies to beta2-glycoprotein I is complement dependent and requires a priming factor, Blood 106 (2005) 2340–2346.

172. G. Kenet, S. Sadetzki, H. Murad, et al., Factor V Leiden and antiphospholipid antibodies are significant risk factors for ischemic stroke in children, Stroke 31 (2000) 1283–1288.

183. R. Diz-Küçükkaya, A. Hacihanefioglu, M. Yenerel, et al., Antiphospholipid antibodies and antiphospholipid syndrome in patients presenting with immune thrombocytopenic purpura: a prospective cohort study, Blood 98 (2001) 1760–1764.

191. C. Frances, S. Niang, E. Laffitte, et al., Dermatologic manifestations of the antiphospholipid syndrome: two hundred consecutive cases, Arthritis Rheum. 52 (2005) 1785–1793.

193. P.A. Nigrovic, R.C. Fuhlbrigge, R.P. Sundel, Raynaud Phenomenon in children: a retrospective review of 123 patients, Pediatrics 111 (2003) 715–721.

194. G. deVeber, M. Andrew, C. Adams, et al., Cerebral sinovenous thrombosis in children, N. Engl. J. Med. 345 (2001) 417–423.

211. R. Cimaz, A. Romeo, A. Scarano, et al., Prevalence of anticardiolipin, anti-β_2 glycoprotein I and anti-prothrombin antibodies in young patients with epilepsy, Epilepsia 43 (2002) 52–59.

230. M.G. Tektonidou, F. Sotsiou, L. Nakopoulou, et al., Antiphospholipid syndrome nephropathy in patients with systemic lupus erythematosus and antiphospholipid antibodies: prevalence, clinical associations, and long-term outcome, Arthritis Rheum. 50 (2004) 2569–2579.

239. R. Cervera, S. Bucciarelli, M.A. Plasin, et al., Catastrophic antiphospholipid syndrome (CAPS): descriptive analysis of a series of 280 patients from the "CAPS Registry," J. Autoimmun. 32 (2009) 240–245.

263. M.-C. Boffa, E. Lachassine, Infant perinatal thrombosis and antiphospholipid antibodies: a review, Lupus 16 (2007) 634–641.

283. M. Motta, G. Chirico, C. Biasini Rebaioli, et al., Anticardiolipin and anti-beta2 glycoprotein I antibodies in infants born to mothers with antiphospholipid antibody-positive autoimmune disease: a follow-up study, Am. J. Perinatol 23 (2006) 247–252.

314. A.V. Kamat, D.P. D'Cruz, B.J. Hunt, Managing antiphospholipid antibodies and antiphospholipid syndrome in children, Haematologica. 91 (2006) 1674–1680.

316. D. Alarcon-Segovia, M.C. Boffa, W. Branch, et al., Prophylaxis of the antiphospholipid syndrome: a consensus report, Lupus 12 (2003) 499–503.

317. W. Lim, M.A. Crowther, J.W. Eikelboom, Management of antiphospholipid antibody syndrome: a systematic review, JAMA. 295 (2006) 1050–1057.

318. G. Ruiz-Irastorza, B.J. Hunt, M.A. Khamashta, A systematic review of secondary thromboprophylaxis in patients with antiphospholipid antibodies, Arthritis Rheum. 57 (2007) 1487–1495.

326. D. Erkan, M.J. Harrison, R. Levy, et al., Aspirin for primary thrombosis prevention in the antiphospholipid syndrome: a randomized, double-blind, placebo-controlled trial in asymptomatic antiphospholipid antibody-positive individuals, Arthritis Rheum. 56 (2007) 2382–2391.

Entire reference list is available online at www.expertconsult.com.

Chapter 23

NEONATAL LUPUS ERYTHEMATOSUS

Jill P. Buyon, Carol B. Lindsley and Earl D. Silverman

Neonatal lupus erythematosus (NLE) is a disease of the developing fetus and neonate defined by characteristic clinical features in the presence of specific maternal autoantibodies. It is considered a model of passively acquired autoimmunity. The transplacental passage of these autoantibodies is necessary but not sufficient to cause the disease. The autoantibodies associated with NLE are directed against a group of small cytoplasmic and nuclear ribonucleoproteins and their associated RNAs, collectively referred to as RoRNP or Ro particle. The most common clinical manifestations of NLE are cardiac, dermatological, and hepatic. The term *neonatal lupus erythematosus* is misleading since the mother may be totally asymptomatic and the affected child does not have systemic lupus erythematosus (SLE).

ETIOLOGY AND PATHOGENESIS

Maternal autoantibodies directed against RoRNP or occasionally against other autoantigens such as U1RNP are required for the development of NLE. However, many mothers with these autoantibodies do not deliver children with NLE. Other candidate factors are required and these likely include genetics and environmental triggers.[1]

Autoantigens

Target antigens (Ags) of the Ro/La system. The candidate Ags and their cognate antibodies (Abs) have been extensively characterized at the molecular level. Initial cloning of 60kD Ro (Ro60) identified a zinc finger and an RNA-binding protein consensus motif.[2-6] It has been suggested that Ro60 may function as part of a novel quality control for ribosome biogenesis since, in addition to binding hY RNA, it binds misfolded 5S rRNA precursors.[7] Xue and colleagues reported that autoimmunity develops in a murine Ro60-knockout model and ultraviolet B (UVB) irradiation results in significantly increased numbers of apoptotic keratinocytes compared to wildtype mice.[8] This model suggested that Ro60 plays a role in preventing autoimmunity, possibly by removing defective ribonucleoproteins from cells, allowing them to escape immune surveillance; thus Ro60 could be involved in cell survival. Furthermore the experiments demonstrating a role for Ro in photosensitivity can occur only if the autoantibody penetrated living cells thus simulating the murine knockout. However, an alternative consistent explanation is that the increased numbers of apoptotic keratinocytes present after photoprovocation represent a defect in clearance of these apoptotic cells, either because anti-Ro60 Abs inhibit phagocytic uptake of apoptotic bodies or the Ro60 ligand for uptake is absent.

Anti-La Abs recognize a 48kD polypeptide (La48) that does not share antigenic determinants with either 52kD Ro (Ro52) or Ro60.[9,10] La facilitates maturation of RNA polymerase III transcripts, directly binds a spectrum of RNAs, and associates at least transiently with Ro60.[11,12]

In addition to the well-characterized Ro60 and La48 autoantigens Ags, another target of the autoimmune response in mothers whose children have congenital heart block (CHB) is Ro52.[13] The full-length protein, 52α, has three distinct domains: an N-terminal region rich in cysteine/histidine motifs containing two distinct zinc fingers; a central region containing two coiled coils with heptad periodicity, one being a leucine zipper; and a C-terminal "rfp-like" domain.[14,15] Analysis by immunoblot of human cell lines, or enzyme-linked immunosorbent assay (ELISA), reveals that between 75% and 100% of sera obtained from mothers whose children have CHB are reactive with recombinant Ro52.[16-20] An alternative 52mRNA transcript (52β) that is derived from the splicing of exon 4 encoding aa168-245 inclusive of the leucine zipper has been identified, which results in a smaller protein[47] with a predicted molecular weight of 45,000.[21] Since 52β expression is maximal at the time of cardiac ontogeny when maternal Abs begin to gain access to the fetal circulation, just prior to the clinical detection of bradyarrhythmia, a role for 52β in the development of CHB is implicated[22] but to date not established. Focus on Ro52 and CHB has been confirmed and extended by Wahren-Herlenius and colleagues.[23,24]

Autoantibodies

The search for a truly pathogenic antibody specificity that could account for the development of CHB has been attempted by many investigative teams. The following paragraphs review the history of some of these efforts. For most reports, the number of patients studied is limited. In addition, many reports compare mothers of affected children with those of unaffected children. The pitfall of this approach is that we now know mothers can have a child with neonatal lupus after having a healthy child.

Anti-La Antibodies

Examination of the fine specificity of the repertoire of maternal anti-La antibodies has revealed the identification of antibodies directed against a small La polypeptide, named DD, that was found by one group to be only in the sera of mothers of children with NLE and not in sera from mothers of unaffected children. Although this finding was specific for NLE, it had only a 30% sensitivity because many mothers without anti-DD antibodies delivered children with NLE, and anti-DD antibodies were present in only 30% of children with NLE.

Anti-52Ro Antibodies

Antibodies to the 52kD SSA/Ro protein are found in >80% of mothers whose children have CHB.[23,24,25,87] Initial epitope mapping of this response revealed an immunodominant region, spanning aa169-291 and containing the leucine zipper, that was recognized by the majority of the CHB-sera, frequently in the context of HLA-DRB1*0301, DQA1*0501, and DQB1*020.[87] The finer specificity of the anti-Ro52 response has been confirmed and extended with current focus on aa200-239 (p200).[23] In an initial evaluation that comprised 9 CHB-mothers and 26 anti-SSA/Ro-positive mothers of healthy children, antibodies to p200 predicted CHB with greater certainty than currently available testing for either 60kD or 52kD SSA/Ro.[23] Recent studies integrating an in vivo rodent model and in vitro culturing system suggest that anti-p200 antibodies bind neonatal rodent cardiocytes and alter calcium homeostasis.[24]

ANTI-P200 ANTIBODIES

To address both the clinical necessity and sufficiency of this newly identified p200 reactivity in the development of CHB, as well as the reduced risk of CHB reportedly associated with antibodies to aa176-196 (p176) and aa197-232 (p197),[23] maternal sera were evaluated from the Research Registry for Neonatal Lupus (RRNL) and the prospective study, PR Interval and Dexamethasone Evaluation (PRIDE) in CHB.[26] In addition, the PRIDE study provided the opportunity to address whether the level of anti-p200 antibodies positively correlated with length of the Doppler mechanical PR interval (> 150 ms corresponds to first degree block). The majority of the 156 Ro52-positive sera tested were reactive with p200 (>3 SD above control), irrespective of clinical status of the child.[27,28] Mean OD values of p200 did not differ significantly among mothers of children with CHB (0.187 ± 0.363 SD), rash (0.176 ± 0.356 SD), or no manifestation of NLE (0.229 ± 0.315 SD). p200 reactivity was found in 80 of 104 (77%) CHB-mothers, 24 of 30 (80%) rash-mothers, and 21 of 22 (95%) mothers who delivered healthy children and had no previous children with NLE ($P = NS$ for all comparisons). Sera from 4 CHB-mothers with varied p200 titers (range OD 0.025 to 1.818) bound the surface of nonpermeabilized apoptotic but not healthy human fetal cardiocytes. These observations suggested that antibodies to pRo52, equivalent to antibodies to full length SSA/Ro, do not bind the surface of fetal cardiocytes unless those cells become apoptotic (p200 is translocated to the membrane). For 32 Ro52-positive women completing the PRIDE study (22 no previous child with NLE, 7 previous child with CHB, 3 previous child with rash) in whom p200 levels were determined during pregnancy, the correlation between level of p200 (OD range 0.000 to 1.170) and maximal fetal PR interval (range 115 to 168 ms) was not significant (Spearman $R = 0.107$, $P = 0.58$).

One other interpretation of these data is that reactivity to p200 is a dominant, but not uniform, anti-Ro52 response in women whose children have CHB and therefore this specificity may be important but not sufficient for the development of CHB. Since exposure to this antibody specificity was observed with a similar frequency in children without CHB born to mothers with anti-Ro52, additional factors are likely necessary to convert risk to disease expression.

Anti-5- serotoninergic 5-Hydroxytryptamine A Receptor Antibodies

Eftekhari and colleagues reported that antibodies reactive with the serotoninergic 5-hydroxytryptamine 5-HT4 receptor, cloned from human adult atrium, also bind to 52kD SSA/Ro.[28] It was subsequently shown that 5-HT4 receptor mRNA was expressed in human fetal atrium and human fetal atrial cells expressed functional 5-HT4 receptors.[29] Moreover, affinity-purified 5-HT4 antibodies antagonized the serotonin-induced L-type Ca channel activation in human atrial cells. Two peptides in the C terminus of 52kD SSA/Ro, aa365-382 and aa380-396, were identified that shared some similarity with the 5-HT4 receptor. The former was recognized by sera from mothers of children with NLE, and was reported to be cross-reactive with peptide aa165-185, derived from the second extracellular loop of the 5-HT4 receptor. These findings are of particular importance, since >75% of sera from mothers whose children have CHB contain antibodies to 52kD SSA/Ro as detected by ELISA, immunoblot, and immunoprecipitation.[25]

Given the intriguing possibility that antibodies to the 5-HT4 receptor might represent the hitherto elusive reactivity directly contributing to AV block, the possibility that the 5-HT4 receptor is a target of the immune response in these mothers was examined.[29] Initial experiments demonstrated mRNA expression of the 5-HT4 receptor in the human fetal atrium. Electrophysiological studies established that human fetal atrial cells express functional 5-HT4 receptors. Sera from 116 mothers enrolled in the RRNL, whose children have CHB, were evaluated: 99 (85%) contained antibodies to SSA/Ro, 84% of which were reactive with the 52kD SSA/Ro component by immunoblot. In summary, none of the 116 sera were reactive with the peptide spanning aa165-185 of the serotoninergic receptor. Rabbit antisera that recognized this peptide did not react with 52kD SSA/Ro. Accordingly, although 5-HT4 receptors are present and functional in the human fetal heart, maternal antibodies to the 5-HT4 receptor are not necessary for the development of CHB.

Most recently, studies have assessed the role of anti-5HT4 antibodies.[29] Sera from 128 patients (101 anti-SSA/Ro52–positive mothers, of whom 74 had children with CHB; 20 anti-SSA/Ro52–negative mothers, of whom 1 had a child with isolated CHB, 6 had children with structural HB, 5 had children who developed HB after birth, 8 had healthy children, and 18 were healthy) were assessed in a single blind test using an ELISA coated with a 5-HT4 receptor–derived peptide. Discrepancies between previous observations could be ascribed to small differences in the set-up of the assay. Of the 74 sera from Ro52 positive mothers of children with CHB, 11 were reactive with the 5-HT4 peptide. Sera from the Ro52-negative mother of a child with CHB, one of 6 Ro52-negative mothers of children with structural HB, 3 of 35 Ro52-positive mothers of unaffected children, and 2 of 18 Ro52-negative controls were also 5-HT4-positive. Although 5-HT4 receptor autoantibodies do not have the predictive value of anti-Ro52 autoantibodies, the presence of these antibodies in a minor subset of mothers whose children have CHB suggests an additional risk factor that may contribute to the pathogenesis of disease.

Anti-Calreticulin antibodies

Although there still is controversy about whether calreticulin is a part of the RoRNP, autoantibodies directed against calreticulin are present in the sera from patients with autoimmune diseases.[22,31-32] Although elevated anticalreticulin antibody levels have been reported in mothers of children with NLE compared with levels in healthy normal subjects, when the anticalreticulin response was compared with that of healthy pregnant women, no differences in the mean titer of these autoantibodies could be demonstrated. However, one report cited differences in anticalreticulin antibody titers when compared with those of normal, healthy control subjects.[33]

Other Autoantibodies

The presence of other antigens on the fetal heart or placenta has been suggested to be important in the development of or protection from the development of cardiac AV block. There is crossreactivity between a subset of anti-La, but not anti-Ro, antibodies and laminin.[34,35] Sera from mothers of infants with CHB may also contain anti–endogenous retrovirus-3 (ERV-3) antibodies. Anti-La, anticalreticulin, and anti–ERV-3 antibodies can bind to the placenta or placental trophoblast or both.[35,36,38] Binding of these autoantibodies to placental tissue may alter the quantity and repertoire of these autoantibodies in the fetal circulation and therefore affect binding to the target fetal tissue.[36-38]

Antilaminin autoantibodies bind to fetal but not adult heart and cardiac tissue, and ERV-3 and laminin are maximally expressed between 11 and 17 weeks' gestation.[33,36,37] Cardiac laminin, calreticulin, or ERV-3 may be targets for maternal autoantibodies, and direct binding to these fetal cardiac proteins may initiate or potentiate inflammation in the fetal heart.[33,36,37]

Antibodies directed against a p57 recombinant protein and α-fodrin have been detected in the sera of mothers of infants with NLE. Anti-p57 antibodies were present in approximately one-third of the sera from mothers of children with NLE and were almost always associated with anti-Ro antibodies.[39] Anti–α-fodrin antibodies were initially reported to be present in sera from patients with Sjögren syndrome (SS) but not in the sera from patients

with rheumatoid arthritis or SLE.[41] Preliminary data in NLE suggested that maternal anti–120-kD α-fodrin antibodies may be an additional serological marker for the risk of development of NLE.[41]

GENETIC BACKGROUND

Specific human leukocyte antigen (HLA) DR and DQ genes are important in the production of anti-Ro and anti-La antibodies. In patients with autoimmune diseases, DR3 was associated with anti–52-kD Ro and anti-La autoantibodies but not anti–60 kD Ro antibodies[42,43] This association is present in most but not all ethnic backgrounds and is independent of the presence of an autoimmune disease and generally differs between patients with primary SS and SLE.[44-52] High-titer anti-Ro antibodies are associated with the DQw1/DQw2 heterozygote.[53,54] In mothers of children with NLE, the HLA profile more closely resembles that present in patients with primary SS than that associated with patients with SLE.[55,56]

It is likely that extended haplotypes are more important than single loci in determining production of anti-Ro and anti-La antibodies. In patients of most ethnic backgrounds, high levels of anti-Ro and anti-La antibodies are associated with all or at least most of the DRB1*0301, DQA1*0501, and DQB1*0201 extended haplotypes, whereas the DQA1*0501 allele is present in other patients.[45,46,56] Glutamine at position 34 of DQA1 and leucine at position 26 of DQB1 are associated with anti-Ro and anti-La antibodies, although the extended haplotype (in linkage disequilibrium) may have the strongest correlation with this autoantibody response.[57,58] The genetic control of anti-RoRNP antibodies is further complicated by the demonstration that response to peptides of the 60-kD Ro protein may be under different genetic control distinct from the HLA associations of the response to the complete 60-kD protein.[59]

In Japanese mothers of children with NLE, the production of anti-Ro and anti-La antibodies was associated with the extended haplotypes DRB1*1101-DQA1*0501-DQB1*0301 and DRB1*08032-DQA1*0103-DQB1*0601, as well as the individual alleles DRB1*1101, DRB1*08032, and DQB1*0301.[60] All of the anti-Ro and anti-La antibody–positive mothers had DRB1 alleles that shared the same amino acid residues at positions 14 to 31 and 71 of DRB1 and were homozygous or heterozygous at DQ6 and DQ3 alleles that shared the same amino acid residues at positions 27 to 36 and 71 to 77 of the hypervariable regions of DQB1.[60] Individual manifestations of NLE may also be influenced by maternal HLA, as the maternal DR5 haplotype DRB1*1101-DQA1*0501-DQB1*0301 and individual class II alleles making up this haplotype, including DQA1 alleles with glutamine at position 34 of the first domain, were significantly associated with cutaneous neonatal lupus erythematosus (C-NLE) but not CHB. DQB1*0602 carried on DR2 haplotypes was associated with CAVB but not C-NLE.[61,62] Although not conclusive, a few studies have suggested that maternal major histocompatibility complex (MHC) class I haplotypes may predispose to the delivery of child with CHB.[55,63,64]

Despite the strong association of maternal HLA antigens with NLE, there generally has not been any association of HLA genes in the offspring with the development of NLE, although there have been exceptions.[61,62,65-68] One study demonstrated that children with NLE tended to have DRB, DQA, and DQB genes identical to those of their mothers.[69] One report suggested that DR3 in the fetus might protect against in utero death, whereas another postulated that DR2 in the infant may be protective (although this was associated with maternal DR2).[52,69] Some data suggest children with NLE are more likely to have a tumor necrosis factor-α (TNF-α) polymorphism, which is associated with high TNF-α production, and tumor growth factor-β (TGF-β) gene polymorphism, which is associated with increased TGF-β production and therefore, may lead to fibrosis.[70] This work suggests that there may be factors in the developing fetus that influence the development of NLE. In addition, multiple genes outside the MHC locus, including T cell receptor genes (in mother or child, or both) can influence the onset and progression of autoimmune diseases.[67,71,72] The same may be true in NLE, particularly with regard to amplifying the pathological cascade to scar (e.g., amplification of apoptosis, macrophage uptake of opsonized cardiocytes, and ultimately fibrosis).

MANIFESTATIONS OF NEONATAL LUPUS ERYTHEMATOSUS

Cardiac Neonatal Lupus Erythematosus

The most clinically significant manifestations of NLE are cardiac, specifically CHB. In most cases, the CHB is isolated, but it may be associated with other cardiac lesions, including ventricular septal defect or patent ductus arteriosus. The first reported case of CHB associated with maternal autoimmune disease (i.e., Mikulicz syndrome or SS) was published in 1901.[73] However, it was not until the 1950s that it was generally recognized that autoantibodies in the mother were associated with NLE. It was another 20 to 30 years until the association with anti-Ro and anti-La antibodies was reported.[74-80]

Epidemiology

It has been estimated that CHB occurs in 1 in 14,000 live births, and at least 90% of the cases of CHB are the result of transplacental passage of maternal autoantibodies. These estimates likely underestimated the true incidence of abnormalities of fetal cardiac conduction, because they were performed at a time that when severe, CHB frequently resulted in intrauterine death.[79-86] In most cases, these deaths occured in fetuses of mothers without a diagnosed autoimmune disease, and the first demonstration of autoantibodies in these mothers occured during the pregnancy or after delivery of a child with NLE. At that time 25% to 50% of pregnancies complicated by fetal CHB resulted in intrauterine death and most mothers did not have an autoimmune disease. It is likely that CHB occurs in more than 1 of 14,000 live births and may be a

factor resulting in death of the fetus in 1 of 7000 to 8000 pregnancies carried only to the late second trimester.

Pathology

Although necropsy studies are few, the characteristic pathological findings in CHB are an absence or a degeneration of the atrioventricular (AV) node with replacement by fibrosis, calcification, or fatty tissue (Fig. 23–1). The distal conducting system may be normal. The few reports of cases of CHB not associated with maternal autoantibodies have demonstrated a normal AV node, but there were other conduction defects.[88] Abnormal histology is present in other areas of the heart; therefore, the inflammation and scarring may be a more generalized process associated with ventricular endomyocardial fibroelastosis (EFE) and an inflammatory cell infiltrate.[75,89] These latter abnormalities suggest the possibility that AV node conduction defects may be the result of the susceptibility of the conduction system to inflammatory damage rather than a specific localization of the autoantibodies to this area of the developing heart. It likely that maternally derived

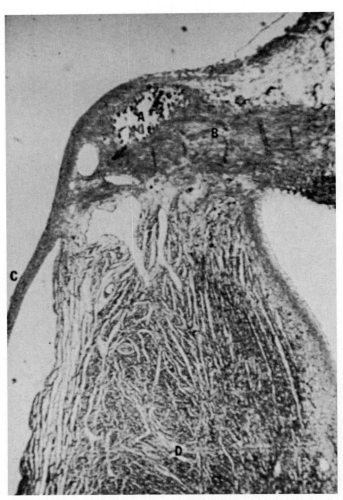

FIGURE 23–1 Section of ventricular septum from the fetus of a mother with systemic lupus erythematosus. The baby died at birth from nonimmune hydrops secondary to complete congenital heart block. **A**, Dystrophic calcification in the region of an atrioventricular node. **B**, Dense fibrosis. **C**, Valve leaflet. **D**, Ventricular septum (Courtesy of Dr. J. Dimmick.)

autoantibodies lead to fetal myocarditis, which can result in EFE and disruption of the conducting system.[89]

The presence of myocardial inflammation has been substantiated by the demonstration of immunoglobulin G (IgG), complement, and fibrin deposition on the myocardium.[75,89-94] Because the fetus is unable to produce this immunoglobulin, the demonstration of IgG deposits on the myocardium implicates maternal immunoglobulin as the likely source of the pathology. In addition to maternally derived IgG, maternal cells have been found in fetal hearts from children with CHB.[95] Studies by the Toronto group suggest a role for the fetal immune system in the inflammatory response and myocardial damage because they have demonstrated IgM and a T cell infiltrate in the myocardium of fetuses who died of CHB and EFE.[89] In vitro experiments have demonstrated that apoptosis of cardiomyocytes leads to expression of Ro and La on the cell surface and that these apoptotic cells can activate production of proinflammatory cytokines, which may lead to scarring.[96-98] Although the Toronto group could not demonstrate evidence of increased apoptosis in the hearts of fetuses who died of CHB and EFE, work by Buyon and Clancy's group has demonstrated significant apoptosis in hearts from fetuses dying with CHB.[94]

One difficulty in identification of a pathogenic effect of an autoantibody is accounting for the heterogeneity of effect. CHB is a stellar example in that not only is the injury rare but the extent of injury is varied. Accordingly, CHB is likely to represent the sum of several components. The maternal component is presumably an autoantibody that, by binding to its cognate antigen, initiates the first step to injury. One of the biological stumbling blocks has been the intracellular localization of the Ag. It is logical to hypothesize that the target is a cardiac surface protein containing a crossreactive epitope recognized by anti–Ro/La Ab. However, a direct pathological consequence to cells by inhibiting function, as in neonatal myasthenia gravis,[100] would predict an even higher recurrence of CHB in subsequent pregnancies than that observed.[101] Alternatively, the candidate antigen might be located intracellularly and translocated to the surface during development of the fetal heart. What is accepted is that without this maternal component, CHB would not ensue, thus the antibody is the requisite but not sufficient factor. Attempts to generate a robust reproducible animal model exploiting the potential pathogenicity of the antibody as an isolated factor have not met with success. A fetal component and environmental component must play some role in the ultimate expression of injury. Since recurrence is almost tenfold the risk in a first pregnancy, the genetics of a particular fetus might be a second reasonable component. The fact that identical twins are more often discordant than concordant for CHB suggests that an environmental factor present in utero might be a third component. In aggregate, the environmental factor would be expected to amplify the extent of injury in susceptible fetuses exposed to Ab generated in susceptible mothers.

If one accepts that the autoantibody is responsible for initiating injury, then understanding the mechanism by which this occurs is important. The first challenge is to explain the mechanism of "necessity,"—i.e. how maternal autoantibody directed to intracellular antigens

binds tissue and perturbs cardiac function. Boutjdir and colleagues extended two previous reports[102,103] regarding arrhythmogenic effects of anti–Ro/La antibodies by demonstrating that affinity-purified anti-Ro52 antibodies induce AV block in an isolated human fetal heart and inhibit inward calcium fluxes through L type calcium channels in human fetal ventriculocytes (whole cell and single channel).[104] Although these observations support the view that maternal antibodies perturb ion flux across the cardiocyte membrane and as such may be a relevant factor in CHB, a molecular basis has yet to be defined (e.g., definitive crossreactivity of anti-Ro/La with calcium channel receptor), particularly with regard to inflammation and subsequent fibrosis. Antibodies to the cardiac 5HT4 serotoninergic receptors (hypothesized to be crossreactive with Ro52) are only rarely present in sera from affected children.[29]

Immunohistological evaluation of hearts from fetuses dying with CHB has revealed exaggerated apoptosis, clusters of macrophages in zones of fibrosis that co-localize with IgG and apoptotic cells, TNF-α and TGF-β mRNA expression in these cells, and extensive collagen deposition in the conducting system.[83] These in vivo observations are supported by in vitro studies. Specifically, the consideration of exaggerated apoptosis as the initial link between maternal autoantibodies and tissue injury led to the observation that cardiocytes are capable of phagocytosing autologous apoptotic cardiocytes and that anti-Ro/La antibodies inhibit this function.[106] Recognizing that this perturbation of physiological efferocytosis might divert uptake to professional FcγR-bearing phagocytes fits well with earlier work demonstrating macrophage secretion of proinflammatory and fibrosing cytokines when coincubated with apoptotic cardiocytes bound by Ro/La antibodies.[106] That macrophages engage Toll-like receptors via binding to the RNA moiety of the target autoantigen is clearly an area that may provide an additional clue to pathogenesis. Finally, building on the premise that fetal genetics contribute to injury, continued genotyping of anti-Ro–exposed affected and unaffected siblings has revealed significant skewing in the frequency of polymorphisms in two genes, FcγR3a (unpublished observation) and TGF-β,[108] whose expressed proteins potentially relate to increased IgG binding to macrophages and fibrosis, respectively. The discordance of disease in monozygotic twins prompted the novel line of research into the role of hypoxia as an amplification factor on the distal fibrosing component. In vitro studies suggest a role of hypoxia in modulating cyclic AMP and promoting a myofibroblast phenotype. Footprints of hypoxic injury comprised expression of hypoxia-inducible factor 1α in affected hearts and increased erythropoietin levels in several cord blood samples of surviving fetuses.[109]

Clinical Approach to CHB, Surveillance of at-Risk Pregnancy, and Treatment of Identified Block

DIAGNOSTIC TECHNIQUES

Most cases of autoimmune CHB are diagnosed in utero, but only when an auscultatory fetal bradycardia is identified. Unfortunately, at this point, the atrioventricular node may already be replaced by extensive fibrosis and thus the bradycardia irreversible. Such late cases of advanced second- or third-degree atrioventricular block may be associated with hydrops fetalis and a high morbidity and mortality rate. Theoretically, one might postulate that there is an orderly disturbance in the fetal conduction system in which initial inflammation precedes subsequent scarring. This would imply that the earliest manifestation of CHB should be a first-degree atrioventricular block manifested as a clinically silent prolonged PR interval. If this is the case, one would predict that a fetal electrocardiogram would be able to demonstrate PR interval prolongation prior to bradyarrhythmia, perhaps at a time when therapy might be effective. However, it is not practical to obtain a noninvasive fetal electrocardiogram.[26] Other common diagnostic modalities of fetal echocardiography with M-mode study have been somewhat difficult to use as a prediction of conduction system disease.

Over the past five years, the "gold standard" for the early noninvasive diagnosis of first-degree atrioventricular block (PR prolongation) has been the fetal echocardiographic Doppler technique known as the *mechanical PR interval*.[110] This technique was first popularized by Friedman and colleagues[111] and was subsequently validated in a multicenter feasibility study in preparation for a prospective clinical trial.[112] The technique has been expanded to include an image-independent measurement of myocardial function as well.[113] This topic was recently reviewed in a paper on CHB that highlighted the role of serial fetal echocardiography with Doppler mechanical PR interval measurement[114] and stressed the therapeutic uncertainty and risks of the use of dexamethasone as treatment for conduction system disease in the fetus. Although it is conceded that the human Doppler mechanical PR interval technique has not been rigorously validated in the human, except with simultaneously derived newborn electrocardiograms, an animal model directly validates the Doppler time intervals of the heart using surface electrocardiography on six exteriorized near-term fetal lambs in normal sinus rhythm.[115]

The technique of measuring the fetal Doppler mechanical PR interval has also been addressed by Sonesson and colleagues,[116] who performed a prospective study using two different methods to measure the mechanical Doppler PR interval. The interval was serially studied in 24 anti-Ro/La antibody–positive women between 18 and 24 weeks of gestation in comparison with 284 control pregnant women. The authors found a surprising 33% (8 of 24) of all pregnancies complicated by statistical prolongation of the PR interval. It is important to note, however, that the PR interval prolongation was transient in all but two of the eight pregnancies: one fetus progressed from a prolonged PR interval (140 ms) to complete block within 6 days; the other fetus had a second-degree block that reversed to first-degree after dexamethasone, but it was not clear whether there was an initial progression through first degree prior to second degree. Subsequent letters to the editor highlighted the difficulty in determining the correct threshold of PR-interval prolongation required to diagnose first-degree heart block.[120]

The U.S.–based PRIDE study (see Autoantibodies) of pregnant women known to have anti-Ro antibodies was initiated several years ago in which echocardiograms were performed serially beginning at 16 weeks of gestation.[26] The primary outcome measure was the mechanical PR interval, defined using the gated-pulsed Doppler technique as the time interval from the onset of the mitral A wave (atrial systole) to the onset of the aortic pulsed Doppler tracing (ventricular systole) within the same left ventricular cardiac cycle. Secondary outcomes included evaluation of myocardial function. The goal was to determine the earliest noninvasive echocardiographic marker of injury.

A total of 118 pregnant women with anti-Ro antibodies were enrolled, with 98 completing an evaluable course. The protocol entailed fetal echocardiograms weekly from 16 to 26 weeks' gestation and biweekly from 26 to 34 weeks. PR intervals >150 ms (mean+3 SD) were considered abnormally prolonged, consistent with first-degree block. 92 fetuses had normal PR intervals throughout the study. Neonatal lupus developed in 10 cases, 4 of which were rash only. Three fetuses had third-degree block, none of whom had a preceding abnormal PR interval, albeit in two more than 1 week elapsed between echocardiographic evaluations. Tricuspid regurgitation preceded complete block in one fetus, and an atrial echodensity preceded the block in a second fetus. Three fetuses had a PR interval greater than 150 ms. Two, each detected before 21 weeks, reversed within 1 week after institution of 4 mg of dexamethasone. Whether dexamethasone was curative or incidental could not be assigned. A third case developed first-degree block at 32 weeks after normal PR intervals in utero, as demonstrated on the ECG performed at birth; the block persisted at age 3 years. No cases of any block developed after a normal EKG at birth. Overall, heart block occurred in 3 (19%) of 16 pregnancies in mothers with a previous CHB child and 3 (5%) of 56 in those with no previously affected children.

In summary, the noninvasive fetal echocardiographic Doppler finding of the mechanical PR interval prolongation, in pregnancies exposed to anti-SSA/Ro antibodies, may serve as a surrogate marker of subclinical disease or a research tool for the pathophysiology of this disease. The two critical issues raised by both the PRIDE and Sonesson studies are: 1) the clinical significance of a prolonged PR interval; and 2) the biological implication with regard to tissue injury. An isolated prolongation of the PR interval may be transient (related to vagal tone or medication use) or reversible injury, or it may be permanent or progress to more marked delay as a result of physical injury to the specialized electrical pathway (e.g., because of inflammation or scarring). It may be that PR prolongation represents a variant of normal and only in retrospect does it have clinical significance if it is either sustained after birth or progresses to more advanced block. A PR interval that exceeds the expected 95% confidence interval of a normal population can be transient, sustained, a normal variant or progressive. Perhaps the final outcome depends on the influence of fetal and environmental factors. These permissive factors might be present in certain fetuses and not others, thus accounting for the rarity of clinical disease. If prolongation of the PR interval does represent tissue injury, regardless of how minimal, it might be so rapid as to go unnoticed. Accurate identification of the fetus in whom first-degree block unambiguously represents a warning sign would be a major advance, since early disease may be reversible. This identification requires a definition that is acceptable to the managing physicians and that has a reasonable probability of being sustained or progressive if left untreated. This task is particularly challenging since dexamethasone and betamethasone have both maternal and fetal risks.

Given the identification of advanced block and severe cardiomyopathy within 1 week of a normal echocardiogram, with the most frequent detection time being at or before 24 weeks of gestation, it would seem appropriate to perform further research studies with weekly monitoring between 16 and 24 weeks. The goal of this monitoring would be to identify a biomarker of reversible injury—such as a PR interval prolongation above 150 ms, moderate/severe tricuspid regurgitation, and/or an atrial echodensity.[121,122]

Other diagnostic tools have been used to detect conduction system disease in the fetus. The technique of magnetocardiology has been described[122] but is not readily available and is not a bedside tool. Other groups have attempted to use tissue velocity imaging, a relatively recently described technique, in the diagnoses of fetal cardiac arrhythmias.[117,118,119] By looking at the simultaneous left atrial, right atrial, and ventricular wall velocities by two-dimensional tissue velocity imaging, Rein and colleagues[123] were able to diagnose arrhythmias and measure noninvasively the fetal cardiac time intervals. Of 31 fetuses examined between 18 and 38 weeks of gestation, one had with complete atrioventricular block. Rein and colleagues were also able to detect atrial premature contractions, ventricular premature contraction, and supraventricular tachycardia.[123]

TREATMENT OF CONGENITAL HEART BLOCK

Even in the ideal world of being able to noninvasively detect the earliest signs of CHB in fetuses at risk, the question of what treatment might be beneficial is still very much unresolved. The use of maternal oral dexamethasone therapy has been popularized by several groups, but its scientific merit and risks are questionable. Saleeb and colleagues[124] investigated the use of this medication in a retrospective chart review of cases from the RRNL. In 28 of 50 pregnancies (in 47 mothers) identified to be carrying a fetus with CHB, treatment was instituted with a fluorinated steroid (dexamethasone or betamethasone). In 21 treated cases with third-degree block at presentation, the third-degree block was not reversible. Three treated fetuses with alternating second- and third-degree block eventually developed permanent third-degree block. There were four interesting cases with second-degree block that had improved to first-degree block at birth. However, long-term follow-up revealed that two of these subsequently progressed to second-degree.[125] In the group of 22 pregnancies in which maternal steroids were not given, 18 had irreversible third-degree heart block, 2 had alternating second- and third-degree block that progressed to third-degree block, and 2 had second-degree block that progressed to third-degree. It was concluded from this retrospective study that there was no difference in mortality, prematurity, or degree of final block or

need for pacemaker for fetuses treated or untreated with steroids. It was noted that the presence of pericardial or pleural effusions as well as ascites and hydrops seemed to improve with the use of steroids. Also, there was a suggestion of reversal of less advanced block, which in theory could forestall the need for a pacemaker. Overall, this study, albeit limited in number of patients and based on retrospectively collected data, helped to popularize the use of fluorinated steroids to treat CHB identified in utero.

Subsequently, the group in Toronto reported the results of their study of transplacental therapy in fetuses in whom complete atrioventricular block without structural heart disease was diagnosed prenatally.[126] This was a single-institution timed series that evaluated the latest standardized treatment approach. Between 1990 and 1996, CHB was diagnosed in 16 pregnancies, of which 4 were treated, resulting in 80% live births and 47% survival at the age of 1 year. Between 1997 and 2003, 21 additional cases of in utero CHB were identified. In these cases the investigators employed a standardized treatment approach of maternal dexamethasone as well as β-adrenergic stimulation for fetuses with a heart rate under 55 beats per minute. Eighteen of these 21 pregnancies were treated, resulting in 95% live-birth and 1-year survival rates. In the entire cohort, (years from 1990–2003), fetuses treated with dexamethasone had a 1-year survival rate of 90%, compared to 46% for untreated fetuses; when dexamethasone treatment was combined with β-stimulation and initiated at diagnosis of CHB, the 1-year survival rate increased to 95%. Notably, in a subgroup of anti–Ro/La-positive pregnancies, immune-mediated conditions (myocarditis, hepatitis, cardiomyopathy) led to death or heart transplant in 4 of 9 live-born babies who received no treatment in utero compared to none of 18 dexamethasone-treated live births. The authors concluded that maternal dexamethasone in conjunction with β-adrenergic stimulation for bradycardia was an effective treatment program.

The Meijboom group[127] reported on a recent case of progression of incomplete atrioventricular block (presumed to be second degree) to complete CHB despite the use of dexamethasone. Moreover, complications of dexamethasone in this case included intrauterine growth retardation, oligohydramnios, prolonged adrenal suppression, and late learning disabilities. Disturbed by this case experience, they reviewed the literature on the use of treatment for CHB. Ninety-three cases were identified in which fetal heart block was treated with maternal steroids. Importantly, complete CHB was always irreversible. Only 3 of the 13 cases of incomplete heart block improved. There were multiple steroid side effects. Fluorinated steroids were the glucocorticoid preparation used, because only betamethasone and dexamethasone cross the placenta unmetabolized, while prednisone and prednisolone are inactivated by placental 11-β-hydroxysteroid dehydrogenase. The steroid side effects included intrauterine growth retardation, oligohydramnios, adrenal suppression, learning disabilities and decreased brain growth, as well as late hypertension and possible diabetes. This European group concluded that maternal dexamethasone therapy as prevention or treatment for CHB is questionable at best and should not be unconditionally recommended.

Other approaches have been reported for the treatment of autoantibody-associated CHB identified in utero. Another European group[128] described two cases at 29 and 30 weeks of gestation of fetal hydrops secondary to CHB treated with maternal steroids as well as thyroid-stimulating hormone and delivered by caesarian section. The newborns were resuscitated with immediate drainage of effusions and then treated with intravenous isoproterenol and temporary pacing. Eventually, permanent epicardial pacemakers were placed and the outcomes were good. Similarly, several groups have described the use of sympathomimetics with the goal of increasing the fetal heart rate. Groves and colleagues[129] treated three cases of complete heart block in this fashion, and the Robinson group[130] used terbutaline for the same purpose. Research data on the efficacy and safety of this therapy are minimal.

Placement of an invasive fetal pacemaker in an attempt to rescue a fetus with hydrops secondary to complete atrioventricular block has been reported,[131] but this was only temporarily effective. Rare case reports have included the use of plasmapheresis[132] and plasma exchange[133] in an attempt to remove maternal antibodies, but such interventions remain rare.

There is a report of the attempt to prophylactically treat pregnancies that are at risk for CHB with maternal prednisone.[134] Although, it was a small study that was underpowered to detect a disease that occurs in only 1%-2% of mothers who have not had a previous child with CHB, the authors recommended that prednisone should be maintained throughout the pregnancy. This recommendation has been seriously discouraged by most groups, given earlier reports of CHB developing in pregnancies during which women were taking prednisone,[135] the apparent inability of prednisone to cross the placenta,[136] the risks of steroids to mother and fetus, and the low risk (1% to 2%) of CHB in pregnancies of antibody-positive women who have not previously had an affected child.

Finally, there is current clinical interest in the possible use of intravenous immune globulin (IVIg) prophylactically to prevent the development of CHB. Such a concept is not novel, and limited success has been reported.[137-140] IVIg has a history of safe and effective use in pregnancies. As noted, prevention of CHB needs to be evaluated in the context of risk for an antibody-positive mother who has never had an affected child. However, in those women who have had a previously affected child, the recurrence rate for CHB is 15-18%. When the chance is nearly one in five that the fetus will be affected with a devastating disease, the risk:benefit ratio is clearly modified. If IVIg can be shown to have a safe therapeutic profile, then it might be an interesting drug to use in a prospective, randomized, and controlled clinical trial. The cost of such an undertaking would need to be strongly considered.

LONG-TERM CARDIAC OUTCOME

Many children require early pacemaker insertion. Most large series suggest a 10-year survival rate of about 80%, with the highest rate of mortality within the first year of life.[141-143] Most cases of CHB leading to postnatal death are associated with EFE. It had been initially suggested that EFE was the result of poor or late pacemaker placement, but later studies have demonstrated that, despite adequate pacing, EFE can lead to a cardiomyopathy that frequently leads to death or the need for cardiac transplantation.[143] The decision to insert a permanent pacemaker early after delivery is determined by the ability of the neonate to tolerate its intrinsic heart rate. The slower the rate, the more likely that early pacemaker insertion will be necessary. Current guidelines suggest that all children should have pacemaker insertion before the end of adolescence.[145-147]

Cutaneous Neonatal Lupus Erythematosus

The rash of C-NLE was first reported in 1954 in a child born to a mother with an autoimmune disease.[148] It was not until 1981, however, that the association of C-NLE and maternal anti-Ro antibodies was described.[149] Similar to mothers of children with CHB, mothers of children with C-NLE are usually clinically well despite the presence of circulating anti-Ro or anti-La antibodies or both. It is likely that a rash is present in 15% to 25% of children with NLE, although it is difficult to determine the true percentage of children born to these mothers who will develop C-NLE because the rash can be easily missed and spontaneously resolves.[150] It was initially reported that there was a female predominance in infants with C-NLE, with a female-to-male ratio of 2:1 to 3:1.[151] The reason for the reported increased incidence in females may be related to the fact that estrogens enhance surface expression of Ro and La proteins on keratinocyte cells (discussed later). It is not clear whether there is a similarly increased risk of CHB in female offspring. It should be noted however, that in the RRNL[153] the female predominance is not as pronounced. Specifically, 168 (57%) of the CHB children are females and 129 (43%) are males. Of the 139 children with rash, 76 (55%) are females and 63 (45%) are males.

The photosensitive nature of the cutaneous lesions has led investigators to examine the effect of ultraviolet irradiation on keratinocyte cell surface expression of the components of RoRNP (these in vivo and in vitro experiments are discussed later).

Clinically, the dermatitis more closely resembles the lesions of subacute cutaneous lupus erythematosus (SCLE) than the malar rash of SLE (Figures 23–2 to 23-4). Most patients with SCLE have anti-Ro or anti-La antibodies or both, and these antibodies are directed against similar proteins on RoRNP, as are the antibodies present in mothers of children with NLE.[153-156] The rash of C-NLE is rarely in a malar distribution, and the lesions are not indurated, whereas follicular plugging or dermal atrophy, typical of discoid lupus erythematosus, is rare; the rash may mimic Langerhans cell histiocytosis.[157] The face and scalp are the most commonly involved areas, but the rash may occur at any site, including the palms and soles. Commonly, it develops around the eyes in a raccoonlike distribution. The rash

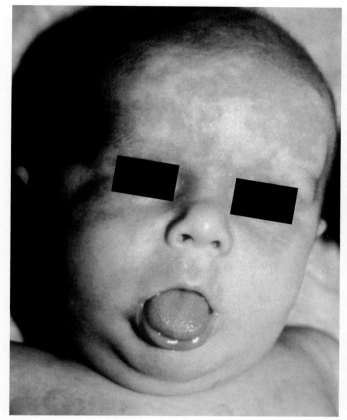

FIGURE 23–2 Neonatal lupus syndrome. This erythematous rash appeared a day after birth, accompanied by thrombocytopenia and leukopenia. (Courtesy of Dr. D.C. Rada and T. Kestenbaum.)

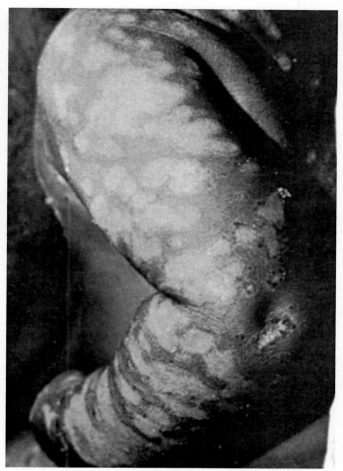

FIGURE 23–3 A child with neonatal lupus syndrome. The rash on this baby is more discoid than the rash on the baby in Figure 23–2. (Courtesy of Dr. D. Kredich.)

tends to consist of discrete, round, or elliptical plaques with a fine scale that has central clearing, and it tends to be papulosquamous or similar to the rash of annular erythema. An infant may have one or both of these typical rashes. In North America, papulosquamous lesions are most commonly described, whereas in Japan, annular erythema is more commonly seen.[158] Bullous lesions may be seen especially on the soles of the feet, and the rash may resemble cutis marmorata telangiectatica, congenita bullous impetigo, primary herpes simplex infection, and erythema multiforme.

The dermatitis of C-NLE may be present at birth but more commonly develops within the first few weeks of life.[150,151,156] The most common age of appearance of the rash is 6 weeks, but it may not be recognized until as late as 12 weeks.[156] New lesions may appear for several months, but they rarely develop beyond 6 months of postnatal life, consistent with the disappearance of maternal antibodies from the infant's circulation. The lesions may be induced or exacerbated by sun exposure, but instances of C-NLE that are present at birth, along with the observations that involvement of the soles of the feet and diaper area occur, illustrate that sun exposure is not absolutely required for development of the rash. Rash appearing after phototherapy for neonatal jaundice has been reported, but it is uncommon. The mean duration of the rash has been reported to be 17 weeks.[156]

The lesions of C-NLE are transient and usually resolve without scarring, although some mild epidermal atrophy may result. Cutaneous telangiectasias, beginning at age 6 to 12 months, occur in approximately 10% of affected infants.[156,159,160] The telangiectasias may occur in areas that were not initially involved with C-NLE and therefore are not just the result of healing of the initial inflammatory rash. The most common area for telangiectasia is at the temples near the hairline, an area not usually affected by the acute lesions. Telangiectasias tend to be bilateral. This lesion may be the presenting feature of C-NLE, although it is not clear in these instances whether the initial rash had been subtle and missed or the telangiectasias had occurred de novo without the characteristic earlier rash.[159] There have been reports of the telangiectasias with atrophy persisting into adolescence.[160,161]

Pathology

Biopsies of the lesions of C-NLE demonstrate the typical histopathology of SCLE, which includes epidermal basal cell damage, a mild mononuclear cell dermal infiltrate, vacuolation of the basal layer, and epidermal colloid bodies. IgG, IgM, and complement are deposited usually at the dermoepidermal junction.[161,162]

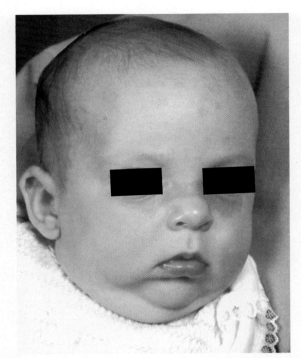

FIGURE 23–4 Neonatal lupus syndrome. Four-month-old girl with the erythematous rash across the bridge of the nose, lower eyelids, and superior forehead. This baby was born at 33 weeks of gestation with complete congenital heart block. Her mother had high titers of anti-Ro antibody.

Table 23–1	
Differential diagnosis of rash of cutaneous NLE	
Polycyclic Lesion	**Annular Erythema**
Urticaria	Erythema annulare
Erythema marginatum	centrifugum
Tinea corporis	Familial annular erythema
Seborrheic dermatitis	Infantile epidermodysplastic
Ichthyosiform genodermatosis	erythema
	Infection with Pityrosporum
	Annular erythema of infancy
	Erythema gyratum atrophicans

Most mothers of infants with C-NLE are anti-Ro antibody positive, often in combination with anti-La antibodies. The percentage of mothers with elevated anti-Ro antibody levels depends on the assay used. A few cases of C-NLE have been reported in association with antibodies to U1RNP in the absence of anti-Ro or anti-La antibody.[163-165] The cutaneous lesions in some of these infants were considered to be atypical in morphological appearance.[165] One infant with C-NLE had anti-U1RNP but not anti-Ro or anti-La antibodies when tested by ELISA.[166] However, anti-La antibodies were identified by immunoblot. In some cases of C-NLE, the antibodies may be directed to epitopes that cannot be detected by ELISA.

Differential Diagnosis

The differential diagnosis of isolated C-NLE includes the other causes of annular and polycyclic lesions.[167-173] When the rash occurs concomitant with CHB, the diagnosis is much easier (see Table 23–1).

Treatment

The usual approach to management of C-NLE is reassurance offered to the parents and continued observation of the child, because the natural history of the skin lesions is spontaneous resolution without scarring; therefore, aggressive treatment is not indicated. However, topical application of a mild glucocorticoid cream may hasten the resolution of the lesions and be used for cosmetic reasons, although it is possible that steroid use increases the risk of developing telangiectasias. Telangiectasias can be treated with pulse dye laser therapy, although they may also spontaneously improve.[159]

Liver Disease

Hepatic dysfunction in NLE is characterized by abnormal levels of liver enzymes and hepatomegaly that were initially ascribed to congestive heart failure, intrauterine hydrops fetalis, disseminated intravascular coagulation, or total parenteral nutrition. It was subsequently suggested that hepatic involvement occurs in approximately 15% of infants with NLE. However, a large, unselected series demonstrated that liver involvement occurred in approximately 25% of all infants with NLE.[150] Liver disease can present as an isolated disorder or in association with C-NLE, CHB, or any other manifestation of NLE. Usually, patients have mild hepatomegaly, with or without splenomegaly, and cholestasis with mildly to moderately elevated transaminases.[174,175] Hepatitis may be the only manifestation of NLE in a mother with anti-Ro and anti-La autoantibodies.[148,150,156] Although a liver biopsy is usually not clinically indicated, histological abnormalities are similar to idiopathic neonatal giant cell hepatitis with mild bile duct obstruction, occasional giant cell transformation, and mild portal fibrosis.[146,175] It is possible in this regard that idiopathic neonatal hepatitis may be another manifestation of NLE. Liver biopsies should be reserved for infants with clinical evidence of severe dysfunction or with persistent, moderate dysfunction.

Abnormalities of liver function usually resolve, although deaths secondary to hepatic failure before age 6 months have been reported.[150,174-178] The only report of a repeat biopsy in an infant with hepatic abnormalities demonstrated persistence of mild fibrosis; the child had a good long-term outcome.[174] There have not been any instances of late liver failure or cirrhosis; however, it has been only since about 1980 that hepatic disease has been identified as part of the syndrome.

Hematological Disease

Thrombocytopenia is the most common hematological manifestation, whereas anemia and neutropenia are less frequently present. Usually, hematological involvement develops in conjunction with other stigmata, but thrombocytopenia, anemia, neutropenia, and pancytopenia have been reported as isolated manifestations of NLE (NLE should therefore be considered in the differential diagnosis of neonatal cytopenias).[150,179-182] Antiplatelet antibodies have been only rarely detected, suggesting that other factors may be responsible for the neonatal thrombocytopenia. The thrombocytopenia and neutropenia may be secondary to anti-Ro or anti-La antibodies because thrombocytopenia in SLE is associated with these autoantibodies and anti-Ro antibodies have been demonstrated to bind to neutrophils.[183-186] In addition, children with chronic immune thrombocytopenic purpura may have anti-Ro antibodies. There have been isolated reports of aplastic anemia and neonatal thrombosis associated with the transplacental passage of maternal autoantibodies.[181,185,187-189] The thrombocytopenia and other hematological manifestations tend to resolve over several weeks and, unless there is bleeding, do not require treatment. However, if the condition is severe or life threatening, high-dose glucocorticoids or intravenous immunoglobulin may be necessary.[189]

Other Manifestations

There have been numerous reports of different diseases of the newborn associated with the transplacental passage of maternal anti-Ro, anti-La, or other autoantibodies, as well as unusual clinical manifestations in neonates with classic NLE. When there is a single case report, it is not clear whether the illness in the neonate is related to the maternal autoantibodies or is a disease coincidentally occurring in offspring of mothers with the candidate autoantibodies. Similarly, when unusual features are identified in children with definite NLE, it is not clear whether the other illness is coincidental or the result of maternal autoantibodies.

Multiple neurological manifestations have been described. A myelopathy with a gait abnormality and spastic paraparesis has been reported in two cases of infants with C-NLE.[190] The neurological disease became apparent in one child at age 1 year and in the other at age 16 months. Although it is possible that there was undiagnosed neonatal thrombocytopenia or vasculitis that resulted in intracerebral hemorrhage or infarction without any other clinical disease, there was no obvious cause other than the presence of anti-Ro antibodies. Other neurological diseases have included an infant with vasculopathy, a nonspecific marker of an insult to the developing blood vessels of the brain; hydrocephalus in two female siblings; and a case of transient neonatal myasthenia gravis.[191-194] Three children with CHB have been identified with cerebral ultrasonography and color Doppler flow imaging studies that demonstrated evidence of a vasculopathy in the area of the thalamus. A short-term follow-up study of these children revealed no signs of progression or neurological impairment. The investigators suggested that when infants are seen with clinical signs and symptoms consistent with a vasculopathy in the gangliothalamic region, they should be examined for other manifestations of NLE, and the mothers should be tested for anti-Ro and anti-La antibodies.[192] There has been one case report of an adolescent with CHB who developed moyamoya disease.[195] A study of 10 consecutive children with other clinical features of NLE demonstrated abnormal computed tomographic (CT) scans or ultrasound findings, or both, in 9. The CT abnormalities included

decreased attenuation of the cerebral white matter, basal ganglia calcifications, ventriculomegaly, and benign macrocephaly of infancy. The ultrasound abnormalities included subependymal cysts, increased echogenicity of the white matter, and echogenic lenticulostriate vessels. The only clinical abnormality in any of these children was one case of macrocephaly. On follow-up, all were developmentally normal.[196] The authors prospectively studied 87 consecutive infants born to mothers with antibodies against the RoRNP and FOUND a significantly increased rate of macrocephaly and hydrocephalus (8%) than predicted in the normal population.[197] Only 1/7 patients with hydrocephalus required a shunt. This group suggested that measuring circumferences should be part of the follow-up of children born to mothers with anti-Ro/La antibodies.

There have been multiple case reports and case series of chondrodysplasia punctata associated with NLE, including one child at our institution with C-NLE and radiographic changes in the hip and ankle consistent with this diagnosis.[198,199] Individual case reports have included congenital nephrotic syndrome in an infant with NLE[200] and a child with C-NLE and Turner syndrome.[201]

COURSE OF THE DISEASE AND PROGNOSIS

Children

NLE is a disease caused by the transplacental passage of maternal autoantibodies and not by the production of these autoantibodies by the fetus or neonate. Skin, liver, and hematological complications generally resolve with minimal sequelae, whereas CHB is permanent; the long-term cardiac outcome of these children is described in the section on CHB.

It was initially reported that children with NLE might be at a high risk for developing SLE in later life.[202,203] The Toronto group has seen SLE develop in 2 of approximately 250 children followed long-term with a history of NLE. A group from Japan reported that 8% of children had persistent or recurrently positive autoantibodies, and one met the American College of Rheumatology classification criteria for SLE.[66] In a second study, 12% of children with NLE developed an autoimmune disease (i.e., juvenile rheumatoid arthritis, Hashimoto thyroiditis, psoriasis, diabetes mellitus, and nephrotic syndrome), although only a minority had autoantibodies, and none had anti-Ro antibodies or SLE.[204] The increased risk of autoimmune disease in these offspring may reflect the genetic predisposition of a child born to a mother with an autoimmune disease, as opposed to a direct delayed consequence of having had NLE. The risk of development of an autoimmune disease in the child with NLE is probably not greater than the risk in any other offspring of anti-Ro antibody–positive women with SLE, and is likely related to the linkage of HLA class II genes to the production of anti-Ro and anti-La antibodies.[48,205-209] Parents of these infants should be counseled that the risk of their offspring developing autoimmune diseases is similar to the risk in children of women with SLE.

Mothers

Initially, NLE was the name of the disorder given to infants born with the characteristic skin or cardiac findings in the presence of maternal connective tissue disease, particularly SLE and SS. All mothers of infants with NLE therefore had an autoimmune disease. However, it rapidly became apparent that CHB and the characteristic rash of C-NLE could be seen in the offspring of mothers who did not have any signs or symptoms of a connective tissue disorder. It was initially surmised that the mothers of children with CHB would develop a connective tissue disease, but only a minority of mothers had a connective tissue disease at the time of delivery of their children with CHB, and at long-term follow-up the majority remained healthy.[210-214] A large study has demonstrated that mothers of children with C-NLE were more likely to have had a diagnosed autoimmune disorder at the time of delivery of the child with NLE and at long-term follow-up than were mothers of children with CHB.[216]

The long-term outcome of the mothers has been addressed in a publication based on a large U.S. cohort.[215] To evaluate autoimmune disease progression in asymptomatic and paucisymptomatic mothers of children with NLE, clinical information on mothers enrolled in the RRNL was obtained from medical records. Of the 321 mothers enrolled, 229 had at least 6 months of follow-up. Twenty-six of the 51 mothers who were asymptomatic at the NLE child's birth progressed: 12 developed pauci-undifferentiated autoimmune syndrome (pauci-UAS), 2 poly-UAS, 7 SS, 4 SLE and 1 SLE/SS. The median time to develop any symptom was 3.15 years. Sixteen of the 37 mothers classified as pauci-UAS at the NLE child's birth progressed: 5 developed poly-UAS, 6 SS, 4 SLE, and 1 SLE/SS. Of the pauci-UAS mothers enrolled within 1 year, the median time to progression was 6.7 years. Four mothers developed lupus nephritis (two asymptomatic, two pauci-UAS). The probability of an asymptomatic mother developing SLE by 10 years was 18.6%, and developing probable/definite SS was 27.9%. Mothers with anti-SSA/Ro and anti-SSB/La were nearly twice as likely to develop an autoimmune disease as mothers with anti-SSA/Ro only. The authors concluded that continued follow-up of asymptomatic NL mothers is warranted since nearly half progress, albeit few develop SLE. These results differ from the findings of the Toronto NLE Cohort as NLE manifestations did not predict disease progression in an asymptomatic mother. Although the anti-SSB/La antibodies may be a risk factor for progression, further work is needed to determine reliable biomarkers in otherwise healthy women with anti-SSA/Ro antibodies identified solely because of an NL child.

Because almost all children with NLE are born to mothers with anti-Ro or anti-La antibodies, or both, it is important to estimate the risk of delivering a child with NLE from mothers with a known connective tissue disease (particularly SLE) or from mothers who have previously delivered a child with NLE. Large series of pregnancies in women with SLE who had anti-Ro or anti-La antibodies, or both, have suggested that the risk of delivering a child with NLE varied between 1% and 10%.[181,217,218,220] Later large, prospective studies have suggested that the risk of delivering a child with NLE in mothers with anti-Ro or anti-La antibodies, or both, was 1% to 2%.[219,221] Retrospective studies have suggested a recurrence rate for CHB of between 8% and 25% in subsequent pregnancies.[182,217-218] Our experience and that of others in pregnancies after the delivery of a child with CHB or C-NLE suggests that the risk is approximately 15% to 20%.[219-221]

ANIMAL MODELS OF NEONATAL LUPUS ERYTHEMATOSUS

The major targets of NLE are the heart, skin, and liver. To better determine the pathogenesis of NLE, in vivo and in vitro models have been established. The in vivo models have used the infusion of human autoantibody–containing sera (passive) or have generated autoantibodies by immunization of mice to generate autoantibodies (active). The in vitro models have used isolated cardiac myocytes or whole organ culture.

In Vitro Experiments

Culture of isolated neonatal, but not adult, rabbit cardiac myocytes with sera from anti-Ro or anti-La antibody–positive women led to changes in the repolarization of these cells.[222] Binding of the maternal sera to rabbit tissue was likely the result of the presence of RoRNP antigen on the surface of fetal hearts.[223,224] However, unlike that which occurs with keratinocytes, the cellular localization of 48-kD La, 52-kD Ro, or 60-kD Ro in fetal cardiac myocytes is not altered by culture in the presence of 17β-estradiol or progesterone.[225]

Calcium channels are important in maintaining cardiac rhythm, and antibodies against these ions therefore are important in CHB. Experiments using cultured human fetal cardiomyocytes have demonstrated that anti-Ro antibodies (particularly anti-52-kD Ro antibodies) alter calcium L-type and T-type channels.[226,227] Affinity-purified antibodies, which recognized both 52-kD Ro isoforms, also recognized the human 5-HT4 receptor and antagonized the serotonin-induced L-type calcium channel activation on isolated human atrial cells. However, as discussed earlier, a study using sera from the RRNL did not show an association of anti-5HT4 receptor antibodies and the development of CHB. Autoantibodies from mothers of children CHB have been shown to bind to and modify the response of muscarinic acetylcholine receptor activation of neonatal, but not adult, rat atria.[228-230] Taken together, it appears that antibodies directed against calcium channels and receptors important in generation of cardiac rhythm, which are present on cardiomyocytes, may play a role in the pathogenesis of CHB.

Skin

Irradiation of keratinocytes enhances the expression of Ro, U1RNP, and Sm antigens.[231-233] Estradiol treatment of keratinocytes can induce a marked increase in mRNA and expression of Ro, U1RNP, and Sm autoantigens.[224,231-234] Other factors, including TNF-α and exposure to viruses, upregulate the surface expression of 52-kD Ro and La on keratinocytes.[237] The direct binding of anti-RoRNP antibodies to skin has been demonstrated.[224,236]

The difference in disease expression in offspring born to the same mother may be at least partially explained by the demonstration that sera from children with C-NLE can be cytotoxic to keratinocytes from patients with NLE but not to cells obtained from normal individuals. This cytotoxicity was enhanced by UVB irradiation. These data suggest that keratinocytes from children with C-NLE may have abnormal surface expression of the Ro and La antigens and that ultraviolet irradiation can further increase that expression.[237] These results are consistent with the demonstration that the rash of C-NLE may be present at birth or later and that it does not occur in all infants born to mothers with autoantibodies directed against RoRNP.

Langendorff Experiments

Initial ex vivo experiments examined the effect of anti-Ro– and anti-La–containing sera on conduction in isolated rabbit hearts. The perfusion of isolated Langendorff preparations of adult rabbit hearts with purified IgG from sera containing anti-Ro and anti-La antibodies induced heart block and altered the peak slow inward current.[238] However, sera from women with SLE or SS without a history of delivering a child with NLE also resulted in heart block in the isolated, whole rabbit heart, although the heart block occurred only with perfusion with affinity-purified anti–52-kD antibodies.[239] These observations are not unique to anti-Ro antibody–containing sera, because similar alterations of cardiac conduction have been observed with sera from patients with conduction defects associated with Chagas disease.[240]

Perfusion of Langendorff preparations of human fetal hearts with affinity-purified anti–52-kD Ro derived from mothers of children with CHB also resulted in the development of complete AV block. At a whole-cell and single-channel level, perfusion experiments with the human heart demonstrated an inhibition of L-type calcium currents. Similarly, when isolated rat hearts were used, a 2:1 AV block followed by complete inhibition of AV nodal action potential was demonstrated, and calcium channels were inhibited in isolated cellular preparations.[241] These results suggested that rodents may be an appropriate species for monitoring the fetal effects of maternal anti-Ro and anti-La antibodies.

In Vivo Experiments

Immunization of female BALB/c mice with recombinant RoRNP proteins generates high-titer antibodies that cross the placenta during pregnancy and are associated with various degrees of atrio-ventricular (AV)-conduction abnormalities in the pups. However, conduction abnormalities were seen in only a low percentage of the offspring born to these mice, and advanced conduction abnormalities rarely developed.[242]

Apoptosis has been proposed as a mechanism for the tissue damage.[243] In human fetal cardiac myocytes, apoptosis results in surface translocation of RoRNP.[244] In vivo murine experiments have supported this hypothesis because the passive transfer of human IgG containing anti-52-kD Ro, anti-60-kD Ro, and anti-La autoantibodies led to the formation of human IgG–apoptotic cell complexes in organs targeted in NLE (i.e., heart, skin, liver, and bone) but not in thymus, lung, brain, or gut. Experiments with affinity-purified antibodies demonstrated that anti-La, but not anti-Ro, antibodies formed these complexes.[243]

It is possible that apoptosis, a normal event during cardiac development, may result in the binding of maternal anti-RoRNP to the apoptotic cells that cause an inflammatory reaction. The neighboring cells may be damaged as bystanders. Initial binding may be by maternal anti–52-kD Ro antibodies or antibodies to isoforms of the La protein, which are maximally expressed early in gestation, with levels decreasing with gestational age until 25 weeks, when adult levels are achieved.[22,245] This hypothesis allows for the selective damage to fetal, but not to maternal, conducting tissue.

REFERENCES

1. R.J. Smeenk, Immunological aspects of congenital atrioventricular block, Pacing Clin. Electrophysiol. 20 (1997) 2093–2097.
2. J. Zhu, Cytomegalovirus infection induces expression of 60 KD/Ro antigen on human keratinocytes, Lupus 4 (1995) 396–406.
3. E. Ben-Chetrit, B.J. Gandy, E.M. Tan, et al., Isolation and characterization of a cDNA clone encoding the 60-kD component of the human SS-A/Ro ribonucleoprotein autoantigen, J. Clin. Invest. 83 (1989) 1284–1292.
4. S.L. Deutscher, J.B. Harley, J.D. Keene, Molecular analysis of the 60-kDa human Ro ribonucleoprotein, Proc. Natl. Acad. Sci. USA 85 (1988) 9479–9483.
5. M.R. Lerner, J.A. Boyle, J.A. Hardin, et al., Two novel classes of small ribonucleoproteins detected by antibodies associated with lupus erythematosus, Science 211 (1981) 400–402.
6. D. Wang, J.P. Buyon, E.K.L. Chan, Cloning and expression of mouse 60 kDa ribonucleoprotein SS-A/Ro, Mol. Biol. Reports 23 (1996) 205–210.
7. H. Shi, C.A. O'Brien, D.J. Van Horn, et al., A misfolded form of 5S rRNA is complexed with the Ro and La autoantigens, RNA 2 (1996) 769–784.
8. D. Xue, H. Shi, J.D. Smith, et al., A lupus-like syndrome develops in mice lacking the Ro 60-kDa protein, a major lupus autoantigen, Proc. Natl. Acad. Sci. USA 100 (2003) 7503–7508.
9. E.K. Chan, A.M. Francoeur, E.M. Tan, Epitopes, structural domains and asymmetry of amino acid residues in SS-B/La nuclear protein, J. Immunol. 136 (1986) 3744–3749.
10. J.C. Chambers, D. Kenan, B.J. Martin, et al., Genomic structure and amino acid sequence domains of the human La autoantigen, J. Biol. Chem. 263 (1988) 18043–18051.
11. E. Gottlieb, J.A. Steitz, Function of the mammalian La protein: evidence for its action in transcription termination by RNA polymerase III, EMBO J. 8 (1989) 851–861.
12. G. Boire, J. Craft, Human Ro ribonucleoprotein particles: characterization of native structure and stable association with the La polypeptide, J. Clin. Invest. 85 (1990) 1182–1190.
13. E. Ben-Chetrit, E.K.L. Chan, K.F. Sullivan, et al., A 52-kD protein is a novel component of the SS-A/Ro antigenic particle, J. Exp. Med. 162 (1988) 1560–1571.
14. E.K. Chan, J.C. Hamel, J.P. Buyon, et al., Molecular definition and sequence motifs of the 52-kD component of human SS-A/Ro autoantigen, J. Clin. Invest. 87 (1991) 68–76.
15. K. Itoh, Y. Itoh, M.D. Frank, Protein heterogeneity in the human Ro/SSA ribonucleoproteins, J. Clin. Invest. 87 (1991) 177–186.
16. J.P. Buyon, R.J. Winchester, S.G. Slade, et al., Identification of mothers at risk for congenital heart block and other neonatal lupus syndromes in their children: Comparison of enzyme-linked immunosorbent assay and immunoblot to measure anti-SS-A/Ro and anti-SS-B/La antibodies, Arthritis Rheum. 36 (1993) 1263–1273.

17. J.P. Buyon, S.G. Slade, J.D. Reveille, et al., Autoantibody responses to the "native" 52-kDa SS-A/Ro protein in neonatal lupus syndromes, systemic lupus erythematosus and Sjögren's syndrome, J. Immunol. 152 (1994) 3675–3684.

18. H. Julkunen, P. Kurki, R. Kaaja, et al., Isolated congenital heart block: long-term outcome of mothers and characterization of the immune response to SS-A/Ro and to SS-B/La, Arthritis Rheum. 36 (1993) 1588–1598.

19. L.A. Lee, M.B. Frank, V.R. McCubbin, et al., Autoantibodies of neonatal lupus erythematosus, J. Invest. Dermatol. 102 (1994) 963–966.

20. E.D. Silverman, J. Buyon, R.M. Laxer, et al., Autoantibody response to the Ro/La particle may predict outcome in neonatal lupus erythematosus, Clin. Exp. Immunol. 100 (1994) 499–505.

21. E.K. Chan, F. DiDonato, J.C. Hamel, et al., 52-kD SS-A/Ro: Genomic structure and identification of an alternatively spliced transcript encoding a novel leucine zipper-minus autoantigen expressed in fetal and adult heart, J. Exp. Med. 182 (1995) 983–992.

22. J.P. Buyon, C.E. Tseng, F. DiDonato, et al., Cardiac expression of 52β, an alternative transcript of the congenital heart block-associated 52-kD SS-A/Ro autoantigen, is maximal during fetal development, Arthritis Rheum. 40 (1997) 655–660.

23. S. Salomonsson, T. Dörner, E. Theander, et al., A serologic marker for fetal risk of congenital heart block, Arthritis Rheum. 46 (2002) 1233–1241.

24. S. Salomonsson, S.E. Sonesson, L. Ottosson, et al., Ro/SSA autoantibodies directly bind cardiomyocytes, disturb calcium homeostasis, and mediate congenital heart block, J. Exp. Med. 201(2005) 11–17.

25. J.P. Buyon, J. Waltuck, K. Caldwell, et al., Relationship between maternal and neonatal levels of antibodies to 48 kDa SSB(La), 52 kDa SSA(Ro), and 60 kDa SSA(Ro) in pregnancies complicated by congenital heart block, J. Rheumatol. 21 (1994) 1943–1950.

26. D.M. Friedman, M.Y. Kim, J.A. Copel, et al., Utility of Cardiac monitoring in fetuses at risk for congenital heart block: The PR Interval and Dexamethasone Evaluation (PRIDE) prospective Study, Circulation 117 (2008) 485–493.

27. R.M. Clancy, J.P. Buyon, K. Ikeda, et al., Maternal antibody responses to the 52-kd SSA/Ro p200 peptide and the development of fetal conduction defects, Arthritis Rheum. 52 (2005) 3079–3086.

28. P. Eftekhari, L. Sallé, F. Lezoualc'h, et al., Anti-SSA/Ro52 autoantibodies blocking the cardiac 5-HT₄ serotoninergic receptor could explain neonatal lupus congenital heart block, Eur. J. Immunol. 30 (2000) 2782–2790.

29. R. Kamel, P. Eftekhari, R. Clancy, et al., Autoantibodies against the serotoninergic 5-HT₄ receptor and congenital heart block: a reassessment, J. Autoimmun. 25 (2005) 72–76.

30. J.P. Buyon, R.J. Winchester, S.G. Slade, et al., Identification of mothers at risk for congenital heart block and other neonatal lupus syndromes in their children: Comparison of ELISA and immunoblot to measure anti-SS-A/Ro and anti-SS-B/La antibodies, Arthritis Rheum. 36 (1993) 1263–1273.

31. L.A. Rokeach, J.A. Haselby, J.F. Meilof, et al., Characterization of the autoantigen calreticulin, J. Immunol. 147 (1991) 3031–3039.

32. L.A. Rokeach, P.A. Zimmerman, T.R. Unnasch, Epitopes of the Onchocerca volvulus RAL1 antigen, a member of the calreticulin family of proteins, recognized by sera from patients with onchocerciasis, Infect. Immun. 62 (1994) 3696–3704.

33. T. Orth, T. Dorner, K.H. Meyer Zum Buschenfelde, W.J. Mayet, Complete congenital heart block is associated with increased autoantibody titers against calreticulin, Eur. J. Clin. Invest. 26 (1996) 205–215.

34. S.H. Chang, M.S. Huh, H.R. Kim, et al., Cross-reactivity of antibodies immunoadsorbed to laminin with recombinant human La (SS-B) protein, J. Autoimmun. 11 (1998) 163–167.

35. J.M. Li, A.C. Horsfall, R.N. Maini, Anti-La (SS-B) but not anti-Ro52 (SS-A) antibodies cross-react with laminin: a role in the pathogenesis of congenital heart block? Clin. Exp. Immunol. 99 (1995) 316–324.

36. A.C. Horsfall, J.M. Li, R.N. Maini, Placental and fetal cardiac laminin are targets for cross-reacting autoantibodies from mothers of children with congenital heart block, J. Autoimmun. 9 (1996) 561–568.

37. J.M. Li, W.S. Fan, A.C. Horsfall, et al., The expression of human endogenous retrovirus-3 in fetal cardiac tissue and antibodies in congenital heart block, Clin. Exp. Immunol. 104 (1996) 388–393.

38. G. Houen, C. Koch, Human placental calreticulin: purification, characterization and association with other proteins, Acta. Chem. Scand. 48 (1994) 905–911.

39. P.J. Maddison, L. Lee, M. Reichlin, et al., Anti-p57: a novel association with neonatal lupus, Clin. Exp. Immunol. 99 (1995) 42–48.

40. S. Miyagawa, K. Yanagi, A. Yoshioka, et al., Neonatal lupus erythematosus: maternal IgG antibodies bind to a recombinant NH₂-terminal fusion protein encoded by human alpha-fodrin, cDNA J. Invest. Dermatol. 111 (1998) 1189–1197.

41. N. Haneji, T. Nakamura, K. Takio, et al., Identification of alpha-fodrin as a candidate autoantigen in primary Sjögren's syndrome, Science 276 (1997) 604–607.

42. D.A. Bell, P.J. Maddison, Serologic subsets in systemic lupus erythematosus: an examination of autoantibodies in relationship to clinical features of disease and HLA antigens, Arthritis Rheum. 23 (1980) 1268–1273.

43. H. Ehrfeld, K. Hartung, M. Renz, et al., MHC associations of autoantibodies against recombinant Ro and La proteins in systemic lupus erythematosus. Results of a multicenter study. SLE Study Group, Rheumatol. Int. 12 (1992) 169–173.

44. H.M. Fei, H. Kang, S. Scharf, et al., Specific HLA-DQA and HLA-DRB1 alleles confer susceptibility to Sjögren's syndrome and autoantibody production, J. Clin. Lab. Anal. 5 (1991) 382–391.

45. P. Lulli, G.D. Sebastiani, S. Trabace, et al., HLA antigens in Italian patients with systemic lupus erythematosus: evidence for the association of DQw2 with the autoantibody response to extractable nuclear antigens, Clin. Exp. Rheumatol. 9 (1991) 475–479.

46. T.O. Kerttula, P. Collin, A. Polvi, et al., Distinct immunologic features of Finnish Sjögren's syndrome patients with HLA alleles DRB1*0301, DQA1*0501, and DQB1*0201. Alterations in circulating T cell receptor gamma/delta subsets, Arthritis Rheum. 39 (1996) 1733–1739.

47. J.M. Martin-Villa, J. Martinez-Laso, M.A. Moreno-Pelayo, et al., Differential contribution of HLA-DR, DQ, and TAP2 alleles to systemic lupus erythematosus susceptibility in Spanish patients: role of TAP2*01 alleles in Ro autoantibody production, Ann. Rheum. Dis. 57 (1998) 214–219.

48. S. Miyagawa, K. Shinohara, M. Nakajima, et al., Polymorphisms of HLA class II genes and autoimmune responses to Ro/SS-A-La/SS-B among Japanese subjects, Arthritis Rheum. 41 (1998) 927–934.

49. J.S. Smolen, J.H. Klippel, E. Penner, et al., HLA-DR antigens in systemic lupus erythematosus: association with specificity of autoantibody responses to nuclear antigens, Ann. Rheum. Dis. 46 (1987) 457–462.

50. W.A. Wilson, E. Scopelitis, J.P. Michalski, Association of HLA-DR7 with both antibody to SSA(Ro) and disease susceptibility in blacks with systemic lupus erythematosus, J. Rheumatol. 11 (1984) 653–657.

51. S. Miyagawa, K. Dohi, H. Shima, et al., HLA antigens in anti-Ro(SS-A)-positive patients with recurrent annular erythema, J. Am. Acad. Dermatol. 28 (1993) 185–188.

52. S. Miyagawa, K. Dohi, H. Shima, et al., Absence of HLA-B8 and HLA-DR3 in Japanese patients with Sjögren's syndrome positive for anti-SSA(Ro), J. Rheumatol. 19 (1992) 1922–1924.

53. R.G. Hamilton, J.B. Harley, W.B. Bias, et al., Two Ro (SS-A) autoantibody responses in systemic lupus erythematosus. Correlation of HLA-DR/DQ specificities with quantitative expression of Ro (SS-A) autoantibody, Arthritis Rheum. 31 (1988) 496–505.

54. A. Fujisaku, M.B. Frank, B. Neas, et al., HLA-DQ gene complementation and other histocompatibility relationships in man with the anti-Ro/SSA autoantibody response of systemic lupus erythematosus, J. Clin. Invest. 86 (1990) 606–611.

55. G. Colombo, A. Brucato, E. Coluccio, et al., DNA typing of maternal HLA in congenital complete heart block: comparison with systemic lupus erythematosus and primary Sjögren's syndrome, Arthritis Rheum. 42 (1999) 1757–1764.

Entire reference list is available online at www.expertconsult.com.

Chapter 24

JUVENILE DERMATOMYOSITIS

Lisa G. Rider, Carol B. Lindsley, and James T. Cassidy

Juvenile dermatomyositis (JDM) is a multisystem disease of uncertain origin that results in chronic inflammation of striated muscle and skin. It is characterized early in its course by perivascular inflammation of varying severity and later by development of calcinosis.

HISTORICAL REVIEW

The clinical presentation of JDM was described by four different investigators in 1887.[1-4] Unverricht[4] clarified the cutaneous and muscular manifestations of the disease, introducing the term *dermatomyositis*. He recognized that the childhood form of the disease was not always fatal, although subsequent reports emphasized the poor prognosis. The clinically distinctive features of JDM were not detailed until some time later.[5-14] Experience with this disease in the era before steroids was reported by Karelitz and Welt (22 children),[5] Scheuermann (47 children),[15] Hecht (5 children),[16] and Selander (22 children).[17] The first postmortem study that described the classic histopathological features of the disease in a child was by Batten in 1912.[18] Pearson[19] recognized the uniqueness of this disorder in children and distinguished it from myositis in adults in his classification in 1966. In 1953, Wedgwood and colleagues[6] reviewed data on 26 children treated with glucocorticoids, and in 1963, Cook and colleagues[20] reported 15 deaths among 50 children and emphasized the therapeutic role of these agents for treatment. Sullivan and colleagues[11,13] in 1972 and 1977, respectively, and Rose[12] in 1974 stressed the importance of an adequately high initial dose of glucocorticoids and sufficiently long therapeutic course to reverse the dismal prognosis of juvenile dermatomyositis.

Definition and Classification

In childhood, the chronic idiopathic inflammatory myopathies are relatively heterogeneous disorders, although most affected children have the characteristic skin and muscle abnormalities of JDM.[21-28] The five criteria of Bohan and Peter in Table 24–1 are applicable to its diagnosis, although their sensitivity and specificity have not been validated in children but are probably 45% to 90%.[21,22] A diagnosis of probable JDM requires the presence of the pathognomonic rash (Gottron papules over the extensor surfaces of the finger joints, elbows, knees or ankles) or the heliotrope rash and two of the other criteria; definite JDM requires the characteristic rash with three other criteria.[29,30] In general, the first two criteria (i.e., proximal muscle weakness and classic rash) are almost always present; criterion 3 (i.e., elevated serum levels of muscle enzymes), 4 (i.e., electromyographic changes), and 5 (i.e., histopathological changes) provide additional laboratory support for the diagnosis. A diagnosis of JDM is not necessarily excluded by failure to meet one or more of these criteria, except that related to the dermatitis. Magnetic resonance imaging (MRI) of the thigh muscles, demonstrating symmetrical muscle edema on fat-suppressed T2-weighted or Short Tau Inversion Recovery (STIR) sequences, has become preferred to electromyography to evaluate patients to confirm a diagnosis of JDM and is sensitive in detecting muscle inflammation, but it is not specific to a diagnosis of myositis because muscular dystrophies and other myopathies may have associated edema on MRI.[31] A muscle biopsy, however, is considered requisite to confirming a diagnosis

---

Table 24–1

Criteria for a diagnosis of juvenile dermatomyositis

1. Symmetrical weakness of the proximal musculature
2. Characteristic cutaneous changes consisting of heliotrope discoloration of the eyelids, which may be accompanied by periorbital edema and erythematous papules over the extensor surfaces of joints, including the dorsal aspects of the metacarpophalangeal and proximal interphalangeal joints, elbows, knees, or ankles (i.e., Gottron papules)
3. Elevation of the serum level of one or more of the following skeletal muscle enzymes: creatine kinase, aspartate aminotransferase, lactate dehydrogenase, and aldolase
4. Electromyographic demonstration of the characteristics of myopathy and denervation, including the triad of polyphasic, short, small motor-unit potentials; fibrillations, positive sharp waves, increased insertional irritability; and bizarre, high-frequency repetitive discharges
5. Muscle biopsy documenting histological evidence of necrosis; fiber size variation, particularly perifascicular atrophy; degeneration and regeneration; and a mononuclear inflammatory infiltrate, most often in a perivascular distribution

Adapted from Bohan A, Peter JB: Polymyositis and dermatomyositis (two parts), *N Engl J Med* 292:344-347, 403-407, 1975.

of polymyositis in the absence of the characteristic skin rashes.[32] A method for scoring muscle biopsies has been shown to be reliable and may help in standardizing biopsy readings.[33]

JDM has many similarities to inflammatory myopathies in adults but also has a number of differences (Table 24–2).[34-36] Other types of inflammatory myopathies exist in children, albeit less frequently than JDM.[37] Polymyositis (i.e., muscle inflammation without cutaneous disease)[38,39] and myositis in association with other connective tissue diseases,[40,41] such as scleroderma (see Chapter 25) and the overlap syndromes (see Chapter 27), occur in approximately 4% to 8%

of affected children.[22,37] Dermatomyositis in association with malignancy is rare in childhood,[42-45] and an evaluation for occult malignancy is only undertaken if the illness is atypical or there are other suggestions of a malignancy, such as depressed peripheral blood cell counts or a palpable mass. Other types of myositis, occurring rarely in children, include inclusion body myositis,[39,46] focal myositis,[47] orbital myositis,[48,49] and eosinophilic myositis.[50] Macrophagic myofasciitis is a newly emerging entity, with focal myositis in the deltoids or quadriceps muscles at the site of injection of aluminum-containing vaccines and a predominantly macrophagic infiltration.[51,52]

Table 24–2

Similarities and differences between juvenile and adult myositis

Factor	Similarities	Differences — Juvenile Myositis	Differences — Adult Myositis
Classification	Same clinical subgroups	JDM most common	DM approximately 30% PM, inclusion body myositis and cancer-associated myositis also common
Epidemiology Clinical features	Female predilection in both Share many clinical features	Peak age at onset 7.6 years Calcinosis, lipodystrophy, and gastrointestinal/cutaneous ulcerations more frequent	Peak age at onset 30-50 years Interstitial lung disease and myocardial involvement more frequent Adult PM and DM patients weaker than JDM and may have more severe disease activity
Autoantibodies	Share same autoantibodies and clinical features associated with autoantibody subgroups	Anti-synthetase autoantibodies less common (seen in 0-5% of juvenile patients)	Antisynthetase autoantibodies among most common, present in 20-25% of adult patients MJ not yet studied in adults, but common in JDM. Other rare autoantibodies found in adults but not yet studied in children include rare antisynthetases, SUMO, and PMS1
Immunogenetic risk factors	Share major immunogenetic risk factors, HLA DRB1*0301-DQA1*0501, as well as TNF-α -308A, PTP N22 R620W and Gm 3 23 5,13 alleles in Caucasians. Share DQA1*01 and motif DQA1 F25 as protective factors	DQA1*0301 is an additional risk factor for JDM in Caucasians Gm phenotypes as additional risk factors and HLA alleles as additional protective factors	Other cytokine polymorphisms not yet studied in adults
Pathogenesis	Share most elements of pathogenesis with adult dermatomyositis, including humoral attack on muscle capillaries, upregulation of MHC class I on myofibers, infiltration of plasmacytoid dendritic cells and type I interferon response	Increased neovascularization of capillaries, increased upregulation of MHC class I on myofibers, increased type I interferon response, especially in JDM and adult dermatomyositis compared to polymyositis.	Polymyositis is mediated primarily by CD8+ T cell attack on nonnecrotic myofibers and cytotoxic granule release resulting in myofiber destruction
Responses to treatment	Prednisone is mainstay of therapy. Agents used to treat JDM similar to adult DM and responses in children similar to adults, but of greater magnitude	Greater magnitude of response to treatment in JDM than adult DM/PM	
Outcomes	Survival and outcomes improving with increased access to immunosuppressive therapies	Lower mortality (≤ 3%), 28-41% with functional disability, 37-41% with monocyclical course	Higher mortality (10-26%) with 10-year survival 53-89%; 35-60% with functional disability; 17-20% with monocyclical course of illness

DM, dermatomyositis; JDM, juvenile dermatomyositis; MHC, major histocompatibility complex; PM, polymyositis.

EPIDEMIOLOGY

Incidence

Estimates of the incidence of JDM are given in Table 24–3.[53-57] Symmons and colleagues[54] calculated a rate of 0.19 cases per 100,000 per year for children younger than 16 years in the United Kingdom and Ireland. Mendez and colleagues[57] calculated an average annual incidence rate of 3.2 cases per 1 million children (95% confidence interval 2.5 to 4.1) for children 2 to 17 years of age diagnosed between 1995 to 1998 in the United States based on data obtained from a national registry. In general, 16% to 20% of patients with dermatomyositis have onset in childhood.[53,58] There are no direct studies of prevalence.

Age at Onset and Sex Ratio

The data of Medsger and coworkers[53] suggested a bimodal distribution of ages at myositis onset with a peak in the 5- to 14-year-old range, and a second, much larger peak in the 45- to 64-year-old range (Fig. 24–1).[53,59] Such a distinctly bimodal distribution underscores the clinical heterogeneity of this disorder and the uniqueness of the childhood form. Data from nine series derived from divergent geographical areas are illustrated in Fig. 24–2. In these pooled data, the female-to-male ratio was 1.7:1. This ratio was 2.7:1 or higher among children with onset at 10 years of age.[38,54,55,60-62] More recent data from two national registries in the United States and United Kingdom suggest a median age at onset of 7 years, with 25% of children < 4 years of age and a female to male ratio of 2.2:1[22,57] The female-to-male ratio was reversed, however, in a review of 25 Arab children.[63] In the Israeli study,[59] the ratio was 3:1 in the youngest cohort and 2:3 in the older one. The average age at onset across studies was 7 years.[11,13,29,64,65] Onset was especially common from the 4th to the 10th year, with two peak ages for girls at 6 years and another at 11 years; for boys the most common age at onset is 6 years. All the boys were younger than 10 years at onset of the disease.[54]

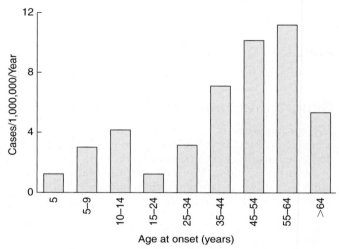

FIGURE 24–1   Incidence of inflammatory myositis.

Table 24–3			
Incidence of juvenile dermatomyositis			
Population	**Study**	**Incidence/100,000 (range)**	**Female/Male**
United States, 1970	Medsger et al[53]		
0-4 yr		0.06	3:1
5-9 yr		0.37	1:1.3
10-14 yr		0.43	4.7:1
United States, 1982	Hanissian et al[38]	0.32	
PM (n = 17)			4.7:1
JDM (n = 26)			
United States, 1990 (Pennsylvania)		0.8 (0.01-1.59)	2.5:1
White female (n = 14)		1.1 (0.01-2.19)	2.8:1
White male (n = 5)		0.4 (0-1.8)	
Black female (n = 1)		0.7 (0-1.4)	1:1
Black male (n = 1)		0.9 (0.01-1.75)	
United Kingdom and Ireland, 1995	Symmons et al[54]		5:1
PM (n = 3)			
JDM (n = 48)		0.19 (0.14-0.26)	
Finland, 1996	Kaipiainen-Seppanen et al[55]		
JDM (n = 4)		0.5	
Japan, 1997	Fujikawa et al[56]		
PM/JDM		0.16	
United States, 1995-1998	Mendez et al[57]	0.32 (0.29-0.34)	2.3:1
White		0.34	
Black		0.33	
Hispanic		0.27	

JDM, juvenile dermatomyositis; PM, polymyositis.

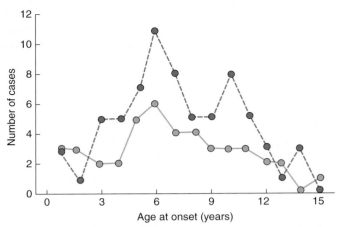

FIGURE 24–2 Age at onset for girls *(dashed line)* and boys *(solid line)*.

Geographical and Racial Distribution

Dermatomyositis is widely distributed throughout the world.[66] Striking racial differences in incidence have been described in adults in the United States, with the incidence of the disease among 55- to 64-year-old black women 10 times that of white women in the same age group.[51] Such differences are less marked in children, and in the data of Mendez and colleagues in the United States,[57] the average 4-year annual incidence rate was comparable for whites and blacks and somewhat lower for Hispanic patients.

ETIOLOGY AND PATHOGENESIS

Environmental risk factors. JDM is thought to be the result of environmental triggers in genetically susceptible individuals, leading to immune dysfunction and specific tissue responses. The potential role of environmental factors in myositis etiology is supported by reports of geographical and seasonal clustering of cases.[21,22,54,63,67,68] Seasonality in the birth distributions of JDM patients who are Hispanic, those with the human leukocyte antigen (HLA) risk factor DRB1*0301 allele, and those with the p155 autoantibody suggests that perinatal or early life exposures may be implicated in these subgroups.[69]

Evidence for the participation of infectious agents is for the most part indirect.[70] In two large cohorts, an antecedent upper respiratory infection or gastrointestinal illness frequently preceded onset of JDM symptoms within 3 months,[65,68] and in a case-control study, children with JDM more frequently reported symptoms of an antecedent illness than healthy control children.[63] Cases of infections with coxsackievirus, influenza, Group A *Streptococcus, Toxoplasmosis,* parvovirus, hepatitis B, *Borrelia,* and *Leishmania* preceding the onset of JDM have been documented.[37,72] Although acute muscle inflammation may result from viral illness, there are no unequivocal data supporting a viral cause for JDM.[73,74] Serological evidence of coxsackievirus B infection was first reported in 83% of children with early JDM, compared with 25% of control subjects,[75] but a second case-control study failed to confirm this association, and enteroviral, herpes virus,

and *Toxoplasma* titers were also not elevated.[63] A search for the presence of viral genome in affected muscle from patients with JDM using the polymerase chain reaction was negative.[76] Acute transitory myositis may occur after influenza infection.[77-84] A case-controlled study suggests elevated titers of influenza A and parainfluenza virus in affected juvenile myositis patients compared to matched controls.[85] Children with JDM have been reported to express IgG antibodies against viral non–syncytium-inducing protein, perhaps induced by persistent parvovirus B19 infection,[86] although a case-controlled study failed to reveal elevation in titers or persistent B19 viral genome in the peripheral blood or muscle of JDM patients compared to matched healthy control children.[87] Group A *Streptococcus* may be more frequent in juvenile polymyositis patients compared to healthy controls.[88] Relapse with β-hemolytic streptococcal disease may be related to molecular mimicry between the M5 protein and skeletal muscle myosin and immune responses to homologous peptide regions.[89-91]

Toxoplasma gondii was demonstrated in muscle in one patient with JDM.[92] Elevated antibody titers to *Toxoplasma* have been reported in some studies,[93,94] but appropriate controls were lacking. A dermatomyositislike disease has been described in a few children with agammaglobulinemia in association with echovirus infection[95,96] and occasionally in patients with selective immunoglobulin A (IgA) deficiency[97,98] or deficiency of the second component of complement (C2), all children in whom an inordinate susceptibility to infection might be anticipated[99] (see Chapter 37).

Electron microscopic examination of muscle has demonstrated tubuloreticular structures within endothelial cells that resembled the myxoviruslike particles identified in patients with systemic lupus erythematosus (SLE). These cytoplasmic tubular array structures are thought to indicate a type I interferon response, which could be induced by viral infections.[64,100,101] This finding, however, may be artefactual and reflect degenerative or regenerative alterations in cytoplasmic constituents of endothelial cells (Fig. 24–3).[102,103] Less information is available on noninfectious environmental exposures related to the onset of JDM. In a large North American registry of JDM patients, 38% of patients reported two or more exposures within 6 months prior to diagnosis, generally a combination of infectious and noninfectious exposures, with variation in the exposures in clinical and serological subgroups of patients.[104]. Noninfectious exposures included medications (18%), a number of which were potentially photosensitizing or myopathic, immunizations (11%), stressful life events (11%), unusual sun exposure (7%), and others including chemicals, animal contact, weight training, and dietary supplement use (< 5% each).[104] Reports of medication exposures prior to onset of juvenile myositis include statins, caine anesthetics, and growth hormone therapy, the latter which is supported by reports of improvement with dechallenge and recurrence upon rechallenge.[37] A number of other medications have been reported in association with adult myositis, including D-penicillamine, statins, zidovudine, hydroxyurea, and interferons.[105,106]

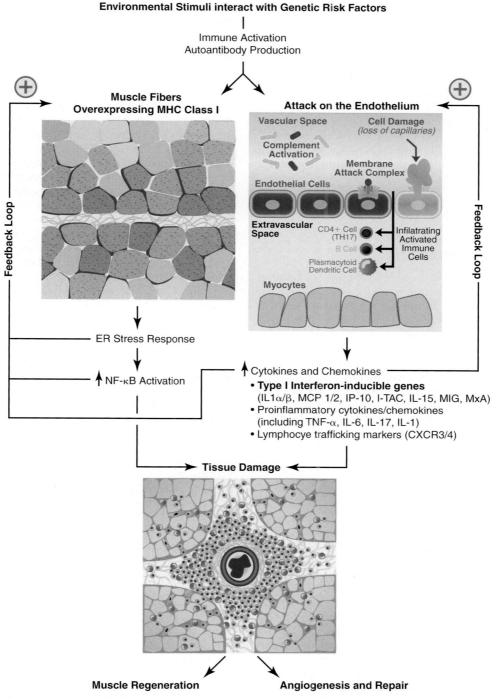

FIGURE 24–3   Key pathogenic events in juvenile dermatomyositis. Note that the initial sequence of events is uncertain and may differ from what is represented in this diagram.

Dermatomyositis has followed immunizations in case reports (e.g., hepatitis B, influenza, rubella, diphtheria, bacillus Calmette-Guérin).[107-113] Such cases are to be distinguished from macrophagic myofasciitis, a recently described condition thought to be the result of aluminium hydroxide–containing adjuvants characterized by muscle weakness at the vaccine injection site (deltoids or quadriceps) accompanied by myalgias, fatigue, arthralgias, and elevated creatine kinase and erythrocyte sedimentation rate. Children with macrophagic myofasciitis may also have hypotonia, developmental delay, and failure to thrive.[114,115] Muscle biopsy shows infiltration of macrophages and CD8+ T lymphocytes in the epimysium, perimysium, and endomysium and, on electron microscopy, presence of aluminium hydroxide in the macrophages.[116]

Although JDM patients frequently have photosensitive skin rashes and some patients anecdotally develop illness after exposure to ultraviolet light, evidence for a role of ultraviolet light in the onset of illness is largely from studies in adult patients. In worldwide population-based studies, the proportion of patients with dermatomyositis (as compared with polymyositis) was directly related to global surface ultraviolet light exposure and not to a number of other geoclimatic variables.[117,118] This association, interestingly, also was found for the proportion of patients with anti–Mi-2 autoantibodies, a DM-specific autoantibody.[117] These findings have also been confirmed in populations of U.S. adult patients, and the association with ultraviolet light is found to be stronger in females and in Caucasian patients.[119]

GENETIC BACKGROUND

Familial Dermatomyositis

There are several reports of the rare occurrence of familial JDM.[6,120-127] In all instances but one, the disease has been typical dermatomyositis. In one daughter-father pair,[122] the daughter had JDM, and the father had polymyositis with positive lupus erythematosus cell preparations. As reported by Harati and associates,[123] monozygotic twin girls developed JDM within 2 weeks of each other after upper respiratory tract infections. A brother-sister pair was reported.[128] There is an increased frequency of other autoimmune diseases in families of children with JDM and an increased frequency of homozygosity at the HLA DQA1 locus.[125]

Human Leukocyte Antigen Relationships

HLA-B*08, DRB1*0301, and DQA1*0501 are parts of an extended ancestral haplotype in the polymorphic MHC class II region that is now confirmed in several case-control studies,[129-135] and in transmission disequilibrium testing,[136] confers risk of myositis in both Caucasians children and adults in (Table 24–4). The DQA1*0301 allele is an additional risk factor for JDM, and DRB1 and DQA1 peptide-binding motifs confer additional risk.[133] The DQA1*0501/DQB1*0301 locus binds poorly to Class II–associated Ii peptide, possibly conferring susceptibility to autoimmunity through access to peptides earlier in antigen processing.[137] HLA-DPB1*0101 also confers independent risk for myositis in both adults and children.[138] The frequency of MHC class II–associated DM molecules (DMA*0103 and DMB*0102) also is increased.[139]

There also are several identified protective alleles for Caucasians, including DQA1*0201, DQA1*0101, and DQA1*0102,[133] that are less frequent in affected patients than in healthy controls and may mechanistically contribute to reduced risk of JDM through binding of self-reactive antigens and elimination of self-reactive T lymphocytes from the thymus. In African Americans, DRB1*0301-DQA1*0501 is also a risk factor,[140,141] and in a small series of Hispanic patients, DQA1*0501 was increased compared to race-matched controls.[140] DRB1*15021 may be the immunogenetic risk factor for

JDM in Japanese patients.[142] A number of distinct HLA associations occur with myositis-specific antibodies.[143,144]

Non-HLA Genetic Risk Factors

Several other polymorphic loci have been shown to be risk factors for JDM, including the cytokine genes TNF-α –308A[145,146] and -238A alleles IL-1α+4845 GT, IL-1β+3953C,[146] IL-1 receptor antagonist intronic polymorphism VNTR A1,[147] the lymphocyte signalling gene PTPN22,[148] and serological polymorphisms of the immunoglobulin heavy chain[149] (see Table 24–4). A number of these loci are potentially proinflammatory, resulting in the production of more stimulated cytokines,[146] less cytokine receptor antagonist,[147] or higher serum IgG3 levels.[149] In these patients, there is also increased production of TNF-α by peripheral blood mononuclear cells in vitro and by regenerating JDM muscle fibers in vivo.[145,150]

A polymorphism in the transcription factor interferon regulatory factor 5 appears to be increased in frequency in patients with JDM and may be associated with elevated type I interferon gene expression.[151] Mannose-binding lectin (MBL) polymorphisms, which are increased in frequency in adult DM, are associated with decreased MBL.[152] Of the cytokine and HLA associations, DRB1*0301 is the strongest risk factor and the IL-1 loci are less strongly associated.[146] It is not clear whether the presence of TNF-308A is independent of the HLA-DRB1 locus[146] or due to linkage disequilibrium with the HLA-B locus.[153]

The TNFα-308A allele is a risk factor for the development of calcinosis and ulcerations[145,146] and is also associated with a prolonged disease course.[145] The IL-1 polymorphism, -889CC, is a possible additional risk factor for the development of calcinosis,[146] as well as photosensitive skin rashes, and IL1β+3953TT is an additional possible risk factor for photosensitivity.[146] The HLA DRB1*0301 allele and other HLA risk factors have not been found to be severity factors for calcinosis, ulcerations, or a chronic course of illness.[133,146,147]

PATHOGENESIS

Most studies suggest that JDM is an autoimmune angiopathy (Fig. 24–3). Although the earliest events in JDM pathogenesis are not entirely clear, the immune attack on muscle capillary endothelium, infiltration of plasmacytoid dendritic cells with a resulting type I interferon response, and upregulation of major histocompatibility (MHC) class I expression on the surface of myofibers appear to be central events, and limited data suggest several of these may be early events. Pathogenic aspects of JDM are largely identical to those of adult dermatomyositis,[154-156] except that these central events of pathogenesis, including the vasculopathy, type I interferon response, and upregulation of MHC class I, appear to be more prominent in JDM.[157,158] Evidence for apoptotic muscle has also not been seen in adult myositis,[159] and microchimerism has not been well studied in adults. Polymyositis, in contrast, is largely a CD8+ T cell– and myeloid dendritic cell–mediated attack on nonnecrotic myofibers, with

Table 24–4

Immunogenetic risk and protective factors for juvenile dermatomyositis

Chromosome	Allele or Binding Motif	Odds Ratio	Comments	References
Risk Factors in Caucasians				
6p21.31	DRB1*0301	3.9	Strongest HLA risk factors in MHC class II region, part of ancestral haplotype (B*08, DRB1*0301, DQA1*0501), also seen in adult DM and PM	156,133,134
6p21.31	DRB1 [9]EYSTS[13]	2.0	Also seen in adult DM and PM	133
6p21.31	DQA1*0501	2.1	Linked to HLA, DRB1*0301, also seen in adult DM and PM	157,158,133,134
6p21.31	DQA1*0301	2.8	Independent of DRB1*0301 DQA1*0501	133
6p21.31	B*08		Linked to HLA DRB1*0301, DQA1*0501	133
6p21.31	DPB1*0101		Also seen in adult DM and PM	138
6p21.3	DMA*0103, DMB*0102			139
6p21.3	TNFα-308A	3.8	Not clear whether independent or in linkage disequilibrium with DRB1*0301, also seen in adult DM and PM	146
6p21.3	TNFα-238GG	3.5	In linkage disequilibrium with TNFα-308A	146
1p13.2	PTPN22 R620W		Also seen in adult DM and PM	148
2q13	IL1RN VNTR A1	2.5		147
2q13	IL1α+4845TT	2.2		146
2q13	IL1β+3953T	1.7		146
14q32.33	GM 13	3.9		149
14q32.33	Gm 1,3,17 5,13,21	2.2		149
14q32.33	Gm 3 23 5,13	2.2	Also seen in adult DM	149
Risk Factors in Other Racial Groups				
6p21.31	DRB1*0301, DQA1*0501	3.9	Associated in African American patients	140, 141
6p21.31	DRB1*15021		Associated in Japanese patients	142
14q32.22	GM 13	4.8	Associated in African American patients	149
2p12	KM 1,1	4.8	Associated in African American patients	149
Protective Factors in Caucasians				
6p21.31	DQA1*0101, *0102, *0201	0.37 – 0.51	DQ1*01 also a protective factor for adult DM	133
6p21.31	DQA1 F[25], S[26], [45](V/A) W(R/K)[47]	0.26– 0.46	F[25] also a protective factor for adult DM	133
6p21.3	TNF-α-308GG	0.26		146
6p21.3	TNF-α-238A	0.29	In linkage disequilibrium with TNF-α-308	146
2q13	IL1α+4845G	0.46		146
2q13	IL1β+3953CC	0.59		146
Severity Factors in Caucasians				
6p21.3	TNF-α-308A	7.0 – 7.3	Associated with chronic illness course, calcinosis, cutaneous and gastrointestinal ulcerations	145, 146
2q13	IL1α-889CC	2.4	Possible risk factor for calcinosis	146
2q13	IL1α-889CC, IL1β+3953TT	2.6 – 9.7	Possible risk factors for photosensitive skin rashes	146

DM, dermatomyositis; JDM, juvenile dermatomyositis; MHC, major histocompatibility complex; PM, polymyositis.

release of cytotoxic perforin and granzyme B granules that mediate muscle cell death.[160-162] Polymyositis does not share a prominent interferon response in the muscle or serum, and infiltrating dendritic cells are myeloid not plasmacytoid.[101,163]

An immune complex–mediated vasculopathy may be an important initiating or perpetuating event.[156,164-168] Complement activation and immune complex deposition have been demonstrated.[167,169] Whitaker and Engel[164] identified immunoglobulin and complement in vessel walls of skeletal muscle in juvenile and adult dermatomyositis, although the frequency and intensity of deposition were more pronounced in children. Immunoglobulin (Ig) G, IgM, the third component of complement (C3), and the membrane attack complex were deposited alone or in combination in this study and others.[166] Capillary loss and membrane attack deposition in the muscle appears to occur early, even prior to other histological changes.[157,168] Angiostatic ELR- CXC chemokines, including IP-10 (CXCL10), monokine induced by γ-interferon (MIG/CXCL9), and interferon γ–inducible T cell α chemoattractant (I-TAC/CXCL11), are expressed at high levels in untreated biopsy specimens, correlating with the degree of capillary loss and mononuclear cell infiltration.[170] Neovascularization of capillaries may then occur later, and this also appears to be of greater intensity in JDM compared to adult dermatomyositis muscle.[171] Both angiogenic and antiangiogenic genes are expressed in juvenile and adult dermatomyositis muscle,[171,172] including leukocyte adhesion molecules that participate in both leukocyte trafficking and angiogenesis.[171] ICAM-1 is selectively upregulated on the capillaries and perimysial large vessels of JDM muscle,[173] compared to adult dermatomyositis and polymyositis.[174] Elevated plasma levels of factor VIII–related antigen,[175] fibrinopeptide A, and C3 provide additional evidence of endothelial cell injury. Some data suggest that increased circulating concentrations of thrombospondin-1, a potent antiangiogenic factor, may play a role in susceptibility to vascular thrombosis in JDM.[176]

Another central, early event in pathogenesis appears to be the upregulation of MHC Class I on the cell surface of muscle fibers, which may also occur prior to the detection of cellular infiltrates.[158,177,178] Normal muscle cells do not express MHC class I antigens, but in dermatomyositis, these antigens are strongly expressed.[158,179-181] This is also evidenced in a transgenic mouse model in which overexpression of MHC class I itself leads to the induction of polymyositis, although the infiltrate is predominantly macrophages.[182] Upregulation of MHC class I on myofibers is associated with the endoplasmic reticulum stress response, the unfolded protein response, and activation of the NF-κB pathway, which can lead to muscle damage.[177]

Following the initial vasculopathy and upregulation of MHC class I on myofibers, a perivascular and perimysial infiltration of predominantly plasmacytoid dendritic cells likely results, accompanied by CD4+ T lymphocytes, including TH-17 cells, B cells, and macrophages.[156,171,183,184] The plasmacytoid dendritic cells and T cells undergo local maturation and develop memory responses locally in extranodal lymphoid follicular structures.[183,185] The predominance of activated plasmacytoid dendritic cells in these lesions results in a characteristic type I interferon response with upregulation of a large number of interferon-regulated genes and chemokines.[70,172,186] Type I interferon–inducible genes are also upregulated in the peripheral blood and correlate with disease activity, perhaps more in the muscle than skin.[186-188] The type I interferon response may perpetuate these processes, leading to upregulation of MHC class I on myofibers, T cell survival, and induction of proinflammatory cytokines and chemokines, including MIG/CXCL9, I-TAC/CXCL11, macrophage inflammatory protein (MIP), monocyte chemoattractant protein (MCP)-1 and MCP-2, that play a role in recruitment of lymphocytes to sites of inflammation and in angiostasis.[156,188] Production of other proinflammatory cytokines and chemokines, including tumor necrosis factor-α (TNF-α) and interleukin-1α (IL-1α) and IL-1β, are also prominently expressed by infiltrating inflammatory cells and by myofibers (TNF-α)[189] and endothelial cells (IL-1α).[190]

Involvement of T cells is apparent through the expression of T helper type 17 (Th17) cells, a subset of CD4+ T lymphocytes. The involvement of Th17 cells also appears to lead to induction of IL-6 and IL-17, which also correlate with the interferon response and with active disease.[188] In a small number of patients, CD8+ T lymphocytes with unique Vβ repertoires were present in the inflammatory infiltrates of muscle, particularly around blood vessels well as peripheral blood, suggesting oligoclonal expansion.[191] Cell-mediated immunity to muscle antigens (i.e., activated T cells) may participate in pathogenesis. Muscle biopsies from JDM patients demonstrate upregulation of heat-shock protein 60 (HSP60), as well as induction of T cell proliferation and production of cytokines in response to HSP60 in the muscle and periphery.[192] Peripheral blood mononuclear cells from JDM patients also demonstrate increased cytotoxicity to potential self-peptides, including the M5 protein of group A streptococcus and human myosin.[91] Response of patients' lymphocytes in vitro to allogeneic or autologous muscle extracts has been described in some reports[193-195] but not all.[196] Some reports have described a cytotoxic effect on muscle monolayers in culture by lymphocytes,[197-202] although the effect has not been reported uniformly.[203] In one study, peripheral blood lymphocytes from four of five children with active disease produced a lymphotoxin that caused necrosis or impaired protein synthesis in monolayers of human fetal muscle in the presence of homogenates of autologous muscle.[198]

Dysregulation of apoptosis in myofibrils may be operative in pathogenesis, as suggested by the observation of overexpression of BCL2 protein in muscle specimens from children with this disease,[204] as well as the expression of TUNEL-positive myonuclei and caspase 3 within the laminin layer.[205]

The role of myositis-specific autoantibodies in disease pathogenesis is unclear, but hints are beginning to emerge. These autoantibodies, specific to patients with myositis, are present prior to the onset of clinical illness, undergo affinity maturation, and may become undetectable when disease enters remission.[206,207] Some of the autoantigens associated with myositis-specific autoantibodies are upregulated in regenerating myoblasts[208] and are cleaved by granzyme B, perhaps resulting in their cell surface expression.[209] They may also have a role in initiating or propagating pathogenic events. Serum from patients with anti-histidyl tRNA synthetase (Jo-1) in the presence of RNA and necrotic material induces type I interferon production and activation of plasmacytoid dendritic cells in muscle tissue,[210] and Jo-1 positive sera also upregulate ICAM-1 expression on lung endothelial cells.[211] Histidyl-tRNA synthetase and asparaginyl-tRNA synthetase are chemotactic for CC chemokine receptor 5 (CCR5)– and CCR3-expressing leukocytes, and in high concentrations induce dendritic cell maturation.[212] Ultraviolet light also upregulates the expression of Mi-2 autoantigen in cell cultures.[213]

Maternal cell chimerism is present in more than 70% of peripheral blood T cells and in muscle tissue in 80% to 90% of children with JDM.[214-217] It was identified in 25% of siblings and 15% of controls in these reports. The phenotypes of the microchimeric cells include B cells and plasmacytoid dendritic cells in the muscle.[184] HLA alleles may control the frequency and potential pathogenic mechanisms of this phenomenon. Reed and colleagues[216] assessed immunological activity in chimeric cells in 60 of 72 children with JDM, in 11 of 48 unaffected siblings, and in 5 of 29 healthy controls. In all groups, chimerism was associated with the maternal HLA-DQA1*0501 allele. Maternal chimeric cells may be autoreactive against the JDM child's cells, producing interferon-γ and a memory T cell response.[216] The HLA maternal genotype influences the fate of the transferred cells and activation of the chimeric cells.

Animal Models

Dermatomyositis- and polymyositis-like diseases have been described in household dogs.[218,219] A familial form of canine dermatomyositis in Collies and Shetland sheep dogs is very similar to human disease, including the presence of skin rashes and vasculopathy.[218-222]

In experimental animal models, antigen-induced models of myositis involve the injection of muscle antigens, including muscle homogenates, purified muscle antigens, viruses, drugs, and DNA constructs, often with an adjuvant to boost the immune response. Recent models of experimental autoimmune myositis include immunization of native C-protein or recombinant skeletal C-protein fragment 2 with complete Freund's adjuvant (CFA) and pertussis toxin into Lewis rats or C57BL6 mice,[223,224] injection of myosin or myosin B with CFA and pertussis toxin into C57BL6, SJL/J or BALB/c mice,[225-227] and immunization of laminin, a muscle structural protein, into rats.[228] Historical animal models of experimental myositis include the induction of myositis by the injection of muscle homogenates in CFA in guinea pigs,[229] rabbits,[230] and rats.[231] Although this disorder was different from JDM, cell-mediated immunity to muscle was detected, and the disease could be transferred by lymphocytes.[232-234]

Experimental induction of a polymyositis like syndrome in neonatal animals has been reported after inoculation of mice with picornaviruses, including coxsackievirus[235-237] and encephalomyocarditis virus.[238] Other viral models include injection of influenza B into juvenile Balb/c mice,[239] as well as infection of mice with the alphaviruse Semliki Forest virus[240] and Ross River virus[241] and rhesus monkeys with retrovirus.[242]

A mouse model of antisynthetase syndrome has been developed by immunization of the murine form of histidyl tRNA synthetase into congenic C57BL/6 or NOD mice. These mice develop clinical features similar to those found in human disease with both lung and muscle inflammation.[181]

Overexpression of class I MHC on the surface of muscle cells in transgenic mice induces muscle inflammation with a macrophagic predominance and a clinical syndrome consistent with polymyositis, including the generation of histidyl-tRNA synthetase autoantibodies in some animals.[243] Overexpression of class I MHC in young mice leads to more rapid and severe muscle weakness and pathological changes, paralleled by a more dramatic and rapid upregulation of a number of genes involved in the endoplasmic reticulum stress response and a decrease in muscle structural genes.[244] A knockout model of myositis involving deletion of suppressor of cytokine signaling-1 (SOCS-1) in mice heterozygous for interferon-γ leads to polymyositis and fatal myocarditis.[245] Cytolytic T lymphocyte–associated antigen (CTLA-4) and transforming growth factor-β knockout mice also develop multifocal inflammation, including involvement of skeletal muscle.[246,247]

PATHOGENESIS OF CALCINOSIS

Studies of the mineral composition of surgically removed calcinosis samples reveal the mineral to be calcium hydroxyappatite or carbonate appatite, with a smaller degree of magnesium also present, which is a mineralization inhibitor. Calcinosis is distinct from bone in its mineral composition and matrix.[248-250] The mineral appears to be deposited in fragments and over time becomes solid.[248,250] Immunohistochemistry reveals a number of SIBLING proteins, including osteocalcin, osteopontin, and matrix gla protein, that promote and inhibit mineralization within the lesions, as well as osteoclasts at the periphery of the lesions that are secondarily infiltrating in an attempt to resolve the calcification.[251] Matrix gla protein, a calcification inhibitor, is expressed at sites of muscle damage and by infiltrating macrophages in the muscle tissue of JDM patients, as well as in the muscle tissue of patients with adult myositis and childhood muscular dystrophies, whereas only phosphorylated matrix gla protein is increased in biopsies of JDM patients who developed calcinosis.[251A] Osteopontin and TNF–α receptor knockout mice on a C57B6 background injected with cardiotoxin in skeletal muscle develop dystrophic calcifications resembling human calcinosis in mineral composition, although these lesions spontaneously resolve.[252]

CLINICAL MANIFESTATIONS

Classic JDM manifest with an insidious progression of malaise, easy fatigue, muscle weakness, fever, and rash that may predate diagnosis by 3 to 6 months (Table 24–5).[10-13,21,22,24,25,27,253-264] There is, however, great variation in the rapidity of evolution of the clinical manifestations. Onset is usually insidious, with development of progressive muscle weakness and pain; a more acute onset occurs in approximately one third of children. Children with myositis-specific and myositis-associated autoantibodies characteristically present with phenotypically distinct disease.[265]

Constitutional Signs and Symptoms

The onset of JDM is often characterized by fever in the range of 38º C to 40º C. An affected child often complains of ease of fatigue, which probably represents muscle weakness. Malaise, anorexia, and weight loss follow. Parents may report that the child had become irritable,

Table 24–5

Frequency of manifestations of juvenile dermatomyositis at onset

Manifestation	Frequency (%)
Easy fatigue	80-100
Malar/facial rash	42-98
Progressive proximal muscle weakness	82-96
Classic rash (heliotrope or Gottron papules)	35-91
Periungual nailfold capillary changes	80-91
Muscle pain or tenderness	25-73
Lymphadenopathy	8-75
Arthralgias	25-66
Fever	16-65
Arthritis	10-65
Dysphagia or dysphonia	17-44
Dyspnea	5-43
Gastrointestinal symptoms	5-37
Edema	11-32
Joint contractures	9-27
Cutaneous ulceration	6-23
Calcinosis	3-23
Hepatomegaly	3-20
Anorexia	18
Splenomegaly	10-15
Nonspecific rash	10-15
Gingivitis	6

Adopted from references 21, 22, 25, 27, 264.

with alterations in gross motor function or regression of motor milestones.

Musculoskeletal Disease

Muscle weakness at onset is predominantly proximal, and complaints related to weakness of the limb girdle musculature of the lower extremities are most common. Weakness of the anterior neck flexors, back, and abdominal muscles leads to inability to hold the head upright or maintain a sitting posture and protrusion of the abdomen. The child may stop walking, be unable to dress or climb stairs, or wash the face or comb hair. The affected child may also complain of moderate muscle pain or stiffness.

Physical examination demonstrates symmetrical weakness that is most pronounced in the proximal muscles of the shoulders and hips, in the neck flexors, and in abdominal musculature.[266] The overlying subcutaneous tissue of affected muscles is occasionally edematous and indurated, and the muscles may be tender. Functional muscle examination may demonstrate that the child is unable to arise from a supine position without rolling over, move from sitting to standing, get out of bed without assistance, or squat or rise from a squatting position without help. *Gowers sign* is often present. The child with weakness of the pelvic girdle musculature has difficulty climbing or descending stairs. The *Trendelenburg sign* indicates weakness of the hip abductors. Later in the disease or in children with an especially severe course, the distal muscles of the extremities may become involved. Occasionally, the disease is so severe that the child is unable to rise from

bed or move at all. Although not as clinically dramatic, the distal muscles of the extremities are involved in many patients.[266] Although muscle weakness may be impressive, the deep tendon reflexes are usually preserved.

Pharyngeal, hypopharyngeal, and palatal muscles are frequently affected. Difficulty swallowing may be related to this involvement or to esophageal hypomotility.[267] Dysphonia (weakness of the voice or a gurgly voice quality) and nasal speech are also frequent signs.[268] Regurgitation of liquids through the nose may be a sign of impending difficulties. The threat of aspiration is increased in these children. Subtle or even asymptomatic dysfunctional swallowing can be demonstrated on barium swallow in up to 80%.[21,269]

Sequential muscle strength examinations including proximal, axial, and distal muscle groups by an experienced physician or physical therapist should be recorded using a standard scale.[266,270,271] The importance of this examination becomes even more critical later in the course of the disease, when serum levels of muscle enzymes may be less dependable indicators of disease activity. Select muscle groups that should generally be evaluated are the neck flexors; shoulder abductors; elbow flexors and extensors; hip flexors, extensors, adductors, and abductors; and knee flexors and extensors. An abbreviated group of muscles that includes neck flexors, deltoids, biceps, wrist extensors, gluteus maximus and medius, quadriceps, and ankle plantar flexors closely approximates a total set of 24 muscles.[272] Assessment of function can also be documented with the Childhood Myositis Assessment Scale, the Childhood Health Assessment Questionnaire, or the Disease Activity Scale (includes skin assessment), which demonstrate decreased endurance and physical dysfunction.[273-278] These and other validated myositis assessment tools, including associated training documents, presentations, and videotapes, are available on the International Myositis Assessment and Clinical Studies Group internet site.[279]

Aerobic and anaerobic exercise capacity is reduced in these patients[280] and correlates with parameters of disease activity, abnormalities on T1-weighted MRI, and disease duration.[281-283]

Some children with JDM have arthralgia or subtle arthritis that is transient and nondeforming, sometimes accompanied by tenosynovitis or flexor nodules. Reports document the presence of arthritis in 35% of 79 children with JDM.[284] Another study identified oligoarthritis in 67% and polyarthritis in 33% of 80 children,[285] frequencies that are much higher than was previously appreciated. Early development of flexion contractures, particularly at the knees, hips, shoulders, elbows, ankles, and wrists, is common and usually represents the effects of myofascial inflammation rather than synovitis. The presence of significant, persistent arthritis in a child with myositis and the skin changes of dermatomyositis also suggests the possibility of an overlap syndrome such as mixed connective tissue disease.

Mucocutaneous Disease

In more than three fourths of the children, the cutaneous abnormalities are pathognomonic of the disease at presentation; a less characteristic rash occurs in the remainder. Often, dermatitis is the first manifestation of the disorder, although asymptomatic (undiagnosed) muscle weakness often occurs in such children. More often, the cutaneous abnormalities become evident in the first few weeks simultaneously with or after the onset of muscle symptoms.[21,22] The three most typical cutaneous manifestations are heliotrope discoloration of the upper eyelids, Gottron papules, and periungual erythema and capillary loop abnormalities.[286] The classic heliotrope rash occurs over the upper eyelids as a violaceous, reddish purple suffusion that often is associated with a malar rash that resembles that of SLE in its distribution but is less well demarcated (Fig. 24–4). Edema of the eyelids and face often accompanies the heliotrope and may be extensive.

The symmetrical changes over the extensor surfaces of joints (i.e., Gottron papules) tend to be associated with shiny, erythematous, scaly plaques (Fig. 24–5). These hypertrophic areas of skin have a bright pink-red appearance. Occasionally, the lesions appear to be thickened and pale early in disease and may represent ischemia as a result of vasculopathy. Gottron papules are especially common over the proximal interphalangeal joints of the hands and less so over the metacarpalphalangeal and distal interphalangeal joints. The skin over the toes is rarely affected. The extensor surfaces of the elbows and knees and, less frequently, the malleoli may also be involved. Characteristic abnormalities of the periungual skin and capillary bed are present in 50% to 100% of JDM patients. The periungual skin is often intensely erythematous, and careful examination with the naked eye,

the 40× lens of an ophthalmoscope as a magnification aid, or a DermLite™ documents the presence of telangiectasias.[287] Dilatation of isolated loops, thrombosis and hemorrhage (often visible), dropout of surrounding vessels,[284] tortuosity, bushy loop formation, and arborized clusters of giant capillary loops are distinctive, if not pathognomonic, for JDM (Fig. 24–6). There is often associated marked cuticular overgrowth. Similar changes occur in other connective tissue diseases,[288] but are seldom as dramatic as those seen in the child with JDM. These abnormalities, like the noninflammatory vasculopathy, correlate with skin disease activity, a longer duration of untreated symptoms, a more severe chronic disease course, cutaneous ulceration, or the development of calcinosis.[278,289-292] The acute nailfold abnormalities may abate and the capillaries may regenerate in patients who experience remission or a unicyclic disease course.[293] Cuticular overgrowth, associated with thickening, hyperkeratosis, and subungual hemorrhage, is a sign of active disease.[281,290,294]

Cutaneous involvement can vary from the slightest erythematous tinge over the knuckles or eyelids to a generalized pruritic, scaly rash. At onset, edema and induration of skin, periorbital regions, and subcutaneous tissues are common; less frequently, the extremities and trunk are affected and severe edema or anasarca is an indicator of severe disease activity.[23,294-296] Rashes may be photodistributed, including malar, facial erythema, V- and shawl-sign rashes, and linear extensor erythema, or they may involve non–sun-exposed skin.[286] Scalp dermatitis, which may be misdiagnosed as seborrhea or psoriasis, has been

FIGURE 24–4 A, Heliotrope discoloration and violaceous suffusion with edema of the upper eyelids in an 11-year-old with acute dermatomyositis. **B,** Erythematous, scaly rash in a malar distribution.

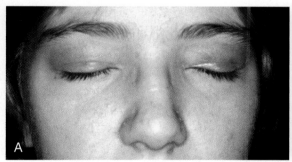
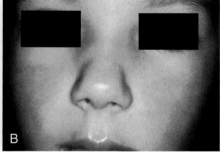

FIGURE 24–5 A, Gottron papules. **B,** Symmetrical, scaly, erythematous papules over the metacarpophalangeal and proximal interphalangeal joints of the hand of an 8-year-old girl (see color insert). **C,** Gottron papules over the proximal interphalangeal joints of the hand in a teenage girl. Note the central porcelain white infarcts, likely the result of vasculopathy.

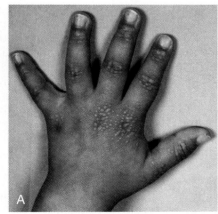
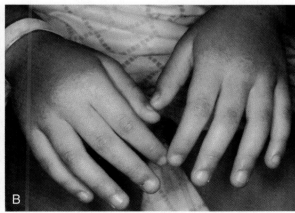

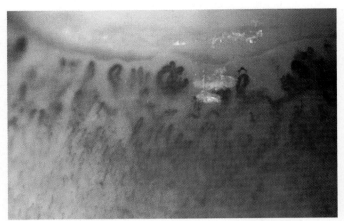

FIGURE 24–6   Advanced changes of the nailfold capillaries, with gross thickening and dropout areas in a child with dermatomyositis. (Courtesy of Dr. Jay Kenik.)

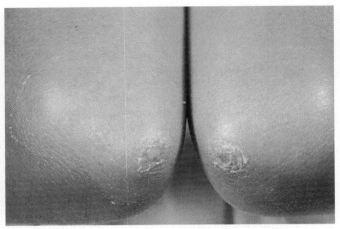

FIGURE 24–7   Acute ulcerations over the olecranon processes in a ⅕-year-old boy with dermatomyositis.

observed in up to 25% of patients.[23] Rashes may also be intradermal, or include panniculitis, with inflammation in the subcutaneous tissue, which may also be the result of an opportunistic infection.[294,296,297] Photosensitivity occurs in up to 50% of patients.[27,257,298,299] Sun exposure has been associated with onset of the disease and exacerbations.[101,119] Gingival and buccal ulcerations develop in 10% to 46% of children and are associated with pain on swallowing.[298,300-302] Oral ulcers may precede or accompany the onset of the disease, and components of the sicca syndrome may be present.

Cutaneous ulceration occurred relatively frequently in the series of Crowe and coworkers[64] and in up to 30% of patients more recently.[22,25,27,294,303] It was associated with severe and prolonged disease in 11 of 42 patients.[64] Vasculitic ulcers at the corners of the eyes, in the axillae, over the elbows or pressure points, and over stretch marks may become a serious problem in management (Figs. 24–7 and 24–8). Children with a generalized rash and cutaneous ulcerations may have the poorest prognosis,[64,304] but this is not always the case.[305]

Late in the course, other cutaneous and subcutaneous changes occur. Thinning and atrophy of the skin and supporting structures may supervene, and alterations in pigmentation become more common. Although individual lesions may be hypopigmented, the child may exhibit generalized hyperpigmentation. Hyperkeratosis is relatively common and may occur in unusual areas such as the palms and the soles and the infrapatellar area.[306,307]

Several tools for assessment of skin disease in JDM have been developed and partially validated, including the Cutaneous Assessment Tool, which comprehensively assesses skin activity and damage,[298,307,308] and the Disease Activity Score, which includes assessment of skin involvement, particularly the vasculopathic manifestations.[275,278] Several tools to assess skin disease in adult DM have also been proposed including the Dermatomyositis Skin Severity Index and the Cutaneous Dermatomyositis Disease Area and Severity Index.[309,310]

Dermatomyositis sine myositis or *amyopathic dermatomyositis* is rare in children,[311-316] although the classic rash of JDM may occur in the absence of clinical muscle

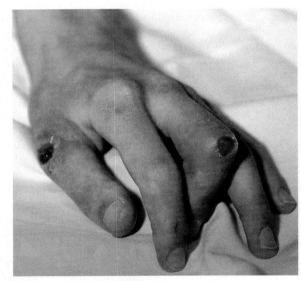

FIGURE 24–8   Vasculitic ulcers on the knuckles of a young boy with severe dermatomyositis. These open ulcerations led to a *Staphylococcus aureus* bacteremia and endocarditis.

involvement[314] or muscle disease may not be initially documented.[317] Do these children eventually develop overt myositis if followed for long enough? In the review by Plamondon and Dent,[317] none of 27 patients developed clinical myopathy at a mean follow-up of 32.8 months, although 2 patients developed calcinosis. In another large series, 18 of 68 patients with juvenile-onset clinical amyopathic DM (26%) evolved to classic JDM after a mean follow-up of 3.9 years.[318] Of patients with a normal serum level of creatine kinase (CK), 3 of 22 patients tested had an abnormal electromyography, 1 of 19 had abnormal muscle biopsy, and 1 of 9 had abnormal MRI. Calcinosis developed in 3 of the 68 patients.[318] In contrast to adult amyopathic dermatomyositis, interstitial lung disease or internal malignancy has not been reported to be associated in the childhood cases of amyopathic DM, suggesting a relatively good prognosis for children.[317,318] Metabolic abnormalities unmasked by exercise as detected by P-31 magnetic resonance spectroscopy—when there is normal muscle strength and serum levels of muscle enzymes and standard MRI—is another sensitive method for detection of muscle abnormalities in patients with amyopathic DM.[319]

Calcinosis

Dystrophic calcification occurs in 12% to 43% of children, sometimes within 6 months of onset but rarely before symptomatic myosis.[25,130,320-322] Calcinosis is less frequently present at diagnosis, reported in only 3% to 23% of patients.[21,22,25] Calcium deposition may occur in subcutaneous plaques or nodules (Table 24–6) (Fig. 24–9), as large tumorous deposits in muscle groups (Fig. 24–10), as calcification within fascial planes, bridging joints, or as an extensive subcutaneous exoskeleton (Fig. 24–11).[304,323] Calcinosis affecting the subcutaneous tissues can result in an accompanying cellulitis that may be difficult to distinguish from a true infection, as well as in painful superficial ulceration of the overlying skin with recurrent extrusion of small flecks or liquefied calcium salts. Calcinosis crossing joint margins may result in flexion contractures, and those lesions entrapping nerves may result in severe pain.[324] These deposits may slowly resolve with time. If deposition is extreme in subcutaneous tissues, along fascial planes, and within muscles, the child may literally be encased within a exoskeleton shell of calcium salts. This type of calcinosis is unlikely to resolve, and results in severe disability. Risk factors for calcinosis include delay to diagnosis and the duration of untreated disease, duration of active disease, inadequate therapy, underlying cardiac or pulmonary disease, and the need for corticosteroid-sparing immunosuppressive therapy, which may be an indicator of severe disease activity.[320,321,325,326] Proinflammatory cytokine polymorphisms of TNF-α and IL-1α are also risk factors for the development of calcinosis.[145,146] Aggressive treatment to achieve rapid and complete control of inflammation, especially early after onset, may minimize calcinosis.[321,327,328]

Vasculopathy

Visceral vasculopathy occurs in a minority of children, usually soon after onset of the disorder, but may also occur later in the illness course.[329] It signifies a poor prognosis and sometimes rapidly leads to death.[29,64,330] This complication is characterized by diffuse, severe, progressive abdominal pain, melena, and hematemesis, which represent vasculopathy of the mucosa of the gastrointestinal tract with resulting tissue ischemia or an acute mesenteric infarction.[331-335] Free intraperitoneal air radiographically indicates the presence of a perforation of the gastrointestinal tract. Multiple perforations of the duodenum are particularly difficult to recognize and may recur.[331,333-335] Vasculitis of the gallbladder, urinary bladder, uterus, vagina, and testes can also occur.[64,336] Anasarca, cholestasis, pancreatitis, hepatitis, and pneumatosis intestinalis have been reported.[294,295,296,337-339] Widespread vascular disease can involve the central and peripheral nervous systems,[64,340] but severe central nervous system involvement is rare.[341,342] Retinal vessel vasculopathy manifesting as cotton-wool spots has been rarely reported.[343]

Table 24–6

Forms of dystrophic calcification

Form	Frequency (%)
Superficial plaques or nodules, usually on the extremities	33
Deep, large, tumorous deposits, generally in the proximal muscles (i.e., calcinosis circumscripta)	20
Intermuscular fascial plane deposition (i.e., calcinosis universalis)	16
Severe, subcutaneous, reticular exoskeleton-like deposits	10
Mixed forms: superficial plaques or nodules, tumorous deposits, intermuscular fascial plane deposition	22

Adapted from reference 304.

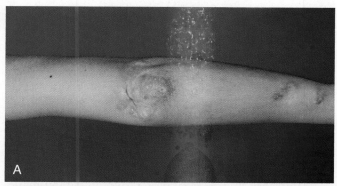
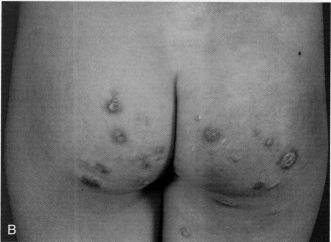

FIGURE 24–9 A, Subcutaneous calcification overlying the elbow, resulting in a flexion contracture, and distal forearm in a 10-year-old girl who had had juvenile dermatomyositis since age 2. **B,** Superficial plaques of calcinosis overlying the buttocks in the same child.

Cardiopulmonary Disease

The most frequently detected cardiac abnormality is nonspecific sinus tachycardia, but murmurs and cardiomegaly with or without electrocardiographic changes may also be seen.[95] Pericarditis has also been described. Serious cardiac involvement (e.g., acute myocarditis, conduction defects, first-degree heart block) is rare but has

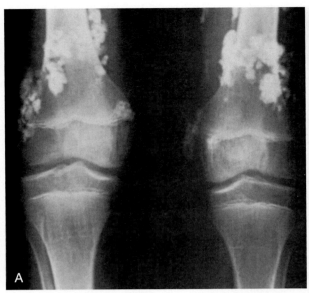
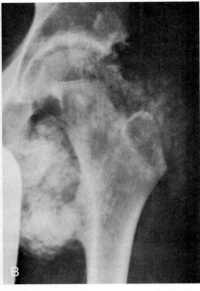

FIGURE 24–10 A, Calcinosis circumscripta can be identified in the supracondylar areas of the knees. **B,** Massive tumorous calcium deposits developed unilaterally around the hip in a 7-year-old boy with the onset of dermatomyositis when he was 3 years old.

been associated with death, and onset may be delayed until years after the initial diagnosis.[64,95] Radioisotopic studies suggest that subclinical involvement of cardiac muscle may be more common than has been appreciated.[344] Hypertension can occur in 25% to 50% of patients, may be severe, and is sometimes associated with or exacerbated by glucocorticoid therapy.[64,345] Raynaud phenomenon is unusual but has been diagnosed in 2% to 15% of patients.[25,64,260]

Respiratory muscle weakness results in symptomatic, restrictive pulmonary disease in most children who are moderately to severely affected. However, asymptomatic pulmonary involvement may occur in up to 50% of children.[346] Interstitial pneumonitis is rare and may be refractory to treatment.[339,347,348] Serum KL-6 levels are elevated in patients with interstitial lung disease, and this may be an early marker.[349,350] Pneumothorax and pneumomediastinum may also rarely occur, presumably due to vasculopathy.[351,352]

Lipodystrophy and Metabolic Abnormalities

Lipodystrophy is a clinically heterogeneous disorder that occurs in acquired and inherited forms.[353] The association of acquired lipodystrophy with JDM may be more common than often appreciated (7% to 50%).[57,354-360] This disorder may be generalized, partial (with fat loss from the extremities), or focal (with a localized fat loss, particularly overlying sites of calcinosis).[358,361] It is characterized by a slow but progressive loss of subcutaneous and visceral fat, often most noticeable over the upper body and face, that is accompanied most frequently by hypertriglyceridemia, as well as by insulin resistance, abnormal glucose tolerance, acanthosis nigricans, hypertension, and nonalcoholic steatohepatitis, with more severe metabolic sequelae and features related to the degree of fat loss (Fig. 24–12).[357-359,362] Patients with generalized lipodystrophy also frequently have hyperandrogenism, with

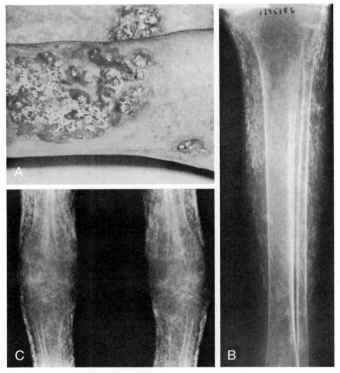

FIGURE 24–11 A, Calcinosis universalis developed in a 15-year-old girl with diffuse cutaneous ulcerations over the legs. Spicules of calcium salts were constantly extruded from these lesions. **B,** Interfascial deposition of calcium salts occurred during the healing phases in the leg of a child with dermatomyositis. **C,** Radiograph of a 12-year-old girl who had the onset of acute, unremitting dermatomyositis at age 10, shows extensive radioopaque deposits of calcium salts throughout the interfascial planes of the musculature of the entire body.

hypertrichosis, hyperpigmentation, clitoral enlargement, and amenorrhea. Pope and colleagues reported that JDM is the most common systemic autoimmune disease associated with lipodystrophy.[357] Lipodystrophy is most often delayed in presentation until several years after onset of

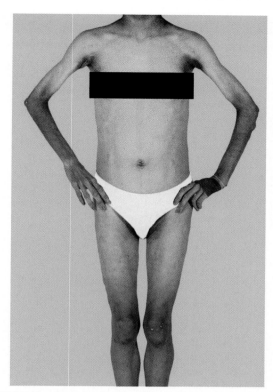

FIGURE 24–12 Generalized lipodystrophy in a teenage girl with longstanding juvenile dermatomyositis. Note loss of body fat from both the extremities and trunk. There is prominent acanthosis nigricans under the axilla and in the neck line. There is generalized hyperpigmentation due to secondary hyperandrogenism. Also note the subcutaneous calcinosis, which is associated with lipodystrophy in juvenile dermatomyositis.

JDM, and duration of untreated disease may be a risk factor for its development.[360] Calcinosis, muscle atrophy, joint contractures, facial rash, greater skin disease activity, and decreased density of periungual nailfold capillaries are the JDM disease features found to be associated with development of lipodystrophy.[358,360] Panniculitis has been associated with focal lipoatrophy while the anti-p155 autoantibody, a newly described myositis-associated autoantibody, is increased in frequency in patients with generalized lipodystrophy.[358] In addition to the metabolic sequelae, loss of fat from the lateral more than medial thigh, on MRI of the thigh muscles, may be an indicator.[358] The etiology of acquired lipodystrophy in patients with JDM remains unclear and does not appear to be related to HLA or TNF alleles, lamin mutations, or complement deficiencies.[358]

Metabolic sequelae in the absence of lipodystrophy are also frequent in patients with JDM, especially in patients with chronic disease. Insulin resistance, hyperlipidemia, hypertension, and an increased body mass index occur in up to 50% of patients, and 25% have the metabolic syndrome, all of which are potential risk factors for the development of early cardiovascular disease.[345,362] Patients with a family history of diabetes mellitus may be at increased risk for glucose abnormalities. Glucose abnormalities are correlated with muscle atrophy, as well as with proinflammatory cytokines, rather than prednisone dose.[345]

Hematological Manifestations and Osteoporosis

Hematological manifestations are rare. They have been described primarily in adult dermatomyositis patients, but occasionally in children, and include macrophage activation syndrome, hemolytic anemia, thrombocytopenia, and thrombotic thrombocytopenic purpura.[363-367] Anemia of chronic disease correlates with disease activity.

The majority of patients studied have frank osteopenia or osteoporosis even prior to initiation of corticosteroid therapy, which is worsened by delay in diagnosis as well as longstanding disease activity and may persist years beyond when the patient enters remission.[368-371] Patients have elevated serum levels of RANKL and decreased osteoprotegrin at the time of diagnosis, resulting in increased osteoclast activity that may result in lower bone mineral density.[371]

PATHOLOGY

The distinctive pathological lesions of JDM involve striated muscles, skin, and the gastrointestinal tract. The severity of clinical disease may correlate with the intensity of the histological findings. Extensive active myopathic changes, including degeneration, vacuolation, sarcoplasmic pallor and necrosis, as well as central nuclei without basophilia, predict a chronic course of illness.[372] Muscle infarction, although not a frequent finding, appears to correlate with a chronic course, gastrointestinal ulceration, and mortality.[372,373] Direct immunofluorescence staining of the muscle arteries also may be associated with a chronic ulcerative course of illness.[372,373] Patients with diffuse infiltrates or lymphocytic aggregates on initial muscle biopsy were responsive to standard therapy with steroids and methotrexate, but those with follicle-like structures, including follicular dendritic cells and high endothelial venules, tended to have severe disease requiring treatment with additional agents.[182] A standardized scoring method to examine histopathological features of JDM biopsies, including immunophenotypes of the inflammatory infiltrates, vascular and muscle fiber changes, and connective tissue fibrosis, has good reliability and appears to be a promising tool to enable future studies of the relationship of muscle pathology with illness outcomes.[33] The histological characteristics of JDM are contrasted with those in muscular dystrophy and neurogenic atrophy in Table 24–7.

Skeletal Muscle

Muscle fibers characteristically demonstrate group atrophy or necrosis at the periphery of the fascicle (Fig. 24–13).[64] This perifascicular atrophy is often associated with a noninflammatory capillaropathy.[64,374] Nonspecific changes include disruption of the myofibrils and tubular systems, central nuclear migration, and prominent nuclei and basophilia.[94,183] Concomitant degeneration and regeneration of muscle fibers occur and result in moderate variations in fiber size. Areas of focal necrosis are replaced during the healing phase by an interstitial proliferation of connective tissue.

Table 24–7

Comparison of muscle histopathology in juvenile dermatomyositis, muscular dystrophy, and neurogenic muscle atrophy

Histopathology	Dermatomyositis	Muscular Dystrophy	Neurogenic Atrophy
Chronic inflammatory infiltrates:			
Endomysial	++	+	−
Perimysial	++	+	−
Perivascular	++	−	−
Fiber degeneration	++	++	−
Fiber regeneration	++	+	−
Perifascicular atrophy	++	−	−
Vasculopathy of blood vessels	++	−	−
Thickened capillaries and capillary loss	++	−	−
Muscle infarction	++	−	−
Endomysial proliferation	++	++	−
MHC class I staining of myocyte	++	±	−
Myofiber necrosis	++	++	−
Phagocytosis of necrotic muscle fibers	+	++	−
Increased perimysial connective tissue	++	+	−
Myofiber size variation	+	++	±
Myofiber hypertrophy	−	++	−
Rounded, hypercontracted myofibers	−	++	−
Muscle fibrosis	±	++	−
Myocytes replaced with fat	±	++	−
Central migration of nuclei	+	++	−
Fiber atrophy	±	+	++
Motor unit atrophy	−	−	++

− absent; ± possible; + present; ++ characteristic.

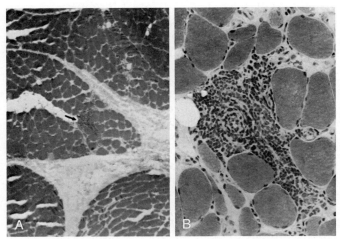

FIGURE 24–13 A. Muscle biopsy (H&E, X40). Scattered foci (*arrow*) of perivascular inflammation and resultant perifascicular atrophy. **B.** Enlargement (H&E, X250) of central area of *A*. Perivascular mononuclear inflammatory infiltrate, arterial wall thickening, and endothelial prominence.

An inflammatory exudate is often present. The inflammatory cells, which are often sparse and consist principally of lymphocytes and mononuclear cells, are located predominantly in the perimysium and perivascularly around the septae or in the fascicles (Fig. 24–14). This infiltrate is not in itself diagnostic because the muscular dystrophies may demonstrate an infiltrate around necrotic fibers. Macrophages, plasma cells, mast cells, and, rarely, eosinophils or basophils are also present. Specialized immunohistochemistry demonstrates plasmacytoid dendritic cells as one of the primary infiltrating immunophenotypes.[185]

Electron microscopy may confirm focal degeneration of the myofibrils, cytoplasmic masses, disorganization of sarcomeres, disruption of the Z lines and Z-disc streaming, actin-myosin filament disorganization, thickening of the capillary basement membranes, mitochondrial abnormalities, or an increase in vacuole formation. Lysosomes are more abundant in inflammatory myopathy than in normal muscle. The relationship of these organelles to muscle necrosis is uncertain.

Immunoglobulins can often be demonstrated on the sarcolemmal membrane by immunofluorescence microscopy, but this finding is of doubtful pathogenic significance.[164,375] Damaged muscle fibers have an increase in calcium content,[376,377] which may explain the uptake of technetium 99m diphosphonate by the muscles in inflammatory myopathy. The regenerative phase probably depends on the mononuclear myoblast that is derived from satellite cells.[378] Regenerating fibers contain increased oxidative enzyme and alkaline phosphatase activities.[379] A number of studies suggest that sarcolemmal overexpression of MHC classes I and II may be specific for myositis and useful in distinguishing JDM from other myopathies and that MHC class I overexpression along the sarcolemma is an early and late event and may remain positive even after initiating corticosteroid therapy.[158,178,380-382] Although overexpression of class I MHC on myofibers has also been occasionally seen in muscular dystrophies, staining appears to be more intense in JDM biopsies.[178,383,384]

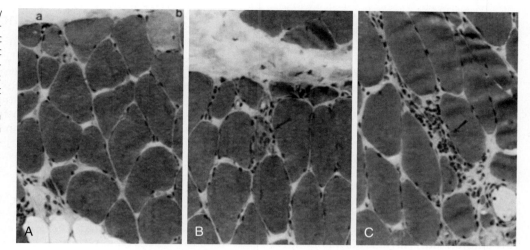

FIGURE 24–14 **A,** Muscle biopsy (hematoxylin and eosin stain; magnification × 250) demonstrates atrophic muscle fibers (a) and a pale necrotic fiber (b). **B,** Muscle biopsy (hematoxylin and eosin stain; magnification × 430) demonstrates a partially necrotic myofiber with phagocytosis (arrow). **C,** Muscle biopsy (hematoxylin and eosin stain; magnification × 250) with an endomysial mononuclear cell inflammatory infiltrate (arrow).

Blood Vessels

JDM should be considered a systemic inflammatory and noninflammatory vasculopathy rather than simply an inflammation of muscle and skin. A nonnecrotizing vasculitis affects arterioles, capillaries, and venules of the striated muscles, gastrointestinal tract, skin, and subcutaneous tissues. Endothelial vessel wall thickening often results, as well as thrombotic changes within the vessel resulting in occlusion and tissue ischemia and infarction.[385] Capillary loss is evident in the muscle, as well as other affected tissues.[157,171] Especially in the gastrointestinal tract, vasculopathy leads to infarction, ulceration, and diffuse bleeding. The early studies of Banker and Victor[330] identified this type of vasculopathy as an important prognostic factor in survival. Investigations by Crowe and associates[64] added distinctive features associated with persistent morbidity to an understanding of this complication. In their patients, muscle infarction and ulceration of the cutaneous and gastrointestinal tissues were associated with a zonal loss of the capillary bed, areas of focal infarction of muscle, nonnecrotizing lymphocytic vasculitis, and noninflammatory endarteropathy (Fig. 24–15). Conversely, severe vasculopathy was absent from the muscle specimens of children with limited disease.[64] This spectrum of capillary endothelial damage had also been suggested in previous studies.[164,330,386] A chronic vasculopathy—with narrowing or complete occlusion of small and medium arteries, subintimal foam cells, fibromyxoid neointimal expansion, luminal compromise, and infiltration of T lymphocytes and macrophages through the muscle layers into the intima—has also been reported, possibly as a later complication.

Capillaries

Widespread capillaropathy leads to intravascular coagulation, microvascular occlusion and infarction, and associated perifascicular myopathy. These capillary changes, although characteristic, are not specific and have been described in other connective tissue diseases, viral and rickettsial infections, malignancy, and normal wound healing.[386,387] Changes in the capillaries can be identified clinically in the nailfolds (see Fig. 24–6) and in tissues by light and electron microscopy.[64,230-232,234,330] Endothelial

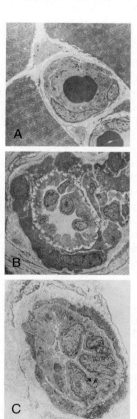

FIGURE 24–15 Electron microscopic sections of a muscle. **A,** Slight degree of endothelial cell swelling in an arteriole (magnification × 63,337). **B,** Increased degree of endarteropathy (magnification × 5200). **C,** Virtual occlusion of the lumen (l) of a small arteriole by extreme swelling of the endothelial cells (magnification × 10,968), although there is no thrombosis or inflammation.

swelling and necrosis, capillary thrombosis and obliteration, and endoplasmic tubuloreticular inclusions occur early in the course of disease.[64,330,386,388-390]

Arterioles

Inflammation of small muscular arteries and infarction of muscle results from an immune complex–mediated vasculitis.[64] Other arterial lesions are unassociated with an inflammatory cell infiltrate. These abnormalities do not always correspond to those present in the capillaries, and severe capillaropathy may not be associated with discernible endarteropathy.

IgM, IgG, and C3 were deposited in the perimysial veins in 9 of 11 patients studied by Whitaker and Engle.[164] IgG may not always be present. Diffuse linear and occasionally granular vascular wall deposits of IgM, C3d, and fibrin were also observed in the areas of noninflammatory vasculopathy.[64] Electron microscopy has not confirmed evidence of subendothelial deposition of immunoglobulins within vessel walls, as might have been expected in classic immune complex disease, although circulating immune complexes and complement activity are often identified in the blood.[95,391]

Veins

Intramural and perivascular mononuclear cell inflammatory infiltrates are frequently identified in the veins and may or may not be associated with immunoglobulin deposition.[64,164]

Skin

A capillary endothelial change similar to that in muscle is usually observed in involved skin.[64] Histopathological examination of the skin demonstrates perivascular inflammation, vascular changes at the dermal-epidermal junction, telangiectasias, hyperkeratosis in the stratum corneal layer, epidermal atrophy, follicular plugging, and basement membrane thickening.[392,393] The H&E skin histopathological changes are not specific to dermatomyositis and are also frequently present in SLE.[394,395] Specialized stains with colloidal iron and periodic acid Schiff demonstrate increased dermal mucin and basement membrane thickening in the majority of adult dermatomyositis skin biopsies.[393] Immunofluorescent stains reveal deposition of C3d, C4d, and the C5b-9 membrane attack complex on blood vessels to a greater degree than in SLE, and immunohistochemistry demonstrates CD123-positive plasmacytoid dendritic cells, primarily in the epidermis in a perivascular distribution, which differs from SLE, where they are primarily dermal.[394-397] Mast cells are also present in increased numbers in lesional skin.[397] An increase in the level of acid mucopolysaccharides has been reported in involved and uninvolved skin in approximately one third of patients.[398] In a study of the histopathology of Gottron papules,[393,399] basal layer vasculopathy, periodic acid–Schiff–positive basement membrane thickening, upper dermal mucin deposition, and a diffuse upper dermal mononuclear infiltrate were frequently identified. Epidermal hyperplasia consisting of acanthosis or papillomatosis often occurred, but epidermal atrophy was rare.

Lobular panniculitis has also been reported, which may result in focal lipoatrophy or calcification.[358,400,401] It may also be associated with infection with *Staphylococcus* or *Mycobacterium*.[400,402]

In the healing phase of the disease, calcium hydroxyappatite or carbonate appatite crystals,[248-250] may be deposited or formed in the skin, subcutaneous tissues, and interfascial planes of the muscle.[403]

Gastrointestinal Tract

Ulceration or perforation resulting from vasculopathy can occur in any part of the gastrointestinal tract, including the esophagus.[64,330] Serious gastrointestinal disease of this type develops in approximately 10% of children with JDM.[95] Pneumatosis intestinalis has been described.[331,404] Constipation, delayed gastric emptying, and prolonged gastrointestinal transit time may occur.[405] Pancreatitis and hepatitis are rare.[143]

Heart

Cardiac muscle is seldom affected by the primary pathological process,[406,407] but its involvement may be more common than clinically appreciated.[344] A few cases of carditis have been described with areas of focal myocardial fibrosis and contraction-band necrosis. Interstitial myocarditis and narrowing of the coronary arteries have been reported.[64]

Pulmonary

Interstitial lung disease is uncommon in children but is a poor prognostic sign. Pathological studies in adults reveal nonspecific interstitial pneumonia to be the most common form of interstitial lung disease.[408] Occasionally bronchiolitis obliterans–organizing pneumonia and interstitial pneumonia may be seen.[408] Diffuse alveolar damage holds a poor prognosis, with rapid progression, frequent respiratory failure, and even death.[409]

Kidneys

Although microscopic hemoglobinuria related to urine myoglobin may be present, especially at onset, histological renal abnormalities are rare. In one report,[9] histopathological findings in five of six renal biopsies were abnormal and included cellular hyperplasia, capillary thickening, capsular adhesions, and hyperplasia involving the small blood vessels. Renal abnormalities have not been commonly cited in postmortem reports.[14,57] Thrombotic microangiopathy related to reduced ADAMTS13 activity has been described.[410]

DIFFERENTIAL DIAGNOSIS

The differential diagnosis includes other forms of idiopathic inflammatory myopathies, including juvenile polymyositis, as well as infectious myopathies, noninflammatory myopathies, other systemic diseases that involve weakness, and mimicking rashes such as psoriasis (Table 24–8). The correct diagnosis is usually straightforward in the presence of the characteristic rash and weak, painful, or tender proximal muscles, whereas patients without characteristic rashes are recommended to undergo a muscle biopsy. Early in the disease course, especially in the absence of the characteristic rash, the differential diagnosis can be challenging (Tables 24–6 through 24–10; Tables 24–9 and 24–10). A future expectation is continued reclassification of the inflammatory and noninflammatory myopathies by identification of specific sets of immune-related genes.[411,412]

Other Forms of Idiopathic Inflammatory Myopathies

Juvenile Polymyositis

Juvenile polymyositis (JPM) is uncommon, with a much lower incidence than JDM and a prevalence of 2% to 8% among the childhood idiopathic inflammatory myopathies.[22,25,38,39,54] Age at onset and the sex ratio are comparable to JDM. Both proximal and distal muscles are often weak, and muscle atrophy is common. There are no associated cutaneous abnormalities; the nailfold capillary pattern is often abnormal and calcinosis occurs infrequently.[25] Arthritis, joint contractures, fevers, dysphagia, and pulmonary disease occur as in JDM.[25,38,39] The disease of most patients pursues a chronic course and is often relatively unresponsive to glucocorticoids. Muscle biopsy is usually necessary for accurate diagnosis to exclude other myopathies.

Myositis with Other Connective Tissue Diseases

Children with systemic scleroderma (see Chapter 25), mixed connective tissue disease (see Chapter 27), or occasionally SLE (see Chapter 22), may have skin and muscle abnormalities at onset that suggest a diagnosis of JDM. The differentiation of these diseases is usually not difficult, however, because clinical features unique to each are almost always present. The overlap of JDM or JPM with another systemic connective tissue disease occurs in 3% to 10% of patients, with scleroderma as perhaps the most common of these overlapping conditions (sharing the HLA DRB1*03-DQA1*05-DQB1*02 haplotype).[22,25,134] The laboratory evaluation provides supportive or definitive diagnostic information in most instances.

The child with JDM may have a malar dermatitis that is similar in distribution to the butterfly rash of SLE, but it often lacks relatively well-defined borders and spares the nasolabial folds. Heliotrope suffusion and periorbital edema are not characteristic of SLE. Periungual capillary abnormalities are present in many connective tissue diseases, but Gottron papules are present only in children with JDM, whereas linear extensor erythema (erythema between the joints) is present in both JDM and SLE. Although early cutaneous abnormalities of scleroderma and JDM are quite different, the skin changes can become similar during the courses of these diseases.

Myositis occurs in systemic scleroderma and mixed connective tissue disease and, to a limited extent, in SLE and juvenile chronic arthritis. The myositis of JDM can be differentiated from that of other connective tissue diseases by its severity, the greater elevation of serum levels of muscle enzymes, and histological examination of muscle obtained by biopsy. In uncomplicated chronic arthritis, acute rheumatic fever, SLE, or scleroderma, muscle biopsy demonstrates focal accumulations of lymphocytes, patchy fiber atrophy, and increased interstitial connective tissue but no significant vasculopathy.[413-415] Muscle fiber degeneration and atrophy, sarcoplasmic

degeneration, and microcyst formation occur in Sjögren syndrome.[416] A necrotizing vasculitis with muscle fiber degeneration and neurogenic atrophy may be identified in polyarteritis. Laboratory evaluation confirms normal or only slightly elevated serum levels of the muscle enzymes in SLE and other connective tissue diseases compared with moderate to marked elevations in JDM. Systemic features of SLE, such as pericarditis and pleural effusions, are rare in JDM. Hepatosplenomegaly and lymphadenopathy occur in fewer than 5% of children with JDM. The arthritis of JDM, although not uncommon, is usually mild; that of SLE occurs more frequently and, although nonerosive, may be quite florid at onset and extremely painful.

Table 24–8

Differential diagnosis of juvenile dermatomyositis

Other forms of idiopathic inflammatory myopathies
  Juvenile polymyositis
  Overlap myositis
  Cancer-associated myositis
  Focal myositis
  Orbital myositis
  Granulomatous myositis
  Eosinophilic myositis
Inflammatory myopathies: Infectious myopathies
  Viral (enterovirus, influenza, Coxsackie, echovirus, parvovirus, hepatitis B, human T lymphotropic virus I)
  Bacterial and parasitic (staphylococcus, streptococcus, toxoplasmosis, trichinosis, lyme borreliosis)
Noninflammatory myopathies*
  Muscular dystrophies
  Congenital myopathies
  Myotonic disorders
  Metabolic myopathies—glycogen storage diseases, lipid myopathies
  Periodic paralyses
  Mitochondrial myopathies
  Endocrinopathies
  Trauma
  Toxins
  Drug-induced myopathies
  Disorders of neuromuscular transmission
Systemic rheumatic diseases (systemic lupus erythematosus, scleroderma, juvenile idiopathic arthritis, mixed connective tissue disease, vasculitis)
Mimicking cutaneous conditions (psoriasis, eczema, allergy)

*For full listing, see Table 24–10.

Table 24–9

Acute myositis associated with influenza B infection

Onset during recovery phase of the viral illness
Predominantly severe bilateral pain and tenderness of the gastrocnemius and soleus muscles
Elevated serum muscle enzyme concentrations (e.g., creatine kinase, aspartate aminotransferase)
Recovery in 3 to 5 days

Table 24–10

Classification of neuromuscular disorders

I. Primary myopathies
  A. Muscular dystrophies
    1. Sex-linked recessive
      a. Duchenne-Becker muscular dystrophy
      b. Emery-Dreifuss muscular dystrophy 3 (Emerin)
    2. Autosomal dominant
      a. Myotonic muscular dystrophy (Steinert)
      b. Facioscapulohumeral muscular dystrophy
      c. Limb-girdle muscular dystrophies
        i. LGMD1A: Myotilin
        ii. LGMD1B: Lamin A/C (Emery-Dreifuss muscular dystrophy 2)
        iii. LGMD1C: Caveolin-3
        iv. LGMDIE: Familial dilated cardiomyopathy with conduction defect and muscular dystrophy E):
        v. LGMD1F
      d. Emery-Dreifuss muscular dystrophies (synaptic nuclear envelope protein 1, synaptic nuclear envelope protein 2)
    3. Autosomal recessive
      a. Limb-girdle muscular dystrophies
        i. LGMD2A: Calpain-3
        ii. LGMD2B: Dysferlin
        iii. LGMD2C: γ-sarcoglycan
        iv. LGMD2D: α-sarcoglycan
        v. LGMD2E: β-sarcoglycan
        vi. LGMD2F: δ-sarcoglycan
        vii. LGMD2G: Telethonin
        viii. LGMD2H: TRIM32
        ix. LGMD2I: FKRP
        x. LGMD2J: Titin
        xi. LGMD2K: POMT1
        xii. LGMD2L: Fukutin
        xiii. LGMD2M: O-Mannose Beta-1, 2-N-acetylglucosaminyl transferase
        xiv. LGMD2N: O-mannosyl transferases-2 (PMOT2)
        xv. Merosin (Laminin α2)
        xvi. Caveolin-3 mutations
        xvii. Myosclerosis: COL6A2
      b. Congenital muscular dystrophy (Fukuyama)
  B. Congenital myopathies
    1. Sex-linked recessive
      a. Myotubular myopathy
      b. Reducing body myopathy
      c. Spheroid body myopathy
    2. Autosomal dominant
      a. Nemaline rod myopathy
      b. Central core disease
      c. Hyaline body myopathy
      d. Actin aggregation myopathy
      e. Cap disease
    3. Autosomal recessive
      a. Nemaline rod myopathy
      b. Central core disease
      c. Hyaline body myopathy
        i. Congenital muscle fiber–type disproportion
  C. Myotonic disorders
    1. Myotonia congenita (Thomsen)
    2. Dystrophia myotonia (Steinert)
    3. Paramyotonia congenita
  D. Metabolic myopathies
    1. Disorders of glycogen metabolism
      a. Sex-linked recessive
        i. Glycogenosis IX (phosphoglycerate kinase deficiency)
      b. Autosomal recessive
        i. Glycogenosis II (Pompe, acid maltase deficiency)
        ii. Glycogenosis V (McArdle, myophosphorylase deficiency)
        iii. Glycogenosis VII (Tarui, phosphofructokinase deficiency)
        iv. Glycogenosis X (phosphoglycerate mutase deficiency)
        v. Glycogenosis XI (lactate dehydrogenase deficiency)
    2. Mitochondrial myopathies
      a. Mitochondrial myopathy (Kearns-Sayre)
      b. Mitochondrial myopathy (MERRF)
      c. Mitochondrial myopathy (MELAS)
    3. Familial periodic paralysis (hyperkalemic and hypokalemic)

Table 24–10—cont'd

Classification of neuromuscular disorders—cont'd

  4. Lipid myopathies
   a. Carnitine palmityl-transferase deficiency 2
   b. Carnitine acyltransferase deficiency
   c. Carnitine deficiency
   d. Carnitine-acylcarnitine translocase deficiency
   e. Multiple acyl–CoA dehydrogenase deficiency (MADD; glutaricaciduria IIA)
   f. Short-chain acyl-CoA dehydrogenase
   g. Medium chain acyl-CoA dehydrogenase deficiency
  5. Secondary to endocrinopathies
   a. Addison disease
   b. Cushing syndrome
   c. Hypopituitarism
   d. Hypothyroidism
  6. Myoadenylate deaminase deficiency
II. Inflammatory diseases
  A. Postinfectious
   1. Viral syndromes
    a. Influenza A/B
    b. Coxsackievirus B
    c. Echovirus
    d. Poliomyelitis
   2. Toxoplasmosis, sarcosporidiosis
   3. Trichinosis, cysticercosis
   4. Septic (staphylococci and other pyogenic organisms)
   5. Tetanus
   6. Gas gangrene
  B. Connective tissue diseases
III. Genetic abnormalities
  A. Osteogenesis imperfecta
  B. Ehlers-Danlos syndrome
  C. Mucopolysaccharidoses
IV. Trauma
  A. Physical (crush, rhabdomyolysis)
  B. Toxic (snakebite)
  C. Drug-induced myopathy
   1. Glucocorticoids
   2. Hydroxychloroquine
   3. Diuretics, licorice
   4. Amphotericin B
   5. Alcohol
   6. Vincristine
   7. D-Penicillamine
   8. Cimetidine
   9. Chronic hemodialysis
V. Neurogenic atrophies
  A. Spinal muscular and anterior horn cell dysfunction
   1. Spinal muscular atrophy (Werdnig-Hoffmann, Kugelberg-Welander)
   2. Familial dysautonomia (Riley-Day)
   3. Arthrogryposis multiplex congenita
   4. Amyotrophic lateral sclerosis
  B. Peripheral nerve dysfunction
   1. Hereditary motor-sensory neuropathy (Charcot-Marie-Tooth, Dejerine-Sottas)
   2. Hereditary motor-sensory neuropathy (axonal type)
   3. Hereditary motor-sensory neuropathy (Charcot-Marie-Tooth-X)
   4. Neurofibromatosis
   5. Guillain-Barré syndrome
  C. Disorders of neuromuscular transmission
   1. Congenital myasthenia gravis
   2. Botulism
   3. Tick paralysis
   4. Organophosphate poisoning

Source: References 253, 255,258: http://neuromuscular.wustl.edu/maltbrain.html.

Other Forms of Idiopathic Inflammatory Myopathies

Cancer-associated myositis has a firm association with adult myositis but is rare in children, so children are not routinely assessed for occult malignancy.[37,262] The associated malignancies include leukemia, lymphoma, and solid-organ tumors, and the dermatomyositis has atypical or unusual features. A number of uncommon forms of myositis have been described, especially in adults,[417] including inclusion body myositis[418-420] and disease restricted to one muscle group or extremity, such as focal myositis,[421-423] orbital myositis confined to the extraocular muscles,[48,49] proliferative myositis,[424] and granulomatous myositis.[425] Inclusion body myositis tends to respond slowly to immunosuppressive therapy. A dermatomyositislike disease has been observed in children[95,97,426-428] with agammaglobulinemia and common variable immune deficiency (see Chapter 42).

Macrophagic myofasciitis, a rare but distinct clinicopathological entity, demonstrates a predominance of macrophagic infiltrates on muscle biopsy, sometimes containing aluminium inclusions, because alum-containing adjuvants in vaccinations may be the etiology.[51] Children with this condition frequently present with shoulder or thigh weakness, myalgias, fatigue, arthralgias, and high levels of creatine kinase. They may also have hypotonia, developmental delay, and failure to thrive.[52]

Some forms of limb girdle muscular dystrophies, including calpain-3 deficiency (LGMD2A) and gamma-sarcoglycanopathy (LGMD2C), may present with eosinophilic myositis,[429,430] but the condition may also be idiopathic or result after drug exposures.[431,432] Infantile polymyositis results from merosin gene mutations, and this entity has been reclassified as a muscular dystrophy.

Inflammatory Myopathies That Are Postinfectious

Acute, transient myositis may follow certain viral infections, especially influenza A and B[78-80] and coxsackievirus B.[73-75] Coxsackievirus B causes epidemic pleurodynia (i.e., Bornholm disease), characterized by fever and sharp pain in the muscles of the chest and abdominal wall. This syndrome is sometimes preceded by a moderate to severe headache, nausea, vomiting, and pharyngitis. The illness is most common in children and adolescents and usually lasts 3 to 5 days. Although myalgia is a characteristic complaint of acute influenza, myositis per se is rare (see Table 24–9).

In 1957, Lundberg[77] described a contagious illness that occurred most commonly in preadolescent boys and was characterized by fever, headache, rhinitis, cough, nausea, and vomiting that lasted 2 to 3 days. This was followed by severe proximal calf pain and tenderness (i.e., myalgia cruris epidemica) that was exacerbated by movement. Complete recovery occurred after approximately 3 days. Laboratory studies demonstrated a slightly elevated erythrocyte sedimentation rate (ESR), moderate leukopenia with relative lymphocytosis, and a concomitant elevation of the serum levels of CK and aspartate aminotransferase (AST). Although no specific infectious agent was identified in this study, subsequent reports have confirmed influenza B as the most common causative agent. Treatment is supportive.

Other infectious causes of myositis include toxoplasmosis; trichinosis; cat-scratch fever; staphylococcal and streptococcal bacteremia; clostridial, mycoplasmal, *Borrelia burgdorferi*, *Salmonella*, or *Serratia* infection; schistosomiasis; trypanosomiasis; and other viral infections, including hepatitis and HTLV. *Candidiasis* and coccidioidomycosis are very uncommon causes. Toxoplasmosis may be associated with a syndrome that resembles dermatomyositis.[92,433,434] Trichinosis, caused by ingestion of the larval cyst of the nematode *Trichinella spiralis*, is characterized initially by fever, diarrhea, and abdominal pain, followed in a week by periorbital edema and swelling and tenderness of muscles, especially those of the face, neck, and chest. Peripheral blood eosinophilia is often striking, and biopsy of affected muscles confirms the presence of the larvae and, later, calcified cysts. Treatment includes glucocorticoids to diminish inflammation and agents such as mebendazole or thiabendazole. Other unusual exposures include *Sarcocystis*, malaria, cysticercosis, echinococcosis, and toxocariasis.

Staphylococcal pyomyositis is an abscess in skeletal muscle that occurs after local muscle injury. It affects patients of all ages and is more common in boys than in girls. Lesions may be solitary or multiple and are usually located in the thigh, calf, buttock, arm, scapular areas, or chest wall. The abscess is tender and, if not too deep, warm. Patients usually have low-grade fever. Symptoms last for up to a week. Ultrasonography or gallium 67 citrate scanning may localize the lesion. Severe pustular acne occasionally may be associated with inflammatory disease of muscle and with arthritis[433] (see Chapter 44).

Rhabdomyolysis may follow an upper respiratory infection, trauma, or extreme muscular exertion.[434] Onset is generally acute and is characterized by profound weakness, myoglobulinuria, very high serum levels of muscle enzymes, and, occasionally, oliguria and renal failure. It may also occur after snakebite, in heat stroke, after certain medications such as lipid lowering agents and zidovudine, in the familial malignant hyperpyrexia syndrome, and in mitochondrial myopathies.[258]

Neuromuscular Diseases and Myopathies

In the absence of characteristic skin changes, the differential diagnosis includes a wide variety of neuromuscular disorders (Tables 24–10 to 24–13).[257] Early in the disease or before the development of cutaneous changes, muscular dystrophy or myotonia may be confused with JDM. In children without the characteristic rashes of JDM, concern about these entities is greater, particularly if chronic inflammation is absent or not prominent on the muscle biopsy. Hypotonia in infancy, often associated with projectile vomiting, is a characteristic of the mitochondrial disorders involving the branched chain amino acids. Paroxysmal myoglobinuria or acute rhabdomyolysis occasionally may be encountered, as well as episodic weakness. Certain drugs or toxins, including alcohol,

Table 24–11

Classification of neuromuscular disorders by course

Acute Disorders
Myasthenia gravis
Carnitine deficiency
Myoglobinuria/rhabdomyolysis
Myositis variants: anti–signal recognition particle autoantibody
Periodic paralysis
Myosin deficiency myopathies
Electrolyte disorders: potassium, magnesium, phosphorous
Guillain-Barré syndrome
Vasculitis
Porphyria
Toxins
Trauma
Infections

Chronic Disorders
Dermatomyositis
Muscular dystrophy (Duchenne, limb-girdle dystrophies, facioscapulohumeral dystrophy)
Central core disease and nemaline myopathy
Congenital hypotonia
Glycogen storage disease
Myoadenylate deaminase deficiency
Endocrine myopathy
Mitochondrial myopathy
Lipid storage myopathies
Nutritional myopathy
Amyloidosis

Episodic Disorders
Paramyotonia congenita
Familial periodic paralysis
Hypokalemia
Myasthenia gravis
Myasthenia of malignancy
Electrolyte disorders
Hyperkalemic periodic paralysis
Hypokalemic periodic paralysis
Hereditary
Ca++ channel
Na+ channel
Renal tubular acidosis, distal
Thyrotoxic
Acquired
K+ wasting
Myoglobinuria/rhabdomyolysis
Myotonia syndromes
Porphyria, acute intermittent

Modified from Washington University Neuromuscular Home Page: http://neuromuscular.wustl.edu/maltbrain.html (ref 258).

Table 24–12

Classification of neuromuscular disorders by predominant site of involvement

Proximal > Distal Involvement
Dermatomyositis
Polymyositis
Steroid myopathy
Thyrotoxic myopathy
Sarcoid myopathy
Muscular dystrophy (Duchenne, Becker, some limb-girdle dystrophies)
Proximal familial neuromuscular diseases
Glycogen storage diseases (Pompe, acid maltase)

Distal > Proximal Involvement
Congenital myopathies (nemaline rod, central core, Bethlem myopathy)
Muscular dystrophies (Emery-Dreifuss, FSH dystrophy, LGMD2A [calpain 3 deficiency]) LBMD2G (telothin)
Myotonic dystrophy
Glycogenoses (acid maltase, debranching enzyme, phosphorylase b kinase)
Inclusion body myositis
Hereditary inclusion body myopathy
Oculopharyngeal distal myopathy
Desmin (myofibrillar) myopathy
Gowers-Laing (myosin heavy chain 7 deficiency)

Proximal or Distal Involvement
Floppy infant syndrome
Myotonia congenita
Dystrophic ophthalmoplegia
Metabolic myopathies
Myasthenia gravis
Periodic paralysis

Modified from Washington University Neuromuscular Home Page: http://neuromuscular.wustl.edu/maltbrain.html (ref 258).

clofibrate, D-penicillamine, glucocorticoids, and hydroxychloroquine, can cause myopathy (see Chapter 6).[435, 436]

The possibility of *muscular dystrophy* is suggested by a family history of myopathy and an insidious onset of slowly progressive, predominantly proximal muscle weakness, and by absence of the normal progression of achievement of developmental landmarks. Patients with dystrophies often have weakness of muscle groups that are not characteristically weak in the idiopathic inflammatory myopathies, including weakness of the scapula, distal muscle groups or facial/ocular muscles. Constitutional signs, muscle tenderness, cutaneous abnormalities, including periungual nailfold capillary changes, arthritis, and a positive antinuclear antibody are absent. In Duchenne muscular dystrophy, there is a characteristic hypertrophy of the calves, a sign that occurs in other myopathies and occasionally in longstanding JDM or JPM. The hereditary nature of Duchenne muscular dystrophy is demonstrated by the presence of markedly elevated levels of serum CK in the patient and the patient's mother. However, approximately one third of these disorders represent new mutations.

Myoadenylate deaminase deficiency (MDD)[437,438] occurs in an autosomal recessive primary form and as an acquired disorder associated with rheumatic and neuromuscular diseases. Data suggest that homozygous MDD is relatively common because 2% of muscle biopsies are deficient in enzyme activity (less than 2% in the primary form, less than 15% in the secondary form). Muscle fatigue, stiffness, and cramping may be noticed after

Table 24–13

Classification of neuromuscular disorders by age at onset

Congenital Onset
Congenital muscular dystrophies
Central core disease
Multicore (minicore) myopathy
Myotubular myopathy
Nemaline myopathy
Bethlem myopathy
Myosin storage myopathy
Congenital myasthenic syndromes
Neonatal perifascicular myopathy
Benign hypotonia
Reducing body myopathies

Childhood Onset
Muscular dystrophy (Duchenne, Becker, limb-girdle dystrophies, Emery Dreifuss dystrophy)
Glycogen storage diseases
Myoadenylate deaminase deficiency
Juvenile dermatomyositis
Polymyositis
Acquired myasthenic syndromes

Late Childhood and Adolescence Onset
Muscular dystrophy (limb-girdle dystrophies, Emery Dreifuss dystrophy, FSH dystrophy)
Periodic paralysis
Juvenile dermatomyositis
Polymyositis
Inclusion body myositis

Any Age at Onset
Steroid and hydroxychloroquine myopathies
Myasthenia gravis
Trichinosis

Modified from Washington University Neuromuscular Home Page: http://neuromuscular.wustl.edu/maltbrain.html (ref 258).

exercise and may begin in childhood (23%) or adolescence (26%), but these features do not occur in all deficient individuals. Patients with MDD may demonstrate a decreased muscle mass, hypotonia, and weakness. With forearm exercise, there is a failure of the plasma ammonia level to rise along with inosine monophosphate. Electromyographic findings are nonspecific. The muscle in primary MDD is normal histologically except for the absence of adenosine monophosphate deaminase. Activity of this enzyme is normal in other tissues.

Other metabolic myopathies, including lipid and glycogen metabolic pathway defects, may present with exercise intolerance, muscle cramping, muscle fatigue, and decreased endurance, with or without progressive muscle weakness and myoglobinuria. Weakness may be exacerbated after fasting or food intake and may be episodic.[439]

Endocrinopathies—especially hyperthyroidism and hypothyroidism, hyperparathyroidism and hypoparathyroidism, diabetes mellitus, and myopathy associated with idiopathic or iatrogenic Cushing syndrome—should be considered in the differential diagnosis of a myopathy without evidence of cutaneous disease. Myasthenia gravis is rare, and the diagnosis is suggested by a decremental response to repetitive nerve stimulation, involvement of ocular and distal muscles, and improvement of the weakness after administration of cholinergic drugs. Primary neurogenic atrophies, including infantile and juvenile spinal muscular atrophy, are associated with proximal muscle weakness and rarely may be confused with inflammatory myopathies.

Miscellaneous Disorders

Fibrodysplasia ossificans progressiva (i.e., myositis ossificans progressiva) is a rare, autosomal dominant inflammatory disorder (usually a new mutation) that results in painful swelling of muscle and fascia (e.g., ligaments, tendons, aponeuroses), followed by fibrosis, calcification, and ossification.[440-446] The gene has been mapped to chromosome 4q27-31.[447] There is a missense mutation, a single nucleotide substitution (c.617G>A) at codon 206 in the glycine-serine activation domain of activin receptor IA (ACVR1) a bone morphogenetic protein type 1 receptor.[448] The patient may present with a spontaneous joint contracture or preosseous soft tissue lesions. The clinical diagnosis is often elusive until calcification and, later, ossification is evident on ultrasound or radiography.[449,450] Biopsy findings of affected sites at an early stage may be misleading and be misinterpreted as malignant sarcoma.[451,455] The back of the neck and posterior trunk are often the sites of the initial tumorlike swellings, followed by the muscles of the limbs. Palmar and plantar fascia may be affected. The great toes are congenitally malformed, usually short and with hallux valgus; the thumbs are sometimes involved. The toe deformity is an early clinical sign to the diagnosis, even before heterotopic ossification occurs.[453] After onset in the first year of life the disease is characterized by exacerbations and remissions and slowly progresses to severe debility, restriction of pulmonary capacity, and reduced life expectancy. There is no therapy for prevention or treatment, although bisphosphonates have been advocated.[454] Early diagnosis can prevent misunderstanding and unnecessary procedures and the associated morbidities. Data on overexpression of bone morphogenic protein-4[455] or osteogenic transcription factor[456] may provide additional modalities of therapy.[457]

LABORATORY EXAMINATION

General Findings and Biomarkers

Nonspecific indicators of inflammation, such as the ESR and C-reactive protein level, tend to correlate with the degree of clinical inflammation and are of diagnostic value in differentiating inflammatory myopathies such as JDM from noninflammatory disorders of muscle such as muscular dystrophy or myotonia.[458,459] Leukocytosis and anemia are uncommon at onset, except in the child with associated gastrointestinal bleeding. Patients may have lymphopenia.[460] Urinalysis is usually normal, although some children at onset have microscopic hematuria.[9] Serum levels of factor VIII–related antigen (i.e., von Willebrand factor) reflect endothelial damage and are often elevated in children with JDM.[136,175,461-464] Although abnormal factor VIII–related antigen levels occur in most children with active disease,[465] particularly with active skin disease,[465] they were not of value in one study in predicting a flare.[175] There are few specific abnormalities of immunoglobulin levels.[466] IgE levels were elevated in one study of 22 Japanese children.[467] Serum acute phase reactants, such as alpha-1 acid glycoprotein, serum albumin, serum amyloid A, ferritin and cystatin C, also correlate with active disease, particularly outside of the muscles.[465]

Flow cytometry of peripheral blood lymphocytes demonstrate increases in CD19+ B lymphocytes and the CD4 (T helper)–to–CD8 (T suppressor) ratio and decreases in CD3– CD16+/CD56+ NK cells in newly diagnosed, untreated JDM patients compared with healthy controls.[468-470] CD19+ B lymphocytes also correlate with disease activity.[471]

Neopterin is a derivative of pyrimidine metabolism, and its serum concentration has been considered a marker of interferon-activated monocytes and macrophages. Levels of neopterin are raised in individuals with inflammation, infections, or malignant diseases. Determination of its concentration has been proposed as a useful laboratory marker of immune activation and disease activity.[464,469] Levels of quinolinic acid, available on a research basis, may be another marker of activity that correlate with macrophage function.[463,472]

Markers in the interferon pathway, important in disease pathogenesis, appear to be promising as biomarkers of disease activity. Serum interferon-α levels correlate with serum levels of muscle enzymes in untreated JDM patients and inversely with disease activity at 36 months.[473] Serum levels of type I interferon–regulated proteins, including IP-10, MCP-1 and MCP-2, also correlate with disease activity in JDM/DM patients.[186]

The serum level of *myoglobin*, a normal constituent of cardiac and skeletal muscle with a molecular mass of approximately 17 kD, is increased in approximately 50% of patients with adult inflammatory myopathies and JPM but is probably less frequently elevated in patients with JDM.[474,475] This elevation does not always correlate with an increase in serum CK levels. Antibodies to myoglobin are present in 70% of patients and may interfere with its quantitation.[476] Although myoglobin is much more nephrotoxic than hemoglobin, myoglobinuria in cases of JDM seldom reaches levels that are associated with renal damage. An adult with 30 kg of muscle mass normally releases 0.3 mg of myoglobin per day.[477,478]

The *creatine/creatinine ratio* is not a practical measure of myopathy in children. Creatine is synthesized in the liver from arginine and glycine by an aminotransferase to form ornithine and guanidinoacetic acid. The latter is transmethylated by interaction with *S*-adenosylmethionine to form creatine and *S*-adenosylhomocysteine. Creatine circulates in the plasma in relatively low concentrations (less than 0.6 mg/dL in adults). It is stored in muscle as creatine phosphate and serves as the reserve energy pool for muscular activity. In muscle, creatine is converted to the anhydride creatinine at a constant rate of approximately 2% per day. Creatinine diffuses passively into the plasma and is excreted by the kidneys. If the body pool of creatine decreases, the creatinine excretion per unit of time is also decreased. Endogenous creatinine excretion is an important index of body creatine stores and total muscle mass. Creatinuria in JDM is not simply a matter of failure of uptake by an inflamed muscle or a decreased muscle mass but rather an inability to maintain normal membrane permeability.

The urinary creatine/creatinine ratio is age related in children with JDM.[479] In those younger than 12 years, it is not a reliable guide to the activity of the myositis. A 24-hour creatinine excretion is an excellent indicator of muscle mass in children between the ages of 3 and 18 years. Boys begin to excrete significantly larger amounts of creatinine than girls at puberty. In males, excretion increases from approximately 0.36 g/day at 5 years of age to 1.6 g/day at 17 years. Creatine excretion, however, is much higher in the younger child; at no age in childhood is there a significant male/female difference in excretion. A 24-hour urine collection would have to document extremely large or infinitesimally low amounts of creatine before a creatine/creatinine ratio could be judged abnormal in young children. Nevertheless, urinary creatine/creatinine is increased in a first-morning urine sample in juvenile myositis patients compared to age- and gender-matched healthy controls, as are other muscle metabolites measured by magnetic resonance spectroscopy, including choline, betaine, glycine, and trimethylamine oxide.[480] Creatinine/creatinine correlates with disease damage, whereas choline correlates with other serum muscle enzyme levels and may be a marker of activity.[481]

Autoantibodies

Rheumatoid factors usually are absent in patients with JDM. Antinuclear antibodies (ANAs) have been reported in a variable frequency of 10% to 85%.[11,13,21,22,481,482] Particularly important are antibodies directed against one of a number of extractable nuclear antigens that are soluble in saline at neutral or acid pH (Table 24–14).[95,483,484] Traditional *myositis-specific autoantibodies* (MSAs), such as those directed to the aminoacyl transfer RNA (tRNA) synthetases, signal recognition particle (SRP), and Mi-2, are seen almost exclusively in myositis patients using validated assays, such as immunoprecipitation. These autoantibodies, however, have been described in a minority of children with myositis.[37,134,149,482,484,485] Recently, however, several autoantibodies, including anti-p155 and anti-MJ, have recently been identified in a large percentage of children with JDM, each present in 13% to 29% of patients.[144,486-488] Although these autoantibodies may be specific for myositis, testing for these autoantibodies in the sera of patients with other conditions has not yet been extensive enough to confirm them as myositis-specific, and so they are currently classified as myositis-associated autoantibodies. *Myositis-associated autoantibodies* (MAAs) occur in JDM, often in association with overlap syndromes. The percentage of children

Table 24–14

Autoantibodies in patients with juvenile idiopathic inflammatory myopathies

Autoantibody	Autoantigen Target	Frequency in Juvenile Patients * %	Clinical Features and Associations in Juvenile Idiopathic Inflammatory Myopathies
Myositis-Specific Autoantibodies			
Anti–Aminoacyl-tRNA synthetases:		1-5	Typically associated with those with moderate to severe weakness and creatine kinase levels, also frequently have nonerosive small joint arthritis, mechanics hands, Raynaud phenomenon, fevers, interstitial lung disease
Anti–Jo-1	Histidyl-tRNA synthetase	2-5	
Anti–PL-12	Alanyl-tRNA synthetase	1-3	
Anti–PL-7	Threonyl-tRNA synthetase	<1	
Anti–EJ	Glycyl-tRNA synthetase	<1	
Anti–OJ	Isoleucyl-tRNA synthetase	<1	
Anti–Mi-2	NuRD helicases: Mi-2α and Mi-2β, histone deacetylases	1-7	Mild JDM, classic rashes, responsive to treatment
Anti-SRP	Signal recognition particle (6 polypeptides and 7SLRNA)	1-3	Associated with severe, refractory polymyositis, acute onset, proximal and distal weakness
Myositis-Associated Autoantibodies			
Anti-p155	Transcriptional intermediary factor (TIF)-1γ	23-29	More severe cutaneous involvement, generalized lipodystrophy
Anti-p140 (MJ)	Nuclear matrix protein NXP2	13-23	Calcinosis, contractures
Anti-Ro	52- or 60-kD ribonucleoproteins (hYRNA)	2-8	
Anti–PM-Scl	Exosome protein: 100 and 75 kD	3-7	Associated with sclerodermatous overlap features; scleroderma usually limited cutaneous
Anti–U1-RNP	U1 small nuclear ribonucleoprotein (snRNP)	5-6	Associated with sclerodermatous overlap features
Anti–U3-RNP	U3 ribonucleoprotein (fibrillarin)	1	Associated with sclerodermatous overlap features
Anti-La	Ribonucleoprotein	1	Associated with anti-Ro
Anti-Ku	DNA binding complex: 70 and 80 kDa heterodimer	1	
Anti-Topo	DNA topoisomerase 1	1	

Based on data from references 133, 148, 491, 489, 490. Certain autoantibodies are more frequent in African American patients, including anti-Jo1, anti-SRP, anti-Ro and anti-URNP.[148] Modified from Wedderburn LR, Rider LG: Juvenile dermatomyositis: new developments in pathogenesis, assessment and treatment. Best Practice and Research in Clinical Rheumatology, 2009; 23: 655-678.

with JDM negative for myositis autoantibodies is currently estimated to be approximately 30% with the availability of more extensive testing for the newly identified autoantibodies.[104] The inclusion of myositis autoantibodies has been proposed for the classification of juvenile and adult dermatomyositis or polymyositis, as well as potentially to aide in their diagnosis.[262,489-491] The titers of these autoantibodies fluctuate with the level of disease activity,[492] and they may become negative when disease enters remission.[206] Testing for MSAs and MAAs using immunoprecipitation is a reliable method available only in a few commercial and research laboratories.

Myositis-Specific Autoantibodies

MSAs are antibodies targeted to cytosolic RNAs or proteins involved in protein synthesis, with autoantibodies in dermatomyositis often directed against nuclear transcription factors and autoantibodies in polymyositis often directed against cellular protein translational machinery. Usually, only one MSA occurs in a patient,

and it often can be detected before onset of the phenotype. Patients with a specific MSA are relatively homogeneous in clinical manifestations and prognosis.[485] MSAs have been uncommon in childhood-onset disease and have only been described in approximately 10% of patients. Their specificities include antibodies to the Jo-1 and other tRNA synthetases, Mi-2, and SRP autoantigens.[493-496]

Antisynthetase autoantibodies usually occur in patients with an acute onset in the spring season and rapid progression of disease, but they have been identified in others with slow progression and in asymptomatic adults.[497,498] The antisynthetases are associated with an increased frequency of the alleles associated with the ancestral haplotype HLA-B*08-DRB1*0301-DQA1*0501-DQB1*0201.[134,138,143,144,499] Anti–Jo-1 is the most common antisynthetase autoantibody. It occurs in approximately 20% of adults and has been described in 1% to 5% of children.[104,134,149] It is specific for histidyl-transfer RNA synthetase, a cytoplasmic enzyme that catalyzes the esterification of histidine to its cognate tRNA. Patients who are anti–Jo-1 positive demonstrate a subset of multisystemic features that have been called the *antisynthetase syndrome*. Patients with this autoantibody have an illness characterized by fever, arthritis, Raynaud phenomenon, and a myositis that is often severe. Interstitial pulmonary fibrosis may become the dominant feature of the course.[497] Although polyarthritis, when it occurs, is generally mild, it can result in erosions and subluxations. A hyperkeratotic nonpruritic fissuring rash of the palms and lateral aspects of the fingers (i.e., mechanic's hands) is another feature of this syndrome, especially in adults. Non-Jo1 antisynthetases, including antialanyl (PL-12) and antithreonyl (PL-7) – tRNA synthetases, have also been reported in children with myositis, but their myositis tends to be milder than patients with Jo-1 autoantibodies.[37] Several other non–Jo1 antisynthetases, including glycyl, isoleucyl, asparagynyl,[500] phenylalanyl, and tyrosyl t-RNA synthetases, have been identified to date only in adults.[501]

Mi-2 is a 218-kD nuclear helicase that is involved in transcriptional activation, and the autoantibody is often associated with HLA-DRB1*0701 and HLA-DQA1*0201.[141] Anti–Mi-2 has been identified in approximately 5% of children with JDM, and in adults, it is strongly associated with a distinct pattern of rash[37,134,488,494,502] and perhaps a more benign course.[496] The areas of most intense involvement often are the V of the neck and the anterior chest area and the shawl area with involvement of the upper back and shoulders. Most children have not displayed this characteristic dermatitis, although they have malar erythema, Gottron papules, and cuticular overgrowth. The disease is responsive to glucocorticoid therapy.

Another subset of patients is associated with autoantibodies to the signal recognition peptide (SRP), which has been identified in approximately 1% of juvenile myositis patients, all exclusively with polymyositis.[37,134,502,503] Onset of disease is often severe and acute with myositis of the proximal and distal muscles. These patients may have severe weakness and a higher frequency of cardiac disease, and they may respond poorly to glucocorticoid therapy.[37,502,504] SRP is a cytoplasmic ribonuclear protein complex that directs the passage of newly synthesized protein from the ribosome to the endoplasmic reticulum. Immunofluorescent tests therefore may demonstrate anticytoplasmic staining. HLA-B*5001 and DQA1*0104 are associated with this autoantibody.[141]

Myositis-Associated Autoantibodies

The MAAs occur in up to 70% of children and consist of several distinct entities.[37,134,149] Anti-p155 autoantibody, which immunoprecipitates a 155-kD band along with a fainter 140-kD band, is present in 23% to 29% of JDM patients studied to date.[486,487] It has also been seen in similar frequencies in adult DM, overlap myositis that is associated with dermatomyositis in adults and children, and in up to 85% of adult DM patients with associated malignancies.[486,505-507] This autoantibody has been detected in the serum of one patient with SLE, but not in polymyositis, muscular dystrophies, or other patients with rheumatoid arthritis, lupus, or scleroderma.[486,505-507] The clinical associations with this autoantibody include extensive

skin rashes, including a wide distribution of Gottron papules and V sign rash, as well as a higher frequency of cutaneous ulcerations and edema.[486,487] It is also seen in high frequency in patients with generalized lipodystrophy who have JDM.[358] The HLA allele associated with this autoantibody is DQA1*0301.[486] The antigenic target has preliminarily been identified as transcriptional intermediary factor 1-γ.[508]

MJ, also known as anti-p140, is found in 13% to 23% of JDM patients, and is not seen in JDM patients with overlap myositis, nor those with JRA, SLE, or scleroderma or in healthy individuals.[104,488,509] It has not yet been studied in adult myositis or other conditions. Patients with anti-MJ autoantibodies have a higher frequency of calcinosis and a lower frequency of truncal rashes.[488] The autoantigen has been preliminarily identified to be nuclear matrix protein NXP-2, a transcription factor and regulator of RNA metabolism.[488,510]

Anti-PM-Scl is suggested by a nucleolar pattern on ANA testing.[35,511,512] It occurs in the overlap syndrome of inflammatory myopathy and systemic scleroderma (i.e., scleromyositis). Clinical features include myositis, arthritis, interstitial lung disease, digital sclerosis, and Raynaud phenomenon.[511,514] The course of the disease is often benign and prolonged but has a good prognosis. This autoantibody is associated with HLA-DRB1*0301-DQA1*0501-DQB1*0201.[134] Anti-U1RNP is characteristic of the overlap syndrome of mixed connective tissue disease (see Chapter 27). It is suggested by the presence of a high-titered ANA speckled pattern. There is a subgroup of patients (1% to 7%) who have autoantibodies to U3RNP.[137,513] Anti-SSA/Ro antibody often occurs in association with anti–Jo-1.[514] The anti-Ku antibody has not often been described in patients from North America[515] but was reported from Japan in approximately 50% of patients with an overlap syndrome. It has been reported in approximately 1% of children with overlap syndromes.[134] The antigen is a protein kinase that is involved in the phosphorylation of a number of transcription factors.

Several autoantibodies have been described in patients with adult myositis, but not yet been identified in JDM. Anti–small ubiquitinlike modifier–activating enzyme is seen in up to 8% of patients with adult DM, including patients with interstitial pneumonia and cancer, but not in other forms of adult myositis.[516] Patients frequently present with skin findings first but progress to involve muscle weakness and a high frequency of dysphagia.[517] CADM-140 has been associated with amyopathic DM and rapidly progressive interstitial lung disease.[518] The autoantigenic target has been identified as the cytoplasmic protein melanoma differentiation–associated gene 5 (MDA5).[519] Autoantibodies to the DNA mismatch repair enzymes, PMS1 and PMS2, also may be myositis-specific and have been identified in 7% of adult myositis patients.[520]

Other Autoantibodies

Anti–annexin XI has been identified frequently in children with JDM and in those with other connective tissue diseases and is not associated with any particular clinical manifestations.[521] It reacts against a 56-kD nuclear protein by Western blotting.

Autoantibodies to endothelial cell antigens have been demonstrated in JDM and adult myositis, particularly in patients with interstitial lung disease,[522,523] although these autoantibodies also occur in other vasculopathies.[524] The frequency of autoantibodies to myosin and muscle is the same for patients with inflammatory myopathy, muscular dystrophy, or denervation atrophy;[525,526] therefore, these autoantibodies may result from muscle damage rather than being a primary phenomenon. One half of the children have circulating immune complexes that may be involved in the pathogenesis of vascular injury.[95,200,527] They may also interfere with the accurate serological detection of autoantibodies and potential antigens, but serum complement determinations are normal.[169,527] Autoantibodies to cardiolipin, found in a minority of children with JDM, may also reflect underlying vasculopathy.[482]

Specific Laboratory Diagnostic Studies

The three laboratory studies that are most useful in substantiating a diagnosis of JDM are measurement of serum levels of the muscle enzymes, MRI and histopathological examination of a muscle specimen obtained by needle or open biopsy (Table 24–15).

Serum Muscle Enzymes

Serum levels of the sarcoplasmic muscle enzymes are important for diagnosis and for monitoring the effectiveness of therapy. Considerable individual variation in the pattern of enzyme elevation is observed; it is therefore recommended that, at least early in disease, AST, CK, lactate dehydrogenase (LDH), and aldolase be measured to obtain a baseline evaluation.[10] The degree of elevation in serum concentration ranges from 20 to 40 times normal for AST or CK. The CK level does not always correlate with disease activity[175]; rarely, some children have normal serum levels of CK during the acute phase of the illness, particularly with a longer duration of untreated disease,[325] and others have a persistent elevation late in the course either associated with ongoing muscle inflammation or, in some cases, without any other clinical indication of muscle inflammation.[21] In the latter instance, evaluation of serum CK levels in family members may suggest an unrelated or unsuspected genetic abnormality. LDH and alanine aminotransferase (ALT)

levels are increased in many children with JDM, and LDH appears to correlate best with measures of disease activity.[528] Although relatively less specific, these enzymes often mirror global disease activity. Elevated ALT and LDH activities may also reflect liver disease associated with lipodystrophy and insulin resistance.[358,362] Serum levels of all muscle enzymes usually decrease 3 to 4 weeks before improvement in muscle strength and rise 5 to 6 weeks before clinical relapse. As a general rule, changes in CK levels occur first, often falling to the normal range within several weeks of instituting therapy; aldolase or LDH levels are the last to respond. Guzman and colleagues[175] reported that flares of disease are best predicted by a combination of AST and LDH and that CK functions poorly as a predictor of exacerbation of myositis.

Creatine Kinase

CK catalyzes the transfer of a phosphoryl group from creatine phosphate to adenosine diphosphate to regenerate adenosine triphosphate in the mitochondria of muscle, brain, and heart. The adenosine triphosphate available to muscle is sufficient to sustain contractile activity for only a fraction of a second. In skeletal muscle, CK constitutes up to 20% of the soluble sarcoplasmic protein, and total CK activity is 225 to 12,000 units per gram of muscle. CK is a dimeric molecule with two subunits: M (muscle) and B (brain). Both consist of 360 amino acids with a molecular mass of 41 kD. Three isoenzymes exist. MM (CK-3) is found in muscle and myocardium, BB (CK-1) in brain, and MB (CK-2) in myocardium but also in regenerating muscle.[529] There may be a persistent elevation of the MB band in muscle inflammation. The adult pattern of isoenzymes is achieved by the age of 4 years.

Serum CK concentration is elevated in many cases of muscle injury, motor neuron diseases, vasculitis, metabolic disorders, endocrinopathies, toxic reactions, and infections. Very high levels are most commonly associated with muscular dystrophy and somewhat less commonly with JDM. Abnormalities of the junctional sites between the T-tubules and the sarcoplasmic reticulum in muscle cells of children with JDM may be the primary sites of leakage of the enzyme. These abnormal anastomoses are far more extensive in the perifascicular than in the centrofascicular myofibers. Enzyme levels are generally not increased in diseases in which there is no loss of sarcolemmal integrity (e.g., glucocorticoid myopathy, disuse atrophy); however, muscle enzyme elevation with glucocorticoid myopathy has been reported.[530]

Transaminases

AST and ALT are cytosolic and mitochondrial enzymes with a wide tissue distribution. AST has two dimeric isoenzymes: one in the cytosol and the other in the mitochondria. The half-life in human plasma is 47 hours for ALT, 6 hours for mitochondrial AST, and 12 to 17 hours for cytosolic AST. Plasma levels decrease to normal adult ranges by 1 year of age.

Aldolase

Aldolase (1,6-diphosphofructoaldolase) is found in myocardium, liver, cerebral cortex, kidneys, and erythrocytes, but it is present in much higher concentration in skeletal

Table 24–15

Specific diagnostic studies performed at the onset of juvenile dermatomyositis

Study	Diagnostic Success (%)
Elevation of serum levels of the muscle enzymes	80-98
Aspartate aminotransferase	48-90
Creatine kinase	64-85
Aldolase	65-75
Lactate dehydrogenase	65-80
Abnormal electromyography	81-95
Abnormal muscle biopsy (inflammation)	80-89

Sources: references 13, 21, 22.

muscle. Aldolase is one of the principal glycolytic enzymes that catalyze the conversion of D-fructose-1,6-diphosphate to dihydroxyacetone phosphate and D-glyceraldehyde-3-phosphate. There are three cytosolic isoenzymes: aldolase A, which predominates in muscle; aldolase B in liver; and aldolase C in brain. Aldolase A is increased in active JDM and in some children with chronic disease.

Lactate Dehydrogenase

LDH is abundant in myocardium and skeletal muscle. There are five isoenzymes: I (30%), II (40%), III (20%), IV (6%), and V (4%). In acute adult polymyositis, there is relatively less isoenzyme I and relatively more II, III, IV, and V. In chronic disease, only isoenzymes I and II are disproportionately elevated. In contrast, patients with active muscular dystrophy exhibit an increase in types I and II and a decrease in III, IV, and V, especially in the younger patient.

Electromyography

Electromyography occasionally is useful in confirming the diagnosis of JDM and in selecting the best site for performing a muscle biopsy. The electromyogram should be evaluated on one side of the body only so that the muscle biopsy, if necessary, can be obtained on the opposite extremity without an artefact created by a needle puncture. Electromyography can be troublesome in the young child, and mild sedation is often necessary. An electromyogram is not mandatory and need not be done unless the diagnosis is in doubt.

The characteristic electromyographic changes of myopathy and denervation (Table 24–16) are associated with membrane instability (e.g., increased insertional activity, fibrillations, positive sharp waves) and random fiber destruction (e.g., decreased amplitude and duration of action potentials). The electrical changes in denervation probably result from segmental myonecrosis of the end plate, although the terminal axons may also be affected. Reinnervation may occur after the acute phase of the disease. Nerve conduction velocities and latencies are normal in JDM, unless severe muscle atrophy is present with a decrease in the number of muscle fibers in a motor unit and with electrical irritability of the sarcolemmal membrane or terminal axonal fibers.

The value of electromyography in identifying continuing inflammatory activity of muscle during the course of JDM has not been adequately documented. Quantitative electromyography may be more informative in this regard.[531-534] In the course of the disease, increasing muscle strength correlates with less spontaneous activity and a decreasing proportion of high-frequency components. During the initial period of treatment, however, a temporary increase in high-frequency signals is expected.

Table 24–16

Electromyography in inflammatory muscle disease

Myopathic motor units, decreased amplitude, short duration, polyphasic

Denervation potentials (positive sharp waves), spontaneous fibrillations, and insertional activity

High-frequency repetitive discharges

Muscle Biopsy

A muscle biopsy is indicated in the initial assessment of a child if the diagnosis is in any way uncertain, including in patients without the characteristic skin rashes of JDM; to evaluate "activity" of the disease, especially late in its course; or if histopathological support for instituting long-term glucocorticoid therapy or immunosuppressive drugs is deemed necessary.[535] Occasionally, a biopsy is indicated in a child who has failed to respond therapeutically to rule out disorders such as dystrophies, metabolic and mitochondrial myopathies, drug-induced myopathies, and inclusion body myositis.[39,46,417,536] A muscle biopsy potentially also provides valuable prognostic information, as discussed above in the section on Pathology.[64,183,330,372,373]

The muscle to be biopsied, usually the deltoid or quadriceps, should be clinically involved, as demonstrated by muscle testing on physical examination, electromyography, or MRI, but it should ideally not be atrophied. MRI can be used to select an area of muscle that is likely to be affected by the disease and thereby increases the probability of obtaining informative tissue.[537,538] If electromyography has been obtained within the previous 6 weeks, the biopsy should be performed on the opposite side of the body.

Care should be taken to prepare the tissue in accordance with the instructions of the pathologist. A generous specimen (12 mm long, 4 mm wide, 2 mm thick) on open muscle biopsy should be obtained in a muscle clamp because muscle involvement is often spotty. The specimen is placed in a transport container and taken immediately to the pathology laboratory. One sample is frozen in isopentane for immunofluorescent and enzyme studies. Another on a separate pediatric clamp is fixed in glutaraldehyde for electron microscopy. The remaining tissue should be stored frozen for additional stains or research studies for situations that are diagnostically unclear. Histopathological results are more likely to be negative or nondiagnostic if the muscle specimen is inadequate in size, obtained from an inappropriate muscle, after the initiation of glucocorticoid or other immunosuppressive therapy, or taken late in the disease when the pathological changes may no longer be specific. Occasionally, there is no evidence of inflammatory change even though characteristic abnormalities such as perifascicular atrophy are present. Although an open biopsy is most often performed, needle biopsy is preferred in some centers.[539] Needle biopsy with a spring-activated, 14-gauge needle may offer a convenient and cost-effective alternative to a surgical procedure.[540] Three or four cores can be obtained with only surface anesthesia by this procedure, although additional frozen tissue for studies is often limited with this approach. The middle deltoid and vastus lateralis are the safest areas to biopsy by this technique from the standpoint of avoiding vascular or neurological damage.

RADIOLOGICAL EXAMINATION

Radiographs in early JDM demonstrate increased soft tissue density caused by edema of the muscle and subcutaneous tissues and, somewhat later, atrophy of muscle.

In chronic disease, areas of calcification in soft tissues can be documented by plain radiographs (see Figs. 24–10 to 24–11). Osteoporosis of long bones and of the vertebral bodies is seen in high frequency and is often extensive (Fig. 24–16).[368] Ultrasound studies of muscle demonstrate increased echogenicity in the muscle and, less frequently, muscle atrophy and increased vascularity on power Doppler, which is more evident on microbubble ultrasound (Fig. 24–17).[541-545] Radionuclide scanning can detect early abnormal changes in blood flow in diseased muscles.[546-549] This technique has limited clinical application, however, and has been superseded by MRI, which is more sensitive for localization of inflamed muscle.

MRI dramatically documents the extent and focal nature of the muscle abnormalities (Fig. 24–18).[541,550-554] The T1-weighted image demonstrates fibrosis, atrophy, and fatty infiltration, which are characteristic of disease damage. The STIR image or T2-weighted MR image with fat suppression demonstrates muscle edema and inflammatory changes by a hyperintense signal,[555-557] and inflammation in skin, subcutaneous tissue, and fascia.[558,559] MRI may be helpful in selecting a site for muscle biopsy[559] but also at selected therapeutic junctures for evaluating the extent and severity of active disease compared to muscle atrophy and fatty infiltration. An increased signal on STIR or T2-weighted MRI of the muscles is seen with inflammation, edema, muscle necrosis and regeneration, rhabdomyolysis, blood, or other proteinaceous material, and it is not specific for idiopathic inflammatory myopathies.[560] Active myositis in general is best documented by STIR or fat-suppressed T2-weighted images, even when serum muscle enzyme elevations or clinical muscle weakness are absent. Although the edema generally enhances after administration of gadolinium as a contrast agent, administration of gadolinium is generally unnecessary because the lesions are adequately visualized without it and some contrast agents carry a risk of nephrogenic systemic fibrosis.[561] Quantitation of T2-weighted images with T2 mapping[562,563] and diffusion-weighted MRI, which suggests decreased capillary perfusion in the muscles of adult myositis patients,[564] are currently research tools. Whole-body MRI is becoming available and may be helpful in revealing the extent of muscle involvement.[565,566] Reversal of these changes occurs in response to treatment, but improvement in MRI may lag behind other indicators.[538,551,558,567] However, exercise-induced changes may mimic active disease.[556]

Investigations have suggested that the course of children with JDM can be monitored with ^{31}P-magnetic resonance spectroscopy (MRS) as an indicator of biochemical defects in energy metabolism.[319,555] Noninvasive ^{31}P-MRS of thigh muscles in children with JDM was studied to characterize metabolic abnormalities during rest, exercise, and recovery.[568] ATP and phosphocreatine levels

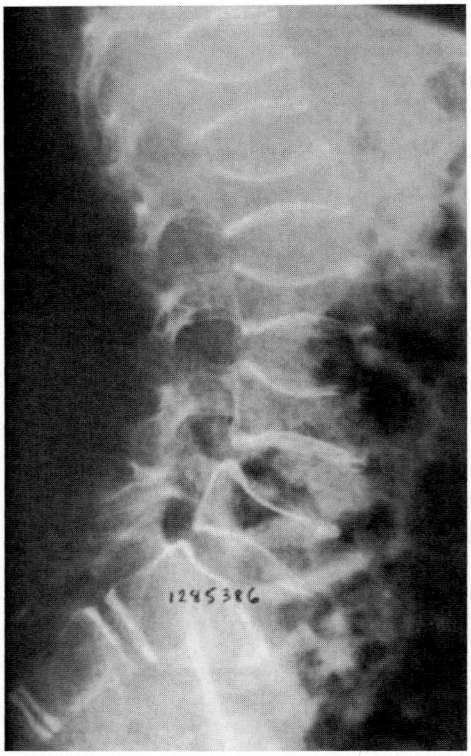

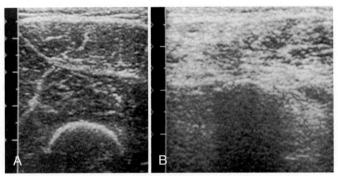

FIGURE 24–17 **A,** Ultrasound view of the midthigh of a normal child. The skin surface is at the *top*; the convex arc is the femoral shaft. Fascial planes are visible in the muscle between the skin and bone. **B,** The same ultrasound view of the midthigh of a child with active dermatomyositis. The convex arc of the femoral shaft is difficult to see, and the fascial planes in the muscle are obliterated because of the intense increase in echogenicity in the inflamed muscle. (Courtesy of Dr. D. Stringer.)

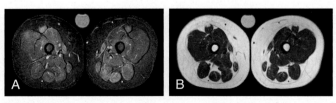

FIGURE 24–18 Cross-sectional magnetic resonance images of the proximal thigh of a child with chronic, severe dermatomyositis. **A,** STIR depicts mild hyperintensity, suggesting edema or increased water content in multiple muscles, most notably in the rectus femoris and sartorius muscles bilaterally, and in the left hamstring musculature. **B,** T1 imaging demonstrates diffuse muscle atrophy in the same distribution and mild fatty infiltration of the muscles.

FIGURE 24–16 Extreme osteopenia of the lumbar spine with multiple vertebral compression fractures in a 15-year-old girl with a long history of chronic polycyclical dermatomyositis and steroid treatment.

were low, as were other measures of mitochondrial oxidative phosphorylation, and they correlated with clinical weakness and fatigue. Low levels of free magnesium and magnesium-ATP were also concordant and in part alleviated by immunosuppressive therapy.[569] Intramyocellular acidification, measured by protocol MRS, is decreased in adult DM/PM patients after exercise compared to healthy controls and patients with mitochondrial mypathies.[570]

Dual energy x-ray absorptiometry has enabled a more accurate assessment of osteopenia and osteoporosis in children with JDM and other chronic rheumatic diseases (see Chapter 49).[368,571] Z scores for these children should be compared with BMC data obtained from healthy, geographic-control children (male and female) with normal values adjusted for height, age, and ethnicity.[572] Alternative evaluation has been proposed by comparisons with data obtained from quantitative calcaneal ultrasound.[573]

TREATMENT

In the presteroid era, approximately one third of children with JDM died, one third recovered, and one third were disabled to a moderate or severe extent.[9,11,20] The introduction of glucocorticoids revolutionized the treatment and prognosis for these children.[6,11-13,254-257,260,261,267,481,574-578] The team approach and general supportive care, including active assisted or passive range of motion exercises early in the disease combined with individualized physical therapy, are essential.[579] There is general agreement that glucocorticoids are always required, but the specifics of management vary considerably from physician to physician and patient to patient.[580]

The response of the child to the treatment program is judged on the basis of systemic signs and symptoms such as fever, general malaise, muscle tenderness, and pain (if present); repeated graded muscle strength and functional examinations by the same observer; sequential serum levels of selected muscle enzymes, acute phase reactants, and other laboratory examinations if indicated (e.g., factor VIII–related antigen);[175,462] and occasionally, other studies, such as MRI of muscle and ultrasonography.[555,556,567] Core set measures of disease activity, including physician and parent global activity assessments, muscle strength and function, extramuscular activity, and enzymes, have been developed and validated by collaborative study groups.[273,276,278,279,555,581-585] Other outcomes including patient-reported outcomes of quality of life and a global index such as the Disease Activity Score, are also included in some core sets.[278,585] Approximately 20% improvement in most measures, although 15% improvement in strength and 30% improvement in enzymes, are considered clinically important change.[528] Indices combining clinically important change in measures of disease activity are being validated.[586,587] Assessment of disease damage related to cumulative changes from previously active disease and other co-morbidities, can now be assessed by the Myositis Damage Index.[588,589] Assessment of protocols of therapy is difficult because appropriately controlled clinical studies have not been performed.

General Supportive Care

The approach to management should be based on the knowledge that the disease is chronic in the majority of patients. It may remit in 2 to 3 years, especially if monophasic, but in a recent study of 84 patients, the median time to remission was 4.7 years.[264] There is no evidence that any therapy is curative; rather, treatment is aimed at suppression of the immunoinflammatory response, maximal preservation of muscle function and joint range of motion, prevention of complications, and maintenance of general health and normal growth and development.

In acute disease, attention must be directed at the adequacy of ventilatory effort and swallowing and occasionally abdominal perforation or myocarditis with severe arrhythmias or congestive heart failure. Occasionally, weakness is so profound that respiratory assistance, nasogastric feeding, and frequent oral suctioning are required. Hypoxia may supervene insidiously. In the older child, vital capacity measurements can be a valuable objective measure of response to therapy. Although respiratory problems occur in approximately one third of severely affected children, ventilatory assistance is seldom required. Profound involvement of the thoracic and respiratory muscles occurs in a few children and leads rapidly to increasing dyspnea at rest, agitation, respiratory insufficiency, aspiration, or death.[590]

Skin care is especially important in children who develop fissures in the axillae and groin or ulcers of the skin over pressure points. Emollients, wound care topical therapies, and padding of pressure areas may help prevent breakdown and ulceration. These ulcerations become sites for secondary infections and abscesses, complications that are abetted by the administration of the glucocorticoid drugs. During the course of the disease, the dermatitis may become markedly photosensitive, and sunblock protective against both ultraviolet A (UV-A) and UV-B wavelengths with high SPF numbers (30 and above) are necessary.[591] The rash may or may not respond to the use of low-potency topical glucocorticoid or tacrolimus/pimecrolimus creams.[592] Long-term use of corticosteroid creams is generally not recommended because of the resulting secondary atrophic effects. Agents to treat pruritus, including antihistamines and emollients, may also be helpful adjuncts in treating skin disease.[593]

Frequent counselling and education of the patient and parents are necessary to help allay anxiety and permit understanding of the necessarily slow pace of treatment and recovery.[594,595] Systemic complications, particularly abdominal pain or gastrointestinal bleeding, require urgent surgical consultation and may be life threatening, especially early in the disease. Attention to nutritional status and intake of potassium and limitation of total caloric and sodium intake may help minimize the side effects of the glucocorticoid drugs.

Glucocorticoid Drugs

Early and adequate treatment with glucocorticoids is probably the single most important factor in improved prognosis during the last 50 years. Acute disease is treated with suppressive doses of the synthetic glucocorticoids

Table 24–17

Medical treatment of juvenile dermatomyositis

*First-Line Therapies**
Prednisone 1-2 mg/kg/day po
Intravenous methylprednisolone 10-30 mg/kg/pulse
Methotrexate 0.4-1 mg/kg/week, or 15 mg/m²
Adjunctive therapies:
   Hydroxychloroquine 3-6 mg/kg/day po divided bid
   Physical therapy
   Photoprotective measures
      Topical therapies for skin rashes—topical corticosteroids,
        tacrolimus, pimecrolimus
      Calcium and vitamin D for bone protection
Second-Line Therapies
Intravenous gammaglobulin 2 g/kg/month
Cyclosporine 2.5-7.5 mg/kg/day po divided bid
Azathioprine 1-3 mg/kg/day
Combinations of the above
Third-Line Therapies
Cyclophosphamide 500-1250 mg/m²/month intravenous pulse
Mycophenolate mofetil 30-40 mg/kg/day po divided bid
Tacrolimus 0.1-0.25 mg/kg/day po divided bid
Rituximab 100 or 375 mg/m² weekly for 2 or 4 weeks
Anti–tumor necrosis factor-α agents—Etanercept: 0.4 mg/kg
   (maximum of 25 mg) SC twice weekly; Infliximab 3-6 mg/
   kg/dose
Combinations of the above

*Agents as first-line therapies are those most often used in the initial treatment of JDM, whereas second- and third-line therapies are most often used in the treatment of refractory patients, patients with severe illness features, or patients with unacceptable medication toxicities. The order in which therapies or combinations of therapies are used is not implied by the listing in this table.
Modified from Wedderburn LR, Rider LG: Juvenile dermatomyositis: new developments in pathogenesis, assessment and treatment. Best Practice and Research in Clinical Rheumatology, 2009; 23: 655-678.

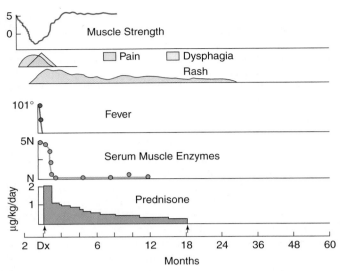

FIGURE 24–19 Course of a 5-year-old girl with an acute onset of dermatomyositis who eventually recovered completely. Dysphagia resolved within the first month, muscle strength returned to normal during the first year, and the rash ultimately subsided by 3 years, as did all other signs of the disease. (Courtesy of Dr. D.B. Sullivan.)

(Table 24–17).[6,11,13] Prednisone is preferred to other analogues, such as dexamethasone or triamcinolone, because these steroids may have a more potent myopathic effect (see Chapter 6). The drug is given in a dosage of approximately 2 mg/kg/day for the first month of the disease and then, if indicated by the clinical response and a fall in the serum levels of the muscle enzymes, reduced by approximately 1 mg/kg/day.[596] For patients with more mild disease, some pediatric rheumatologists prefer a lower starting dose, and for patients with moderate to severe disease, some prefer to administer prednisone initially in two divided doses for the first month of therapy.[596] For many pediatric rheumatologists, factors that contribute to using an initial dose of oral prednisone at the higher end of the range include length of delay to diagnosis, severity of illness at diagnosis, extramuscular manifestations (presence of dysphagia, gastrointestinal involvement, interstitial lung disease, cutaneous ulcerations) and periungual nailfold capillary dropout that may reflect gastrointestinal vasculopathy and contribute to decreased absorption of oral prednisone.[597] Thereafter, the drug is gradually tapered as permitted by careful monitoring of improvement in muscle weakness, skin rashes, and other symptoms and by assay of serum levels of the

muscle enzymes. Alternate-day glucocorticoid therapy is generally not recommended because disease control is often inadequate. It is axiomatic that satisfactory clinical control is not attained until all of the serum enzymes have returned to normal or near-normal levels and have remained there during continued tapering of the steroids and a gradual increase in the physical activity of the child. It is necessary to maintain some children on very low dose glucocorticoids even many years after "clinical control" of myositis. It is difficult to be certain when glucocorticoids can be discontinued without risking an exacerbation of the disease, and this partly appears to depend on initiation of adequate therapy at the time of diagnosis,[321] as well as a gradual reduction in dose that is commensurate with the patient's clinical improvement.

The clinical response of the child to glucocorticoids is not entirely predictable. The fever should abate within a few days, and the serum levels of muscle enzymes should appreciably decrease in the first 1 to 2 weeks of therapy (Figs. 24–19 and 24–20). There may be no significant improvement in muscle strength for 1 to 2 months. Improvement in the dermatitis is unpredictable. Of note, the course of the rash does not necessarily parallel that of the muscle disease, and both aspects of illness must be fully treated. An extensive rash at onset or a generalized progression of the dermatitis is, however, a poor prognostic sign, as is persistence of Gottron papules and periungual nailfold capillary abnormalities.[13,264,293]

Children who require high-dose steroids for long periods develop severe osteopenia and osteoporosis, often with vertebral compression fractures.[571] It is unsettled whether supplementation with dietary calcium and vitamin D can prevent this complication. The efficacy and long-term safety of bisphosphonates are being evaluated, and therefore this therapy is only recommended for patients with recurrent fractures, painful spinal compression fractures, or reduced bone density.[598,599] Cushing

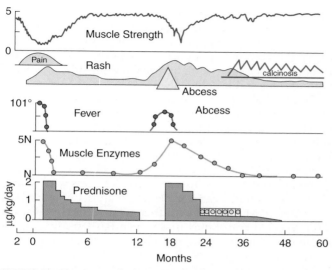

FIGURE 24–20 Course of an 8-year-old boy who initially responded to steroid treatment that was discontinued after 12 months. At 18 months, a gluteal abscess developed and an acute relapse occurred that required combined immunosuppressive therapy because of the development of clinically significant steroid toxicity. ◎, immunosuppression (Courtesy of Dr. D.B. Sullivan.)

Table 24–18

Characteristics of steroid-induced myopathy

Insidious onset
Hip flexor weakness and atrophy
Normal serum concentrations of muscle enzymes
Minimal myopathic changes on electromyography
Thigh muscle atrophy without increased muscle edema on magnetic resonance imaging
Type II fiber atrophy on muscle biopsy

---

syndrome and growth retardation result in any child placed on suppressive doses for a period of months. The dosage of the glucocorticoid drug and duration of its use should therefore be kept as low as possible, commensurate with the clinical and laboratory responses to therapy. Steroid myopathy, which is common in mild form but rarely severe, may be misinterpreted as an exacerbation of the basic disease process (Table 24–18) (see Chapter 6). The manifestations of this syndrome are insidious onset of hip flexor weakness and atrophy with normal assays of the serum muscle enzymes and minimal myopathic changes on electromyography.[530] MRI may show atrophy of the proximal thigh muscles on T1 axial images but no muscle edema on STIR or fat-suppressed T2-weighted images.

Intravenous pulse glucocorticoid therapy has been proposed to gain rapid control of muscle inflammation while minimizing the exposure of the child to long-term, high-dose daily steroids.[37,600-606] An initial publication by Laxer and associates[603] indicated a satisfactory response in six children; subsequently, two additional patients were treated. Both were boys who had mild early disease; a single intravenous pulse of methylprednisolone (30 mg/kg) led to a decrease in the enzyme levels and improved

muscle strength over 2 months. There may be a subgroup of children with JDM in whom this initial approach to management will be successful and abrogate the need for long-term daily glucocorticoid treatment. The majority of North American pediatric rheumatologists include intravenous pulse methylprednisolone as part of the initial therapy of patients with moderate to severe illness. Pachman[60] advanced the concept that early use of intravenous pulse therapy reduces future disability and the extent of calcinosis. The bioavailability of pulse methylprednisolone may be better than that of oral prednisone, particularly in patients with vasculopathy and periungual nailfold capillary density.[597] As with any form of therapy, this approach to glucocorticoid administration is not always effective and may not impact long-term outcome.[607,608] Pulse therapy may be combined advantageously with methotrexate as part of the initial therapeutic regimen, resulting in less calcinosis, increased frequency of remission and reduced likelihood of flare later in the illness course in data from uncontrolled studies.[321,328,605] Intravenous pulse therapy may also be of benefit for acute or life-threatening manifestations, such as myocarditis or severe dysphagia, or pneumatosis intestinalis.

Hydroxychloroquine

Hydroxychloroquine has been recommended as a steroid-sparing agent and as a drug that is effective in treating the dermatitis of JDM.[609] Olson and Lindsley[610] reported significant improvement of the rash following 3 months and of muscle weakness after 6 months of treatment in a dose of 2 to 5 mg/kg/day in nine children. Anecdotal experience suggests that the addition of hydroxychloroquine to a glucocorticoid regimen is warranted but has modest efficacy. As such, it tends to be included as part of the therapy of patients with mild to moderate disease.[596] It is alleged that patients with dermatomyositis may be prone to non–life-threatening cutaneous reactions from the antimalarial agents.[611]

Immunosuppressive Therapy

Primary indications for the use of immunosuppressive drugs include *glucocorticoid resistance or dependence*. In steroid-resistant disease, there is inadequate improvement in muscle strength and a persistence of elevated serum levels of muscle enzymes in response to a closely monitored glucocorticoid program (prednisone, 1 to 2 mg/kg/day for at least 3 to 4 months). Steroid dependence occurs later in the course of the disease and is characterized by failure of the clinical manifestations of disease to remain suppressed during a gradual reduction of the glucocorticoid dose to an acceptable level, recurrence of progressive muscle weakness despite continuing therapy, or unacceptable steroid toxicity.

Several immunosuppressive drugs have been employed in resistant disease: methotrexate,[606,612-617] azathioprine,[616,618] and cyclosporine[43,44,61,619-624] have been used most commonly as second-line agents (Table 24–17). Mycophenolate mofetil,[625-627] tacrolimus,[628,629] and cyclophosphamide[64,630,631] are used most often as third-line agents due to less experience with them (Table 24–17). The efficacy of these drugs is difficult to evaluate because, as with glucocorticoids or hydroxychloroquine, there have been no controlled trials to date. Of the immunosuppressive drugs, weekly oral or subcutaneous methotrexate is the preferred agent among pediatric rheumatologists in North America, with a minimal initial dose of 0.35 mg/kg/week, reaching a maximum 1 mg/kg/week. Careful monitoring of dosage and potential toxicity relative to age, height, and weight is mandatory. Benefit is usually evident within 2 to 3 months. No controlled study has been published on the consistency of response; however, a report of 12 JDM patients suggested a favorable improvement in all over 3 to 78 weeks after initiating therapy without major toxicity or hepatic disease.[614] Recent reports suggest early introduction of methotrexate (often subcutaneously) may be associated with reduced steroid toxicity, better growth velocity and overall reduction in duration and cumulative dose of steroids.[321,328,615] Many North American pediatric rheumatologists now use methotrexate as part of the initial therapy of JDM, regardless of illness severity.[594]

There have been several case reports and series of successful cyclosporine therapy.[37,619-624] Some investigators have suggested that this drug should be considered first-line therapy in the treatment of inflammatory muscle disease,[632] and it is often the preferred second medication for patients receiving treatment in Europe. Except for renal impairment, cyclosporine has less long-term toxicity than the traditional immunosuppressive drugs, and for this reason, its use should perhaps be considered earlier in the child who is nonresponsive to steroids or steroid dependent or who has evidence of interstitial lung disease.[633,634] The efficacy of cyclosporine in the treatment of steroid-resistant or steroid-dependent disease has been reported by Heckmatt and associates.[621] In this study, 14 children who had failed to respond fully to glucocorticoids and immunosuppressives were given a dose of 2.5 to 7.5 mg/kg/day (younger children require an increased dosage because drug clearance is age dependent). The investigators reported considerable benefit, with reduced prednisolone requirements in all, including discontinuation of glucocorticoid in 6. Two of 3 nonambulatory patients were able to walk after treatment, and 6 with limited ambulation subsequently regained good independent ambulation. Muscle strength improved but remained significantly reduced. The only notable side effects were hypertension and reversible decreases in renal function.[635] The ongoing PRINTO randomized controlled study compares prednisone alone versus prednisone combined with methotrexate versus prednisone in combination with cyclosporine as initial therapy for JDM.[636]

There is little published experience with azathioprine or cyclophosphamide. Crowe and colleagues[64] first recommended cyclophosphamide in children with a chronic ulcerative course that was unresponsive to glucocorticoids. An open label study of intravenous monthly pulse cyclophosphamide in severe or treatment-refractory JDM patients demonstrated significant improvements in 10 of 12 patients after 6 months.[631] Many of these patients had severe weakness, dysphagia, skin or gastrointestinal ulcerations, or central nervous system disease that improved after the initiation of therapy. This therapy may also be of benefit in patients with interstitial lung disease.[4] Intravenous cyclophosphamide therapy, however, is not always successful, particularly in adult patients with chronic stable active disease.[637]

Open-label reports in adult myositis support use of mycophenolate mofetil for patients with severe or recalcitrant disease, resulting in improvement in strength, skin rashes, and muscle enzymes and an ability to reduce the steroid dose in the majority.[625,626] Seven treatment-refractory JDM patients in an open-label study improved their skin and muscle Disease Activity Scores with mycophenolate mofetil treatment.[627] The majority of adult DM and three JDM patients with treatment-refractory disease who received tacrolimus in an open-label study demonstrated improvement, supporting use in the treatment of refractory patients.[628,629] Tacrolimus also appears to be beneficial for the treatment of refractory interstitial lung disease.[634,638]

Combinations of drugs as initial therapy for JDM, including prednisone, methotrexate, and intravenous pulse methylprednisolone, followed by cyclosporine and intravenous immunoglobulin (IVIg), may increase the frequency of remission and decrease the frequency of calcinosis.[321] An experimental protocol in adults that consisted of comparing combination oral methotrexate and azathioprine to high dose intravenous methotrexate (500 mg/m^2) suggests that the combination regimen may be superior to methotrexate alone.[639] Case reports in adult patients support other combinations, including cyclosporine or azathioprine with cyclophosphamide,[640,641] as well as cyclosporine or cyclophosphamide with IVIg.[642,643] The Childhood Arthritis and Research Alliance has developed consensus protocols that include combinations of prednisone and methotrexate with or without IVIg as part of the initial treatment of JDM.[598]

Intravenous Immunoglobulin

A number of studies and anecdotal reports describe the efficacy of IVIg (Table 24–17).[644-649] Clinical experience in children has been summarized in several reviews on JDM therapy.[37] Lang and coworkers[644] reported results of administration of IVIg to five children who were steroid resistant or steroid dependent. All patients exhibited improved muscle strength and diminished rash over the 9-month period with infusions every 4 weeks of 1 g/kg/day on each of 2 consecutive days. A follow-up report in a retrospective review of 18 patients confirmed reduction in disease activity and ability to reduce corticosteroid dose in the majority.[649]

Controlled studies enrolling adult DM and PM patients provide additional information.[650-652] In these reports, IVIg was of significant benefit, particularly if used early in the disease course and especially with respect to the skin changes. However, without controlled clinical trials of this therapeutic approach in children, no firm conclusions can be reached regarding efficacy. Of note, JDM patients receiving IVIg frequently develop fever, lethargy, malaise, nausea and vomiting, apparently related to the immunoglobulin A concentration present in the IVIg preparation.[653]

Biological Agents and Stem Cell Transplantation

All seven refractory adult DM patients receiving rituximab (four weekly infusions of 100 mg/m² or 375 mg/m²) responded, beginning 4 to12 weeks in parallel with depletion of peripheral blood B lymphocytes, with a maximal response at 12 to 36 weeks, and response duration of 24 to > 52 weeks (Table 24–17).[654] In four patients with refractory JDM, three had marked clinical responses with rituximab therapy and one developed disease worsening.[655] Little improvement in skin disease activity was noted in one study of refractory adult DM.[656] Results of a randomized clinical trial are expected.[657] The TNF-α inhibitors, including recombinant soluble human TNF-α receptor (p75)–Fc fusion protein and chimeric monoclonal antibodies to TNF-α have been used with promising results in a few patients.[582] In one trial of etanercept,[658] 9 of 10 children improved in activity, skin, and muscle scores and in functional ability, but one child's rash had a severe flare. In five severe JDM cases treated with infliximab (3 mg/kg every 8 weeks to 6 mg/kg every 4 weeks), all improved in disease activity after 8 to 30 months, and in some cases calcinosis also improved, with no serious side effects reported.[659] Responses to anti–TNF-α therapy have been mixed in adult DM/PM,[660] with disease progression in some patients.[661] Results of a randomized trial of etanercept in early adult DM are anticipated.[662]

Experience with autologous hemopoietic stem cell transplantation for JDM is limited, but it has been successful in a few patients with refractory disease. However, these children are at high risk for developing severe viral infections.[663,664] A preliminary study of alemtuzumab in inclusion body myositis suggests slowing of disease progression, improvement in strength of some patients, and reduction in endomysial inflammation, warranting studies in other forms of myositis.[665] A trial of anti–interferon-α is in progress in adult DM patients.[666]

Plasmapheresis

Plasmapheresis has been of benefit in a few children with severe, life-threatening disease refractory to other therapies.[667-670] Studies suggest that there is no therapeutic effect in adults, based on a randomized controlled trial.[671] A report of a single patient with JDM who was treated by extracorporeal photopheresis (i.e., ultraviolet activation of methoxsalen to covalently crosslink lymphocyte DNA) is an experimental approach of interest.[672]

Physical and Occupational Therapy

Physiotherapy should be initiated at the time of diagnosis. Although skeletal muscles are actively inflamed, the focus of attention should be on preventing loss of range of motion by giving twice- to thrice-daily active assisted or passive range of motion exercises to all joints, with the use of gentle stretching to regain lost range.[579] Splinting of knees, elbows, or wrists at night or during periods of rest helps to achieve these goals. During the healing phase, the physical therapy program is increased to normalize function as nearly as possible and to minimize development of contractures from muscle weakness or atrophy. Isometric muscle strengthening should be added to the exercise program only after clinical evidence of acute inflammation has subsided. Later, when disease activity is mild, isotonic strengthening and graded aerobic activity are included.[579] Exercise therapy does not appear to worsen myositis disease activity, and studies in adults suggest improved strength and functional outcomes following strengthening programs.[673]

MANAGEMENT OF CALCINOSIS

None of many approaches to the treatment of calcinosis has been consistently effective, and no randomized controlled trials have been performed to adequately evaluate such therapies.[403,674-691] Therapy has included colchicine, aluminum hydroxide, probenecid, alendronate and diphosphonates, diltiazem, intravenous ethylenediaminetetraacetic acid, and warfarin. Colchicine may suppress local and systemic signs of inflammation associated with calcinosis.[682] Lithotripsy may decrease associated pain in patients with stable calcinosis.[690] There is general agreement that early aggressive therapy with glucocorticoids and other medications results in decreased frequency and severity of calcinosis.[60,321,328] Experimental data suggest that TNF blockade may be beneficial because overexpression of the TNF-α308A allele is associated with a long duration of active disease and pathological calcifications.[145] Surgical excision of calcifications that mechanically interfere with function or have resulted in breakdown of skin may be indicated,[690] although recurrence of calcinosis and infections in such sites are a risk.[691]

The natural history of many of these calcific deposits is that they spontaneously begin to regress after months or years, coincident with inactivity of the muscle disease and increasing mobility of the patient. However, the one fourth of children who develop calcinosis in interfascial planes tend to have persistent lesions.[304] Hypercalcemia and hypercalciuria have been reported during spontaneous resolution of calcinosis.[593,693]

MANAGEMENT OF LIPODYSTROPHY

Recent data have emphasized the role of leptin deficiency in the abnormalities characteristic of generalized lipodystrophy and the potential role of replacement therapy in treating this complication of dermatomyositis. This adipocyte hormone is critical in energy homeostasis and glycemic control.

Oral and colleagues[694-696] administered escalating doses of recombinant methionyl human leptin to nine female patients with leptin levels less than 4 ng/mL (0.32 nmol/mL) subcutaneously twice daily for 4 months. With treatment, triglyceride and hemoglobin A1C levels decreased along with hepatic volume, and the resting metabolic rate improved. Observations extended to several additional patients confirmed a marked improvement in insulin sensitivity in the liver and muscle and in whole-body insulin-stimulated glucose metabolism,[695] as well as in hepatic steatosis.[696]

COURSE OF THE DISEASE AND PROGNOSIS

The course of JDM can be divided into four clinical phases (Table 24–19).[305] The early prodromal phase is supplanted by a period of progressive muscle weakness and rash that then stabilizes for 1 to 2 years before recovery (Table 24–19). Thirty-seven percent to 60% of children pursue this type of a uniphasic course.[11,13,36,264,293,303,322,713] The entire disease duration can be as brief as 8 months with complete recovery, or it can last 2 or more years with a chronically active disease and a continuing requirement for treatment with glucocorticoids. From a national U.S. registry of 136 children with JDM, 47% had persistent rashes, 18% weakness, and 8% arthritis; 12.5% had both rash and weakness at 36 month reevaluation[697] (Table 24–20). Family interviews of patients enrolled in this registry documented the persistence of symptoms for at least 25% of 229 children at 36 months after diagnosis,[698] and 54% were still receiving medication for JDM.[699] Acute exacerbations and remissions without any stabilization of the initial course of the disease have occurred in up to 20% of children.[25] There has been a significant improvement in outcome over the past 3 decades (Table 24–21).

Four Canadian centers evaluated functional outcome in 80 children treated between 1984 and 1995 (46 girls and 19 boys) with a mean follow-up of 7.2 years (range, 3.2 to 13.9 years).[322] A monocyclical course was characteristic of 37% and a chronic continuous or polycyclical one in 63%. Favorable outcomes were predominant: only 8% had moderate to severe disability, 34% had developed calcinosis, and there was one death. However, persistent rash was seen in 40%, 23% had ongoing weakness, and 35% were continuing to take medications more than 3 years after disease onset.

In examining long-term sequelae of disease using sensitive measures such as the Myositis Damage Index, almost 80% of patients exhibited measurable damage, including cutaneous scar, contractures, persistent weakness, and muscle dysfunction, and calcinosis was present in 23% to 30% of patients after a median of 6.8 years from diagnosis.[593] In a multicenter, cross-sectional study of 490 JDM patients from Europe and Latin America with a mean disease duration of 7.7 years, 41% to 53% had reduced muscle strength, although only 10% had moderate to severe impairment, 41.2% to 60.5% had persistently active disease, and 69% had measurable damage.[326] Items of damage present in 10% to 44% of patients included cutaneous scarring, muscle atrophy, calcinosis and joint contractures, muscle dysfunction, persistent weakness, and hirsutism.[326] Disease course was monocyclic in 41% of patients and chronic polycyclical or continuous in 59%.[326] JDM patients, as adults, may be at increased risk of early atherosclerosis, as seen by increased carotid intimal medial thickness and brightness in young adulthood; patients with calcinosis and more severe disease activity may be at particularly increased risk.[700]

Predictors of disease course based on early illness features have been difficult to identify.[264,322] (Table 24–22) Persistence of rash within the first 6 months after diagnosis, including Gottron papules and periungual nailfold capillary changes, may be predictive of a longer

Table 24–20

Clinical features of juvenile dermatomyositis during the course of the disease

Feature	%
Muscle weakness	90-100
Dysphagia or dysphonia	13-40
Muscle atrophy	10
Muscle pain and tenderness	30-83
Skin lesions	85-100
Heliotrope rash of eyelids	66-83
Gottron papules	57-91
Erythematous rash of malar/facial area	42-100
Periungual capillary changes	80
Photosensitive rash	5-42
Ulcerations	22-30
Calcinosis	12-30
Lipodystrophy	11-14
Raynaud phenomenon	2-15
Arthritis and arthralgia	22-58
Joint contractures	26-27
Fever	16-46
Gastrointestinal signs and symptoms	8-22
Restrictive pulmonary disease	4-32
Interstitial lung disease	1-7
Cardiac involvement	0-3

From references 22, 24, 25, 27.

Table 24–19

Clinical phases of juvenile dermatomyositis

1. Prodromal period with nonspecific symptoms (weeks to months)*
2. Progressive muscle weakness and rash (days to weeks)
3. Persistent weakness, rash, and active myositis (up to 2 years or longer)
4. Recovery with or without residual muscle atrophy, contractures, and calcinosis

*Durations of the clinical phases in part depend on treatment.
Adapted from reference 305.

Table 24–21

Prognosis of juvenile dermatomyositis

Outcome	% of Patients
Normal to good functional outcome	65-80
Minimal atrophy or contractures	25-30
Calcinosis*	12-40
Wheelchair dependence	5
Death	1-2

*Children with calcinosis were also included in the other categories.

Table 24-22

Factors that adversely influence outcome

Disease-Related Factors

Rapid onset and extensive weakness

Cutaneous vasculopathy with ulceration

Gastrointestinal vasculopathy/ulceration

Severe endarteropathy and infarction in muscle biopsy specimen

Persistent disease activity, including skin activity

Therapy-Related Factors

Delay in diagnosis and institution of therapy

Inadequate dose or duration of glucocorticoid therapy

Minimal initial or sustained response to glucocorticoid therapy

Inconsistent or nonadherence to medical therapy

time to remission.[264,293] Risk factors for a poor prognosis include unremitting severe disease activity, cutaneous ulcerations, extensive calcinosis, dysphagia or dysphonia, advanced nail fold capillary abnormalities, a high serum creatine kinase level, a noninflammatory vasculopathy on muscle biopsy, and the presence of certain MSAs (such as antisynthetase and anti–signal recognition particle autoantibodies). Delays in treatment and inadequate treatment are also important risk factors.[701] Determinants of physical function are receiving further elucidation.[282]

The studies of Crowe and associates[64] identified a group of children with noninflammatory vasculopathy who had extensive and chronic ulcerative cutaneous disease. These children and a similar group reported earlier by Banker and Victor[7] were characterized by significant systemic complications, including fatal gastrointestinal hemorrhage. At a minimum, children with severe generalized erythroderma and cutaneous ulcerations often develop extensive calcinosis and significant overall functional impairment.[320] Approximately 5% of children eventually develop a clinical disease that is more typical of systemic vasculitis.[64,330] A small number of children late in the course of disease may assume more of the characteristics of scleroderma with sclerodactyly and cutaneous atrophy, develop an overlap connective tissue disease,[13,36] or experience a recurrence of arthritis.

Late progression has been reported with a recurrence of active disease after a prolonged remission[701,702] or smoldering, persistent activity many years after onset with multiple physical or dermatological sequelae.[703-705] Of interest in this regard is the risk from pregnancy in women who have had or have JDM.[706-708] Depending on the activity of the disease, residual muscle weakness, calcinosis, and disability, pregnancy may be high risk for both mother and baby.

Calcinosis

Historically, 12% to 40% of children with JDM have developed calcinosis (see Tables 24-6 and 24-21).[13,25,36,130,304,320,321,322,326,592,699,700] Children with extensive calcinosis were often those who had suffered from a severe and unremitting course.[304] In those children and to a lesser extent in others, calcinosis was responsible

for more long-term disability with limitation of movement of involved muscles or contiguous joints than the residual effects of myositis.[322] Calcinosis appears to be decreased in frequency and extent in those children treated earlier after symptom onset and those treated with adequate doses of steroids or other immunosuppressives as part of the initial therapy of disease.[321,328,700] Calcific deposits may develop as early as 6 months or as late as 10 to 20 years after disease onset. Calcinosis is occasionally present at first presentation of the child to a physician. In this situation, it is surmised that the child had a prolonged but mild and therefore undiagnosed myositis before development of the calcinosis.[709] Rarely, calcinosis is accompanied by hypercalcemia.[681] Trauma may play a role in the generation of calcific deposits because they also tend to occur in surgical incisions and over pressure points. A study by Moore and coworkers[692] concluded that calcinosis was associated with preceding staphylococcal infection and high levels of IgE and IgE antistaphylococcal antibodies. Granulocyte chemotaxis to staphylococci was depressed, an effect that was mediated by unidentified serum factors.

Functional Disability

In children with a typical uniphasic course, functional outcome is usually excellent, although minor flexion contractures and residual skin changes may persist (see Table 24-21). In others in whom the disease remains active beyond 3 years, there may be smoldering myositis and dermatitis with deposition of calcium salts and progressive loss of function. Adverse factors that influence outcome are listed in Table 24-22. Early and adequate steroid treatment has the greatest impact on a favorable outcome.[10,13] Functional outcome appears best in children who have been diagnosed shortly after onset and treated vigorously, perhaps with initial steroid-pulse administration.[321,328,612,700] Most survivors are able to function independently as adults, although some have flexion contractures and residual atrophy of skin or muscle.[322,704]

In a multicenter study, 72% of patients had no or minimal disability an average of 7 years after onset.[322] In the large cross-sectional multicenter study from Europe and Latin America, 41% had measurable functional disability with a mean follow-up of 7.7 years, although only 6% of patients had severe impairment.[326]

Psychosocial Outcome

A study by Miller and associates[710] suggested that a number of children who enter adulthood continue to have psychological problems and learning disabilities based on unrecognized cerebral abnormalities that occurred at onset of disease. Another review of late outcome in JDM indicated that the educational achievements and employment status of 18 patients were better than those of the general adult population or a comparable group who had had chronic arthritis.[711] Significant disability related to calcinosis or contractures developed in 3 patients, 6 had persistent muscle weakness, and 7 had recurrent rash. Huber and colleagues reported 3 of 80 patients experienced school delay of 1 year due to illness, but the population otherwise experienced no educational impairment or difficulty working.[322] In measuring health-related quality of life, the crosssectional European/Latin American study of Ravelli and colleagues indicates 14% have mild and 4% more substantial psychosocial impairment. [326]

Death

Long-term survival is better than 95%; in the presteroid era, this disease was associated with a mortality rate that approached 40%.[13,64,710,711] Children who survived often had devastating residual problems of contractures and muscular atrophy. Fatalities most often occur within 2 years of onset and are often associated with progressive involvement of skin or muscle that is unresponsive to steroids. This observation suggests that the basic nature of the inflammatory disease, its early treatment and response, the presence of widespread vasculitis, and involvement of other organ systems (e.g., gastrointestinal tract, lungs) are major factors that should be assessed in estimating prognosis. Death most often results from respiratory insufficiency or interstitial lung disease, myocarditis, or from acute gastrointestinal ulceration with intestinal perforation or bleeding. Surgical intervention in the latter group of children may be successful.

There were six deaths in the Ann Arbor series of 71 children.[13] One young girl died 5 years after onset as a result of cardiorespiratory collapse. Necropsy examination documented no active myositis. Three patients died at 2 months, 6 months, and 4 years after onset from gastrointestinal hemorrhage. Another girl died from a subdural hematoma caused by a fall from a wheelchair. A boy succumbed shortly after onset of disease from respiratory insufficiency and hypoxia. In the series of Spencer and colleagues,[305] 7 of 66 patients died. Five deaths occurred early (1 to 11 months from diagnosis) and were related to sepsis (1), gastrointestinal perforation (2), and unresponsive muscle weakness and pneumonitis (2). One patient died of pulmonary fibrosis with cor pulmonale 9 years after disease onset, and one patient committed suicide 16 years after onset.

In the report of 39 patients by Miller and associates,[710] there were 10 deaths (26%); 8 of these were children seen before 1972. No child who had received intensive glucocorticoid treatment (and azathioprine in some cases) died. All deaths were associated with bowel perforation or aspiration pneumonitis and occurred an average of 2.5 years after onset. The improved outcome rate since 1972 (98% survival rate) is related to early and appropriate steroid regimens and use of adjunctive medications, better clinical assessment, follow-up with sequential serum muscle enzyme determinations, and optimal management of complications.[712]

From the Canadian inception cohort of 80 children diagnosed between 1984 and 1995 with a median of 7.2 years of follow-up, one child died of myocardial infarction.[322] In the European/Latin American multicenter cross-sectional study with patients diagnosed between 1980 to 2004, the mortality rate was 3.1%.[326] None of the 38 children with JDM treated in Hungary died, with a median follow-up of 3 years.[36]

REFERENCES

22. L.J. McCann, A.D. Juggins, S.M. Maillard, et al., The Juvenile Dermatomyositis National Registry and Repository (UK and Ireland)—clinical characteristics of children recruited within the first 5 yr, Rheumatology 45 (2006) 1255–1260.

25. A.V. Ramanan, B.M. Feldman, Clinical features and outcomes of juvenile dermatomyositis and other childhood onset myositis syndromes, Rheum. Dis. Clin. North Am. 28 (2002) 833–857.

37. L.G. Rider, F.W. Miller, Classification and treatment of the juvenile idiopathic inflammatory myopathies, Rheum. Dis. Clin. North Am. 23 (1997) 619–655.

57. E.P. Mendez, R. Lipton, R. Ramsey-Goldman, et al., US incidence of juvenile dermatomyositis, 1995-1998: results from the National Institute of Arthritis and Musculoskeletal and Skin Diseases Registry, Arthritis Rheum. 49 (2003) 300–305.

65. L.M. Pachman, R. Lipton, R. Ramsey-Goldman, et al., History of infection before the onset of juvenile dermatomyositis: results from the National Institute of Arthritis and Musculoskeletal and Skin Diseases Research Registry, Arthritis Rheum. 53 (2005) 166–172.

70. Z. Tezak, E.P. Hoffman, J.L. Lutz, et al., Gene expression profiling in DQA10501* children with untreated dermatomyositis: a novel model of pathogenesis, J. Immunol. 168 (2002) 4154–4163.

72. A.M. Reed, S.R. Ytterberg, Genetic and environmental risk factors for idiopathic inflammatory myopathies, Rheum. Dis. Clin. North Am. 28 (2002) 891–916.

133. G. Mamyrova, T.P. O'Hanlon, J.B. Monroe, et al., Immunogenetic risk and protective factors for juvenile dermatomyositis in Caucasians, Arthritis Rheum. 54 (2006) 3979–3987.

134. L.R. Wedderburn, N.J. McHugh, H. Chinoy, et al., HLA class II haplotype and autoantibody associations in children with juvenile dermatomyositis and juvenile dermatomyositis-scleroderma overlap, Rheumatology 46 (2007) 1786–1791.

146. G. Mamyrova, T.P. O'Hanlon, L. Sillers, et al., Cytokine gene polymorphisms as risk and severity factors for juvenile dermatomyositis, Arthritis Rheum. 58 (2008) 3941–3950.

147. L.G. Rider, C.M. Artlett, C.B. Foster, et al., Polymorphisms in the IL-1 receptor antagonist gene VNTR are possible risk factors for juvenile idiopathic inflammatory myopathies, Clin. Exp. Immunol. 121 (2000) 47–52.

156. A.M. Reed, T.A. Griffin, The inflammatory milieu: cells and cytokines, in: L.J. Kagen (Ed.), The inflammatory myopathies, Humana Press, New York (2009) 29–53.

183. C.M. Lopez De Padilla, A.N. Vallejo, D. Lacomis, et al., Extranodal lymphoid microstructures in inflamed muscle and disease severity of new-onset juvenile dermatomyositis, Arthritis Rheum. 60 (2009) 1160–1172.

185. C.M. Lopez de Padilla, A.N. Vallejo, K.T. McNallan, et al., Plasmacytoid dendritic cells in inflamed muscle of patients with juvenile dermatomyositis, Arthritis Rheum. 56 (2007) 1658–1668.

186. E.C. Baechler, J.W. Bauer, C.A. Slattery, et al., An interferon signature in the peripheral blood of dermatomyositis patients is associated with disease activity, Mol. Med. 13 (2007) 59–68.

243. K. Nagaraju, N. Raben, L. Loeffler, et al., Conditional up-regulation of MHC class I in skeletal muscle leads to self-sustaining autoimmune myositis and myositis-specific autoantibodies, Proc. Natl. Acad. Sci. 97 (2000) 9209–9214.

251. A.L. Urganus, Y.D. Zhao, L.M. Pachman, Juvenile dermatomyositis calcifications selectively displayed markers of bone formation, Arthritis Rheum. 61 (2009) 501–508.

258. Washington University Neuromuscular Home Page: http://neuromuscular.wustl.edu/maltbrain.html

262. B.M. Feldman, L.G. Rider, A.M. Reed, L.M. Pachman, Juvenile dermatomyositis and other idiopathic inflammatory myopathies of childhood, Lancet 371 (2008) 2201–2212.

263. L.G. Rider, L.M. Pachman, F.W. Miller, H. Bollar (Eds.), Myositis and you: a guide to juvenile dermatomyositis for patients, families and health care providers, The Myositis Association, Washington, DC, 2007.

264. E. Stringer, D. Singh-Grewal, B.M. Feldman, Predicting the course of juvenile dermatomyositis: significance of early clinical and laboratory features, Arthritis Rheum. 58 (2008) 3585–3592.

276. A.M. Huber, B.M. Feldman, R.M. Rennebohm, et al., Validation and clinical significance of the Childhood Myositis Assessment Scale for assessment of muscle function in the juvenile idiopathic inflammatory myopathies, Arthritis Rheum. 50 (2004) 1595–1603.

278. R.L. Smith, J. Sundberg, E. Shamiyah, et al., Skin involvement in juvenile dermatomyositis is associated with loss of end row nail-fold capillary loops, J. Rheumatol. 31 (2004) 1644–1649.

279. International Myositis Assessment and Clinical Studies Group (IMACS) internet site (assessment tools and training materials): http://www.niehs.nih.gov/research/resources/collab/imacs/disease activity.cfm; http://www.niehs.nih.gov/research/resources/collab/imacsforms.cfm; http://www.niehs.nih.gov/research/resou rces/collab/imacs/othertools.cfm; and http://www.niehs.nih.gov/research/resources/collab/imacs/diseasedamage.cfm

286. E.M. Dugan, A.M. Huber, F.W. Miller, et al., Photoessay of the idiopathic inflammatory myopathies, Dermatol. Online J. 15 (2009) 1.

293. S. Christen-Zaech, R. Seshadri, J. Sundberg, et al., Persistent association of nailfold capillaroscopy changes and skin involvement over thirty-six months with duration of untreated disease in patients with juvenile dermatomyositis, Arthritis Rheum. 58 (2008) 571–576.

304. S.L. Bowyer, C.E. Blane, D.B. Sullivan, et al., Childhood dermatomyositis: factors predicting functional outcome and development of dystrophic calcification, J. Pediatr. 103 (1983) 882–888.

321. S. Kim, M. El-Hallak, F. Dedeoglu, et al., Complete and sustained remission of juvenile dermatomyositis resulting from aggressive treatment, Arthritis Rheum. 60 (2009) 1825–1830.

322. A.M. Huber, B. Lang, C.M. LeBlanc, et al., Medium- and long-term functional outcomes in a multicenter cohort of children with juvenile dermatomyositis, Arthritis Rheum. 43 (2000) 541–549.

324. L.G. Rider, Calcinosis in juvenile dermatomyositis: pathogenesis and current therapies, Pediatr. Rheum. Online. J. 1 (2003) 2. Accessed at http://www.pedrheumonlinejournal.org/April/calinosis.htm.

326. A. Ravelli, L. Trail, C. Ferrari, et al., Long-term outcome and prognostic factors of juvenile dermatomyositis: a multinational, multicenter study of 490 patients, Arthritis Care Res. 62 (2010) 63–72.

358. A. Bingham, G. Mamyrova, K.I. Rother, et al., Predictors of acquired lipodystrophy in juvenile-onset dermatomyositis and a gradient of severity, Medicine 87 (2008) 70–86.

372. L. Miles, K.E. Bove, D. Lovell, et al., Predictability of the clinical course of juvenile dermatomyositis based on initial muscle biopsy: a retrospective study of 72 patients, Arthritis Rheum. 57 (2007) 1183–1191.

473. T.B. Niewold, S.N. Kariuki, G.A. Morgan, et al., Elevated serum interferon-alpha activity in juvenile dermatomyositis: associations with disease activity at diagnosis and after thirty-six months of therapy, Arthritis Rheum. 60 (2009) 1815–1824.

486. I.N. Targoff, G. Mamyrova, E.P. Trieu, et al., A novel autoantibody to a 155-kd protein is associated with dermatomyositis, Arthritis Rheum. 54 (2006) 3682–3689.

487. H. Gunawardena, L.R. Wedderburn, J. North, et al., Clinical associations of autoantibodies to a p155/140 kDa doublet protein in juvenile dermatomyositis, Rheumatology 47 (2008) 324–328.

488. H. Gunawardena, L.R. Wedderburn, H. Chinoy, et al., Autoantibodies to a 140-kd protein in juvenile dermatomyositis are associated with calcinosis, Arthritis Rheum. 60 (2009) 1807–1814.

501. H. Gunawardena, Z.E. Betteridge, N.J. McHugh, Myositis-specific autoantibodies: their clinical and pathogenic significance in disease expression, Rheumatology (Oxford) 48 (2009) 607–612.

558. R.J. Hernandez, D.B. Sullivan, T.L. Chenevert, et al., MR imaging in children with dermatomyositis: musculoskeletal findings and correlation with clinical and laboratory findings, Am. J. Roentgenol. 161 (1993) 359–366.

584. L.G. Rider, Outcome assessment in the adult and juvenile idiopathic inflammatory myopathies, Rheum. Dis. Clin. North Am. 28 (2002) 935–977.

586. L.G. Rider, E.H. Giannini, H.I. Brunner, et al., International consensus outcome measures for patients with idiopathic inflammatory myopathies: preliminary definitions of improvement for adult and juvenile myositis, Arthritis Rheum. 50 (2004) 2281–2290.

589. L.G. Rider, P.A. Lachenbruch, J.B. Monroe, et al., Damage extent and predictors in adult and juvenile dermatomyositis and polymyositis using the myositis damage index, Arthritis Rheum. 60 (2009) 3425–3435.

596. A.M. Huber, E. Giannini, S.L. Bowyer, et al., Protocols for the initial treatment of moderately severe juvenile dermatomyositis: results of a Children's Arthritis and Rheumatology Research Alliance Consensus Conference. Arthritis Care Res. 62 (2010) 219–225.

608. R. Seshadri, B.M. Feldman, N. Ilowite, et al., The role of aggressive corticosteroid therapy in patients with juvenile dermatomyositis: a propensity score analysis, Arthritis Rheum. 59 (2008) 989–995.

616. L.C. Miller, B.A. Sisson, L.B. Tucker, et al., Methotrexate treatment of recalcitrant childhood dermatomyositis, Arthritis Rheum. 35 (1992) 1143–1149.

617. A.V. Ramanan, N. Campbell-Webster, S. Ota, et al., The effectiveness of treating juvenile dermatomyositis with methotrexate and aggressively tapered corticosteroids, Arthritis Rheum. 52 (2005) 3570–3578.

624. A. Reiff, D.J. Rawlings, B. Shaham, et al., Preliminary evidence for cyclosporin A as an alternative in the treatment of recalcitrant juvenile rheumatoid arthritis and juvenile dermatomyositis, J. Rheumatol. 24 (1997) 2436–2443.

631. P. Riley, S.M. Maillard, L.R. Wedderburn, et al., Intravenous cyclophosphamide pulse therapy in juvenile dermatomyositis: a review of efficacy and safety, Rheumatology (Oxford) 43 (2004) 491–496.

649. S.M. Al Mayouf, R.M. Laxer, R. Schneider, et al., Intravenous immunoglobulin therapy for juvenile dermatomyositis: efficacy and safety, J. Rheumatol. 27 (2000) 2498–2503.

697. L.M. Pachman, R. Ramsey-Goldman, R. Lipton, et al., The NIAMS Juvenile Dermatomyositis (JDM) Research Registry: a preliminary analysis of physician data at 36 months after JDM diagnosis, Arthritis Rheum. 46 (2002) S491.

Entire reference list is available online at www.expertconsult.com.

Chapter 25

THE SYSTEMIC SCLERODERMAS AND RELATED DISORDERS

Francesco Zulian and James T. Cassidy

The word *scleroderma* means "hard skin." The diseases grouped under this term mean much more, although hardening of the skin is a feature that is common to all types of the disorder and is the most signal characteristic of these entities. A classification of the systemic and localized sclerodermas is summarized in Table 25–1. Systemic sclerosis is subdivided by the extent of the skin disease into *diffuse cutaneous systemic sclerosis* (dSSc) and *limited cutaneous systemic sclerosis* (lSSc), previously designated as the CREST syndrome (Calcinosis cutis, Raynaud phenomenon, Esophageal dysfunction, Sclerodactyly, Telangiectasia). The localized forms of the disease, such as morphea or linear scleroderma, often are regarded as more dermatological than rheumatological (see Chapter 26). Systemic sclerosis is rare in childhood. Many generalizations have been based primarily on the adult literature, and dSSc and lSSc are often discussed together in publications or inadequately separated.

HISTORICAL REVIEW

The early literature presents a confusing picture of scleroderma in a child because many cases were more compatible with a diagnosis of scleredema. In 1895, Lewin and Heller[1] reviewed 505 cases of scleroderma, mainly from the European literature. Goodman[2] observed that 88 occurred in children from birth to 19 years but that most cases were examples of circumscribed disease. Only 1 of 12 children reported as diffuse scleroderma was compatible with current concepts, with the rest being the "acute form," probably scleredema.[3] Another survey concluded that only 12 children with generalized scleroderma had been reported in the world literature through 1960.[4] In 1961, the Mayo Clinic added 63 additional pediatric cases in summarizing experience with 727 patients.[5] A survey (Padua database) of members of the Pediatric Rheumatology European Society and other pediatric rheumatology centers around the world (67 centers in 28 countries) reviewed 153 children with systemic sclerosis, and other American authors reported a series of 111 childhood-onset SSc patients followed at one center.[6,7]

Pathological studies lagged behind clinical reports, and there were no comprehensive descriptions until 1924, when Kraus[8] described pulmonary and cardiac fibrosis in a patient with scleroderma, and Matsui[9] detailed necropsy findings in five patients with scleroderma and cutaneous histological characteristics in another. In 1969, D'Angelo and colleagues[10] reported postmortem abnormal involvement as percentages in excess of control subjects: skin, 98%; esophagus, 74%; lungs, 59%; kidneys, 49%; small intestine, 46%; pericardium, 41%; large intestine, 39%; pleura, 29%; and myocardium, 26%. Other organs with less frequent involvement were the adrenal glands, lymph nodes, thyroid, and peripheral arteries.

DIFFUSE CUTANEOUS SYSTEMIC SCLEROSIS

dSSc is a chronic, multisystem connective tissue disease characterized by sclerodermatous skin changes and widespread abnormalities of the viscera. Rodnan[11] defined dSSc as a disorder in which "symmetrical fibrous thickening and hardening (sclerosis) of the skin is combined with fibrous and degenerative changes in synovium, digital arteries, and certain internal organs, most notably the esophagus, intestinal tract, heart, lungs, and kidneys."

Systemic sclerosis sine scleroderma has been described in adults as a variant of limited cutaneous involvement and not a separate or distinct disorder.[12,13] Other than the absence of skin thickening, this disease has no significant differences in internal organ involvement, laboratory abnormalities, serum autoantibodies, or survival rate compared with lSSc.

Classification

According to classification criteria of the American College of Rheumatology for adults,[14] definite dSSc requires the presence either of the major criterion

Table 25–1

Classification of systemic and localized sclerodermas and scleroderma-like disorders

Systemic Sclerosis
Cutaneous scleroderma
Diffuse
Limited

Overlap syndromes
Sclerodermatomyositis or with other connective tissue diseases
Mixed connective tissue disease

Localized scleroderma
Circumscribed morphea
Generalized morphea
Pansclerotic morphea
Linear morphea
Mixed subtype

Graft-versus-host disease
Chemically induced scleroderma-like disease
Polyvinyl chloride
Bleomycin
Pentazocine
Toxic oil syndrome
Adjuvant disease

Pseudosclerodermas
Phenylketonuria
Syndromes of premature aging
Localized idiopathic fibroses
Scleredema
Diabetic cheiroarthropathy
Porphyria cutanea tarda

Table 25–2

Preliminary criteria for the classification of systemic sclerosis (scleroderma)

Major Criterion
Proximal scleroderma: typical sclerodermatous skin changes (tightness, thickening, and nonpitting induration) involving areas proximal to the metacarpophalangeal or metatarsophalangeal joints

Minor Criteria
Sclerodactyly: sclerodermatous skin changes limited to digits
Digital pitting scars resulting from digital ischemia
Bibasilar pulmonary fibrosis not attributable to primary lung disease

From Subcommittee for Scleroderma Criteria of the American Rheumatism Association Diagnostic and Therapeutic Criteria Committee: Preliminary criteria for the classification of systemic sclerosis (scleroderma), *Arthritis Rheum* 23:581-590, 1980.

Epidemiology

dSSc has been reported worldwide and in all races.[17-25] It has an estimated annual incidence of 0.45 to 1.9 cases per 100,000 persons in the general population and a prevalence of approximately 24 cases per 100,000.[17,19,24-26] The frequency of this disorder increases with age and is highest in the 30- to 50-year age group. Prevalence has been estimated at 27.6 cases per 100,000 adults (95% CI: 24.5–31.0). The disease is more frequent in African Americans and in Choctaw Native Americans.[25] African American women are more likely to develop diffuse disease, be diagnosed at a younger age, and have a poorer survival rate.[24]

Onset in childhood is uncommon. Children younger than 10 years account for less than 2% of all cases, and patients between 10 and 20 years of age for only 1.2% to 9%.[20-23,27-34] It has been estimated that approximately 3% of all patients had onset in childhood.[35] dSSc constitutes 0.2% to 0.9% of the major connective tissue disorders in pediatric rheumatology clinics. There is no racial predilection or peak age at onset determined for children.

There are several small series and case reports of children with dSSc totaling just over 115 patients, although there are undoubtedly many unreported cases.[3,4,30,35-53] An additional 153 patients in the Padua database are included.[6] dSSc occurs with equal frequency in boys and girls younger than 8 years old, whereas girls outnumber boys 3 to 1 when disease onset occurs in children who are older than 8 years. Among adults, the female-to-male ratio in the childbearing years is 3:1 to 5:1, whereas in an older age group (older than 45 years) it is 1.8:1.[54] One hypothesis is that factors such as the hormonal milieu, pregnancy-related events, or reproductive-specific exposures are responsible for these differences in disease susceptibility.

Etiology and Pathogenesis

The cause of dSSc is unknown, despite significant advances in understanding of potential pathogenetic mechanisms.[55] The disease can be represented as a tripartite process in which dysfunction of the *immune system, endothelium,* and *fibroblasts* gives rise to a heterogeneous phenotype that is characterized prominently by fibrosis (Fig. 25–1).

(fibrosis/induration involving areas proximal to the metacarpophalangeal (MCP) or metatarsophalangeal (MTP) joints) or of two minor criteria (sclerodactyly, digital pitting scars, bibasilar pulmonary fibrosis) (Table 25–2). Subsequently, the widespread use of nailfold capillary microscopy, the more precise autoimmune serological tests, and the early detection of Raynaud phenomenon in patients who, years later, developed SSc, have raised the need for a more comprehensive classification.

Leroy and Medsger proposed a new set of criteria[15] to identify patients with vascular abnormalities and serological changes typical of scleroderma but who do not yet fulfill criteria for dSSc or lSSc. Patients who exhibit Raynaud phenomenon, and either nailfold capillary abnormalities or an antibody profile characteristic of dSSc or lSSc, are classified as having the limited form of scleroderma. More recently, an ad hoc International Committee on Classification Criteria for Juvenile Systemic Sclerosis developed new classification criteria to help standardize the conduct of clinical, epidemiological, and outcome research for this rare pediatric disease.[16] According to these criteria, a patient, age less than 16 years, shall be classified as having dSSc if the one major (presence of skin sclerosis/induration proximal to MCP or MTP) and at least two of the 20 minor criteria listed in Table 25–3 are present. This set of classification criteria has a sensitivity of 90%, a specificity of 96%, and a kappa statistic value of 0.86.

Table 25–3

Preliminary classification criteria for juvenile systemic sclerosis

Major Criterion
Sclerosis/induration of the skin proximal to the metacarpophalangeal or metatarsophalangeal joints

Minor Criteria
Skin
Sclerodactyly
Vasculopathy
Raynaud phenomenon
Nailfold capillary abnormalities
Digital tip ulcers

Gastrointestinal
Dysphagia
Gastroesophageal reflux

Renal
Renal crisis
New-onset arterial hypertension

Cardiac
Arrhythmias
Heart failure

Respiratory
Pulmonary fibrosis (HRCT/x-ray)
DL$_{CO}$
Pulmonary hypertension

Musculoskeletal
Tendon friction rubs
Arthritis
Myositis

Neurological
Neuropathy
Carpal tunnel syndrome

Serology
Antinuclear antibodies
SSc selective autoantibodies (anticentromere,
antitopoisomerase I, antifibrillarin, anti-PM-Scl, antifibrillin
or anti-RNA polymerase I or III)
A patient, aged less than 16 years, shall be classified as having
juvenile systemic sclerosis if 1 major and at least 2 of the 20
minor criteria are present. This set of classification criteria
has a sensitivity of 90%, a specificity of 96%, and kappa
statistic value of 0.86.

DL$_{CO}$, carbon monoxide diffusing capacity ; HRCT, high-resolution
computed tomography; SSc, systemic sclerosis.
From PRES/ACR/EULAR ad hoc Committee on Classification Criteria for
JSSc, The Pediatric Rheumatology European Society/American College
of Rheumatology/European League Against Rheumatism Provisional
Classification Criteria for Juvenile Systemic Sclerosis, *Arthritis Rheum*
57:203-212, 2007.

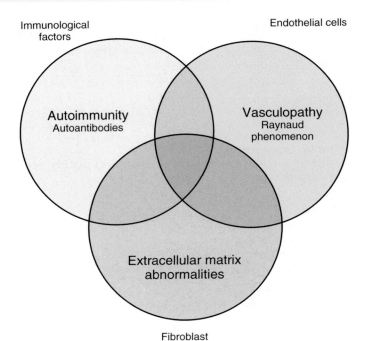

FIGURE 25–1   Possible pathogenic mechanisms in scleroderma.

Table 25–4

Cytokines and growth factors involved in the regulation of the biological behavior of fibroblasts

Biological Effect	Cytokine or Growth Factor
Increased collagen synthesis	TGF-β, PDGF, IL-1, IL-4, IL-6
Decreased collagen synthesis	IFN-β, IFN-γ, TNF-α, β
Fibroblast proliferation	IFN-β, IFN-γ, TGF-β, PDGF, TNF, IL-1, IL-4
Chemoattraction	IFN-γ, TGF-β, PDGF, TNF, IL-4
Glycosaminoglycan synthesis	TGF-β, TNF, IL-1
Fibronectin synthesis	TGF-β, IL-4
Endothelial cell injury	IFN-γ, TNF-α, β, IL-2, NK cell, granzyme A
Reduction of collagen synthesis	TGF-β
Collagenase gene induction	TNF-α

IFN, interferon; IL, interleukin; NK, natural killer cell; PDGF, platelet-
derived growth factor; TNF, tumor necrosis factor; TGF, transforming
growth factor.

fibrosis as the result of increased synthesis and deposition of extracellular matrix proteins. These three areas
of abnormal function, although apparently unassociated
with each other, are closely linked by several immunological alterations.

Immunological Factors

Many reports suggest that cellular immunity plays a major
role in the initiation of scleroderma. These factors include
the presence of mononuclear cell (MNC) infiltrates in
early lesions, altered function of helper T and NK cells,
and release of cytokines, chemokines, and growth factors
(Table 25–4). MNC infiltration in various organ systems

Autoimmunity is evident by the elaboration of circulating disease-specific autoantibodies and multiple
abnormalities of T-cell function. Raynaud phenomenon,
capillary dropout, endothelial injury, and abnormalities
in vascular tone are manifestations of endothelial cell
dysfunction. Fibroblast dysfunction is represented by

occurs early and consists of lymphocytes, plasma cells, and fibroblast-histiocytic cells around small blood vessels, eccrine sweat glands, and subcutaneous tissue.[56] Activated T lymphocytes are prominent as evidenced by the expression of surface human leukocyte antigen (HLA) class II molecules.[57]

The early infiltrates of MNCs release a number of cytokines and chemokines that affect endothelial cells and fibroblasts. Several growth factors have also been identified in scleroderma skin, including transforming growth factor-β (TGF-β), connective tissue growth factor (CTGF), and adhesion molecules. TGF-β has pleomorphic cellular actions principally on fibroblasts and endothelial cells.[58] In vitro, it stimulates the synthesis of the extracellular matrix, including types I and III collagen.[59] It also promotes fibrosis indirectly by inhibiting collagenase activity.[60] Fibroblasts from scleroderma skin express in vivo and in vitro increased levels of TGF-β1 and TGF-β2 receptor proteins compared with controls.[61,62] Blockade of TGF-β1 signaling with monoclonal antibodies inhibits upregulation of collagen synthesis in scleroderma fibroblasts.[61] Polymorphisms of the TGF-β1 gene have been reported in Japanese patients.[63] CTGF levels are greatly elevated in the dermis of patients with scleroderma and down-regulated by iloprost infusion.[64] Although TGF-β1 is known to initiate fibrosis, CTGF may play a greater role in maintaining and promoting fibrosis.[65,66]

Levels of a number of cytokines (e.g., interleukin [IL]-1, IL-2, IL-4, IL-6, IL-8) are increased in the serum.[67-69] Several interleukins (e.g., IL-4, IL-6, IL-8) have also been demonstrated in scleroderma skin. Serum levels and spontaneous production of IL-12, a potent inducer of type 1 helper (Th1) T cells, were increased in patients with renal vascular damage.[70] Specific cytokines promote fibrosis; others, such as interferon-γ (IFN-γ), are potent suppressors of collagen synthesis. The effects of some cytokines are mixed. Tumor necrosis factor (TNF) decreases fibroblast production of types I and III collagen while promoting collagenase gene induction.[58] This cytokine also stimulates the proliferation of some fibroblasts and increases endothelial cell expression of adhesion molecules (i.e., E-selectin, intracellular adhesion molecule-1 [ICAM-1] and vascular cell adhesion molecule-1 [VCAM-1]) and release of endothelin-1. The level of circulating soluble VCAM-1 correlates with impaired left ventricular diastolic function.[71] Serum CD44 (sCD44), another adhesion molecule that regulates the migration of leucocytes, was elevated in scleroderma patients, particularly in those with limited cutaneous disease.[72] Genetic predispositions are being clarified: for example, the TNF-863A allele is associated with anticentromere antibody seropositivity.[73]

Chemokines are operative in the recruitment of specific types of leukocytes to involved skin and tissue. Serum levels of MCP-1, which attracts MNCs, and MIP-1, which attracts monocytes and helper T cells, are elevated.[74] A constitutive overexpression of MCP-1 mRNA has been identified in scleroderma skin.[75] Treatment with antibodies to MCP-1 results in reduced chemotactic activity, indicating that this chemokine may be an important agent in the initiation of cutaneous inflammation.[76] Levels of chemokines IL-8 and growth-regulated oncogene-α (GRO-α), potent chemoattractants and activators of neutrophils, were found to be elevated in scleroderma and GRO-α correlated particularly with pulmonary involvement.[77] Cell-mediated immunity to laminin, a constituent of basement membrane and to a lesser extent to type IV collagen, has also been demonstrated in patients with dSSc.[78]

Vascular Factors

According to some authorities, endothelial cell injury is the central pathogenic event and predates fibrotic changes. The endothelial cell may be damaged by protease-dependent mechanisms that are independent of complement and immunoglobulin. Abnormalities of cutaneous mast cell number and type and of mast cell activation as a prefibrotic event have been documented.[79] Damage to the endothelial cell results in increased vascular permeability, which is responsible for the edematous phase of the illness, leading to activation of fibroblasts, increased collagen production, and resultant fibrosis. It also initiates activation of the coagulation pathway, contributing to an accumulation of platelets that release factors leading to proliferation and migration of myointimal cells.

Endothelial Cell Factors

Evidence that the endothelial cell is damaged is provided by studies of the histology of the lesions in dSSc and by demonstration of elevated levels of factor VIII–related antigen,[80] although this has not been a consistent observation.[81] Reduced plasma angiotensin-converting–enzyme activity may be an additional marker of endothelial injury.[82] Endothelial cell apoptosis is accelerated.[83] The microvascular injury leads to arteriolar intimal fibrosis and narrowing of the vascular lumen, which results in ischemic damage.[84] Anti–endothelial cell antibodies are also present[85,86] and lead to endothelial damage, vascular hyperpermeability, and myointimal cell proliferation.

The link between vascular alterations and cellular immunity is represented by adhesion molecules. Three major families have been defined: selectins, integrins, and members of the immunoglobulin gene superfamily. Selectins mediate the initial contact of leukocytes with endothelial cells. Overexpression of E-selectin and P-selectin has been found in sera[87,88] and in endothelial cells of the skin and minor salivary glands of scleroderma patients.[89] Integrins, a family of heterodimeric transmembrane glycoprotein molecules, serve as a means of communication between extracellular matrix molecules (e.g., collagen, laminin, fibronectin) through the cell membrane to the intracellular compartment. Expression of integrins VLA-2, VLA-4, and LFA-1 is increased on endothelial cells, MNCs, fibroblasts, and dendritic cells in scleroderma skin.[89] ICAM-1 and VCAM-1, members of the immunoglobulin gene superfamily on endothelial cells, and LFA-1 and VLA-4, integrin receptors on lymphocytes, play a significant role in the interaction between lymphocytes and endothelial cells or fibroblasts. These molecules are increased on endothelial cells and fibroblasts in sclerodermatous skin[90,91] and facilitate MNC damage to endothelial cells and fibroblasts.

Abnormalities of Collagen

Excessive accumulation of collagen in affected skin led to the hypothesis that there might be abnormalities of collagen type or metabolism.[25,92] There is an increased number of collagen-producing fibroblasts in the skin[93]; however, the ratios of various collagen types are normal.[94] Although reduced collagenase activity was found in one study,[95] it was normal in another.[96] Abnormalities of glycosylation[97] and hydroxylation[95] of the collagen molecule may prevent normal feedback mechanisms from being effective in controlling synthesis and permit excessive deposition of collagen. A defect in the regulation of genes controlling apoptosis of fibroblasts (for example caspase 6, Bcl2, and elastin) has been reported.[99]

Genetic Background

The rare familial occurrence of dSSc has been confirmed in a mother and her 6-year-old son,[44] in a second family with two affected sisters ages 12 and 16 years,[100] and in monozygotic twins.[101]

There is little agreement about the potential associations of histocompatibility antigens with dSSc. Initial studies indicated associations with class I alleles HLA-A9,[102] HLA-B8,[103,104] and HLA-Bw35[105] and class II alleles HLA-DR3,[104] HLA-DR5,[106] and HLA-DRw15.[107] Associations with HLA-DR and HLA-DQ alleles (DQB3.1, DQB1.1, DQB1.2, DQB1.3) have been reviewed by Whiteside and colleagues[108] and Fox and Kang.[109] DRB1*1104 and DRB1*1101 confer odds ratios of 3.5 and 2.3 for the disease in adults.[110]

Prolonged persistence of fetal progenitor cells and microchimerism in T cells has been associated with DQA1*0501.[111,112] Microchimerism, the presence within one individual of a very low level of cells derived from a different individual, was postulated as a possible cause of scleroderma from studies of chronic graft-versus-host disease (GVHD), a chimeric disorder in which donor T cells or NK cells react against the HLAs of the recipient.

Microchimerism occurs in women who had previous pregnancies, individuals who have had blood transfusions, and children with cells from the mother or a twin. Maternal cells can persist in an immunocompetent offspring even in adult life, and fetus-derived hemopoietic cells have persisted in the maternal circulation for many years postpartum.[113] Fetal DNA persists for even longer periods.[114] Although microchimerism can be identified in normal subjects and in other diseases, it has been proposed as an important factor in pathogenesis of autoimmune diseases.[115] In scleroderma, chimeric cells are increased in number and, compared with normal subjects, are more similar to the maternal cells. Quantitative analysis of microchimerism has been reported in sclerodermatous skin.[116] Nelson and coworkers[114] studied 40 mothers and documented high, persistent concentrations of male DNA in cells of the vascular compartment years after giving birth to a son. HLA class II compatibility of the child was more common in dSSc patients than in control subjects. An investigation by Artlett and colleagues[117] also concluded that fetal antimaternal graft-versus-host reactions might be involved in pathogenesis. Although this theory of a chronic graft-versus-host reaction is attractive, studies offer no data to explain the occurrence of scleroderma in men or women who have never had children.

Clinical Manifestations

Early Signs and Symptoms

Presenting signs and symptoms of dSSc in children are in Table 25–5. Onset of the disease is usually insidious and the course prolonged, punctuated by periods of inactivity or episodes of severe systemic complications, occasionally ending in remission or more often in chronic disability or death.[118] The onset is often characterized by the development of Raynaud phenomenon; tightening, thinning, and atrophy of the skin of the hands and face; or the appearance of cutaneous telangiectasias about the face, upper

Table 25–5

Presenting signs and symptoms in children with systemic scleroderma

	Jaffe et al (n=5) 1961	Goel et al (n=4) 1974	Cassidy et al (n=13) 1977	Kornreich et al (n=13) 1977	Larrègue et al (n=3) 1983	Suarez-Almazor et al (n=4) 1985	Lababidi et al (n=5) 1991	Martini et al (n=153) 2006	Total %*
Skin tightening	4	4	15	13	3	4	3	74	82.2
Raynaud phenomenon	5	2	11	5	3	4	3	75	70.4
Soft tissue contracture	2	1	10	—	2	4	3	—	61.1
Arthralgia	—†	3	9	—	2	1	6	26	28.2
Muscle weakness and pain	—	1	4	—	—	2	2	12	15.2
Subcutaneous calcification	—	—	3	—	—	1	—	9	10.2
Dysphagia	—	—	3	—	—	1	2	10	13.5
Dyspnea	—	—	3	—	—	1	2	10	12.9

*Percentage calculated only on series in which detailed information was provided.
†Dash indicates that information was not provided.

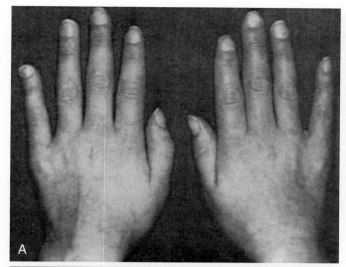

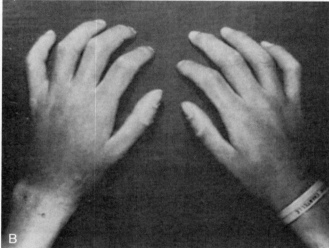

FIGURE 25–2 A, The hands of a 9-year-old girl with diffuse cutaneous systemic scleroderma. The skin over the dorsa of the fingers is taut and shiny. **B,** Five years later, the tightening is more evident, and flexion contractures have developed. (Courtesy of Dr. K. Oen.)

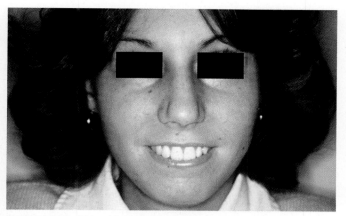

FIGURE 25–3 Shiny skin on the face.

SCLEROSIS

During the sclerotic phase, the skin develops a waxy texture and becomes tight, hard, and bound to subcutaneous structures. This is particularly noticeable in skin of the dorsal surface of the digits, so-called acrosclerosis (Fig. 25–2), and face (Fig. 25–3); the characteristic immobile, expressionless, unwrinkled appearance of the skin may be the first clue to the diagnosis. The absence of forehead wrinkling and the presence of circumoral furrowing or diminished aperture of the mouth are particularly characteristic. Sclerotic changes usually follow a temporal sequence of development, beginning with bilateral, symmetrical acrosclerosis, followed by involvement of the face, and finally by changes in the skin of the trunk and proximal limbs.

ATROPHY

The long-term consequence of edema and sclerosis is atrophy of skin and adnexa. These superficial abnormalities result in a shiny appearance of the skin accompanied by areas of hypo- or hyperpigmentation and often by deposition of calcium salts in the subcutaneous tissues. Cutaneous lesions in all stages of evolution may be observed simultaneously in the same child.

TELANGIECTASIAS

Telangiectasias, fine macular dilatations of cutaneous or mucous membrane blood vessels, are characteristic (Fig. 25–4). Unlike "spider" angiomata that fill rapidly from central arterioles, telangiectatic vessels fill slowly and lack the characteristic central vessel. The periungual nailfold is often the most obvious early location of abnormal vessels (Fig. 25–5), and examination with an ophthalmoscope, at +40 dioptre, demonstrates capillary dropout, tortuous dilated loops, and occasionally distorted capillary architecture (Fig. 25–6).[47,120,121] There is usually redundant cuticular growth; dystrophic changes in the nails have also been reported.[122] Digital pitting, sometimes with ulceration and gangrene, occurs in the pulp of the fingertips as a result of ischemia and is one of the minor diagnostic criteria (Fig. 25–7).

CALCINOSIS

Subcutaneous calcification, especially over the elbows, metacarpophalangeal joints, and knees, may occur,

trunk, and hands. There is often a diagnostic delay of years because of the subtle nature of this presentation. A comprehensive general review of the assessment of patients with systemic sclerosis has been published.[119]

Skin Disease

The onset of cutaneous abnormalities may be especially insidious, but these changes characteristically evolve in a sequence beginning with edema, followed by induration and sclerosis resulting in marked tightening and contractures, and eventually resulting in atrophy.

EDEMA

Tense, nonpitting swelling of the skin and subcutaneous tissues of the digits, hands, arms, and face, or localized areas on the trunk, may be the initial manifestation of the disease. Edematous areas may be warm and tender with an erythematous border, but are often asymptomatic. Swelling may persist for weeks or months before subsiding or being replaced by sclerosis.

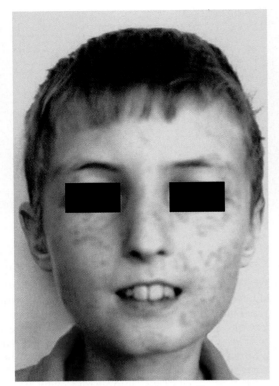

FIGURE 25–4   Telangiectasias.

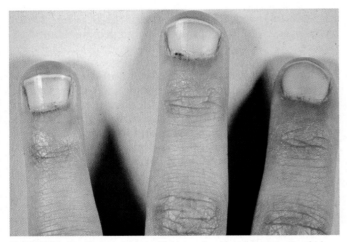

FIGURE 25–5   Changes in the nailfold vessels with visible tortuosity, thickening, and pigmentary extrusion onto the cuticles.

FIGURE 25–6   **A,** There is a reduction in the number of nail fold capillaries and tortuosity of the remaining vessels in the microvasculature viewed with a microscope (magnification × 100). **B,** Normal vessels. (Courtesy of Dr. J. Kenik.)

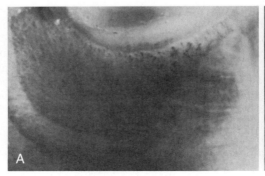
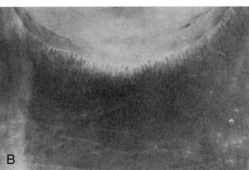

sometimes with ulceration of surrounding skin. Extensive periarticular calcification (i.e., calcinosis circumscripta) may be a late complication (Fig. 25–8). These lesions, if extensive, lead to a severe reduction in joint mobility. Small, hard, subcutaneous nodules sometimes occur over the extensor surfaces of joints of the fingers and differ histologically from rheumatoid nodules by the absence of fibrinoid necrosis.[123]

Raynaud Phenomenon

Raynaud phenomenon occurs in 90% of children with dSSc and is often the initial symptom of the disorder, preceding other manifestations in some instances by years.[124,125] Raynaud phenomenon represents the first manifestation of the disease in 70% of children with dSSc and in 10% is complicated by digital infarcts. During the overall course of the disease, Raynaud phenomenon is also the most frequently reported symptom.[6] Raynaud phenomenon is covered extensively in Chapter 29.

Musculoskeletal Disease

Musculoskeletal symptoms are common and characteristically occur at or near onset. Among the 153 children with dSSc included in the Padua database, 36% had musculoskeletal symptoms during the course of the disease.[6] Morning stiffness and pain of the small joints of the hands, knees, and ankles may also be initial manifestations of the disease. Movement of a thickened tendon through its sheath, which is covered with fibrinous deposits, can often be palpated or detected with a stethoscope as an audible, coarse crepitus.

Joint pain is usually mild and transient. Joint contractures of insidious onset and limitation of motion are most common at the proximal interphalangeal joints and elbows, but other joints can be affected. Objective evidence of articular inflammation is absent or mild in most instances, although small, bland synovial effusions occur. Muscle inflammation characterized by pain and tenderness occurs in up to one fifth of children, and proximal or distal muscle atrophy may be marked.

Gastrointestinal Disease

Gastrointestinal involvement affects one third of the patients during the course of the disease; proximal disease usually precedes distal involvement.[6] Lesions of the mouth include mucosal telangiectasias, reduced

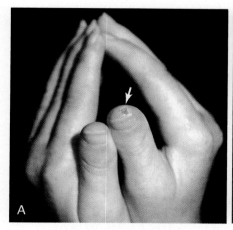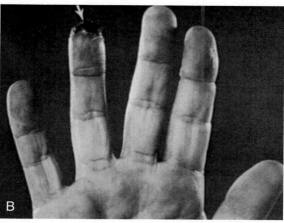

FIGURE 25–7 **A,** Digital pitting of the fingertips. Notice the ulceration of tip of the right thumb *(arrow)* and shiny, tightly stretched skin over the fingertips bilaterally with pronounced flexion contractures at the metacarpophalangeal joints. **B,** Digital gangrene of the fourth right finger *(arrow)*.

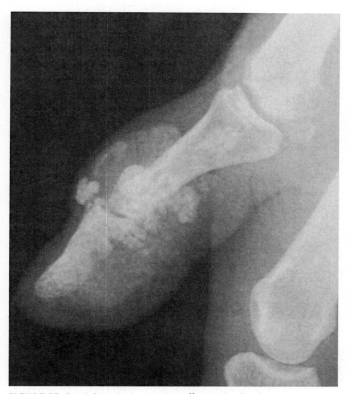

FIGURE 25–8 Calcinosis circumscripta affecting the thumb.

interincisor distance caused by skin thickening and tightness, parotitis as part of the sicca syndrome, and loosening of the teeth because of changes in the periodontal membrane. The esophagus is involved, often quite early in the disease, and dysphagia may be one of the presenting signs. Although many patients are asymptomatic, symptoms (in order of decreasing frequency) include heartburn with postural aggravation, dysphagia, delayed emptying, regurgitation with reflux into the throat, nocturnal aspiration, and cough with swallowing. Esophagitis with persistent ulceration and stricture along with progressive weight loss because of voluntary restriction of food intake may follow. Dilatation of the stomach or duodenum occurs uncommonly. At least in adults, gastric arteriovenous ectasia ("watermelon stomach")

may develop. Small-bowel involvement usually develops in association with esophageal or colonic disease.[10] Abdominal distention and pain with nausea and vomiting result from gut hypotonia that may occasionally be so severe that pseudoobstruction occurs.[126] Pneumatosis intestinalis may develop. Malabsorptive diarrhea and delayed colon transit, when present, reflect longstanding disease.[127] Malabsorption in SSc is primarily due to small bowel bacterial overgrowth and should be treated with rotating oral antibiotics (antibiotic change every 4 weeks) since continuous therapy with one agent may result in the emergence of resistant organisms and an increased relapse rate.

Large-bowel disease, although not uncommon, is usually asymptomatic; however, it may cause severe constipation, bloating, or diarrhea. Primary biliary cirrhosis has not been reported in children.

Cardiac Disease

Cardiopulmonary disease, although not common at presentation, is a leading cause of morbidity.[50,128,129] Pericardial effusions are usually small and asymptomatic, although fever and retrosternal pain may accompany acute disease.[130] Changes in cardiac hemodynamics reflected by the presence of pedal edema, jugular venous distension, hepatomegaly, pulsus paradoxus, and pulsus alternans may be present in patients with chronic effusions. Tamponade from pericardial constriction and severe cardiomyopathy are, however, rare, although they can be one of the causes of early death and require prompt and aggressive immunosuppressive treatment.[128]

Cardiac ischemia may result from the equivalent of Raynaud phenomenon of the coronary arteries and is a potential precursor of myocardial fibrosis. Although coronary artery disease is uncommon, electrocardiographic changes and even angina pectoris may occur as a result of disease of the myocardial microvasculature.[131] Systemic and pulmonary hypertension may contribute to myocardial ischemia.

Pulmonary Disease

Pulmonary parenchymal disease is frequently asymptomatic; a minority of patients have a dry, hacking cough or dyspnea on exertion.[132] Occasionally, rales or a pleural friction rub are present. Clinical predictors of end-stage disease have been evaluated in adults.[133,134]

Pulmonary vascular disease results in progressive dyspnea with preserved lung volumes on pulmonary function testing. It can result from pulmonary fibrosis; however, the isolated form of this complication has a much worse prognosis. It can occasionally complicate dSSc associated with antifibrillin autoantibodies and is typical also of the lSSc subset of patients.[135] Interstitial pulmonary fibrosis, long recognized as a devastating complication, is being reclassified to reflect differences in histopathology and outcome. It has been postulated that fibrosis also results from pulmonary vascular hyperreactivity similar to Raynaud phenomenon.

Furst and associates[136] demonstrated decreased pulmonary perfusion as measured by krypton 81m scans after cold challenge to the hands. Fahey and colleagues[137] noticed a low carbon monoxide diffusing capacity (DL_{CO}) in patients with dSSc and Raynaud phenomenon but failed to demonstrate a decrease with cold challenge as found in patients with idiopathic Raynaud disease. Increased pulmonary uptake of gallium 67 occurred in most patients with early disease, a finding that suggested an inflammatory process. Vesely and colleagues[138] measured serum concentrations of KL-6, high–molecular-weight, mucinlike glycoprotein expressed on type II pneumonocytes in alveoli and bronchiolar epithelial cells, in 6 children with and 6 without interstitial lung disease, and compared their results with 20 healthy controls. KL-6 was significantly higher in the children with pulmonary involvement and served as a clinically useful marker of fibrosis.

Renal Disease

Overt renal disease is one of the most ominous features of dSSc.[139] Although little information is available, it is an impression that children may do better than adults in this regard.[4,35,50,129] In the Padua database, 5% of the children had renal involvement (as increased urinary protein excretion or raised creatinine level), and one developed renal crisis.[6] Medsger and colleagues[140] indicated that almost 50% of adult patients who developed renal disease did so within the first year after disease onset and that presence of anti-topoisomerase I antibody and rapidly progressing skin involvement are predictors of early and often fatal renal and cardiac involvement.[134]

A significant relationship between the use of high-dose steroids and the development of scleroderma renal crisis in adult patients has been reported by several authors.[141,142] Although no study regarding this issue in pediatric patients has been published, a close monitoring of blood pressure and renal function in patients treated with steroids is recommended, particularly in early diffuse SSc with rapidly progressing skin involvement.

Systemic hypertension occurs in up to one half of adult patients and is usually associated with proteinuria.[143,144] The degree of hypertension ranges from mild or moderate in most patients to malignant hypertension in approximately 25%. This complication often begins during the colder months of the year[143] and may be heralded by the development of microangiopathic hemolytic anemia.[145] Onset is followed rapidly in most patients by death within a few weeks in the absence of intensive intervention. Renal or prerenal azotemia occurs in at least 25% of patients in the presence or absence of hypertension or proteinuria.[144]

Renovascular Raynaud phenomenon, demonstrated by decreased cortical blood flow, may be induced by immersion of the hands in cold water.[143] Even in the absence of angiographic evidence of vascular disease, xenon 133–demonstrated cortical blood flow may be impaired.[143] These reversible changes are mediated by the renin-angiotensin system, and plasma renin levels correlate with the presence of malignant hypertension.[146]

Central Nervous System Disease

The most frequently described central nervous system (CNS) abnormality is cranial nerve involvement, especially of the sensory branch of the trigeminal nerve.[147-149] In contrast, peripheral neuropathies are uncommon (1.6%).[150] A more subtle abnormality, diminished perception of vibration, probably reflects the damping effect of cutaneous sclerosis on the transmission of the vibrations of a tuning fork.[151] Clinical involvement of the CNS is usually a reflection of renal or pulmonary disease; however, cerebral arteritis has been described.[152]

Sicca Syndrome (Sjögren Syndrome)

Xerostomia (i.e., dry mouth) and *keratoconjunctivitis sicca* (i.e., dry eyes) are common in dSSc (see Chapter 28). Histological evidence of salivary gland involvement was uniformly demonstrable in lip biopsies in a prospective study of Sjögren syndrome in 17 adult patients with dSSc and 8 patients with lSSc.[153] Xerostomia and salivary gland enlargement were present in 84%. Scintigraphy of the salivary glands was abnormal in 88%, and sialography abnormal in 75%. Ocular symptoms of dryness or a foreign-body sensation occurred in 76%. Results of Schirmer test were abnormal for 40%, and rose bengal staining of the cornea was positive in 55%.

SIMILARITIES AND DIFFERENCES BETWEEN CHILDREN AND ADULTS WITH SSC

As compared with adults, at diagnosis children show a significantly less frequent involvement of all organs, except for the prevalence of arthritis.[6,7,154] Differences with adults become less evident during follow-up with the exception of interstitial lung involvement, gastroesophageal dysmotility, renal involvement, and arterial hypertension, which are significantly much more common in adults. Other differences with SSc in adults can be seen in the prevalence of arthritis and muscle inflammation, which are slightly more common in children, whereas Raynaud phenomenon and skin sclerosis are fairly less frequent in the pediatric age.[6,154] Another interesting feature is that in children the limited cutaneous form, which is the far most frequent in adults, is rare. However, it has now been shown that a substantial number of patients with childhood-onset SSc have their diagnosis made either during adolescence or as young adults.[7] Indeed, it is possible that the limited cutaneous subset might be underdiagnosed in younger children because of the lack of a full clinical picture.

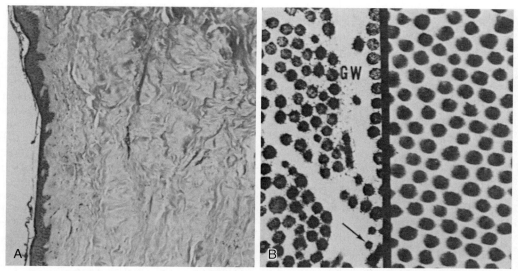

FIGURE 25–9 **A,** The classic histopathological features of the cutaneous disease are visible in this full-thickness section of skin from a patient with diffuse cutaneous systemic scleroderma. The epidermis is thin, and there is atrophy of the dermal appendages. The rete pegs are relatively obliterated (hematoxylin and eosin stain; magnification × 480). **B,** Electron microscopic studies indicate a relative reduction in the fiber size of newly synthesized collagen. Transverse sections of collagen fibers *(left)* are from the skin of a patient. A marked variation in fiber size is apparent when compared with healthy skin *(right).* Many smaller collagen fibers are observed *(arrow)* (normal diameter × 1200). The fine granular and whiskery material (GW) surrounding the sclerodermal collagen probably represents mucopolysaccharides, and their visibility is enhanced by staining with ruthenium red, lead citrate, and uranyl acetate (magnification × 38,610). (Courtesy of Dr. C. R. Wynne-Roberts.)

Pathology

An angiitis is regarded as the basic initial lesion, with activated lymphocytes infiltrating around small blood vessels. There are increased numbers of T lymphocytes, plasma cells, and macrophages in the deep dermis and subcutaneous tissue and around small blood vessels, nerves, the pilosebaceous apparatus, and sweat glands.[56] Marked hyalinization of blood vessel walls and proliferation of endothelium occur later. Raynaud phenomenon, renal crisis, and pulmonary hypertension are all associated with a distinctive arteriosclerotic fibrotic lesion.[155] Another characteristic finding is mast cell hyperplasia in skin and viscera.[156] Hydrophilic glycosaminoglycan in the dermis may account in part for the accumulation of edema.[157]

Later in the course, biopsies document homogenization of collagen fibers with loss of structural detail and an increased density and thickness of collagen deposition (Fig. 25–9A).[78,158] With electron microscopy, the collagen appears embryonic with narrow fibrils and an immature cross banding pattern (Fig. 25–9B).[159] The histological characteristics of the skin in late disease include thinning of the epidermis, and loss of the rete pegs and atrophy of dermal appendages, often with a persistent inflammatory infiltrate of T lymphocytes. The synovial membrane histologically resembles that of rheumatoid arthritis except for the abundance of fibrin and dense fibrosis.[103,160,161]

Biopsy specimens of muscle are abnormal in approximately one half of the patients.[162] The most prominent abnormalities are increased deposition of collagen and fat in interstitial perivascular sites of the perimysium and epimysium and focal, predominantly lymphocytic, perivascular infiltration. There is a relative loss of type II fibers.[163] Blood vessels are thickened and vessel lumens

are narrowed. Immunofluorescence studies have demonstrated no abnormalities.[163]

Histopathological changes in the vasa nervorum, neural dysfunction from fibrosis, and smooth muscle atrophy and fibrosis are similar throughout the gastrointestinal tract but are most prominent in the esophagus, where atrophic muscle is replaced by fibrous tissue. The smooth muscle of the lower two thirds of the esophagus is most commonly affected, but in some patients, striated muscle of the upper third may also be involved. The lamina propria and Auerbach plexus are infiltrated with mononuclear cells. Arterial walls are thickened.

One half of patients in one necropsy series had evidence of myocardial fibrosis that was unrelated to coronary artery disease (Fig. 25–10).[164] Other findings included contraction band necrosis (i.e., myofibrillar degeneration) from transient ischemia in 31% (possibly the equivalent of Raynaud phenomenon of the coronary arteries and a precursor to myocardial fibrosis). Necropsies in adults have demonstrated effusions or fibrous, fibrinous, and adhesive pericarditis in approximately 40%,[165] a frequency similar to that detected by echocardiography.[166] Convincing clinical evidence of pericarditis was present in only 3% to 16% of patients.[165]

The main histological abnormality in the lungs is diffuse alveolar, interstitial and peribronchial fibrosis. The thickened walls lead to a reduction of alveolar space (i.e., compact sclerosis). Rupture of alveolar septae results in small areas of bullous emphysema (i.e., cystic sclerosis) (Fig. 25–11). Extensive bronchiolar hyperplasia, arteriolar endothelial proliferation, fibrous pleuritis, and pleural adhesions are also present. Young and Mark[167] reported that 14 of 30 patients had moderate or marked abnormalities in the pulmonary vasculature at necropsy and postulated that malignant pulmonary hypertension analogous to malignant renal hypertension was the cause of

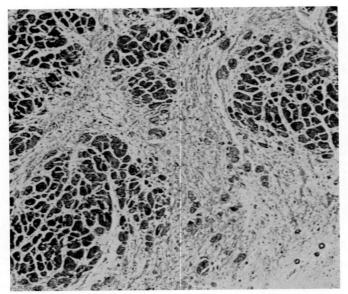

FIGURE 25–10 Fibrosis of the myocardium (hematoxylin and eosin stain; magnification × 480).

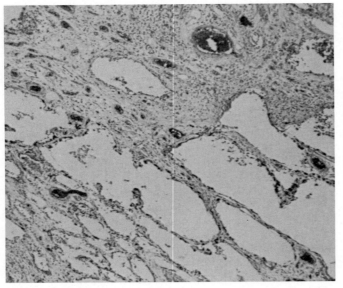

FIGURE 25–11 Biopsy of a lung reveals striking fibrosis and disruption of the alveoli (hematoxylin and eosin stain; magnification × 480).

the rapidly progressive pulmonary failure that culminated in the death of three patients.

The characteristic histopathological change in the renal vasculature is concentric intimal proliferation of the interlobar and arcuate arteries, together with cortical infarcts and fibrinoid necrosis of the media. Vasculitis (other than the changes of malignant hypertension) is uncommon. The glomeruli exhibit a wide spectrum of abnormalities (Fig. 25–12), ranging from acute ischemic necrosis to thickening and sclerosis of the basement membrane. Swelling of the endothelial cells results in vascular narrowing.[168] Deposition of immunoglobulin and complement in the renal vasculature has been reported[168-170] but is generally sparse. On electron microscopy, intimal thickening of the vessels is associated with the presence of myointimal cells resembling those of smooth muscle, but with the capability to produce collagen and elastin.[171]

Differential Diagnosis

Because dSSc usually involves internal organs, muscles, and skin, the differential diagnosis includes many disorders such as juvenile dermatomyositis (see Chapter 24), mixed connective tissue disease, and other undifferentiated connective tissue diseases (see Chapter 27).[172-175]

Chronic Graft-Versus-Host Disease

Chronic GVHD is a complication of allogeneic bone marrow transplantation for the treatment of marrow aplasia, leukemia, or malignant diseases. GVHD results from the interaction between immunocompetent T lymphocytes from the donor and host cells bearing histocompatibility antigens that are recognized as foreign. The graft attempts to "reject" the host because, under the circumstances of the transplantation, the recipient is rendered immunologically incompetent by immunosuppression and x-irradiation. The resulting scleroderma-like disease may follow acute GVHD or occur de novo up to 100 days after transplantation. It is characterized by dermatitis, usually beginning with erythema of the face, palms, soles, and other regions that are distal in location, or is sometimes generalized, involving only one side of the body in a harlequin-type syndrome. Hyperpigmentation and hypopigmentation follow. A hidebound skin and extreme tightening of the tendons, subcutaneum, and

FIGURE 25–12 Necropsy specimen from a patient who died of renal failure and hypertension during the first few months of the disease. **A,** Virtual obliteration of the lumen of an arteriole by subintimal proliferation, thrombus formation, and mucoid hyperplasia of the media. **B,** Glomerulus from the same patient, showing fibrinoid necrosis and effacement of capillary loops without significant inflammatory cell infiltration (hematoxylin and eosin stain; magnification × 480).

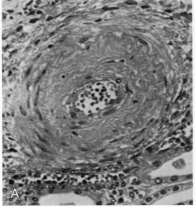

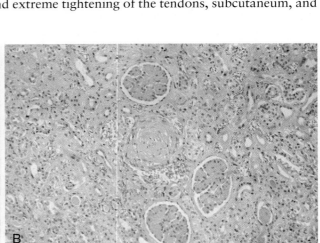

periarticular structures may severely limit motion. Gastrointestinal disease with severe diarrhea and hepatitis is common. Other SSc features, such as Raynaud phenomenon and respiratory or esophageal involvement, are less frequent in GVHD. The histology in these two conditions is similar but not identical.[176] D-penicillamine may be beneficial for some patients. Extracorporeal photopheresis after sensitization of host leukocytes by methoxypsoralen, a procedure successfully used for the treatment of T-cell lymphoma, has therapeutic promise.[177] However, modifications of the chemotherapeutic preparation of the graft recipient may offer some hope of prevention of this complication.[178]

Nephrogenic Systemic Fibrosis

Nephrogenic systemic fibrosis (NSF) is a recently identified fibrosing disorder seen only in patients with kidney failure. It is characterized by thickening and hardening of the skin overlying the extremities and trunk and marked expansion and fibrosis of the dermis in association with CD34-positive fibrocytes.[179]

NSF was originally named *nephrogenic fibrosing dermopathy* because of the characteristic skin findings.[180] However, subsequent studies showed that some patients had fibrosis of deeper structures including muscle, fascia, lungs, and heart.[179]

NSF is characterized by skin involvement in all patients and systemic involvement in some.[179] Among patients with gadolinium exposure, the latent period between exposure and disease onset is usually 2 to 4 weeks.[181,182] However, the reported range is as short as 2 days and as long as 18 months.[183]

Skin disease in NSF typically manifests as symmetrical, bilateral fibrotic indurated papules, plaques, or subcutaneous nodules that may or may not be erythematous.[179,180] In the majority of cases, the lesions first develop on the feet and hands and then move proximally to involve the thighs, forearms, and, less often, the trunk or buttocks. The head is spared. The lesions are often preceded by edema and may initially be misdiagnosed as cellulitis. The edema usually resolves and the involved skin retains a thickened and firm texture.[179] The lesions may be pruritic and accompanied by sharp pain or a burning sensation. Movement of the joints may be quite limited by the fibrosis. Unlike autoimmune sclerosing conditions, Raynaud phenomenon and livedo reticularis are not features of NSF. Late in the disease course, hyperpigmentation, hairlessness, and epidermal atrophy have been described.[184]

The prevalence of systemic involvement is unknown, but a number of different organ system manifestations have been described. Muscle induration may be seen, but strength is normal or only slightly reduced.[185] Joint contractures are common in advanced disease, but the limitation in motion appears to be due to periarticular skin thickening, because there is no evidence of synovitis or arthritis. Computed tomography shows fibrosis of the fascia and muscles in the most severely affected patients. Fibrosis has also been identified in the lungs (reduced DL_{CO}) and diaphragm (respiratory failure),[186-188] myocardium,[186,188,189] pericardium and pleura,[187] and dura mater.[189] Yellow asymptomatic scleral plaques may be seen. Patients with systemic disease may have marked elevations in erythrocyte sedimentation rate and serum C-reactive protein.[190]

The diagnosis of NSF is based upon histopathological examination of a biopsy of an involved site. A deep incisional biopsy should be performed since the typical changes can extend into the subcutaneous fat, fascia, and muscle.[191]

On microscopic examination, there is a subtle proliferation of dermal fibroblasts in early lesions and florid proliferation of fibroblasts and dendritic cells in more advanced disease. Inflammatory infiltrates are usually absent. Collagen bundles with surrounding clefts are prominent, and dermal mucin and elastic fibers are variably increased. Electron microscopy confirms these findings, which in some cases resemble a sarcomatous process.

The evaluation of possible NSF should include asking if the patient has had a recent MR imaging procedure that might have involved gadolinium administration. Gadolinium is a non–tissue-specific contrast agent that is primarily administered during magnetic resonance imaging (MRI). For patients with end-stage renal disease, the half-life is as long as 34 hours, and its accumulation in the body seems to be responsible of this syndrome.

Support for the pathogenic role of gadolinium comes from the demonstration of gadolinium deposition in tissue specimens of some patients with NSF.[192-194] In addition, observational clinical studies from the United States and Europe show a link between NSF and exposure to gadodiamide (Omniscan), a form of gadolinium that is the only approved MRI contrast agent in Europe.

In case series from Austria and Denmark, NSF developed in end-stage renal disease patients who received gadodiamide (Omniscan) for MRI 2 to 4 weeks after exposure.[195,196] There was no correlation with age, sex, underlying renal disease, drug therapy, dialysis modality, or comorbid conditions. Of note, around one half of the patients had been previously exposed to gadolinium without developing NSF. These initial observations have been confirmed in review of 75 cases of NSF in the United States performed by the FDA[183] and by the International NSF Registry.[197] However, there is some suggestive evidence that the risk may vary with the different gadolinium preparations. According to the most recent recommendations, if a gadolinium preparation must be given in patients with end stage renal failure, gadoteridol in the lowest possible dose is the preferred agent.[198,199]

Chemically Induced Scleroderma-like Disease

Several chemicals have been implicated in the induction of scleroderma.[200] Polyvinyl chloride, initially used as an anesthetic agent,[201] caused a scleroderma-like disease among workers. It is characterized by Raynaud phenomenon; localized papular skin lesions, especially on the fingers and hands, excluding the face and trunk; and osteolysis of the distal phalanges. Bleomycin, an antineoplastic agent, causes skin changes resembling scleroderma[202] and pulmonary fibrosis.[203] This syndrome is not accompanied by Raynaud phenomenon and may improve on cessation of the drug.[204] Pentazocine, a nonnarcotic analgesic drug, has been reported to cause cutaneous sclerosis with or without ulceration.[205] Predisposing factors may include diabetes mellitus and alcohol abuse.

The toxic-oil syndrome, caused by ingestion of rapeseed cooking oil that contained unidentified contaminants, occurred in epidemic proportions in Spain in early 1981.[206-207] It affected approximately 20,000 persons and resulted in at least 350 deaths.[208] A report of 21 children indicated that complications may have been less severe in the younger group and that the F/M sex ratio was closer to equal (2.5:1) than in adults (6:1).[209] Onset of the disease was characterized by fever, eosinophilia, dyspnea caused by pulmonary edema, a pruritic rash, and malaise. Sclerodermatous skin lesions, alopecia, conjunctivitis sicca, Raynaud phenomenon, myositis, neuropathy, joint contractures, dysphagia, and liver disease evolved over a period of months.

Adjuvant disease, a systemic scleroderma-like condition, has followed cosmetic surgery involving injection of paraffin or silicone.[210,211] An inflammatory reaction in surrounding tissue occurs when silicone gel leaks from implants used for augmentation mammoplasty. A granulomatous reaction can also be demonstrated in regional lymph nodes. Silicone synovitis is well documented in patients after arthroplasty.[212] A variety of atypical "connective tissue diseases," principally, scleroderma-like conditions with chronic fatigue, myalgia, arthralgia, and arthritis, had been reported in women who had silicone breast implants. Causality had been based on extrapolation of epidemiological data.[213] Although there was concern about a possible relationship between silicone exposure, primarily in breast implant recipients, and SSc or SSc-like disease, a large epidemiological study and a meta-analysis failed to provide evidence supporting a causative role.[214,215] A recent report has raised new doubts about this possible relationship.[216]

Pseudosclerodermas

The term *pseudoscleroderma* describes a diverse group of disorders that are characterized by scleroderma-like fibrotic changes in the skin in association with other nonrheumatic diseases. This discussion is restricted to disorders of significance in the pediatric population.

PHENYLKETONURIA

A minority of children with phenylketonuria (i.e., phenylalanine hydroxylase deficiency) develop sclerodermatous skin lesions.[217-220] These lesions, which usually appear within the first year of life, are symmetrical, poorly demarcated, and resemble morphea. They occur most frequently on the lower extremities and trunk. The lesions may regress on introduction of a low-phenylalanine diet.[221,222] Although no differences in serum phenylalanine or tryptophan levels were found in children with phenylketonuria who did or did not have sclerodermatous changes, urinary excretion of 5-hydroxyindoleacetic acid, indoleacetic acid, and tryptamine was much higher in affected children.[221] The relationship of these biochemical abnormalities to the pathogenesis of the accompanying skin lesions or to that of scleroderma per se is unclear. The experimental use of a low-phenylalanine diet in patients with dSSc produced inconclusive results.[221]

SYNDROMES OF PREMATURE AGING

Two rare autosomal recessive disorders accompanied by dwarfing, premature aging, and early death from atherosclerotic heart disease are associated with sclerodermatous skin changes. In *progeria*, the cutaneous changes usually develop before 1 year of age and are characterized by thickened, bound-down skin on the abdomen, flanks, proximal thighs, and upper buttocks.[223-225] During the second year of life, the skin becomes thinner, subcutaneous vascularization is more evident, and alopecia and nail dystrophy develop. *Werner syndrome* most often presents in adolescence with generalized atrophy of muscle and subcutaneous tissue, graying of the hair, baldness, and scleroderma-like skin changes and ulcers involving the extremities.[224,226,227] The histological features of this disorder mimic those of scleroderma. Metastatic calcification may also develop.[228]

LOCALIZED IDIOPATHIC FIBROSES

Several relatively rare disorders in children result in fibrosis of specific organs or structures.[229-231] Keloids are an obvious example. Retroperitoneal fibrosis usually occurs in the region of the sacral promontory and affects vital structures such as the great vessels and ureters. It is more common in males than in females and occurs in children and adults. The syndrome may be idiopathic or associated with administration of the serotonin inhibitor methysergide. An association with spondyloarthropathies has been reported.[232] Retractile mesenteritis, mediastinal fibrosis, fibrosing pericarditis, fibrosing carditis, and peritoneal fibrosis may represent similar disorders that have been related in some instances to administration of certain drugs, notably methysergide and some antihypertensives and anticonvulsants.[233,234]

Some variants of fibromatosis restricted to childhood are distinctive pathologically.[229,235-237] *Congenital torticollis* or *fibromatosis colli* affects the lower sternomastoid muscle and is present at birth or shortly thereafter. It is associated with other anomalies such as congenital dislocations of the hip. *Fibromatosis hyalinica multiplex* is a morphologically distinctive type of *familial multiple fibromatosis* affecting children but not present at birth. *Infantile digital fibromatosis* affects predominantly the distal fingers or toes. A distinctive microscopic abnormality is the presence of eosinophilic cytoplasmic inclusions. *Infantile myofibromatosis* presents as solitary or multiple nodules limited to superficial soft tissues or associated with internal organ involvement. This disorder probably represents an inborn error of metabolism with possible autosomal dominant transmission. It is characterized microscopically by hyalinization of connective tissues of the skin, oral cavity, joint capsules, and bones. Microscopically, areas that resemble smooth muscle alternate with hemangiopericytomalike foci with a more typical fibroblastic configuration. Central necrosis and intravascular growth may be present.

Gardner syndrome is a form of fibromatosis associated with multiple colonic polyps and osteomas. The fibrosis has a tendency to involve intraabdominal structures, such as the omentum and mesentery or to occur after an operative procedure. *Dupuytren contracture* is a nodular thickening of the palmar fascia and flexion contractures of the digits. Unassociated with disorders such as diabetes, it is rare in children. *Lipogranulomatosis subcutanea of Rothmann-Makai* produces scleroderma-like changes in the skin of the lower extremities with subcutaneous nodules. Morphea or linear scleroderma may be the initial diagnostic consideration. Systemic involvement is absent. The *stiff-skin syndrome* represents congenital scleroderma-like indentations of fascia, predominantly of the buttocks and thighs.

Scleromyxedema is characterized by papular cutaneous lesions with induration of underlying subcutaneous tissues. The lesions occur predominantly on the hands, forearms, trunk, face, and neck. Histological characteristics include a prominent fibrohistiocytic infiltrate and dense acid mucopolysaccharide deposits in the upper dermis. The disease in adults has been associated with monoclonal gammopathies.

Scleredema

Scleredema, a nonsuppurative disorder that is primarily of historical interest, follows β-hemolytic streptococcal infection and is characterized by edematous induration of the face, neck, shoulders, thorax, and proximal extremities, but not the hands.[238,239] Onset is characteristically insidious, and resolution spontaneously occurs after 6 to 12 months. Cardiac abnormalities suggesting the concurrence of acute rheumatic fever have been reported. Diagnosis is based on documentation of nonpitting, indurated edema or stiffness of the skin in the typical locations. Dysphagia may be present, but Raynaud phenomenon and telangiectasias are not. Histologically, the dermis is thickened; there are multiple fenestrations between swollen collagen bundles, a scant perivascular lymphocytic infiltrate, and minimal deposits of acid mucopolysaccharides within the fenestrations. Immunofluorescent staining is negative. Although some children with scleredema have poorly controlled insulin-dependent diabetes, the disorder is presumably distinct from diabetic cheiroarthropathy.

Diabetic Cheiroarthropathy

Diabetic cheiroarthropathy, a syndrome of juvenile-onset diabetes mellitus, causes short stature and tightening of the skin and soft tissues, leading to contractures of the finger joints in as many as 29% of children (see Chapter 41).[240]

Porphyria Cutanea Tarda

The development of scleroderma in adults with porphyria cutanea tarda has been reviewed.[241,242] Plaquelike skin changes occurred predominantly on the face, neck, upper chest, and back. Some patients had features of other connective tissue diseases such as discoid lupus. There are no reports of this association in children.

Laboratory Examination

Anemia, although uncommon, occurs in approximately one fourth of patients and is characteristic of the anemia of chronic disease or, less commonly, reflects vitamin B_{12} or folate deficiency resulting from chronic malabsorption. Microangiopathic hemolysis[243] or bleeding from mucosal

telangiectasias may also occur. Autoimmune hemolytic anemia is rare.[243] Leukocytosis is not prominent but correlates in degree with advanced visceral or muscle disease. Eosinophilia occurs in approximately 15% of patients.[244] Synovial fluid analysis was reported in one study to exhibit increased protein content and high numbers of polymorphonuclear leukocytes that had inclusions similar to those seen in rheumatoid arthritis.[245] Pericardial fluid has the characteristics of an exudate.[246]

High-titers of ANAs are frequently identified; the predominant patterns on HEp-2 cell substrate are speckled and nucleolar. ANA seropositivity in two large pediatric series was 81% to 97%, a frequency similar to that reported in adults.[6,7] Antitopoisomerase I (anti–Scl-70) autoantibodies are present in 28% to 34% of patients, whereas the prevalence of anticentromere antibodies is lower in children as compared with adults.

In contrast, a large study of adults with dSSc indicated that 26% had anti–Scl-70 antibodies and 22% anticentromere antibodies.[247] No patient had reactivity to both antigens, an observation also confirmed by Kikuchi and Inagaki.[248] Antibody to Scl-70, which occurred most frequently in patients with dSSc, was associated with peripheral vascular disease, digital pitting, pulmonary interstitial fibrosis, renal involvement, and high rate mortality.[249,134] Anticentromere antibody occurred almost exclusively in patients with lSSc in association with calcinosis and telangiectasias.

Anti–PM-Scl and anti–U1RNP antibodies correlate with scleroderma in overlap syndromes with musculoskeletal involvement. Anti–RNA-polymerase III antibodies are very unusual, in parallel with the rarity of renal involvement in juvenile SSc.[7] The frequency of occurrence of rheumatoid factor and antiphospholipid antibodies is similar in adults and children with SSc.[6,154]

Serological and genetic markers help to predict particular complications. Patients with anti–Scl-70 autoantibodies or the HLA-DR52a genotype are at increased risk for developing interstitial pulmonary fibrosis, irrespective of their apparent clinical subset.[250] In contrast, anti-RNA polymerase I or III antibodies are associated with renal involvement.[251] Anticentromere antibodies in lSSc are an indicator of risk for isolated pulmonary hypertension and severe gastrointestinal involvement,[252] and in at least one study in children, they were a marker of Raynaud phenomenon.[253] An association between the presence of antibody to Scl-70 and malignancy has been observed in adults.[254] Antibodies that are specific for a 70-kD mitochondrial antigen have been described in a small proportion of patients.[255] The associations of antibodies to the PM-Scl antigen have been reviewed.[256] Antineutrophil cytoplasmic antibodies have been reported with specificities to bactericidal or permeability protein and cathepsin G.[257]

Cardiac Function

Electrocardiographic abnormalities include first-degree heart block, right and left bundle branch block, premature atrial and ventricular contractions, nonspecific T-wave changes, and evidence of ventricular hypertrophy.[258] The most frequent cardiac arrhythmias in children are of supraventricular origin, whereas ventricular arrhythmias do not occur very often.[259]

Thallium 201 radionuclide scans will often document abnormalities of myocardial perfusion, ventricular wall motion, chamber size, and left ventricular ejection fraction.[260] Echocardiographic abnormalities in addition to effusions include thickening of the left ventricular wall in 57% and diminished left ventricular compliance in 42%.[261] Ultrasonic videodensitometric analysis has been introduced as an additional mechanism for evaluation.[262]

Pulmonary Function

Characteristic findings of involvement of the respiratory tract include a decrease in timed vital capacity and forced expiratory flow, an early decrease in diffusion, and an increase in functional residual volume.[263,264,265] In one series, 11 of 15 children with dSSc had diminished pulmonary diffusion.[35] The two-dimensional echocardiogram is important in confirming early pulmonary hypertension by documentation of a dilated right ventricle with thickening of the ventricular wall and straightening of the septum. One-dimensional (M-mode) echocardiography is characterized by changes in the midsystolic movement of the pulmonary valve. Right heart catheterization provides definitive confirmation but is often unnecessary.

Steen and colleagues[266] reported that only 38% of 77 adults with dSSc and 28% of 88 with lSSc had normal pulmonary function studies. Restrictive lung disease and isolated reduction of DL_{CO} were the most common abnormalities, occurring in 34 dSSc patients (18%) and 23 (26%) patients with lSSc. The earliest change was a decrease in the forced vital capacity with an FEV_1/FVC less than 70%. This abnormality was present in 8% of patients with diffuse disease and 16% of those with limited disease. Guttadauria and associates[267] also found a high prevalence of small airways disease (42%), usually in the absence of symptoms, chest radiographic changes, or other abnormalities of pulmonary function.

Renal Function

Renal plasma flow is decreased in most patients, especially in the cortex, although normal glomerular filtration may be preserved by intrarenal shifts in blood flow.[268] Even in patients without clinical evidence of renal disease, plasma renin levels correlate with the degree of histological abnormality of the renal arteries and arterioles.[268] Renal arteriography may document irregular arterial narrowing, tortuosity of the interlobular and arcuate arterioles, cortical hypoperfusion, and other changes of malignant hypertension. Kidney size is small to normal.

Skin Scoring

One of the most used scoring systems for the skin involvement is the modified Rodnan Skin Score (mRSS).[269] According to this score the body surface is divided into 17 regions and the skin thickness is assessed on a 0- to 3-point scale (0, normal; 1, thickened skin; 2, decreased ability; 3, unable to pinch or move skin). The score ranges from 0 to 51. The mRSS, routinely used in adult SSc, is the only instrument available and it used also in pediatric patients. However, it has been shown that mRSS in children correlates with the body mass index and the Tanner stage and it should be corrected for these two parameters.[270]

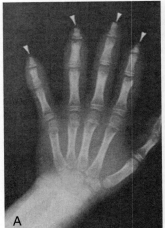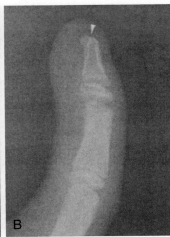

FIGURE 25–13 **A,** Radiograph of a boy with early resorption of the tufts of the distal phalanges *(arrowheads).* **B,** Magnified view of acroosteolysis of the index finger *(arrowhead).*

Radiological Examination

The most characteristic radiological findings in the hands are a marked decrease in soft tissue and resorption of the tufts of the distal phalanges (acroosteolysis), particularly in patients with severe Raynaud phenomenon (Fig. 25–13). Resorption of the distal tufts is particularly common in children.[35,271] Resorption may also occur in ribs, clavicles, distal radius and ulna, and other sites. An increase in the thickness of the periodontal membrane results in radiolucent widening between the teeth and the jaw.[272] Periarticular or subcutaneous calcification, especially in the dominant hand, occurs in 15% to 25% of patients (see Figure 25–8).[35] Bony erosions can also develop at the distal interphalangeal and proximal interphalangeal joints. Involvement of the first carpometacarpal joint is particularly characteristic of dSSc.[273]

Radiological studies of the gastrointestinal tract often demonstrate characteristic abnormalities even in the absence of symptoms. A cine-esophagogram may document decreased or absent peristalsis in the lower part of the esophagus with distal dilatation and, frequently, a hiatal hernia with stricture and shortening of the esophagus (Fig. 25–14). The presence of air in the distal esophagus on the lateral chest radiograph suggests the diagnosis. Esophageal motility studies by manometry and pH probe monitoring of the distal esophagus for 12 to 24 hours provide more sensitive indicators of diminished lower sphincter tone and the presence of reflux.[274] The most frequent radiographic changes in the small bowel are dilatation of the second and third parts of the duodenum and the proximal jejunum (Fig. 25–15). Abnormalities in the colon are characterized by loss of colonic haustrations[275] and the presence of wide-mouthed diverticula or pseudosacculations on the antimesenteric border. Colonic transit is delayed.[127]

Radiographic changes on chest x-ray films correlate poorly with pulmonary function. Bibasilar pulmonary fibrosis is one of the minor criteria for classification of dSSc (Fig. 25–16). It may be accompanied by rib notching

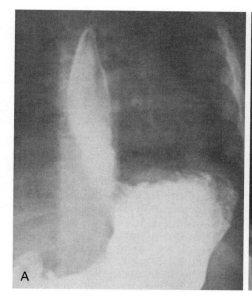
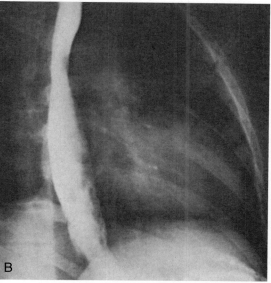

FIGURE 25–14 Barium-contrast examinations of the esophagus illustrate moderate dilatation and lack of a normal peristaltic pattern. **A,** Supine anteroposterior view. **B,** Lateral view.

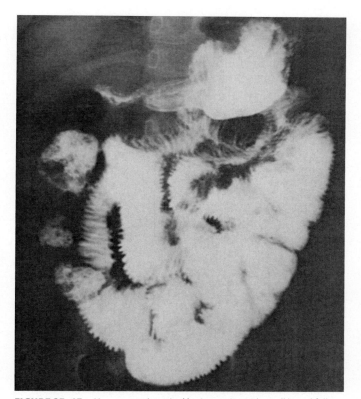

FIGURE 25–15 Upper gastrointestinal barium series with small bowel follow-through in a 3-year-old girl with dilatation of the jejunum and closely approximated valvulae conniventes (the "closed accordion" sign) caused by thickening of the ileal mucosa.

and calcified pulmonary "granulomata" in lSSc.[266] High-resolution computed tomography (HRCT) may confirm pulmonary disease despite a normal chest radiograph.[276,277] In children, the most frequent HRCT findings are (in order) ground-glass opacification, subpleural micronodules, linear opacities, and "honeycombing."[278]

Assessment of Disease Activity and Severity

Assessment of disease activity or severity is difficult. Regular follow-up and clinical review are the cornerstones of monitoring activity and progression. Serological markers of activity have long been sought, and those which may be useful include soluble adhesion molecules such as sICAM-1, collagen propeptides,[279] products of type I collagen breakdown,[280] and immunological markers such as sIL-2 receptor, neopterin, or vascular activation markers (e.g., E-selectin, thrombomodulin, von Willebrand factor). [281] For organ-based complications such as pulmonary fibrosis, pulmonary hypertension, or renal involvement, objective assessment is easier. Sequential skin scores can be recorded. To provide a more global index of severity, a scoring system has been proposed in adults.[282]

Modified health assessment questionnaires have been developed in the United States[283] and Europe.[284-286] They will undoubtedly be of considerable value, particularly because constitutional symptoms and functional impairment are among the most troublesome consequences of this disorder. The European Scleroderma Study Group has developed three different 10-point indices of disease activity, one for scleroderma as a group, one for dSSc, and one for lSSc.[286] These assessments require further validation. No such tool exists for scleroderma in children.

Treatment

Management of dSSc presents one of the most difficult and frustrating challenges in all of rheumatology because no uniformly effective therapy is available.[287] Disease severity ranges from mild and stable to rapidly progressive and fatal. Management can be divided into two general areas: general supportive measures and therapy directed at controlling the underlying disease process and complications (e.g., fibrosis, immunological abnormalities, vasculopathy).

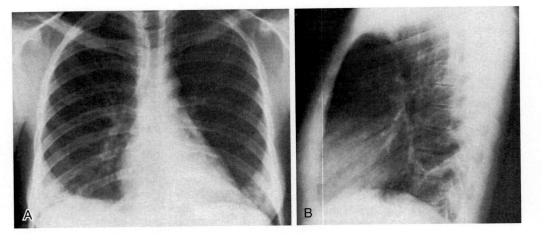

FIGURE 25–16 A, Posteroanterior radiograph of the chest illustrates a fine reticular pattern in both lower lobes. **B,** Lateral view of the chest.

General Supportive Measures

Supportive therapy is of utmost importance in managing a chronic, unpredictable, and potentially debilitating or fatal disease. Education of the child and parents should be undertaken early in an attempt to prevent unnecessary psychological uncertainty and trauma. In general, "optimistic veracity" regarding complications, outcome, and treatment is appropriate. Patient support groups may be helpful and important, albeit difficult to assemble for such a rare disease. Patients should be instructed to avoid cold and trauma. Especially in cold climates, the family should keep the child warm by maintaining a satisfactory household temperature and by use of appropriate clothing, including well-insulated mittens (not gloves), boots, and a hat. The child should avoid excessive sun exposure and heat in the summer because of the susceptibility to hyperpigmentation of the skin and a relative inability to dissipate heat through sclerotic skin.

General skin care should include avoidance of drying or irritating substances and daily application of lanolin or water-soluble cream as an emollient. The child should be encouraged to be as physically active as possible within the constraints of the disease. Active range of motion and gentle passive range of motion are essential to preserve maximal function. Dynamic splints may be necessary to treat or prevent contractures. Nonsteroidal antiinflammatory drugs may relieve some of the musculoskeletal symptoms but may be detrimental to renal function. Subcutaneous calcifications, if ulcerating, may require incision and drainage.

Therapy of the Disease Process and Complications

Few of the drugs used as disease-modifying agents have undergone placebo-controlled evaluation, and the results from those that have are often disappointing. No drug has been of unequivocal benefit, and even if such data were available, therapeutic gain must be carefully balanced against toxicity and considered in the context of the natural history of the disorder.

The treatment of dSSc is mainly symptomatic and focuses on clinical manifestations, and organ involvement. The EULAR Scleroderma Trials and Research (EUSTAR) group has recently established a group of evidence-based recommendations to be used in clinical practice. Following EULAR's standard operating procedures, an ad hoc expert committee was established by EULAR and EUSTAR.[288]

The main aim of these recommendations is to provide guidance to adult and pediatric rheumatologists to correctly approach and choose the treatment for SSc patients. Possible combinations of these approaches to treatment are suggested in Table 25–6.

DIGITAL VASCULOPATHY

Raynaud Phenomenon (see also Chapter 29). In addition to avoidance of precipitating circumstances such as cold or emotional stress, specific treatment of Raynaud phenomenon may be necessary. Pharmacological side effects are often dose limiting, responses to individual vasodilators are idiosyncratic, and substantial placebo responses and lack of mechanisms for objective assessment confound therapeutic trials. The most commonly used vasodilator agents are the calcium channel blockers (CCBs). Nifedipine is the most widely recommended agent. It has been well tolerated in several controlled trials, has reduced the frequency and severity of Raynaud phenomenon, and has promoted healing of cutaneous ischemic ulcers.[289-292] One meta-analysis involving 109 SSc adult patients indicates that CCBs reduce the frequency and severity of ischemic attacks in SSc-related Raynaud phenomenon.[293] Nifedipine induces a reduction of ischemic attacks of more than 35% as compared with placebo.[293]

Another meta-analysis, including the results of five randomized clinical trials (RCTs) with intravenous iloprost and one with oral iloprost, indicates that iloprost is effective in reducing the frequency and severity of SSc-related Raynaud phenomenon.[294] Iloprost, given intravenously (0.5 to 2 ng/kg/min for 3 to 5 consecutive days sequentially) or orally (50 μg to 150 μg twice daily) significantly reduced the frequency of ischemic attacks and improved the Raynaud phenomenon severity score in comparison with placebo. Oral prostanoids seem to be generally less effective than intravenous iloprost in the treatment of SSc-related Raynaud phenomenon, although some beneficial effects could be seen with higher doses.[294] Iloprost has been reported to be safe and effective in treatment of ischemic digits in children with dSSc and other connective

Table 25-6

Treatment approach for systemic sclerosis for children

General supportive measures	Avoid cold and trauma with appropriate clothing, avoid excessive sun exposure and heat in the hot seasons. General skin care: daily application of lanolin or water-soluble cream as an emollient. Rehabilitation program to preserve maximal function and dynamic splints to treat or prevent contraclures. Patient support groups.	
Organ-based treatment	**Raynaud Phenomenon**	CCBs, iloprost, sildenafil
	Digital ulcers	CCBs, iloprost, bosenian
	Fibrosing alveolitis	cyclophosphamide, corticosteroids
	Pulmonary arterial hypertension	bosentan, sitaxsentan, sildenafil, prostanoids
	Gastro-oesophageal reflux	PPIs, prokinetics
	Midgut disease	Rotating antibiotics
	Muscoloskeletal involvement	low-dose corticosteroids, MTX
	Renal disease	ACE inhibtors
	Skin involvement	MTX, MMF

CCBs: calcium channel blockers, PPIs: proton pump inhibitors, CPM: cyclohosphamide, ERAs: endothelin receptor antagonists, ACEi: angiotensin-converting enzyme inhibitors, MMF: Mycophenolate mofetil, HSCT: autologous hemopoietic stem cell transplantation.

tissue diseases.[295] It may be combined with another agent for enhanced therapeutic effect. In view of costs and feasibility, CCBs should be considered the first-line therapy in the treatment of SSc-related RP. Intravenous prostanoids should be used when CCBs fail and there is severe ischemia.

Other agents include drugs that inhibit or suppress the sympathetic nervous system, thereby indirectly promoting vasodilation, and those that act directly on the smooth muscle of the vessel wall, such as reserpine, methyldopa, and ketanserin.[296-301] One drug may be effective in one patient, whereas a different agent is effective in another. It is therefore worth trying several, one at a time, until the desired effect is obtained. Griseofulvin has been beneficial in a few resistant patients, as have surgical sympathectomy and prostaglandin E$_1$ infusions.[302-306]

Sildenafil, a selective type 5 phosphodiesterase inhibitor, may be beneficial in treatment of SSc-related vasculopathy by reducing symptoms of Raynaud phenomenon and improving digital ulcer healing.[307] However, the small number of RCTs with low numbers of SSc patients and the lack of pediatric data represent the main limitations for its wide recommendation in children.

Digital Ulcers. Digital ulcers (DU) are another severe and disabling complication of dSSc. Intravenous iloprost (0.5 to 2 µg/kg/min for 3 to 5 consecutive days) significantly reduces the number of DU and improves DU healing in comparison with placebo in two distinct RCTs.[308,309]

During the past decade, targeting mediators of immune or vasoactive reactions has been an innovative step in the treatment of connective tissue diseases. Endothelin-1, a potent vasoconstrictor and smooth muscle mitogen, is a possible target in patients with DU. Bosentan, a dual endothelin receptor antagonist, was evaluated in two placebo-controlled RCTs involving 210 SSc patients in total.[310,311] Bosentan, at an oral dose of 62.5 mg twice daily for 4 weeks followed by 125 mg twice daily for another 12 weeks, significantly reduced the number of new DU by 48% as compared with placebo.[310] The efficacy of bosentan in preventing new DU formation was corroborated by the results of the recent RAPIDS-2 study. In these patients, bosentan

caused 61% reduction of DU over 16 weeks, especially in dSSc, whereas in lSSc the mean reduction was 38%.[311]

Both trials indicate that bosentan is not superior to placebo in healing of SSc-related DU.[310,311] There are two major concerns related to the use of bosentan: potential liver injury and teratogenicity. Elevated liver aminotransferases have been reported in 11% to 14% of bosentan-treated patients, but these abnormalities were reversible after drug discontinuation.[310,311] All endothelin receptor antagonists including bosentan are considered to be teratogenic.[312] Accordingly, pregnancy must be excluded before the start of treatment and prevented thereafter by the use of reliable contraceptive measures.[313]

The available evidence concerning CCBs and prostanoids in the prevention of new DU in SSc patients is far less comprehensive and robust than that of bosentan, but their toxicity pattern is milder, and long-term clinical experience suggests a good safety profile. In view of overall risk-to-benefit considerations, CCBs and prostanoids should be used as first-line therapy in SSc-related DU. If the clinical response is unsatisfactory, bosentan should be considered as an adjunct treatment, aiming at the prevention of new DU rather than for healing DU.

Interstitial Lung Disease. Pulmonary complications are very serious, and there may be no effective long-term therapeutic approach to fibrosing alveolitis or primary pulmonary hypertension. Alveolitis is predominant early, and later progresses to fibrosis. Generally, cyclophosphamide is recommended when there is evidence of active alveolitis or interstitial lung disease (ILD)—usually determined by a ground-glass HRCT scan or by the presence of neutrophils in bronchoalveolar lavage. The efficacy and safety of cyclophosphamide in the treatment of SSc-ILD were evaluated in two RCTs.[314,315] The first, involving 158 SSc patients with active alveolitis, demonstrated that cyclophosphamide, given orally at a dose of 1 to 2 mg/kg/d, improved lung function tests, dyspnea score, and quality of life over a 12-month period, compared with placebo. Cyclophosphamide was not effective in increasing the lung diffusing capacity for carbon monoxide (DL$_{CO}$) but showed improvement in the HAQ disability index and the vitality- and health-transition domains of the SF36. Oral cyclophosphamide was associated with leucopenia and neutropenia (p<0.05 versus placebo).[314]

The second trial evaluated cyclophosphamide (dose of 600 mg/m²/month IV) versus placebo in 45 SSc patients with SSc-ILD. The mean-adjusted between-group difference in FVC was 4.2% in favor of cyclophosphamide, which just missed statistical significance (p=0.08). DL_{CO} and other outcome measures did not improve.[315]

Although the efficacy of cyclophosphamide was considered moderate, it is currently the only drug with proven efficacy in SSc-ILD and should be considered the drug of choice in progressive SSc-ILD. Toxicity related to cumulative cyclophosphamide doses suggests an intravenous regimen.

Pulmonary Arterial Hypertension. One of the most lethal complications is pulmonary arterial hypertension (PAH), which can occur in the context of established interstitial fibrosis or without it in lSSc.

During the past decade, targeting mediators of immune or vasoactive reactions has been an innovative step in the treatment of connective tissue diseases. Endothelin-1, a potent vasoconstrictor and smooth muscle mitogen, is a possible target in patients with primary or secondary PAH. The efficacy of endothelin receptor antagonists (ERAs), namely bosentan and sitaxsentan, for the treatment of PAH has been summarized in a meta-analysis of five RCTs evaluating 482 patients, mainly with idiopathic PAH (iPAH), of whom 85 (18%) were patients with SSc-PAH.[316] ERAs, tested for a period of 12 to 16 weeks against placebo, significantly improved exercise capacity in 6-minute walk test (6MWT), pulmonary artery pressure (PAP) and cardiac index. The oral formulation and the potential use of these agents for other vascular complications represent important arguments for its potential value in pediatric patients with dSSc.

Two placebo-controlled RCTs showed that bosentan (62.5mg twice daily during 4 weeks, followed by 125 to 250 mg twice daily) significantly improved the 6MWT after 12 and 16 weeks in a heterogeneous population of PAH patients.[317,318] Indeed, the long-term extension of these studies suggested that bosentan may improve survival in SSc-PAH in comparison with historical controls (1-, 2- and 3-year survival rates: 82%, 67% and 64%, respectively, versus 45%, 35% and 28%).[319]

Two RCTs including 423 patients with different forms of PAH, among whom 116 patients had CTD-related PAH,[320,321] showed that sitaxsentan, administered orally at a dose of 100 mg/day or 300 mg/day for 12 to 18 weeks, significantly improved exercise capacity and hemodynamics, with both dosage regimens. However, in view of a comparable efficacy of the two regimens and the fact that the higher dose is associated with greater toxicity (increased prothrombin time and elevation of liver enzyme levels), sitaxsentan at a dose of 100 mg/day is suggested in the treatment of PAH.

For similar reasons, sitaxsentan may also represent an alternative to bosentan in patients with SSc-related PAH. An open-label extension study suggested that sitaxsentan may be safer than bosentan with regard to the frequency of liver test abnormalities (3% versus 18%) and premature discontinuation (20% versus 57%).[322] Moreover, sitaxsentan administered at 100 mg/day improved the clinical status in more than one third of PAH patients in whom bosentan was ineffective.[323]

Sildenafil significantly improves 6MWT results, functional class, and hemodynamics in PAH of different origin.[324] In a subgroup of 84 patients with CTD-PAH (including 38 SSc-PAH patients), sildenafil significantly improved walking distance, functional class, and mean PAP in comparison to placebo.[325]

Sildenafil is generally well tolerated and the majority of adverse events are mild to moderate. However, because the amount of data confirming the efficacy and safety of sildenafil in SSc-PAH is scarce, it should be considered only for patients in whom ERAs have been ineffective or cannot be used for safety reasons.

Intravenous infusion of epoprostenol (starting dose 2 µg/kg/min IV, increased based on clinical symptoms and tolerability) in combination with conventional therapy improves exercise capacity, functional status, and hemodynamic measures in severe SSc-PAH, as compared with conventional therapy.[326]

Treatment with parenteral prostanoids is associated with frequent adverse events (mainly vascular reactions and gastrointestinal symptoms). Because of its very short half-life, epoprostenol is administered through a permanent indwelling central venous catheter, which may cause adverse events, including infections, pneumothorax, and hemorrhage. Sudden disruption/withdrawal of intravenous epoprostenol (due to catheter/vein thrombosis and/or patient's decision) may lead to life-threatening PAH rebound. Based on overall risk-to-benefit considerations, intravenous epoprostenol is recommend as treatment of choice in severe, therapy-resistant SSc-PAH.

Skin Involvement. In two RCTs involving 29 and 73 SSc patients with early dSSc or lSSc, respectively, methotrexate showed a trend towards improvement of the Total Skin Score.[327,328]

Adverse events associated with methotrexate included oral ulcers, liver toxicity, and pancytopenia.[327] In view of these results, methotrexate should be considered as an option in early dSSc not requiring other immunosuppressants for internal organ involvement.

Renal Disease. Until recently, prognosis for renal crisis was uniformly dismal. Immediate and effective lowering of the blood pressure in patients with malignant hypertension is mandatory. Any sudden change in plasma volume should be avoided because marked reductions in renal blood flow may precipitate acute clinical deterioration. The introduction of angiotensin-converting enzyme inhibitors (ACEi) (e.g., captopril or enalapril) brought about a remarkable improvement in the outlook for prevention of vascular damage, effective long-term control of blood pressure, and stabilization of renal function.[329-332]

Despite the lack of RCTs, ACEi are indicated for the treatment of scleroderma renal crisis (SRC). Prospective analysis of 108 patients with SRC has suggested that patients on ACEi had a significantly better survival rate at 1 year (76%) and 5 years (66%) compared with patients not on ACEi (15% at 1 and 10% at 5 years, respectively).[331,333-334]

In cases of irreversible renal failure or uncontrollable hypertension, some success has followed the use of hemodialysis with or without bilateral nephrectomy and transplantation.[335] Dialysis may lead to improvement in the cutaneous abnormalities.

Musculoskeletal Involvement. The treatment of musculoskeletal involvement (myositis, arthritis, and tenosynovitis) includes the use glucocorticoids, preferably prednisone, at a dosage of 0.3 to 0.5 mg/kg per day. Because several studies suggest that the use of steroids, particularly in patients with a high skin score and joint contractures, is associated with a higher risk of scleroderma renal crisis (43% versus 21% of patients without steroids),[142] patients on steroids should be carefully monitored for blood pressure and renal function. Attention should be paid especially to patients with early dSSc and high or rapidly progressing skin score.

Gastrointestinal Disease. Few studies in children address the most effective management for gastrointestinal disease. Except for symptomatic approaches, definitive therapy is materially lacking. Treatment of erosive esophagitis often is characterized by considerable delay in healing with the standard approaches of small, more frequent meals, with the last well before bedtime, and elevation of the head of the bed. Acid reflux and esophageal hypomotility are also complementary factors for the development of pulmonary fibrosis.[336]

Despite the lack of specific RCTs, proton pump inhibitors (PPIs) represent the drugs of choice for prevention of SSc-related gastroesophageal reflux disease (GERD), esophageal ulcers, and strictures. The efficacy of PPIs in the treatment of GERD in the general population is well documented in meta-analyses of RCTs.[337-338] Considering the efficacy of PPIs in the management of GERD in the otherwise healthy population and the high frequency of esophageal involvement in SSc patients, PPIs should be used, even in the early phase, for the prevention of SSc-related upper gastrointestinal involvement.

Several nonrandomized or uncontrolled studies in adults suggest that prokinetic drugs may improve gastrointestinal signs and symptoms (dysphagia, early satiety, bloating, pseudoobstruction) in SSc patients.[339-341]

Arteriovenous ectasia of the stomach may require multiple attempts at argon plasma coagulation. Malabsorption is difficult to manage. Diarrhea and bloating are most often caused by bacterial overgrowth and are treated by rotating antibiotics, because continuous therapy with one agent may result in the emergence of resistant organisms. The choice of antibiotic is usually empirical and includes amoxicillin with clavulanate or oral cephalosporins. In refractory cases, metronidazole can be added for 5 to 7 days to treat anaerobic flora.

Hyperalimentation may be necessary but has not been demonstrated to be a wise long-term choice.

Experimental Therapy

Mycophenolate mofetil (MMF) has been successfully used for early diffuse scleroderma and lung disease.[342] The apparent safety and tolerability of this drug was confirmed in a recent retrospective study.[343] Data from 109 patients with diffuse cutaneous systemic sclerosis treated with MMF were compared with those of 63 control subjects receiving other immunosuppressive drugs. MMF was discontinued because of disease stabilization in 9%, side effects in 8%, or no effects on disease activity in 14%. A lower frequency of clinically significant pulmonary fibrosis and better 5-year survival from disease onset were reported. According to the authors' conclusion, MMF appears to be at least as effective as the other current therapies for diffuse SSc, and this provides support for further evaluation in prospective clinical trials.

One of the most aggressive approaches to therapy is immunoablation followed by reconstitution with hematopoeitic stem cell transplantation (HSCT).[344] The rationale for this therapy is similar to that in other autoimmune diseases. If scleroderma is driven by an autoimmune process, ablation of self-reactive lymphocyte clones may block pathogenesis. If the immune system is reconstituted in the presence of the neoantigens responsible for autoimmunity, tolerance will be reestablished. However, even if such tolerance does not occur, the intensive immunosuppression may be directly beneficial. A multicenter study reported that HSCT improved the skin score for 69% of patients, did not affect lung function, but halted pulmonary hypertension.[345,346] However, disease progression occurred in 19%, and 17% died of complications related to the procedure. Because of this high mortality rate, HSCT must be carefully considered for pediatric patients,[347] and unfortunately, it may only be rational therapy early in disease course (3 years or less from the first non-Raynaud sign or symptom) before unmodifiable damage has resulted (e.g., fibrosis).

Course of the Disease and Prognosis

The systemic nature of dSSc cannot be stressed too strongly, because the ultimate prognosis of the child depends primarily on the extent and nature of visceral involvement. The outcome has been poor but may be improving. Skin tightness and joint contractures inevitably lead to severe disability in some patients (Fig. 25–17).[348] It is a curious but often-repeated observation that the skin may eventually soften years after onset. Progressive gastrointestinal involvement is typical, however, starting with the esophagus and proceeding distally, although the disease may stabilize in some patients for long periods (Table 25–7). Gastrointestinal complications and inanition may also become severe. Cardiac arrhythmias may result from myocardial fibrosis. Congestive heart failure is often a terminal event. Pulmonary interstitial disease and vascular lesions are probably universal, even if not clinically evident. Renal failure or acute hypertensive encephalopathy supervenes as a potentially fatal outcome in a few children. At least in adults, this event seems more likely to occur early in the course of the disease.

A recent study investigating clinical and genetic variables, at initial presentation, that predict survival, showed that age >65 years and forced vital capacity <50% predicted clinically significant arrhythmia on ECG, absence of anticentromere antibodies, hypertension, chest radiograph suggestive of pulmonary fibrosis, and low

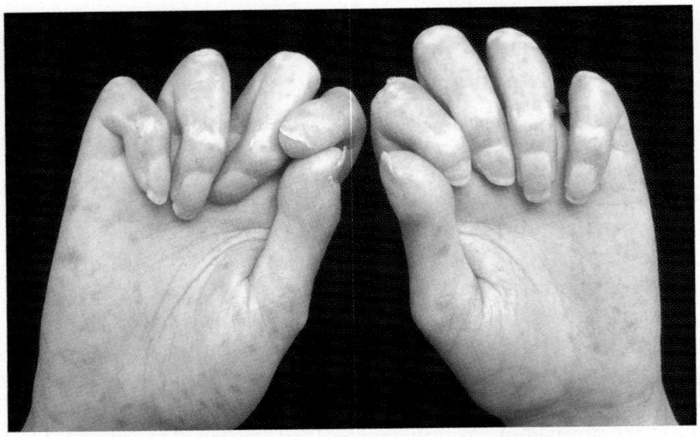

FIGURE 25–17 Hands of a 27-year-old woman with diffuse cutaneous systemic scleroderma that began in childhood. There was essentially no movement possible in these fingers because of joint contractures. Notice the extensive telangiectasias.

body mass index were significant predictors of mortality.[349] In addition, some of the HLA genes associated with SSc susceptibility, namely DRB1*0802 and DQA1*0501, are useful for predicting SSc outcome.

Survivorship has not been determined in any large series of children because of the rarity of this disease. The age-specific mortality rate in one epidemiological study for the 0- to 14-year age group was 0.04 per million person-years.[350] Recent studies showed that the prognosis of SSc in children appears better than in adults. The survival rates of childhood-onset SSc at 5, 10, 15, and 20 years after diagnosis were 89%, 80% to 87.4%, 74% to 87.4%, and 69% to 82.5%, respectively. These rates are significantly higher than for those in adult-onset disease.[7,129,351]

The most common causes of death in children are related to the involvement of cardiac, renal, and pulmonary systems (Table 25–8). Indeed, cardiomyopathy is a leading cause of early death, especially in children.[128,129] This complication is rare and usually associated with diffuse cutaneous disease and features of polymyositis. An aggressive immunosuppressive treatment has been effective for muscle, skin, and lung involvement but does not impair progression of myocardial dysfunction.

In children with poor prognosis, diagnosis is often made earlier, probably because clinical manifestations have been clear since the onset of the disease and severe enough to lead rapidly to death, as shown by the fact that most of the deaths occurred in the first 5 years after diagnosis.[129] Therefore, in children SSc may have two possible evolutions: some children have a rapid development of internal organ failure leading to severe disability and eventually to death, while most patients experience a slow, insidious course of the disease with lower mortality.

Compared with studies in adults in which the diffuse cutaneous SSc subset is considered a risk factor for higher mortality[352,353] this does not appear so relevant in children.[7,129,351] This observation is influenced by the fact that in children a clear-cut differentiation between the various subsets is difficult because the limited cutaneous form is rare.[6] Similarly, in adult series the presence of antitopoisomerase I and anti-RNA polymerase III antibodies and the male sex have been associated with

Table 25-7

Organ system involvement during the course of systemic sclerosis in children

	No. with Involvement/No. Observed			
Organ System	**Cassidy et al[32]**	**%**	**Martini et al[6]**	**%**
Skin				
Subcutaneous calcification	4/15	27	28/151	18
Ulcerations	9/15	60	60/150	40
Telangiectasias	4/15	27	—	
Pigmentation	3/15	20	—	
Digital arteries (Raynaud phenomenon)	11/15	73	128/152	84
Musculoskeletal System				
Contractures	11/15	73	—	
Resorption of digital tufts	9/11	82	—	
Muscle weakness	6/15	40	37/152	24
Muscle atrophy	6/15	40	—	
Gastrointestinal Tract				
Abnormal esophageal motility	11/15	73	45/150	30
Dilatation of duodenum	1/15	7	—	
Colonic sacculations	3/5	60	—	
Lungs				
Abnormal DL_{CO}	11/15	73	40/150	27
Abnormal vital capacity	10/15	67	63/150	42
Heart				
Cardiomegaly	2/15	13	—	
Electrocardiographic abnormalities	4/15	27	15/153	10
Congestive heart failure	2/15	13	11/150	7

poorer survival, whereas in children no clear relationship was found between serological features, age at onset, sex, and mortality.[129]

As children with dSSc live into adulthood, complications associated with pregnancy become a concern.[354,355]

Mortality rates for adults were significantly increased in a study from Denmark (standardized mortality ratio [SMR] = 4.5; 95% CI: 3.5–5.7) and even more in patients younger than 35 years (SMR =13; 95% CI: 2.7–37).[356] This study and another from Spain[357] identified the extent of cutaneous sclerosis as an important determining factor in prognosis. Another report cited a 7-year survival rate from diagnosis of 72.5% for black women and 77.6% for white women.[24]

Mortality seemingly increases throughout life and is higher for males than females and for nonwhites than whites.[26] Studies of patients of all ages demonstrated mean survival rates of 70% to 94% at 1 year, 34% to 73% at 5 years, and 35% to 74% at 10 years.[140] Cardiac and renal disease were the most common contributors to mortality. Outcomes of 48 adults with "early" scleroderma indicated that survivorship was 92% at 1 year, 75% at 3 years, and 68% at 5 years.[358] In another report, 20-year mortality rates for patients with renal involvement was

Table 25–8

Causes of death in children with systemic sclerosis

Study	Sex	Age at Onset (yr)	Disease Duration	Cause of Death
Kornreich et al[30]	M	4	10 yr	Cerebral hemorrhage due to thrombocytopenia
	F	6	9 yr	Cardiac failure
	M	7	23 mo	Renal failure
	F	10	15 mo	Cardiac failure
	F	10	22 mo	Pulmonary emboli
	F	15	5 mo	Cardiac failure
Cassidy et al[35]	F	12	6 mo	Cardiac failure
	F	11	10 yr	Cardiac failure
	F	8	9 yr	Central nervous system disease, hypertension
Bulkley[164]	M	13	2 yr	Pulmonary hypertension
	F	16	1 yr	Pulmonary hypertension
Suárez-Almazor et al[50]	M	10	2 yr	Cardiac failure
Martini et al[129]	5M, 10F	5-15	0.5 m 0-18 yr	Cardiac failure (10)
				Renal failure (2)
				Respiratory failure (2)
				Infection (2)

60%, compared with 10% for those without renal disease.[141] An overall 10-year survival rate close to 90% was reported for a group of 106 patients from Italy who were predominantly female.[22] Median survival in the Detroit tricounty area was approximately 11 years.[26]

LIMITED CUTANEOUS SYSTEMIC SCLERODERMA

Definition

lSSc is the designation for patients previously classified as having the CREST syndrome. Winterbauer[359] first described this syndrome as a variant of systemic scleroderma. Very few instances of lSSc in children have been reported.[6,48-50] Whether it is a relatively mild form of dSSc or an entirely separate, although related, disorder is uncertain.[11,360] The combination of scleroderma and calcinosis was designated as *acrosclerosis* in the older literature, or has been referred to as the *Thibierge-Weissenbach syndrome*.[361]

Epidemiology

Overall, lSSc accounts for approximately one third to one half of the adult patients with scleroderma.[362] Limited disease is more common among women and tends to occur at an earlier age than dSSc. A long interval between the onset of Raynaud phenomenon and diagnostic skin changes is characteristic.

Clinical Manifestations

Calcinosis is usually more severe in patients with lSSc than in dSSc (Fig. 25–18), Raynaud phenomenon is more frequently complicated by digital ulceration and gangrene, and telangiectasias are more widespread.[359] LSSC is by no

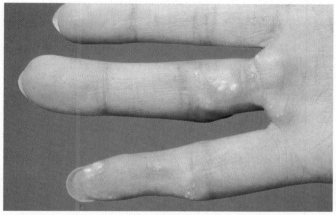

FIGURE 25–18 Striking subcutaneous calcification with extrusion of calcaneous material.

means a mild disease, however, and severe systemic involvement, especially pulmonary fibrosis and hypertension, occurs, although renal disease is less frequent than in dSSc.

Diagnosis

Cutaneous sclerosis is restricted to the distal segments of the digits, and telangiectasias, Raynaud phenomenon, and calcinosis are prominent. Isolated proximal scleroderma supports a diagnosis of dSSc rather than limited disease. In other ways, however, these two syndromes closely resemble each other, and *clinical separation of these disorders may be entirely artificial.*

Immunological Characteristics

Antibody to centromere has been described as the serological hallmark of lSSc, and its discovery historically supported the rationale for clinical differentiation of the

CREST syndrome from dSSc.[360,363] This antibody specificity is directed at the kinetochore of components of the mitotic spindle. It is evident, however, that anticentromere antibody is associated with diseases other than lSSc,[364] notably with primary biliary cirrhosis; occasionally with dSSc, Sjögren syndrome, or isolated Raynaud phenomenon; and rarely with rheumatoid arthritis, systemic lupus erythematosus, and other connective tissue diseases. Other ANAs (e.g., anti-ssDNA, anti-RNP) occasionally may be present.[365] Elevated levels of soluble CD31 were reported in patients with a relatively early age at onset and a lower frequency and severity of pulmonary fibrosis. Because this marker is associated with an antiinflammatory effect by inhibiting transendothelial migration of leukocytes, it could represent a protective factor for the development of cutaneous and pulmonary fibrosis.[366]

Treatment

The management of children with lSSc is not materially different from that for diffuse disease, modified according to each patient's specific organ involvement and severity (see Table 25–6).

Course of the Disease and Prognosis

It was initially believed that patients with this variant of scleroderma had a more benign course and lower mortality rate than those with dSSc, but this distinction has not been entirely substantiated. The mortality rate for lSSc, although somewhat less than in dSSc, is substantial, with a 10-year survival rate of approximately 75% in adults.[357]

REFERENCES

6. G. Martini, I. Foeldvari, R. Russo, et al., Systemic sclerosis in childhood: clinical and immunological features of 153 patients in an international database Arthritis Rheum. 54 (2006) 3971–3978.
7. K. Scalapino, T. Arkachaisri, M. Lucas, et al., Childhood onset systemic sclerosis: classification, clinical and serologic features, and survival in comparison with adult onset disease, J. Rheumatol. 33 (2006) 1004–1013.
12. H. Poormoghim, M. Lucas, N. Fertig, et al., Systemic sclerosis sine scleroderma: demographic, clinical, and serologic features and survival in forty-eight patients, Arthritis Rheum. 43 (2000) 444–451.
14. Preliminary criteria for the classification of systemic sclerosis (scleroderma), Subcommittee for scleroderma criteria of the American Rheumatism Association Diagnostic and Therapeutic Criteria Committee, Arthritis Rheum. 23 (1980) 581–590.
15. E.C. LeRoy, T.A. Medsger Jr., Criteria for the classification of early systemic sclerosis, J. Rheumatol. 28 (2001) 1573–1576.
16. F. Zulian, P. Woo, B.H. Athreya, et al., The PRES/ACR/EULAR Provisional Classification Criteria for Juvenile Systemic Sclerosis, Arthritis Rheum. 57 (2007) 203–212.
25. M.D. Mayes, Scleroderma epidemiology, Rheum. Dis. Clin. North Am. 29 (2003) 239–254.
53. R. Vancheeswaran, C.M. Black, J. David, et al., Childhood-onset scleroderma: is it different from adult-onset disease, Arthritis Rheum. 39 (1996) 1041–1049.
55. S.A. Jimenez, C.T. Derk, Following the molecular pathways toward an understanding of the pathogenesis of systemic sclerosis, Ann. Intern. Med. 140 (2004) 37–50.
57. A.D. Roumm, T.L. Whiteside, T.A. Medsger Jr., et al., Lymphocytes in the skin of patients with progressive systemic sclerosis: quantification, subtyping, and clinical correlations, Arthritis Rheum. 27 (1984) 645–653.

101. F. De Keyser, I. Peene, R. Joos, et al., Occurrence of scleroderma in monozygotic twins, J. Rheumatol. 27 (2000) 2267–2269.
109. R.I. Fox, H.I. Kang, Genetic and environmental factors in systemic sclerosis, Curr. Opin. Rheumatol. 4 (1992) 857–861.
113. S.E. Burastero, S. Galbiati, A. Vassallo, et al., Cellular microchimerism as a lifelong physiologic status in parous women: an immunologic basis for its amplification in patients with systemic sclerosis, Arthritis Rheum. 48 (2003) 1109–1116.
114. J.L. Nelson, D.E. Furst, S. Maloney, et al., Microchimerism and HLA-compatible relationships of pregnancy in scleroderma, Lancet 351 (1998) 559–562.
117. C.M. Artlett, J.B. Smith, S.A. Jimenez, Identification of fetal DNA and cells in skin lesions from women with systemic sclerosis, N. Engl. J. Med. 338 (1998) 1186–1191.
120. H.R. Maricq, G. Spencer-Green, E.C. LeRoy, Skin capillary abnormalities as indicators of organ involvement in scleroderma (systemic sclerosis), Raynaud's syndrome and dermatomyositis, Am. J. Med. 61 (1976) 862–870.
128. P. Quartier, D. Bonnet, J.C. Fournet, et al., Severe cardiac involvement in children with systemic sclerosis and myositis, J. Rheumatol. 29 (2002) 1767–1773.
129. G. Martini, F. Vittadello, Ö. Kasapçopur, et al., Factors affecting survival in Juvenile Systemic Sclerosis, Rheumatology (Oxford.) 48 (2009) 119–222.
133. C. Morgan, C. Knight, M. Lunt, et al., Predictors of end stage lung disease in a cohort of patients with scleroderma, Ann. Rheum. Dis. 62 (2003) 146–150.
134. A. Perera, N. Fertig, M. Lucas, et al., Clinical subsets, skin thickness progression rate, and serum antibody levels in systemic sclerosis patients with anti-topoisomerase I antibody, Arthritis Rheum. 56 (2007) 2740–2746.
141. V.D. Steen, T.A. Medsger Jr., Case-control study of corticosteroids and other drugs that either precipitate or protect from the development of scleroderma renal crisis, Arthritis Rheum. 41 (1998) 1613–1619.
150. P. Lee, J. Bruni, S. Sukenik, Neurological manifestations in systemic sclerosis (scleroderma), J. Rheumatol. 11 (1984) 480–483.
154. A. Della Rossa, G. Valentini, S. Bombardieri, et al., European multicentre study to define disease activity criteria for systemic sclerosis. I. Clinical and epidemiological features of 290 patients from 19 centres, Ann. Rheum. Dis. 60 (2001) 585–591.
162. T.A. Medsger Jr., G.P. Rodnan, J. Moossy, et al., Skeletal muscle involvement in progressive systemic sclerosis (scleroderma), Arthritis Rheum. 11 (1968) 554–568.
168. D. Lapenas, G.P. Rodnan, T. Cavallo, Immunopathology of the renal vascular lesion of progressive systemic sclerosis (scleroderma), Am. J. Pathol. 91 (1978) 243–258.
179. A. Galan, S.E. Cowper, R. Bucala, Nephrogenic systemic fibrosis (nephrogenic fibrosing dermopathy), Curr. Opin. Rheumatol. 18 (2006) 614–617.
206. E.M. Kilbourne, J.G. Rigau-Perez, C.W. Heath Jr., et al., Clinical epidemiology of toxic-oil syndrome: manifestations of a new illness, N. Engl. J. Med. 309 (1983) 1408–1414.
209. M. Izquierdo, I. Mateo, M. Rodrigo, et al., Chronic juvenile toxic epidemic syndrome, Ann. Rheum. Dis. 44 (1985) 98–103.
215. E.C. Janowsky, L.L. Kupper, B.S. Hulka, Meta-analyses of the relation between silicone breast implants and the risk of connective-tissue diseases, N. Engl. J. Med. 342 (2000) 781–790.
217. H.K. Kornreich, K.N. Shaw, R. Koch, et al., Phenylketonuria and scleroderma, J. Pediatr. 73 (1968) 571–575.
224. R. Fleischmajer, J.L. Pollock, Progressive systemic sclerosis: Pseudoscleroderma, Clin. Rheum. Dis. 5 (1979) 243.
226. C.J. Epstein, G.M. Martin, A.L. Schultz, et al., Werner's syndrome a review of its symptomatology, natural history, pathologic features, genetics and relationship to the natural aging process Medicine (Baltimore.) 45 (1966) 177–221.
230. V. Falanga, Fibrosing conditions in childhood, Adv. Dermatol. 6 (1991) 145–158.
240. A. Grgic, A.L. Rosenbloom, F.T. Weber, et al., Joint contracture-common manifestation of childhood diabetes mellitus, J. Pediatr. 88 (1976) 584–588.
242. J.A. Doyle, S.J. Friedman, Porphyria and scleroderma: a clinical and laboratory review of 12 patients, Australas. J. Dermatol. 24 (1983) 109–114.

251. C.C. Bunn, C.P. Denton, X. Shi-Wen, et al., Anti-RNA polymerases and other autoantibody specificities in systemic sclerosis, Br. J. Rheumatol. 37 (1998) 15–20.

256. C.V. Oddis, Y. Okano, W.A. Rudert, et al., Serum autoantibody to the nucleolar antigen PM-Scl: clinical and immunogenetic associations, Arthritis Rheum. 35 (1992) 1211–1217.

259. J. Wozniak, R. Dabrowski, D. Luczak, et al., Evaluation of heart rhythm variability and arrhythmia in children with systemic and localized scleroderma, J. Rheumatol. 36 (2009) 191–196.

263. B.Z. Garty, B.H. Athreya, R. Wilmott, et al., Pulmonary functions in children with progressive systemic sclerosis, Pediatrics 88 (1991) 1161–1167.

265. K.M. Antoniou, A.U. Wells, Scleroderma lung disease: evolving understanding in light of newer studies, Curr. Opin. Rheumatol. 20 (2008) 686–691.

269. G. Valentini, S. D'Angelo, R.A. Della, et al., European Scleroderma Study Group to define disease activity criteria for systemic sclerosis. IV. Assessment of skin thickening by modified Rodnan skin score, Ann. Rheum. Dis. 62 (2003) 904–905.

270. I. Foeldvari, A. Wierk, Healthy children have a significantly increased skin score assessed with the modified Rodnan skin score, Rheumatology (Oxford) 45 (2006) 76–78.

278. D.M. Koh, D.M. Hansell, Computed tomography of diffuse interstitial lung disease in children, Clin. Radiol. 55 (2000) 659–667.

282. T.A. Medsger Jr., Assessment of damage and activity in systemic sclerosis, Curr. Opin. Rheumatol. 12 (2000) 545–548.

286. G. Valentini, R.A. Della, S. Bombardieri, et al., European multicentre study to define disease activity criteria for systemic sclerosis. II. Identification of disease activity variables and development of preliminary activity indexes, Ann. Rheum. Dis. 60 (2001) 592–598.

287. I. Foeldvari, N. Wulffraat, Recognition and management of scleroderma in children, Paediatr. Drugs 3 (2001) 575–583.

293. A.E. Thompson, B. Shea, V. Welch, et al., Calcium-channel blockers for Raynaud's phenomenon in systemic sclerosis, Arthritis Rheum. 44 (2001) 1841–1847.

294. J. Pope, D. Fenlon, A. Thompson, et al., Iloprost and cisaprost for Raynaud's phenomenon in progressive systemic sclerosis, The Cochrane Library 1 (2007) 1–16. (review).

295. F. Zulian, F. Corona, V. Gerloni, et al., Safety and efficacy of iloprost for the treatment of ischaemic digits in paediatric connective tissue diseases, Rheumatology (Oxf) 43 (2004) 229–233.

307. R. Fries, K. Shariat, H. von Wilmowsky, et al., Sildenafil in the treatment of Raynaud's phenomenon resistant to vasodilatory therapy, Circulation 112 (2005) 2980–2985.

308. F.M. Wigley, R.A. Wise, J.R. Seibold, et al., Intravenous iloprost infusion in patients with Raynaud phenomenon secondary to systemic sclerosis: a multicenter, placebo-controlled, double-blind study, Ann. Intern. Med. 120 (1994) 199–206.

310. J.H. Korn, M. Mayes, M. Matucci-Cerinic, et al., Digital ulcers in systemic sclerosis; prevention by treatment with bosentan, an oral endothelin receptor antagonist, Arthritis Rheum. 50 (2004) 3985–3993.

314. D.P. Tashkin, R. Elashoff, P.J. Clements, et al., Scleroderma Lung Study Research Group: cyclophosphamide versus placebo in scleroderma lung disease, N. Engl. J. Med. 354 (2006) 2655–2666.

315. R.K. Hoyles, R.W. Ellis, J. Wellsbury, et al., A multicenter, prospective, randomized, double-blind, placebo-controlled trial of corticosteroids and intravenous cyclophosphamide followed by oral azathioprine for the treatment of pulmonary fibrosis in scleroderma, Arthritis Rheum. 54 (2006) 3962–3970.

316. C. Liu, J. Chen, Endothelin receptor antagonists for pulmonary arterial hypertension, Cochrane. Database. Syst. Rev. 3 (2006) CD004434.

322. K.B. Highland, C. Strange, R. Girgis, et al., Comparison of sitaxentan and bosentan in pulmonary arterial hypertension associated with connective tissue diseases, Ann. Rheum. Dis. 65 (suppl. 2) (2006) 393.

328. J.E. Pope, N. Bellamy, J.R. Seibold, et al., A randomized, controlled trial of methotrexate versus placebo in early diffuse scleroderma, Arthritis Rheum. 44 (2001) 1351–1358.

343. S.I. Nihtyanova, G.M. Brough, C.M. Black, et al., Mychophenolate Mofetil in diffuse cutaneous systemic sclerosis- a retrospective analysis, Rheumatology 46 (2007) 442–445.

345. J.M. van Laar, D. Farge, A. Tyndall, Stem cell transplantation: a treatment option for severe systemic sclerosis? Ann. Rheum. Dis. 67 (suppl. 3) (2008) 35–38.

349. D. Del Junco, K. Sutter, et al., Clinical and genetic factors predictive of mortality in early systemic sclerosis, Arthritis Rheum. 61 (2009) 1403–1411.

352. L. Scussel-Lonzetti, F. Joyal, J.P. Raynauld, et al., Predicting mortality in systemic sclerosis: analysis of a cohort of 309 French Canadian patients with emphasis on features at diagnosis as predictive factors for survival, Medicine 81 (2002) 154–167.

360. M.J. Fritzler, T.D. Kinsella, The CREST syndrome: a distinct serologic entity with anticentromere antibodies, Am. J. Med. 69 (1980) 520–526.

Entire reference list is available online at www.expertconsult.com.

Chapter 26

LOCALIZED SCLERODERMAS

Francesco Zulian and Ronald M. Laxer

The unifying characteristic of all types of scleroderma is an excessive accumulation of collagen.[1,2] The localized sclerodermas (LS) are a group of disorders whose manifestations are mostly confined to the skin and subdermal tissues. LSs, with some exceptions, do not affect internal organs. They are rare conditions, even in childhood, in which *linear scleroderma* is the most common. There is no accepted uniform terminology; dermatologists typically use the term "morphea," and rheumatologists tend to use the term "localized scleroderma" to refer to the same group of conditions.

DEFINITION AND CLASSIFICATION

LS includes a number of conditions often grouped together. The classification used most widely currently divides LS into five general types: plaque morphea, generalized morphea, bullous morphea, linear scleroderma, and deep morphea.[3] Some conditions, such as atrophoderma of Pasini Pierini, eosinophilic fasciitis, or lichen sclerosus et atrophicus are sometimes included, but this aspect is still controversial. The classification does not include the mixed forms of LS, where different lesions occur in the same individual. The mixed form is more common than previously recognized, accounting for 15% of patients.[4] Recently the Pediatric Rheumatology European Society (PRES) proposed a new classification for LS.[5] It includes five subtypes: circumscribed morphea, linear scleroderma, generalized morphea, pansclerotic morphea, and the new mixed subtype where a combination of two or more of the previous subtypes is present[5] (Table 26-1).

Circumscribed morphea (CM) is characterized by oval or round circumscribed areas of induration with a central waxy, ivory colour surrounded by a violaceous halo (Figure 26-1). The superficial variety is usually confined to the dermis. Very rarely lesions are small, less than 1 cm in diameter (guttate). In the deep variety the entire skin feels thickened, taut, and bound down and the primary site of involvement is the panniculus or subcutaneous tissue. CM lesions occur most frequently on the trunk and less often on the extremities. The face is usually spared.

Guttate morphea is much less common; lesions are small, and oval areas are less than 1 cm in diameter.

Sometimes, as in morphea profunda, the entire skin feels thickened, taut, and bound down, or, as in subcutaneous morphea, the primary site of involvement is the panniculus or subcutaneous tissue. These two conditions, distinct in previous classifications, are now part of the CM deep subtype.

Generalized morphea (GM), is diagnosed when four or more individual plaques are larger than 3 cm, become confluent and involve at least two of seven anatomical sites (head-neck, right upper extremity, left upper extremity, right lower extremity, left lower extremity, anterior trunk, posterior trunk, a diagnosis of *generalized morphea (GM)* is made). Unilateral GM has been proposed as an extreme variant, usually beginning in childhood.[6]

Linear scleroderma is the most common subtype in children and adolescents.[4,7,8] It is characterized by one or more linear streaks that typically involve an upper or lower extremity. With time, the streaks become progressively more indurated and can extend through the dermis, subcutaneous tissue, and muscle to the underlying bone (Fig. 26-2). The lesions frequently follow Blaschko lines[9] and are unilateral in 85% to 95% of cases.[4,8]

The face or scalp may also be involved, as in the *en coup de sabre* variety *(ECDS)*. This term was applied historically because the lesion was reminiscent of the depression caused by a dueling stroke from a sword (Fig. 26-3). Progressive hemifacial atrophy may occur with or without ECDS. The *Parry Romberg syndrome (PRS)*, characterized by a progressive hemifacial atrophy of the skin and tissue below the forehead, with mild or absent involvement of the superficial skin, is considered the severe end of the spectrum of ECDS, and, for this reason, is included in the linear head subtype.[5,10] Evidence for this close relationship is the presence of associated disorders, including seizures and dental and ocular abnormalities, reported with similar prevalence in both conditions.[11-16]

In both circumscribed and linear morphea subtypes, deep variants where the entire skin feels thickened, taut, and bound down can be present.[17,18]

Disabling pansclerotic morphea of children, first described in 1980 by Diaz-Perez and colleagues,[19] is an extremely rare but severe disorder characterized by generalized full-thickness involvement of the skin of the trunk, extremities, face, and scalp with the sparing of the

Table 26–1

Classification of juvenile localized scleroderma

Main group	Subtype	Description
1. *Circumscribed morphea*	a. Superficial	Oval or round circumscribed areas of induration, limited to the epidermis and dermis, often with altered pigmentation and violaceous, erythematous halo (lilac ring). They can be single or multiple.
	b. Deep	Oval or round circumscribed deep induration of the skin, involving subcutaneous tissue, extending to fascia, and may involve underlying muscle. The lesions can be single or multiple. Sometimes the primary site of involvement is in the subcutaneous tissue without involvement of the skin.
2. *Linear scleroderma*	a. Trunk/limbs	Linear induration involving dermis, subcutaneous tissue, and sometimes muscle and underlying bone, and affecting the limbs and/or the trunk.
	b. Head	En coup de sabre (ECDS). Linear induration that affects the face and/or the scalp and sometimes involves muscle and underlying bone. Parry Romberg syndrome or progressive hemifacial atrophy. Loss of tissue on one side of the face that may involve the dermis, subcutaneous tissue, muscle, and bone. The skin is mobile.
3. *Generalized morphea*		Induration of the skin starting as individual plaques (four or more and larger than 3 cm) that become confluent and involve at least two out of seven anatomical sites (head-neck, right upper extremity, left upper extremity, right lower extremity, left lower extremity, anterior trunk, posterior trunk)
4. *Pansclerotic morphea*		Circumferential involvement of limb(s) affecting the skin, subcutaneous tissue, muscle, and bone. The lesion may also involve other areas of the body without internal organs involvement.
5. *Mixed morphea*		Combination of two or more of the previous subtypes. The order of the concomitant subtypes, specified in brackets, will follow their predominant representation in the individual patient (i.e., mixed [linear-circumscribed])

Data from Consensus Conference, Padua (Italy), 2004.
Associated conditions: eosinophilic fasciitis, bullous morphea, lichen sclerosus et atrophicus, and atrophoderma of Pasini and Pierini can be concomitant, or can precede or follow each of the localized scleroderma subtypes, but are not included in the classification.

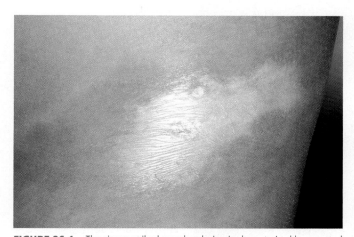

FIGURE 26-1 The circumscribed morphea lesion is characterized by a central area of induration with a waxy, ivory-colored area surrounded by inflammation and hyperpigmentation.

fingertips and toes. The involvement of the entire body without internal organ involvement helps differentiate this from systemic scleroderma (SSc). Recent reports have raised awareness on the possible evolution of chronic ulcers, frequently complicating pansclerotic morphea, to squamous cell carcinoma, a threatening complication already reported in SSc.[20-22]

The *mixed subtype* results from a combination of two or more of the previous subtypes. The order of the concomitant subtypes, specified in brackets, follows their predominant representation in the individual patient (i.e., mixed [linear-circumscribed]).[5]

Associated Conditions

Other disorders have been included in earlier classifications but are not included in the more recent classification of LS.[5] They can precede, follow, or be concomitant with LS.

Lichen sclerosus et atrophicus is characterized by shiny white plaques often preceded by violaceous discoloration with some predilection for anogenital area, wrists, and ankles. The superficial layers of the skin are usually involved.

Atrophoderma of Pasini and Pierini is characterized by asymptomatic hyperpigmented atrophic patches, usually located on the trunk with well-demarcated, so-called cliff-drop borders. These lesions lack the typical inflammatory changes of CM and represent the end-stage of the disease.

Bullous morphea can occur with most subtypes, including typical CM. The bullous lesions may possibly result from localized trauma or may be related to lymphatic obstruction from the sclerodermatous process.[23,24]

Eosinophilic fasciitis was described in 1974 by Shulman,[25,26] and in 1975 by Rodnan and colleagues,[27] who called the condition "diffuse fasciitis with eosinophilia" and observed that these patients typically had hypergammaglobulinemia and eosinophilia. The fascia is the predominant site of involvement. These lesions typically involve the extremities, but spare the hands and feet, and

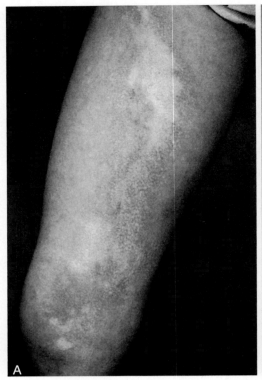
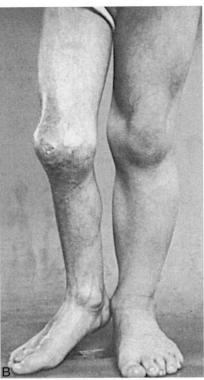

FIGURE 26-2   A, Typical lesion of linear scleroderma involving the lower extremity. The skin changes are characterized by a waxy induration with surrounding inflammation and hyperpigmentation distributed in a linear pattern. **B,** Linear scleroderma results in undergrowth of the leg, taut, shiny skin, and shortening of the extensor tendon to the second toe on the right foot.

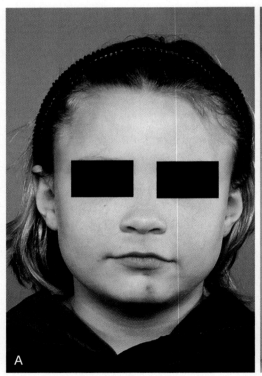
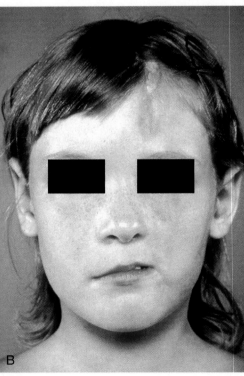

FIGURE 26-3   A, En coup de sabre linear scleroderma of approximately two years' duration affects the chin just to the left of midline, resulting in a depression and mild asymmetry of the jaw. **B,** En coup de sabre linear scleroderma involves the left face with hyperpigmentation, atrophy of subcutaneous tissues, and early hemifacial atrophy.

have an appearance that is described as "peau d'orange." Histological changes similar to eosinophilic fasciitis are found in most of the subtypes of LS, strengthening the conjecture that this disorder is a subtype of LS. In the pediatric literature, eosinophilic fasciitis is frequently described as involving the hands and feet, which is a departure from the syndrome in adults. Some of these pediatric cases may be more consistent with subcutaneous morphea or morphea profunda rather than eosinophilic fasciitis.

EPIDEMIOLOGY

LS is more frequent than SSc but is still a rare condition.[28-32] In the general population, where systemic disease is estimated to have an incidence of 0.45 to 1.9 cases per 100,000,[33,34] the incidence of the LSs is 2.7 cases per 100,000.[8] In a population-based study of LS,[8] CM accounted for 56%, GM for 13%, linear morphea for 20%, and deep morphea for 11%. Linear morphea and CM coexisted in 11% of the patients. Referral-based studies of LS include a higher proportion of linear scleroderma.[4,7] The female-to-male ratio of LS is 2.4:1, whereas in linear scleroderma, it is 2.1:1.[4] In children there are no differences in the mean age at onset for the various LS subtypes.[4]

Linear scleroderma is predominantly a pediatric disease. In a population-based study covering patients of all ages,[8] 67% of those with linear scleroderma are diagnosed before they reach 18 years old. The prevalence of morphea in children 17 years old or younger is estimated to be 50 per 100,000. The mean age at onset of LS in the pediatric population is approximately 7.3 years old.[4]

The disease can start as early as at birth.[30] It can be misdiagnosed as skin infection, nevus, or salmon patch, and this may lead to a consistent delay in diagnosis.

Uziel and colleagues[31] reported 30 patients with LS over a 7-year period and observed that this patient group numbered approximately the same as those with juvenile dermatomyositis and about 50% of those with systemic lupus erythematosus (SLE) seen during the same time. A study by Woo and colleagues[32] reported that 2% of the patients attending their pediatric rheumatology clinic had LS.

ETIOLOGY AND PATHOGENESIS

The cause and pathogenesis of the LS are unknown. The focus of much investigation is on abnormalities of regulation of fibroblasts, production of collagen, and immunological abnormalities. In morphea, the collagen fibers become thickened and hyalinized.[33] Multiple studies have demonstrated increased levels of cytokines and other molecules that influence fibroblasts and collagen synthesis.[34] Autoimmunity, environmental factors, infection, and trauma have all been associated with localized disease. It appears certain that autoimmunity is important to the cause, because of the multiplicity of abnormal serum antibodies[4] that occur in patients with LS, and because of the association of similar cutaneous abnormalities in patients with chronic graft-versus-host disease.[35,36]

The clinical and histopathological similarities of LS with chronic graft-versus-host disease have suggested that nonself cells or chimerism may be involved in the pathogenesis of the disease.[37] A great number of chimeric infiltrating cells, mainly epithelial or dendritic cells, have been found from biopsies of LS patients. The presence of immature chimeric cells in LS lesions suggests a possible role for chimerism in the pathogenesis of this disease, similar to other autoimmune diseases, such as juvenile dermatomyositis, neonatal lupus, and systemic sclerosis.

A number of drugs and environmental toxins have resulted in scleroderma-like reactions, including bleomycin, ergot, bromocriptine, pentazocine, carbidopa, and vitamin K1.[38] A toxin contained in some lots of L-tryptophan was incriminated in 1990 during a large epidemic of a syndrome similar to eosinophilic fasciitis and morphea, called the *eosinophilia-myalgia syndrome*.[39,40]

A number of investigations have examined a putative association of morphea and *Borrelia burgdorferi*, the spirochete that causes Lyme disease. Since this association was first reported in 1985,[41] many studies have documented evidence of infection with *B. burgdorferi* in patients with morphea who live in areas endemic for Lyme disease or who have a history of tick bites;[42,43] however, patients with morphea who do not live in endemic areas have no evidence of prior exposure to *B. burgdorferi*.[44-46] In the evaluation of patients with morphea, serological testing for Lyme disease is not likely to be positive unless the patient has been in an endemic area.

Trauma or physical exertion has been implicated in the initiation of lesions, particularly with the onset of eosinophilic fasciitis.[4,18] A review of childhood-onset scleroderma reported a history of trauma at the site of the lesion in 67 of 750 patients;[4] a similar history was not obtained in adults with morphea.[32] The investigators also observed that three patients had developed typical lesions at the site of their measles, mumps, and rubella vaccination. Morphea has also been reported after irradiation of malignant tumors in adults at the site of irradiation and at a distance from the site.[47,48]

CLINICAL MANIFESTATIONS

The onset of LS is subtle. The earliest manifestation is usually a localized area of erythema or waxy induration with a surrounding halo of erythema. A few patients have systemic symptoms such as arthralgias, synovitis, joint contractures, and carpal tunnel syndrome.[4,8] Commonly, patients present with lesions that show changes of chronicity, such as cutaneous atrophy and hyperpigmentation.

Most patients with GM have bilateral involvement, whereas unilateral lesions are most frequent in circumscribed and linear disease. Calcinosis has rarely been noted in areas involved with linear scleroderma.[49,50]

The en coup de sabre type may be associated with a set of manifestations unique to this group, including progressive hemifacial atrophy, ipsilateral uveitis, and various dental abnormalities, such as separation of the teeth and involvement of the eyebrows and eyelashes.[51,52] Hemiatrophy of the tongue and palatal growth changes are common for PRS. Central nervous system (CNS) disorders, including seizures and manifestations of CNS vasculitis, have been reported;[53-55] 13% to 47% of patients with craniofacial involvement may have neurological abnormalities.[16,55]

One-fifth of patients with LS present with extracutaneous manifestations and 4% may have multiple features.[56,57] Extracutaneous findings are more frequent in patients with linear scleroderma and consist essentially of arthritis (19%), neurological findings (4%), or other autoimmune conditions (3%). In these patients, organ impairment is milder and not life-threatening compared with systemic sclerosis. This may indicate that LS and SSc could represent two ends of a continuous spectrum of disease, or conversely that a third intermediate subtype, with mild extracutaneous features, stands in the middle between LS and SSc and possibly has a different pathogenesis.

Articular involvement is the most frequent extraarticular feature and is more common in patients with linear scleroderma. The joint involved may be completely unrelated to the site of the skin lesion. Children with LS who develop arthritis often have a positive rheumatoid factor (RF) test and sometimes an elevated erythrocyte sedimentation rate (ESR) and circulating autoantibodies.[56] These children tend to have an accelerated course with predominant musculoskeletal disease, including rapid development of contractures.

The most frequent neurological conditions are seizures and headaches, although behavioral changes and learning disabilities also have been described.[53,57,58] Abnormalities on magnetic resonance imaging (MRI), such as calcifications, white matter changes, vascular malformations, and changes consistent with CNS vasculitis have also been reported.[59,60] Many of the imaging abnormalities have no clinical relevance, and therefore imaging patients without clinical signs or symptoms is probably not warranted. Biopsy findings can include sclerosis, fibrosis, gliosis, and vasculitis.[61] Gastroesophageal reflux is the only gastrointestinal complication reported.[4,62,63] In a cohort of 14 consecutive patients, esophageal involvement was found in 8 (57%), 7 had pathological pH test findings, and in 4 of them, concomitant esophageal dysmotility was also present.[63]

Ocular involvement has been reported in 3.2% of patients affected by LS.[52] As expected, two-thirds of the patients with ocular manifestations have the ECDS subtype, but, interestingly, the other one-third have no facial skin lesion. The most frequent lesions (42%) are on eyelids and eyelashes; one-third of lesions consist of anterior segment inflammation, such as anterior uveitis or episcleritis, with the remaining being mainly CNS-related abnormalities. While extracutaneous manifestations should be considered in all patients, routine screening for internal organ manifestations (other than uveitis in facial morphea) is generally not recommended.

PATHOLOGY

The histological abnormalities of LS and SSc are considered by most investigators to be indistinguishable. Before fibrosis, there may be an intense inflammatory infiltrate with lymphocytes, plasma cells, macrophages, eosinophils, and mast cells. Subsequently, there is an increase in collagen and fibroblasts that leads to escalating sclerosis. In advanced stages, the entire dermis may be replaced by compact collagen fibers.

The depth of involvement is important in differentiating the various morphea subtypes (Fig. 26–4).[3] CM is more superficial, with principal involvement of the dermis and occasionally the panniculus, whereas linear morphea

involves the dermis, subcutaneous tissue, muscle, and underlying bone. Deep morphea syndromes tend to spare the superficial dermis and involve the deep dermis, subcutaneous tissue, fascia, or superficial muscle. PRS is an example of such deep involvement, which ends up in skin atrophy.

Eosinophilic fasciitis involves the deep subcutaneous tissues with sclerosis and inflammatory infiltrates while sparing the dermis.

Torres and colleagues[64] reviewed 51 skin biopsy specimens submitted to their laboratory from 1993 to 1995 from patients with a diagnosis of scleroderma, and they classified the cases into SSc or localized disease. They concluded that localized and SSc could be differentiated by the thickness of the dermis and amount of inflammatory infiltrate, both of which were greater in LS.

DIFFERENTIAL DIAGNOSIS

It is important to differentiate LS from systemic disease; this is often the main concern of parents when they come to the clinic. In the most common form, linear scleroderma, the lesions are discrete, limited to a single extremity, and easily differentiated from systemic disease. The more difficult diagnostic challenge is to differentiate SSc from the diffuse and deep forms of morphea with distal involvement. These patients, in contrast to those with SSc, rarely have Raynaud Phenomenon and do not develop symptomatic evidence of internal organ involvement. Occasionally, the deep forms of morphea may be confused with juvenile idiopathic arthritis in that they can present with contractures of the hands, arthralgias, and sometimes synovitis and may have a positive RF test result. In these cases, further testing frequently documents the presence of antinuclear antibodies, antihistone antibodies (AHA), hypergammaglobulinemia, and eosinophilia typical of the deep varieties of LS. Erosive joint disease does not occur.

Other conditions may mimic LS (Table 26–2).[3] Morphea has been reported to coexist with systemic sclerosis. Soma and colleagues[65] observed morphea in 9 (6.7%) of 133 patients who presented with systemic sclerosis. They considered morphea to be a part of the skin involvement of this disease.

LABORATORY EXAMINATION

The diagnosis of LS is established on clinical grounds, usually by the physical appearance of the lesions and sometimes aided by biopsy of skin or subcutaneous tissues. No laboratory abnormality is diagnostic. Results of routine laboratory tests, such as a complete blood cell count, blood chemistries, and urinalysis are normal. The ESR may be elevated with active inflammation, particularly in eosinophilic fasciitis. Eosinophilia and hypergammaglobulinemia are hallmarks of this disorder but also occur in the other deep subtypes. Eosinophilia and hypergammaglobulinemia tend to be markers of active disease, and levels normalize as the disease becomes less active.[4,5,66] RFs are present in

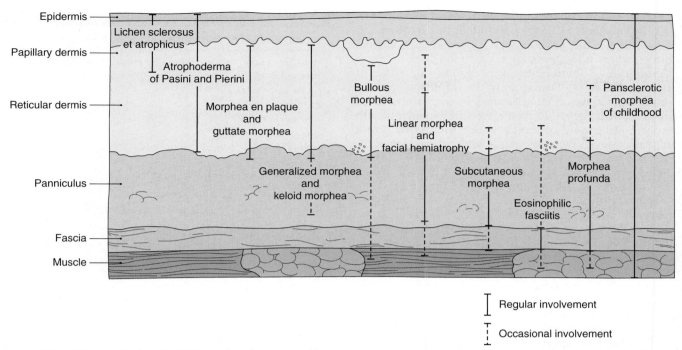

Epidermis

Papillary dermis

Lichen sclerosus et atrophicus

Atrophoderma of Pasini and Pierini

Reticular dermis

Morphea en plaque and guttate morphea

Bullous morphea

Pansclerotic morphea of childhood

Linear morphea and facial hemiatrophy

Panniculus

Generalized morphea and keloid morphea

Subcutaneous morphea

Morphea profunda

Eosinophilic fasciitis

Fascia

Muscle

Regular involvement

Occasional involvement

FIGURE 26-4 Schematic diagram of a full-thickness skin biopsy sample, demonstrating location of tissue involvement by the subtypes of localized scleroderma. (Courtesy of Dr. W. P. Daniel Su.)

Table 26–2

Conditions that mimic Morphea

Eosinophilia-myalgia syndrome
Graft-versus-host disease
Agents that induce sclerodermalike diseases
  Vinyl chloride
  Bleomycin
  Pentazocine
  L-Tryptophan
Scleredema adultorum
Scleromyxedema
Premature aging (Werner's syndrome)
Poikiloderma
Acrodermatitis chronica atrophicans
Diabetic cheiroarthropathy
Polyneuropathy, Organomegaly, Endocrinopathy, M protein, and Skin changes (POEMS syndrome)
Winchester syndrome
Pachydermoperiostosis
Phenylketonuria
Localized idiopathic fibrosis
Acromegaly
Progeria
Porphyria cutanea tarda
Amyloidosis
Carcinoid syndrome
Connective tissue hamartomas
Growers panatrophy
Connective tissue panniculitis
Focal lipoatrophy

25% to 40% of patients.[4,31] The presence or absence of RF seropositivity does not correlate significantly with any particular clinical finding, although higher titers are usually associated with more severe cutaneous and articular involvement.[4,66]

Autoantibodies are found in many patients with LS. Antinuclear antibodies can be present in any of the LS subtypes, with a frequency ranging from 23% to 73%.[4,31] In a large cohort of 750 pediatric patients, Zulian and colleagues found antinuclear antibodies in 42% of patients with LS[4] with no significant variations among the various subtypes or different disease course.[4]

AHA have been detected in 47% of patients with LS with a different prevalence in the various subtypes, e.g., higher in GM, lower in CM.[67] AHA are associated with more extensive localized disease,[68] and monitoring AHA titers may be helpful in assessing disease activity.[69]

In a study by Rosenberg and colleagues,[70] antibodies to denatured DNA were present in 56% of children; 41% had antibodies to high-mobility-group proteins, and 15% had AHA. Yamane and colleagues[71] identified anti-U1RNP antibodies in 3% of patients with LS.

Anti-topoisomerase I antibodies (anti-Scl 70), a marker of SSc in adults, were found to be present in 2% to 3% of children with LS but not in adults with LS.[4,67] Conversely, anticentromere antibodies were found in 12% of adults with LS but only in 1.7% of children.[4,72] Anti-DNA topoisomerase IIα (anti-topo IIα) were detected in 76% of patients with LS and in 85% of those with GM.[73] Immunoblotting showed no crossreactivity of anti-topo IIα with anti-topo I autoantibodies, which are almost exclusively detected in SSc. Anti-topo IIα, however, is not completely specific for LS, because it is also present in 14% of the patients with SSc, in 8% of those with SLE, and even in those with dermatomyositis (10%). Sato and colleagues reported that 46% of the patients with LS have anticardiolipin antibodies (aCL), and 24% exhibit lupus anticoagulant, whereas β2-glycoprotein I antibodies were absent.[74] In children, aCL were found in 14 out of 111 tested patients (12.6%).[4] Although this frequency is lower than in adult patients, it is higher than in normal subjects, where it ranges from 1.5% to 9.4%.[75]

Antifibrillin-1 antibodies were found in 28% of patients with LS.[76,77] Deficiency of the second component of complement has been described in patients with en coup de sabre lesions.[78] In their review of 76 patients with morphea, Dehen and colleagues[56] also found that serum complement levels were frequently lower than normal.

RF has been detected, at low titre, in 25–40% of LS patients and was correlated with the presence of arthritis.[4,21] In adults, immunoglobulin M RF is present in 30% of patients with LS, particularly in those with GM, and seems to be correlated with the disease severity.[79]

Elevations of serum aldolase levels in the presence of normal concentrations of creatine kinase have been observed in patients with eosinophilic fasciitis.[80,81] These levels of enzymatic activity may correlate with activity of the disease.[80] Serum concentrations of soluble interleukin-2 receptor have been increased in cases of LS and may differentiate active from inactive disease,[82,83] although this finding is not supported by all studies.[32] Table 26–3 lists the immunological abnormalities that have been reported in patients with LS.[84-109]

DISEASE MONITORING

During recent years, various methods for the clinical monitoring of LS have been developed; however, none of these methods has been validated in a large cohort of patients.

Semiquantitative scoring methods, such as the Localized Scleroderma Severity Index (or the Modified Skin Score, have been proposed.[110,111] According to these scores, the body surface is divided into several regions, and skin thickness, inflammation, and extension area are scored on a 0 to 3-point scale. These methods are quite subjective and do not evaluate the real size of the lesions. A computerized skin score method for the measurement of circumscribed lesions in LS has recently been proposed,[112] it consists in the demarcation of hyperemic and indurated borders of the scleroderma lesions on an adhesive transparent film, transfer over a cardboard, scanning, and recording in a computer. Calculation of the affected area, performed by computer software, takes into account the child growth, and in this way allows the longitudinal monitoring of the lesions.

Infrared thermography (IT) has been valuable in the detection of active LS lesions in children with high sensitivity (92%) but low specificity (68%).[113] The false positive results are related to old lesions with marked atrophy of skin, subcutaneous fat, and muscle, with increased heat conduction from deeper tissues.

More recently, laser Doppler flowmetry (LDF), a noninvasive method for the measurement of cutaneous microcirculation, was applied to the evaluation of scleroderma lesions.[114] Blood flow, measured by LDF, was significantly increased in clinically active lesions with high sensitivity and specificity. LDF and IT can be complementary tools in evaluating LS: IT may reveal active hidden

Table 26–3

Immunological abnormalities in localized scleroderma

Elevated Levels of Circulating Cytokines or Receptors, or Both
Interleukin 13[84]*
Tumor necrosis factor[84, 85]
Interleukin-1[85]
Interleukin-6[85, 86]
Interleukin-6 receptor[87]
Interleukin-2[86]
Interleukin-4[86]
Interleukin-2 receptor[83, 82]
Interleukin-8[88]

Elevated Levels of Soluble Cell Surface Molecules
CD4[89]
CD8[89]
CD 23[90]
CD 30[91]

Elevated Levels of Circulating Adhesion Molecules
ICAM-1[92]
VCAM-1[93]

Endothelial Activation
Serum E-selectin[93]

Autoantibodies
Antinuclear antibody[4, 70, 94–98]
Anticentromere[94, 99]
Antihistone[67, 70, 94, 100, 101]
Antihigh mobility group protein[70]
Antiheat shock protein[70, 102]
Anti-Fc gamma receptor[103]
Antimitochondrial 2-oxo-acid dehydrogenase complexes[104]
Anti-DNA topoisomerase II alpha[105]
Antiphospholipid[74]
Lupus anticoagulant[74]
Anti-U3SnRNP[106]
Anti-U1RNP[71]
Anti-Th/T0 RNP[107]
Antifibrillin[76]
Anti-single-stranded DNA[70, 95, 97, 108]
Rheumatoid factor[98, 109]

*Reference numbers are given in parenthesis.

lesions, while LDF can confirm the presence of active lesions or exclude activity in atrophic lesions, falsely positive with IT.

Skin imaging with high-frequency ultrasound has been found to be useful in monitoring therapy in a preliminary study.[115] Ultrasonography can detect several abnormalities, such as increased blood flow, increased echogenicity due to fibrosis, and loss of subcutaneous fat. The main limits of this tool are its operator dependency and the lack of standardization.[116]

MRI is clearly indicated when CNS or orbital involvement are suspected[117] and is able to demonstrate the true depth of soft tissue lesions in other sites, particularly in deep morphea and GM,[118] or it is able to show the clinical improvement in eosinophilic fasciitis.[119–121] The two main disadvantages are the need for sedation in younger patients and the presence of possible artifacts.

TREATMENT

There is very little good evidence on which to base treatment recommendations, as most studies have been uncontrolled, and standardized outcome measures have not been consistently applied.

CM is generally of cosmetic concern only, and treatments with potentially significant toxicity are not justified. In general, these lesions spontaneously remit with residual pigmentation and minimal cutaneous atrophy as the only abnormalities. Treatment should primarily focus on topical therapies, such as moisturizing agents, topical glucocorticoids, or calcipotriene.[122]

Good results have been recently reported with topical imiquimod, a novel immunomodulator, which upregulates interferon-α and -γ, and inhibits the collagen production by fibroblasts, likely by downregulating TGF-β.[123] This method appears particularly effective in the more indurated lesions. The use of vitamin D or its analogues (topically and systemically) has been reported in several case series with encouraging results;[124] however, in the only randomized controlled trial, oral treatment was no more effective than placebo.[125]

Phototherapy with ultraviolet (UV) represents another possible therapeutic choice for LS.[126-130] Treatments with UVA1 at low, medium, and high doses, with or without psoralens, appear to be effective clinically, although high doses seem to be most effective. UV phototherapy works in a variety of ways, and these include causing an increase in matrix metalloproteinase 1 (collagenase) activity, an increase expression of interferon-γ (INF-γ), and a decrease in TGF-β.[128] This approach seems to be much more effective for superficial lesions than for the subtypes with deeper involvement, such as linear or generalized scleroderma.[126-130] Since the rate of relapse after UV phototherapy discontinuation is not known, the need for prolonged maintenance therapy, which leads to a high cumulative dosage of irradiation, and the increased risk for potential long-term effects, such as skin aging and carcinogenesis, are clear limitations for its use in the pediatric age group.[131,132]

When there is a significant risk for disability, such as in linear and deep subtypes, systemic treatment with methotrexate (MTX) in combination with corticosteroids should be considered.[133-136] The treatment protocol usually consists in a combination of oral prednisone (0.5 to 1 mg/kg/day) or intravenous methylprednisolone (IVMP 20 to 30 mg/kg/day for three consecutive days, monthly) and MTX (oral or subcutaneous, 10 to 15 mg/m²/week). Most patients show a response within two to four months, and the side effects are usually mild and are associated more with corticosteroid use rather than with the MTX treatment. Unfortunately, the difficulty in measuring the lesion size and the lack of a control group represent evident limits for the interpretation of these studies. Patients who do not respond to this treatment approach may also be treated with mycophenolate mofetil.[137]

Bosentan, an orally active dual endothelin (ET_A/ET_B) receptor antagonist, acting as inhibitor of the endothelin overexpression, appears to be a promising treatment for disabling pansclerotic morphea, especially for refractory skin ulcers.[138] This very severe form of disease has also been treated with autologous stem cell transplantation with excellent results in several anecdotal cases. A double-blind, placebo-controlled study of intralesional IFN-γ concluded that this agent was ineffective.[139]

In eosinophilic fasciitis, corticosteroid treatment is indicated when there is evidence of active disease by laboratory measures, such as eosinophilia, hypergammaglobulinemia, or an elevated ESR.[25,133]

Patients with significant involvement from one of the forms of LS should have physical therapy directed at counteracting the development of flexion contractures. Surgical reconstruction may be considered, but usually after the active phase of the disease has abated, and the child's growth is complete.[140-143] In cases of depressed atrophic scars of the face, autologous fat transplantation should be considered, although this technique seems to be more effective for corrections of the forehead than for the nose, infraorbital area, and chin.[144]

COURSE OF THE DISEASE AND PROGNOSIS

In contradistinction to SSc, the prognosis for LS is usually benign. The course is that of an early inflammatory phase, with progression to multiple or extensive lesions, then stabilization, and finally improvement with softening of the skin and increased pigmentation about the lesions. In most instances, the mean duration of activity of disease is 3 to 5 years.[7,8]

In a population-based study of LS,[8] 50% of the patients had documented skin softening of 50% or more, or they had disease resolution by 3.8 years after the diagnosis. The 50% resolution point occurred at 2.7 years in the plaque groups, 5 years in the generalized and linear subtype groups, and 5.5 years in the deep groups. A small number of patients had active disease for more than 20 years. Prolonged disease activity was associated preponderantly with the linear type. During follow-up, 25% of patients with linear scleroderma and 44% of those with deep morphea had developed significant disability. In this series, none of the patients progressed to systemic scleroderma; such progression occurs rarely.[7,43,49,118]

Farrington and colleagues[81] reported the long-term outcome of 21 pediatric patients with biopsy-proven eosinophilic fasciitis. Two-thirds of these patients developed residual cutaneous fibrosis. Children younger than 7 years old had a twofold greater risk for progression to cutaneous fibrosis. All of the 14 patients who progressed to cutaneous fibrosis had involvement of three or four extremities; six had truncal involvement.[145]

A survey of patients seen between 1996 and 2006 concluded that JLS Juvenile LS patients have some impairment in skin disease-specific health-related quality of life (HRQOL) when compared with healthy controls, but the impairment was not as severe as that seen in patients with atopic dermatitis, and the overall HRQOL was as good as healthy controls.[146] Similar findings had been reported earlier, including reassuring findings that patients had normal self-esteem.[147] However, these studies, based on voluntary surveys, have included patients with benign subtypes of LS, such as CM, with limited numbers of patients with the potentially most disfiguring and disabling lesions, such as pansclerotic morphea or linear scleroderma of the face.

LS should be viewed as a usually benign and self-limited condition with minimal risk of progression to SSc.[148] The spectrum of LS and SSc may be likened to that of discoid lupus erythematosus and SLE. It is important to identify the subtypes at risk for disability and to intervene early with appropriate antiinflammatory medication and physical therapy to minimize the possibility of long-term disability.

REFERENCES

16. M.M. Toffelson, P.M. Witman, En coup de sabre morphea and Parry-Romberg syndrome: a retrospective review of 54 patients, J. Am. Acad. Dermatol. 56 (2007) 257–263.

17. W.P. Su, J.R. Person, Morphea profunda: a new concept and a histopathologic study of 23 cases, Am. J. Dermatopathol. 3 (1981) 251–260.

19. J.L. Diaz-Perez, S.M. Connolly, R.K. Winkelmann, Disabling pansclerotic morphea in children, Arch. Dermatol. 116 (1980) 169–173.

24. W.P. Su, S.L. Greene, Bullous morphea profunda, Am. J. Dermatopathol. 8 (1986) 144–147.

25. L.E. Shulman, Diffuse fasciitis with hypergammaglobulinemia and eosinophilia: a new syndrome? J. Rheumatol. 1 (Suppl. 1) (1974) 46.

30. F. Zulian, C. Vallongo, S.K.F. de Oliveira, et al., Congenital localized scleroderma, J. Pediatr. 149 (2006) 248–251.

31. Y. Uziel, B.R. Krafchik, E.D. Silverman, et al., Localized scleroderma in childhood: a report of 30 cases, 23 (1994) 328–340.

32. R. Vancheeswaran, C.M. Black, J. David, et al., Childhood-onset scleroderma: is it different from adult-onset disease? Arthritis Rheum. 39 (1996) 1041–1049.

34. B. Liu, M.K. Connolly, The pathogenesis of cutaneous fibrosis, Semin. Cutan. Med. Surg. 17 (1998) 3–11.

37. K.T. McNallan, C. Aponte, R. el-Azhary, et al., Immunophenotyping of chimeric cells in localized scleroderma, Rheumatology (Oxford) 46 (2007) 398–402.

38. U.F. Haustein, B. Haupt, Drug-induced scleroderma and sclerodermiform conditions, Clin. Dermatol. 16 (1998) 353–366.

39. R.W. Martin, J. Duffy, A.G. Engel, et al., The clinical spectrum of the eosinophilia-myalgia syndrome associated with L-tryptophan ingestion. Clinical features in 20 patients and aspects of pathophysiology, Ann. Intern. Med. 113 (1990) 124–134.

41. E. Aberer, R. Neumann, G. Stanek, Is localised scleroderma a Borrelia infection? Lancet 2 (1985) 278.

46. B. Weide, B. Schittek, T. Klyscz, et al., Morphoea is neither associated with features of Borrelia burgdorferi infection, nor is this agent detectable in lesional skin by polymerase chain reaction, Br. J. Dermatol. 143 (2000) 780–785.

47. M.H. Gollob, J.G. Dekoven, M.J. Bell, et al., Post-radiation morphea, J. Rheumatol. 25 (1998) 2267–2269.

52. M.E. Zannin, G. Martini, B.H. Athreya, et al., Ocular involvement in children with localized scleroderma: a multicenter study, Br. J. Ophthalmol. 91 (2007) 1311–1314.

53. I. Kister, M. Inglese, R.M. Laxer, et al., Neurologic manifestations of localized scleroderma: a case report and literature review, Neurology 71 (2008) 1538–1545.

57. F. Zulian, C. Vallongo, P. Woo, et al., Localized scleroderma in childhood is not just a skin disease, Arthritis Rheum. 52 (2005) 2873–2881.

58. M. Blaszczyk, L. Krolicki, M. Krasu, et al., Progressive facial hemiatrophy: central nervous system involvement and relationship with scleroderma en coup de sabre, J. Rheumatol. 30 (2003) 1997–2004.

60. D.E. Flores-Alvarado, J.A. Esquivel-Valerio, M. Garza-Elizondo, et al., Linear scleroderma en coup de sabre and brain calcification: is there a pathogenic relationship?, J. Rheumatol. 30 (2003) 193–195.

63. G. Guariso, S. Conte, F. Galeazzi, et al., Esophageal involvement in juvenile localized scleroderma: a pilot study, Clin. Exp. Rheumatol. 25 (2007) 786–789.

64. J.E. Torres, J.L. Sanchez, Histopathologic differentiation between localized and systemic scleroderma, Am. J. Dermatopathol. 20 (1998) 242–245.

65. Y. Soma, T. Tamaki, K. Kikuchi, et al., Coexistence of morphea and systemic sclerosis, Dermatology 186 (1993) 103–105.

68. K. Takehara, S. Sato, Localized scleroderma is an autoimmune disease, Rheumatology (Oxford) 44 (2005) 274–279.

70. A.M. Rosenberg, Y. Uziel, B.R. Krafchik, et al., Antinuclear antibodies in children with localized scleroderma, J. Rheumatol. 22 (1995) 2337–2343.

72. A. Ruffatti, A. Peserico, S. Glorioso, et al., Anticentromere antibody in localized scleroderma, J. Am. Acad. Dermatol. 15 (1986) 637–642.

73. I. Hayakawa, M. Hasegawa, K. Takehara, et al., Anti-DNA topoisomerase IIα autoantibodies in Localised Scleroderma, Arthritis Rheum. 50 (2004) 227–232.

74. S. Sato, M. Fujimoto, M. Hasegawa, et al., Antiphospholipid antibody in localised scleroderma, Ann. Rheum. Dis. 62 (2003) 771–774.

77. T. Arkachaisri, N. Fertig, S. Pino, et al., Serum autoantibodies and their clinical associations in patients with childhood- and adult-onset linear scleroderma. A single-center study, J. Rheumatol. 35 (2008) 2439–2444.

81. M.L. Farrington, J.E. Haas, V. Nazar-Stewart, et al., Eosinophilic fasciitis in children frequently progresses to scleroderma-like cutaneous fibrosis, J. Rheumatol. 20 (1993) 128–132.

82. Y. Uziel, B.R. Krafchik, B. Feldman, et al., Serum levels of soluble interleukin-2 receptor. A marker of disease activity in localized scleroderma, Arthritis Rheum. 37 (1994) 898–901.

101. S. Sato, H. Ihn, Y. Soma, et al., Antihistone antibodies in patients with localized scleroderma, Arthritis Rheum. 36 (1993) 1137–1141.

105. I. Hayakawa, M. Hasegawa, K. Takehara, et al., Anti-DNA topoisomerase II alpha autoantibodies in localized scleroderma, Arthritis Rheum. 50 (2004) 227–232.

112. F. Zulian, D. Meneghesso, E. Grisan, et al., A new computerized method for the assessment of skin lesions in localized scleroderma, Rheumatology (Oxford) 46 (2007) 856–860.

113. G. Martini, K.J. Murray, K.J. Howell, et al., Juvenile-onset localized scleroderma activity detection by infrared thermography, Rheumatology (Oxford) 41 (2002) 1178–1182.

114. L. Weibel, K.J. Howell, M.T. Visentin, et al., Laser Doppler flowmetry for assessing localized scleroderma in children, Arthritis Rheum. 56 (2007) 3489–3495.

116. S.C. Li, M.S. Liebling, K.A. Haines, Ultrasonography is a sensitive tool for monitoring localized scleroderma, Rheumatology (Oxford) 46 (2007) 1316–1319.

118. M. Horger, G. Fierlbeck, J. Kuemmerle-Deschner, et al., MRI findings in deep and generalized morphea, Am. J. Roentgenol. 190 (2008) 32–39.

122. B.B. Cunningham, I.D. Landells, C. Langman, et al., Topical calcipotriene for morphea/linear scleroderma, J. Am. Acad. Dermatol. 39 (1998) 211–215.

123. M. Dytoc, P.T. Ting, J. Man, et al., First case series on the use of imiquimod for morphea, Br. J. Dermatol. 153 (2005) 815–820.

126. M. Kerscher, M. Volkenandt, C. Gruss, et al., Low dose UVA phototherapy for treatment of localized scleroderma, J. Am. Acad. Dermatol. 38 (1998) 21–23.

130. A. Kreuter, J. Hyun, M. Stucker, et al., A randomized controlled study of low-dose UVA1, medium-dose UVA1, and narrowband UVB phototherapy in the treatment of localized scleroderma, J. Am. Acad. Dermatol. 54 (2006) 440–447.

133. Y. Uziel, B.M. Feldman, B.R. Krafchik, et al., Methotrexate and corticosteroid therapy for pediatric localized scleroderma, J. Pediatr. 136 (2000) 91–95.

134. A. Kreuter, T. Gambichler, F. Breuckmann, et al., Pulsed high-dose corticosteroids combined with low-dose methotrexate in severe localized scleroderma, Arch. Dermatol. 141 (2005) 847–852.

136. L. Weibel, M.C. Sampaio, M.T. Visentin, et al., Evaluation of methotrexate and corticosteroids for the treatment of localized scleroderma (morphea) in children, Br. J. Dermatol. 155 (2006) 1013–1020.

137. G. Martini, A.V. Ramanan, F. Falcini, et al., Successful treatment of severe or methotrexate-resistant juvenile localized scleroderma with mycophenolate mofetil, Rheumatology (Oxford) 48 (2009) 1410–1413.

138. R. Roldan, G. Morote, C. Castro Mdel, et al., Efficacy of bosentan in treatment of unresponsive cutaneous ulceration in disabling pansclerotic morphea in children, J. Rheumatol. 33 (2006) 2538–2540.

140. M. Sengezer, M. Deveci, N. Selmanpakoglu, Repair of "coup de sabre," a linear form of scleroderma, Ann. Plast. Surg. 37 (1996) 428–432.

144. M.R. Roh, J.Y. Jung, K.Y. Chung, et al., Linear scleroderma-induced facial atrophic scars, Dermatol. Surg. 34 (2008) 1659–1665.

145. J.J. Miller 3rd, The fasciitis-morphea complex in children, Am. J. Dis. Child. 146 (1992) 733–736.

146. N.M. Orzechowski, D.M. Davis, T.G. Mason 3rd, et al., Health-related quality of life in children and adolescents with juvenile localized scleroderma, Rheumatology (Oxford) 48 (2009) 670–672.

147. Y. Uziel, R.M. Laxer, B.R. Krafchik, et al., Children with morphea have normal self-perception, J. Pediatr. 137 (2000) 727–730.

Entire reference list is available online at www.expertconsult.com.

Chapter 27

MIXED CONNECTIVE TISSUE DISEASE AND UNDIFFERENTIATED CONNECTIVE TISSUE DISEASE

Peri H. Pepmueller, Carol B. Lindsley, and James T. Cassidy

Connective tissue diseases (CTD) are inflammatory conditions with characteristic signs and symptoms defining specific disorders. Classification criteria developed by the American College of Rheumatology have provided guidelines for diagnosis in adult patients and have been used to some extent in children. The criteria were developed initially to ensure diagnoses for clinical investigations. Some children, however, present simultaneously with signs and symptoms characteristic of two or more of the major rheumatic disorders, such as juvenile rheumatoid arthritis (JRA), systemic lupus erythematosus (SLE), juvenile dermatomyositis (JDM), cutaneous systemic scleroderma (CSS), and vasculopathy. Children with these disorders are often difficult to categorize under existing classification criteria and are properly referred to as having overlap syndromes. The most studied of these conditions is *mixed connective tissue disease (MCTD)*, which will be further discussed in this chapter.

MIXED CONNECTIVE TISSUE DISEASE

Definition and Classification

MCTD was initially described by Sharp and colleagues in 1972[1] in 25 adults as a disorder with an excellent initial response to relatively low-dose glucocorticoid therapy and a favorable prognosis. The syndrome included clinical features of rheumatoid arthritis (RA), scleroderma, SLE, and dermatomyositis in conjunction with a high antibody titer to an extractable nuclear antigen (ENA). However, reassessment of the original patients indicated that the inflammatory manifestations (e.g., arthritis, serositis, fever, myositis) tended to become less evident over time, whereas sclerodactyly and esophageal disease, less responsive to treatment with glucocorticoids, persisted and began to dominate the clinical picture.[2] Severe renal disease continued to remain an unusual feature. Although the concept of MCTD as a clinical entity separate from the other CTDs has remained controversial, classifications employing more precise serological criteria and human leukocyte antigen (HLA) typing have confirmed the uniqueness of this disorder (Table 27–1).[3-6]

Criteria for MCTD have been evaluated for adults but not for children (Table 27–2).[7-10] These criteria are summarized in the review by Smolen and colleagues.[11] Shen and coworkers[12] studied 50 patients from China during a 2- to 8-year period and indicated that the criteria of Sharp[7] were the most reliable for the diagnosis of MCTD. Among 23 patients fulfilling these criteria, only one (4.3%) developed scleroderma. Among 23 patients satisfying the criteria of Kasukawa and colleagues,[8] seven (30.4%) developed another CTD. Of the 27 who met the criteria of Alarcon-Segovia and colleagues,[9] 12 (44%) fulfilled classification criteria for another major rheumatic disease. The frequencies of HLA-DR4 and -DR5 were significantly higher among the patients whose disease fulfilled Sharp's criteria.[7] Different conclusions were reached, however, in a comparative study of four diagnostic criteria from France by Amigues and coworkers.[13] These investigators analyzed the criteria of Sharp,[7] Kasukawa and colleagues,[8] Alarcon-Segovia and coworkers,[9] and Kahn and associates[10] in 45 patients with anti-uridine rich (U1) ribonucleoprotein (RNP) antibodies who were classified as having MCTD. They found that the criteria of Alarcon-Segovia and coworkers[9] had the highest sensitivity (62.5%) and specificity (86.2%), with an overlap of 16% with other major CTDs. These results were comparable with those obtained with the criteria of Kahn and associates.[10]

Epidemiology

MCTD is one of the least common disorders in a pediatric rheumatology clinic. It had a frequency of 0.1% in a Finnish nationwide prospective study[14] and 0.3% in

Table 27–1

Clinical characteristics of mixed connective tissue disease

Clinical Signs of at Least Two of the Following Diseases
Juvenile rheumatoid arthritis
Systemic lupus erythematosus
Juvenile dermatomyositis
Systemic scleroderma

Positive Serological Findings
High-titer of antibodies to U1snRNP and the 70-kD A and C polypeptides
Anti-U1RNA antibodies

Presence of HLA-DR4 or DR2

HLA, human leukocyte antigen; U1RNA, U1 ribonucleic acid; U1snRNP, uridine-rich small nuclear ribonucleoprotein.

the U.S. Pediatric Rheumatology Database.[15] Data from the British Pediatric Rheumatology Association Disease Registry[16] and the Canadian Pediatric Rheumatology Association Disease Registry[17] showed frequencies of 0.5% and 0.2% respectively. The median age at onset was approximately 11 years (range, 4- to 16-years). MCTD occurred three times more frequently in girls than in boys.[15] There was one report of this disorder occurring in siblings.[18]

Immunogenetic Background

In studies from several continents including North and South America, Japan, and Europe, the predominant HLA class II specificity associated with MCTD has been DR4; association with HLA-DR2 is less well established.[5,11,19-25] Patients with DR4 or DR2 have a region of homology of seven amino acids (numbers 26, 28, 30, 31, 32, 70, and 73) in the highly polymorphic antigen-binding segment of the DRB1 gene *(HLA-DRB1)*.[25,26] These HLA specificities are also linked to antibodies to the uridine-rich small nuclear ribonucleoprotein (U1sn-RNP) that are characteristic of the disorder. It is notable that MHC haplotypes most commonly associated with CSS (DR5) or SLE (DR3) are uncommon.

Etiology and Pathogenesis

MCTD is characterized immunologically by the presence of autoantibodies and T cells reactive with U1-RNP and polypeptides of the spliceosomes complex, including their associated uridine-rich (U) small nuclear ribonucleic acids (RNAs). A number of immunological factors have been associated with MCTD and may contribute to disease pathogenesis.[27,28] The 70-kD peptide of the U1-RNP antigen appears to be a dominant autoantigen in MCTD and consists of a 437 residue polypeptide, which noncovalently associates with U1-RNA through an RNA binding domain on the polypeptide spanning residues 92-202.[29] There are a variety of potential and proven structural modifications, which occur to the U1 70-kD polypeptide and RNP, especially those occurring during apoptosis and oxidative cleavage, any of which might influence antigenicity

of the RNP complex.[30,31] The apoptotically modified 70-kD has been shown to be antigenically distinct from intact 70-kD, which may have clinical implications in breaking immune tolerance to the autoantigen.[32-34] One study reported that autoantibodies reactive with apoptotic 70-kD are superior markers to those against intact 70-kD for MCTD.[33]

Various independent observations over the years have led to the conclusion that the innate and adaptive immune systems play a central role in the development of many systemic autoimmune diseases, including MCTD.[35-37] In MCTD, B and T cell epitope mapping studies led to observations that the dominant epitopes recognized on the 70-kD polypeptide resided within the RNA binding domains of the peptide. These observations coincided with the discovery of a series of pathogen-associated pattern recognition receptors, including the Toll-like receptors (TLR), especially those that recognize double-stranded RNA or single-stranded RNA and normally play a vital role in host defense through their recognition of bacterial and viral cell products. These findings led to a series of studies examining TLR in autoimmunity. Studies have shown that U1-RNA can activate cells of a TLR3 using U1-RNA and TLR-deficient mutant endometrial cell lines.[38]

Autoantibodies are widely recognized as a hallmark of many of the rheumatic diseases, including MCTD.[39] Two studies have supported a role for anti-RNP antibodies in the pathogenesis of MCTD by providing linkage between the emergence of antibodies and clinical disease.[40,41] B cells can function in several other key immunological pathways beyond antibody production including functioning as antigen presenting cells, secreting pathological cytokines, and mediating tissue injury through a variety of antibody directed mechanisms.[27]

T cells appear to have a central role in the pathogenesis of MCTD. RNP-reactive CD4+ T cells have been identified from peripheral blood of MCTD patients. Both anti-RNP and anti-U-RNA antibodies found in patients' sera have, in most instances, undergone isotope switching to Immunoglobulin G (IgG) subtypes. Also, there is dense lymphocyte infiltration with many T cells found in the sites of tissue injury at autopsy and in biopsy specimens from patients. Findings have also shown that human RNP reactive T cells can provide B cell help in vitro to anti-RNP autoantibody production.[27,39] A murine model for MCTD has been developed, and it will assist in advancing preclinical and translational research in MCTD.[42]

Clinical Manifestations

MCTD has been recognized with increasing frequency in childhood.[23,43-59] These children present with features of more than one CTD, a speckled antinuclear antibody (ANA) pattern, and high titers of antibody to ribonucleoprotein (RNP) (see Table 27–1). The condition characteristically evolves over time from a more limited presentation of clinical disease to one with overlapping features of JRA, SLE, CSS, or JDM. Manifestations develop sequentially, but not in any predictable order or over any circumscribed period. The rashes of

Table 27–2

Classification criteria for mixed connective tissue disease (MCTD)

Sharp	Alarcón-Segovia	Kasukawa	Kahn
Criteria			
Major	1. **Serological**	1. **Common Symptoms**	1. **Serological**
a Severe myositis	a Anti-RNP at hemaggluti-	a Raynaud Phenomenon	a High-titer anti-RNP cor-
b Lung involvement:	nation titer >1:1,600	b Swollen fingers	responding to speckled
DLCO<70% and/or pulmo-	2. **Clinical Criteria**	2. **Anti-RNP Ab**	ANA at titer >1:2,000
nary hypertension and/	b Swollen hands	3. **Symptoms**	2. **Clinical**
or proliferative vascular	c Synovitis		a Raynaud Phenomenon
lesions on biopsy	d Biologically or histologi-	*SLE*	b Synovitis
c Raynaud Phenomenon or	cally proven myositis	a Polyarthritis	c Myositis
esophageal hypomotility	e Raynaud Phenomenon	b Adenopathies	d Swollen fingers
d Swollen hands or	f Acrosclerosis with or	c Malar rash	
sclerodactyly	without proximal sys-	d Pericarditis or pleuritis	
e Anti-ENA ≥1:10,000 with	temic sclerosis	e Leukopenia or	
anti-RNP+ and anti-S–		thrombocytopenia	
Minor		*SSc*	
a Alopecia		a Sclerodactyly	
b Leukopenia <4000		b Pulmonary fibrosis or	
c Anemia		restrictive changes in lung	
d Pleuritis		function or reduced DLCO	
e Pericarditis		c Hypomotility or esophageal	
f Arthritis		dilation	
g Trigeminal neuralgia			
h Malar rash		*PM*	
i Thrombocytopenia		a Muscle weakness	
j Mild myositis		b Elevated muscle enzymes	
k History of swollen hands		c Myogenic signs on EMG	
Diagnosis			
MCTD Certain	*MCTD*	*MCTD*	*MCTD*
4 major criteria, no anti-Sm,	If serological criterion above	If presence of at least 1 of	If serological criteria fulfilled,
anti-U1-RNP >1:4000	is met, and at least 3 clinical	the 2 common symptoms,	and Raynaud Phenomenon,
	criteria are identified (if a, d,	anti-RNP antibodies, *and* the	*and* at least 2 of the 3 fol-
	and e are present, b or c are	presence of at least 1 sign of	lowing signs are present:
	also required)	at least 2 of the following	synovitis, myositis, and
		connective tissue diseases:	swollen fingers.
		SLE, SSc, and PM.	
MCTD Probable			
3 major criteria and no anti-			
Sm, or 2 major criteria and			
1 minor criterion, anti-U1-			
RNP >1:1000			

Adapted from reference 13.
DLCO, Diffusing capacity for carbon monoxide; EMG, electromyography; PM, polymyositis; SSc, systemic sclerosis; Sm, Smith antigen.

SLE or JDM are common at onset. Sclerodermatous skin changes are slow to develop but may become the most prominent feature of the disease late in its course. Moderately asymptomatic involvement, such as myositis with minimal weakness, mild atrophy, and minimal to moderate increases in the serum muscle enzyme concentrations, is common. Dysphagia and bowel dysmotility also may occur. Manifestations of the sicca syndrome with xerostomia, keratoconjunctivitis sicca, or parotid gland enlargement occur in one third of the children.[109] Although children do not usually complain of shortness of breath (depending on cognitive development or unconsciously self-imposed restriction of activity), they often have pulmonary functional impairments.

Clinical characteristics of children from selected studies are summarized in Table 27–3. Polyarthritis (93%) and Raynaud Phenomenon (85%) are the most common manifestations at onset (Fig. 27–1). The arthritis may be relatively painful; erosive disease is uncommon, but deformity may develop with flexion contractions or swan-neck deformities. The arthritis is often associated with rheumatoid factor (RF) seropositivity that is often present early in approximately two thirds of the children. Cutaneous changes include scleroderma-like disease in one half, the rash of SLE in one third, and the rash of of JDM in one third of MCTD patients. Nailfold capillary abnormalities are similar to those in CSS.[61-63] Cardiopulmonary disease and esophageal

Table 27–3

Disease characteristics of children with mixed connective tissue disease

Characteristic	No. Reported*	No. Present†	Percent
Arthritis	72	67	93
Raynaud Phenomenon	72	61	85
Sclerodermatous skin	67	33	49
Rash of systemic lupus erythematosus	67	22	33
Rash of dermatomyositis	67	22	33
Fever	61	34	56
Abnormal esophageal motility	56	23	41
Cardiac disease	67	20	30
Pericarditis	67	18	27
Muscle disease	72	44	61
Sicca syndrome	66	24	36
Central nervous system disease	61	14	23
Lung			
Abnormal diffusion	56	24	43
Restrictive disease	56	8	14
Hypertension	56	4	7
Effusion	56	13	23
Radiographic changes only	56	1	2
Splenomegaly	63	18	29
Hepatomegaly	68	19	28
Renal disease	72	19	26
Anti-dsDNA positive	64	13	20
Anti-Sm positive	58	6	10
Anti-RNP positive	72	72	100
Rheumatoid factor positive	57	39	68

Data from 10 reports with a total of 72 children: references 1, 43, 44, 45, 46, 47, 50, 51, 60, 68

dsDNA, double-stranded DNA; RNP, ribonucleoprotein; Sm, Smith antigen 60, 68.

*The number of children in whom the characteristic was identified.
†The number in whom the abnormality was present.

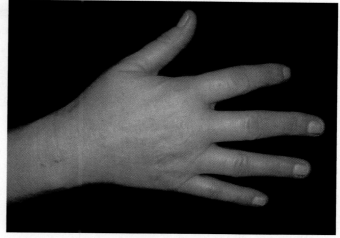

FIGURE 27–1   The hand of a patient with MCTD demonstrating swelling and mild skin rash. The second digit is shortened due to a history of digital ischemia with autoamputation.

dysmotility occur more frequently than clinical symptoms indicate.[64] Vasculitis can occur and be severe (i.e., transverse myelopathy). Although nephritis occurs in about one fourth of the patients with MCTD, it is less common and is usually less severe than in those with SLE. However, children with MCTD may have more frequent and more severe renal disease, more hematological complications, such as thrombocytopenia, and less pulmonary hypertension than adults with MCTD have.[56,58,65]

Pulmonary disease is a major source of morbidity and mortality among adults who have MCTD. In a prospective longitudinal study, 31 of 34 adults with high titers of RNP antibody had typical MCTD in which pulmonary disease, often initially asymptomatic, was common.[66] Pulmonary hypertension was the most frequent serious complication. Pulmonary disease is common among pediatric patients, although it is more varied in type. Restrictive pulmonary disease has been seen in up to 35% of patients in some studies,[58] and abnormal carbon monoxide diffusion in up to 42%.[58] These prevalences reflect retrospective data and may represent a select patient population. Pulmonary fibrosis, pleural effusions, and pulmonary hypertension are also seen.

Pathology

Widespread intimal proliferation and medial hypertrophy of vascular walls have been described in four children with MCTD who died.[67] Renal biopsies in eight additional patients confirmed abnormalities of the glomerular basement membrane or vascular sclerosis. These investigators commented that, although the histopathology of MCTD resembled that of CSS, the extent of fibrosis was less, and intimal vascular abnormalities in larger vessels such as the aorta and the coronary, pulmonary, and renal arteries, were more prominent. Another study reported pulmonary hypertension and proliferative vasculopathy in the virtual absence of interstitial fibrosis in patients with MCTD, in contrast to those with CSS.[66]

Laboratory Examination

Very high titers of ANAs are usually present initially, often in a speckled pattern on HEp-2 cell substrate. These antibodies react specifically with an RNAse-sensitive component of ENA and RNP. Anti-RNP antibodies in high titers have been the serological hallmark of MCTD, but these antibodies may be present in low titers in other diseases, such as SLE.[11,39,44,60] Further investigations confirmed that the most characteristic specificities of the anti-RNP antibodies in MCTD were directed against a uridine-rich (U1), small nuclear RNP (snRNP) complex (U1snRNP) of the splicesome consisting of U1RNA and the associated 70-kD A and C polypeptides (Fig. 27–2).[27,39,68-72] The anti-U1snRNP profile of patients

Table 27–4

Clinical findings of childhood MCTD at presentation, cumulative over time, and at most recent evaluation.

	Hoffman et al[19]		Mier et al[58]			Tiddens et al[80]	
	Presentation (%)	Cumulative (%)	Presentation (%)	Cumulative (%)	Most Recent Evaluation (%)	Present During Disease Course (%)	Most Recent Evaluation (%)
Raynaud Phenomenon	9 (82)	9 (82)	81	94	88	13 (93)	12 (86)
Polyarthropathy	11 (100)	11 (100)	91	94	48	10 (71)	7 (50)
Swollen hands	6 (55)	9 (82)	65	68	19	11 (79)	6 (43)
Sclerodactyly	4 (36)	7 (64)	12	26	24	12 (86)	12 (86)
Proximal muscle weakness	4 (36)	6 (55)	34	–	9	7 (70)	7 (50)
Pleuritis/pericarditis	4 (36)*	5 (45)*	–	12/16		3 (21)	0 (0)
Esophageal dysmotility	3 (27)+	6 (55)+	25	21†	33	–	10/10 (100)+
Pulmonary dysfunction	3 (27)x	9 (82)x	22/21§	35/42±	64/58»	9 (64)⁻	7/2 (53/15)=
Leukopenia/ lymphopenia	1 (9)	4 (36)	–	36	–	7 (50)	9 (64)
Thrombocytopenia	1 (9)	2 (18)	–	18	–	3 (21)	1 (7)

*Pleural effusion
+Determined by barium esophagography, manometry, or both
xDecreased carbon monoxide (CO) diffusion
†Documented objectively
§Restrictive lung disease, 22; Decreased CO diffusion, 21
±Restrictive lung disease, 35; Decreased CO diffusion, 42
»Restrictive lung disease, 64; Decreased CO diffusion, 58
⁻Restrictive lung disease
=Restrictive lung disease, 7/13; Decreased CO diffusion, 2/13

Table 27–5

Clinical findings of 47 adult MCTD patients (23% with childhood onset) at presentation, cumulative over time, and at most recent evaluation

	Burdt and colleagues [93]		
	At Diagnosis (%)	Cumulative (%)	Most Recent Evaluation (%)
Raynaud Phenomenon	89	96	60
Polyarthropathy	85	96	38
Swollen hands	60	66	17
Sclerodactyly	34	49	43
Myositis	28	51	6
Pleuritis/ pericarditis	34	43	6
Esophageal dysmotility	47	66	34
Pulmonary dysfunction	43	66	47
Leukopenia/ lymphopenia	30	53	13
Pulmonary Hypertension	9	23	21
Skin rash	30	53	11

with MCTD is characterized by a high-titer antibody response, predominantly or solely of IgG antibodies, and specificity for an epitope different from that of SLE sera;[11] a false-positive anti-U1snRNP antibody response may be observed in cases of SLE.[73] Later reports indicate that antibodies to U1RNA are even more closely associated clinically with disease activity during the course of MCTD than are U1RNP antibodies,[74-76] although assays for U1-RNA themselves are poorly standardized and of limited availability to clinicians in most areas; this makes this observation primarily one of research relevance.

Substantial advances have been made in employing specific autoantibody activities against the U1snRNP polypeptides for classification of disease.[11,77] In contrast to patients with CTDs who did not demonstrate these antibody activities, there were significant clinical associations with Raynaud Phenomenon, swollen hands, sclerodactyly, telangiectasia, and abnormal esophageal motility among adult patients with high titers of autoantibodies against the U1-70kD antigen.[24] In the study by DeRooij and colleagues,[23] all five children who had antibodies against the U1-70kD antigen had clinical disease characterized by arthralgia or arthritis, swollen hands, Raynaud Phenomenon, and abnormalities of pulmonary function.

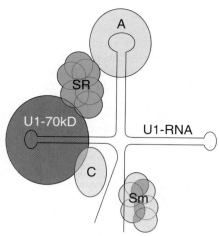

FIGURE 27–2 The U1-RNP. The U1-RNP is composed of an RNA backbone, U1-RNA, three proteins highly specific for the U1-RNP (the U1-A, U1-C, and U1-70kD proteins), and a series of additional proteins common to multiple U-RNP and RNA splicing macromolecules (Sm and SR). From Greidinger EL, Hoffman RW: Autoantibodies in the pathogenesis of mixed connective tissue disease, *Rheum Dis Clin N Am* 31:437-450, 2005.

Children with antibodies against the 70-kD polypeptide uncommonly develop diffuse glomerulonephritis, cardiac disease, widespread cutaneous sclerosis or central nervous system (CNS) disease. Clinical renal disease occurred, however, in three of 11 patients reported by Hoffman and colleagues[19] and was confined to a subset of children who had IgG autoantibodies against the D polypeptide of U1snRNP. All of these children were HLA-DR2 positive and were the same patients who developed an adverse or fatal outcome associated with anti-dsDNA antibodies. Children with anti-Sm antibodies may develop reactivity to the D polypeptide and clinically important renal disease. Their course may be accompanied by hypocomplementemia and other features of nephritis more characteristic of SLE. Their sera may not be positive for anti-Sm antibodies by the relatively insensitive techniques of double immunodiffusion or counterimmunoelectrophoresis.

Some MCTD sera, including those from patients without renal disease, also react with B/B' polypeptides, but probably to one or more epitopes different from those characteristic of the anti-Sm antibody activity found in SLE.[77,78]

In a prospective investigation of 11 children with MCTD,[19] antibodies to U1snRNP polypeptides were compared sequentially during the course of the disease. All patients had high-titer anti-ENA antibodies determined by hemagglutination (>1:1,000,000) and positive anti-RNP reactivity by immunodiffusion. Antigenic specificity identified by immunoblot analysis and enzyme-linked immunosorbent assay was to the 70-kD polypeptide in 11, A in 10, C in 2, B/B' in 9, and D in 3 patients. Four children had both IgG and IgM antibodies to the 70-kD protein, 5 to the A peptide, 2 to B/B', and only 1 to D. One patient developed low-titer anti-Sm antibodies, and three developed low-titer, transient anti-dsDNA seropositivity. Three had anti-Ro/SS-A antibodies. Anti-ENA titers and 70-kD reactivity decreased in patients

during prolonged remission; positive reactions remained in those with continuing active disease and in patients receiving only symptomatic treatment. The predominant HLA antigens were DR2 in six of nine and DR4 in four of nine; all patients were either DR2 or DR4 positive, similar to findings in adults with MCTD.

Hematological abnormalities are seen in childhood MCTD. Anemia in up to 64%[80] and leukopenia in 9% to 58%[11,57,58,79] have been reported. Thrombocytopenia in 40% was emphasized in early series of children with MCTD;[44] however, later series have reported 9% to 21%.[11,58,60,79,80] When it occurs, it can be severe and resistant to conventional therapy.[44,60] Hypocomplementemia has been reported in 10% to 30% of patients.[57-59,60] RF is commonly seen, as are elevated muscle enzymes. Hypergammaglobulinemia is noted to be common when it is reported.[81] Some patients have marked elevations of serum Ig levels, especially of IgG.[45-50] Two children with selective IgA deficiency have been reported.[43,60]

In a study of adults with MCTD,[82] 48 anti-U1-70kD antibody–positive patients with MCTD were compared with 59 anti-U1-70kD antibody–negative patients with classic SLE. Although levels of antiphospholipid antibodies were increased in the patients with MCTD compared with control subjects, levels of these antibodies were even higher in the patients with SLE who had clinical manifestations of the antiphospholipid antibody syndrome in which deep vein thrombosis, pulmonary embolism, recurrent fetal loss, chorea, livido reticularis, severe thrombocytopenia, and avascular necrosis occurred.

Treatment

There is no specific treatment for MCTD. Management should address the predominant problems of the child, such as arthritis, cutaneous disease, or visceral involvement. Many children respond satisfactorily to low-dose glucocorticoids, nonsteroidal antiinflammatory drugs, hydroxychloroquine, or a combination of these medications.[58,60,80] Raynaud Phenomenon should be treated with nonpharmacological measures, such as avoidance of cold and emotional stress. Patients should be instructed to keep the entire body warm, not only the hands. Vasodilating agents, most commonly calcium channel blockers, are used in severe cases. Nifedipine is the most extensively studied agent. Patients with severe myositis, renal, or visceral disease generally require high-dose glucocorticoids and sometimes require cytotoxic drugs (cyclophosphamide), especially for life-threatening complications, such as pulmonary hypertension.[83] In recent years, several new agents have emerged for the treatment of pulmonary hypertension in adults, including prostacyclin analogues[84-86] and endothelin receptor antagonists.[81, 86,87] Experience with use of these agents in children is promising but limited.[88] Methotrexate has been advocated;[58,89] authors have also reported the use of mycophenolate mofetil, etanercept, azathioprine, cyclosporine, and infliximab in children with MCTD.[58,80] Case studies have reported use of imatinib and immunoadsorption.[90,91] Autologous hemopoietic stem-cell transplantation has been attempted for refractory, life-threatening disease.[92]

Course of the Disease and Prognosis

The long-term outcomes of children with MCTD are varied and unpredictable.[56,57,60,80,79] Deaths have been reported from disease resembling that of SLE accompanied by renal failure. In contrast to SLE, however, morbidity and mortality in MCTD are more often associated with development of pulmonary hypertension (7%)[48,51,66,60,93] or gradually evolving restrictive disease (15%) with minimal fibrosis.[44,48,65] Pulmonary dysfunction may be underestimated clinically, because it tends to develop insidiously.[66] Another ominous development is severe thrombocytopenia (20%), which is often resistant to conventional therapy. This complication is more common in children than in adults.[60]

In a retrospective review, Tiddens and colleagues[80] (see Table 27–4) reported 14 children with MCTD who met the criteria of Kasukawa and coworkers,[8] with a mean follow-up of 9.3-years (range, 3.8- to 14.1-years) and a mean age at onset of 10.6 years (range, 5.2- to 15.6-years). Features of the disease characteristic of SLE and JDM tended to disappear over time, whereas those of CSS, Raynaud Phenomenon, and JRA persisted. At follow-up, thrombocytopenia persisted in three children; four had extensive limitation of range of joint movement, all had abnormal esophageal function, and none had active renal disease. No pulmonary hypertension was documented, although one-half had restrictive disease on function studies. Glucocorticoids were judged successful in managing MCTD but were associated with osteonecrosis in three children and growth retardation in one child.

The outcomes of children with MCTD were evaluated in a study in three U.S. Midwestern clinics[60] (Fig. 27–3). There were 21 girls and 6 boys, with a mean age at onset of 13-years (range, 5- to 18-years) and a mean duration of disease of 8-years (range, 1- to 18-years). Organ systems predominantly involved at onset and at follow-up at 8-years or more were the joints (24 and 11 patients, respectively), muscles (8 and 9), skin (16 and 8), lungs (10 and 13), heart (7 and 4), gastrointestinal tract (5 and 5), and kidneys (3 and 4). A characteristic onset involved Raynaud Phenomenon, arthritis, swollen hands, myositis, and the cutaneous features of JDM or SLE. Cutaneous disease, esophageal dysfunction, myositis, and arthritis were prominent during the entire course of the disease. These clinical features were similar to those of adults with MCTD, with less frequent and less severe pulmonary disease, and only one instance of pulmonary hypertension. Five patients developed severe thrombocytopenia. All patients had positive immunodiffusion results for anti-RNP antibodies. Anti-ENA antibodies were found in titers up to 1:16,000,000 by hemagglutination and were often maintained at high levels for many years, but concentrations ultimately declined if the course stabilized or the patient entered remission. Transient, low-titer anti-dsDNA antibodies were present in eight patients. Hypocomplementemia occurred in eight patients, and high titers of RF in seven patients.12 patients had good or stable outcomes, and five had prolonged remissions. Seven developed progressive disease, and four died of renal disease, diffuse intravascular coagulation, or cardiopulmonary failure.

Michels[79] reviewed the course of MCTD in 224 children reported until 1996, including 33 patients from the Rheumakinderklinik in Garmisch-Partenkirchen, Germany. Because this review involved a number of studies over many years that were often retrospective and without serological or genetic characterization by current standards, it predominantly reflects the clinical classifications and historical conclusions of the various centers. Nevertheless, this meta-analysis indicated that most of the children improved over time, and that remissions occurred in 3% to 27% of the series. Raynaud Phenomenon and scleroderma-like skin changes were reported in up to 86%. Long-term problems included loss of range of joint motion in 29%, renal disease in up to 47%, pulmonary restrictive disease in up to 57%, and esophageal dysmotility in up to 29%. Cardiovascular disease included cardiomyopathy, pericarditis, and pulmonary hypertension. CNS involvement was rare but could be severe. 17 (7.6%) of the 224 patients died of sepsis (seven patients), cerebral disease (three patients), heart failure (two patients), pulmonary hypertension (two patients), renal failure (two patients), or gastrointestinal bleeding (one patient). It was concluded that this mortality rate was in the range of that for other major systemic CTDs and that otherwise the long-term problems in patients who survived were minor.

Mier and colleagues reviewed several reports of pediatric MCTD[56,59,80,79] and supplemented the data with information collected by the authors from 34 pediatric patients with MCTD from seven pediatric rheumatology centers.[58] Similar to other studies, they noted in their series that manifestations of inflammation, such as muscle weakness, arthritis, and hand swelling, were present more often at disease onset, and they decreased in frequency over time, whereas scleroderma-like manifestations increased in frequency. In the authors' cohort, 3% had achieved remission, 82% exhibited a favorable outcome, and 15% exhibited an unfavorable outcome. Other features of the authors' cohort are shown in Table 27–4.

Kotajima and colleagues[56] compared two groups of Japanese patients with MCTD, one with onset when patients were younger than 16-years-old and another with onset when patients were 16-years-old or older. Signs typical of SLE, such as facial erythema, photosensitivity, the presence of lupus erythematosus cells, lymphadenopathy, and cellular casts, were more common in the juvenile-onset group. Conversely, scleroderma-like symptoms, such as esophageal dysmotility, sclerodactyly, and pulmonary disease, were more common in the older group. The investigators also found that swelling of the hands occurred less frequently in children. The mortality rate was approximately 2.8% for the juvenile onset group. Compared with other CTDs, these outcomes were interpreted as relatively favorable.

The long-term outcomes of 47 adults and children with MCTD who met the criteria of Kasukawa and coworkers[8] and were followed for 3 to 29 years were studied by Burdt and colleagues[93] (see Table 27–5). In 23% of the patients, the disease began during childhood. All patients had antibodies to the 70-kD polypeptide of U1RNP, 81% to A, 79% to B/B', 48% to C, and 14% to D. Anti-U1RNA was positive in 89% of the patients, and these

Disease characteristics of MCTD

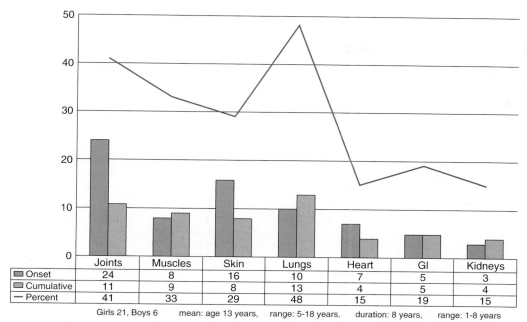

	Joints	Muscles	Skin	Lungs	Heart	GI	Kidneys
Onset	24	8	16	10	7	5	3
Cumulative	11	9	8	13	4	5	4
Percent	41	33	29	48	15	19	15

Girls 21, Boys 6   mean: age 13 years,   range: 5-18 years,   duration: 8 years,   range: 1-8 years

FIGURE 27–3   Characteristics of MCTD at disease onset and cumulative for 27 children from three U.S. Midwestern clinics. Data from Cassidy JT, Hoffman RW, Wortmann DW et al: Long-term outcome of children with mixed connective tissue disease (MCTD) *J Rheumatol* 27:100, 2000

antibody levels correlated with the activity of the disease. Initially, epitope spreading was observed as a feature of active MCTD, and with time, antibody reactivity was selectively reduced in patients in remission (i.e., epitope contraction). HLA-DR4 and HLA-DR2 were present in 23 (85%) of 27 patients. Inflammatory features of the disease, such as Raynaud Phenomenon and esophageal hypomotility, diminished over time, whereas pulmonary hypertension and CNS disease persisted despite treatment. Sclerodactyly was frequent (49%), but diffuse sclerosis occurred in only 19% of patients. Antibodies to centromere, Scl-70, and PM-1/PM-Scl antigens were not detected. Renal disease developed in five patients (11%: World Health Organization class III in two, class IV in two, and classes III and V in one). 11 patients died three to 25 years after the onset of MCTD, with pulmonary hypertension the major contributory factor in nine deaths and often associated with the presence of anticardiolipin antibodies. A favorable outcome was documented in 62% of the patients, with 17% in remission (11 off therapy) leading normal lives without functional disabilities at the time of the study.

UNDIFFERENTIATED CONNECTIVE TISSUE DISEASE AND OVERLAP SYNDROMES

A number of patients present with some features of CTD, but lack adequate clinical or diagnostic features to fit a recognizable clinical syndrome. The term undifferentiated connective tissue disease (UCTD) is often used to designate such patients. The term was first used by Leroy

and colleagues in 1980 to describe an early phase of CTDs when the findings were nonspecific and indistinct.[94] Subsequent authors have used the term, although uniform criteria have not been determined. The patient's characteristics may range from the presence of a single clinical or laboratory finding, such as a positive ANA to the presence of a number of clinical or serological features. There may be evolution of the disease initially classified as UCTD into a clinically recognizable rheumatic disease or the condition may remain with inadequate features for classification as a well recognized rheumatic disease. Several reports of adult cohorts have been published.[94-103] Alarcon and colleagues have published a series of studies examining the evolution of UCTD and classification of the rheumatic diseases. Their studies indicate that a moderate percentage of patients will evolve into recognizable disease, although many remain characterized as UCTD.[95-100] Observations by Bombardieri indicated that patients with UCTD in their cohort did not progress into distinctively recognizable rheumatic diseases.[101-102]

The term overlap syndrome is sometimes confused with the term undifferentiated connective tissue disease. The term overlap syndrome is typically applied to patients who have two or more distinctly recognizable rheumatic diseases. Although the concept seems uncomplicated, classification remains somewhat controversial, e.g., a patient with features of RA and systemic lupus may represent a distinct clinical entity or may reflect the coexistence of two rheumatic conditions in a patient, which is based on chance rather than a specific entity. There may also be some question, e.g., of an erosive arthritis occurring in systemic lupus, whether it is the coexistence of RA or the fact that erosive arthritis could be a feature of systemic lupus at times. The precise relationship of such coexisting conditions ultimately awaits a more complete understanding of the genetics and pathogenesis of autoimmunity and the CTDs.

One approach to classification of rheumatic diseases is the use of antibodies as disease markers. There are several overlap syndromes identifiable by the presence of specific autoantibodies, such as MCTD. These conditions are clinically defined by the presence of characteristics of two or more defined rheumatic diseases and the presence of specific autoantibodies. In addition to MCTD, other well-defined overlap syndromes associated with specific autoantibodies include synthetase syndromes associated with antibodies to aminoacyl transfer-RNA synthetases and clinically associated with myositis, arthritis, and pulmonary involvement. Patients with PM-Scl autoantibodies have features of polymyositis and limited scleroderma.[104-106] These overlap syndromes have been described in children.[107-108]

REFERENCES

1. G.C. Sharp, W.S. Irvin, E.M. Tan, et al., Mixed connective tissue disease—an apparently distinct rheumatic disease syndrome associated with a specific antibody to an extractable nuclear antigen (ENA), Am. J. Med. 52 (1972) 148–159.
2. S.H. Nimelstein, S. Brody, D. McShane, et al., Mixed connective tissue disease: a subsequent evaluation of the original 25 patients, Medicine (Baltimore) 59 (1980) 239–248.
5. R.W. Hoffman, G.C. Sharp, Is anti-U1-RNP autoantibody positive connective tissue disease genetically distinct? J. Rheumatol. 22 (1995) 586–589.
7. G.C. Sharp, Diagnostic criteria for classification of MCTD, in: R. Kasukawa, G.C. Sharp (Eds.), Mixed Connective Tissue Disease and Anti-Nuclear Antibodies, Excerpta Medica, Amsterdam, 1987, 23–32.
8. R. Kasukawa, T. Tojo, S. Miyawaki, et al., Preliminary diagnostic criteria for classification of mixed connective tissue disease, in: R. Kasukawa, G.C. Sharp (Eds.), Mixed Connective Tissue Disease and Anti-Nuclear Antibodies, Excerpta Medica, Amsterdam, 1987, 41–48.
9. D. Alarcon-Segovia, M. Villarreal, Classification and diagnostic criteria for mixed connective tissue disease, in: R. Kasukawa, G.C. Sharp (Eds.), Mixed Connective Tissue Disease and Anti-Nuclear Antibodies, Excerpta Medica, Amsterdam, 1987, 33–40.
11. J.S. Smolen, G. Steiner, Mixed connective tissue disease: to be or not to be? Arthritis Rheum. 41 (1998) 768–777.
13. J.M. Amigues, A. Cantagrel, M. Abbal, et al., Comparative study of 4 diagnosis criteria sets for mixed connective tissue disease in patients with anti-RNP antibodies Autoimmunity Group of the Hospitals of Toulouse, J. Rheumatol. 23 (1996) 2055–2062.
15. S. Bowyer, P. Roettcher, Pediatric rheumatology clinic populations in the United States: results of a 3 year survey, Pediatric Rheumatology Database Research Group, J. Rheumatol. 23 (1996) 1968–1974.
19. R.W. Hoffman, J.T. Cassidy, Y. Takeda, et al., U1-70-kd autoantibody-positive mixed connective tissue disease in children: a longitudinal clinical and serologic analysis, Arthritis Rheum. 36 (1993) 1599–1602.
23. D.J. de Rooij, T. Fiselier, L.B. van de Putte, et al., Juvenile-onset mixed connective tissue disease: clinical, serological and follow-up data, Scand. J. Rheumatol. 18 (1989) 157–160.
24. R.W. Hoffman, L.J. Rettenmaier, Y. Takeda, et al., Human autoantibodies against the 70-kd polypeptide of U1 small nuclear RNP are associated with HLA-DR4 among connective tissue disease patients, Arthritis Rheum. 33 (1990) 666–673.
27. R.W. Hoffman, M.E. Maldonado, Immune pathogenesis of mixed connective tissue disease: A short analytical review, Clinical. immunology 128 (2008) 8–17.
28. R.W. Hoffman, E.L. Greidinger, Mixed connective tissue disease, Curr. Op. Rheumatol. 12 (2000) 386–390.
36. A. Marshak-Rothstein, Toll-like receptors in systemic autoimmune disease, Nat. Rev. Immunol. 6 (2006) 823–835.
39. E.L. Greidinger, R.W. Hoffman, Autoantibodies in the pathogenesis of mixed connective tissue disease, Rheum. Dis. Clin. N. Am. 31 (2005) 437–450.
40. M.R. Arbuckle, M.T. McClain, M.V. Rubertone, et al., Development of autoantibodies before the clinical onset of systemic lupus erythematosus, N. Engl. J. Med. 349 (2003) 1526–1533.
43. D.Y. Sanders, C.C. Huntley, G.C. Sharp, Mixed connective tissue disease in a child, J. Pediatr. 83 (1973) 642–645.
44. B.H. Singsen, H.K. Kornreich, K. Koster-King, et al., Mixed connective tissue disease in children, Arthritis Rheum. 20 (1977) 355–360.
45. A. Fraga, J. Gudino, F. Ramos-Niembro, et al., Mixed connective tissue disease in childhood. Relationship to Sjögren's syndrome, Am. J. Dis. Child 132 (1978) 263–265.
46. M. Rosenthal, Juvenile sharp syndrome (mixed connective tissue disease), Helv. Paediatr. Acta. 33 (1978) 251–258.
47. S.A. Peskett, B.M. Ansell, P. Fizzman, et al., Mixed connective tissue disease in children, Rheumatol. Rehabil. 17 (1978) 245–248.
50. W.J. Oetgen, J.A. Boice, O.J. Lawless, Mixed connective tissue disease in children and adolescents, Pediatrics 67 (1981) 333–337.
51. K. Eberhardt, H. Svantesson, B. Svensson, Follow-up study of 6 children presenting with a MCTD-like syndrome, Scand. J. Rheumatol. 10 (1981) 62–64.
56. L. Kotajima, S. Aotsuka, M. Sumiya, et al., Clinical features of patients with juvenile onset mixed connective tissue disease: analysis of data collected in a nationwide collaborative study in Japan, J. Rheumatol. 23 (1996) 1088–1094.
57. S. Yokota, T. Imagawa, S. Katakura, et al., Mixed connective tissue disease in childhood: a nationwide retrospective study in Japan, Acta. Paediatr. Jpn. 39 (1997) 273–276.
58. R.J. Mier, M. Shishov, G.C. Higgins, et al., Pediatric-onset mixed connective tissue disease, Rheum. Dis. Clin. N. Am. 31 (2005) 483–496.
59. S. Yokota, Mixed connective tissue disease in childhood, Acta. Paediatr. Jpn. 35 (1993) 472–479.
60. J.T. Cassidy, R.W. Hoffman, D.W. Wortmann, et al., Long-term outcome of children with mixed connective tissue disease (MCTD), J. Rheumatol. 27 (2000) 100.
66. W.D. Sullivan, D.J. Hurst, C.E. Harmon, et al., A prospective evaluation emphasizing pulmonary involvement in patients with mixed connective tissue disease, Medicine (Baltimore) 63 (1984) 92–107.
67. B.H. Singsen, V.L. Swanson, B.H. Bernstein, et al., A histologic evaluation of mixed connective tissue disease in childhood, Am. J. Med. 68 (1980) 710–717.
69. I. Pettersson, G. Wang, E.I. Smith, et al., The use of immunoblotting and immunoprecipitation of (U) small nuclear ribonucleoproteins in the analysis of sera of patients with mixed connective tissue disease and systemic lupus erythematosus: cross-sectional, longitudinal study, Arthritis Rheum. 29 (1986) 986–996.
77. Y. Takeda, G.S. Wang, R.J. Wang, et al., Enzyme-linked immunosorbent assay using isolated (U) small nuclear ribonucleoprotein polypeptides as antigens to investigate the clinical significance of autoantibodies to these polypeptides, Clin. Immunol. Immunopathol. 50 (1989) 213–230.
78. M. Takano, S.S. Golden, G.C. Sharp, et al., Molecular relationships between two nuclear antigens, ribonucleoprotein and Sm: purification of active antigens and their biochemical characterization, Biochemistry 20 (1981) 5929–5936.
79. H. Michels, Course of mixed connective tissue disease in children, Ann. Med. 29 (1997) 359–364.
80. H.A. Tiddens, J.J. van der Net, E.R. Graeff-Meeder, et al., Juvenile-onset mixed connective tissue disease: longitudinal follow-up, J. Pediatr. 122 (1993) 191–197.
82. G.R. Komatireddy, G.S. Wang, G.C. Sharp, et al., Antiphospholipid antibodies among anti-U1-70 kDa autoantibody positive patients with mixed connective tissue disease, J. Rheumatol. 24 (1997) 319–322.
83. X. Jais, D. Launay, A. Yaici, et al., Immunosuppressive therapy in lupus- and mixed connective tissue disease-associated pulmonary arterial hypertension: a retrospective analysis of twenty three cases, Arthritis Rheum. 58 (2008) 521–531.
85. R.J. Barst, L.J. Rubin, W.A. Long, et al., A comparison of continuous intravenous epoprostenol (prostacyclin) with conventional therapy for primary pulmonary hypertension: The Primary Pulmonary Hypertension Study Group, N. Engl. J. Med. 334 (1996) 296–302.

86. T.M. Bull, K.A. Fagan, D.B. Badesch, Pulmonary vascular manifestations of mixed connective tissue disease, Rheum. Dis. Clin. N. Am. 31 (2005) 451–464.
87. L.J. Rubin, D.B. Badesch, R.J. Barst, et al., Bosentan therapy for pulmonary arterial hypertension, N. Engl. J. Med. 46 (2002) 896–903.
88. S.G. Haworth, A.A. Hislop, Treatment and survival in children with pulmonary arterial hypertension: the UK Pulmonary Hypertension Service for Children 2001-2006, Heart 95 (2009) 312–317.
89. S. Nakata, K. Uematsu, T. Mori, et al., Effective treatment with low-dose methotrexate pulses of a child of mixed connective tissue disease with severe myositis refractory to corticosteroid, Nihon. Rinsho. Meneki. Gakkai. Kaishi. 20 (1997) 178–183.
93. M.A. Burdt, R.W. Hoffman, S.L. Deutscher, et al., Long-term outcome in mixed connective tissue disease: longitudinal clinical and serologic findings, Arthritis Rheum. 42 (1999) 899–909.
95. G.S. Alarcon, G.V. Williams, J.Z. Singer, et al., Early undifferentiated connective tissue disease. I. Early clinical manifestation in a large cohort of patients with undifferentiated connective tissue diseases compared with cohorts of well established connective tissue diseases, J. Rheumatol. 18 (1991) 1332–1339.
98. H.J. Williams, G.S. Alarcon, R. Joks, et al., Early undifferentiated connective tissue disease (CTD). VI. An inception cohort after 10 years: disease remissions and changes in diagnoses in well established and undifferentiated CTD, J. Rheumatol. 26 (1999) 816–825.
100. J. Calvo-Alen, H.M. Bastian, K.V. Straaton, et al., Identification of patient subsets among those presumptively diagnosed with, referred, and/or followed up for systemic lupus erythematosus at a large tertiary care center, Arthritis Rheum. 38 (1995) 1475–1484.
101. M. Mosca, R. Neri, S. Bombardieri, Undifferentiated connective tissue diseases (UCTD: a review of the literature and a proposal for preliminary classification criteria, Clin. Exp. Rheumatol. 17 (1999) 615–620.
102. M. Mosca, A. Tavoni, R. Neri, et al., Undifferentiated connective tissue diseases: the clinical and serological profiles of 91 patients followed for at least 1 year, Lupus 7 (1998) 95–100.
108. L.G. Rider, F.W. Miller, I.N. Targoff, et al., A broadened spectrum of juvenile myositis. Myositis-specific autoantibodies in children, Arthritis Rheum. 37 (1994) 1534–1538.

Entire reference list is available online at www.expertconsult.com.

Chapter 28

SJÖGREN SYNDROME

Lori B. Tucker

The syndrome of chronic inflammation of the exocrine glands, principally the salivary and lacrimal glands, was first described by Henrik Sjögren, a Swedish ophthalmologist, who published the first complete description of a disorder he named keratoconjunctivitis sicca in 1933.[1] He reported that the disorder occurred most often in menopausal women, and that arthritis was a prominent feature of the disease, as well as raised erythrocyte sedimentation rate (ESR), anemia, and fever. This disease has been considered to be rare in children and adolescents; however, it has almost certainly been underdiagnosed, and it may be more common than previously realized. It is now recognized that this disorder can affect children and adolescents, and that the presentation may be different from that in adults with this condition, which contributes to the low recognition of the disorder.

DEFINITION

Sjögren Syndrome (SS) is defined as a chronic autoimmune disease characterized by inflammation of the exocrine glands. The principal inflammatory targets are the salivary and lacrimal exocrine glands, resulting in dryness of the mucosal surfaces of the mouth and eyes. However, there can be more extensive exocrinopathy involving skin, the respiratory tract, and urogenital tracts. Extraglandular or systemic features can also be part of the disorder. Table 28–1 outlines the principal clinical manifestations of SS.

CLASSIFICATION

SS is described as *primary Sjögren Syndrome (pSS)* when there is no association with other autoimmune disease, and as *secondary Sjögren Syndrome (sSS)* when there is another autoimmune disease present, most commonly systemic lupus erythematosus (SLE) or rheumatoid arthritis.

None of the proposed classification criteria sets for pSS in adults has gained universal acceptance.[2] The American-European Consensus Group (AECG) criteria, revised in 2002, are shown in Table 28–2, and have been validated in adults with SS in whom they have sensitivity of 89.5% and specificity of 95.2%.[3,4] More recently, Bartunkova and colleagues[5] have proposed a set of criteria for the

diagnosis of pSS in children, but these have not been validated (Table 28–3). The proposed pediatric criteria include parotid enlargement or recurrent parotitis, and additional laboratory tests (elevated amylase, evidence of renal tubular acidosis (RTA), leukopenia, elevated ESR, antinuclear antibodies (ANA), rheumatoid factor (RF), and hypergammaglobulinemia). These criteria, not included in any of the adult criteria sets, seem to occur with increased frequency in pediatric SS. Houghton and colleagues[6] compared the usefulness of the AECG adult criteria and the proposed pediatric criteria in a group of six patients in British Columbia, and 128 cases found on literature review. The adult criteria were fulfilled by 14% of the local cases and 39% of reported pediatric cases, whereas the proposed pediatric criteria were fulfilled by 71% of the local cases and 76% of the reported pediatric cases. The conclusion of this study was that, although the new proposed pediatric criteria improved the diagnostic accuracy considerably, neither set of criteria was sensitive when compared with the gold standard of pediatric rheumatologist clinical diagnosis.

CLINICAL MANIFESTATIONS

Oral Manifestations

One of the principal clinical findings of SS is dryness of the oral mucosa (xerostomia), which is described in 90% of adults with SS.[7] Poor oral salivary flow can result in difficulty in swallowing dry food, a change in taste, halitosis and an increase in dental caries. These symptoms may be difficult to elicit from children or youth.[8] On examination of the mouth, one may see dry "sticky"-appearing mucosa, dental caries, or atrophy of the filiform papillae on the dorsum of the tongue.

Parotid enlargement is described in two-thirds of adults with pSS, but it may be a more frequent feature in children diagnosed with SS. Review of the reported cases of pediatric SS demonstrates that parotitis is the most common presenting feature, present overall in 50% to 70% of children.[8,9] In many cases, the sole presenting complaint may be recurrent parotitis. Parotitis may be unilateral but frequently becomes bilateral and may be painful or painless. It is most often episodic but may be chronic in some patients. Children with recurrent episodes of parotid swelling are

Table 28-1

Clinical manifestations of Sjögren Syndrome

Dry eyes (xerophthalmia, keratoconjunctivitis sicca)
Dry mouth (xerostomia)
Parotid swelling
Extraglandular manifestations
    Fatigue
    Arthritis
    Purpura
    Pulmonary involvement
        Interstitial pulmonary disease
        Small airways disease
    Nephritis
    Neurological involvement
        Central nervous system disease
        Peripheral neuropathy
    Neonatal lupus in babies whose mothers have SS

Table 28-2

American-European consensus group classification criteria for Sjögren Syndrome (Revised 2002)

Ocular symptoms (positive answer to at least one of the following):
1. Have you had daily, persistent, troublesome dry eyes for more than 3 mos?
2. Do you have a recurrent sensation of sand or gravel in the eyes?
3. Do you use tear substitutes more than 3 times a day?

Oral symptoms (positive answer to at least one of the following):
1. Have you had a daily feeling of dry mouth for more than 3 mos?
2. Have you had recurrently or persistently swollen salivary glands as an adult?
3. Do you frequently drink liquids to aid in swallowing dry food?

Ocular signs (objective finding, positive result on at least one of the following):
1. Schirmer test, without anesthesia (≤5 mm in 5 min)
2. Rose Bengal score (≥ 4)

Histopathology: focal lymphocytic sialadenitis from a minor salivary gland biopsy, evaluated by an expert histopathologist, with a focus score of ≥1 (defined as a number of lymphocytic focuses adjacent to normal mucous acini and containing >50 lymphocytes per 4 mm^2 of glandular tissue)

Salivary gland involvement: objective evidence of salivary gland involvement defined as a positive result for at least one of the following diagnostic tests:
1. Unstimulated whole salivary flow (≤ 1.5 mL in 15 min)
2. Parotid sialography showing the presence of diffuse sialectasis, without evidence of obstruction in the major ducts
3. Salivary scintigraphy showing delayed uptake, reduced concentration, and/or delayed excretion of tracer

Autoantibodies: presence in the serum of antibodies to Ro (SSA) or La (SSB) antigens, or both

For diagnosis of primary SS:
Presence of 4 of 6 items, provided either histopathology or serology are positive
Presence of 3 of 4 objective items (ocular signs, histopathology, salivary gland involvement, or autoantibodies)

For diagnosis of secondary SS:
In patients with a potentially associated disease, presence of either ocular or oral symptoms, plus any 2 of ocular signs, histopathology, or salivary gland involvement

From Vitali C, Bombardieri S, Jonsson R et al: Classification criteria for Sjögren's Syndrome: a revised version of the European criteria proposed by the American-European Consensus Group, *Ann. Rheum. Dis.* 61:554-558, 2002.

Table 28-3

Proposed criteria for juvenile primary Sjögren Syndrome

I. Clinical symptoms
  1. Oral (dry mouth, recurrent parotitis, or enlargement of parotid glands)
  2. Ocular (recurrent conjunctivitis without obvious allergic or infectious etiology, keratoconjunctivitis sicca)
  3. Other mucosal (recurrent vaginitis)
  4. Systemic (fever of unknown origin, noninflammatory arthralgias, hypokalemic paralysis, abdominal pain)
II. Immunological abnormalities (presence of at least 1 of: anti-SSA, anti-SSB, high titer ANA, RF)
III. Other laboratory abnormalities or additional investigations
  1. Biochemical (elevated serum amylase)
  2. Hematological (leucopenia, high ESR)
  3. Immunological (polyclonal hyperimmunoglobulinemia)
  4. Nephrological (renal tubular acidosis)
  5. Histological proof of lymphocytic infiltration of salivary glands or other organs
  6. Objective documentation of ocular dryness (Bengal red staining, Schirmer test)
  7. Objective documentation of parotid gland involvement (sialography)
IV. Exclusion of all other autoimmune diseases
  Presence of 4 or more criteria

From Bartunkova J, Sediva A, Vencovsky J et al: Primary Sjögren's Syndrome in children and adolescents: Proposal for diagnostic criteria, *Clin Exp Rheumatol* 17:381-386, 1999.

Table 28-4

Differential diagnosis of recurrent parotitis in children

Juvenile recurrent parotitis
Diffuse infiltrative lymphocytosis (associated with HIV)
Streptococcal or staphylococcal infection
Hemangioma
Neoplastic (benign or malignant)
    Viral infection
        Epstein-Barr
        Cytomegalovirus
        Parvovirus
        Paramyxovirus
Unilateral parotitis:
    Bacterial infection
    Sialothiasis

generally seen by a pediatrician or pediatric otolaryngologist for diagnosis. The differential diagnosis of recurrent parotid swelling in childhood (Table 28–4) includes infection, juvenile recurrent parotitis,[10] lymphoma, hemangiomas, and other rare inflammatory conditions.[11] PSS should be strongly considered in the differential diagnosis of a child with recurrent parotid swelling, and a complete diagnostic evaluation should be performed.[9,12,13] The reason that SS has been considered a 'rare' disease in pediatrics is almost certainly the lack of recognition of SS as a potential cause of recurrent parotid swelling in children.

Ocular Manifestations

Patients with SS may experience a decrease in tear production, due to inflammation of the lacrimal glands, which leads to damage to the corneal and bulbar epithelium (keratoconjunctivitis sicca). The symptoms of ocular involvement in SS include burning sensations in the eye, a feeling of having a foreign body in the eye, "sandy" or scratchy feeling under the lids, itchiness, erythema of the eyes, or photosensitivity. These symptoms may be difficult to elicit from children. On examination, one may find pericorneal irritation, dilation of conjunctival vessels, or enlargement of the lacrimal glands.

Other Glandular Involvement

Less commonly, dryness can affect the upper respiratory tract or oropharynx, resulting in hoarseness, bronchitis, or pneumonitis. The skin may be dry, and there may be loss of exocrine function in other glands, resulting in pancreatic dysfunction and hypochlorhydria.

Extraglandular Manifestations

Extraglandular manifestations of childhood SS may be less common than those in adults. However, general systemic complaints, such as fatigue, low grade fever, myalgias, and arthralgias are frequent, particularly at the time of parotitis attacks.

Extraglandular manifestations can be considered in two different pathophysiological groups:

1. Peripheral organ involvement due to lymphocytic invasion in the epithelia of organs other than the exocrine glands, e.g., interstitial nephritis or obstructive bronchiolitis
2. Extraepithelial involvement secondary to immune complex deposition and subsequent inflammation

The types of extraglandular manifestations which may be seen in SS are shown in Table 28–1, with further details on more common findings below.

Skin Manifestations

Raynaud phenomenon is reported to be relatively common among individuals with SS, and it may precede sicca complaints by years. Purpura or pernio have been reported in SS, and they may be signs suggesting a poor prognosis.

Arthritis

Adults with SS commonly complain of arthralgia, and inflammatory arthritis is reported in approximately 20% of patients.[14] The presence of arthritis has rarely been commented on in case series of children with SS, and it is difficult to determine how often it occurs.

Pulmonary Involvement

Pulmonary manifestations in patients with pSS are common and may be present in as many as 75% of patients.[15] Dryness of the epithelium of the trachea can result in a dry cough. Small airway obstructive disease and airway hyperactivity may result from lymphocytic infiltration around bronchi and bronchioles.

Interstitial lung disease occurs in approximately 8% of adults with pSS, and has the appearance of lymphocytic interstitial pneumonitis in many cases.[16,17] Patients with lung disease may present with cough and/or dyspnea, although some are asymptomatic early in their course. Chest x-rays may be abnormal, showing interstitial changes in 27% (pSS) to 75% (sSS) of asymptomatic patients. A high resolution computerized tomography scan can detect abnormalities not seen on plain radiographs. Abnormalities detected in 65% of asymptomatic patients include inter- and intralobular thickening and ground glass appearance in lower lung fields. Pulmonary function tests may demonstrate decreased peak flows or diffusing capacity. Less commonly, pulmonary arterial hypertension has been reported.[18] If hilar and/or mediastinal adenopathy or lung nodules are found, an evaluation to rule out lymphoma should be conducted. Houghton and colleagues reported fraternal twin girls with pSS, one of whom presented with mild dyspnea and was found to have large pulmonary nodules.[19] Biopsy of these nodules substantiated the diagnosis of pSS, with lymphocytic interstitial pneumonitis. Five years after the diagnosis of pSS, clinical worsening prompted reinvestigation, and repeat biopsy demonstrated a mucosa associated lymphoid tissue (MALT) lymphoma.

Renal Involvement

Renal involvement in patients with SS is not common, but patients may develop interstitial nephritis or glomerulonephritis. Distal RTA, with hyposthenuria, reflects interstitial lymphocytic infiltration. One report reviewed 12 cases of RTA in children with SS.[20] In this small series, RTA was more frequently seen in pSS in childhood than in adults. Clinically significant hypokalemia was seen in the majority, and some patients had proximal or mixed RTA. Other more rare manifestations in patients with SS include proximal tubular acidosis, membranous or membranoproliferative glomerulonephritis, tubulointerstitial nephritis,[21] and interstitial cystitis.

Neurological Involvement

The spectrum of neurological manifestations associated with SS is broad and includes meningitis, myelopathy, cranial neuropathy, sensorimotor polyneuropathy, and mononeuritis multiplex.[22,23] A syndrome of purely sensory neuropathy is said to be relatively unique to SS among the rheumatic diseases,[22] and has been reported in childhood.[24] A peripheral neuropathy may precede the appearance of sicca symptoms in many patients. There have been reports of optic neuropathy in pediatric onset SS.[25] Other central nervous system (CNS) manifestations include hemiparesis, movement disorders, brainstem, motor neuron, and cerebellar syndromes.[26,27] The CNS manifestations reported in SS overlap with those seen in patients with CNS lupus, making the differentiation between these disorders difficult.

Connection between Neonatal Lupus and Sjögren's Syndrome

Neonatal lupus syndrome, including congenital heart block, can occur in offspring of women who have anti-Ro and/or anti-La antibodies during their pregnancy (see Chapter 23). These autoantibodies are those most commonly found in women with SS.[28] Among mothers of infants with neonatal lupus, SS is as common as lupus.[29] Counseling older adolescents with SS and anti-Ro/La antibodies about the risk of neonatal lupus in future pregnancies is advisable; more intensive pregnancy screening should take place for teenagers with SS who become pregnant.

PATHOLOGY

The primary pathological finding in SS is of lymphocytic infiltration of affected tissues. Salivary gland biopsies show focal aggregates of lymphocytes, plasma cells, and macrophages; there may be larger foci with the appearance of germinal centers. This appearance is characteristic of chronic lymphocytic sialadenitis. A minor salivary gland biopsy is said to be specific for the diagnosis of SS if it is obtained through normal appearing mucosa, has 5 to 10 glands present but separated by surrounding connective tissue with focal lymphocytic infiltration, and with all or most of the glands abnormal.[30]

PATHOGENESIS

The proposed model of the pathogenesis of SS is that genetically predisposed individuals are exposed to environmental factors, such as viral infection, which lead to a protracted autoimmune response focused in the epithelial cells of exocrine glands.[31-33] However, the specifics of these pathways are not well understood, and the pathogenic relationship between initial autoimmune disease in exocrine glands and further extraglandular disease is unknown. To date, there have been relatively few gene association studies of large SS patient groups, and no genome wide association studies. The few genetic association studies done demonstrate a set of genes as potential risk alleles, including STAT 4 and IRF 5, which are also susceptibility genes for SLE.[34] Larger genetic studies are required to identify the more specific genetic associations of this disease.

Autoantibodies

Patients with SS have a variety of autoantibodies, which include RF, ANA most commonly directed against the extractable nuclear antigens Ro/SSA and La/SSB, and others directed against organ specific antigens such as thyroid cells or gastric mucosa. At least three pieces of evidence support the possibility that autoantibodies against Ro and La may have a pathogenic role: They are present in the saliva of patients with SS; there is increased messenger RNA for La in conjunctival epithelial cells in SS; B cells infiltrating salivary glands in SS have intracytoplasmic immunoglobulin directed against Ro and La.[35]

More recently, autoantibodies directed against the cytoskeletal protein β-fodrin and muscarinic receptor M3

have been described,[35] have been described although their pathogenic roles are not yet known.

Potential Viral Triggers of Sjögren's Syndrome Autoimmunity

Although both clinical and experimental observations suggest a role for viruses as triggers for SS, no specific infectious agent has been identified. Several retroviruses have been associated with pSS, including human T lymphotropic virus Type 1, human retrovirus 5, hepatitis C virus, and Coxsackie virus.[31,36] Viral activation of the innate immune system may play a role in inciting SS, with a maladaptive response leading to autoimmunity.

Immunopathological Mechanism of Disease

The majority of lymphocytes infiltrating the affected glandular tissue are activated CD4+ T cells and activated B cells. The involvement of the innate immune system in the pathogenesis of SS is increasingly an area of study, with a focus on the potential role of interferon (IFNα) and a possible role for B cell activating factor (BAFF).[32]

There is increased expression of IFN-regulated genes in salivary glands of SS patients,[37,38] and plasmacytoid dendritic cells, known to be a major source of IFNα, are present.[38] In addition, this IFN signature was found in peripheral blood mononuclear cells of SS patients, and correlated with anti-SSA and anti-SSB levels.[39]

In addition to IFN genes, which are markers for innate immunity, an increase in BAFF, one of the cytokines upregulated by IFNα, has been demonstrated in salivary glands, saliva, and serum of SS patients.[40] BAFF promotes B cell survival, and BAFF deficient mice develop a lupus-like disease with infiltrates in the salivary glands and decreased salivary flow.[41] These data suggest a pathogenic role for BAFF in SS; however, the specifics of this role are not currently known.

LABORATORY EXAMINATION

Laboratory testing in SS is important, although not specific. Patients frequently have a very elevated ESR, although this is likely related to significant hypergammaglobulinemia seen in nearly 100% of patients.[5,6,42] The majority of patients with SS also have ANA; RFs are found in 57% to 87.5% of pediatric patients.[5,6,42] Approximately 20% of adults with SS are reported to have cryoglobulins in their serum,[7] which is a poor prognostic factor, identifying patients at higher risk of developing more organ involvement and at higher potential for lymphoma. Autoantibodies to nuclear antigens Ro/SSA and La/SSB are considered the "hallmark" feature of this disease; however, these autoantibodies are found in only 60% to 90% of patients. The presence of anti-Ro and anti-La has been reported to be associated with a higher prevalence of systemic, hematological, and immunological abnormalities.[43]

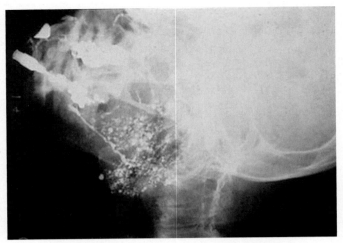

FIGURE 28–1   Typical sialogram in Sjögren's Syndrome.

RADIOLOGIC STUDIES

Salivary flow can be measured by sialometry, but this procedure is difficult to do, particularly in younger children; in addition, there are no appropriate age-matched normal values for children. Sialography is a radiocontrast method of examining the anatomical detail of the parotid ductal system. In SS, sialectasis can be demonstrated on sialography. The radiographic features found in sialograms in 21 pediatric patients with either pSS or sSS ranged from punctuate or globular ectasia sialectasis (Fig. 28–1) to considerable narrowing of the ductal system and destroyed parenchyma.[8] The authors of the study suggested that sialography provided highly accurate and sensitive findings in children with suspected SS.

Parotid Scintigraphy and Ultrasound

Salivary gland scintigraphy assesses salivary gland function, using 99Tc-pertechnetate injection, and demonstration of uptake and distribution of the isotope. In patients with SS, the uptake and secretion of isotope is delayed or absent. Abnormal parotid scintigraphy is included as one of the criteria the AECG diagnostic criteria for SS, with abnormal results classified into grades 1-4 (1 least severe, 4 most severe) by an accepted system proposed by Schall et al.[44] A prospective study of 405 adult patients with SS who had scintigraphy performed at disease diagnosis demonstrated that severe scintographic findings early in disease were significantly associated with a higher risk of systemic features, progression to lymphoma and lower survival rate over a mean 7 year follow-up.[45]

Ultrasound can also be used to demonstrate abnormal salivary gland architecture, with the benefit of being noninvasive. A comparative study of salivary gland ultrasound, scintigraphy and salivary gland biopsy in 107 adult patients demonstrated that ultrasound was highly accurate as a diagnostic test, with 90.8% specificity and 87.1% sensitivity. There have been no studies of salivary gland ultrasound in children, but this may be a useful and accurate non-invasive diagnostic test.[46]

Schirmer test is a standardized valid method of testing the amount of tear secretion. A small specially measured strip of filter paper is slipped under the inferior lid of the eye for five minutes; the wet length of paper is measured. If the tear secretion is less than 5 millimeters, a significant decrease in tear secretion is demonstrated. Although this is a simple test, it may be difficult to apply in many children. In these cases, Rose Bengal staining, which dyes the corneal and conjunctival epithelium damaged secondary to low tear output, may be performed by an ophthalmologist.

Minor Salivary Gland and Parotid Biopsy

Biopsy of the minor salivary glands of the lower lip has been used widely as a diagnostic tool, particularly for adults with a presumptive diagnosis of SS. The AECG diagnostic criteria include the finding of focal sialadenitis from a minor salivary gland biopsy as a major diagnostic parameter. Histological findings diagnostic for SS from the minor salivary gland biopsy are periductal lymphocytic infiltration or chronic sialadenitis. However, in some cases, these biopsies may be nondiagnostic or may not provide adequate glandular tissue for diagnostic confirmation. In one retrospective single center study, Caporali and colleagues studied the usefulness of a minor salivary gland biopsy in 435 adult patients who underwent the procedure as part of the diagnostic evaluation for possible SS.[47] The procedure was safe with no major adverse events, and only 1% of samples had inadequate material for testing. 93 patients (24.5%) had a positive biopsy, and, in 51 patients, the minor salivary gland biopsy results were essential in making the diagnosis definitively. In a study of 23 children with pSS and sSS, 20 patients had typical pathological findings of SS, which was important information substantiating the diagnosis, as reported symptoms of xerostomia or xerophthalmia were not reliable particularly in younger children.[8] These data give support to the view that in a child or youth with suspected SS, a minor salivary gland biopsy can be a very useful and important procedure to determine a definite diagnosis.

Parotid biopsy is suggested by some as a more definitive diagnostic procedure. McGuirt and colleagues reported six pediatric patients (6 to 12 years old),[42] four of whom underwent parotid biopsy to confirm the diagnosis of SS.[43] In all four, parotid swelling was present, but the minor salivary biopsy was normal. The authors suggest that the parotid biopsy is a minor procedure, which can be a safe method of confirming the diagnosis of SS in the pediatric population.

MANAGEMENT

For the majority of patients with SS, the management of their disease is focused on symptom relief of dry eyes and dry mouth or episodic treatment of parotitis. Compared with many other of the rheumatic conditions, such as SLE, the disease course is more indolent, and it less frequently requires immunosuppressive therapy.

The treatment of dry eyes is generally application of topical artificial tears as necessary. Avoidance of conditions that may add to dry eyes, such as smoking or medications that may have anticholinergic side effects, may also be helpful.[14] In some patients, topical cyclosporine has been reported to improve tear production and decrease ocular symptoms. For younger children who may not complain of dry eyes, annual ocular screening should be considered to look for keratitis or scarring.

The treatment of dry mouth may be challenging, but luckily this symptom is rare in pediatrics. The use of sugar-free lozenges or chewing gum may help to stimulate salivary flow. Good dental hygiene and more frequent dental check-ups are very important for patients with SS to prevent or detect caries. Pilocarpine hydrochloride may be useful in some individuals to increase salivary secretion.[14]

Hydroxychloroquine is widely prescribed for patients with SS, and may be helpful in treating constitutional symptoms, arthralgias, or fatigue associated with disease. One study evaluating the effect of hydroxychloroquine on xerostomia in adults with pSS showed a significant increase in saliva production after six months of treatment.[48] There have been conflicting results from other reported studies, with some suggestions of improvement in ocular or oral symptoms in many patients but with few studies demonstrating improvements in laboratory parameters.[49]

Immunosuppressive agents are not uniformly required in patients with SS. However, patients with extraglandular organ manifestations, severe ocular or mucosal symptoms, or disabling constitutional problems may require more aggressive treatment. Corticosteroids do not seem to stop the progression of SS or to improve salivary flow, but they have been demonstrated in one randomized trial to result in a decrease in episodes of parotid swelling and improvement in systemic complaints of fatigue and arthralgia.[50] Based on these results, corticosteroid treatment may be beneficial to treat troublesome recurrent parotid swelling and constitutional symptoms. Although not frequently recommended for patients with SS, methotrexate was shown to result in clinical symptom improvement and decreased parotid gland swelling in one trial in adults with pSS.[51]

More recently, there has been interest in the effects of biologic agents in the treatment of SS. There have been several publications describing the use of anti-tumor necrosis factor agents, etanercept and infliximab, in the treatment of SS. One trial using etanercept did not show clinically significant effectiveness for treating oral or ocular symptoms of SS or in improving salivary or lacrimal flow by specific testing.[52] Infliximab was shown to be effective in reducing global and local disease manifestations in a small open-label pilot study of 16 patients with pSS, with sustained improvement over a one year period.[53]

Rituximab, a chimeric monoclonal antibody directed against CD20 molecules present on the surface of mature B cells, has been tested in a small number of studies of patients with pSS (10 case reports and six studies); the results of these studies have been carefully reviewed by Isaksen and colleagues.[54] There has been a universal lack of objective effect on the sicca phenomenon, but significant improvement in systemic complaints, such as fatigue, arthritis, arthralgia, and cryoglobulin-associated vasculitis, has been shown. In some case reports, patients have had good results with rituximab, despite failure of other immunomodulating drugs. Adverse events have been generally transient and mild, usually related to infu-sions; some patients developed later serum sickness-like reactions. Of 12 patients reported with pSS-related lymphoma treated with rituximab, seven went into a full remission, three remained stable, and only two did not respond, suggesting an important role for this medication in treating this serious complication of pSS.

PROGNOSIS AND OUTCOME

Despite a significantly increased risk for B cell lymphoma in some patients with SS, outcome in most adult patients with SS is very good, with many patients having a stable and benign course of disease. Long-term outcome of pediatric patients with SS has not been studied. Skopouli and colleagues[7] analyzed outcomes of 261 adult Greek patients with SS and determined that overall mortality in SS was only increased in the presence of particular predictive factors. Factors associated with an adverse outcome included purpura, glomerulonephritis, low C4, or a mixed monoclonal cryoglobulinemia. Patients who developed arthritis, Raynaud phenomenon, interstitial nephritis, or lung or liver involvement had a more favorable outcome. In general, serological profiles of patients did not change over time.

Progression to Lymphoma

It has been well-demonstrated that patients with SS are at high risk of developing malignancy; they have a 44 times relative risk for development of lymphoma, compared with age matched peers.[55] Although this is well-reported in adult patients, lymphoma in pediatric SS patients has not been reported in the literature. This may be because the development of lymphoma may take years to become clinically apparent, and therefore is not "revealed" in the pediatric patients. The majority of the lymphomas are non-Hodgkin lymphoma, with the most common being extranodal B cell lymphomas of the MALT cell type. The salivary glands are the most commonly affected site, but other organs can be involved. Lymphoma development in SS is thought to be driven by a combination of factors, including chronic antigenic stimulus, lymphocyte persistence due to defective apoptosis, and additional oncogenic events involving oncogenes.[55]

There have been a number of clinical and laboratory findings felt to be predictive of highest risk for lymphoma development. Clinical features include persistent enlargement of parotid glands, lymphadenopathy, splenomegaly, or palpable purpura.[56] Laboratory features include the presence of a mixed monoclonal cryoglobulinemia, low level of C4, or monoclonal bands in the serum or urine.[55] Patients with SS should be examined for these risk factors, and patients with any of these findings warrant closer follow-up.

REFERENCES

1. H. Sjögren, Keratoconjunctivitis sicca, Acta. Ophthalmol. (Suppl. 2) (1933) 1–145.
2. M.P. Novljan, B. Rozman, M. Jerse, et al., Comparison of the different classification criteria sets for primary Sjögren's Syndrome, Scand. J. Rheumatol. 35 (2006) 463–467.

3. C. Vitali, S. Bombardieri, R. Jonsson, et al., Classification criteria for Sjögren's Syndrome: a revised version of the European criteria proposed by the American-European Consensus Group, Ann. Rheum. Dis. 61 (2002) 554–558.

4. C. Vitali, S. Bombardieri, H.M.G. Moutsopoulos, et al., Preliminary criteria for the classification of Sjögren's Syndrome, Arthritis Rheum. 36 (1993) 340–347.

5. J. Bartunkova, A. Sediva, J. Vencovsky, et al., Primary Sjögren's Syndrome in children and adolescents: Proposal for diagnostic criteria, Clin. Exp. Rheumatol. 17 (1999) 381–386.

6. K. Houghton, P. Malleson, D. Cabral, et al., Primary Sjögren's Syndrome in children and adolescents: are proposed diagnostic criteria applicable? J. Rheumatol. 32 (2005) 2225–2232.

7. F.N. Skopouli, J. Dafni, J.P. Ioannidis, et al., Clinical evolution, and morbidity and mortality of primary Sjögren's Syndrome, Semin. Arthritis Rheum. 29 (2000) 296–304.

8. M. Stiller, W. Golder, E. Doring, et al., Primary and secondary Sjögren's Syndrome in children-a comparative study, Clin. Oral Investig. 4 (2000) 176–182.

9. M. Civilibal, N. Canpolat, A. Yurt, et al., A child with primary Sjögren's Syndrome and a review of the literature, Clin. Pediatr. 46 (2007) 738–742.

10. C.M. Leerdam, H.C. Martin, D. Isaacs, Recurrent parotitis of childhood, J. Paediatr. Child Health 41 (2005) 631–634.

11. G.L. Wright, R.J.H. Smith, C.D. Katz, et al., Benign parotic diseases of childhood, Laryngoscope 95 (1985) 915–920.

12. H.A. Cohen, S. Gross, M. Nussinovitch, et al., Recurrent parotitis, Arch. Dis. Child 67 (1992) 1036–1037.

13. T. Hara, M. Nagata, Y. Mizuno, et al., Recurrent parotid swelling in children: clinical features useful for differential diagnosis of Sjögren's Syndrome, Acta. Paediatr. 81 (1992) 547–549.

14. P.J. Venables, Management of patients presenting with Sjögren's Syndrome, Best Prac. Res. Clin. Rheumatol. 20 (2006) 791–807.

15. A.L. Parke, Pulmonary manifestations of primary Sjögren's Syndrome, Rheum. Dis. Clin. N. Am. 34 (2008) 907–920.

16. P. Gardiner, C. Ward, A. Allison, et al., Pleuropulmonary abnormalities in primary Sjögren's Syndrome, J. Rheumatol. 20 (1993) 831–837.

17. V. Dalvi, E.B. Gonzalez, L. Lovett, Lymphocytic interstitial pneumonia in Sjögren's Syndrome: a case report and a review of the literature, Clin. Rheumatol. 26 (2007) 1339–1343.

18. D. Launay, E. Hachulla, P.Y. Hatron, et al., Pulmonary arterial hypertension: a rare complication of Sjögren's Syndrome: report of 9 new cases and review of the literature, Medicine 86 (2007) 299–315.

19. K. Houghton, D. Cabral, R. Petty, et al., Primary Sjögren's Syndrome in dizygotic adolescent twins: one case with lymphocytic interstitial pneumonia, J. Rheumatol. 32 (2005) 1603–1606.

20. F. Pessler, H. Emery, L. Dai, et al., The spectrum of renal tubular acidosis in paediatric Sjögren's Syndrome, Rheumatology (Oxford) 45 (2006) 85–91.

21. S. Johnson, S.A. Hulton, M.A. Brundler, et al., End-stage renal failure in adolescence with Sjögren's Syndrome autoantibodies, Pediatr. Nephrol. 22 (2007) 1793–1797.

22. B. Segal, A. Carpenter, D. Walk, Involvement of nervous system pathways in primary Sjögren's Syndrome, Rheum. Dis. Clin. N. Am. 34 (2008) 885–906.

23. S.I. Meligren, L.G. Goransson, R. Omdal, Primary Sjögren's Syndrome associated neuropathy, Can. J. Neurol. Sci. 34 (2007) 280–287.

24. K. Kumon, A. Satake, M. Mizumoto, et al., A case of sensory neuropathy associated with childhood Sjögren's Syndrome, Eur. J. Pediatr. 159 (2000) 630–631.

25. J. Rojas-Rodriguez, M. Garcia-Carrasco, E.S. Ramirez, et al., Optic neuropathy in a child with primary Sjögren's Syndrome, Rev. Rhum. Engl. Ed. 65 (1998) 355–357.

26. J.A. Gottfried, T.H. Finkel, J.V. Hunter, et al., Central nervous system Sjögren's Syndrome in a child: case report and review of the literature, J. Child Neurol. 16 (2001) 683–685.

27. I. Kobayashi, H. Furuta, A. Tame, et al., Complications of childhood Sjögren's Syndrome, Eur. J. Pediatr. 155 (1996) 890–894.

28. A.L. Parke, Sjögren's Syndrome: a women's health problem, J. Rheumatol. 61 (2000) 4–5.

29. A.R. Neiman, L.A. Lee, W.L. Weston, et al., Cutaneous manifestations of neonatal lupus without heart block: characteristics of mothers and children enrolled in a national registry, J. Pediatr. 137 (2000) 674–680.

30. R. Amarasena, S. Bowman, Sjögren's Syndrome, Clin. Medicine 7 (2007) 53–56.

31. N. Delaleu, M.V. Jonsson, S. Appel, et al., New concepts in the pathogenesis of Sjögren's Syndrome, Rheum. Dis. Clin. N. Am. 34 (2008) 833–845.

32. N.P. Nikolov, G.G. Illei, Pathogenesis of Sjögren's Syndrome, Curr. Opin. Rheumatol. 21 (2009) 465–470.

33. G. Nordmark, G.V. Alm, L. Ronnblom, Mechanisms of disease: primary Sjögren's Syndrome and the type I interferon system, Nat. Clin. Pract. Rheumatol. 2 (2006) 262–269.

34. R.H. Scofield, Genetics of systemic lupus erythematosus and Sjögren's Syndrome, Curr. Opin. Rheumatol. 21 (2009) 448–453.

35. J.G. Routsias, A.G. Tzioufas, Sjögren's Syndrome: study of autoantigens and autoantibodies, Clin. Rev. Allergy Immunol. 32 (2007) 238–251.

36. A. Triantafyllopoulou, H.M. Moutsopoulos, Persistent viral infection in primary Sjögren's Syndrome: Review and perspectives, Clin. Rev. Allergy Immunol. 32 (2007) 210–214.

37. J.E. Gottenberg, N. Cagnard, C. Lucchesi, et al., Activation of IFN pathways and plasmacytoid dendritic cell recruitment in target organs of primary Sjögren's Syndrome, Proc. Natl. Acad. Sci. USA 103 (2006) 2770–2775.

38. T.O. Hjelmervik, K. Petersen, I. Jonassen, et al., Gene expression profiling of minor salivary glands clearly distinguishes primary Sjögren's Syndrome patients from healthy control subjects, Arthritis Rheum. 52 (2005) 1534–1544.

39. E.S. Emamian, J.M. Leon, C.J. Lessard, et al., Peripheral blood gene expression profiling in Sjögren's Syndrome, Genes Immunol. 10 (2009) 285–296.

40. F. Lavie, C. Miceli-Richard, M. Ittah, et al., B-cell activating factor of the tumour necrosis factor family expression in blood monocytes and T cells from patients with primary Sjögren's Syndrome, Scand. J. Immunol. 67 (2008) 185–192.

41. M. Ittah, C. Miceli-Richard, J.E. Gottenberg, et al., Viruses induce high expression of BAFF by salivary gland epithelial cells through TLR- and type-I IFN-dependant and independent pathways, Eur. J. Immunol. 38 (2008) 1058–1064.

42. W.F. Mcguirt Jr., C. Whang, W. Moreland, The role of parotid biopsy in the diagnosis of pediatric Sjögren's Syndrome, Arch. Otolaryngol Head Neck Surg. 128 (2002) 1279–1281.

43. M. Ramos-Casals, R. Solans, J. Rosas, et al., Primary Sjögren's Syndrome in Spain: clinical and immunologic expression in 1010 patients, Medicine 87 (2008) 210–219.

44. G.L. Schall, L.G. Anderson, R.O. Wolf, et al., Xerostomia in Sjögren's Syndrome. Evaluation by serial salivary scintigraphy, JAMA 216 (1971) 2109–2116.

45. M. Ramos-Casals, P. Brito-Zeron, M. Perez-de-lis, et al., Clinical and prognostic significance of parotid scintigraphy in 405 patients with primary Sjögren's Syndrome, J. Rheumatol. 37(3) (2010) 585–591.

46. V.D. Milic, RR. Petrovic, I.V. Boricic, et al., Diagnostic value of salivary gland ultrasonographic scoring system in primary Sjögren's Syndrome: a comparison with scintigraphy and biopsy, J. Rheumatol. 36(7) (2009) 1495–1500.

47. P. Caporali, E. Bonacci, O. Epis, et al., Safety and usefulness of minor salivary gland biopsy: Retrospective analysis of 502 procedures performed at a single center, Arthritis Rheum. 59 (2008) 714–720.

48. M. Rihl, K. Ulbricht, R.E. Schmidt, et al., Treatment of sicca symptoms with hydroxychloroquine in patients with Sjögren's Syndrome, Rheumatology (Oxford) 48 (2009) 796–799.

49. S.E. Carsons, Issues relating to clinical trials of oral and biologic disease-modifying agents for Sjögren's Syndrome, Rheum. Dis. Clin. N. Am. 34 (2008) 1011–1023.

50. P.C. Fox, M. Datiles, J.C. Atkinson, et al., Prednisone and piroxicam for treatment of primary Sjögren's Syndrome, Clin. Exp. Rheumatol. 11 (1993) 149–156.

51. F.N. Skopouli, P. Jagiello, N. Tsifetaki, et al., Methotrexate in primary Sjögren's Syndrome, Clin. Exp. Rheumatol. 14 (1996) 555–558.

52. V. Sankar, M.T. Brennan, M.R. Kok, et al., Etanercept in Sjögren's Syndrome: a twelve-week randomized, double-blind, placebo-controlled pilot clinical trial, Arthritis Rheum. 50 (2004) 2240–2245.

53. S.D. Steinfeld, P. Demols, I. Salmon, et al., Infliximab in patients with primary Sjögren's Syndrome: a pilot study, Arthritis Rheum. 44 (2001) 2371–2375.

54. K. Isaksen, R. Jonsson, R. Omdal, Anti-CD20 treatment in primary Sjögren's Syndrome, Scand. J. Immunol. 68 (2008) 554–564.

55. M. Voulgarelis, F.N. Skopouli, Clinical, immunologic, and molecular factors predicting lymphoma development in Sjögren's Syndrome patients, Clin. Rev. Allergy Immunol. 32 (2007) 265–274.

56. S.S. Kassan, T.L. Thomas, H.M. Moutsopoulos, et al., Increased risk of lymphoma in sicca syndrome, Ann. Intern. Med. 89 (1978) 888–892.

Chapter 29

RAYNAUD PHENOMENON AND VASOMOTOR SYNDROMES

Robert C. Fuhlbrigge

Episodic color changes of the hands and feet in response to cold or stress, known as Raynaud Phenomenon (RP), are a frequent complaint among patients presenting to pediatric rheumatology clinics. The first description of vasomotor instability triggered by cold exposure, or "local asphyxia of the extremities," is ascribed to A.G. Maurice Raynaud, a French medical student, whose name has become synonymous with this disorder.[1] Despite 150 years of clinical observation and basic research, only recently have significant inroads been established to explain the biological basis for this condition and to establish evidence-based therapeutic interventions.

CLINICAL PRESENTATION

The classic presentation of RP includes recurrent episodes of pallor and/or cyanosis of the hands and feet associated with cold exposure or emotional stress.[2] Episodes typically occur as sudden attacks, often triggered by changes in the relative ambient temperature or contact of the extremities with cold surfaces. An RP attack typically begins in a single finger and then spreads to other digits, symmetrically involving both hands and/or feet (Fig. 29-1). RP involving the fingers and toes is characteristically sharply demarcated and can be accompanied by sensations of pins and needles, numbness, and/or clumsiness of the hands and aching pains. The index, middle, and ring fingers are the most frequently involved digits, while the thumb is often spared. Patients with RP commonly report symptoms of cutaneous vasospasm at other sites, including the ears, nose, face, knees, and, rarely, the nipples, and patients can display livedo reticularis involving the distal arms and legs.[3] Vascular spasm within viscera, such as the esophagus and coronary arteries, may accompany peripheral symptoms, particularly in patients with systemic sclerosis (SSc).

The symptoms of RP reflect transient arterial vasospasm, leading to restricted blood supply to the skin (pallor) and subsequent extraction of oxygen from stagnant or slow flowing blood (cyanosis). Episodes can last from minutes to hours and are typically readily reversed by mechanical warming measures. Upon warming, blood flow is often exaggerated, the skin appears reddened or flushed, and the digits may swell or itch. In severe RP, tender red subcutaneous nodules (pernio) and ulcerations of the fingers and toes may result from local tissue ischemia (Fig. 29-2).

The triggers of RP in children are similar to those described in adults, with cold, emotional stress, and exercise as the most commonly reported initiators.[3-5] Although exposure to absolute cold (e.g., air temperature below freezing) is readily recognized as a stimulus, provocation may also occur during relative shifts from warmer to cooler temperatures. Thus, mild cold exposures, such as entering an air-conditioned space or handling cold food, may cause an attack. A general body chill can also trigger an episode, even if the hands or feet are kept warm. In some patients, RP occurs after nonspecific stimulation of the sympathetic nervous system (e.g., periods of intense emotional stress, startle response).

Primary RP, Raynaud sign, or idiopathic Raynaud disease are terms used to describe those patients without a definable cause for their symptoms beyond nonspecific vascular hyperreactivity (Table 29-1).[6] In this setting, RP is considered an exaggeration of the normal vasoconstriction response to cold exposure, the clinical features are generally benign, and the symptoms are reversible with rewarming. Use of the word "disease" in this context may cause undue concern, and many clinicians prefer the term "primary RP" for otherwise healthy individuals. Secondary RP, or Raynaud syndrome, refers to patients in whom an associated disease or known cause of vascular injury drives the frequency and severity of symptoms.[7,8]

EPIDEMIOLOGY

Estimates of the prevalence of RP range from 5% to 20% in women and 4% to 14% in men.[2,6,9] The large variation between studies reflects, in part, the ethnic balance of the populations studied and the climate of the regions where the study patients live.[10,11] A study of children 12- to 15-years old in Manchester, United Kingdom, reported an overall prevalence of 18% in females and 12% in males, with values increasing with age in this population.[12] In general, RP is more common among women, younger age groups, and family members of patients with RP.[9,13] For obvious reasons, patients living in colder climates are more likely to present for evaluation and at younger ages.[10] Although the large majority of patients with RP do not have, nor will they develop, an associated rheumatological

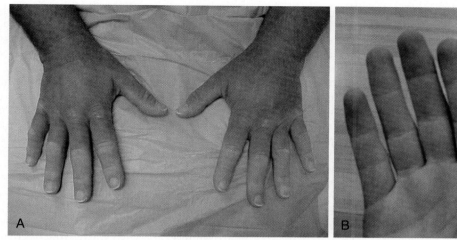

FIGURE 29–1 **A,** Classic presentation of Raynaud Phenomenon with symmetrical, sharply demarcated pallor affecting all fingers and sparing the thumbs. **B,** Cyanosis associated with Raynaud Phenomena typically follows after pallor and represents deoxygenation of slow flowing blood. **A** from: www.clevelandclinic.org/arthritis/treat/facts/Raynaud.htm. **B** from: www.weisshospital.com/medical-services/excellence-centers/vascular/news/09-05-01/May_2009_Cold_Hands_Warm_Heart_Understanding_Cold_Hand_Diseases.aspx.

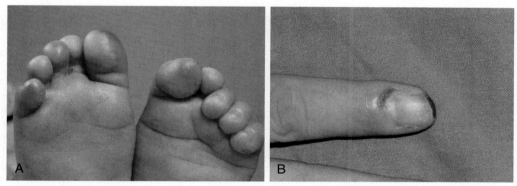

FIGURE 29–2 **A,** Digital ischemia secondary to Raynaud Phenomenon, resulting in painful erythematous plaques (pernio) on the tips of affected toes. **B,** Necrosis of the finger tip and the proximal periungual area associated with Raynaud Phenomenon. **A** from http://emedicine.medscape.com/article/1087946-media. B http://asps.confex.com/asps/2006am/techprogram/paper_10931.htm

Table 29–1

Clinical features of primary and secondary Raynaud Phenomenon

Primary Raynaud Phenomenon
  Episodic vasospastic attacks precipitated by cold or emotional stress
  Symmetrical involvement of distal extremities
  No evidence of peripheral vascular disease
  Absence of tissue necrosis, digital pitting, or gangrene
  Normal nailfold capillary examination
  Negative antinuclear antibody (ANA) test and normal erythrocyte sedimentation rate (ESR)
Secondary Raynaud Phenomenon
  Older age at onset
  Male gender
  Painful, asymmetric attacks with signs of digital ischemia (pernio or ulceration)
  Ischemia proximal to the fingers or toes
  Abnormal nailfold capillary examination with enlarged or distorted capillary loops
  Abnormal laboratory parameters suggesting vascular or autoimmune disease (e.g., elevated ESR or CRP, autoantibodies (ANA, antitopoisomerase, anti-Smith antigen, antiphospholipid), decreased complement levels

or vascular disorder, it is important to recognize that RP may herald significant rheumatic disease. RP occurs at high frequency (80% to 90%) in children with SSc or mixed connective tissue disease (MCTD) and is often the initial symptom of these disorders, preceding other manifestations of disease in some instances by years.[4] New onset RP should, therefore, prompt consideration and examination for signs and symptoms of systemic disease and, potentially, further rheumatological evaluation.

ETIOLOGY/PATHOGENESIS

In his thesis published in 1862, Raynaud ascribed the features he saw to "increased irritability of the central parts of the cord presiding over the vascular innervations."[1,14] Observing that local sympathectomy did not cure RP, Sir Thomas Lewis proposed in 1929 that RP was due to a "local fault," rather than a defect in the central nervous system (CNS).[15] Current data support this view, suggesting that RP primarily represents excessive activation of normal local physiological vasomotor responses to cold temperature (i.e., lowering of blood flow to the skin, thereby reducing the loss of body heat and preserving core body temperature) and/or emotional stress.[2,16-19] In broad terms, blood flow volume is regulated by an interactive system involving neural signals, cellular mediators, circulating hormones, and soluble vasoactive compounds.[20,21] The inherent tone, or contractile activity, of vascular smooth muscle varies substantially between different arterial structures, ranging from relatively high basal tone in the coronary circulation to low or absent in the pulmonary circulation, and it can increase or decrease dramatically.[20] Numerous mechanisms participate in the regulation of vascular tone, including both intrinsic functions of vascular smooth muscle and endothelial cells, and extrinsic effects of nerves, adjacent tissues, circulating cells, and soluble factors (Table 29–2).[21]

The pathophysiological mechanisms influencing RP can be segregated into three broad headings: vascular, neural, and intravascular abnormalities.[22] Vascular dysfunction in primary RP is, by definition, fully reversible, whereas secondary RP may combine defective function and structural abnormalities. Endothelial cells play an active role in regulating vascular tone. Depending on their state of activation, endothelial cells can produce both potent vasodilating agents (e.g., prostacyclin and nitric oxide [NO]) and potent vasoconstricting agents (e.g., endothelins and angiotension). Endothelial NO production, for example, has a large effect on vascular tone, regulating vascular smooth muscle contraction, proliferation, and migration. NO also stimulates platelet disaggregation and hinders the adhesion of platelets, lymphocytes, and neutrophils to the endothelial surface, which can have secondary effects on vascular function. SSc-associated RP fundamentally differs from primary RP because of its associated vasculopathy, involving fibrous intimal proliferation with associated intravascular thrombi. Endothelin-1 and angiotension are potent vasoconstrictors with profibrotic activities that have been shown to be overexpressed in the skin of patients with SSc and other forms of secondary RP.[22] These are but a few examples from a long list of agents and functions proposed to contribute to the pathogenesis of vascular abnormalities in SSc.[16]

Neurotransmitters from both autonomic and sensory afferent nerves also alter digital vascular tone. Blood vessels can receive innervation from three main classes of neurons: sympathetic vasoconstrictor neurons, sympathetic or parasympathetic vasodilator neurons, and sensory neurons that can mediate vasodilation. While the sympathetic nervous system, via release of norepinephrine, is considered a major mediator of vasoconstriction in the skin, local nerve endings also sense the microenvironment and release both vasodilating (substance P, vasoactive intestinal peptide, calcitonin gene-related peptide, neurokinin A) and vasoconstricting (somatostatin, neuropeptide Y) neuropeptides that contribute to the balance of vascular function.[23] Although central mechanisms alone cannot account for the characteristic features of RP, many patients report stress-induced vasospasm, suggesting influence of the CNS on local vasospasm. Studies investigating the differential effects of mental stress on vascular tone and finger perfusion in patients with RP have produced mixed results and have failed to clarify the role of the sympathetic nervous system in the pathogenesis of this disorder.[24] Vascular reactivity is also affected by shear stress, vasoactive substances released by platelets (thromboxane, serotonin), changes in blood viscosity, and changes in the rheological properties of blood (e.g., altered red blood cell deformability), highlighting the complexity of regulatory mechanisms involved.[17,20]

The marked sensitivity to cold in both primary and secondary RP appears to be mediated, at least in part, by an abnormal or enhanced response to stimulation of alpha adrenergic receptors in the digital and cutaneous vessels.[17,21,25] Alpha adrenergic receptors are increased in small vessels relative to larger vessels in normal subjects, and are particularly numerous in cutaneous arteries and veins relative to other tissue beds.[17] In humans, the administration of "selective" alpha-1 and alpha-2 adrenergic agonists causes a reduction in skin or finger blood flow.[26] Cold exposure has been shown to amplify selectively the vascular smooth muscle constriction response to norepinephrine mediated through alpha adrenergic receptors.[17] Estrogen has recently been shown to increase expression of alpha-2 adrenergic receptors in vascular smooth muscle and to increase cold sensitivity, which may explain the greater prevalence of RP among postpubertal women.[27-29] Within the alpha-2 adrenergic receptor family, individual subtypes (e.g., alpha 2a, 2b, and 2c) have been shown to display differing sensitivity to cold in both humans and mice.[30,31] Under normal conditions (37°C), alpha 2c-adrenoreceptors in cutaneous arteries are stored within the Golgi apparatus. Cooling induces activation of a Rho/Rho kinase signaling pathway, prompting translocation of alpha 2c-adrenoreceptor from Golgi complex to the plasma membrane and augmenting sensitivity of contractile proteins to calcium ions.[32] One trigger for Rho/Rho kinase signaling may be a rapid increase of reactive oxygen species (ROS) seen in smooth muscle cells following cold exposure (28°C).[33] Ischemia and reperfusion

---

Table 29–2

Factors influencing vascular reactivity

Arterial smooth muscle cells
  Transmural pressure (autoregulation)
  Oxygen tension/ischemia
  Temperature (decreased temperature selectively increases
    response to norepinephrine)
Endothelial cell products
  Nitric oxide (vasodilation)
  Prostacyclin (vasodilation)
  Endothelin-1 (vasoconstriction)
Sympathetic nervous system
  Norepineprine (vasoconstriction)
Neuropeptides
  Substance P (vasodilation)
  Vasoactive intestinal peptide (vasodilation)
  Calcitonin gene-related peptide (vasodilation)
  Neurokinin A (vasodilation)
  Somatostatin (vasoconstriction)
  Neuropeptide Y (vasoconstriction)
Other
  Shear stress
  Platelet products (thromboxane, serotonin)
  Blood viscosity
  Blood cell deformability
  Estrogen

associated with RP may, in turn, induce production of additional ROS by mitochondria, leading to further activation of the Rho/Rho kinase pathway and provoking repeated or persistent cycles of vasospasm. Selective inhibition of the alpha-2 adrenergic receptor abolishes cold-induced vasoconstriction of isolated blood vessels in vitro,[30] and inhibition of the Rho kinase signaling pathway prevents translocation of the alpha-2 adrenoreceptor from the Golgi to the cell surface on cooling.[32]

Increased contractile protein responses to alpha 2-adrenergic agonists and cooling, and the associated increased Rho/Rho kinase and protein tyrosine kinase activity, are observed in both primary and secondary RP subjects compared to healthy controls. These findings provide a possible unifying explanation for cold-induced vascular reactivity in primary and secondary RP, supply a target of mutations that may contribute to familial and ethnic clustering, and highlight opportunities for the development of new therapeutics.[34,35]

A large number of diseases, disorders, drugs, and environmental exposures have been associated with secondary RP, presumably reflecting a common endpoint of vascular injury and the complex nature of the mechanisms responsible for control of vessel reactivity (Table 29–3).[2,21,36] As noted previously, unique changes in the microvascular system develop in association with intimal fibrosis and endothelial dysfunction in SSc. Changes in endothelial cell function appear to occur at an early stage and are associated with increased platelet adhesion, decreased storage of von Willebrand factor, and decreased adenosine uptake.[22,37-39] Ischemic reperfusion injury results in increased production of ROS, which then alters smooth muscle adrenoreceptor expression and vascular function.[40] However, not all increased vascular reactivity in patients with SSc can be attributed to endothelial injury or fibrosis. These mechanisms may occur with, or even induce, the increase in alpha-2 adrenergic receptor reactivity discussed previously.[41] Other observations in SSc include enhanced endothelial cell proliferation, reduced activity of NO, increased circulating levels of endothelin-1, and increased expression of endothelin receptors.[16,38,42] It is beyond the scope of this chapter to consider the range of potential mechanisms of injury that may affect the vasculature of patients with SSc, and the reader is directed to detailed discussions of these diseases elsewhere in this text.

Intravascular or circulating factors have also been implicated either in the pathogenesis or in the exacerbation of RP, especially when associated with SSc. Platelet activation, defective fibrinolysis, and oxidant stress have all been reported. Although their actions are not fully understood, these intravascular factors may exacerbate the effect of digital vasospasm by reducing basal blood flow in the microvasculature.

DIAGNOSIS

History

The complaint of cold hands or feet is very common and must be distinguished from RP, which involves both cool skin and cutaneous color changes. Normal individuals

Table 29–3
Conditions associated with secondary Raynaud Phenomenon in children

Rheumatological disorders
  Systemic sclerosis
  Mixed connective tissue disease (MCTD)
  Systemic lupus erythematosus (SLE)
  Juvenile dermatomyositis (JDMS)
  Vasculitides
  Sjögren syndrome
  Antiphospholipid syndrome
Primary vasospastic disorders
  Migraine
Mechanical/obstructive disorders
  Primary vasculopathies
  Recurrent trauma/frostbite
  Thoracic outlet syndrome
  Repetitive motion injury/carpal tunnel syndrome
Hyperviscosity/thromboembolic disorders
  Cryoglobulinemia
  Polycythemia
  Sickle cell disease
  Essential thrombocythemia
  Hyperlipidemia
Endocrine disorders
  Carcinoid
  Pheochromocytoma
  Hypothyroidism
Infectious disorders
  Parvovirus B19
  Helicobacter pylori
Chemical/drug exposures
  Chemotherapeutic agents (bleomycin, vinblastine)
  Vasoconstrictive agents (amphetamines, antihistamines, pseudoephedrine, phenylephrine)
  CNS stimulants/ADHD therapeutics (methylphenidate, dextroamphetamine)
  5-hydroxtryptamine receptor antagonists (ergotamine, methysergide)
  Polyvinyl chloride
  Mercury
  Street drugs (cocaine, LSD, ecstasy, psilocybin)
Other
  Down syndrome
  Arteriovenous malformation
  Anorexia nervosa
  Reflex sympathetic dystrophy

may have cool skin and show skin mottling on cold exposure. However, unlike RP, the recovery phase of vascular flow is not delayed, and there is no prolonged or sharp demarcation of color changes in skin. A diagnosis of RP may be made if the patient provides a history of the sudden onset of symptoms characteristic of a Raynaud episode; history alone is accepted as diagnostic in general practice, since no simple clinical test consistently triggers an attack. If necessary, digital arteriolar blood flow can be documented by Doppler flow studies.[43] Characteristic changes have also been reported by plethysmography and arteriography, although the latter is not usually necessary or indicated in patients with severe RP and is performed with some danger of precipitating acute catastrophic arteriolar spasm. In practice, digital artery ultrasound is readily available and depicts the same anatomical structures as angiography; it is cheaper, faster, and noninvasive. While measurement of digital blood pressure, digital blood flow, or skin temperature responses to cooling may be predictive in a research setting, attempts to induce and measure attacks in an office setting are not consistent, even in those with definite RP.[44-47] A simple approach employing the use of standard questionnaires and color photos of actual attacks has proven useful in clinical trials and epidemiological studies.[48,49]

A detailed patient history should be collected and should include affected sites; frequency, severity, and duration of attacks; color pattern; triggers; seasonality; and associated symptoms (i.e., numbness, paresthesia, pain). Patients should also be questioned for any history suggestive of connective tissue disease (CTD). such as unexplained fever, fatigue, rash, morning stiffness, arthralgia, myalgia, dysphagia, peripheral edema, lymphadenopathy, or oral ulcers; about changes in digits, such as pits, ulcers, or poor healing; and about the incidence of infection. They should also be asked about possible associated or precipitating factors including frostbite, drug or toxin exposure, infection, vibration injury, personal and family history of RP or CTDs, migraines, weight loss or eating disorders, and cardiovascular diseases.

Clinical Criteria

Specific criteria for the diagnosis of RP were first proposed in 1932.[50] Several modifications designed to improve the differentiation of primary and secondary RP have been proposed and validated (see Table 29–1).[48,51] The diagnosis of RP is fundamentally based on a history of episodic vasospastic attacks precipitated by cold or stress. Characteristic features include sharply demarcated lesions, bilateral symptoms, and white, blue, and/or red color changes, although the spectrum of symptoms observed is broad.[18] Maricq and colleagues have reported that, among adults who were cold sensitive, only 1% had triphasic color changes, and 37% had white or blue color only.[10] In a retrospective review of 123 pediatric patients, Nigrovic and colleagues reported that 24% of children with primary RP and 19% of children with secondary RP reported triphasic color changes, while 40% to 50% had only monophasic color changes.[5] An interesting crosssectional study of patients in the Netherlands indicated that reactive hyperemia at the end of an attack and discoloration of the earlobes and nose were more likely to be associated with primary RP than with secondary RP.[52]

Significant factors differentiating primary from secondary RP are the absence of evidence for vascular disease by clinical examination (including blood pressure, pulses, and nailfold capillaroscopy) in primary RP, and the presence of abnormal nailfold capillaries and/or laboratory studies suggesting systemic disease in secondary RP. Primary RP attacks typically involve all fingers in a symmetrical pattern and are not commonly associated with significant pain. Asymmetrical finger involvement and severe pain, in contrast, are suggestive of an underlying pathology and should prompt a more vigorous evaluation. Although patients with primary RP are, by definition, generally healthy, comorbid conditions, including hypertension, atherosclerosis, cardiovascular disease, and diabetes mellitus, can increase the frequency or severity

of symptoms (see Table 29–3). Anatomical variants of normal, such as incomplete palmar arterial arch (clinical Allen test) can augment vasospasm, leading to earlier and more severe presentations.[53] An issue important in the evaluation of children with RP is the use of stimulants for attention deficit disorder, which may exacerbate vascular dysfunction.[54]

As indicated previously, the regulation of regional blood flow is complex and susceptible to a variety of insults. Also, the number of disorders associated with RP is extensive (see Table 29–3).[2] As research progresses, the border between idiopathic and "disease"-associated symptoms blurs. Ultimately, primary RP is a diagnosis of exclusion supported by lack of progression to development of an associated disorder over time. While extensive special testing is not always necessary, every patient with a diagnosis of RP should be carefully evaluated for features that suggest a concurrent or incipient disease. Among these, the rheumatological diagnoses most often associated with secondary RP are SSc, MCTD, and other CTDs (e.g., systemic lupus erythematosus, overlap syndromes, polymyositis, dermatomyositis, Sjogren syndrome, and vasculitis). Other disorders that must be considered include occlusive vascular disease, drug effects, hematological abnormalities, and other vasospastic syndromes (see Table 29–3 and later discussion).[2,55] Standard clinical tests, such as chest radiography, pulmonary function tests, electrocardiography, echocardiography, high-resolution lung computerized tomography scanning, or gastrointestinal (GI) evaluation, may be needed to evaluate a patient for associated rheumatic and nonrheumatic disorders.

Nailfold Capillary Microscopy

Nailfold capillary microscopy is a simple, yet powerful diagnostic tool shown to improve significantly the predictive power of clinical evaluation.[51,56-60] The examination can be performed at the bedside using a handheld magnifier or with a low power microscope (Fig. 29–3). Enlarged or distorted capillary loops, telangiectasias, and a relative paucity or loss of capillary loops strongly suggests a concurrent or incipient CTD. The presence of these features in a patient with RP should prompt a quick and vigorous search for related findings.

Laboratory Testing

If the history and physical examination, including nailfold capillary microscopy, are not suggestive of a cause for secondary RP, a diagnosis of primary RP may be made, and there is no need for further specialized testing. In particular, blood tests, such as the erythrocyte sedimentation rate and antinuclear antibody (ANA), are not necessary and may be misleading. If, however, there is a moderate or high clinical suspicion of a secondary cause of RP, then special testing is appropriate as indicated by the clinical assessment. Recommended laboratory testing for possible connective tissue disorders includes a complete blood count, a general blood chemical analysis with tests of renal and liver function, urinalysis, complement (C3 and C4), and ANA. If the ANA is

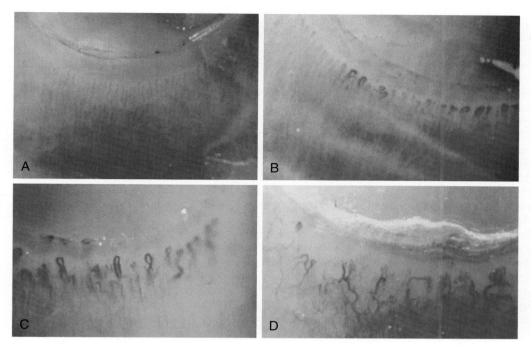

FIGURE 29-3 Nailfold capillaroscopy. **A,** Normal nailfold capillary size and distribution. **B,** Early changes of scleroderma showing dilation, tortuosity, and disorganization. **C,** Active stage scleroderma showing increasingly disorganized architecture, giant capillaries and hemorrhage, decreased number of vessels, and increased frequency of abnormal vessels. **D,** Late stage scleroderma showing severe dropout and abnormal vessels with arborization. From www.hakeem-sy.com/main/node/20196.

positive, tests for specific autoantibodies may assist with formulating a diagnosis (e.g., anti-double stranded DNA, anti-SSA [Ro], anti-SSB [La], anti-ribonucleoprotein, anti-topoisomerase (anti-Scl 70), and anti-phospholipid antibodies). Anticentromere pattern ANA and anti-Scl 70 antibodies have the highest sensitivity for predicting evolution to SSc and the risk for development of digital ischemia, including ulcers and digit loss.[18,61,62] It is important to recognize that while most pediatric patients with secondary RP will have a positive ANA (85% to 100%), a significant number of pediatric patients with primary RP also have a positive ANA without evidence for an associated rheumatic disorder.[4,5,63,64] Conversely, in a cohort of 1039 adult patients monitored prospectively, only 6.3% of patients with negative autoantibody studies developed CTD over more than 10 years of follow-up, while nearly 60% of patients with RP and a positive ANA were ultimately diagnosed with a CTD.[65] About 30% of pediatric patients with primary or secondary RP were also found to have antiphospholipid antibodies, although none of the patients had features of antiphospholipid syndrome.[5]

Although anticentromere or anti-topoisomerase antibodies are associated with development of SSc,[62] the combination of autoantibodies and nailfold capillary microscopy may be more informative than either test alone. In a 20-year prospective study of 586 patients with RP who had no known CTD at enrollment, the overall incidence of limited (CREST variant) or diffuse SSc was 13%.[66] In patients with one or more related autoantibodies or abnormal nailfold capillary microscopy, the incidence of SSc was 47%, while in those with both an autoantibody and abnormal nailfold capillary microscopy, the incidence of SSc was nearly 80%. Further discussion of the clinical evaluation of systemic rheumatologic disorders and the significance of autoantibodies in the prognosis of SSc is included elsewhere in this text (Chapter 25).

Differential Diagnosis

The differential diagnosis for RP should include consideration of the extensive list of conditions in Table 29–3. In patients who present with prolonged peripheral vasoconstriction, it is particularly important to distinguish whether they are experiencing a thrombotic event rather than transient ischemia. Although an exhaustive discussion of these possibilities is beyond the scope of this chapter, the following paragraphs represent disorders commonly considered in the differential diagnosis of nonclassic RP.

Acrocyanosis is an uncommon, painless, vasospastic disorder causing persistent coldness and bluish discoloration of the hands (and less commonly of the feet).[42] Patients with acrocyanosis have cold and diffusely cyanotic color changes that can involve the entire hand and foot, extending proximally without a sharp demarcation between affected and unaffected tissue. Mild diaphoresis may be present, creating a clammy feel to the extremities. Mild abnormalities may exist but do not show the avascular regions or giant capillaries found in patients with scleroderma.[67] Both acrocyanosis and RP are more common in individuals with low body weight or who have anorexia nervosa.[68] Evaluation for cyanotic heart disease, eating disorders, or GI malabsorption should be considered.

Perniosis, or chilblains, is a cold-induced condition marked by the appearance of painful, erythematous, papular, or nodular lesions, usually located on the fingers, toes, thighs, and buttocks.[69,70] As with RP, perniosis may present as an idiopathic process or in association with systemic disease (i.e. SLE). It is distinguished from RP by the lack of blanching. Although clinically and histologically distinct from RP, the treatment paradigms are similar and based primarily on nonpharmacological lifestyle modifications. Although definitive data are lacking, many of the other agents used for RP can be considered if pharmacological intervention is necessary.

Frostbite is relatively common in cold climates and can have prolonged sequelae including persistent cold sensitivity. In a study of 30 patients who had suffered moderate (second degree) frostbite, Ervasti and colleagues reported subjective symptoms at 4 to 11 years after injury in 63% of the subjects, including hypersensitivity to cold, numbness, and decreased touch sensitivity. Cold air provocation testing revealed an increased tendency for vasospasm in these patients, including white fingers in 20%.[55]

Carpal Tunnel Syndrome is relatively rare in children and is more often idiopathic or secondary to lysosomal storage disorders, rather than related to overuse as is seen in adults.[71] Symptoms are more characteristically numbness and reduced manual dexterity, rather than color changes, and are generally not related to cold exposure. Although the wrist-flexion test (Phalen maneuver) and the nerve compression or percussion test (Tinel sign) can be informative, they are often nondiagnostic in pediatric patients, and electrophysiological testing is indicated to confirm a diagnostic suspicion.

Brachial or lumbosacral plexus neuropathies are also rare in children, outside of those related to birth injury, but may present in older adolescents and young adults seen in pediatric clinics.[72] The typical presentation of idiopathic brachial plexus neuritis (Parsonage-Turner syndrome) or lumbosacral plexopathy includes acute onset of shoulder or proximal leg pain, respectively, associated with weakness and muscle wasting in the extremity and without restricted passive range of motion. Numbness and color changes in the extremity are variable, but fixed and less prominent a complaint than pain and neuromuscular symptoms. Idiopathic plexus neuropathies often follow an upper respiratory infection and may be recurrent. Electromyographic findings are characteristic and diagnostic. Prognosis is generally good, though recovery may be protracted and may require intensive physical therapy to reduce contractures and restore muscle strength.

Erythromelalgia is a rare condition of paroxysmal vasodilation. Erythromelalgia can be thought of as the opposite of RP. Symptoms manifest as episodic burning pain accompanied by erythema, warmth and swelling of the hands and/or feet; they are often brought on by heat, exercise, or friction, and affected patients report dramatic relief with application of ice or cold water. Erythromelalgia also presents in both primary and secondary forms. Primary erythromelalgia presents in childhood and can be familial (autosomal dominant) or sporadic. It affects girls more than boys, symptoms are most often symmetrical, and it is frequently resistant to treatment. Recent studies have attributed a majority of both familial and sporadic cases to gain-of-function mutations of SCN9A, the gene that encodes the voltage-gated sodium channel $Na(v)1.7$.[73] Loss-of-function mutations in the same gene are associated with congenital insensitivity to pain. Secondary erythromelalgia is more common and typically presents in older children and adults. The majority of cases are associated with essential thrombocytosis and are characteristically responsive to low dose aspirin therapy.[74] Erythromelalgia can also develop in patients with small fiber neuropathies of many sources, including multiple sclerosis, hypercholesterolemia, mercury and other heavy-metal poisoning, and a variety of autoimmune diseases. These patients are not responsive to aspirin, but the condition typically responds to treatment of the underlying disorder. Management of erythromelalgia includes avoidance of triggers (heat, friction) and application of cold during acute attacks. If aspirin or treatment of associated conditions is unsuccessful, a variety of attempts at interventions have been reported. Although controlled studies are lacking, case studies have reported successful use of a range of pharmacological (e.g., nifedipine, verapamil, propranolol, nitroprusside), non-pharmacological (e.g., biofeedback, hypnosis), and surgical (sympathectomy, amputation, stereotactic destruction of regions of the hypothalamus) approaches.

Complex regional pain syndrome (CRPS), or reflex sympathetic dystrophy, will often present with altered coloration of the involved extremity.[75] Patients with CRPS usually have unilateral distal limb involvement, with the affected area showing differences in temperature (warmer or colder) and color (red, pale, or mottled) compared with the unaffected side. These patients typically describe severe diffuse allodynia; paresthesia, causalgia or other abnormal sensations; refusal to move the affected region; and unusual positioning of the affected extremity. A detailed discussion of CRPS can be found elsewhere in this text (Chapter 48).

TREATMENT

Recent insights into pathogenesis have led to promising new therapies that affect the treatment algorithm for RP. Treatment choices depend on the severity of digital ischemia and the presence of underlying disease. Patients with primary RP do not generally report significant disability, although quality of life may be affected by symptoms and the need for cold avoidance. Spontaneous remission or improvement is also common. In a prospective survey of a middle-aged white population with new onset RP, remissions occurred in 64% of both women and men over a seven-year period.[9] Thus, a conservative, non-pharmacological approach is often sufficient and most appropriate for these patients. By comparison, patients with secondary RP are more likely to have more severe attacks and to require pharmacological agents to achieve symptomatic control.[2,76,77] Treatment of these patients is often problematic, because pharmacological side-effects are often dose-limiting, responses to vasodilators are idiosyncratic, and there is lack of agreement as to measures of objective improvement. Clinical trials also consistently demonstrate a high rate of improvement (10% to 40%) among placebo-treated patients with either primary or secondary RP. This not only supports the recommendation that general education is an important factor in controlling attacks, but it emphasizes the importance of placebo-controlled trials in evaluating the efficacy of specific therapies.

General Measures

Patients with either primary or secondary RP benefit from education regarding the common triggers of Raynaud attacks, and simple interventions to help prevent and terminate an episode (Table 29–4).[2,78] Nonpharmacological therapeutic interventions include avoidance of cold temperatures, stress, and vasoconstrictors; the use of warm/layered clothing; and techniques to terminate an attack, such as massage, windmill motions of the arms, and immersion in warm water. Since sympathetic tone and sensitivity to sympathetic mediators are enhanced in patients with RP, reduction of emotional stress and anxiety are important treatment goals.[79]

Behavioral Therapy

A variety of behavioral therapies (e.g., biofeedback, autogenic training, classic conditioning) have been employed in patients with RP.[78] Multiple studies have demonstrated that normal subjects can voluntarily control peripheral blood flow and skin temperature.[80,81] Studies exploring the use of these techniques in RP vary greatly in their methodological rigor. Many lack no-treatment controls and, in general, they report an effect size similar to that of placebo-response seen in other trials. In one well-controlled randomized study of primary RP, the authors found no benefit with temperature or electromyogenic biofeedback, and they reported that sustained release nifedipine was superior to either behavioral method.[82] Similarly, a study of biofeedback in 24 scleroderma patients failed to demonstrate either symptomatic improvement or increased finger temperature in response to voluntary control or cold stress.[83] Although controlled trials have not shown dramatic effects, behavioral therapies and education can be helpful to reduce stress related triggers and to improve compliance with both pharmacological and nonpharmacological interventions. Thus, while behavioral therapies alone are unlikely to be sufficient to control symptoms in secondary forms of RP, they can provide substantial benefit as an adjunct to medical interventions. Overall, these approaches appear to be safe.

Pharmacological Measures

A variety of agents have been used to treat RP with varying degrees of support from controlled trials (Table 29–5).[2,61,84] *Calcium channel blockers* (CCB) are the most commonly prescribed agents, and their efficacy has been well-proven in controlled trials with both pediatric and adult patients.[85] Use of alternative vasodilator agents as first-line therapy for the treatment of even severe RP is not recommended, since CCB have been shown to be effective and are often better tolerated. However, because individual responses may be idiosyncratic, patients who do not tolerate or who fail to respond adequately to CCB can be treated with other vasoactive agents alone or, more commonly, in combination with a CCB.[2] Many other vasoactive drugs have been reported in the treatment of RP.[61,84] A brief summary of major findings is included below, and algorithms for management of primary or mild RP and complex RP with digital ischemia are shown in Figures 29–4 and 29–5. For patients with uncomplicated primary RP, medical therapy should only be considered in patients who fail vigorous application of nonpharmacological measures. In these cases, a long acting CCB, such as controlled-release nifedipine or amlodipine, is the initial

treatment of choice. Titrating to lowest effective dose and use of medications only during periods of expected cold exposure (e.g., winter months) can help to minimize medication exposure in patients with minimal risk (primary RP and mild secondary RP).[2,121] Due to their condition, patients with secondary or more severe RP are likely to require more aggressive therapy. In these patients, it is unlikely that medical therapy will completely terminate attacks, and it is not useful to use this as the primary goal or measure of effectiveness of treatment. Instead, the major goals of treatment in secondary RP are to reduce the frequency of attacks and to prevent new digital ulceration.

Table 29–4

General measures for the management of the Raynaud Phenomenon

Avoid sudden cold exposure
Minimize emotional stress
Dress warmly (layered clothing, long sleeves and pants, socks, thermal underwear, and heat conserving hats)
Keep hands/feet warm (e.g., mittens, electric or chemical hand/foot warmers)
Use warming methods to terminate attacks, e.g., place hands under warm water or in a warm body fold (e.g., axillae), rotate arms in a windmill pattern or swing-arm maneuver (forceful side-to-side swinging motion)
Avoid rapidly changes in temperature, such as quickly moving from a hot to cool environments, cool breezes, or humid cold air.
Avoid cigarette smoking and exposure to secondhand smoke
Avoid sympathomimetic drugs and central nervous system stimulants (e.g., decongestants, amphetamines, diet pills, methylphenidate, and dextroamphetamine)

Table 29–5

The Pharmacological treatment of Raynaud Phenomenon

Calcium channel blockers
  Nifedipine, amlodipine, diltiazem, felodipine, nisoldipine, and isradipine
Direct vasodilators
  Nitroglycerin, nitroprusside, hydralazine, papaverine, minoxidil, niacin, and nitric oxide (via a generating system)
Indirect vasodilators
  Angiotension converting enzymes inhibitor (captopril)
  Angiotensin receptor blockers (losartan)
  Endothelin-1 inhibitors (bosentan)
  Phosphodiesterase inhibitors (sildenafil, pentoxifylline)
  Serotonin reuptake inhibitors (fluoxetine)
Sympatholytic agents (alpha-adrenergic receptor blockers)
  Methyldopa, reserpine, phentolamine, and prazosin
Prostaglandins
  Prostaglandin E_1 (PGE_1) (aloprostadil)
  Prostacyclin (PGI2) (epoprostenol)
Antioxidant agents
  Zinc gluconate
  N-acetylcysteine
Anticoagulation, antithrombotic and thrombolytic agents
  Aspirin
  Dipyridamole
  Heparin
  Tissue plasminogen activator
Other
  Botulinum toxin A

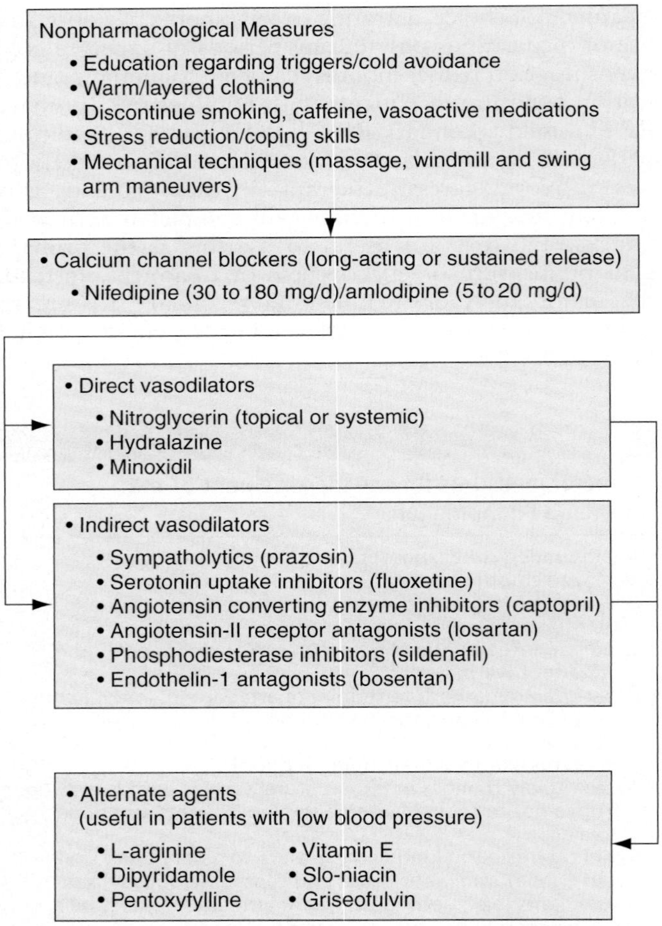

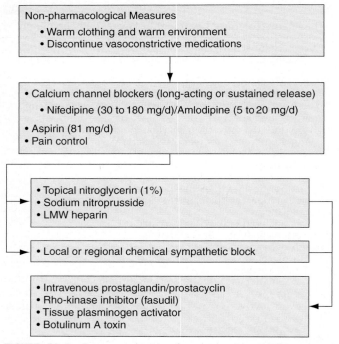

Nonpharmacological Measures
- Education regarding triggers/cold avoidance
- Warm/layered clothing
- Discontinue smoking, caffeine, vasoactive medications
- Stress reduction/coping skills
- Mechanical techniques (massage, windmill and swing arm maneuvers)

- Calcium channel blockers (long-acting or sustained release)
  - Nifedipine (30 to 180 mg/d)/amlodipine (5 to 20 mg/d)

- Direct vasodilators
  - Nitroglycerin (topical or systemic)
  - Hydralazine
  - Minoxidil

- Indirect vasodilators
  - Sympatholytics (prazosin)
  - Serotonin uptake inhibitors (fluoxetine)
  - Angiotensin converting enzyme inhibitors (captopril)
  - Angiotensin-II receptor antagonists (losartan)
  - Phosphodiesterase inhibitors (sildenafil)
  - Endothelin-1 antagonists (bosentan)

- Alternate agents
  (useful in patients with low blood pressure)
  - L-arginine   - Vitamin E
  - Dipyridamole   - Slo-niacin
  - Pentoxyfylline   - Griseofulvin

FIGURE 29–4   Treatment algorithm for uncomplicated Raynaud Phenomenon.

Non-pharmacological Measures
- Warm clothing and warm environment
- Discontinue vasoconstrictive medications

- Calcium channel blockers (long-acting or sustained release)
  - Nifedipine (30 to 180 mg/d)/Amlodipine (5 to 20 mg/d)
- Aspirin (81 mg/d)
- Pain control

- Topical nitroglycerin (1%)
- Sodium nitroprusside
- LMW heparin

- Local or regional chemical sympathetic block

- Intravenous prostaglandin/prostacyclin
- Rho-kinase inhibitor (fasudil)
- Tissue plasminogen activator
- Botulinum A toxin

FIGURE 29–5   Treatment algorithm for complex Raynaud Phenomenon/digital ischemia.

Calcium Channel Blockers

CCB are the most widely used class of drugs in the treatment of RP. In addition to their vasodilating properties, CCB have biological effects, including inhibitions of platelet activation that are beneficial in management of RP.[86] Among the different pharmacological classes, the dihydropyridine group (nifedipine, amlodipine, felodipine) is the least cardioselective and appears to be the most efficacious. Variability of reported responses occurs, in part, because patients with secondary RP (particularly SSc) are less likely to benefit from nifedipine and other CCB than those with primary RP, and not all trials clearly segregate primary and secondary RP populations. Two metaanalyses of randomized, double-blind, placebo-controlled trials assessing efficacy of CCB (primarily nifedipine) in primary and secondary (SSc-associated) RP have reported benefit, with a significant reduction in mean number of attacks and in severity of symptoms in both groups.[85,87] Results were more significant for secondary RP than primary RP. Primary RP patients generally have lower degrees of severity and were treated with lower doses of CCB, which may have lowered the measured effectiveness in these studies. Therapeutic benefit in practice, therefore, may be even greater than predicted from these results. For the management of nonurgent RP, slow release or long-acting preparations of nifedipine (30 to 180 mg daily) or amlodipine (5 to 20 mg daily) are recommended to improve compliance, reduce the incidence of adverse effects, and potentially achieve more sustained vascular improvement. Adverse effects, including headache and lower extremity edema, require discontinuation or dose modification in approximately 15% of patients and can be minimized by initiating therapy at a low dose with a sustained-release preparation.

Angiotensin Inhibitors

Angiotensin converting enzyme inhibitors and angiotensin II receptor antagonists have experienced a sharp increase in interest based on increasing awareness of their effects on endothelial function and vascular remodeling, though only limited trials have been completed.[84] A randomized, parallel-group, controlled trial of losartan, an angiotensin II receptor antagonist, significantly reduced the frequency and severity of vasoconstrictive episodes in patients with primary and SSc-related RP, and its effects were comparable with sustained-release nifedipine.[88] Although these results are promising, further investigation is needed to establish the role of these agents in the treatment of RP.

Serotonin Receptor Inhibitors

Selective Serotonin Receptor Inhibitors such as fluoxetine and ketanserin, have engendered strong interest due to their potential effects on both local and CNS-mediated mechanisms regulating vasoconstriction. Although there are many anecdotal reports of benefit,[84] there have been few well-designed, placebo-controlled studies of their use in RP, and results have been mixed. Further studies are required before recommendations related to their use in daily management can be made.

Phosphodiesterase Inhibitors

Phosphodiesterase Inhibitors, including sildenafil, have been promoted based on their effectiveness in improvement of peripheral and pulmonary circulation in other conditions. Although studies reported to date are suggestive, additional work is needed to assess adequately the role of these agents in primary and secondary RP.[17,61,84,89]

Endothelin Inhibitors

Bosentan, an oral, nonpeptide endothelin receptor antagonist, has been shown to be effective in the treatment of both idiopathic and SSc-related pulmonary hypertension.[17,61] Two placebo-controlled randomized clinical trials among SSc patients (RAPIDS-1 and RAPIDS-2) have demonstrated the efficacy of bosentan in preventing new digital ulcers, although, there was no reduction in frequency or intensity of RP attacks, and no improvement in the healing of existing digital ulcers.[90] Endothelin receptor antagonists, including bosentan, are considered teratogenic and should be used only when appropriate measures to prevent pregnancy are in place.[91]

Antioxidants

Increased awareness of the importance of oxidative stress in the pathogenesis of RP has stimulated interest in antioxidant therapy; however, evidence of benefit from controlled studies is lacking. In a pilot study of 22 patients with SSc, treatment with intravenous N-acetylcysteine improved the frequency and severity of RP episodes and reduced the number of unhealed ulcers.[92] A randomized, parallel group study of 40 patients with primary and secondary RP treated with probucol, a cholesterol lowering and antioxidant agent, showed only a modest effect on the frequency and severity of Raynaud attacks,[93] and a double-blind, placebo-controlled study of 33 patients with SSc-associated RP demonstrated no benefit after 20 weeks of treatment with micronutrient antioxidants (selenium, beta-carotene, vitamin C, vitamin E, and methionine) and allopurinol (which blocks superoxide).[94] It is possible that antioxidant therapy must be started early to be effective, but the current data do not support a substantial benefit.

Nitric Oxide

Although the specific role NO plays in the pathophysiology of RP remains to be elucidated, there is considerable interest in its therapeutic use. Supplementation of NO has been explored in several ways, including administration of its precursor, L-arginine, and treatment with NO donors, including topical glyceryl trinitrate and parenteral sodium nitroprusside. Small studies of topical glyceryl trinitrate (1%) significantly reduced the number and severity of Raynaud attacks in both primary and secondary RP when compared with placebo.[95,96] Oral L-arginine supplementation for 28 days did not produce any benefits in RP, but intraarterial L-arginine and sodium nitroprusside both significantly improved the response to an acute cold challenge in patients with SSc.[97-99] Further studies are needed to explore the potential benefits of NO therapy.

Calcitonin gene related peptide

Calcitonin gene related peptide (CGRP), a neuropeptide found in sensory nerves, has been shown to be present in lower concentrations in patients with RP when compared with controls. In one study of patients with severe RP, intravenous CGRP improved hand and digital blood flow, skin temperature, and hand rewarming, compared to saline, and it resulted in healing of digital ulcers in four of five patients.[100]

Alpha-Adrenergic Blockade

As highlighted previously, it is increasingly clear that sympathetic adrenergic stimulation, particularly of the alpha-2 adrenergic receptors on the digital arteries, plays an important role in the pathogenesis of RP.[2] Although a variety of sympatholytic drugs have been tried in RP patients, few controlled studies are available to define the role of these agents, and there is some evidence that patients become refractory with prolonged use. In a placebo-controlled trial, the alpha-1 adrenergic receptor antagonist prazosin provided modest improvement in SSc-associated RP, but frequent side effects were noted.[101] Preclinical studies and early trials of more selective alpha-adrenergic blockers, including selective alpha-2c adrenergic receptor antagonists, have stimulated new interest in evaluating the digital vascular effects of agents in this drug class.[102,103]

Rho-Kinase Inhibition

Recent data indicating that Rho-kinases are directly involved in cold-induced vasoconstriction has prompted increasing interest in inhibition of this pathway.[104] Fasudil, a Rho-kinase inhibitor, has been shown to have significant acute vasodilator effects in patients with pulmonary hypertension and other vasospastic conditions.[105-107] Rho-kinase inhibitors represent an innovative and distinct set of therapeutic agents for RP that merit further clinical investigation.

Botulinum Toxin-A

Botulinum toxin-A (Botox®) inhibits acetylcholine signaling, causing flaccid paralysis and inhibition of signaling through C-type pain fibers. In a case series of 11 patients with vasospasm who failed aggressive medical therapy, all patients treated with perivascular injections of botulinum toxin-A experienced significant pain reduction, and 9 of 11 patients reported digital ulcer healing and decreased severity and frequency of vasospastic episodes.[108]

Prostanoids

Prostanoids can be predicted to have a number of beneficial effects in patients with RP, including vasodilation, inhibiting platelet aggregation, suppressing profibrotic cytokines, connective tissue growth factors, and affecting vascular remodeling. Limited availability of nonparenteral agents and significant side-effects of therapy have limited use primarily to treatment of severe refractory RP and ischemic digital ulcers. In these patients, a variety of studies have examined the efficacy of preparations of prostaglandin E1 (PGE1),[109] prostacyclin (PGI2),[110] and iloprost (a PGI2 analog).[111-114] Mixed results have been obtained so far, since these agents are generally only considered in exceptionally refractive cases involving digital ulceration or ischemia. Intravenous iloprost has been shown to be beneficial in children with RP, but it is not available in the United States. An inhalation product (Ventavis) is available in the United States with an indication for treatment of pulmonary hypertension, though experience with its use for RP is limited.[115] Epoprostenol has also been reported as beneficial in pediatric patients with severe RP with digital ischemia, although cost and the need for continuous intravenous infusion limit clinical use.[116] New oral and transdermal agents are approaching the market, and it will be interesting to study their effectiveness in patients with severe RP.[117]

Antithrombotic agents

Antithrombotic agents are commonly considered in patients with RP in whom ulceration and thrombosis have occurred, although published data are largely case-based and limited.[118] Antiplatelet therapy with aspirin (75 or 81 mg/day) should be considered in patients with secondary RP who have a history of ischemic ulcers or other thrombotic events; however, aspirin could theoretically worsen vasospasm via reduction in the production of vasodilating prostaglandins, such as prostacyclin. Similarly, dipyridamole has been used for its antiplatelet and vasodilating properties, but this agent does not appear to have a major impact in patients with severe RP. Anticoagulation or thrombolytic therapy can be considered during the acute phase of an ischemic event, but controlled trials are lacking, and these treatments are best limited to acute care of embolic or vascular occlusive disease associated with new thrombosis.[118] A small placebo controlled study of long-term therapy with low molecular weight heparin was associated with a reduction in the severity of RP after four and 20 weeks.[119] Small studies have also suggested that thrombolytic therapy, such as tissue plasminogen activator, may be helpful in patients with RP and scleroderma.[120] However, controlled studies will need to be performed before it is known if this approach will reverse acute ischemia in severe RP.

Other measures

Sympathectomy

Sympathectomy has been used to treat RP for more than 50 years.[2,76] Temporary local (digital or wrist block) or regional (cervical or lumbar) chemical sympathectomy to reverse vasoconstriction can be performed with lidocaine or bupivacaine (without epinephrine). This form of sympathectomy may not have a long-lasting benefit, but it is sometimes successful in reversing severe acute vasospasm (e.g., critical digital ischemia) that is slowly or poorly responsive to medical therapy.[121] Localized microsurgical digital sympathectomy has been introduced as an alternative to proximal sympathectomy.[122] Although case series have reported successful responses and few complications, sympathectomy's role has not been defined by controlled investigations. Differences in causes of ischemia, surgical technique, and outcome measures make interpretation of the reported series difficult. It is also unclear if benefits of sympathectomy persist over time. The available data suggest variable rates of benefit at one year and high rates of relapse.[121] At present, it appears these procedures should be limited to patients who have failed medical treatment and who have ischemia or severe RP.

Vascular Reconstruction

Occlusion of a major artery can occur in patients with secondary RP. Microsurgical revascularization of the hand and digital arterial reconstruction may improve digital vascular perfusion and heal digital ulcers when proximal arterial occlusion is associated with digital vasospasm. As an example, in patients with SSc, arterial occlusion most commonly occurs in the ulnar artery and the proper digital arteries. Revascularization of the ulnar artery in this setting may improve RP and improve healing of digital ulcers.[123]

Management of Digital Ischemia

The keys to success in the setting of critical digital ischemia are early intervention and rapid escalation (Figure 29–5). Patients with severe digital ischemia, uncontrolled pain, or impending digital amputation should be hospitalized and kept warm and quiet. Pain due to severe ischemia may be intense, and adequate pain control may require the use of narcotic analgesics or a regional nerve block. All complex cases should be fully evaluated for reversible processes that may be causing or aggravating the crisis, including correctable macrovascular disease, vasculitis, or hypercoagulable states. Angiography can be helpful in distinguishing reversible from nonreversible obstruction and in directing diagnostic and therapeutic decisions.

Hospitalized patients should receive aggressive vasodilator therapy with either extended release nifedipine or amlodipine (at the highest tolerated dose) and antiplatelet therapy with aspirin as initial therapy. Antibiotics should be considered if the area of ischemia appears infected. If normal blood flow is not restored within a few hours, then combination therapy, such as addition of transdermal nitroglycerin or a sympatholytic agent is suggested. Treatment with heparin for a period of 24 to 72 hours is suggested if digital ischemia progresses during vasodilator therapy, and/or the onset of arterial occlusion is thought to be secondary to acute thrombosis or embolization, but no trials have assessed this treatment. Temporary chemical sympathectomy should be considered when oral and/or topical vasodilator therapy does not quickly result in improvement in digital blood flow. If temporary chemical sympathectomy succeeds in reversing vasospasm and relieving critical ischemia, it suggests that the structural arterial disease is not advanced. If ischemia recurs as the effects of chemical sympathectomy wane, despite the ongoing use of vasodilator therapy, surgical sympathectomy or perivascular injections of botulinum toxin A can be considered. If these measures do not reverse the ischemia, or if the clinical presentation is severe (e.g., multiple ischemic digits, limb threatening ischemia), an intravenous infusion of a prostaglandin (PGE1) or prostacyclin (PGI2) analogue may be beneficial.[109,111-114,124] Intravenous iloprost, in particular, has been reported to be safe and effective in the treatment of ischemic digits in children with SSc and other CTDs.[125] In patients with late stage ischemia or severe structural arterial disease who cannot vasodilate in response to medical therapy, pain control and surgical amputation may be the only options.

FUTURE DIRECTIONS

RP is a common presenting feature among patients seen in pediatric clinics and should be evaluated with an eye toward identification of causes of secondary RP. Both primary and secondary RP patients will benefit from education and nonpharmacological control measures. This is often all that is required for primary RP, while patients with secondary RP more often require medical therapy. First-line drug therapy for RP is most commonly a long acting CCB, given during symptomatic periods or seasons. A variety of agents are available, and they can be used in combination with CCB therapy for patients requiring more aggressive care. Severe or critical digital ischemia requires immediate evaluation to identify reversible vascular and coagulation defects and aggressive intervention to restore blood flow. Consideration should be given to pain control, vasodilatation, anticoagulation, and chemical or surgical sympathectomy in management of these patients.

The complexity involved in conducting clinical trials of RP and the lack of standard outcome measures remain a challenge to investigators. However, advances in the understanding of the pathogenesis of RP and the development of complementary therapeutics continue to provide improved outcomes for patients, particularly for those with severe disease. The indications that primary RP reflects a fundamental vascular disorder with a genetic basis is an area ripe for future investigation. Preliminary results with novel vasoactive therapies suggest many opportunities exist for development of even more effective therapies on the horizon.

REFERENCES

2. R. Bakst, J.F. Merola, A.G. Franks Jr., et al., Raynaud Phenomenon: pathogenesis and management, J. Am. Acad. Dermatol. 59 (2008) 633–653.
3. B.H. Athreya, Vasospastic disorders in children, Semin. Pediatr. Surg. 3 (1994) 70–78.
4. C.M. Duffy, R.M. Laxer, P. Lee, et al., Raynaud syndrome in childhood, J. Pediatr. 114 (1989) 73–78.
5. P.A. Nigrovic, R.C. Fuhlbrigge, R.P. Sundel, Raynaud Phenomenon in children: a retrospective review of 123 patients, Pediatrics 111 (2003) 715–721.
6. F.M. Wigley, Clinical manifestations and diagnosis of the Raynaud Phenomenon, in: J. Axford (Ed.), UpToDate, Medical Resource, Waltham, MA, 2009.
8. E.C. LeRoy, T.A. Medsger Jr., Raynaud Phenomenon: a proposal for classification, Clin. Exp. Rheumatol. 10 (1992) 485–488.
9. L.G. Suter, J.M. Murabito, D.T. Felson, et al., The incidence and natural history of Raynaud Phenomenon in the community, Arthritis Rheum. 52 (2005) 1259–1263.
10. H.R. Maricq, P.H. Carpentier, M.C. Weinrich, et al., Geographic variation in the prevalence of Raynaud Phenomenon: a 5 region comparison, J. Rheumatol. 24 (1997) 879–889.
12. G.T. Jones, A.L. Herrick, S.E. Woodham, et al., Occurrence of Raynaud Phenomenon in children ages 12-15 years: prevalence and association with other common symptoms, Arthritis Rheum. 48 (2003) 3518–3521.
16. N.A. Flavahan, S. Flavahan, S. Mitra, et al., The vasculopathy of Raynaud Phenomenon and scleroderma, Rheum. Dis. Clin. North. Am. 29 (2003) 275–291.
17. F. Boin, F.M. Wigley, Understanding, assessing and treating Raynaud Phenomenon, Curr. Opin. Rheumatol. 17 (2005) 752–760.
18. F.M. Wigley, Clinical practice. Raynaud Phenomenon, N. Engl. J. Med. 347 (2002) 1001–1008.
19. C. Sunderkotter, G. Riemekasten, Pathophysiology and clinical consequences of Raynaud Phenomenon related to systemic sclerosis, Rheumatology (Oxford) 45 (2006) iii33–35.
21. F.M. Wigley, Pathogenesis of Raynaud Phenomena, in: J. Axford (Ed.), UpToDate, Medical Resource, Waltham, MA, 2009.
22. A.L. Herrick, Pathogenesis of Raynaud Phenomenon, Rheumatology (Oxford) 44 (2005) 587–596.
30. M.A. Chotani, S. Flavahan, S. Mitra, et al., Silent alpha(2C)-adrenergic receptors enable cold-induced vasoconstriction in cutaneous arteries, Am. J. Physiol. Heart Circ. Physiol. 278 (2000) H1075–H1083.
31. M.A. Chotani, S. Mitra, B.Y. Su, et al., Regulation of alpha(2)-adrenoceptors in human vascular smooth muscle cells, Am. J. Physiol. Heart Circ. Physiol. 286 (2004) H59–H67.
32. S.R. Bailey, A.H. Eid, S. Mitra, et al., Rho kinase mediates cold-induced constriction of cutaneous arteries: role of alpha2C-adrenoceptor translocation, Circ. Res. 94 (2004) 1367–1374.
34. P.B. Furspan, S. Chatterjee, M.D. Mayes, et al., Cooling-induced contraction and protein tyrosine kinase activity of isolated arterioles in secondary Raynaud Phenomenon, Rheumatology (Oxford) 44 (2005) 488–494.
36. J.A. Block, W. Sequeira, Raynaud Phenomenon, Lancet 357 (2001) 2042–2048.
39. M.B. Kahaleh, Raynaud Phenomenon and the vascular disease in scleroderma, Curr. Opin. Rheumatol. 16 (2004) 718–722.
40. M. Matucci Cerinic, M.B. Kahaleh, Beauty and the beast. The nitric oxide paradox in systemic sclerosis, Rheumatology (Oxford) 41 (2002) 843–847.
42. J.P. Cooke, J.M. Marshall, Mechanisms of Raynaud disease, Vasc. Med. 10 (2005) 293–307.
43. W.A. Schmidt, A. Krause, B. Schicke, et al., Color Doppler ultrasonography of hand and finger arteries to differentiate primary from secondary forms of Raynaud Phenomenon, J. Rheumatol. 35 (2008) 1591–1598.
47. S. Kim, H.O. Kim, Y.G. Jeong, et al., The diagnostic accuracy of power Doppler ultrasonography for differentiating secondary from primary Raynaud Phenomenon in undifferentiated connective tissue disease, Clin. Rheumatol. 27 (2008) 783–786.
48. P. Brennan, A. Silman, C. Black, et al., Validity and reliability of three methods used in the diagnosis of Raynaud Phenomenon. The UK Scleroderma Study Group, Brit. J. Rheumatol. 32 (1993) 357–361.
50. E. Allen, G. Brown, Raynaud disease: A critical review of minimal requisites for diagnosis, Am. J. Med. Sci. 183 (1932) 187.
51. M. Hudson, S. Taillefer, R. Steele, et al., Improving the sensitivity of the American College of Rheumatology classification criteria for systemic sclerosis, Clin. Exp. Rheumatol. 25 (2007) 754–757.
52. H. Wollersheim, T. Thien, The diagnostic value of clinical signs and symptoms in patients with Raynaud Phenomenon. A cross-sectional study, Neth. J. Med. 37 (1990) 171–182.
54. W. Goldman, R. Seltzer, P. Reuman, Association between treatment with central nervous system stimulants and Raynaud syndrome in children: a retrospective case-control study of rheumatology patients, Arthritis Rheum. 58 (2008) 563–566.
56. F. Ingegnoli, P. Boracchi, R. Gualtierotti, et al., Prognostic model based on nailfold capillaroscopy for identifying Raynaud Phenomenon patients at high risk for the development of a scleroderma spectrum disorder: PRINCE (prognostic index for nailfold capillaroscopic examination), Arthritis Rheum. 58 (2008) 2174–2182.
58. S. Pavlov-Dolijanovic, N. Damjanov, P. Ostojic, et al., The prognostic value of nailfold capillary changes for the development of connective tissue disease in children and adolescents with primary raynaud Phenomenon: a follow-up study of 250 patients, Pediatr. Dermatol. 23 (2006) 437–442.
60. M. Cutolo, W. Grassi, M. Matucci Cerinic, Raynaud Phenomenon and the role of capillaroscopy, Arthritis Rheum. 48 (2003) 3023–3030.
61. J.E. Pope, The diagnosis and treatment of Raynaud Phenomenon: a practical approach, Drugs 67 (2007) 517–525.
63. P. Navon, A. Yarom, E. Davis, Raynaud features in childhood. Clinical, immunological and capillaroscopic study, J. Mal. Vasc. 17 (1992) 273–276.

64. M. Hirschl, K. Hirschl, M. Lenz, et al., Transition from primary Raynaud Phenomenon to secondary Raynaud Phenomenon identified by diagnosis of an associated disease: results of ten years of prospective surveillance, Arthritis Rheum. 54 (2006) 1974–1981.

65. G.J. Landry, J.M. Edwards, R.B. McLafferty, et al., Long-term outcome of Raynaud syndrome in a prospectively analyzed patient cohort, J. Vasc. Surg. 23 (1996) 76–85. discussion 85-76.

73. S.D. Dib-Hajj, Y. Yang, S.G. Waxman, Genetics and molecular pathophysiology of Na(v)1.7-related pain syndromes, Adv. Gen. 63 (2008) 85–110.

76. M. Garcia-Carrasco, M. Jimenez-Hernandez, R.O. Escarcega, et al., Treatment of Raynaud Phenomenon, Autoimmun. Rev. 8 (2008) 62–68.

77. O. Kowal-Bielecka, R. Landewe, J. Avouac, et al., EULAR recommendations for the treatment of systemic sclerosis: a report from the EULAR Scleroderma Trials and Research group (EUSTAR), Ann. Rheum. Dis. 68 (2009) 620–628.

78. F.M. Wigley, Nonpharmacologic therapy for the Raynaud Phenomenon, in: J. Axford (Ed.), UpToDate, Medical Resource, Waltham, MA, 2008.

84. S. Henness, F.M. Wigley, Current drug therapy for scleroderma and secondary Raynaud Phenomenon: evidence-based review, Curr. Opin. Rheumatol. 19 (2007) 611–618.

85. A.E. Thompson, J.E. Pope, Calcium channel blockers for primary Raynaud Phenomenon: a meta-analysis, Rheumatology (Oxford) 44 (2005) 145–150.

87. A.E. Thompson, B. Shea, V. Welch, et al., Calcium-channel blockers for Raynaud Phenomenon in systemic sclerosis, Arthritis Rheum. 44 (2001) 1841–1847.

88. M. Dziadzio, C.P. Denton, R. Smith, et al., Losartan therapy for Raynaud Phenomenon and scleroderma: clinical and biochemical findings in a fifteen-week, randomized, parallel-group, controlled trial, Arthritis Rheum. 42 (1999) 2646–2655.

102. R.A. Wise, F.M. Wigley, B. White, et al., Efficacy and tolerability of a selective alpha(2C)-adrenergic receptor blocker in recovery from cold-induced vasospasm in scleroderma patients: a single-center, double-blind, placebo-controlled, randomized crossover study, Arthritis Rheum. 50 (2004) 3994–4001.

115. A. Pakozdi, K. Howell, H. Wilson, et al., Inhaled iloprost for the treatment of Raynaud Phenomenon, Clin. Exp. Rheumatol. 26 (2008) 709.

116. G. Zandman-Goddard, N. Tweezer-Zaks, Y. Shoenfeld, New therapeutic strategies for systemic sclerosis—a critical analysis of the literature, Clin. Dev. Immunol. 12 (2005) 165–173.

121. F.M. Wigley, Pharmacologic and surgical treatment of the Raynaud Phenomenon, in: J. Axford (Ed.), UpToDate, Medical Resource, Waltham, MA, 2008.

125. F. Zulian, F. Corona, V. Gerloni, et al., Safety and efficacy of iloprost for the treatment of ischaemic digits in paediatric connective tissue diseases, Rheumatology (Oxford) 43 (2004) 229–233.

Entire reference list is available online at www.expertconsult.com.

Chapter 30

VASCULITIS AND ITS CLASSIFICATION

James T. Cassidy and Ross E. Petty

The term *vasculitis* indicates the presence of inflammation in a blood vessel wall. The inflammatory infiltrate may be one that is predominantly neutrophilic, eosinophilic, or mononuclear. *Perivasculitis* describes inflammation around the blood vessel wall but without mural involvement. *Vasculopathy*, a broader term, indicates an abnormality of blood vessels that may be inflammatory, degenerative, or may result from intimal proliferation.

CLASSIFICATION

The vasculitides are the most difficult of all rheumatic diseases to classify. A number of attempts have been made, and none has completely succeeded. In part, this has resulted from inconsistent use of definitions of individual disorders, a problem addressed by a committee of the American College of Rheumatology (ACR) in 1990.[1] Subsequently, the Chapel Hill Consensus Conference in 1994 refined and modified the ACR classification (Table 30–1).[2] In these classifications, diseases are grouped by the size of the vessel affected. Neither of these classifications specifically addressed vasculitis in childhood, and, from a practical point of view, they have limited usefulness in pediatrics.[3,4]

Using Delphi and nominal group techniques, an international consensus meeting in 2005 resulted in a suggested classification of childhood vasculitides (Table 30–2) and pediatric-appropriate definitions of individual vasculitides.[5] This classification is based on predominant vessel size and the presence or absence of granulomatous vasculitis, similar to that suggested by Savage and colleagues in 1997 (Table 30–3).[6] It is recognized that the consistency of histopathological findings within any clinical diagnostic category is often limited.[7] Some disorders, such as Henoch-Schönlein purpura (HSP) and Kawasaki disease (KD), have consistent pathological pictures; however, in polyarteritis nodosa, microscopic polyarteritis, granulomatous vasculitides, and giant cell arteritides, the histological picture is often mixed, with lesions of different histologies occurring in patients with similar clinical syndromes. Classification due to the presence or absence of antineutrophil cytoplasmic antibodies has been suggested.[8] In practice, the classification of vasculitis is very much dependent on the clinical presentation. The term *polyangiitis overlap syndrome* has been suggested in recognition of the high frequency (40%) of patients who exhibit features of more than one distinct vasculitic syndrome.[9] The subject has been recently reviewed by Jennette and Falk.[10] The classification used in this book accommodates the most significant histopathological and clinical findings of the common vasculitides of childhood.

GENERAL CLINICAL ASPECTS OF VASCULITIS

Childhood vasculitis is a complex and fascinating area of pediatric rheumatology. It is a clinical field often shared with other pediatric subspecialists, such as dermatologists, cardiologists, and nephrologists, a reflection of the multisystem nature of these diseases. The type of pathological change, site of involvement, size of vessel, and systemic extent of the vascular injury determine the clinical expression of the disease and its severity. Table 30–4 summarizes features that suggest a vasculitic syndrome. The onset of some vasculitides (e.g., HSP, KD) is usually abrupt, and diagnostic characteristics of the disease become apparent in a few days to a week. In many of the vasculitides, however, presentation is more indolent, and various signs and symptoms developing over weeks to months are characteristic. In this case, the diagnosis is often difficult and delayed, and it requires a high index of suspicion and a thorough investigation

---

Table 30–1

Chapel Hill consensus conference on nomenclature of systemic vasculitis

*Large-Vessel Vasculitis**

Giant cell (temporal) arteritis	Granulomatous arteritis of the aorta and its major branches with a predilection for the extra-cranial branches of the carotid artery. *It often involves the temporal artery. Usually occurs in patients older than 50-years-old and is often associated with polymyalgia rheumatica.* [†]
Takayasu arteritis	Granulomatous inflammation of the aorta and its major branches. *Usually occurs in patients much younger than 50-years-old.*

*Medium-Vessel Vasculitis**

Polyarteritis nodosa	Necrotizing inflammation of medium-sized or small arteries without glomerulonephritis or vasculitis in arterioles, capillaries, or venules.
Kawasaki disease	Arteritis involving large, medium-sized, and small arteries associated with the mucocutaneous lymph node syndrome. *Coronary arteries are often involved. Aorta and veins may be affected. Usually occurs in children.*

*Small-Vessel Vasculitis**

Wegener granulomatosis[‡]	Granulomatous inflammation involving the respiratory tract associated with necrotizing vasculitis affecting small to medium-sized vessels. *Necrotizing glomerulonephritis is common.*
Churg-Strauss syndrome[‡]	Eosinophilic and granulomatous inflammation involving the respiratory tract accompanied by necrotizing vasculitis affecting small- to medium-sized vessels associated with asthma and eosinophilia.
Microscopic polyangiitis[‡]	Necrotizing vasculitis with few or no immune deposits, affecting small vessels. *Necrotizing arteritis involving small- and medium-sized arteries may be present. Necrotizing glomerulonephritis is common. Pulmonary capillaritis often occurs.*
Henoch-Schönlein purpura	Vasculitis characterized by Immunoglobin A-dominant immune deposits affecting small vessels. *Typically involves skin, gut, and glomeruli. Arthralgias and arthritis are common.*
Essential cryoglobulinemic vasculitis	Vasculitis with cryoglobulin immune deposits affecting small vessels associated with cryoglobulinemia. *Skin and glomeruli are often involved.*
Cutaneous leukocytoclastic angiitis	Vasculitis. Isolated cutaneous leukocytoclastic angiitis without systemic vasculitis or glomerulonephritis.

*Large vessels: aorta and its larger branches directed toward major anatomic regions; medium vessels: renal, hepatic, coronary, and mesenteric arteries; small vessels: venules, capillaries, arterioles, and intraparenchymal distal arteries and arterioles.
[†]Essential components are in normal type; *italicized type* represents usual, but not essential, components.
[‡]Strongly associated with antinuclear cytoplasmic antibodies.
Adapted from Jennette JC, Falk RJ, Andrassy K, et al.[2]

Table 30–2

EULAR/PReS classification of childhood vasculitis

I. Predominantly large vessel vasculitis
   Takayasu arteritis
II. Predominantly medium-sized vessel vasculitis
   Childhood polyarteritis nodosa
   Cutaneous polyarteritis
   Kawasaki disease
III. Predominantly small-sized vessel vasculitis
   A. Granulomatous
      Wegener granulomatosis
      Churg-Strauss syndrome
   B. Nongranulomatous
      Microscopic polyangiitis
      Henoch-Schönlein purpura
      Isolated cutaneous leucocytoclastic vasculitis
      Hypocomplementic urticarial vasculitis
IV. Other vasculitides
   Behçet disease
   Vasculitis secondary to infection (including hepatitis B-associated polyarteritis nodosa), malignancies, and drugs (including hypersensitivity vasculitis)
   Vasculitis associated with connective tissue diseases
   Isolated vasculitis of the central nervous system
   Cogan syndrome
   Unclassified

From Ozen et al.[5]

Table 30–3

Classification of Primary Systemic Vasculitis by Vessel Size and the Presence of Granulomata

Vessel Size	Granulomatous Forms	Nongranulomatous Forms
Large	Temporal arteritis	
	Takayasu arteritis	
Medium		Polyarteritis nodosa
		Kawasaki disease
Small	Wegener granulomatosis	Microscopic polyangiitis
	Churg-Strauss syndrome	Henoch-Schönlein purpura
		Cutaneous leukocytoclastic vasculitis
		Essential cryoglobulinemic vasculitis

From Savage COS, Harper L, Adu D.[6]

of symptomatic and asymptomatic (but potentially affected) organs, such as the heart, lungs, liver, brain, and kidneys. Definitive diagnosis frequently requires a biopsy of one or more sites, magnetic resonance angiography, or arteriography. Table 30–5 compares the clinical and pathological characteristics of the vasculitides in childhood discussed in greater detail in subsequent chapters.

EPIDEMIOLOGY

The incidence and prevalence of vasculitis in children are unknown. In the pediatric population, the most common vasculitides are HSP and KD. All others are very uncommon or rare. There are striking geographic differences in relative disease frequency. KD and Takayasu arteritis are most prevalent in Japan. Without doubt, KD and HSP are the most common disorders in North America and Europe. Comprehensive studies of the frequencies of the vasculitides in other parts of Asia are not available, but it is probable that KD and Takayasu arteritis constitute a larger proportion of vasculitis in that area of the world. Polyarteritis nodosa and cutaneous polyarteritis may also be more common in Japan and Turkey. In a multicenter survey in Turkey, Ozen and colleagues[11] noted that HSP was much more common than KD, that polyarteritis nodosa was possibly increased relative to other vasculitides, and that Wegener granulomatosis, which appears to be more common in western Europe and North America, is rare in the Turkish population. Isolated vasculitis of the central nervous system has only recently been recognized in childhood,[12] and its classification and relative frequency have yet to be established. Studies in African populations have not been reported.

In national diagnostic registries, the various forms of vasculitis account for 1% to 6% of pediatric rheumatic diseases.[13-15] The proportions of children from three registries that identified specific vasculitides are in Table 30-6. The wide differences in frequencies probably reflect referral patterns rather than determinable geographic differences.

Table 30–4

Features that suggest a vasculitic syndrome

Clinical Features

Fever, weight loss, fatigue of unknown origin
Skin lesions (palpable purpura, vasculitic urticaria, livedo reticularis, nodules, ulcers)
Neurological lesions (headache, mononeuritis multiplex, focal central nervous system lesions)
Arthralgia or arthritis, myalgia or myositis, serositis
Hypertension
Pulmonary infiltrates or hemorrhage

Laboratory Features

Increased erythrocyte sedimentation rate or C-reactive protein level
Leukocytosis, anemia
Eosinophilia
Antineutrophil cytoplasmic antibodies
Elevated factor VIII-related antigen (von Willebrand factor)
Cryoglobulinemia
Circulating immune complexes
Hematuria

Table 30–5

Clinical and pathological characteristics of some vasculitides in childhood

Syndrome	Frequency	Vessels Affected	Pathology
Polyarteritis			
Polyarteritis nodosa	Rare	Medium and small muscular arteries and sometimes arterioles	Focal segmental (often near bifurcations); fibrinoid necrosis; gastrointestinal, renal microaneurysms; lesions at various stages of evolution
Kawasaki disease	Common	Coronary and other muscular arteries	Thrombosis, fibrosis, aneurysms, especially coronaries
Leukocytoclastic Vasculitis			
Henoch-Schönlein purpura	Common	Arterioles and venules, often small arteries and veins	Leukocytoclasis; mixed cells, eosinophils; Immunoglobulin A deposits in affected vessels (gastrointestinal tract)
Hypersensitivity angiitis	Rare	Arterioles and venules	Leukocytoclastic or lymphocytic, varying eosinophils, occasionally granulomatous; widespread lesions at same stage of evolution
Granulomatous Vasculitis			
Wegener granulomatosis	Rare	Small arteries and veins, occasionally larger vessels	Upper and lower respiratory tract; necrotizing granulomata; glomerulonephritis
Churg-Strauss syndrome	Rare	Small arteries and veins, often arterioles and venules	Necrotizing extravascular granulomata; lung involvement; eosinophilia
Giant Cell Arteritis			
Takayasu arteritis	Uncommon	Muscular and elastic arteries	Granulomatous inflammation, giant cells; aortic arch and branches; aneurysms, dissection
Temporal arteritis	Rare	Medium and large arteries	Granulomatous inflammation, giant cell arteritis; carotid artery and branches

Table 30–6

Relative frequencies of vasculitides in childhood

Vasculitides	U.S.A.* N = 434	%	Canada† N = 225	%	Turkey# N = 376	%
Kawasaki disease	97	22.4	147	65.3	78	9.0
Henoch-Schönlein purpura	213	49.1	38	16.9	218	81.6
Wegener granulomatosis	6	1.4	5	2.2	1	0.4
Polyarteritis nodosa	14	3.2	4	1.8	60	5.6
Behçet disease	—	—	2	0.9	5	1.9
Takayasu arteritis	8	1.8	2	0.9	14	1.5
Unclassified	96	22.1	27	12.0	—	—

*Data from Bowyer S, Roettcher P: Pediatric rheumatology clinic populations in the United States: results of a 3 year survey, *J Rheumatol* 23:1968-1974, 1996.
†Data from Malleson PN, Fung MY, Rosenberg AM, *J Rheumatol* 23:1981-1987, 1996.
#Data from Ozen et al Clin Rheumatol 2007.

Although childhood vasculitis is uncommon, it is an important component of referrals to pediatric rheumatology clinics, and these children often require disproportionately large amounts of time and expertise. Diagnosis can be difficult, monitoring disease activity is problematic, and the outcome for some of the vasculitides may be serious or fatal.

REFERENCES

1. G.G. Hunder, W.P. Arend, D.A. Bloch, et al., The American College of Rheumatology 1990 criteria for the classification of vasculitis. Introduction, Arthritis Rheum. 33 (1990) 1065–1067.
2. J.C. Jennette, R.J. Falk, K. Andrassy, et al., Nomenclature of systemic vasculitides. Proposal of an international consensus conference, Arthritis Rheum. 37 (1994) 187–192.
3. P.A. Brogan, M.J. Dillon, Vasculitis from the pediatric perspective, Curr. Rheumatol. Rep. 2 (2000) 411–416.
4. A. Yalcindag, R. Sundel, Vasculitis in childhood, Curr. Opin. Rheumatol. 13 (2001) 422–427.
5. S. Ozen, N. Ruperto, M. Dillon, et al., EULAR/PReS endorsed consensus criteria for the classification of childhood vasculitides, Ann. Rheum. Dis. 65 (2006) 936–941.
6. C.O. Savage, L. Harper, D. Adu, Primary systemic vasculitis, Lancet 349 (1997) 553–558.
7. G.S. Hoffman, L.H. Calabrese, Vasculitis 2003, Clin. Exp. Rheumatol. 21 (2003) S1–S139.
8. S.L. Hogan, R.J. Falk, P.H. Nachman, et al., Various forms of life in antineutrophil cytoplasmic antibody-associated vasculitis, Ann. Intern. Med. 144 (2006) 317–318.
9. R.Y. Leavitt, A.S. Fauci, Polyangiitis overlap syndrome. Classification and prospective clinical experience, Am. J. Med. 81 (1986) 79–85.
10. J.C. Jennette, R.J. Falk, Nosology of primary vasculitis, Curr. Opin. Rheumatol. 19 (2007) 10–16.
11. J.C. Jennette, R.J. Falk, Small-vessel vasculitis, N. Engl. J. Med. 337 (1997) 1512–1523.
12. S. Ozen, A. Bakkaloglu, R. Dusunsel, et al., Childhood vasculitides in Turkey: A nationwide survey, Clin. Rheumatol. 26 (2007) 196–200.
13. S. Benseler, E. Silverman, R. Aviv, et al., Primary central nervous system vasculitis in children, Arthritis Rheum. 54 (2006) 1291–1297.
14. S. Bowyer, P. Roettcher, Pediatric rheumatology clinic populations in the United States: results of a 3 year survey. Pediatric Rheumatology Database Research Group, J. Rheumatol. 23 (1996) 1968–1974.
15. P.N. Malleson, M.Y. Fung, A.M. Rosenberg, The incidence of pediatric rheumatic diseases: results from the Canadian Pediatric Rheumatology Association Disease Registry, J. Rheumatol. 23 (1996) 1981–1987.

Chapter 31

LEUKOCYTOCLASTIC VASCULITIS

Paul Brogan and Arvind Bagga

Necrotizing vasculitis affecting small blood vessels, especially the postcapillary venules, capillaries, and arterioles, often caused by immune complex deposition, may show *leukocytoclastic vasculitis* on histology (Fig. 31–1 and Table 31–1).[1-3] The term *leukocytoclasis* refers to the infiltration of polymorphonuclear leukocytes into vessel walls, resulting in necrosis with scattered nuclear debris, and thus is not a diagnosis in itself. This is the predominant inflammatory reaction in Henoch-Schönlein purpura (HSP), hypersensitivity angiitis and mixed cryoglobulinemia. It is also observed in the ANCA associated vasculitides and the vasculitis of other connective tissue diseases, such as systemic lupus erythematosus (SLE). Leukocytoclastic vasculitis is sometimes observed as a sequel of drug hypersensitivity, infectious endocarditis, and hematological malignancies.

HENOCH-SCHÖNLEIN PURPURA

Definition and Classification

HSP is one of the most common vasculitides of childhood.[4-8] It is characterized by nonthrombocytopenic purpura, arthritis and arthralgia, abdominal pain and gastrointestinal hemorrhage, and glomerulonephritis. This syndrome has a long history with early references by Willan[9] and Heberden.[10] A diagnostic triad of purpuric rash, arthritis, and abnormalities of the urinary sediment was proposed by Schönlein in 1837,[11] and Henoch described the association of purpuric rash, abdominal pain with bloody diarrhea, and proteinuria in 1874.[12] The term *anaphylactoid purpura* was applied by Gairdner in 1948.[13]

Epidemiology

HSP is predominantly a disease of childhood, although a similar syndrome has been reported in adults.[14-17] It occurs most frequently between the ages of three and 15 years and is more common in boys than in girls (1.5:1).[17,18] The condition is rare in children younger than two-years.[19] Recently collected prospective data from an international cohort of 827 patients with HSP showed a mean age at onset of 6.9±3 (range 1 to 16.2) years, and at diagnosis 7±3-years, 408 (49%) were girls.[20]

An incidence of 13.5 cases per 100,000 children per year was observed in an unselected childhood population in Belfast, Northern Ireland.[21] An incidence of 0.2 to 10 was estimated by Farley and colleagues.[22] In the latter study, incidence was highest among Hispanic children and children in lower socioeconomic groups. In a study from Britain, although the combined incidence was 20.4, it was 70.3 in the 4- to 6-year-old age group.[23] Striking seasonal variations have been observed,[22] with most cases occurring in winter, often preceded by an upper respiratory tract infection (30% to 50%).[24,25]

Etiology and Pathogenesis

Many reports have implicated infection as a potential trigger for this disease, particularly with β-hemolytic streptococci.[13,26-28] Some investigators have, however, doubted this association.[24,25,29] Other preceding coincidences have been described, including vaccination,[30,31] viral infection[32-35] (e.g., varicella,[36-38] rubella, rubeola, hepatitis A and B),[39,40] *Mycoplasma pneumoniae*,[41,42] *Bartonella henselae*,[43] and *Helicobacter pylori*.[44]

As the term *anaphylactoid purpura* suggests, allergy has been regarded by some as the basis for development of this disease after insect bites[4] and exposure to drug and dietary allergens.[45] The characteristic vascular deposition of immunoglobulin A (IgA) suggests that HSP is an IgA-mediated dysregulated immune response to antigen and may operate through the alternative complement pathway.[46] In a recent study,[47] serum levels of IgA anticardiolipin antibodies were elevated during the acute stage of the disease, along with transforming growth factor-β secreting T cells. Although the pathogenetic mechanisms of nephritis are still not delineated, studies suggest that galactose-deficient IgA1 is recognized by antiglycan antibodies, leading to the formation of circulating immune complexes and their mesangial deposition, which results in renal injury in HSP.[48]

Disorders of coagulation and its activation are also associated with the development of HSP or an HSP-like

483

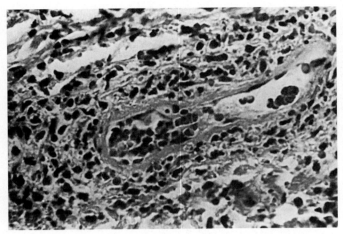

FIGURE 31–1 Histopathological demonstration of leukocytoclastic vasculitis. The characteristic "nuclear dust" is seen as granular, dark-stained material in the vessel wall. Hematoxylin and eosin stain.

Table 31–1

Conditions associated with leukocytoclastic vasculitis

Henoch-Schönlein purpura
Hypersensitivity angiitis
Hypocomplementemic urticarial vasculitis
Mixed cryoglobulinemia
Cutaneous polyarteritis
ANCA-associated small-vessel vasculitis*
Goodpasture syndrome
*Rheumatic disorders**
   SLE, juvenile dermatomyositis, MCTD, scleroderma, JIA
   Mucha-Habermann disease
   Relapsing polychondritis
   Köhlmeier-Degos syndrome
   Antiphospholipid antibody syndrome
Malignancy-associated disease
   Sweet syndrome
Cronkhite-Canada syndrome
Stevens-Johnson syndrome
Erythema elevatum diutinum

*Leukocytoclastic vasculitis may occur in cutaneous lesions in some patients with ANCA-associated vasculitis and collagen vascular diseases
ANCA, Antineutrophil cytoplasmic antibody; JIA, juvenile idiopathic arthritis; MCTD, mixed connective tissue disease; SLE, systemic lupus erythematosus.

vasculitis.[49] It is recognized that disease activity may be linked to a rapid decline in factor XIII, particularly in patients with severe abdominal involvement.[50-52] This may be useful as a prognostic or diagnostic marker because the decline occurs before classic skin rash and thus could allow early diagnosis of HSP, where abdominal symptoms and signs predominate. Anecdotal reports of factor XIII replacement to treat severe abdominal symptoms are described.[52] Factor XIII also declines prior to recurrence of HSP.

One study concluded that oxidant stress, especially lipid peroxidation, was involved in the origin of renal injury.[53] Vasculitis may develop after antirheumatic therapy, including administration of methotrexate[54] and antitumor necrosis factor agents.[55]

Genetic Background

Familial clusters of the disease may occur, with siblings affected simultaneously or sequentially.[22,56,57] Investigations from Spain have presented preliminary data on genetic associations. The frequency of HLA-B35 increased in patients who developed nephritis.[58] The incidence of HLA-DRB1*01 also increased compared with matched controls, and HLA-DRB1*07 decreased.[59] A study on unselected children with HSP from Turkey showed that HLA A2, A11, and B35 antigens were associated with a significantly increased risk, whereas HLA A1, B49, and B50 antigens were associated with decreased risk for the disease.[60]

Although there were no general associations with the expression of intercellular adhesion molecule 1 in patients compared with controls, a K/E polymorphism at codon 469 was significantly decreased in those who did not develop severe gastrointestinal manifestations (and possibly in patients without renal sequelae).[61] In studies from Israel and Turkey, mutations in the familial Mediterranean fever (MEFV) gene were frequent in patients with HSP.[62,63] Other genetic polymorphisms have also been implicated.[64] HSP has also been described in a number of patients with heterozygous C2 complement component deficiency.

Several polymorphisms relating to disease susceptibility, severity, and/or risk of renal involvement have recently been described. Studies of this nature have been hampered by relatively small patient numbers and thus lack the power to be definitive or necessarily applicable to all racial groups. It is, however, increasingly apparent that the genetic contribution is complex and probably polygenic in nature.

Clinical Manifestations

Clinical characteristics of HSP are presented in Table 31–2.[15,65-68] The onset is often acute with the principal manifestations appearing sequentially over several days to weeks. Nonspecific constitutional signs, such as a low-grade fever or malaise, are often present.[7]

Cutaneous Involvement

The presence of *palpable purpura* is essential to the diagnosis.[15,69,70] This rash is most prominent on dependent or pressure-bearing surfaces, especially the lower extremities and buttocks, but it may occur in other areas. The cutaneous lesions range from small petechiae to large ecchymoses to rare hemorrhagic bullae; they tend to occur in crops and progress in color from red to purple to brown (Figs. 31–2 and 31–3). Ulceration may occasionally develop in large ecchymotic areas. The rash is often preceded by maculopapular or urticarial lesions. Subcutaneous edema over the dorsa of the hands and feet and around the eyes, forehead, scalp, and scrotum may occur early in the disease, particularly in the very young child.

Gastrointestinal Disease

Gastrointestinal manifestations occur in approximately two thirds of children, usually within a week after onset of the rash and almost always within 30 days; in 14%

Table 31-2

Clinical features of Henoch-Schönlein purpura (percent patients)

Clinical Feature	Emery et al, 1977[65] N=43	Rosenblum, Winter, 1987[66] N=43	Bagga et al, 1991[67] N=47	Saulsbury, 1999[69] N=100	Nong, et al, 2007[68] N=107	Average (%)
Purpura	100*	97	96	100*	95	96
Arthralgia, arthritis	79	65	47	82	47	64
Abdominal pain	63	100*	64	63	72	66
Gastrointestinal bleeding		26	26	33		28
Renal involvement	37		51	40	28	39
Subcutaneous edema	63		21			42
Orchitis			6	4		5

*Criterion used for inclusion in the series

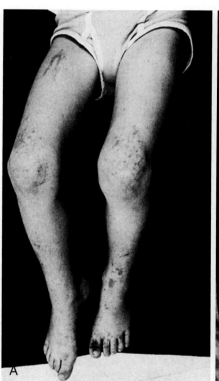
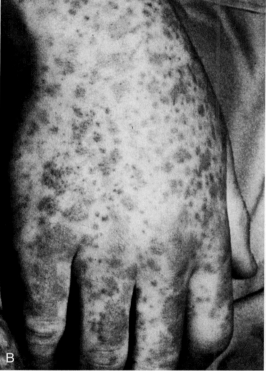

FIGURE 31-2 Henoch-Schönlein purpura. **A,** These purpuric lesions appeared on the lower extremities of a 10-year-old boy who had an acute, self-limited illness characterized by fever, arthritis, melena, and transient hematuria. Notice the periarticular swelling around the ankles and knees. **B,** Purpura on dorsum of the hand of a 14-year-old-boy with Henoch-Schönlein purpura.

to 36% of cases, abdominal pain precedes other manifestations.[66,71-73] Edema and submucosal and intramural hemorrhage resulting from vasculitis of the bowel wall occasionally lead to intussusception (usually confined to the small bowel), gangrene, or overt perforation. Less common involvement includes acute pancreatitis,[74] hepatobiliary involvement,[75] ulcerative colitis, other forms of enteropathy,[76] and steatorrhea.

In one study, abdominal pain was usually intermittent, colicky, and periumbilical.[66] Rebound tenderness was uncommon. Vomiting occurred in 60%, hematemesis in 7%, and melena in 19% of children, although occult blood was present in the stools of one half of the patients. Massive gastrointestinal hemorrhage or intussusception occurred in less than 5% of children, but it could develop suddenly without preceding abdominal symptoms.

Renal Disease

Glomerulonephritis affects up to one third of the children, but in less than 10% it is a serious and potentially life-threatening complication.[4,21,22,25,36,77] In the Belfast study of 155,000 unselected children, 55 of 270 patients had evidence of nephritis at onset.[21] Renal disease, like abdominal pain, seldom precedes the purpura, and, in most instances, serious renal disease develops within four to six weeks of the onset of the rash. The spectrum of manifestations range from microscopic hematuria and mild proteinuria to the less common nephrotic syndrome, acute nephritic syndrome, hypertension, or renal failure. Age at onset of more than 7-years, persistent purpuric lesions, severe abdominal symptoms, and decreased factor XIII activity are associated with an increased risk of nephritis.[78-80] The severity of renal

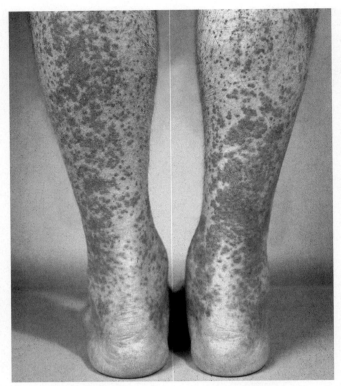

FIGURE 31–3 Palpable purpuric lesions involve the heels and ankles of a patient with Henoch-Schönlein purpura.

symptoms at onset determines the intensity of glomerular lesions.[81]

The initial three months are critical in determining the eventual extent of the illness. In a few children, however, nephritis may not occur until much later in the course, sometimes after a number of recurrences of the purpura. Renal involvement characteristically develops early, but end-stage disease may not be obvious for a number of years. In a small number of children, renal abnormalities occur alone and clinically and immunopathogenically resemble IgA nephropathy in adults.

In a systematic review involving 1133 select patients with HSP, renal manifestations (proteinuria, hematuria) were found in 34.2%. These features developed in 85% of cases within four weeks of the diagnosis of HSP, in 91% within six weeks, and in 97% within six months.[77] Permanent renal impairment never developed after normal urinalysis; it occurred in 1.6% of those with isolated urinary abnormalities and in 19.5% of those who developed nephritic or nephrotic syndrome. Based on these findings, it is recommended that patients with HSP should be followed up for a minimum of six months to detect renal involvement.

Arthritis

Arthralgia or arthritis involving only a few joints occurs in 50% to 80% of children with HSP. Large joints, such as the knees and ankles, are most commonly affected, but other areas, including the wrists, elbows, and small joints of the fingers, may be involved. Characteristic findings include periarticular swelling and tenderness, usually occurring without erythema, warmth, or effusions,

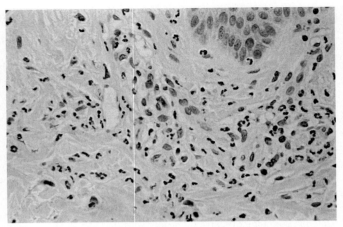

FIGURE 31–4 Leukocytoclastic vasculitis in the skin of a patient with Henoch-Schönlein purpura. Hematoxylin and eosin stain; magnification X 480.

but with considerable pain and limitation of motion. The joint disease is transient, although usually not migratory, and resolves within a few days to a week without residual abnormalities. Occasionally, arthritis may precede the appearance of the rash by one or two days.[65]

Other Manifestations

Other manifestations of HSP include an isolated central nervous system vasculitis, seizures, coma, and hemorrhage;[82] Guillain-Barré syndrome;[83] ataxia and central and peripheral neuropathy;[84] ocular involvement;[66,85] intramuscular, subconjunctival, or pulmonary hemorrhages;[86-88] interstitial pneumonitis;[89] recurrent epistaxis; parotitis;[25] carditis;[4,90,91] and stenosing ureteritis.[92] Scrotal pain and swelling are frequent, occurring in 13% (range 2% to 38%)[69,93-96] of boys evaluated for HSP.

Pathology

The pathological lesion essential for diagnosis is leukocytoclastic vasculitis (Fig. 31–4).[1,25,97,98] In the skin, this is demonstrated in the dermal capillaries and postcapillary venules. Deposition of IgA (principally IgA$_1$) in these lesions is characteristic.[15,46,99,100] It is possible to fail to detect IgA deposition in vascular tissue in some cases of HSP, especially if the biopsy was obtained from the middle of a lesion where the presence of proteolytic enzymes can result in negative staining for IgA.[101]

In the kidneys, proliferative glomerulonephritis ranges from focal and segmental lesions to severe crescentic disease (Fig. 31–5).[99,102] Group A streptococcal antigen (i.e., nephritis-associated plasmin receptor) was identified in the mesangium of 10 of 33 children by immunofluorescent microscopy.[28] Levy and coworkers[25] provided a comprehensive review of the renal pathology. The principal lesion is an endocapillary proliferative glomerulonephritis with an increase in endothelial and mesangial cells. All gradations of severity may be present in the same biopsy. There may be marked interstitial inflammatory disease, but vasculitis per se is usually not present. Fluorescence microscopy confirms deposits of Ig, principally IgA,[46,100,103] but it is often accompanied by IgG, fibrin, C3, and properdin in most involved

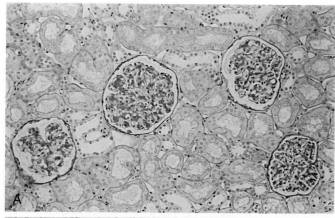

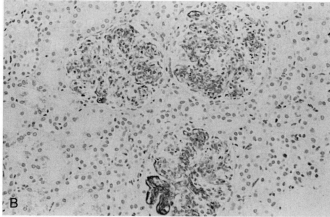

FIGURE 31–5 A, Diffuse, mesangial, proliferative nephritis in Henoch-Schönlein purpura. Hematoxylin and eosin stain. **B,** Mesangial and capillary wall deposition of immunoglobulin A (immunoperoxidase stain) in Henoch-Schönlein purpura.

Table 31–3

Criteria for the classification of Henoch-Schönlein purpura

Criterion	Definition
Palpable purpura	Slightly raised, "palpable" hemorrhagic skin lesions not related to thrombocytopenia
Age ≤20 yr at onset	Patient ≤20 yr old at onset of first symptoms
Bowel angina	Diffuse abdominal pain that is worse after meals or the diagnosis of bowel ischemia, including bloody diarrhea
Wall granulocytes on biopsy	Histological changes showing granulocytes in the walls of arterioles or venules

For purposes of classification, a patient is said to have Henoch-Schönlein purpura if at least two of these criteria are present. The presence of any two or more criteria had a diagnostic sensitivity of 87.1% and specificity of 87.7%.

From Mills JA, Michel BA, Bloch DA, et al: The American College of Rheumatology 1990 criteria for the classification of Henoch-Schönlein purpura, *Arthritis Rheum* 33:1114-1121, 1990.

glomeruli. These deposits are invariably in mesangial cells, but peripheral capillary loops also are involved in more severe cases. Dense deposits in the mesangium and occasionally in the subendothelial and paramesangial regions are present on electron microscopy. Thickening and splitting of the basement membrane, caused by the interposition of mesangial cell cytoplasmic material, are notable.

Differential Diagnosis

The American College of Rheumatology (ACR) criteria are listed in Table 31–3.[70] These criteria were derived by comparing 85 patients with HSP to 722 controls with other vasculitides and had a diagnostic sensitivity of 87.1% and specificity of 87.7%.[70] In 2005 the vasculitis working group of the Pediatric Rheumatology European Society (PRES) proposed new classification criteria for pediatric vasculitides, endorsed by the European League Against Rheumatism (EULAR),[104] which required palpable purpura with lower limb predominance (as mandatory criteria) plus at least one among the following four features: diffuse abdominal pain, biopsy showing typical leukocytoclastic vasculitis or proliferative glomerulonephritis with predominant IgA deposition, arthritis/arthralgia, and renal involvement (any hematuria and/or

proteinuria). In case of purpura with atypical distribution, a demonstration of IgA deposit in a biopsy is required.[104] The EULAR criteria have been prospectively validated through an international, web-based prospective data that included 827 patients with HSP and 356 with other vasculitides. The sensitivity and specificity of the new classification criteria were 100% and 87% respectively with a kappa-agreement of 0.90 (95% CI 0.84-0.96).[20] Table 31–4 summarizes the new criteria.

HSP must be distinguished from immune thrombocytopenic purpura, acute poststreptococcal glomerulonephritis,[2 9] SLE, septicemia, disseminated intravascular coagulation, the hemolytic-uremic syndrome, the papular-purpuric gloves-and-socks syndrome,[105] and other types of vasculitis.[6,106-108] MEFV can also mimic or occur in association with HSP in areas where this is endemic.[109,110]

The more common causes of an acute surgical abdomen with abdominal pain and gastrointestinal tract bleeding must be considered. A tender abdominal mass may indicate intussusception, and abdominal tenderness with an elevated serum amylase level may suggest acute pancreatitis. Punch biopsy of a cutaneous lesion may assist in the diagnosis of difficult cases by demonstrating a leukocytoclastic vasculitis characterized by deposition of IgA and C3.[46] A renal biopsy is indicated only in children with persistent or significant renal manifestations.[25] Indications for diagnostic renal biopsy in children with HSP are:[111]

- Nephritic/nephrotic presentation
- Raised creatinine, hypertension, or oliguria
- Heavy proteinuria (Ua:Ucr persistently >100 mg/mmol) on an early morning urine sample at four weeks. Serum albumin not necessarily in the nephrotic range.
- Persistent proteinuria (not declining) after four weeks
- Impaired renal function (GFR <80 mL/min/1.73 m^2)

Table 31–4

2010 Classification criteria for Henoch Schönlein purpura

Criterion	Definition	Sensitivity	Specificity
Purpura (mandatory)	Purpura (palpable, in crops) or petechiae, with lower limb predominance,* not related to thrombocytopenia	89%	86%
And at least 1 out of 4 of the following			
Abdominal pain	Diffuse, acute, colicky pain. May include intussusception and gastrointestinal bleeding.	61%	64%
Histopathology	Leukocytoclastic vasculitis with predominant IgA deposit; or proliferative glomerulonephritis with predominant IgA deposit	93%	89%
Arthritis or arthralgias	Arthritis. Acute joint swelling or pain with limitation on motion Arthralgia. Acute joint pain without joint swelling or limitation on motion	78%	42%
Renal involvement	Proteinuria. >0.3 g/24 hr; spot urine albumin to creatinine ratio >30 mmol/mg; or ≥ 2+ on dipstick Hematuria, red cell casts. Urine sediment showing >5 red cells per high power field or red cell casts	33%	70%

*If purpura with atypical distribution, demonstration of IgA deposit on biopsy is required
The sensitivity and specificity of the above classification for HSP is 100% and 87% respectively.
Adapted from: Ozen S et al. The EULAR/PRINTO/PRES criteria for Henoch-Schönlein purpura, Ann Rheum Dis, *in press*, 2010.

Infantile Acute Hemorrhagic Edema

Infantile acute hemorrhagic edema (Finkelstein-Seidlmayer syndrome) affects infants between 4- and 24-months-old with an acute onset of fever, purpura, ecchymoses, and inflammatory edema of the limbs, ears and face.[112-116] Although spontaneous remission in one to three weeks and a benign course are characteristic, attacks may recur. Involvement of viscera (e.g., kidneys, gastrointestinal tract) is rare. Histopathology is typical of a leukocytoclastic vasculitis with occasional demonstration of perivascular IgA deposition.[117] This disorder in older children overlaps clinically with HSP.

HSP in Adults

HSP is uncommon in adults, with a reported incidence of 0.12 cases per 100,000 persons. Males are affected as commonly as females.[14,16,118-121] In a study of clinical features and outcomes in an unselected population of 46 adults and 116 children with HSP,[122] cutaneous lesions were the principal initial manifestation in both groups. However, adults had a lower frequency of abdominal pain and fever and a higher frequency of joint symptoms and severe renal involvement. Adults often required aggressive therapy with glucocorticoids or cytotoxic agents, or both.

Outcome was relatively good in both age groups, with a complete recovery in 94% of children and 89% of adults. Another study indicated that leukocytosis, thrombocytosis, and elevated levels of serum C-reactive protein were more common in children, whereas elevated serum IgA and cryoglobulin levels were more common in adults.[119] HSP in adults may represent a more severe form of the disease with a higher frequency of significant renal involvement and risk of progressive kidney disease, but without the other manifestations of HSP.[119-123]

Laboratory Examination

There are no diagnostic laboratory abnormalities.[65,69,70] The platelet count is normal or increased, differentiating this form of purpura from that caused by thrombocytopenia.

A moderate leukocytosis of up to 20,000 white blood cells/mm^3 (20 x 10^9/L) with a left shift is identified in some children. Normochromic anemia is often related to gastrointestinal blood loss, confirmed by a positive stool guaiac examination in 80% of the children who have abdominal complaints. Antinuclear antibody (ANA) and rheumatoid factor (RF) are not characteristic.

Although renal disease may occur in the absence of overt urinary findings and minimal abnormalities, such as hematuria, are not necessarily associated with a severe glomerular lesion, these laboratory abnormalities usually demonstrate a direct correlation with the severity of the proliferative changes. Patients occasionally have decreased concentrating ability and creatinine clearance. Proteinuria, sometimes severe enough to result in hypoalbuminemia, may occur.[65,124]

Although levels of C1q, C3, and C4 are usually normal,[125] activation of the alternative complement pathway is demonstrated in one half of the children during the acute illness by the presence of C3d, low levels of total hemolytic complement, and decreased concentrations of properdin and factor B in the serum.[125,126] Plasma levels of von Willebrand factor antigen are elevated, indicating endothelial cell damage.[127,128]

Circulating IgA-containing immune complexes[129,130] and cryoglobulins[131] may be present. Serum IgA and IgM concentrations are increased in one half of the patients during the acute phase of the disease.[132] An increased number of circulating IgA-producing cells was found in one study in definite HSP cases but not in other forms of leukocytoclastic vasculitis.[133] ANCAs are absent, except rarely in adult patients with severe symptoms.

Radiological Examination

Plain radiographs delineate decreased bowel motility with dilated loops of bowel in children with abdominal involvement. Ultrasound studies can identify specific gastrointestinal abnormalities in children with abdominal complaints,[71] and magnetic resonance imaging and magnetic resonance angiography can define the extent of cerebral vasculitis.[134-136] Occasionally, intussusception is identified on a barium study and is relieved by it if performed early in the course.[69,137] Epididymal enlargement, subcutaneous swelling or hydrocele, or rarely, testicular torsion can be confirmed if necessary by scrotal ultrasonography.

Treatment

Treatment is supportive with maintenance of good hydration, nutrition, and electrolyte balance, and with control of pain with simple analgesics, such as acetaminophen and, if necessary, control of hypertension.[138] Although glucocorticoids dramatically decrease the severity of joint and cutaneous disease, they are not usually indicated for management of these manifestations.[15] Short-term glucocorticoid therapy is effective in relieving the pain of severe orchitis. Prednisone has been advocated in children with severe gastrointestinal disease or hemorrhage.[26,66,139,140] The severity of disease may occasionally prompt the use of intravenous corticosteroids.[140,141] However, studies do not demonstrate a clear advantage of prednisone over supportive therapy (e.g., nasogastric suction, parenteral nutrition, antibiotics). Pulmonary hemorrhage is an extremely rare and sometimes fatal complication, which requires aggressive immunosuppressive treatment, combining IV methylprednisolone and cyclosporin (or another immunosuppressive agent) and supportive care.[88]

Management of HSP Nephritis

The management of HSP nephritis has recently been reviewed by Zaffanello and Fanos.[142] The authors highlighted that currently prescribed treatments for HSP nephritis are not adequately guided by evidence obtained in robust randomized placebo-controlled trials with outcome markers related to the progression to end stage renal disease.

TREATMENT TO PREVENT RENAL DISEASE

Various treatment strategies to prevent the occurrence of HSP nephritis have been reported with variable effect. The efficacy of corticosteroids to prevent complications, such as abdominal pain is debated.[143,144] Chartapisak and colleagues recently systematically reviewed all published randomized controlled trials (RCTs) for the prevention or treatment of renal involvement in HSP.[145] Metaanalyses of four RCTs, which evaluated prednisone therapy at presentation of HSP, showed that there was no significant difference in the risk of development or persistence of renal involvement at one, three, six, and twelve months with prednisone compared with placebo or no specific treatment. Findings from this review suggest that prophylactic therapy with corticosteroids does not prevent the onset of HSP nephritis.

That said, there could still be a role for early use of corticosteroids in patients with severe extrarenal symptoms and in those with renal involvement, as suggested by Ronkainen and colleagues.[144] Prednisone (1 mg/kg/day for 2 weeks, with weaning over the subsequent two

weeks) was effective in reducing the intensity of abdominal pain and joint pain. Prednisone did not prevent the development of renal symptoms but was effective in treating them if present; renal symptoms resolved in 61% of the prednisone patients after treatment, compared with 34% of those receiving placebo.[144]

TREATMENT OF RAPIDLY PROGRESSIVE GLOMERULONEPHRITIS

There are good data indicating that crescents in >50% of glomeruli and nephrotic range proteinuria carry an unfavorable prognosis, thus highlighting the need for an effective intervention. To date, there is only one RCT evaluating the benefit of treatment, which shows no difference in outcome using cyclophosphamide versus supportive therapy alone.[146] However, this study did not examine combined therapy with cyclophosphamide and steroids, a regimen used in most other severe small vessel vasculitides. For patients with rapidly progressive glomerulonephritis with crescentic changes on renal biopsy, uncontrolled data suggest that treatment may comprise aggressive therapy with intravenous methylprednisolone,[147-150] cyclophosphamide, and plasma exchange,[142] as for other causes of crescentic nephritis. Warfarin and heparin have been used with disputable effect, as have cyclosporine,[16,151-153] azathioprine,[142] intravenous Ig, and plasma exchange.[16,154,155] Shenoy and colleagues reported on 14 children with severe HSP nephritis treated successfully with plasma exchange alone.[156] These treatment options, while potentially important in select cases, are not yet supported by RCTs.

TREATMENT OF HSP NEPHRITIS, THAT IS NOT RAPIDLY PROGRESSIVE

Such patients may exhibit the following features: less than 50% crescents on renal biopsy; suboptimal GFR; or heavy proteinuria, which is not necessarily nephrotic range.[111] There are no robust clinical trials to guide therapy of this type of presentation, though many physicians would advocate corticosteroids. Others advocate the addition of cyclophosphamide to corticosteroids in HSP nephritis with biopsy showing diffuse proliferative lesions or sclerosis, but with <50% crescentic change who have ongoing heavy proteinuria. A typical regimen would comprise 8 to 12 weeks of oral cyclophosphamide (2 mg/kg/day) with daily prednisolone, converting to alternate day prednisolone and azathioprine for 12 months.[111] The published evidence for the efficacy of this approach is lacking, but it may be a reasonable option for selected patients. In patients with greater than six months' duration of proteinuria, an angiotensin converting enzyme inhibitor may be indicated to limit secondary glomerular injury, although again the evidence to support this therapy is lacking.[142]

Renal transplantation has been successful in some children with renal failure.[157-159] In pooled data,[157,159] there was a 35% risk of recurrence five years after transplantation and an 11% risk of graft loss. A recent study on the long-term outcome of renal transplantation in adult patients with HSP, showed 15 year patient and graft survival of 80% and 64% respectively.[160] Forty percent of patients, particularly those with necrotizing or crescentic glomerulonephritis of the native kidneys, developed recurrent HSP nephritis resulting in graft loss in one-half.

Course of the Disease and Prognosis

In two thirds of children, HSP runs its entire course within four weeks of onset.[138,161,162] Younger children generally have a shorter course and fewer recurrences than older patients do. One third to one half of the children have at least one recurrence that commonly consists of a rash and abdominal pain, with each episode usually being similar but briefer and milder than the preceding one.[15] Most exacerbations take place within the initial six-week period but may occur as late as two years after onset. They may be spontaneous or coincide with repeated respiratory tract infections. The severity of the cutaneous leukocytoclastic vasculitis does not correlate with visceral involvement.[98]

Prognosis is excellent for most children.[163,164] Significant morbidity or mortality is associated with gastrointestinal tract lesions in the short term and with nephritis in the long term.[14,165] The development of major indications of renal disease within the first six months after onset or the occurrence of numerous exacerbations associated with nephropathy suggests a poor prognosis for renal function.[102,166] Additional poor prognostic factors[166] are decreased factor XIII activity; hypertension; renal failure at onset; and, if a renal biopsy had been performed, an increased number of glomeruli with crescents; macrophage infiltration; and tubulointerstitial disease.

The reported outcome of children with renal disease are highly variable.[167] With minimal lesions, more than 75% recover within two years; in contrast, two thirds of children with crescentic glomerulonephritis in more than 80% of glomeruli progress to renal failure within the first year. The worst outcome is associated with the presence of the nephrotic or nephritic syndrome at onset.[77,161,168] Almost one half of such children have active renal disease or renal insufficiency at follow-up periods of six or more years. Thus, the extent of the renal disease has been the ultimate determinant of long-term outcome.

Overall, less than 5% of children progress to end-stage renal failure. HSP accounts for less than 1% of children with renal failure from all causes. In a follow-up evaluation of 64 children,[169] the renal survival rate at 10 years was 73%, and initial renal insufficiency was the best predictor of the future course of nephritis. Similar results were found in a multicentric study on 443 patients with HS nephritis from Turkey, in which 87% patients had a favorable and 13% an unfavorable outcome; 1.1% children showed end-stage renal disease at follow-up.[170] All patients who showed end-stage renal disease had nephritic-nephrotic syndrome at presentation and >50% crescents on renal biopsy.[170]

Patients who have had clinical nephritis should be followed closely for at least five years.[161,166,167] In one study, 8 of 12 patients had mesangial IgA deposition at follow-up of two to nine years, despite an apparent clinical remission of their renal disease. Later, 16 of 44 pregnancies in adults were complicated by proteinuria or hypertension, even in the absence of active renal disease.[167] Of 18 patients in the Belfast study who had a nephrotic or nephritic syndrome at onset[21] and who were followed a mean of

8.3 years, one had died and three had persistent urinary abnormalities but no azotemia. The overall mortality rate was less than 1%, and the morbidity rate was 1.1%. This somewhat optimistic outcome is tempered by a study of 16 children from Minnesota that indicated the longer a child was followed, the more likely it was that renal disease would become clinically evident.[171]

HYPERSENSITIVITY ANGIITIS

Vascular inflammation in hypersensitivity angiitis occurs more typically in smaller vessels than in those involved in the classic form of polyarteritis nodosa and, in this regard, resembles HSP. Previously, it was the most frequently encountered form of vasculitis after the administration of therapeutic antisera.[172] The Chapel Hill International Consensus Conference did not use the term *hypersensitivity vasculitis*.[173] It was proposed instead that *microscopic polyarteritis* and *cutaneous leukocytoclastic vasculitis* were best equated with the common usage of this designation. The terminology used to describe leukocytoclastic vasculitis resulting from an allergic reaction remains confusing. The ACR criteria define hypersensitivity vasculitis (Table 31–5)[174] as palpable purpura, with or without a maculopapular rash precipitated by a medication or other agent, and a biopsied lesion characterized by a neutrophilic perivascular or extravascular infiltration in small vessels (like those affected in HSP).[175,176] The new pediatric vasculitis classification suggested by Ozen and colleagues refers to hypersensitivity vasculitis under the subheading "other vasculitis."[104]

A report of serum sickness-like arthritis in Finland estimated its frequency at 4.7 cases per 100,000 children younger than 16-years, establishing it as one of the most common causes of acute arthritis in childhood.[177] In this study, the arthritis was transient, usually lasting only a few weeks, and most commonly affected the ankles,

Table 31–5	
Criteria for the diagnosis of hypersensitivity vasculitis	
Criterion	**Definition**
Age at onset >16 yr	Development of symptoms after age 16 yr
Medication at disease onset	Medication that may have been a precipitating factor was taken at the onset of symptoms
Palpable purpura	Slightly elevated purpuric rash over one or more areas; does not blanch with pressure and not related to thrombocytopenia
Maculopapular rash	Flat and raised lesions of various sizes over one or more areas of the skin
Biopsy, including arteriole and venule	Histological changes showing granulocytes in a perivascular or extravascular location

For purposes of classification, a patient is said to have hypersensitivity vasculitis if at least three of these criteria are present. The presence of any three or more criteria has a diagnostic sensitivity of 71.0% and specificity of 83.9%. The age criterion is not applicable for children.
From Calabrese LH, Michel BA, Bloch DA et al: The American College of Rheumatology 1990 criteria for the classification of hypersensitivity vasculitis, *Arthritis Rheum* 33:1108-1113, 1990.

metacarpophalangeal joints, wrists, and knees (Fig. 31–6). Occasionally, pulmonary, renal, and other vasculature systems were affected (Fig. 31–7).

Leukocytosis usually occurs in cases of hypersensitivity angiitis and is sometimes accompanied by eosinophilia and circulating immune complexes.[177] *The erythrocyte sedimentation rate is often normal.* IgG antibodies to the putative antigen may be demonstrable. Synovial fluid examination in one report demonstrated 8800 to 59,000 leukocytes/mm³ (8 to 59 x 10⁹/L), of which 38% to 80% were polymorphonuclear leukocytes.[177] Biopsy of a cutaneous lesion confirms that small venules and capillaries are the predominantly involved vessels. Inflammatory lesions are at a similar stage of development in all areas of involvement, and the cellular infiltrate contains large numbers of neutrophils and eosinophils.

Systemic treatment is directed at the relief of symptoms, because the course, although often acute and variable, is self limited. Removal of the precipitating agent, if identified, is the first step in treatment. In the absence of systemic features, management is usually symptomatic. Antihistamines and nonsteroidal antiinflammatory drugs (NSAIDs) alleviate cutaneous symptoms and arthralgias. Glucocorticoid therapy may be indicated in children with severe cutaneous symptoms or systemic vasculitis.

Historically, serum sickness, a classic example of immune complex-mediated disease in humans, was encountered after the administration of heterologous antiserum to treat or prevent specific infections such as diphtheria and tetanus. Although current indications for use of heterologous antiserum are uncommon, it has been superseded as a cause of serum sickness by myriad drugs, notably cefaclor, penicillin, quinolones, allopurinol, thiazide diuretics, NSAIDs, phenytoins, antithyroid drugs, and, rarely, streptokinase, recombinant human growth hormone, cytokines, and monoclonal antibodies.

The clinical syndrome begins 7 to 14 days after primary exposure to the antigen and is characterized by fever, arthralgia, frank arthritis (sometimes), myalgia, lymphadenopathy, and a rash that may be purpuric, linear, urticarial, or ecchymotic and distributed predominantly over the lower legs, although the trunk and arms may be involved (Fig. 31–8). Kunnamo and colleagues[177] described a patchy discoloration over the affected joints, with urticaria predominantly on the trunk. With the use of equine antithymocyte globulin in the treatment of bone marrow failure, 30 of 35 patients developed serum sickness characterized by malaise, headache, fever, cutaneous eruptions, arthralgias, arthritis, myalgias, gastrointestinal complaints, and lymph node enlargement, beginning seven to nine days after infusion and lasting 10 to 14 days.[172]

A study that compared the clinical features of HSP and hypersensitivity angiitis found that transient arthralgias and oligoarthritis, myalgias, cutaneous nodules, ulcerations, livido, gangrene, and eosinophilia were common in patients with hypersensitivity angiitis. Gastrointestinal bleeding, hematuria, and palpable purpura were frequent in those with HSP.[175]

HYPOCOMPLEMENTEMIC URTICARIAL VASCULITIS

This form of vasculitis is currently classified under the heading "predominantly small vessel vasculitis, nongranulomatous forms."[104] Children, usually girls, with this rare syndrome have recurrent episodes of urticaria associated with pruritus and a burning sensation. The urticaria resolves over two to four days, leaving residual pigmentation (Fig. 31–9).[178,179] Other skin lesions include purpura, papules, and vesicles. Fever, nausea, vomiting,

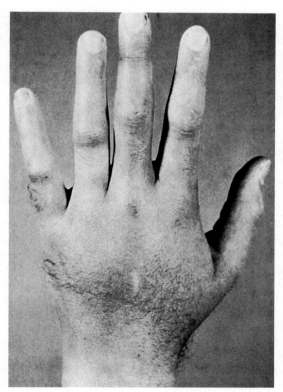

FIGURE 31–6   Diffuse and periarticular swelling of the hand in a boy with acute serum sickness.

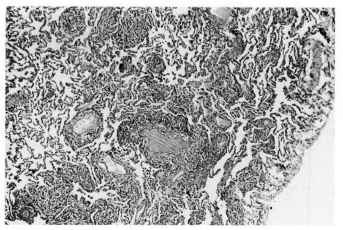

FIGURE 31–7   Hypersensitivity angiitis is demonstrated in a lung biopsy specimen from a young drug addict with a short history of increasing dyspnea on exertion and purpura. This section shows prominent infiltration by inflammatory cells and eosinophils of the alveolar walls and around blood vessels. Hematoxylin and eosin stain.

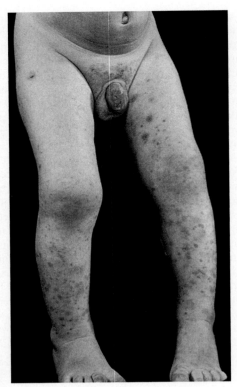

FIGURE 31–8 Skin lesions of a patient with hypersensitivity vasculitis.

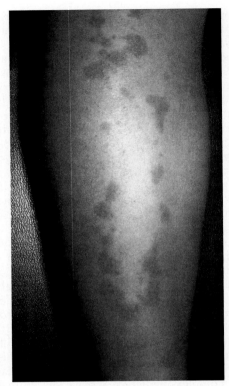

FIGURE 31–9 Linear bands of urticarial lesions in a 6-year-old girl with hypocomplementemic urticarial vasculitis. These lesions were transient and recurrent.

and abdominal pain may accompany each cutaneous exacerbation. Arthralgias occur in approximately 60%, and arthritis, usually of small joints, in 30% of patients. The arthritis has a brief duration and has no long-term residua. Abdominal and chest pain occur in 25% patients, pulmonary disease (e.g., cough, dyspnea, hemoptysis) in 30%, and glomerulonephritis in 15%. Less commonly, uveitis and episcleritis, fever, angioedema, Raynaud Phenomenon, pseudotumor cerebri, and seizures may be associated. Rapidly progressive glomerulonephritis and pulmonary hemorrhage have been described.[180]

Hypocomplementemic urticarial vasculitis (HUV) has also been associated with SLE,[181,182] Sjögren syndrome, hepatitis B and C antigenemia, drug reactions, and excessive exposure to sun.[183] A separate group of patients with urticarial vasculitis have normal complement levels.[179,181] Patients with hypocomplementemia tend to have more severe systemic symptoms.[178]

The pathogenesis of this type of vasculitis is unknown, but an immune complex process with activation of the classic complement pathway is suggested by lesional deposits of Igs and complement and circulating immune complexes.[184] Levels of early and late components of the complement cascade may be depressed, with the degree of hypocomplementemia paralleling the severity of the disease. ANA, RF, and cryoglobulins are usually absent. An IgG antibody to the collagenlike region of C1q has been described (HUV, 100%; SLE, 35%).[184] Levels of C3, C4, and C1q are reduced in 18% to 50%. Skin biopsy documents a leukocytoclastic vasculitis, predominantly a venulitis, with abundant neutrophilic and occasionally eosinophilic infiltrates.[178,181,183] Immunofluorescence

microscopy confirms the deposition of IgM and C3 in affected vessels. A mild membranoproliferative glomerulonephritis may accompany the cutaneous disease.

Management consists of supportive measures and treatment of any associated disorders. Antihistamines, dapsone, hydroxychloroquine, colchicine, and indomethacin have been used with variable success.[178] Systemic glucocorticoids or other immunosuppressive drugs may be required in severely involved children. The course of the disease is usually benign but may vary depending on the associated disorders and extent of systemic involvement.

MIXED CRYOGLOBULINEMIA

Vasculitis with essential mixed cryoglobulinemia (types II and III) clinically resembles other leukocytoclastic vasculitides. This disease is defined by the Chapel Hill Consensus Conference as vasculitis with immune deposits in capillaries, venules, or arterioles of the skin and kidney associated with cryoglobulins in the serum.[173] Mixed cryoglobulinemic vasculitis would be considered under the heading "other vasculitis" using the recently described pediatric classification criteria.[104] Purpura on the distal extremities, often precipitated by exposure to cold, is accompanied by arthralgia, with or without frank arthritis,[185] and by glomerulonephritis in up to one half of the patients.[186] Patients also may have pulmonary involvement. High levels of mixed cryoglobulins (i.e., IgG and IgM that reversibly precipitate on cooling), sometimes with hepatitis B[186] or coccidioidin antigen,[187] are the serological hallmark of the disorder.

Cryoglobulinemic vasculitis is rare in children[185] and results in an acute vascular inflammation after localization of mixed cryoglobulins in vessel walls. Low levels of C4 with normal or slightly low C3 levels are distinctive. Infection with hepatitis B or C virus must always be excluded.[186,188] Progressive renal disease that resembles membranoproliferative glomerulonephritis is the principal cause of long-term morbidity.[187] Outcome is related to severity of the systemic disease. Treatment with combinations of glucocorticoids, cyclophosphamide, plasmapheresis, and intravenous Ig may benefit some patients.[189]

OTHER LEUKOCYTOCLASTIC AND PERIVASCULITIC SYNDROMES

In several other types of vasculitis, the histopathology shows a leukocytoclastic element. Some of these disorders, such as cutaneous polyarteritis and sarcoidosis, are discussed later.

The differential diagnosis of systemic vasculitis is often challenging in that other forms of secondary vasculitis and vasculitic mimics, such as thromboangiitis obliterans (Buerger disease) and infectious angiitis (including syphilis and Lyme disease), must be considered. Other syndromes are more difficult to classify: vasculitis associated with retroperitoneal fibrosis, inflammatory bowel disease, primary biliary cirrhosis, and transplant rejection. Children may present with a vasculopathy from ergot poisoning, neurofibromatosis, coarctation-hypoplasia-dysplasia, and embolism. Vasculitis has also been observed (anecdotally) in the skin following trauma in the context of accidental or nonaccidental injury.[190]

Antineutrophil Cytoplasmic Antibody-Associated Small-Vessel Vasculitis

Antibodies to neutrophil cytoplasmic antigens (ANCAs) are described in more detail in Chapter 34. ANCAs are associated with three major vasculitides, all uncommon in children: Wegener granulomatosis, microscopic polyangiitis (and the likely *forme fruste* variant of this renal limited vasculitis) and the Churg-Strauss syndrome.[191,192] Wegener granulomatosis and the Churg-Strauss syndrome are characterized by granulomatous inflammation involving the respiratory tract and necrotizing vasculitis affecting small- and medium-sized vessels (i.e., capillaries, venules, arterioles, veins, and arteries).[193,194] Cutaneous involvement is common and consists of petechiae, palpable purpura, skin ulcers, papules, and nodules.[191,195] Skin lesions rarely precede the appearance of other features of these illnesses. Rapid diagnosis of ANCA-associated vasculitis is important because appropriate immunosuppressive treatment often limits life-threatening injury to vital organs.

Goodpasture Syndrome

Goodpasture syndrome is characterized by pulmonary hemorrhage and severe crescentic proliferative glomerulonephritis. Constitutional symptoms occur in one fourth of patients, and pulmonary complaints (e.g., dyspnea, weakness, chest pain, wheezing) are common.[196] Pulmonary hemorrhage is often the initial manifestation and may precede renal abnormalities anywhere from weeks to years, or clinical progression may be rapid. Serum antibodies to the alpha 3 chain of type IV collagen (NCI domain) in alveolar and glomerular basement membranes are diagnostic.[197] These antibodies can be demonstrated as linear staining of the basement membranes in lung tissue and glomeruli by immunofluorescence microscopy.

This disease predominantly affects young men and has only occasionally been reported in children or adolescents.[196,198-200] In children, idiopathic pulmonary hemosiderosis, Wegener granulomatosis, hemolytic-uremic syndrome, and SLE are considerations in differential diagnosis. Goodpasture syndrome has occurred after therapy with D-penicillamine, in cases of heavy metal poisoning, and in patients with a variety of rheumatic diseases.

Treatment includes the prompt use of glucocorticoids, plasmapheresis, and immunosuppressive agents.[198,199,201] Nonetheless, the survival rate is low. Death is caused by asphyxia, pulmonary hemorrhages, or uremia.

Vasculitis Associated with Connective Tissue Disorders

Leukocytoclastic vasculitis may occur in SLE, usually presenting as palpable purpura or urticaria,[202] and in dermatomyositis, mixed connective tissue disease, and scleroderma. Vascular involvement is particularly well recognized in juvenile dermatomyositis, in which small-vessel vasculitis has been identified in striated muscle, skin, subcutaneous tissue, and the gastrointestinal tract.[107,203]

Familial Mediterranean Fever and Behçet Disease

A number of reports describe the occurrence of vasculitis in patients with MEFV.[204,205] In some patients, the onset of vasculitis may be the first indication of this disorder. Similarly, patients with Behçet disease develop papular or pustular lesions that may ulcerate from a vasculitis with a predominant lymphocytic infiltrate, but a leukocytoclastic vasculitis may be present. Also see Chapters 36 and 43.

Mucha-Habermann Disease

Mucha-Habermann disease (or pityriasis lichenoides et varioliformis acuta [PLEVA]), is a form of cutaneous vasculitis of unknown origin. At presentation, the dermatitis has the appearance of chronic or recurrent chickenpox-like lesions that become atrophic and scarred. The rash is accompanied by fever and joint pain and swelling (Fig. 31–10). Histologically, the lesions are characterized by a lymphocytic inflammation of capillaries and venules of the upper dermis. PLEVA has been described in two children with chronic arthritis resembling juvenile idiopathic arthritis, one of whom developed severe acrosclerosis and scleroderma late in her course.[206] A third patient with similar cutaneous findings was reported previously.[207]

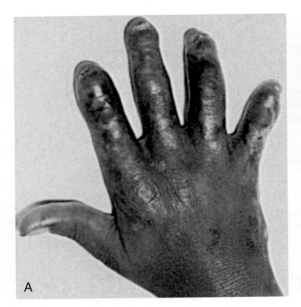

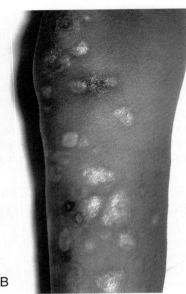

FIGURE 31–10 An 11-year-old, black girl with destructive acrosclerosis and Mucha-Habermann disease. **A,** Hand. **B,** Forearm. The characteristic cutaneous lesions of Mucha-Habermann disease are visible, along with advanced ischemic digital changes.

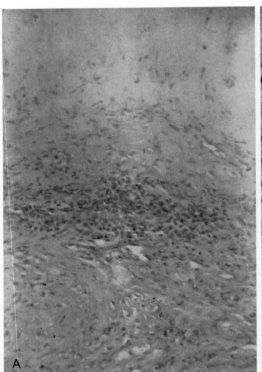

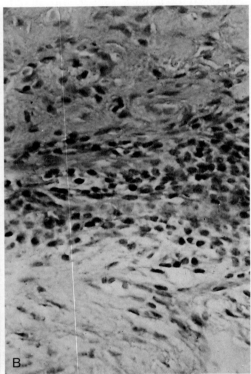

FIGURE 31–11 Histopathology of relapsing polychondritis. **A,** Biopsy specimen of ear cartilage. Hematoxylin and eosin stain. **B,** Close-up view. Hematoxylin and eosin stain. Acute inflammation and perichondritis are evident, with numerous lymphocytes and plasma cells and smaller numbers of polymorphonuclear cells. The edge of the aural elastic cartilage is being destroyed by the cellular exudate.

Relapsing Polychondritis

Relapsing polychondritis is a rare, idiopathic, and widespread inflammation of cartilage associated with uveitis, deafness, vestibular involvement, and aortic valve insufficiency.[208] It has seldom been observed in children.[209,210] Differential diagnosis includes Wegener granulomatosis and a variety of infections. Inflammation affects the cartilage of the ear or hyaline cartilage of the joints and then spreads to involve cartilage of the upper respiratory tract, including the nose, trachea, and bronchi (Fig. 31–11).

Episodic oligoarthritis occurs in approximately 80% of affected patients. The synovial fluid is noninflammatory, and the synovial membrane demonstrates minimal inflammation.[210]

The course is initially episodic but becomes progressive in most patients. Relapsing polychondritis has been described in one patient with HSP.[211] Intrauterine transmission has been suggested in another, but this association appears to be exceptional.[212] Glucocorticoids suppress the disease, and death is often the result of respiratory obstruction.[209]

Köhlmeier-Degos Syndrome

Köhlmeier-Degos syndrome (malignant atrophic papulosis; progressive arterial occlusive disease) is a rare, often fatal occlusive vasculopathy of cutaneous, gastrointestinal, and central nervous system small- and medium-sized arteries, which results in progressive occlusion by fibrosis, leading to infarction.[213] It occurs almost exclusively in young- to middle-aged men and has been reported in teenage boys,[213,214] although very young children have been described.[215,216] Some investigators regard it as a lupus variant,[217] although this view is controversial.

Antiphospholipid Antibody Syndrome

Patients with the antiphospholipid antibody syndrome have repeated episodes of intravascular coagulation and thrombosis. In the absence of identifiable systemic disease, these patients may be erroneously diagnosed as having idiopathic vasculitis (see Chapter 22).[218,219]

Atrial myxoma may simulate vasculitis by embolization[220,221] and should be considered in the diagnosis of an obscure vasculitis-like syndrome. This phenomenon is rarely reported in children or adolescents.[222] Echocardiography demonstrates the lesion and surgical removal is curative. Infectious endocarditis produces a similar but not identical clinical syndrome.

Vasculitis Associated with Malignancy

Lymphoproliferative disease rarely is accompanied by a leukocytoclastic vasculitis limited to the skin. Lymphocytic lymphoma and Waldenström macroglobulinemia, both rare in children, can result in a cryoglobulinemic vasculitis.[223] Lymphoma may also be associated with Wegener granulomatosis, Sjögren syndrome, and HSP. Occasionally, vasculitis precedes the diagnosis of a lymphoproliferative syndrome.

Sweet Syndrome

Acute febrile neutrophilic dermatosis (Sweet syndrome) is rare in children and consists of an inflammatory perivasculitis (with a dermal infiltrate of mature neutrophils) characterized clinically by spiking fever and tender, raised, pseudovesicular, erythematous plaques or nodules on the face and extremities and sometimes on the trunk.[224,225] Arthritis occurs in one third of adult patients[226] and has been described in an 8-month-old boy.[225] Musculoskeletal pain, including arthritis or multifocal osteomyelitis, has also been reported in children.[225,227,228] This syndrome may be secondary to malignancy and its treatment, Behçet syndrome, or miscellaneous disorders.

Cronkhite-Canada Syndrome

Juvenile gastrointestinal polyposis is rarely associated with a widespread vasculitis of small- and medium-sized arteries, the Cronkhite-Canada syndrome.[229] The syndrome is characterized by cutaneous anergy, skin hyperpigmentation, alopecia, onychatrophia, intestinal polyps, and malabsorption. This disorder has a poor prognosis, and few affected children live more than two years.[230] The differential diagnosis includes *infantile necrotizing enterocolitis*, which also may be associated with a vasculitis.[231]

Stevens-Johnson Syndrome

The Stevens-Johnson syndrome is a severe, systemic, widespread form of mucocutaneous *erythema multiforme* and merges into *toxic epidermal necrolysis* (depending on the surface area involved). Numerous erosive, vesiculobullous, hemorrhagic, and papular lesions develop acutely on the mucosa and skin of the face, hands, trunk, and feet (Fig. 31–12). Anal, genital, and ocular orifices are often affected, and scarring may result. Onset is usually abrupt and is associated with fever, profound constitutional symptoms, and the appearance of periarticular swelling and pain or frank arthritis. The respiratory and gastrointestinal tracts can be involved in severe disease.

Histopathological studies demonstrate a perivasculitis that results in stomatitis, conjunctivitis, or corneal ulcerations, with no evidence of a necrotizing vasculitis. The cause of the syndrome is unknown, but a preceding infectious illness, particularly with *Mycoplasma pneumoniae*, is frequently documented.[232] Antibiotics, especially trimethoprim-sulfamethoxazole[233] and cefaclor, NSAIDs, and anticonvulsant medications have also been implicated.[234]

Expert supportive care is usually the sole treatment necessary for this self-limited disease. Extensive mucosal and cutaneous disease is best managed in a burn unit. In severe cases, glucocorticoids may be considered necessary, but they increase the risk of infection.[235]

Erythema Elevatum Diutinum

Erythema elevatum diutinum is a rare form of chronic, localized, cutaneous leukocytoclastic vasculitis, characterized by edematous papules and plaques (e.g., yellow, red, purple) occurring mainly over extensor surfaces. A similar lesion, *granuloma faciale*, is localized to the face. Fibrinoid necrosis of the upper and middle dermal vessels develops in both conditions.[236] Systemic involvement is

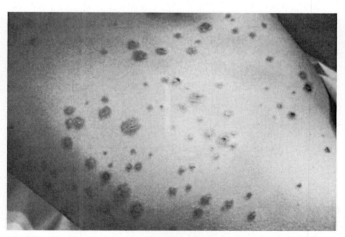

FIGURE 31–12 Vesicular erythematous lesions of erythema multiforme occurred in a young boy with Stevens-Johnson syndrome. The characteristic bullous lesions also developed around body orifices.

unusual.[237] Treatment with dapsone or intralesional steroids may be beneficial.[238]

Livedoid Vasculopathy

Livedoid vasculopathy (or livedoid vasculitis as it is sometimes mistakenly called) is characterized by ulceration of the lower extremities.[239] In its late stages, it can progress to the cutaneous features described as atrophie blanche. The condition can mimic leukocytoclastic vasculitis clinically, but histologically an occlusive vasculopathy is observed with thrombosis within dermal blood vessels and endothelial proliferation. The disease is more common in middle-aged females but is also described in children. Sometimes a defined prothrombotic state is identified, such as factor V Leiden mutation, decreased protein C or S, lupus anticoagulant, and/or anticardiolipin antibodies, although this is by no means a universal feature of the condition. Corticosteroids are usually ineffective and may even worsen the condition. Treatment is aimed at prevention of thrombosis with low molecular weight heparin, warfarin, or antiplatelet agents, such as dipyridamole or low dose aspirin. Vasodilators, such as calcium channel blockers, may be useful to maintain perfusion in the superficial skin vessels.

REFERENCES

1. J.T. Lie, Illustrated histopathologic classification criteria for selected vasculitis syndromes. American College of Rheumatology Subcommittee on Classification of Vasculitis, Arthritis Rheum. 33 (1990) 1074–1087.
2. A. Yalcindag, R. Sundel, Vasculitis in childhood, Curr. Opin. Rheumatol. 13 (2001) 422–427.
3. S. Ozen, The spectrum of vasculitis in children, Best. Pract. Res. Clin. Rheumatol. 16 (2002) 411–425.
4. O. Kobayashi, H. Wada, K. Okawa, et al., Schönlein-Henoch's syndrome in children, Contrib. Nephrol. 4 (1975) 48–71.
5. E.J. Tizard, Henoch-Schönlein purpura, Arch. Dis. Child. 80 (1999) 380–383.
6. N.S. Murali, R. George, G.T. John, et al., Problems of classification of Henoch Schönlein purpura: an Indian perspective, Clin. Exp. Dermatol. 27 (2002) 260–263.
7. S. Ballinger, Henoch-Schönlein purpura, Curr. Opin. Rheumatol. 15 (2003) 591–594.
8. S. Mrusek, M. Kruger, P. Greiner, et al., Henoch-Schönlein purpura, Lancet 363 (2004) 1116.
9. R. Willan, On cutaneous diseases, J Johnson, London, 1808.
10. Heberden W: Commentaries on the history and cure of diseases, London, 1896.
11. J.L. Schönlein, Allegemeine und Specielle Pathologie und Therapie, ed 3, Literatur-Comptoir, Herisau, Germany, 1837.
12. E.H. Henoch, About a peculiar form of purpura, Berlin. Reprinted in Am. J. Dis. Child. 128 (1974) 78–79.
13. D. Gairdner, The Schönlein-Henoch syndrome (anaphylactoid purpura), Q. J. Med. 17 (1948) 95.
14. P. Rieu, L.H. Noel, Henoch-Schönlein nephritis in children and adults. Morphological features and clinicopathological correlations, Ann. Med. Interne. (Paris) 150 (1999) 151–159.
15. F.T. Saulsbury, Henoch-Schönlein purpura in children. Report of 100 patients and review of the literature, Medicine (Baltimore) 78 (1999) 395–409.
16. G. Rostoker, Schönlein-Henoch purpura in children and adults: diagnosis, pathophysiology and management, Bio. Drugs 15 (2001) 99–138.
17. F.T. Saulsbury, Epidemiology of Henoch-Schönlein purpura, Cleve. Clin. J. Med. 69 (2002) SII87–SII89.
18. M.C. Calvino, J. Llorca, C. Garcia-Porrua, et al., Henoch-Schönlein purpura in children from northwestern Spain: a 20-year epidemiologic and clinical study, Medicine (Baltimore) 80 (2001) 279–290.
19. M. Al Sheyyab, H. El Shanti, S. Ajlouni, et al., The clinical spectrum of Henoch-Schönlein purpura in infants and young children, Eur. J. Pediatr. 154 (1995) 969–972.
20. S. Ozen, A. Pistorio, M. Iusan, et al., The EULAR/PRINTO/PRES criteria for Henoch-Schonlein purpura. Abstract presentation at EULAR, June 2009, Ann. Rheum. Dis. (2009) In press.
21. M. Stewart, J.M. Savage, B. Bell, et al., Long term renal prognosis of Henoch-Schönlein purpura in an unselected childhood population, Eur. J. Pediatr. 147 (1988) 113–115.
22. T.A. Farley, S. Gillespie, M. Rasoulpour, et al., Epidemiology of a cluster of Henoch-Schönlein purpura, Am. J. Dis. Child. 143 (1989) 798–803.
23. J.M. Gardner-Medwin, P. Dolezalova, C. Cummins, et al., Incidence of Henoch-Schönlein purpura, Kawasaki disease, and rare vasculitides in children of different ethnic origins, Lancet 360 (2002) 1197–1202.
24. S.R. Atkinson, D.J. Barker, Seasonal distribution of Henoch-Schönlein purpura, Br. J. Prev. Soc. Med. 30 (1976) 22–25.
25. M. Levy, M. Broyer, A. Arsan, et al., Anaphylactoid purpura nephritis in childhood: natural history and immunopathology, Adv. Nephrol. Necker. Hosp. 6 (1976) 183–228.
26. D.M. Allen, L.K. Diamond, D.A. Howell, Anaphylactoid purpura in children (Schönlein-Henoch syndrome): review with a follow-up of the renal complications, Am. J. Dis. Child. 99 (1960) 833–854.
27. M. Al Sheyyab, A. Batieha, H. El Shanti, et al., Henoch-Schönlein purpura and streptococcal infection: a prospective case-control study, Ann. Trop. Paediatr. 19 (1999) 253–255.
28. M. Masuda, K. Nakanishi, N. Yoshizawa, et al., Group A streptococcal antigen in the glomeruli of children with Henoch-Schönlein nephritis, Am. J. Kidney. Dis. 41 (2003) 366–370.
29. H. Matsukura, A. Ohtsuki, T. Fuchizawa, et al., Acute poststreptococcal glomerulonephritis mimicking Henoch-Schönlein purpura, Clin. Nephrol. 59 (2003) 64–65.
30. P.A. Courtney, R.N. Patterson, R.J. Lee, Henoch-Schönnlein purpura following meningitis C vaccination, Rheumatology (Oxford) 40 (2001) 345–346.
31. E.M. Lambert, A. Liebling, E. Glusac, et al., Henoch-Schönlein purpura following a meningococcal vaccine, Pediatrics 112 (2003) e491.
32. Y. Minohara, Studies on the relationship between anaphylactoid purpura and human parvovirus B19, Kansenshogaku Zasshi 69 (1995) 928–933.
33. T. Watanabe, Y. Oda, Henoch-Schönlein purpura nephritis associated with human parvovirus B19 infection, Pediatr. Int. 42 (2000) 94–96.
34. E.M. Eisenstein, Lack of evidence for herpesvirus, retrovirus, or parvovirus infection in Henoch-Schönlein purpura, Clin. Exp. Rheumatol. 20 (2002) 734.
35. E.D. Heegaard, E.B. Taaning, Parvovirus B19 and parvovirus V9 are not associated with Henoch-Schönlein purpura in children, Pediatr. Infect. Dis. J. 21 (2002) 31–34.
36. S.R. Meadow, E.F. Glasgow, R.H. White, et al., Schönlein-Henoch nephritis, Q. J. Med. 41 (1972) 241–258.
37. F.K. Pedersen, E.A. Petersen, Varicella followed by glomerulonephritis. Treatment with corticosteroids and azathioprine resulting in recurrence of varicella, Acta. Paediatr. Scand. 64 (1975) 886–890.
38. M. Kalyoncu, E. Odemis, N. Yaris, et al., Association of Henoch-Schönlein purpura with varicella zoster, Indian Pediatr. 40 (2003) 274–275.
39. G. Maggiore, A. Martini, S. Grifeo, et al., Hepatitis B virus infection and Schönlein-Henoch purpura, Am. J. Dis. Child. 138 (1984) 681–682.
40. I. Islek, A.G. Kalayci, F. Gok, et al., Henoch-Schönlein purpura associated with hepatitis A infection, Pediatr. Int. 45 (2003) 114–116.
41. S.W. Liew, I. Kessel, Mycoplasmal pneumonia preceding Henoch-Schönlein purpura [letter], Arch. Dis. Child. 49 (1974) 912–913.
42. K. Kaneko, S. Fujinaga, Y. Ohtomo, et al., Mycoplasma pneumoniae-associated Henoch-Schönlein purpura nephritis, Pediatr. Nephrol. 13 (1999) 1000–1001.
43. E.M. Ayoub, J. McBride, M. Schmiederer, et al., Role of Bartonella henselae in the etiology of Henoch-Schönlein purpura, Pediatr. Infect. Dis. J. 21 (2002) 28–31.
44. C. Hoshino, Adult onset Schonlein-Henoch purpura associated with Helicobacter pylori infection, Intern. Med. 48 (2009) 847–851.

45. J.F. Ackroyd, Allergic purpura, including purpura due to foods, drugs and infections, Am. J. Med. 14 (1953) 605–632.
46. J. Giangiacomo, C.C. Tsai, Dermal and glomerular deposition of IgA in anaphylactoid purpura, Am. J. Dis. Child. 131 (1977) 981–983.
47. Y.H. Yang, M.T. Huang, S.C. Lin, et al., Increased transforming growth factor-beta (TGF-beta)-secreting T cells and IgA anti-cardiolipin antibody levels during acute stage of childhood Henoch-Schönlein purpura, Clin. Exp. Immunol. 122 (2000) 285–290.
48. K.K. Lau, H. Suzuki, J. Novak, et al., Pathogenesis of Henoch-Schönlein purpura nephritis, Pediatr. Nephrol. 25 (2010) 19–26.
49. K. Brendel-Muller, A. Hahn, R. Schneppenheim, et al., Laboratory signs of activated coagulation are common in Henoch-Schönlein purpura, Pediatr. Nephrol. 16 (2001) 1084–1088.
50. T.S. Gunasekaran, J. Berman, M. Gonzalez, Duodenojejunitis: is it idiopathic or is it Henoch-Schönlein purpura without the purpura? J. Pediatr. Gastroenterol. Nutr. 30 (2000) 22–28.
51. H. Kamitsuji, K. Tani, M. Yasui, et al., Activity of blood coagulation factor XIII as a prognostic indicator in patients with Henoch-Schönlein purpura. Efficacy of factor XIII substitution, Eur. J. Pediatr. 146 (1987) 519–523.
52. K. Kawasaki, H. Komura, Y. Nakahara, et al., Factor XIII in Henoch-Schönlein purpura with isolated gastrointestinal symptoms, Pediatr. Int. 48 (2006) 413–415.
53. G. Demircin, A. Oner, Y. Unver, et al., Erythrocyte superoxide dismutase activity and plasma malondialdehyde levels in children with Henoch-Schönlein purpura, Acta. Pediatr. 87 (1998) 848–852.
54. A. Yoruk, F. Cizmecioglu, H. Yukselgungor, et al., Methotrexate-induced systemic vasculitis, Med. Pediatr. Oncol. 38 (2002) 139–140.
55. P.A. Livermore, K.J. Murray, Anti-tumour necrosis factor therapy associated with cutaneous vasculitis, Rheumatology (Oxford) 41 (2002) 1450–1452.
56. F. Levy-Khademi, S.H. Korman, Y. Amitai, Henoch-Schönlein purpura: simultaneous occurrence in two siblings, Pediatr. Dermatol. 17 (2000) 139–140.
57. V. Grech, C. Vella, Henoch-Schönlein purpura with nephritis in two siblings following infectious mononucleosis, Ann. Trop. Paediatr. 22 (2002) 297–298.
58. M.M. Amoli, W. Thomson, A.H. Hajeer, et al., HLA-B35 association with nephritis in Henoch-Schönlein purpura, J. Rheumatol. 29 (2002) 948–949.
59. M.M. Amoli, W. Thomson, A.H. Hajeer, et al., HLA-DRB1*01 association with Henoch-Schönlein purpura in patients from northwest Spain, J. Rheumatol. 28 (2001) 1266–1270.
60. H. Peru, O. Soylemezoglu, S. Gonen, et al., HLA class 1 associations in Henoch Schönlein purpura: increased and decreased frequencies, Clin. Rheumatol. 27 (2008) 5–10.

Chapter 32

POLYARTERITIS NODOSA AND CUTANEOUS POLYARTERITIS NODOSA

Michael J. Dillon and Seza Ozen

Polyarteritis nodosa (PAN) is a necrotizing vasculitis associated with aneurysmal nodules along the walls of medium-sized muscular arteries. It was classically described by Kussmaul and Maier in 1866,[1] although there were earlier reports in the literature, e.g., Michaelis and Matani in 1755 quoted by Lamb in 1914,[2] Pelletan in 1810,[3] and Rokitansky's case of 1852 quoted by Eppinger in 1887.[4] By 1932, 23 cases had been described in children,[5] and by 1939 44 cases had appeared in the literature.[6] In the presteroid era, mortality was high, and the diagnosis was almost exclusively made postmortem. Circumstances now are very different, and the outlook is much improved, but there is still a high morbidity and, in very severe cases, a consequential mortality. Historically it has been difficult to distinguish clearly between PAN and other types of vasculitis. Currently, in spite of some overlap with smaller vessel disease, PAN appears to be a separate entity. However, an issue remains as to whether systemic disease and disease localized to the skin, cutaneous PAN, are manifestations of the same condition or separate disorders. In this account, they will be described under separate headings.

POLYARTERITIS NODOSA

Definition and Classification

In the Chapel Hill Consensus Conference held for the nomenclature and definition of vasculitides, classical PAN was defined as necrotizing inflammation of medium- or small-sized arteries without vasculitis in arterioles, capillaries, or venules.[7] The group has separated PAN from the distinct group of microscopic polyangiitis (MPA), which they defined as necrotizing vasculitis with few or no immune deposits affecting small vessels. MPA is predominantly a renal disease and usually presents, in childhood, as rapidly progressive, crescentic, glomerulonephritis associated with antineutrophil cytoplasmic antibodies (ANCA).

The widely accepted classification criteria for PAN have been the American College of Rheumatology (ACR) criteria, which were introduced in the 1990s and based solely on an adult registry.[8] There have been two attempts to introduce specific pediatric criteria for PAN, one by Ozen and colleagues in 1992[9] and one by Brogan and colleagues in 2002.[10] These criteria were based on the pediatric practice and experience in children with PAN, although neither was tested for specificity, and there were no attempts at validation.

In 2006, the first true childhood criteria were published with the endorsement of the European League against Rheumatism (EULAR) and the Paediatric Rheumatology European Society (PRES) with the participation of the European Society of Paediatric Nephrology (ESPN) and the ACR.[11] These criteria were established in two steps: initially opinions were gathered from pediatric rheumatologists and nephrologists worldwide through a Delphi technique. Subsequently the final criteria were agreed on in a consensus conference with ten experts, using the nominal group technique. The criteria were hoped to be widely accepted, based on the reliable techniques used and the international and multispecialist character of the expert group involved.

For the validation of these criteria, a large international web-based registry for childhood vasculitides was formed. The 2006 criteria were revised and validated based on this international registry and the consensus of an expert panel. After minor revisions, the final criteria with the highest sensitivity and specificity for childhood PAN were agreed on (Table 32–1).[12]

The involvement of other organ systems were not separate criteria but were to be reflected in the histopathology or angiographic findings. The aforementioned criteria have been validated and revised based on pediatric data only. It is hoped that they will be widely accepted and used for future collaborative studies. However, it should be emphasized that these are classification criteria and not diagnostic criteria, although they are often used as such.

Epidemiology and Genetics

We lack data describing the epidemiology of childhood PAN. In adults, at least in Europe and the United States, an estimated annual incidence ranges from 2.0 to 9.0/million.[13] Although PAN is comparatively rare in childhood,

Table 32–1

Classification criteria for childhood PAN

Evidence of necrotizing vasculitis in medium- or small arteries or an angiographic abnormality showing aneurysm, stenosis, or occlusion of a medium- or small-sized artery (histopathology or angiography mandatory), plus 1 out of 5 of the following criteria:

1. Skin involvement (livedo reticularis, skin nodules or infarcts)
2. Myalgia or muscle tenderness
3. Hypertension (systolic/diastolic blood pressure greater than 95th percentile for height)
4. Peripheral neuropathy (sensory peripheral neuropathy or motor mononeuritis multiplex)
5. Renal involvement (proteinuria >0.3 g/24 hours or >30 mmol/mg of urine albumin/creatinine ratio on a spot morning sample; hematuria or red blood cell casts, >5 red blood cells/high power field, red blood cells casts in the urinary sediment, or = 2+ on dipstick; or impaired renal function, measured or calculated glomerular filtration rate (Schwartz formula) <50% normal.)

From Ozen S, Pistorio A, Iusan SM et al. Ann. Rheum. Dis. (In press 2010).

it appears, in some series to be the most common systemic vasculitis after Henoch-Schönlein Purpura (HSP) and Kawasaki Disease (KD), although worldwide Takayasu Arteritis is the third most common childhood vasculitic disease.[14,15] Childhood PAN seems to be of worldwide distribution, with no sex bias and with the majority of cases presenting in mid-childhood, although with a wide spectrum of ages affected.

In a multinational survey registering 110 childhood PAN patients, the majority of patients were from the eastern Mediterranean and South America, areas where *Streptococci* are still frequent.[16] Since not all countries are represented in this survey, there is a certain bias involved, and future studies are needed to define whether there is a true geographic or even ethnic difference.

PAN is probably a multifactorial disease. A number of childhood cases have been reported; genome wide search has not been performed, probably because of the low number of patients in individual centers. However, there are probably genetic predisposing factors that may make individuals vulnerable to develop PAN, an assumption that has also been considered for other vasculitides.

Recently, an association of childhood PAN with mutations in the familial Mediterranean fever (MEFV) gene has been shown with a significantly increased MEFV mutation carrier rate in Turkish children with PAN.[17,18] This suggests that at least in certain populations where the MEFV mutations are frequent, these mutations may be acting as one of the susceptibility factors for PAN. Additionally, there are three reports of PAN occurring in siblings within families, which may add weight to the genetic hypothesis, although no detailed genetic studies have been undertaken to prove the link.[19-21]

Etiopathogenesis

The etiology of PAN remains unclear. Classic PAN with hepatitis B is an immune complex disease; however, this association is extremely rare in childhood.[16,22-24]

There are reports of a higher exposure frequency to parvovirus B19 and cytomegalovirus in PAN patients compared to control populations.[25-28] In adults and children, HIV has also been implicated,[28-30] and PAN-like illnesses have been reported in association with cancers and hematological malignancies.[31] However, in childhood, these associations between PAN and infections or other conditions are less clear cut. Recently, evidence has emerged suggesting that bacterial superantigens may play a role in some cases.[32,33] In terms of pathogenetic mechanisms, it seems likely that the immunological processes involved are similar to those in other systemic vasculitides, and they include immune complexes, complement, possibly autoantibodies, cell adhesion molecules, cytokines, growth factors, chemokines, neutrophils, and T cells.[34,35]

Clinical Manifestations

The main clinical features of PAN are malaise, fever, weight loss, skin rash, myalgia, abdominal pain, and arthropathy.[9,36-46] In addition, children present with ischemic symptoms of the affected organ systems due to the severe vessel inflammation: ischemic heart and testicular pain; renal manifestations, such as hematuria, proteinuria, and hypertension[42,47,48]; and neurological features, such as focal defects, hemiplegia, visual loss, mononeuritis multiplex, and organic psychosis.[49-51] Skin lesions are variable and may masquerade as those of HSP or multiform erythema, but they can also be necrotic and be associated with peripheral gangrene (Figs. 32–1 and 32–2).[52,53] Livedo reticularis is also a characteristic feature, and occasionally subcutaneous nodules overlying affected arteries are present.[52,53] System involvement is variable, but the skin, the musculoskeletal system, the kidneys, and the gastrointestinal tract are most prominently affected with cardiac, neurological, and respiratory manifestations occurring less frequently.[9,10,37,39,40,42,45,54] If the condition is untreated, widespread infarction can occur in affected viscera (Fig. 32–3). In some patients, rupture of arterial aneurysms can cause peritoneal bleeding with perirenal hematomata being a recognized manifestation of this phenomenon (Fig. 32–4).[55] This feature has been noted a number of times in Turkey where it has occurred in patients with the well recognized association of PAN and familial Mediterranean fever (FMF).[56,57] However, clinical manifestations (and investigation findings) can be very confusing with absence of conclusive diagnostic evidence, certainly in the early phase and sometimes the late phase of the illness.[58]

Laboratory and Radiological Data

Leukocytosis and thrombocytosis are frequent, along with elevated erythrocyte sedimentation rate and CRP levels.[16] Mild anemia may occur as well. Antineutrophil cytoplasmic antibodies (ANCA) are not a part of the work-up for childhood PAN. In a multicenter study recruiting 110 PAN patients from 21 pediatric centers worldwide, only six of the 47 childhood patients tested for ANCA had mild or nonspecific staining, and none had elevated ELISA titers for either myeloperoxidase (MPO)-ANCA

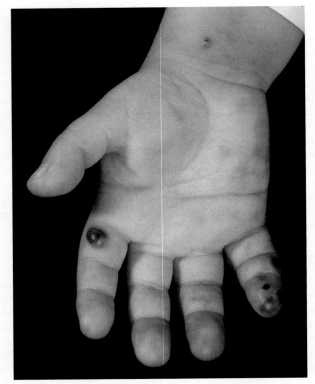

FIGURE 32–1   Lesions on the hand of a 2-year-old girl with PAN. The biopsy revealed severe necrotizing vasculitis. (Courtesy of Dr. P.A. Brogan)

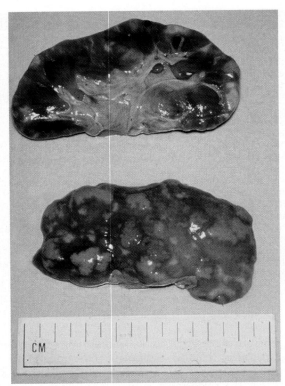

FIGURE 32–3   Postmortem appearances of the kidneys from a child with widespread aggressive PAN, showing extensive areas of infarction secondary to the renal arterial necrotizing vasculitis.

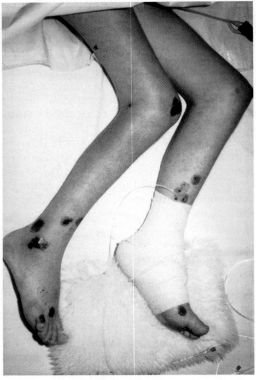

FIGURE 32–2   Necrotic lesions on the legs of a child with PAN. Livedo reticularis also present. (From reference 44 by permission of Oxford University Press)

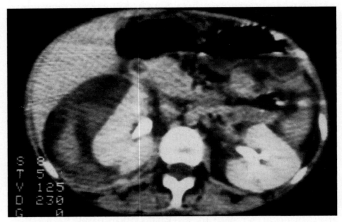

FIGURE 32–4   Abdominal CT scan undertaken on a teenager with long-standing PAN that was resistant to treatment, showing bilateral perirenal hematomata due to rupture of affected renal vessels.

or proteinase 3 (PR3)-ANCA.[16] However, for microscopic polyarteritis/polyangiitis patients, ANCA is a crucial part of the work-up since it plays a major role in the pathogenesis of the disease.[59] In MPA, ANCA is often against the myeloperoxidase of the neutrophils and is detected by ELISA tests for MPO. Other autoantibodies, such as antinuclear antibody (ANA), are negative. Markers of endothelial inflammation, such as factor

VIII-related antigen, may be elevated.[60] Recently there has also been some interest in measurement of circulating endothelial microparticles and circulating endothelial cells as markers of endothelial inflammatory damage in PAN and other vasculitides,[61-67] and circulating endothelial progenitor cells that might point to evidence of endothelial repair.[65,68] Urinalysis findings may reflect renal involvement. Proteinuria, hematuria, and decrease in renal function may occur.[68] Demonstration of aneurysms reflecting the necrotizing vasculitis of renal, celiac, mesenteric, or arteries in other parts of the body is a part of the diagnosis (Fig. 32–5).[10,47,70-72] Brogan and colleagues have shown that changes other than aneurysms may also suggest a diagnosis of PAN.[10] The most reliable nonaneurysmal signs were perfusion defects, the presence of collateral arteries, lack of crossing of peripheral renal arteries, and delayed emptying of small renal arteries. The authors indicated that the sensitivity of the diagnosis of PAN increased with the use of these features; magnetic resonance and especially computerized tomography (CT) angiography have emerged as alternative noninvasive techniques to delineate vasculitic lesions in PAN.[73] A number of patients have been diagnosed with these techniques. However, the sensitivity of these techniques is hampered in small aneurysms and smaller affected vessels. Furthermore, the radiation dose of CT angiography is rather high. Conventional angiogram remains the overall gold standard, though future progress in imaging may improve the sensitivity of noninvasive imaging.

Indirect evidence of the presence of medium-sized vessel vasculitis affecting the renal arteries may be obtained by demonstrating patchy areas within the renal parenchyma of decreased isotope uptake on Tc99m-dimercaptosuccinic acid scanning of the kidneys.[54,74] These findings are not specific for vascular ischemia but in the context of a vasculitic illness, they are very suggestive, particularly if there is no history or evidence of another cause.

Pathology

Biopsy is one of the criteria in the new classification of the disease. The characteristic pathological lesion is necrotizing arteritis with the formation of nodules along the walls of medium- and small-sized muscular arteries, hence the name. However, PAN may also affect the arterioles and venules, although the predominant manifestation is medium and small artery disease. The lesions tend to be focal and segmental or sectoral.[75] Thrombosis and fibrinoid necrosis may accompany the necrotizing vasculitis, and the sectoral involvement may produce blow-out type of aneurysms (Fig. 32–6). Arteries in any organ system can be involved. Biopsies of the muscle, sural nerve, kidney, liver, testis, or the GI tract may provide the diagnostic lesion. Immunofluorescence studies usually reveal no immune deposition.

Treatment

For many years the treatment of PAN has involved the administration of high dose steroid with an additional cytotoxic agent, such as cyclophosphamide, to induce remission.[76-81] Steroid in the form of prednisolone might be given orally in a dose of 1 to 2 mg/kg/day for four weeks, weaning over the next six to eight weeks (depending on response) to 0.3-0.7 mg/kg on alternate days or as IV methyl prednisolone 30 mg/kg (maximum 1 G) for three consecutive days, followed by oral prednisolone that should be tapered soon after. Cyclophosphamide might be administered in a dose of 2 mg/kg/day orally for two to three months or as 500-1000 mg/m² IV monthly for six months with dose reduction if renal or hepatic failure is present, although this is often maintained in children for shorter periods if remission is clearly achieved. Empirically, aspirin, or dipyridamole if aspirin is contraindicated, has also been given as an antiplatelet agent by some groups.[82] Once remission is achieved, maintenance therapy with daily or alternate day prednisolone and oral azathioprine in a dose of 2 mg/kg/day is

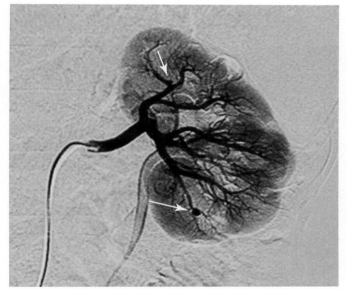

FIGURE 32–5 Aneurysms in branches of the renal artery in an angiogram from a child with PAN. (Courtesy of Dr. B. Peynircioglu)

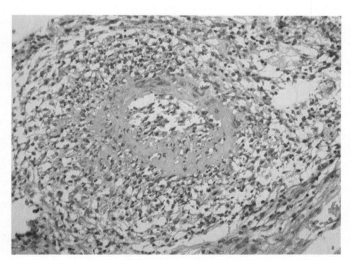

FIGURE 32–6 Biopsy of an intestinal wall artery in PAN showing transmural fibrinoid necrosis and inflammatory infiltrate (H & E, original magnification x 200). (Courtesy of Dr. D. Orhan)

frequently used for up to 18 months.[81,83] Alternative maintenance agents, e.g., methotrexate or mycophenolate mofetil, have been used when azathioprine has failed or has not been tolerated.[82] However, in PAN, no randomized controlled trial has been undertaken in adults or children to establish which agent is preferable, although, in ANCA-associated vasculitis, adult data favor the use of azathioprine.[84] Adjunctive plasma exchange can be used in life-threatening situations,[81,85,86] and, at times, intravenous immunoglobulin (IVIG) has been beneficially administered.[87] More recently, successful treatment with biological agents, such as infliximab or rituximab, has been reported.[82,88–91] When all therapeutic measures fail, treatment by immunoablation and autologous stem cell transplantation may be life-saving.[92]

PAN associated with hepatitis B infection requires a different approach since conventional treatment with glucocorticoids and cyclophosphamide allows the virus to replicate, facilitating evolution towards chronic hepatitis and liver cirrhosis. The recommended approach is to combine plasma exchange and antiviral treatment with steroids to control acute manifestations, then to stop the steroids to enhance immunological clearance of hepatitis B virus-infected hepatocytes, and to favor seroconversion from positive hepatitis B e antigen to a positive anti-hepatitis B e antigen.[53]

Prognosis/Outcome

In comparison to the almost 100% mortality rates in the presteroid era,[93] mortality rates are now remarkably low at approximately 1% in a recent retrospective multicenter analysis.[16] Other reports describe similarly good results.[36,39,69] However, although the prognosis has dramatically improved, PAN remains a life-threatening systemic vasculitis in need of early diagnosis and aggressive treatment. In tertiary referral centers seeing more severe cases, mortality rates of up to 10% are still recorded.[94] Recurrences are less frequent in childhood PAN compared to adult series but unlike with some other vasculitides, such as Wegener granulomatosis, PAN in childhood appears to be a condition where permanent remissions can be achieved.

Late morbidity can occur years after childhood PAN from chronic vascular injury, causing diffuse endothelial dysfunction[95] and increased arterial rigidity.[96] This remains a concern and is an area of ongoing active research.

CUTANEOUS POLYARTERITIS NODOSA

Cutaneous PAN is a form of vasculitis affecting small- and medium-sized vessels essentially limited to the skin.[97] It is characterized by the presence of fever, subcutaneous nodular, painful, nonpurpuric lesions with or without livedo reticularis (Fig. 32–7) occurring predominantly in the lower extremities, and with no systemic involvement (except for myalgia, arthralgia, and nonerosive arthritis).[97,98] It is well recognized in childhood, and there are a number of reports in the literature.[16,99–101] In a recent international survey of childhood vasculitis,

approximately one third of children identified as having PAN were categorized as not having systemic disease but instead cutaneous PAN.[16] The clinical course is characterized by periodic exacerbations and remissions that may persist for many years and occasionally throughout childhood.[97] Skin biopsy shows necrotizing nongranulomatous small- and medium-sized vessel vasculitis; tests for ANCA are usually negative, and the condition is often associated with serological or microbiological evidence of streptococcal infection.[102–104] Nonrecurring cutaneous PAN has been observed in neonates born to mothers with chronic cutaneous PAN.[97,105–107] There has been much discussion as to whether the condition should be classed as a separate entity or as a part of the spectrum of PAN.[96] The condition remains essentially localized to the skin,[97,108] although a proportion of cases appear to evolve into full blown PAN in time, and clinicians need to be mindful of this possibility.[109] The distinction is difficult, and cases with more extensive clinical involvement or lack of response to standard treatment may need to be further evaluated and possibly treated as if they had PAN.[110] In spite of the previous discussion, some clincians feel their data support the view that cutaneous PAN does not progress to PAN.[111]

Treatment

The condition may respond to nonsteroidal antiinflammatory drugs[99,112,113] but can require oral steroids in moderate doses to achieve remission.[97] When streptococcal infection is implicated, penicillin may be effective.[104,114] Some clinicians recommend continuing prophylactic penicillin throughout childhood, since relapses are common and occur in up to 25% of cases in association with further streptococcal infections.[104,115]

In circumstances where there has been lack of response to standard treatment or concerns about possible steroid toxicity, IVIG has been used.[116,117] Some success has also been reported with the use of methotrexate,[118] colchicine and dapsone,[119] cyclophosphamide,[101] pentoxifylline,[120] and chloroquine.[121]

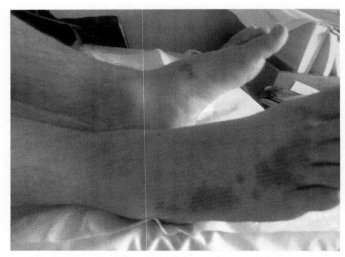

FIGURE 32–7 Cutaneous PAN: painful purpuric and nodular lesions on the feet and a livedo pattern on the legs.

Outcome

Many, but not all, patients experience a persistence of cutaneous lesions throughout childhood, but it is uncommon for the condition to progress to PAN.[97] However, it is mandatory for such patients to remain under surveillance to detect any evidence of developing systemic disease that would be an indication for intensification of treatment along the lines of that required for PAN.

PAN Associations

Hepatitis B antigen related PAN is an immune complex disease where the pathogenesis is known. The disease often presents in the form of "classic PAN" as described by the adult literature, especially with renal artery involvement. There have been four cases reported in the aforementioned survey[16]; all, however, were diagnosed before mandatory vaccination schedules. With effective hepatitis B vaccinations, this subtype has become extinct in our pediatric practice. PAN associated with FMF has become an important topic in the eastern Mediterranean, where FMF is frequent. In a large nationwide study, an increased rate of PAN has been noted among patients with FMF.[122] On the other hand, PAN patients have an increased rate of MEFV mutations, as discussed previously. In a joint series from Turkey and Israel, certain characteristics of patients with FMF and PAN have been highlighted, such as younger age at onset and overlap of disease presentation.[57] The association may simply be due to the increased inflammatory milieu in patients with one or two mutations of the MEFV gene.[17] In fact, both patients and carriers have higher acute phase reactants as compared to normals, and they encounter more inflammatory diseases.[17,123]

CONCLUSION

PAN and its localized form, cutaneous PAN, are well recognized forms of vasculitis affecting children. Developments in investigative procedures and therapeutic approaches have resulted in improvements in diagnosis and treatment such that currently the outlook for the majority of affected children is good. However, those diagnosed late or with severe systemic disease still have a consequential morbidity and mortality. Hopefully, newer characterization of the etiopathogenetic mechanisms and genetic predispositions may lead to a better understanding of the processes involved and hence to more focused treatment options such that therapeutic bullets, not bombs, will become the mainstay of management.

REFERENCES

5. J.L. Rothstein, S. Welt, Progress in pediatrics. Periarteritis nodosa in infancy and in childhood. Report of two cases with necropsy observations; abstracts of cases in the literature, Am. J. Dis. Child. 45 (1933) 1277–1308.
7. J.C. Jennette, R.J. Falk, K. Andrassy, et al., Nomenclature of systemic vasculitides: Proposal of an international consensus conference, Arthritis Rheum. 37 (1994) 187–192.
8. R.W. Lightfoot Jr., B.A. Michel, D.A. Bloch, et al., The American College of Rheumatology 1990 criteria for the classification of polyarteritis nodosa, Arthritis Rheum. 33 (1990) 1088–1093.
9. S. Ozen, N. Besbas, U. Saatci, et al., Diagnostic criteria for polyarteritis nodosa in childhood, J. Pediatr. 120 (1992) 206–209.
10. P.A. Brogan, R. Davies, I. Gordon, et al., Renal angiography in children with polyarteritis nodosa, Pediatr. Nephrol. 17 (2002) 277–283.
11. S. Ozen, N. Ruperto, M.J. Dillon, et al., EULAR/PRES endorsed consensus criteria for the classification of childhood vasculitides, Ann. Rheum. Dis. 65 (2006) 936–941.
12. S. Ozen, A. Pistorio, S.M. Iusan et al: The EULAR/PRINTO/PRES criteria for Henoch-Schönlein purpura, childhood polyarteritis nodosa, childhood Wegener granulomatosis and childhood Takayasu arteritis: Ankara 2008. Part II. Final classification criteria. Ann. Rheum. Dis. (In Press 2010).
13. R.A. Watts, D.G.I. Scott, Epidemiology of vasculitis, in: G.V. Ball, S.L. Bridges (Eds.), Vasculitis, ed 2, Oxford University Press, Oxford, 2008.
15. S. Ozen, A. Bakkaloglu, R. Dusunsel, et al., Childhood vasculitides in Turkey: a nationwide survey, Clin. Rheumatol. 26 (2007) 196–200.
16. S. Ozen, J. Anton, N. Arisoy, et al., Juvenile polyarteritis: results of a multicenter survey of 110 children, J. Pediatr. 145 (2004) 517–522.
17. S. Ozen, A. Battaloglu, E. Yilmaz, et al., Mutations in the gene for familial Mediterranean fever: do they predispose to inflammation, J. Rheumatol. 30 (2003) 2014–2018.
18. F. Yalcinkaya, Z.B. Ozcakar, O. Kasapcopur, et al., Prevalence of the MEFV gene mutations in childhood polyarteritis nodosa, J. Pediatr. 151 (2007) 675–678.
22. L. Guillevin, A. Mahr, P. Callard, et al., French Vasculitis Study Group: Hepatitis B virus-associated polyarteritis nodosa: clinical characteristics, outcome, and impact of treatment in 115 patients, Medicine (Baltimore) 84 (2005) 312–322.
32. P.A. Brogan, V. Shah, A. Bagga, et al., T cell Vbeta repertoires in childhood vasculitides, Clin. Exp. Immunol. 131 (2003) 517–527.
33. P.A. Brogan, What's new in the aetiopathogenesis of vasculitis, Pediatr. Nephrol. 22 (2007) 1083–1094.
34. G.V. Ball, S.L. Bridges, Pathogenesis of vasculitis, in: G.V. Ball, S.L. Bridges (Eds.), Vasculitis, ed 2, Oxford University Press, Oxford, 1998.
37. C.W. Fink, Polyarteritis and other diseases with necrotizing vasculitis in childhood, Arthritis Rheum. 20 (1977) 378–384.
38. R.E. Petty, D.B. Magilavy, J.T. Cassidy, et al., Polyarteritis in childhood. A clinical description of eight cases, Arthritis Rheum. 20 (1977) 392–394.
41. M.J. Dillon, B.M. Ansell, Vasculitis in children and adolescents, Rheum. Dis. Clin. North Am. 21 (1995) 1115–1136.
42. M. Maeda, M. Kobayashi, S. Okamoto, et al., Clinical observation of 14 cases of childhood polyarteritis nodosa in Japan, Acta. Paediatr. Jpn. 39 (1997) 277–279.
43. M.J. Dillon, Childhood vasculitis, Lupus 7 (1998) 259–265.
44. M.J. Dillon, Primary vasculitis in children, in: P.J. Maddison, D.A. Isenberg, P. Woo, et al. (Eds.), Oxford textbook of rheumatology, ed 2, Oxford University Press, Oxford, 1998.
45. J.T. Cassidy, R.E. Petty, Polyarteritis nodosa and related vasculitides, in: J.T. Cassidy, R.E. Petty (Eds.), Textbook of pediatric rheumatology, ed 5, Saunders, Philadelphia, 2007.
46. D. Elefthereou, M.J. Dillon, P.A. Brogan, Advances in childhood vasculitis, Curr. Opin. Rheumatol. 21 (2009) 411–418.
47. N. Besbas, S. Ozen, U. Saatci, et al., Renal involvement in polyarteritis nodosa: evaluation of 26 Turkish children, Pediatr. Nephrol. 14 (2000) 325–327.
53. L. Guillevin, C. Pagnoux, L. Teixeira, Polyarteritis nodosa, in: G.V. Ball, S.L. Bridges (Eds.), Vasculitis, ed 2, Oxford University Press, Oxford, 2008.
54. M.J. Dillon, Vasculitic syndromes, in: P. Woo, P.H. White, B.M. Ansell (Eds.), Paediatric rheumatology update, Oxford University Press, Oxford, 1990.
57. S. Ozen, E. Ben-Chetrit, A. Bakkaloglu, et al., Polyarteritis nodosa in patients with Familial Mediterranean Fever (FMF): a concomitant disease or a feature of FMF, Semin. Arthritis Rheum. 30 (2001) 281–287.
59. A. Bakkaloglu, S. Ozen, E. Baskin, et al., The significance of antineutrophil cytoplasmic antibody in microscopic polyangiitis and classic polyarteritis nodosa, Arch. Dis. Child. 85 (2001) 427–430.
62. P.A. Brogan, V. Shah, C. Brachet, et al., Endothelial and platelet microparticles in vasculitis of the young, Arthritis Rheum. 50 (2004) 927–936.

63. U. Erdbruegger, M. Grossheim, B. Hertel, et al., Diagnostic role of endothelial microparticles in vasculitis, Rheumatology (Oxford) 47 (2008) 1820–1825.

66. M. Haubitz, A. Woywodt, Circulating endothelial cells and vasculitis, Intern. Med. 43 (2004) 660–667.

69. R. Handa, J.P. Wali, S.D. Gupta, et al., Classical polyarteritis nodosa and microscopic polyangiitis—a clinicopathological study, J. Assoc. Phys. India. 49 (2001) 314–319.

70. E.A. Ewald, D. Griffin, W.J. McCune, Correlation of angiographic abnormalities with disease manifestations and disease severity in polyarteritis nodosa, J. Rheumatol. 14 (1987) 952–956.

71. P. Hekali, H. Kajander, R. Pajari, et al., Diagnostic significance of angiographically observed visceral aneurysms with regard to polyarteritis nodosa, Acta. Radiol. 32 (1991) 143–148.

72. S. Saddekni, L. Horesh, R. Leonardo, et al., Angiography and percutaneous interventions, in: G.V. Ball, S.L. Bridges (Eds.), Vasculitis, ed 2, Oxford University Press, Oxford, 2008.

73. W.A. Schmidt, Use of imaging studies in the diagnosis of vasculitis, Curr. Rheumatol. Rep. 6 (2004) 203–211.

75. J.T. Lie, Illustrated histopathological classification criteria for selected vasculitis syndromes American College of Rheumatology Subcommittee on Classification of Vasculitis, Arthritis Rheum. 33 (1990) 1074–1087.

76. P.A. Brogan, M.J. Dillon, Vasculitis from a paediatric perspective, Curr. Rheumatol. Rep. 2 (2000) 411–416.

77. P.A. Brogan, M.J. Dillon, The use of immunosuppressive and cytotoxic drugs in non-malignant disease, Arch. Dis. Child. 83 (2000) 259–264.

80. D. Jayne, Current attitudes to the therapy of vasculitis, Kidney Blood Press. Res. 26 (2003) 231–239.

81. M.J. Dillon, Vasculitis treatment—new therapeutic approaches, Eur. J. Pediatr. 165 (2006) 351–357.

82. D. Eleftheriou, M. Melo, S.D. Marks, et al., Biologic therapy in primary systemic vasculitis of the young, Rheumatology (Oxford) 48 (2009) 978–986.

84. D. Jayne, N. Rasmussen, K. Andrassy, et al., A randomized trial of maintenance therapy for vasculitis associated with antineutrophil cytoplasmic antibodies, N. Engl. J. Med. 349 (2003) 36–44.

96. Y.F. Cheung, P.A. Brogan, C.B. Pilla, et al., Arterial distensibility in children and teenagers: normal evolution and the effect of childhood vasculitis, Arch. Dis. Child. 87 (2002) 348–351.

97. H.M. Bastian, Cutaneous polyarteritis nodosa, in: G.V. Ball, S.L. Bridges (Eds.), Vasculitis, ed 2, Oxford University Press, Oxford, 2008.

98. M.S. Daoud, K.P. Hutton, L.E. Gibson, Cutaneous periarteritis nodosa: a clinicopathological study of 79 cases, Brit. J. Dermatol. 136 (1997) 706–713.

101. L. Kumar, B.R. Thapa, B. Sarker, et al., Benign cutaneous polyarteritis nodosa in children below 10 years of age—a clinical experience, Ann. Rheum. Dis. 54 (1995) 134–136.

104. J. David, B.M. Ansell, P. Woo, Polyarteritis associated with streptococcus, Arch. Dis. Child. 69 (1993) 685–688.

115. C.W. Fink, The role of the streptococcus in post streptococcal reactive arthritis and childhood polyarteritis nodosa, J. Rheumatol. 29 (1991) 14–20.

122. M. Tunca, S. Akar, F. Onen, et al. and the Turkish FMF Study-Group. Familial Mediterranean fever (FMF) IN Turkey: results of a nationwide multicenter study, Medicine (Baltimore) 84 (2005) 1–11.

Entire reference list is available online at www.expertconsult.com.

Chapter 33

KAWASAKI DISEASE

Robert P. Sundel and Ross E. Petty

HISTORICAL BACKGROUND

Kawasaki disease (KD) is one of the most common vasculitides of childhood. It has the potential to cause severe complications, significant morbidity, and even mortality. Expeditious treatment can largely prevent these complications, underscoring the importance of early and accurate diagnosis. The diagnosis is based on clinical criteria (Table 33–1), and correct identification of KD can still be as exacting a challenge today as it has been for more than 40 years.

This vasculitis bears the eponym *Kawasaki disease* because of the painstaking description of this illness in 50 children by Tomisaku Kawasaki in 1967.[1] Scattered case reports of young children who died of ruptured or thrombosed coronary artery aneurysms or infantile polyarteritis nodosa[2,3] have appeared in the medical literature since 1871. A clinical syndrome comprising most of the components of what is today recognized as KD was described by Munro-Faure in 1959[4] and by Itoga in 1960.[5]

DEFINITION AND DIAGNOSTIC CRITERIA

KD is a self-limited vasculitis of unknown origin, characterized by fever, rash, conjunctivitis, changes in the oral mucosa, changes in the extremities, cervical lymphadenopathy, and in a proportion of cases, dilatation or aneurysms of the coronary and other arteries.

The 1967 guidelines for the diagnosis of KD are shown in Table 33–1. Slightly modified criteria were commonly applied in studies from the U.S., in which fever was a required criterion. Four of the other five criteria were also needed for diagnosis. Recently proposed criteria require fever as mandatory, include perineal rash with changes in the extremities, and recognize that, in the presence of fever and coronary artery changes demonstrated by echocardiography, fewer than four criteria are required to make the diagnosis of KD.[6] Muta and colleagues[7] showed that fever for four or fewer days in the presence of four other criteria increased the sensitivity of the criteria. There have been no studies comparing the sensitivity and specificity of these varying formulations.

None of these guidelines has 100% sensitivity and specificity for the diagnosis of KD. If a child has the characteristic clinical features and develops coronary artery aneurysms, the diagnosis is certain. Children who do not meet the criteria may have an incomplete or atypical form of KD (discussed later). Alternatively, some patients who fulfill all criteria may have other conditions. In a study of patients referred because of possible KD, Burns and colleagues[8] found that the standard clinical diagnostic criteria for KD were fulfilled in 18 (46%) of 39 patients in whom other diagnoses were established. Up to one-third of children with KD also have an identifiable infection,[9] including Group A streptococcal tonsillitis, viral illnesses, pneumonia, and gastroenteritis.

More concerning from the perspective of trying to prevent disease sequelae is that many children who develop coronary artery aneurysms never meet criteria for KD.[10] A review of 127 patients treated for KD found that 36% did not meet criteria. Further, the proportion developing aneurysms was higher among this group than among those who had the full clinical syndrome.[11]

The youngest patients are most likely to have atypical features and to develop aneurysms—up to 60% of children younger than 12 months old developed aneurysms in one series.[12] The diagnosis of KD should be considered for any infant with prolonged, unexplained fever. Treating KD is seldom an emergency, especially when patients present after only five or six days of fever. Observation of children who do not fulfill criteria may be the best course of action. The mean duration of fever in children with untreated KD is 12 days,[13] much longer than typical viral illnesses, so persistence of fever or development of additional signs of KD favors treatment for KD.

EPIDEMIOLOGY

Although worldwide in distribution, the incidence of KD is highest in Japan, where, by 2002, more than 186,000 cases of KD had been registered since 1967.[14] The incidence has been steadily increasing in Japan,[15] reaching 212 per 100,000 males and 163 per 100,000 females 0-4 years old in 2006. Children of Japanese descent who reside outside Japan also face a higher risk of KD than do Caucasian children.[16] Rates in Korea, Taiwan, and China are also high.[17] As assessed by hospital admissions, in the U.S., children of Asian or Pacific Island ancestry have the highest incidence (39/100,000 < 18 years). The incidence

Table 33–1
Criteria for the diagnosis of Kawasaki disease
Fever for more than five days (four days if treatment with intravenous immunoglobulin eradicates fever) plus at least four of the following clinical signs not explained by another disease process: • Bilateral conjunctival injection (80% to 90%)*   • Changes in the oropharyngeal mucous membranes, including one or more of injected and/or fissured lips, strawberry tongue, injected pharynx (80% to 90%)   • Changes in the peripheral extremities, including erythema and/or edema of the hands and feet (acute phase) or periungual desquamation (convalescent phase) (80%)   • Polymorphous rash, primarily truncal; nonvesicular (>90%)   • Cervical lymphadenopathy with at least one node >1.5 cm (50%)

*Numbers in parentheses indicate the approximate percentage of children with Kawasaki disease who demonstrate the criterion.

*Modified from Centers for Disease Control: *Revised diagnostic criteria for Kawasaki disease, MMWR Morb Mortal Wkly Rep* 39:27-28, 1990.

was intermediate for African-Americans (19.7) or children of Hispanic origin (13.6), and lowest for whites (11.4).[18] In one large area of Great Britain, the annual incidence rate was 5.5 cases per 100,000 for children younger than 5 years old; the incidence for children of Asian ancestry was more than double that for Caucasian and African or Afro-Caribbean children.[19]

KD is an illness of early childhood; 85% of affected patients are younger than 5 years old, with an average age of approximately 2 years old,[18] although there are reports of KD occurring in older children[20] and adults.[21] KD is more common in boys than in girls (male:female ratio of 1.36:1 to 1.62:1).[22,23]

In Japan, the highest incidence occurs between 9 and 11 months old in boys, and between 3 and 8 months old in girls.[23] In North America, the peak age at onset of KD is between 2 and 3 years old. In an Australian study, only 20% of children were younger than 1 year old at diagnosis, and 25% were older than 5 years old. The reasons for the geographic differences in age at onset are unclear.[24]

Several reports document a seasonal incidence of KD.[24,25] In Japan, the disease occurs most frequently in January, June, and July, with a nadir in October. This pattern was observed every year for the 14 years of the study in Japan.[25] This bimodal distribution was not noted in Taiwan, where the highest incidence was in the summer.[17] In North America, cases have tended to occur between November and May.[26] Clustering of cases in time and geographic area further suggests an unrecognized vector. Kao and colleagues[27] demonstrated a temporal and spatial clustering of disease in San Diego County, California, U.S.A. Although epidemics of KD were documented in Japan up to 1987, none has occurred since then.[28]

In Japan, siblings of affected children have a risk of contracting KD that is approximately 10 times higher than the risk in the general population,[29] but cases among children sharing the same home in other countries are uncommon.[25] Dergun and colleagues[30] reported 18 families in the U.S. with 24 affected members, including nine sibling pairs. Second and even third attacks have been reported in from 1.5% to 3% of cases.[17]

ETIOLOGY AND PATHOGENESIS

The cause of KD remains unknown. Many of its epidemiological and clinical manifestations suggest an infectious origin. If an infectious agent does indeed cause KD, the putative organism would appear to be of very low communicability, or predominantly responsible for subclinical infections. Repeated attempts to identify a particular infectious trigger have been unsuccessful.[31] It is possible that vasculitis in KD is caused by either conventional antigens or by superantigens that trigger an immune response to endothelial cells, rather than by direct infection of the vessels.[32] Superantigens are produced by several bacteria, notably certain strains of *Staphylococcus* and *Streptococcus*, and are capable of stimulating large numbers of T cells in an antigen-nonspecific manner by interaction with the β chain of the T cell receptor. Overrepresentation of T cells bearing Vβ2 among lymphocytes in coronary artery aneurysms, intestinal mucosa,[33,34] and peripheral blood[35] from patients with KD supports the hypothesized role of superantigens in the pathogenesis. A variety of additional circumstantial evidence[30–32,36–38] and a murine model of *Lactobacillus casei*-induced vasculitis lend credence to this theory. Further, children with KD have unique reactions to mycobacterial antigens,[39–41] which may also function as superantigens, including recall reactions at the site of a previous bacillus Calmette-Guérin immunization.[39] Nonetheless, the only human illness definitively ascribed to superantigens is toxic shock syndrome, and other researchers have failed to identify evidence of a role for superantigens in the pathogenesis of KD.[42] Thus, whether these findings represent a specific response to superantigens or crossreactivity with other antigens is not clear.

A predominance of immunoglobulin A (IgA)-secreting plasma cells in the blood vessel walls of children with fatal KD has suggested to Rowley and colleagues that an organism that gained entry through mucosal surfaces underlies the disease.[43] No single pathogen is regularly demonstrable, although associations with Epstein-Barr virus,[43] rotavirus,[44] and other viruses[45–47] and with bacteria[48,49] have been reported. An association with a coronavirus[50] has not been confirmed.[51] It is nonetheless a possibility that the vascular injury in KD may be the result of a direct cell-mediated attack on endothelial cells that are infected with an unidentified pathogen.[52]

Additional clues to the cause of KD come from the humoral factors, including antiendothelial cell antibodies, circulating immune complexes, and antineutrophil cytoplasm antibodies (ANCAs) that are demonstrated in a large proportion of patients.[53] Serum levels of tumor necrosis factor alpha (TNF-α) and interleukin-6 (IL-6),[54] and growth factors, such as vascular endothelial growth factor,[55] are elevated, generally in proportion to the severity of the illness. In the absence of confirmed evidence of a single etiological agent, a reasonable working hypothesis is that KD represents a stereotyped, pathological immune response to one or a variety of environmental or infectious triggers. Presumably, certain individuals are predisposed by virtue of their genetic constitution. The predilection for childhood onset may reflect the presence of developmental antigens that are targets for the inflammatory response only early in life, subtle maturational defects in immune responsiveness,[56] or the timing of exposure to environmental triggers.

GENETIC BACKGROUND

In Japan, approximately 1% of patients with KD have a history of an affected sibling,[57] and concordance for KD was 13.3% in dizygotic twins and 14.1% in monozygotic twins.[58] Similarly, in Japan, there is a significantly increased frequency of a history of KD in the parents of children with the disease.[59] These observations indicate that there is a genetic predisposition to this disease, although the fact that affected twin pairs became ill within two weeks of each other also suggests an important role for (an) environmental agent(s).

The exact genetic factors that may underlie the disorder are unknown. Reported genetic associations have been reviewed by Hata and Onouchi.[60] Candidate genes include those at the histocompatibility locus and those for other proteins involved in immunoregulation. Human leukocyte antigen (HLA) genes for B5, B44, Bw51, DR3, and DRB3*0301 have been associated with KD in Caucasians; Bw54, Bw15, and Bw35 in Japanese; and Bw51 in Israelis.[61] However, Onouchi and colleagues[62] concluded that HLA polymorphisms contributed little to the pathogenesis of KD. There has been no reported association of any HLA antigen with the risk of coronary artery disease.[63]

Polymorphisms of the TNF-α gene *(TNF),*[64] the IL 18 gene,[65] the HLA E gene,[66] and the gene for angiotensin converting enzyme[67,68] have been associated with KD, but their pathogenic significance is disputed. A recent report implicated polymorphisms of the mannose binding lectin (MBL) in the pathogenesis of KD.[69] MBL binds to n-acetyl glucosamine and mannose present on the surface of many microbes. This interaction results in activation of complement (C3) independent of antibody. Levels of MBL are determined by polymorphisms of the MBL 2 gene and its promoters. Higher expression of MBL is associated with lower incidence of coronary artery lesions in patients under 1 year old, but it has the opposite effect in older patients. This apparent paradox is congruent with the belief that MBL is important in protecting the very young child from infectious diseases.[69]

The gene controlling expression of inositol 1,4,5-triphosphate 3-kinase (ITPKC) has recently been identified as a susceptibility gene not only for KD, but also for coronary artery disease.[70] This enzyme is strongly expressed by peripheral blood mononuclear cells and has an important role in inflammation by decreasing IL-2 expression. The functional polymorphism ITPKC 3 is significantly increased in patients with KD and coronary artery disease in Japanese and American populations.[71] Neither studies of individual genes nor genome-wide association studies[72] have revealed consistent markers of disease susceptibility. Thus, to the extent that certain children are predisposed to developing KD, the effect is likely due to small contributions from multiple genetic loci.

CLINICAL MANIFESTATIONS

Disease Course

The course of untreated KD may be divided into three phases (Fig. 33–1): An acute, febrile period lasting for 10-14 days is followed by a subacute phase of approximately two to four weeks. This ends with a return to normal of the platelet count and erythrocyte sedimentation rate (ESR). The subsequent convalescent or recovery period lasts months to years, during which time vessels undergo healing, remodeling, and scarring.

Acute Febrile Phase

The onset of fever in KD is characteristically abrupt, often preceded by symptoms of an upper respiratory or gastrointestinal illness. Baker and colleagues[72] studied the symptoms in the 10 days prior to diagnosis of KD in 198 patients, and reported that irritability occurred in 50%, vomiting in 44%, decreased food intake in 37%, diarrhea in 26%, and abdominal pain in 18%. Cough was reported in 28%, and 19% had rhinorrhea. In addition, 19% reported weakness, and 15% reported arthralgia or arthritis. Over the next three to four days, cervical adenitis, conjunctivitis, changes in the buccal and oral mucosa, a pleomorphic rash, and erythema and edema in the hands and feet develop (in no particular order). Perineal desquamation may be another early sign of KD.[73] Untreated, these manifestations subside after an average of 12 days. If carditis occurs, it often does so early and may be manifested by tachycardia, an S3 gallop, and subtle or occasionally marked signs of congestive heart failure.[74] Pericarditis, abdominal pain, ascites, and hydrops of the gallbladder may occur at this time.

Subacute Phase

After the acute phase, the child may be entirely asymptomatic if given intravenous immunoglobulin (IVIG). Untreated, fever, mucositis, and conjunctivitis usually resolve entirely by the third or fourth week. During this period, desquamation of the skin of the digits[75] may be the only clinically apparent residual feature. Up to one in 13 children develops arthritis of one or several joints during the late acute and subacute phases.[76] Coronary artery aneurysms most commonly first develop during the subacute phase, occasionally earlier, but rarely later in children treated with IVIG.

Convalescent Phase

Most children are asymptomatic during the convalescent phase. The acute phase response has usually returned to normal, unless there are complications. Horizontal ridging of the nails (Beau lines), characteristic of many acute inflammatory conditions, may appear during this period.

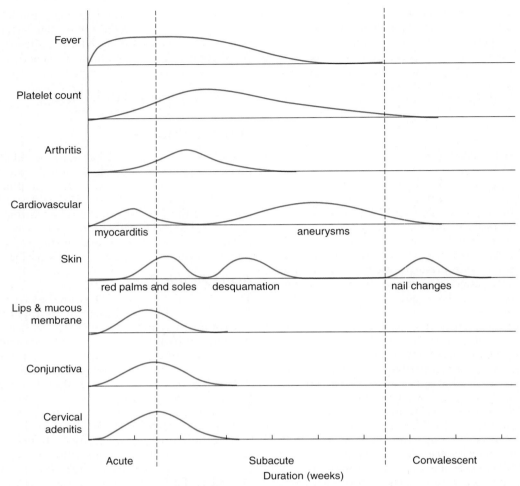

FIGURE 33–1 Kawasaki disease can be viewed as an illness with acute, subacute, and recovery phases. The temporal characteristics outlined here are typical of the course of the disease. (Adapted from ref. 1.)

Clinical Characteristics of the Classification Criteria

Fever

Fever, often exceeding 40°C, is the most consistent manifestation of KD. The fever is typically persistent and minimally responsive to antipyretic agents, tending to remain above 38.5° C during most of the acute phase of the illness. It reflects elevated levels of TNF-α and IL-1, which are thought to mediate the underlying vascular inflammation.[77] The diagnosis must be suspect in the absence of fever.

Conjunctivitis

Bilateral, nonexudative bulbar conjunctivitis occurs in more than 85% of patients with KD. Conjunctival injection typically spares the limbus, which is the zone immediately around the cornea. Inflammation of the palpebral conjunctiva is not prominent. Purulent discharge is especially unusual[78] and suggests an alternative diagnosis.

Other ocular abnormalities may also occur, although they are not part of the diagnostic criteria (Table 33–2).

Table 33–2	
Frequency of ocular signs and symptoms in Kawasaki disease	
Ocular Sign or Symptom	**Frequency (%)**
Injection of bulbar conjunctivae	89
Nongranulomatous iridocyclitis	78
Superficial punctate keratitis	22
Vitreous opacities	12
Papilledema	11
Subconjunctival hemorrhage	3

Data from Kumagai N, Ohno S: Kawasaki disease. In Pepose JS, Holland GM, Wilhelmus KR, editors: *Ocular immunity and infection*, St. Louis, 1996, Mosby.

During the first week of illness, about three-fourths of children are photophobic, an effect of anterior uveitis,[79] which peaks between five and eight days of illness and is more common in children over 2 years old. Ocular inflammation usually resolves without specific therapy or sequelae. Exceptionally, there may be posterior synechiae, conjunctival scarring,[80] changes in the retina and vitreous,[81] or blindness.[82]

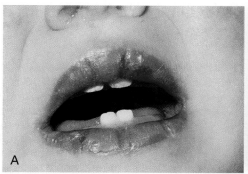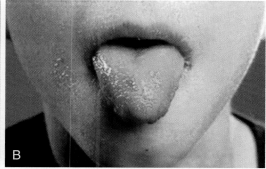

FIGURE 33–2 **A,** The intense reddening, swelling, and vertical cracking of the lips are characteristic of Kawasaki disease (KD). **B,** The strawberry tongue of acute KD with hypertrophied papillae on an erythematous base and the peeling of the facial skin.

Changes in the Lips and Oral Mucosa

Swollen, vertically cracked red lips and a strawberry tongue are characteristic; the latter is caused by sloughing of filiform papillae and prominence of the large hyperemic fungiform papillae (Fig. 33–2). Vesicles, ulcers, or tonsillar exudate suggest a viral or bacterial infection rather than KD.

Exanthem

The cutaneous manifestations of KD are protean. Although the rash usually begins on the trunk, there is often a perineal confluence during the first days of the illness, followed by desquamation in the diaper area by day six in most cases.[73] Macular, morbilliform, or targetoid lesions of the trunk and extremities are most characteristic. The rash is seldom pruritic, and vesicular or bullous lesions are rare (Fig. 33–3). Psoriasis has been reported in several children with KD.[83]

Lymphadenopathy

Anterior cervical lymphadenopathy occurs during the acute phase of the disease, is usually unilateral, and may appear to involve only a single node. However, ultrasound or computed tomographic imaging of the neck typically reveals grapelike clusters of enlarged nodes similar to those seen in Epstein-Barr virus infections rather than the isolated adenopathy typical of bacterial adenitis.[84] Occasionally, a node enlarges rapidly and may be mistaken for bacterial infection. After three or four days, it usually shrinks with or without specific therapy. Diffuse lymphadenopathy and splenomegaly are not typical of KD and should raise suspicions of a viral illness.

Extremity Changes

Indurated edema of the dorsum of the hands and feet and a diffuse red-purple erythema of the palms and soles occur early and last for one to three days. Sheet-like desquamation typically occurs 10 days or more after the start of the fever. It characteristically begins at the tips of the fingers (less commonly the toes), just below the distal edge of the nails (Fig. 33–4). Flaky desquamation may occur elsewhere, but peripheral skin peeling usually occurs late in the course of KD and may be absent or inapparent.[75] Consequently, it is useful more for retrospective confirmation of the diagnosis than for making therapeutic decisions.

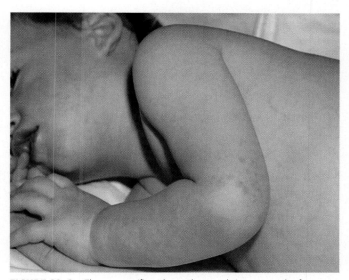

FIGURE 33–3 The nonspecific polymorphous rash is seen on the face arms and chest of this 2-year-old boy with acute KD.

Incomplete Kawasaki Disease

Signs, symptoms, and outcome in children who do not meet criteria for KD tend to parallel those of children who fulfill the diagnostic criteria. In a Japanese study, 25 of 242 patients hospitalized for KD failed to meet diagnostic criteria.[85] Only one patient ultimately developed transient dilatation of a coronary artery. A particularly high level of suspicion is needed in infants younger than 1 year old. In a retrospective review of 45 cases of KD, 5 (45%) of 11 infants had incomplete disease, compared with 4 (12%) of 33 older children.[86] Unfortunately, infants are the group at the highest risk for developing coronary artery aneurysms, and in this study, coronary artery complications occurred in seven infants (64%), compared with three older children (9%), including all five infants with incomplete disease.[86]

In view of these data, the American Heart Association (AHA) has suggested additional markers for identification of children not meeting classical criteria for KD who might nonetheless be at increased risk of developing coronary artery aneurysms.[87] Early reports suggest that the algorithm recommended by the AHA committee performs well in decreasing the number of children who are not treated for KD and yet ultimately develop aneurysms.[88]

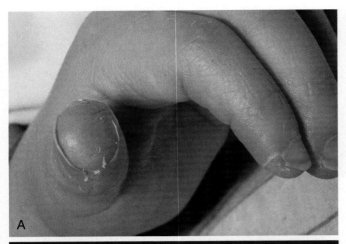

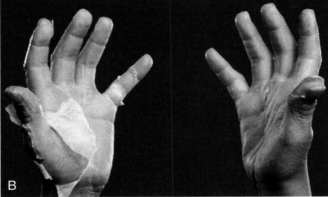

FIGURE 33–4 **A,** Desquamation of the skin of the tips of the thumb and finger seen during the subacute phase of Kawasaki disease. **B,** Desquamation of the skin of the hand occurs later in the subacute and early recovery phase of the disease. In many children, the degree of desquamation is much less than is depicted here.

Other Clinical Manifestations of Kawasaki Disease (Table 33–3)

Cardiovascular Disease

At onset, there is usually a tachycardia commensurate with the degree of fever. "Early myocarditis occurs in at least one-third[89] to one-half[90] of patients, and pericarditis also may occur. Myocardial involvement often leads to decreased contractility, commonly manifested by an S3 gallop that may become more prominent with hydration. Such children may be misdiagnosed with viral myocarditis. In more severe cases, myocardial involvement may progress to dysrhythmias and signs of congestive heart failure.[91] Children with prominent KD-associated myocarditis tend to respond less briskly to treatment with IVIG, but long-term abnormalities of cardiac contractility are nonetheless very uncommon in children treated appropriately during the acute phase of KD.[92]

The most significant and characteristic complication of KD, the development of coronary artery aneurysms in up to 25% of untreated patients, makes KD the leading cause of acquired heart disease among children in the developed world (Figs. 33–5 and 33–6). Treatment with IVIG decreases the incidence of giant aneurysms (internal diameter >8 mm) by more than 95% and the overall incidence of aneurysms by 85%. Despite treatment, however, one retrospective survey reported that 8.5% of patients younger than 12 months old developed coronary artery abnormalities, compared with 1.8% of those 12 months old or older.[93] Overall, the odds ratio for development of cardiac sequelae in infants younger than 1 year old was 1.54.[94]

Coronary aneurysms may cause morbidity early in the course due to rupture or thrombosis, resulting in sudden death or myocardial infarction.[95] Development of *de*

Table 33–3

Manifestations of Kawasaki Disease

Organ System	Common	Uncommon	Finding Suggests Alternate Diagnosis
Skin	Targetoid, urticarial, morbilliform rashes, livedo reticularis	Psoriasiform rash	Pustular, vesicular rashes
Lungs	Pleural effusion	Nodules, interstitial infiltrates	
Urinary tract	Urethritis, pyuria	Hematuria, proteinuria, orchitis	
Nervous system	Irritability, lethargy, anterior uveitis, sensorineural hearing loss	Seizure, stroke, cranial nerve palsy	
Gastrointestinal system	Diarrhea, vomiting, hydrops of gallbladder, hepatomegaly	Intestinal hemorrhage, ruptured viscus	
Hematological system	Anemia, thrombocytosis, leukocytosis	Thrombocytopenia, consumptive coagulopathy, hemophagocytic syndrome	Lymphocytosis*
Reticuloendothelial system	Anterior cervical lymphadenopathy	Posterior cervical, axillary lymphadenopathy	Diffuse lymphadenopathy, splenomegaly
Mucosa	Mucositis, glossitis, conjunctivitis		Discrete oral lesions, exudative conjunctivitis
Musculoskeletal system	Extremity edema, arthritis	Raynaud Phenomenon	
Cardiac system	Tachycardia, gallop rhythm, myocarditis, pericarditis	Coronary artery aneurysm, aortic root dilatation, valvulitis	

*Except during the convalescent phase.

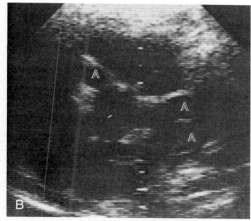

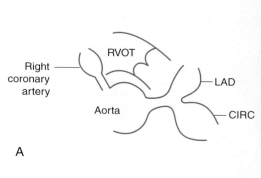

FIGURE 33–5 Echocardiographic demonstration of aneurysms of three coronary arteries in a child with Kawasaki disease. A, aneurysms; CIRC, circumflex; LAD, left anterior descending coronary artery; RVOT, right ventricular outflow tract. (Courtesy of Dr. Dennis Crowley.)

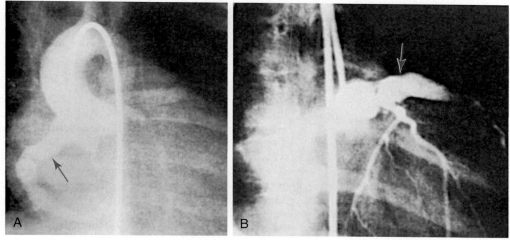

FIGURE 33–6 **A,** Angiography of the coronary vessels in a 7-month-old boy with Kawasaki disease shows a huge aneurysmal dilatation of the right coronary artery *(arrow).* **B,** Aneurysm of the left coronary artery in a 3-year-old girl with Kawasaki disease *(arrow).* (**A** and **B,** Courtesy of Dr. Zuidi Lababidi.)

novo coronary artery abnormalities more than two weeks after the end of the acute illness is unusual, although ongoing scarring of existing vascular lesions may result in progressive coronary insufficiency. Approximately one-half of coronary artery aneurysms demonstrated by echocardiogram ultimately resolve, usually those smaller than 6 mm in diameter,[96] but persistent vasodilatory abnormalities have been observed in arteries where aneurysms have resolved.[97] Giant coronary artery aneurysms, with an internal diameter larger than 8 mm, are associated with the highest risk of morbidity and mortality. Up to one-third of such aneurysms become obstructed, leading to myocardial infarction, dysrhythmias, or sudden death.[98]

Although involvement of the coronary arteries is the most characteristic manifestation of the vasculitis of KD, other medium-sized muscular arteries also may be involved. Aneurysms of brachial and femoral arteries may be palpable clinically or demonstrable angiographically (Fig. 33–7). In severe cases, peripheral arterial obstruction may lead to ischemia and gangrene. Visceral arteries are usually spared, although there are reports of gastrointestinal obstruction[99] and acute abdominal

catastrophe[100] occurring because of vasculitis. Such complications generally arise in children with other signs of severe vasculitis, including aneurysms in coronary and peripheral arteries.

Central Nervous System Complications

One of the most consistent clinical observations of children with KD, particularly infants and very young children, is their extreme irritability. This probably represents the effect of aseptic meningitis and associated headache.[101] Cerebrovascular accident[102] and facial nerve paralysis[103] also have been reported.

Musculoskeletal Disease

Arthritis was observed by Gong and colleagues[76] in 7.5% of 414 children with KD. Arthritis was oligoarticular in 55% and polyarticular in 45%. Joints most commonly affected were (in order of decreasing frequency) knee, ankle, wrist, elbow, and hip. Joint pain was often severe, but responded to IVIG and high dose aspirin in most instances. It may occur at any time during the disease course but has been described most commonly during the

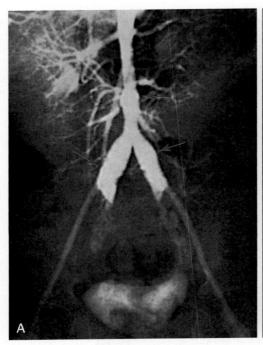 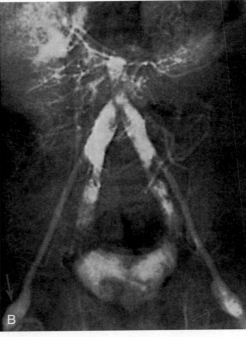

FIGURE 33–7 Angiographic study of a 2-year-old boy with severe Kawasaki disease resulting in multiple aneurysms of the coronary, axillary, iliac, and femoral arteries. The study revealed large aneurysms of the aorta and iliac (**A**) and femoral (**B**) arteries (*arrows*). Aneurysms that were palpable in the axilla and groin in this patient later resolved. (**A** and **B**, Courtesy of Dr. G. Culham.)

recovery phase. Arthritis in KD ultimately resolves, leaving no residua.

Respiratory Tract Disease

Cough, coryza, or hoarseness, and otitis media frequently occur early in the course of the disease and suggest a viral upper respiratory tract infection. Approximately one-third of children have some degree of sensorineural hearing loss when tested within 30 days of fever onset. Salicylate toxicity may be responsible for transient cases, but sensorineural hearing loss of unclear etiology may persist.[104,105]

Gastrointestinal Tract Disease and Other Abnormalities

Abdominal pain is common, and approximately one-fourth of children with KD have profuse, watery diarrhea during the acute febrile period. Abdominal distention may mimic mesenteric vasculitis or intussusception. Segmental bowel wall thickening has been described in children with KD and abdominal pain, presumably reflecting visceral arteritis.[106] The relatively common occurrence of hydrops of the gallbladder demonstrated by ultrasonography[107] may aid in the diagnosis of incomplete or atypical KD. Occasionally, the gallbladder becomes large enough to be seen as a bulge in the anterior abdominal wall. The specificity of gallbladder distension is limited, however, and a dilated, engorged gallbladder may be seen in cases of streptococcal and staphylococcal infections, among other mimics of KD. Hepatosplenomegaly may occur in the absence of heart disease or may reflect cardiac failure.

Genitourinary Tract Involvement

A study of 50 children with KD from Taiwan[108] revealed hematuria (>5 RBC/HPF) in six patients, proteinuria (>100 mg/dL) in five, and leukocyturia (>10 white blood cells per high power field) in 19. Renal ultrasonography was abnormal in five patients, and DMSA SPECT revealed inflammatory lesions in 26 children. Although renal function remained normal, scarring was demonstrated in 46% on repeated DMSA SPECT.

Scrotal pain and swelling due to testicular inflammation are characteristic of pediatric vasculitides, including Henoch-Schönlein purpura, polyarteritis nodosa, and KD. Meatitis and dysuria also occur frequently during the acute phase of KD, and priapism has been described.[109] Hemolytic-uremic syndrome, immune complex-mediated glomerulonephritis, and acute interstitial nephritis have each been reported in a few cases.[110,111] Acute renal failure is a rare complication most commonly ascribed to complications of treatment with certain preparations of IVIG.[112]

DIFFERENTIAL DIAGNOSIS

KD is often difficult to differentiate from viral exanthems of childhood, particularly early in the disease course or in children with incomplete KD (Table 33-4). The differential diagnosis includes poststreptococcal scarlet fever, toxic shock syndrome, drug reactions, and systemic-onset juvenile idiopathic arthritis. Viral illnesses such as measles (especially when atypical or occurring after vaccination), Epstein-Barr virus, and adenovirus infections share many of the signs of mucocutaneous involvement, but they typically have less evidence of systemic inflammation and generally lack the extremity changes of KD. Toxin-mediated illnesses, especially scarlet fever and toxic shock syndrome, lack the ocular and articular involvement typical of KD. Drug reactions, such as those in Stevens-Johnson syndrome or serum sickness, may mimic KD but have subtle differences in the ocular

Table 33–4

Differential diagnosis of Kawasaki Disease

Infectious Conditions
Adenovirus
Measles
Parvovirus
Human herpesviruses (HHV) (e.g., herpes simplex virus,
   cytomegalovirus, HHV-6, HHV-7)
Rocky Mountain spotted fever
Leptospirosis
Streptococci
Staphylococci
Immune Reactions
Stevens-Johnson syndrome
Serum sickness
Rheumatic Diseases
Systemic-onset juvenile idiopathic arthritis
Polyarteritis nodosa

and mucosal manifestations. In particularly severe or prolonged KD, the possibility of a chronic vasculitis such as polyarteritis nodosa must be considered carefully.

PATHOLOGY

The signs and symptoms of KD are due to a systemic necrotizing vasculitis with fibrinoid necrosis of the medium-sized muscular arteries; the coronary arteries are the predominant sites of involvement.[113] Disruption of the lamina elastica is characteristic of the aneurysms. An early neutrophilic infiltrate occurs in all layers of the heart, including the valves. Inflammation begins in the microvasculature (i.e., arterioles, capillaries, vasa vasorum, and venules) and subsequently spreads to larger vessels, especially the coronary arteries.[114] In these lesions, infiltrating cells are mostly macrophages and IgA-secreting plasma cells,[42] findings that may be unique to KD.[115] Endothelial cells express a variety of markers of activation, presumably as a result of the high levels of proinflammatory cytokines that characterize the acute phase of disease.[116] Some children have a lymphocytic myocarditis, with endomyocardial biopsy demonstrating cellular infiltrates or myofibrosis that may persist for years in untreated cases.[117]

Evolution of the cardiac lesions is detailed in the study of Fujiwara and Hamashima.[114] Coronary artery vasculitis predominated early in the disease but was absent in those who died after 28 days of illness. Aneurysms, thrombosis, and stenosis did not appear until 12 days of disease or later. Pericarditis, myocarditis, and endocarditis were universal findings early in the disease, but diminished as fibrosis of the myocardium became the predominant lesion in children whose death occurred 40 days or more after onset. In a study of 262 children, Suzuki and colleagues[118] documented an equal frequency of aneurysms in right and left coronary arteries, but a higher propensity for development of segmental stenosis and occlusions in the right coronary artery.

LABORATORY EXAMINATION

There are no specific diagnostic tests for KD, but at onset, evidence of inflammation is manifested by elevation of C-reactive protein (CRP) and ESR, leukocytosis, and a left shift in the white blood cell (WBC) differential count. Toxic granulation of neutrophils is more frequent in children with KD than in those with other febrile illnesses.[119] Occasionally, significant neutropenia occurs early[120]; this may be a marker for particularly severe disease. Thrombocytopenia and anemia may herald the onset of macrophage activation syndrome (see Chapter 45).[121] Although platelet counts may be abnormally low at disease onset, by the second week of illness they characteristically rise and may reach 1,000,000/mm^3 (reactive thrombocytosis) in the most severe cases. Children with KD often present with a normocytic, normochromic anemia; hemoglobin concentrations greater than two standard deviations below the mean for age are found in one half of patients within the first two weeks of illness.[8]

Sterile pyuria is of urethral origin and therefore is missed on urinalyses obtained by bladder aspiration or catheterization. The WBCs are mononuclear and are not detected by dipstick tests for leukocyte esterase. Measurement of liver enzymes often reveals elevated transaminase levels or mild hyperbilirubinemia due to intrahepatic congestion. A few children develop obstructive jaundice from hydrops of the gallbladder or hepatic vasculitis.

Cerebrospinal fluid (CSF) analysis typically displays a mononuclear pleocytosis with normal glucose and protein. In a chart review of 46 children with KD, 39% were documented to have elevated CSF WBC counts.[101] The median count was 22.5 cells/mm^3 with 6% neutrophils and 91.5% mononuclear cells, although cell counts as high as 320/mm^3 with up to 79% neutrophils were reported. Arthrocentesis of involved joints typically demonstrates synovial fluid WBC counts of 50 to 300,000 WBC/mm,^{3} consisting primarily of neutrophils.

Children with KD develop significant perturbations in serum lipid profiles beginning during the subacute phase of illness. These abnormalities include elevated concentrations of triglycerides and low-density lipoproteins and depressed levels of high-density lipoproteins.[122] They are most likely caused by widespread endothelial injury. As with other sequelae of KD, normalization may take years in untreated children but typically occurs within weeks or months after IVIG therapy.

ANCAs[123] and antibodies to endothelial cells[124] may be present late but not early in the disease.[125] Consequently, they have unclear pathological significance and are of little diagnostic value. Other autoantibodies are usually absent. Elevated levels of von Willebrand factor antigen indicate the presence of damaged endothelium.[126] Activation products of C3 and C4 have been demonstrated on erythrocytes (C3g) and in the plasma (C4d),[127] suggesting the participation of complement in at least some of the manifestations of the disease.

TREATMENT

General Approach

The child with suspected or definite KD should be admitted to the hospital for observation, monitoring of cardiac status, and management of systemic manifestations (Table 33–5). Initial evaluation of the heart should include an electrocardiogram to identify dysrhythmias, signs of ischemia, or myocarditis; and a baseline echocardiogram to detect coronary artery vasculitis, ectasia, or aneurysms. If the diagnosis is relatively certain (even if diagnostic criteria are not met), and other diagnoses have been considered and excluded, treatment should be initiated with aspirin and IVIG without further delay.

Goals of Therapy

In addition to control of the acute inflammation and its symptoms, the goal of therapy is to prevent long-term sequelae and, most importantly, coronary artery abnormalities. The consequences of failure to treat a child appropriately with KD are so important that, within reason, after very careful evaluation, error on the side of premature or unnecessary therapy is preferable to delayed or missed therapy for a child for whom the diagnosis is uncertain. The American Academy of Pediatrics and the AHA recommend that children with KD should be treated with aspirin and IVIG during the first 10 days of the illness.[87,128] Subsequent management remains controversial, however, and depends on the presence or absence of coronary artery abnormalities.

The Japanese Ministry of Health criteria[129,130] use angiography or echocardiography to define coronary arteries as abnormal if the internal lumen diameter is greater than 3 mm in children younger than 5 years old or greater than 4 mm in children at least 5 years old. In addition, vessels are considered aneurysmal if the internal diameter of a segment measures at least 1.5 times that of an adjacent segment or the coronary artery lumen is clearly irregular. Although coronary artery dimensions in normal children have been shown to increase linearly with body surface area (BSA) or length,[131] these criteria are not based on body size. Evaluation of coronary arteries in KD using age-, size-, and sex-adjusted indices suggests that the incidence of abnormalities is higher than was generally recognized.[132] Among patients classified as having normal coronary arteries by the Japanese Ministry of Health criteria, 27% had at least one BSA-adjusted coronary artery dimension more than two standard deviations above the mean. Even children whose vessel dimensions are within the "normal" range may demonstrate a decrease in coronary artery diameter as they convalesce from KD.[133]

Treatment strategies also depend on the implications of coronary artery dilatation. Long-term outcome studies are somewhat reassuring. Fifty percent of coronary artery aneurysms regress angiographically, and among such children, at least one longitudinal study demonstrated no increase in morbidity or mortality rates, even after more than two decades.[98] Nonetheless, abnormalities of

Table 33-5

Initial Evaluation and Management of Kawasaki Disease

Evaluate	Treat
General physical exam	
Cardiac status (ECHO, ECG)	Aspirin
CNS status	If patient is febrile:
Hematologic and inflammatory parameters (CBC, differential, platelet count, ESR, CRP)	80–100 mg/kg/day in 4 doses
	If patient is afebrile:
	3–5 mg/kg/day in 1 to 4 doses
Fluid and electrolyte status (AST, ALT, bilirubin, electrolytes, BUN, creatinine)	IVIG: 2 g/kg
Urinalysis	
Ophthalmologic status	
Monitor cardiac status	Keep in hospital until afebrile for 24 hr or if there are complications.
Monitor CRP (ESR) and platelet count at 2-week intervals until stable, then 1-month intervals until normal	If fever persists, repeat IVIG once.
	If no clinical response, consider intravenous methylprednisolone: 30 mg/kg
Repeat echocardiogram at 6-8 weeks	Maintain low-dose aspirin until ESR and platelet count are normal if there have been no coronary artery abnormalities; for 2 years if coronary abnormalities have resolved; "forever" if coronary artery disease persists.

CNS, central nervous system; ECG, electrocardiogram; ECHO, echocardiogram; ESR, erythrocyte sedimentation rate; IVIG, intravenous immunoglobulin, CRP, c-reactive protein; AST, aspartate transaminase; ALT, alanine transaminase; BUN, blood urea nitrogen.

more subtle markers of endothelial health are a matter of concern. Vessels show histological[134] and functional[135] abnormalities at the sites of healed aneurysms, and vascular reactivity to endogenous vasodilators is abnormal in children who have had KD, regardless of whether they have detectable coronary artery abnormalities.[136] This lends credence to the report of an increased long-term standardized mortality ratio of 2.35 among male patients with cardiac sequelae.[137] Acute phase reactants and platelet counts do not return to normal for up to 2 months after apparently successful treatment, suggesting that vasculitis and endothelial inflammation may not fully resolve, even when fever is controlled. It is reasonable to ask whether persistent KD requires additional therapy and whether initial treatment should be more robust than IVIG alone, at least for some children, aiming for anatomically and functionally normal vessels in everyone.

Aspirin

Aspirin was the first medication to be used for treatment of KD because of its anti-inflammatory and antithrombotic effects.[138] Anti-inflammatory regimens using high-dose (>80 mg/kg/day) or lower-dose (30 mg/kg/day) aspirin have been recommended during the acute phase of the illness. After the fever resolves, the dose is usually reduced to an antiplatelet range of 3 to 5 mg/kg/day. These doses, well below the anti-inflammatory level, have the effect of inhibiting platelet adhesion to endothelium by curtailing platelet release of thromboxane A_2 without suppressing prostacyclin production by endothelial cells.[139] This effect is believed to be beneficial in preventing thrombosis when platelet counts are elevated, although no studies have demonstrated such a benefit clinically, and aspirin does not appear to reduce the frequency of coronary artery abnormalities.[140] In the event of aspirin sensitivity, another antiplatelet agent, such as dipyridamole, should be considered. Unless coronary artery abnormalities are detected by echocardiogram, aspirin is discontinued after results of laboratory studies return to normal, usually within 2 months of disease onset.

There have been no published comparisons of aspirin with other anti-inflammatory agents, and it is unclear whether salicylates are uniquely efficacious in this condition. A metaanalysis found that high-dose and lower-dose aspirin regimens were associated with a similar incidence of coronary artery abnormalities at 30 and 60 days after disease onset.[140] Although the necessity of using high-dose aspirin might be questioned because of the rapid response to IVIG, all of the trials showing the benefit of IVIG were conducted with children who also were receiving anti-inflammatory doses of aspirin. For other effects, such as treatment of prolonged arthritis, alternative anti-inflammatory agents may be used. The AHA warns against prescribing ibuprofen because it antagonizes the antiplatelet effects of low dose aspirin.[87,141]

The risks of aspirin appear to be similar to those reported in other settings: chemical hepatitis, transient hearing loss, and, rarely, Reye syndrome.[142] These risks may be increased in KD. Aspirin binding studies have suggested that the hypoalbuminemia of children with KD predisposes them to toxic levels of free salicylate, despite measured (bound) values within the therapeutic range.[143]

Intravenous Immunoglobulin

Furusho and coworkers[144] first reported that high-dose IVIG appeared to decrease the incidence of coronary artery abnormalities. Newburger and colleagues[13] verified these findings in a 19-month-long, randomized, controlled clinical trial in 168 children with KD. One-half received IVIG (400 mg/kg/day on four consecutive days) plus high-dose aspirin (100 mg/kg/day), and one-half received aspirin alone. IVIG reduced the incidence of coronary artery abnormalities by 78%, and no child suffered serious adverse effects from the therapy, confirming the remarkable therapeutic potential of IVIG.

The initial IVIG treatment regimen was based on then-current protocols for treating immune thrombocytopenic purpura. The question of whether this protocol was optimal for KD was addressed in 1991.[145] Children were randomized to receive the traditional four-dose regimen or a single dose of 2.0 g/kg of IVIG infused over 8 to 12 hours. Children receiving the larger, single dose fared better. Meta-analyses have documented a dose-response benefit of IVIG therapy in the range between 200 mg/kg and 2 g/kg.[146]

Although standard therapy with IVIG and aspirin given within the first 10 days of illness greatly reduces the risk of coronary artery involvement, approximately 5% of children still develop coronary artery aneurysms, according to Japanese Ministry of Health criteria, and a larger number demonstrate coronary artery ectasia. In general, younger patients, especially infants younger than 6 months old, are at higher risk.[147] Stockheim and colleagues[148] reported that older children also were at additional risk. In their retrospective series, 21% of patients over 8 years old had coronary artery abnormalities. They attributed this increased incidence to a delay in diagnosis and treatment among older children in whom KD is rare and is therefore often not considered. A change in the biology of KD with age (analogous to the increased risk of renal involvement in adults with HSP) cannot be excluded.

In a retrospective series from Japan, Fukunishi and colleagues[149] found higher serum levels of CRP, lactate dehydrogenase, and bilirubin to be predictive of failure to respond to IVIG. More recently, Kobayashi and colleagues reported that hyponatremia and high levels of hepatic transaminase at presentation were associated with decreased responsiveness to IVIG.[150] In a Canadian study, Han and colleagues[151] could not identify any difference in laboratory parameters between responders and non-responders. Confirming the importance of controlling inflammation in KD, Mori and coworkers[152] reported that a rise in the WBC count and CRP level after IVIG infusion are independent predictors of coronary artery abnormalities.

IVIG is most effective in reducing the risk of coronary artery disease when administered within 10 days of the onset of fever. Unfortunately, the diagnosis may remain in doubt as this deadline approaches. In ambiguous cases, the physician may be guided by the epidemiology of the disease. More than 50% of infants with KD present atypically (i.e., do not fulfill diagnostic criteria), and they have a very high incidence of aneurysms. Thus, empiric treatment in very young children is worthy of consideration.

The mechanism of action of IVIG is uncertain, with recent studies adding induction of neutrophil apoptosis[153] and reversal of inhibited lymphocyte apoptosis[154] to a long list of immunomodulatory effects of IVIG (Table 33-6). The response is generally prompt, and temperature returns to normal in most children even before the end of the IVIG infusion, with rapid clearing of the rash, mucositis, and conjunctivitis. Irritability and emotional lability, however, may persist for up to several weeks before resolving.

The greatest long-term concern about IVIG use is potential transmission of blood-borne pathogens. Technical deficiencies in production led to more than 100 cases of hepatitis C in recipients of a single brand of IVIG in 1994, although none was a child with KD.[155] No cases of IVIG-transmitted infections have been reported since the institution of current purification and processing practices in 1995, and no cases of IVIG-transmitted HIV have ever been reported. Overall, cost-benefit analysis documents that IVIG treatment of KD is one of the most cost-effective medical therapies available, leading to impressive short- and long-term savings.[156]

Table 33–6

Potential effects of Intravenous Immunoglobulin in Kawasaki Disease

Specific Effects

- Provides antibodies against infectious agent
- Provides antibodies against circulating toxin
- Provides anti-idiotypic antibodies

Nonspecific Effects

- Blockades Fc receptors
- Accelerates clearance of activated complement fragments
- Alters solubility characteristics of circulating immune complexes
- Decreases soluble adhesion molecules (e.g., E-selectin, ICAM-1)
- Upregulates activity of natural killer cells
- Reverses immunoregulatory abnormalities by increasing suppressor T cells and decreasing helper T cells and circulating B cells
- Downregulates transcription of cytokine genes
- Neutralizes activity of proinflammatory cytokines
- Causes feedback inhibition of autoantibody synthesis
- Reverses inhibited lymphocyte apoptosis
- Induces neutrophil apoptosis

Infusion reactions (fever, rash, nausea, and hypotension) occasionally accompany IVIG administration and are best managed by slowing the rate of infusion and treating with diphenhydramine. With no viable alternative therapies, aggressive premedication with corticosteroids, or even use of a different brand of IVIG, is preferable to foregoing immunoglobulin. Rarely, a child might develop congestive heart failure during or after infusion of the IVIG because of the high solute load and subsequent increase in intravascular volume. Slowing the infusion rate and administration of furosemide are usually the only treatments required. Ultimately the improvement in myocardial contractility associated with IVIG treatment is almost invariably adequate therapy.[87] Hemolysis is uncommon, but occasionally it may be severe, requiring transfusion. Headache up to 72 hours after the infusion is common, especially in older patients. Such children may require low-dose opiates for relief.[157]

Virtually all data concerning the role of IVIG are limited to treatment during the first 10 days of illness. This is not to say that treatment after 10 days of illness is ineffective or contraindicated; it is merely inadequately studied. In a report of 16 children with coronary artery aneurysms treated a mean of 17 days after onset of fever, there was a trend toward increased resolution of abnormalities by echocardiogram.[158] The American Academy of Pediatrics cautiously recommends IVIG for children beyond the 10th day of illness with "manifestations of continuing inflammation," and such an approach appears prudent.[128] Questions have arisen concerning the efficacy of very early treatment of KD. Tse and colleagues,[159] on the other hand, reported that IVIG given on or before the fifth day of illness resulted in fewer coronary artery abnormalities at the 1-year follow-up assessment. Thus, decisions about the optimal date for treating with IVIG are best made based on a patient's clinical status and the certainty of the diagnosis of KD.

Glucocorticoids

Glucocorticoids, the preferred initial treatment for other forms of vasculitis, had been considered unsafe in KD. This is based primarily on a study,[160] which demonstrated an extraordinarily high incidence of coronary artery aneurysms (11 of 17 patients) in a group that received oral prednisolone at a dose of 2 to 3 mg/kg/day for at least two weeks, followed by 1.5 mg/kg/day for an additional two weeks. Interestingly, seven patients in the same study received prednisolone plus aspirin, and none developed aneurysms. In fact, no subsequent study has indicated that corticosteroids are harmful when used either with IVIG or as an alternative to IVIG therapy. If they are not contraindicated, then what, if any role might steroids have for treating KD?

Potential benefits of corticosteroids are supported most convincingly as "rescue therapy." Initially, two retrospective analyses supported the use of corticosteroids in children who were unresponsive to two doses of IVIG or who relapsed after such therapy.[161,162] Hashino and colleagues[163] also found a beneficial effect of glucocorticoids in KD in a prospective trial. Children who had failed to respond to two doses of IVIG were randomized to receive a third dose of IVIG or pulse-dose methylprednisolone. Patients who received methylprednisolone had a significantly shorter duration of fever, and although transient coronary artery dilatation was associated with glucocorticoid therapy, there was no overall difference in the incidence of coronary artery abnormalities between groups. Based on these studies, IVMP has become the mainstay of "rescue" therapy in children who are unresponsive to IVIG.[93]

Might steroids also have a role to play earlier in the course of KD? Shinohara and colleagues[164] retrospectively reviewed the results in almost 300 patients with acute KD seen between 1982 and 1998 who were treated before the 10th day of illness. All patients received aspirin, dipyrimidole, and propranolol. The addition of prednisolone therapy, either alone or with IVIG, was associated with a significantly shorter duration of fever and a lower prevalence of coronary artery aneurysms. No adverse reactions were recorded for any therapy. A prospective study was suggestive of benefit as well; Inoue[165] reported that the frequency of coronary artery abnormalities in children treated with IVIG plus prednisolone 2 mg/kg/d was lower than in those treated with IVIG alone. Three other studies[161,166,167] have shown that children treated with IVMP (or dexamethasone) plus IVIG had faster resolution of fever, more rapid improvement in markers of inflammation, and shorter length of hospitalization than those receiving IVIG alone. Two of these studies had insufficient statistical power to detect a potential benefit of glucocorticoid therapy on coronary artery outcomes. The third trial, by Newburger and colleagues, found no significant difference in the frequency or severity of coronary artery lesions between treatment groups at one week or five week followup. Interestingly, however, *post hoc* analysis suggested that children who ultimately failed to respond to an initial dose of IVIG were less likely to develop coronary artery aneurysms if their initial therapy had included IVMP.

Following up on this finding, the Osaka Kawasaki Disease Study Group[168] conducted a comparative trial of IVIG vs. IVIG plus IVMP in children with KD regarded as being at high risk for nonresponse to IVIG.[169] High risk was defined as the presence of at least two of the following: CRP ≥7 mg, total bilirubin ≥0.9 mg, or aspartate transaminase ≥200 I.U./L. Patients were given heparin (10 U/kg/hr) for 48 hours beginning two hours before receiving IVMP (30 mg/kg), followed by IVIG (2 g/kg). Aspirin (30 mg/kg/d) was started at the end of the heparin infusion and reduced to 10 mg/kg/d after resolution of fever. Therapy was effective in 44% of those given IVIG alone compared to 66% of those receiving both IVIG and IVMP. The disease was refractory in 56% of those receiving IVIG alone and 11% of those receiving IVIG and IVMP, although a rebound fever was observed in 23% of those treated with IVIG and IVMP, but not in the group receiving IVIG alone. Coronary artery abnormalities, including aneurysms, were significantly less frequent in the IVIG plus IVMP group (24%) compared to the IVIG alone group (46%). In a meta-analysis of eight studies, Wooditch and Aronson concluded that the incidence of coronary artery aneurysms was reduced by the addition of corticosteroids to aspirin-containing therapeutic regimens.[162]

While it is clear that corticosteroids are not a substitute for IVIG in the treatment of KD, a case may be made for the inclusion of corticosteroids in the initial management of children with KD who are high risk of being refractory to IVIG. Studies to date have shown a decrease in the frequency of coronary artery abnormalities in some children who received IVIG plus corticosteroids as initial therapy, in comparison to those who received IVIG alone. The toxicity associated with combination therapy appears to be higher than that seen with IVIG alone, although reactions are generally not severe. Further, with the addition of pulsed dose methylprednisolone, the systemic manifestations of KD (fever, rash, etc.) appear to resolve more quickly, and the duration of hospitalization is, on average, shortened. Clinical and biological markers to identify such high-risk children are improving[170] and ongoing trials are examining the effects of other adjunct therapies for treatment with IVIG. These studies should refine attempts to optimize the treatment of KD.

Anti-TNF Agents

Levels of TNFα are markedly increased in children with KD, especially in those who develop coronary artery lesions.[171,172] The use of monoclonal antibodies to TNFα inhibits actions of this cytokine. An anecdotal series reported the results of the use of infliximab, an anti TNFα monoclonal antibody, in 17 children with KD who had either persistent arthritis or persistent or recurrent fever 48 hours or more after treatment with IVIG (2 g/kg) and high dose aspirin.[173] All had received at least two doses of IVIG, six had received three or more doses of IVIG, and eight had received one to three doses of intravenous methylprednisolone (30 mg/kg/dose). One patient had persistent fever, 15 had persistent fever and arthritis, and one had persistent severe arthritis; symptoms lasted for from eight to 53 days before infliximab was administered.

Coronary artery abnormalities were present in 12 patients (including three with aneurysms and five with ectasia). A single infusion of infliximab (5 mg/kg) was given to 15 patients; two patients received 10 mg/kg. The fever responded promptly in 14 of 16 febrile patients, and levels of CRP fell. The effect on coronary artery abnormalities was not described in detail.

A prospective randomized multicenter comparison of the effectiveness of IVIG and infliximab in children who had not responded to an initial infusion of IVIG[174] showed that both agents were equally effective and well-tolerated. Hirono and colleagues[175] also found that infliximab was effective in controlling fever, but did not completely prevent coronary artery changes, although single case reports document resolution of aneurysms following infliximab therapy in some patients.[176,177] A retrospective comparison of patients at two institutions treated with either methylprednisolone or infliximab for KD resistant to initial treatment with IVIG found no differences in responses.[178] The role of infliximab in treatment of KD, either as initial therapy or as treatment for resistant disease, remains uncertain.

Other Therapeutic Approaches

Therapies that are effective in other forms of vasculitis have been used in KD. Pentoxifylline was alleged to be effective in preventing coronary artery aneurysms,[179] but demonstration of flaws in the analysis of the data in this study[180] lead to the conclusion that it is ineffective. Similarly, the human trypsin inhibitor, Ulinastatin, has been the subject of studies from Japan. Its efficacy in preventing coronary artery disease in KD is not convincing.[181]

A dramatic response to plasmapheresis has been reported,[182] but the technical limitations and potential hazards of this therapy are considerable. It should be reserved for children with active inflammation who have failed all available medical interventions, including multiple doses of IVIG, intravenous methylprednisolone, and TNF inhibition. There have been conflicting reports of the efficacy of abciximab, a monoclonal antibody that inhibits platelet glycoprotein IIb/IIIa receptor. In one study,[183] there was an increased resolution of aneurysms in patients with KD who received abciximab compared to those who received conventional treatment. However, a second study[184] could not duplicate these findings.

The role for immunosuppressive agents in KD, such as cyclophosphamide[185] or cyclosporine,[186] is extremely limited, but they may have a role in cases with persistent active disease unresponsive to conventional therapy. In addition, alternative diagnoses including chronic vasculitides, such as PAN, should be considered.

TREATMENT OF RELAPSES

Fever returns within 48 hours of treatment with IVIG in 10% to 20% of children, indicating failure to suppress the underlying inflammatory process. Because prolonged fever is an independent risk factor for the development of coronary artery aneurysms, these children should be retreated with a second dose of IVIG (2 g/kg). Those who fail to respond to a second dose—up to one-third of patients in some studies[93]—are at extremely increased risk of developing coronary artery aneurysms. They should be treated in rapid succession with intravenous methylprednisolone (30 mg/kg/day for one to three days)[151] or with infliximab (5 mg/kg). Treatment should continue until fever resolves and the CRP is normal, and frequent evaluations of the coronary arteries should be pursued until children have fully recovered.

PREVENTION AND MANAGEMENT OF THROMBOSES

The risk of thrombosis of coronary or other arteries depends on the degree of vascular damage. In all patients with KD, irrespective of the demonstration of coronary artery abnormalities, low-dose (3 to 5 mg/kg/day) aspirin should be continued until the ESR and platelet counts have normalized. Children with coronary artery abnormalities demonstrated by echocardiography are often treated with antithrombotic agents, such as low-dose aspirin, for as long as the abnormalities persist (Table 33–7). Children with large aneurysms are anticoagulated with warfarin. Trials with low-molecular-weight heparin are ongoing.

When injured coronary arteries become obstructed (risk level V) in addition to anticoagulation, various therapies have been attempted to restore circulation. Control of vascular inflammation with sufficient IVIG and other agents is an essential prerequisite to arterial reperfusion. Thereafter, treatments may include thrombolytic therapy for arterial thrombosis or vasodilators if tissue viability is primarily threatened by vasospasm. Urokinase, streptokinase, and tissue-type plasminogen have all been used for

Table 33–7

Recommendations for Long-term Follow-up

Risk Level	Pharmacological Therapy	Physical Activity	Follow-Up and Diagnostic Testing	Invasive Testing
I (no coronary artery changes at any stage of illness)	None beyond 1st 6-8 weeks	No restrictions beyond 1st 6-8 weeks	Cardiovascular risk assessment counseling at 5 yr intervals	None recommended
II (transient coronary artery ectasia disappears within 1st 6-8 weeks)	None beyond 1st 6-8 weeks	No restrictions beyond 1st 6-8 weeks	Cardiovascular risk assessment counseling at 3 to 5 yr intervals	None recommended
III (1 small-medium coronary artery aneurysm/major coronary artery)	Low-dose aspirin (3-5 mg/kg aspirin/day), at least until aneurysm regression documented	For patients <11 yrs old, no restriction beyond 1st 6-8 weeks; patients 11-20 yrs old, physical activity guided by biennial stress test, evaluation of myocardial perfusion scan; contact or high-impact sports discouraged for patients taking antiplatelet agents	Annual cardiology follow-up with echocardiogram + ECG, combined with cardiovascular risk assessment, counseling; biennial stress test/evaluation of myocardial perfusion scan	Angiography, if noninvasive test suggests ischemia
IV (≥1 large or giant coronary artery aneurysm, or multiple or complex aneurysms in same coronary artery, without obstruction)	Long-term antiplatelet therapy and warfarin (target International normalized ratio 2.0-2.5) or low-molecular-weight heparin (target: antifactor Xa level 0.5-1.0 U/mL) should be combined in giant aneurysms	Contact or high-impact sports should be avoided because of risk of bleeding; other physical activity recommendations guided by stress test/evaluation of myocardial perfusion scan outcome	Biannual follow-up with echocardiogram + ECG; annual stress test/evaluation of myocardial perfusion scan	1st angiography at 6-12 mo or sooner if clinically indicated; repeated angiography if noninvasive test, clinical, or laboratory findings suggest ischemia; elective repeat angiography under some circumstances
V (coronary artery obstruction)	Long-term low-dose aspirin; warfarin or low-molecular-weight heparin if giant aneurysm persists; consider use of β-blockers to reduce myocardial O_2 consumption	Contact or high-impact sports should be avoided because of risk of bleeding; other physical activity recommendations guided by stress test/myocardial perfusion scan outcome	Biannual follow-up with echocardiogram and ECG; annual stress test/evaluation of myocardial perfusion scan	Angiography recommended to address therapeutic options

From Newburger JW, Takahashi M, Gerber MA et al: Diagnosis, treatment and long-term management of Kawasaki disease: a statement for health professionals from the committee on rheumatic fever, endocarditis and Kawasaki disease. Council on Cardiovascular Disease in the Young: American Heart Association, *Pediatrics* 114:1708-1733, 2004.

the lysis of coronary artery thromboses. Similarly, peripheral arterial obstruction may be corrected by thrombolysis, after which perfusion is maintained with heparin followed by a chronic oral anticoagulant regimen. If these treatments fail, a variety of invasive approaches have been suggested, including percutaneous transluminal coronary angioplasty[187] and coronary artery bypass grafting.[188] A small number of children with particularly severe coronary artery disease due to KD have required cardiac transplantation.[189]

MONITORING CARDIAC STATUS

There is no universal agreement about the timing and frequency of echocardiographic monitoring of patients with KD. Most protocols take into account the development of coronary artery aneurysms, which occur most frequently between the second and the eighth weeks after the onset of fever. It is recommended[190] that the initial echocardiogram should be obtained at the time a diagnosis of KD is suspected and that each child with KD should have a second echocardiogram obtained six to eight weeks after onset of the disease. Patients should also have repeated clinical examinations during the first 2 months to detect dysrhythmias, congestive heart failure, valvular insufficiency, or myocarditis.[191] Further follow-up is individualized, with more frequent studies performed in children with demonstrated coronary artery abnormalities (see Table 33–7).

Children whose coronary arteries have always been normal (risk level I) or are normal by echocardiographic criteria one to two months after the acute illness (risk level II) are regarded as healthy, and no further intervention is recommended after the eight-week follow-up assessment. In view of the chronic abnormalities in endothelial function, however, many physicians consider a history of KD to be a risk factor for the development of coronary artery disease later in life.[192] They counsel modification of other risk factors and continue to monitor children once every 5 years.

Single small- to medium-sized aneurysms (risk level III) usually resolve as determined by echocardiographic criteria, although this is not always the case. Healing occurs by fibrointimal proliferation, often accompanied by calcification, and vascular reactivity does not return to normal despite a grossly normal appearance.[136] This point is highlighted by a report of sudden death in a 3.5-year-old child three months after dilated coronary arteries had regained a normal echocardiographic appearance.[194] Autopsy revealed obliteration of the lumen of the left anterior descending coronary artery due to fibrosis, with evidence of ongoing active inflammation in the epicardial arteries. Such reports emphasize the need for confirmation of complete response to therapy in children who have had KD.

Giant aneurysms with an internal diameter of at least 8 mm represent a significant risk for morbidity and mortality, including a 35% chance of infarction (risk level IV).[98] These children are followed more closely and are treated with more aggressive antithrombotic and anticoagulation regimens.

DISEASE COURSE AND PROGNOSIS

Although standard therapy with IVIG and aspirin given within the first 10 days of illness greatly improves outcomes, approximately 5% of children still develop coronary artery aneurysms, and more children demonstrate coronary artery ectasia.[105] The mortality rate has dropped steadily as the diagnosis and treatment have improved. Currently the rate is about 0.1% in the U.S. and Japan.[194,195]

Recurrent disease after full recovery from a first episode of KD is rare but does occur. In Japan, the recurrence rate is 2.9%, with a higher incidence of cardiac complications during the second episode.[165] In the U.S., the rate of recurrence is lower.

REFERENCES

1. T. Kawasaki, Acute febrile mucocutaneous syndrome with lymphoid involvement with specific desquamation of the fingers and toes in children, Arerugi 16 (1967) 178–222.
6. S. Ozen, N. Ruperto, M.J. Dillon, et al., EULAR/PReS endorsed consensus criteria for the classification of childhood vasculitides, Ann. Rheum. Dis. 65 (2006) 936–941.
8. J.C. Burns, W.H. Mason, M. Glode, et al., Clinical and epidemiologic characteristics of patients referred for evaluation of possible Kawasaki disease. United States Multicenter Kawasaki Disease Study Group, J. Pediatr. 118 (1991) 680–686.
9. S.M. Benseler, B.W. McCrindle, E.D. Silverman, et al., Infections and Kawasaki disease: implications for coronary artery outcome, Arthritis Rheum. 48 (2003) S516.
12. E.A. Rosenfeld, K.E. Corydon, S.T. Shulman, Kawasaki disease in infants less than one year of age, J. Pediatr. 126 (1995) 524–529.
13. J.W. Newburger, M. Takahashi, J.C. Burns, et al., The treatment of Kawasaki syndrome with intravenous gamma globulin, N. Engl. J. Med. 315 (1986) 341–347.
26. J.C. Burns, D.R. Cayan, G. Tong, et al., Seasonality and temporal clustering of Kawasaki syndrome, Epidemiology 16 (2005) 220–225.
30. M. Dergun, A. Kao, S.B. Hauger, et al., Familial occurrence of Kawasaki syndrome in North America, Arch. Pediatr. Adolesc. Med. 159 (2005) 876–881.
36. P.A. Brogan, V. Shah, N. Klein, et al., V beta-restricted T-cell adherence to endothelial cells: A mechanism for superantigen-dependent vascular injury, Arthritis Rheum. 50 (2007) 589–597.
38. T.T. Duong, E.D. Silverman, M.V. Bissessar, et al., Superantigenic activity is responsible for induction of coronary arteritis in mice: an animal model of Kawasaki disease, Int. Immunol. 15 (2003) 79–89.
43. A.H. Rowley, S.T. Shulman, B.T. Spike, et al., Oligoclonal IgA response in the vascular wall in acute Kawasaki disease, J. Immunol. 166 (2001) 1334–1343.
53. C.O. Savage, J. Tizard, D. Jayne, et al., Antineutrophil cytoplasm antibodies in Kawasaki disease, Arch. Dis. Child 64 (1989) 360–363.
69. M. Biezefeld, J. Geissler, G. Weverling, et al., Polymorphisms in the mannose binding lectin of determinants of age-defined risk of coronary aneurysms artery lesions in Kawasaki disease, Arthritis Rheum. 54 (2006) 369–376.
70. Y. Ounouchi, T. Gunji, J.C. Burns, et al., ITPKC functional polymorphism associated with Kawasaki disease susceptibility and formation of coronary aneurysms, Nat. Gen. 40 (2008) 35–42.
71. D. Burgner, S. Davila, W.B. Breunis, et al., A genome-wide association study identifies novel and functionally related susceptibility Loci for Kawasaki disease, PLoS Genet. 5 (2009) e1000319.
72. A.L. Baker, M. Lu, L. Minich, et al., Associated symptoms in the ten days before diagnosis of Kawasaki disease, J. Pediatr. 154 (2009) 592–595.
76. G.W.K. Gong, B. McCrindle, J.C. Ching, et al., Arthritis presenting during the acute phase of Kawasaki disease, J. Pediatr. 148 (2006) 800–805.

85. J. Fukushige, N. Takahashi, Y. Ueda, et al., Incidence and clinical features of incomplete Kawasaki disease, Acta Paediatr. 83 (1994) 1057–1060.

87. J.W. Newburger, M. Takahashi, M.A. Gerber, et al., Diagnosis, treatment and long-term management of Kawasaki disease: a statement for health professionals from the Committee on Rheumatic Fever, Endocarditis and Kawasaki Disease, Council on Cardiovascular Disease in the Young. American Heart Association, Pediatrics 114 (2004) 1708–1733.

88. E.S Yellen, K. Gauvreau, M. Takahashi, et al., Performance of 2004 American Heart Association recommendations for treatment of Kawasaki disease, Pediatrics 125 (2) (2010 Feb) e234–e241. Epub 2010 Jan 25.

91. J.W. Newburger, S.P. Sanders, J.C. Burns, et al., Left ventricular contractility and function in Kawasaki syndrome. Effect of intravenous gamma-globulin, Circulation 79 (1989) 1237–1246.

92. A. Moran, J.W. Newburger, S.P. Sanders, et al., Abnormal myocardial mechanics in Kawasaki disease: rapid response to gamma globulin, Am. Heart J. 139 (2000) 217–223.

93. J.C. Burns, E.V. Capparelli, J.A. Brown, et al., Intravenous gamma-globulin treatment and retreatment in Kawasaki disease. US/Canadian Kawasaki Syndrome Study Group, Pediatr. Infect. Dis. J 17 (1998) 1144–1148.

95. H. Kato, E. Ichinose, T. Kawasaki, Myocardial infarction in Kawasaki disease: clinical analyses in 195 cases, J. Pediatr. 108 (1986) 923–927.

102. B. Tabarki, A. Mahdhaoui, H. Selmi, et al., Kawasaki disease with predominant central nervous system involvement, Pediatr. Neurol. 25 (2001) 239–241.

104. R.P. Sundel, S.S. Cleveland, A.S. Beiser, et al., Audiologic profiles of children with Kawasaki disease, Am. J. Otol. 13 (1992) 512–515.

107. E.A. Suddleson, B. Reid, M.M. Woolley, M. Takahashi, Hydrops of the gallbladder associated with Kawasaki syndrome, J. Pediatr. Surg. 22 (1987) 956–959.

108. J.N. Wang, Y.Y. Chiou, N.T. Chiu, et al., Renal scarring sequelae in childhood Kawasaki disease, Pediatr. Nephrol. 22 (2007) 684–689.

114. H. Fujiwara, Y. Hamashima, Pathology of the heart in Kawasaki disease, Pediatrics 61 (1978) 100–107.

128. American Academy of Pediatrics. Kawasaki disease, in: L.K. Pickering, C.J. Baker, S.S Long, J.A. McMillan (Eds.), Red Book: 2006 Report of the Committee on Infectious Diseases, 27th ed, American Academy of Pediatrics, Elk Grove, Village, IL, 2006, pp. 414.

130. Report of the Subcommittee on Standardization of Diagnostic Criteria and Reporting of Coronary Artery Lesions in Kawasaki Disease, Ministry of Health and Welfare, Tokyo, Japan, 1984.

133. M.A. Crystal, C. Manlhiot, R.S. Yeung, et al., Coronary artery dilation after Kawasaki disease for children within the normal range, Int. J. Cardiol. 136 (2009) 27–32.

136. R. Dhillon, P. Clarkson, A.E. Donald, et al., Endothelial dysfunction late after Kawasaki disease, Circulation 94 (1996) 2103–2106.

139. T. Akagi, H. Kato, O. Inoue, et al., Salicylate treatment in Kawasaki disease: high dose or low dose? Eur. J. Pediatr. 150 (1991) 642–646.

141. F. Catella-Lawson, M.P. Reilly, S.C. Kapoor, et al., Cyclooxygenase inhibitors and the anti-platelet effects of aspirin, New. Engl. J. Med. 345 (2001) 1809–1817.

145. J.W. Newburger, M. Takahashi, A.S. Beiser, et al., A single intravenous infusion of gamma globulin as compared with four infusions in the treatment of acute Kawasaki syndrome, N. Engl. J. Med. 324 (1991) 1633–1639.

149. M. Fukunishi, M. Kikkawa, K. Hamana, et al., Prediction of non-responsiveness to intravenous high dose gamma-globulin therapy in patients with Kawasaki disease at onset, J. Pediatr. 137 (2000) 172–176.

150. T. Kobayashi, Y. Inoue, K. Takeuchi, et al., Prediction of intravenous immunoglobulin unresponsiveness in patients with Kawasaki disease, Circulation 113 (2006) 2606–2612.

151. R.K. Han, E.D. Silverman, A. Newman, et al., Management and outcome of persistent or recurrent fever after initial intravenous gamma globulin therapy in acute Kawasaki disease, Arch. Pediatr. Adolesc. Med. 154 (2000) 694–699.

152. M. Mori, T. Imagawa, K. Yasui, et al., Predictors of coronary artery lesions after intravenous gamma-globulin treatment in Kawasaki disease, J. Pediatr. 137 (2000) 177–180.

155. J.S. Bresee, E.E. Mast, P.J. Coleman, et al., Hepatitis C virus infection associated with administration of intravenous immune globulin. A cohort study, JAMA 276 (1996) 1563–1567.

157. Y. Sherer, Y. Levy, P. Langevitz, et al., Adverse effects of intravenous immunoglobulin therapy in 56 patients with autoimmune diseases, Pharmacology 62 (2001) 133–137.

158. M. Marasini, G. Pongiglione, D. Gazolo, et al., Late intravenous gamma globulin treatment in infants and children with Kawasaki disease and coronary artery abnormalities, Am. J. Cardiol. 68 (1991) 796–797.

159. S.M. Tse, E.D. Silverman, B.W. McCrindle, et al., Early treatment with intravenous immunoglobulin in patients with Kawasaki disease, J. Pediatr. 140 (2003) 450–455.

161. R.P. Sundel, A.L. Baker, D.R. Fulton, et al., Corticosteroids in the initial treatment of Kawasaki disease: report of a randomized trial, J. Pediatr. 142 (2003) 611–616.

162. A.C. Wooditch, S.C. Aronoff, Effect of initial corticosteroid therapy on coronary artery aneurysm formation in Kawasaki disease: A meta-analysis of 862 children, Pediatrics 116 (2005) 989–995.

163. K. Hashino, M. Ishii, M. Iemura, et al., Re-treatment for immune globulin-resistant Kawasaki disease: a comparative study of additional immune globulin and steroid pulse therapy, Pediatr. Int. 43 (2001) 211–217.

165. Y. Inoue, Y. Okada, M. Shinohara, et al., A multicenter randomized trial of corticosteroids in primary therapy for Kawasaki disease: Clinical course and coronary artery outcome, J. Pediatr. 149 (2006) 336–341.

167. J.W. Newburger, L.A. Sleeper, B.W. McCrindle, et al., Randomized trial of pulsed corticosteroid therapy for primary treatment of Kawasaki disease, New Engl. J. Med. 356 (2007) 664–675.

169. T. Sano, S. Kurotobi, K. Matsuzaki, et al., Prediction of non-responsiveness to standard high-dose gamma globulin-therapy in patients with acute Kawasaki disease before starting initial treatment, Eur. J. Ped. 166 (2007) 131–137.

170. S. Ogata, Y. Ogihara, K. Nomoto, et al., Clinical score and transcript abundance patterns identify Kawasaki disease patients who may benefit from addition of methylprednisolone, Pediatr. Res. 66 (2009) 577–584.

173. J.C. Burns, W.H. Mason, S.B. Hauger, et al., Infliximab treatment for refractory Kawasaki syndrome, J. Pediatr. 146 (2005) 662–667.

174. J.C. Burns, B.M. Best, A. Mejias, et al., Infliximab treatment of intravenous gamma globulin-resistant Kawasaki disease, J. Pediatr. 153 (2008) 833–838.

175. K. Hirono, Y. Kemmotsu, H. Wittkowski, et al., Infliximab reduces the cytokine-mediated inflammation but does not suppress the cellular infiltration of the vessel wall in refractory Kawasaki disease, Pediatr. Res. 65 (2009) 696–701.

178. M.B. Son, K. Gauvreau, L. Ma, A.L. Baker, et al., Treatment of Kawasaki disease: analysis of 27th US pediatric hospitals from 2001 to 2006, Pediatrics 124 (2009) 1–8.

188. N. Gotteiner, C.V. Mavroudis, C.L. Backer, et al., Coronary artery bypass grafting for Kawasaki disease, Pediatr. Cardiol. 23 (2002) 62–67.

189. P.A. Checchia, E. Pahl, R.E. Shaddy, et al., Cardiac transplantation for Kawasaki disease, Pediatrics 100 (1997) 695–699.

190. A.S. Dajani, K.A. Taubert, M. Takahashi, et al., Guidelines for long-term management of patients with Kawasaki disease. Report from the Committee on Rheumatic Fever, Endocarditis, and Kawasaki Disease, Council on Cardiovascular Disease in the Young, American Heart Association, Circulation 89 (1994) 916–922.

192. Y.F. Cheung, T.C. Yung, S.C. Tam, et al., Novel and traditional cardiovascular risk factors in children after Kawasaki disease: implications for premature atherosclerosis, J. Am. Coll. Cardiol. 43 (2004) 120–124.

193. M.E. McConnell, D.W. Hannon, R.D. Steed, et al., Fatal obliterative coronary vasculitis in Kawasaki disease, J. Pediatr. 133 (1998) 259–261.

195. Y. Nakamura, H. Yanagawa, T. Ojima, et al., Cardiac sequelae of Kawasaki disease among recurrent cases, Arch. Dis. Child 78 (1998) 163–165.

Entire reference list is available online at www.expertconsult.com.

Chapter 34

GRANULOMATOUS VASCULITIS, MICROSCOPIC POLYANGIITIS AND PRIMARY ANGIITIS OF THE CENTRAL NERVOUS SYSTEM

David Cabral and Susanne Benseler

Granulomatous vasculitis is a subset of vasculitis that includes Wegener granulomatosis (WG), Churg Strauss syndrome (CSS), giant cell arteritis (GCA), Takayasu arteritis (TA), and primary angiitis of the central nervous system (PACNS). Microscopic polyangiitis (MPA) characteristically does not have granulomatous inflammation but is often described with both WG and CSS, because of the shared predominant pathological involvement of small- to medium-sized blood vessels, clinically overlapping features, and the association with antineutrophil cytoplasmic antibodies (ANCAs). Classic GCA affecting the temporal artery, as described in adults, probably does not occur in children. Although PACNS has been described as a necrotizing granulomatous vasculitis, this does not pathologically characterize the large majority of children diagnosed with this disorder. All of these conditions are rare in childhood and adolescence, and consequently most knowledge about these diseases comes from a few small case series, or it has been adapted from studies of adults.

WEGENER GRANULOMATOSIS

WG is a chronic systemic vasculitis predominantly involving small- to medium-sized arteries. It is characterized by granulomatous inflammation of the upper and lower respiratory tracts and necrotizing, pauciimmune glomerulonephritis, but vasculitis may frequently involve other organs. It is usually associated with ANCA. McBride first described the condition in 1897 as a midfacial granuloma syndrome,[1] but the complete picture was not described until the 1930s.[2,3] It is now known that the disease can often be organ- or life-threatening. The peak incidence is in the fourth to sixth decades;[4-6] like all types of chronic primary systemic vasculitis,[7,8] WG is rare in childhood, but it may be one of the most common forms seen by pediatric rheumatologists.[9]

Classification

The 1990 American College of Rheumatology (ACR) classification criteria[10] may not be optimal for classifying children with vasculitis. One third of 17 children with WG diagnosed by expert opinion never fulfilled these criteria in a long term follow up.[10] Both the ACR classification criteria[11] and the subsequent Chapel Hill consensus conference (CHCC) disease definitions,[12] although used in children, were based largely on adult data. Recently, a consensus committee of pediatric rheumatology and nephrology experts, under the auspices of the European League Against Rheumatism (EULAR) and the Pediatric Rheumatology European Society (PRES), proposed a system of classification for vasculitis that took into account existing pediatric knowledge and experience.[13] The resulting proposed system of classification and criteria (EULAR/PRES criteria) for WG have yet to be validated in a cohort of children with vasculitis. EULAR/PRES and ACR criteria for WG are compared in Table 34–1. One study comparing the criteria for WG among children with unclassified and ANCA-associated vasculitis showed only small differences in the ability to classify additional children.[14] While the EULAR/PReS criteria now include features that may be more frequent or characteristic for children, the requirement for fulfillment of an additional criterion (three out of six criteria) excludes children from being classified as having WG who would otherwise be included using two out of four criteria required by the ACR classification.

Epidemiology

Population studies from Norway,[4] the United Kingdom (U.K.)[6] Sweden,[15] and Finland,[16] comparing consecutive periods from the 1970s to the 1990s, all describe an increasing incidence of WG rising from 0.2 to 1.2 per 100,000 persons per year. The Swedish study[15] spanning 26 years (1975 to 2001) estimates an incidence in three consecutive

Table 34–1

Comparison of the ACR[10] and proposed EULAR/ PReS[13] criteria for classification of Wegener Granulomatosis (with difference shown in bold face italics)

ACR	EULAR /PReS
A patient is said to have WG when two of the following four criteria are present:	A patient is said to have WG when three of the following six criteria are present:
1 Nasal or oral inflammation	1 Nasal, oral inflammation or *sinus inflammation*†
2 Abnormal chest radiograph	2 Abnormal chest radiograph or *chest CT scan*†
3 Abnormal urinalysis	3 Abnormal urinalysis including *significant proteinuria*†
4 Granulomatous inflammation on biopsy	4 Granulomatous inflammation on biopsy or *Necrotizing pauciimmune GN on biopsy*†
	5 *Subglottic, tracheal, or endobronchial stenosis*†
	6 *PR3 ANCA or cANCA staining*†

Additional Descriptors Provided with ACR Criteria

Nasal or oral inflammation	Painful or painless oral ulcers or purulent or bloody nasal discharge
Abnormal chest X-ray	Nodules, fixed infiltrates or cavities
Abnormal urinalysis	Microhematuria: >5 RBC/high-power field
Granulomatous inflammation on biopsy	Granulomatous inflammation within wall of artery or in perivascular or extravascular area of artery or arteriole

ACR, American College of Rheumatology; EULAR, European League against Rheumatism; PReS, Pediatric Rheumatology European Society

periods rising from 0.3 to 0.8 to 1.2. This study concludes that increased disease recognition resulting from the availability of ANCA testing is an incomplete explanation of the rising incidence. Regional differences of WG are described with higher incidences in both Norway[17] and areas of U.K.,[18] compared to Spain. A study in New Zealand similarly describes a higher incidence in higher latitudes.[19] Much less is known about the incidence of WG in children and adolescents. American[5] and Norwegian[4] population studies from the 1980s and 1990s estimate incidences of 0.6 and 0.8 per 100,000 persons per year. In these studies, 3.3% and 7% of patients had disease onset before reaching 20 years of age or 16 years of age respectively, for calculated annual incidences of 0.02 and 0.06. In the pediatric population, most studies concur that WG is generally a disease of the second decade of life with a caucasian and female preponderance,[10,20,21] although in adults, males outnumber females 1.6:1.[4] In the largest pediatric study of 65 children from United States (U.S.) and Canada, 69% were caucasian, 63% were female, the median age at WG diagnosis was 14.2 (range 4 to 17) years, and the median interval from symptom onset to diagnosis was 2.7 months (range 0 to 49).[14]

Etiology, Pathogenesis, and Role of Antineutrophil Cytoplasmic Antibodies

The cause of WG is unknown, although it is likely a multifactorial disease. Theories of causation and mechanisms of pathogenesis have included hypersensitivity reactions to unknown antigens, sensitization of the respiratory tract to bacterial pathogens, and likely a "mosaic of autoimmunity."[22] Putative roles for ANCA in the pathogenic process continue to evolve. Associations of WG with antigens of the histocompatibility system (human leukocyte antigen [HLA]) have been limited and inconsistent, but the most consistent finding has been a decrease in the frequency of HLA-DR13/DR6.[23,24] Epidemiological studies describing Caucasian predisposition[14,25] suggest genetic factors play some role; however, the infrequently reported familial occurrences[26-29] relatively late mean age-of-onset of WG in the general population, and the variations in incidence related to season or latitude argue for the importance of environmental and nongenetic factors. Since WG was first described,[2,3] researchers have unsuccessfully looked for exogenous agents that might stimulate granuloma formation in the airway. An association between primary systemic vasculitis, or WG and crystalline silica exposure, and farming has been shown by some studies,[30,31] but not by others.[32] An environmental predisposition may be mediated through nasal carriage of *Staphylococcus aureus*[33] Several mechanisms for its pathogenic role have been proposed.[22]

ANCAs are a heterogeneous group of autoantibodies characteristic of WG. Their additional association with CSS and MPA has resulted in these diseases being collectively described as the ANCA-associated vasculitides (AAV). ANCAs are directed against enzymes contained within the granules of polymorphonuclear cells (PMNs). They may be detected on immunofluorescence microscopy[34] in predominantly cytoplasmic (cANCA), perinuclear (pANCA), or indeterminate or atypical fluorescence patterns (Fig. 34–1). The target antigen of cANCA is proteinase-3 (PR-3), and, although it is highly sensitive and specific for WG, it is also found in MPA and CSS. The predominant target antigen of pANCA is myeloperoxidase (MPO), but others include elastase, cathepsin G, lactoferrin, lysozyme, and beta-glucuronidase. pANCA is strongly associated with MPA and CSS but may also be found in about 10% of patients with WG.[35,36] The AAV are characterized by the presence of necrotizing vasculitis of small vessels, frequent involvement of the kidneys, and a paucity of immune deposits in the vessel wall.[37] WG is distinguished among the AAV by the PR3-ANCA specificity and by the presence of granulomas.

The role of PR3-ANCA in the pathogenesis of WG is not clear. Attempts to develop a PR3-ANCA vasculitis animal model similar to the MPO-ANCA animal model[38] have been unsuccessful. Membrane expression of PR-3 on neutrophils appears to be genetically determined.[39] Patients with WG have an increased percentage of neutrophils expressing PR-3 on their membranes compared to healthy individuals,[40] and among patients with WG, membrane expression of PR-3 is associated

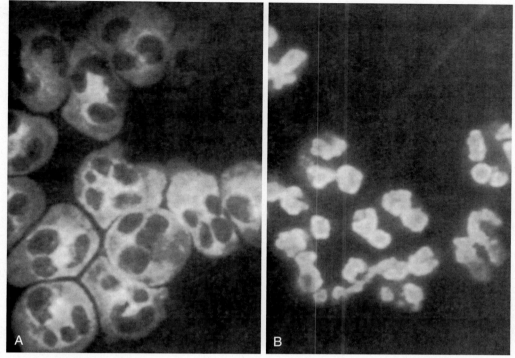

FIGURE 34–1   Indirect immunofluorescence microscopy staining patterns produced by antibodies directed at neutrophil cytoplasmic antigens (ANCAs) with a cytoplasmic staining pattern (cANCAs) **(A)** and those with a perinuclear staining pattern (pANCAs) **(B)** on alcohol-fixed neutrophils. (**A** and **B**, from Jennette JC, Falk RJ: Antineutrophil cytoplasmic autoantibodies and associated diseases: a review, *Am J Kidney Dis* 15:517, 1990.)

with severity[41] or rate of relapse.[42] Studies of the association of active WG and relapse with rising titers of C-ANCA or PR3-ANCA show conflicting results.[43,44] Limited success in some pilot studies of B cell depletion therapy with rituximab argues for a pathogenic role of autoantibodies;[45] however, in other studies, efficacy of this therapy was poor.[46] Although autoantibodies probably play some role in WG pathogenesis, the characteristic presence of granulomas[47] suggest a more complex process with a predominance of Th-1 cells in the cell-mediated hypersensitivity model of disease.[48] Arguably, inflammation of the upper airways by *S. aureus*,[33,49,50] other pathogens, or environmental exposure induces cytokine production. These cytokines assist in upregulating PMN membrane expression of PR-3,[51] induce expression of adhesion molecules, and allow interaction of PMNs and endothelium, notably in the kidney.[52] In binding to PR-3, ANCA blocks α_1-antitrypsin, its natural inhibitor, and potentiates inflammation. Monocytes, primed by tumor necrosis factor (TNF) α can be activated by ANCA or by ANCA-opsonized PMNs to produce TNFα, interferon (IFN) γ,[53] and chemokines integral to granuloma formation. These monocytes can be found in nasal[54] and renal tissues[55] of patients with WG. PR3-ANCA also interacts with Fcγ receptors, and polymorphisms of this receptor explain variation in expression or severity of WG in some studies but not others.[56-59] Elucidation of the intricate immune pathways and processes continues, and recently a role for Th-17 cells in the pathogenesis of WG and other autoimmune disease has been proposed.[60,61]

Clinical Manifestations

The triad of upper and lower respiratory tract inflammation and renal disease is characteristic of WG as described in the four largest pediatric cohorts.[10,14,20,21] At onset, nonspecific complaints of fever, malaise, fatigue, and weight loss are very common (89%). The next most common presenting features by organ system, as described in the largest series comprising 65 patients,[14] were pulmonary (80%); ear, nose, and throat (80%); and renal (75%) manifestations (Table 34–2). A large majority of children with WG present with multiple organ involvement. In contrast to the adult experience[25,62] and two smaller pediatric series,[63,64] so-called limited WG defined by the absence of kidney disease would appear to the relatively infrequent in children at presentation[14,20,21] and even less frequent in follow-up as the frequency of renal disease may increase with time.[20]

The spectrum of presenting pulmonary manifestations in the A Registry for Children with Vasculitis: e-entry (ARChiVe) cohort[14] included shortness of breath or chronic cough in just over half of the patients. Oxygen therapy was required for 18%, and 11% required mechanical ventilation. Pulmonary function tests were abnormal in 42% of patients tested. Upper respiratory tract signs and symptoms at presentation were as common as lower respiratory tract features and, in follow-up, are reported in 91% and 96% of patients.[20,21] Subglottic stenosis has been noted in some reports to occur more frequently in pediatric onset WG compared to adults, and this feature has been included in the EULAR/PReS classification criteria. In the ARChiVe cohort subglottic

Table 34–2

Presenting manifestations of Wegener Granulomatosis in childhood

Clinical Feature	ARChiVe§ (n=65)	HSC‡ (n=25)	
	Onset	Onset	Any time
Constitutional/General	**89**	**96**	**96**
Malaise, fatigue	89	NR	NR
Fever	54	72	76
Weight loss	43	56	60
Pulmonary	**80**	**80**	**84**
Hemoptysis/alveolar hemorrhage	45	44	48
Nodules	42**	44	52
Abnormal pulmonary function tests	77††	NR	NR
Fixed pulmonary infiltrates	23**	16	24
Oxygen dependency	18	NR	NR
Pleurisy	23	8	8
Requiring ventilation	11	16	20
Renal	**75**	**88**	**88**
Abnormal urinalysis	75	88	88
Biopsy proven glomerulonephritis	52	64	64
Elevated serum creatinine	42	28	44
Ear, nose, throat	**80**	**84**	**96**
Nasal involvement	65	40 ‡‡	60
Sinusitis	60	44	56
Otitis/mastoiditis	14	24	24
Subglottic involvement	14	4	4
Hearing loss	11	16	16
Oral ulcers	9	28	32
Eyes	**37**	**52**	**60**
Non-specific red-eye	15	NR	NR
Conjunctivitis	9	44	56
Scleritis	5	12	12
Cutaneous	**35**	**32**	**48**
Palpable purpura/petechiae	23	32	40
Gastrointestinal	**42**	**12**	**16**
Nonspecific abdominal pain	32	NR	NR
Chronic nausea	17	NR	NR
Musculoskeletal	**57**	**NR**	**NR**
Arthralgia/myalgia	54	64	76
Arthritis	20	32	44
Nervous System	**25**	**8**	**12**
Severe headache	14	NR	NR
Dizziness	12	NR	NR
Cardiovascular	**0**	**12†**	**16**
Venous thrombosis	0	12	16

§A Registry for Children with Vasculitis: e-entry (ARChiVe), patients met two or more of the American College of Rheumatology classification criteria for WG.

§§Arthralgias and arthritis at disease onset were not reported separately.

**From 62 children who underwent chest imaging.

†No cardiovascular features described.

††From 35 children who had pulmonary function tests done.

‡Hospital for Sick Children, Toronto, Canada.

‡‡Nasal involvement features were reported separately, with epistaxis occurring in 40% and nasal ulcers in 24% of children at disease onset.

NR, Frequency not reported.

stenosis was no more frequent than otitis/mastoiditis or hearing loss, and less frequent than nasal and sinus involvement. Nonetheless, it has a much narrower differential diagnosis than other upper respiratory complaints. Damage to the nasal cartilage, characteristic of long-standing disease, may result in a saddle-nose deformity, suggesting the possible diagnosis of relapsing polychondritis (Fig. 34–2). In the ARChiVe and Toronto cohorts[14,21] significantly elevated serum creatinine, was found in 42% and 28%, and renal dialysis was necessary in 11% and 20% respectively. End-stage renal disease was present in one ARChiVe patient. The frequency of other clinical features at presentation according to organ system as described in the two most recent and largest pediatric series are listed in Table 34–2.

Diagnosis

The diagnosis of WG is based on a combination of clinical features (e.g., pulmonary-renal vasculitis syndrome), the presence of serological markers (specifically antibodies to PR-3 ANCA), and characteristic histopathological findings (pauci-immune granulomatous inflammation of predominantly small- to medium-sized arteries, capillaries, small veins, or pauci-immune glomerulonephritis). If WG is suspected and is apparently limited to a single organ system, it is crucial to take a careful and specific history of upper respiratory tract involvement. Since one-third of adult patients initially have asymptomatic renal and pulmonary involvement, it is crucial to examine the urinary sediment and to look for pulmonary changes radiographically and by pulmonary function testing. A decrease in the diffusion capacity of carbon monoxide (DL_{CO}) may be the earliest sign of pulmonary hemorrhage. If the disease is limited to a single organ system, tissue diagnosis is desirable to confirm the diagnosis and exclude other diseases. The differential diagnoses include infections (notably mycobacteria, fungi, or helminths, which may also be associated with granulomatous vasculitis[65]), neoplastic disease,[66] sarcoidosis,[67] and, in young children, chronic granulomatous disease. Pulmonary manifestations of ANCA-positive ulcerative colitis patients have also mimicked WG.[68] Other forms of vasculitis that can manifest as pulmonary-renal syndromes, such as Goodpasture syndrome, systemic lupus erythematosus (SLE), mixed connective tissue disease, or microscopic polyarteritis nodosa (PAN), should also be considered. Guided kidney biopsy is now a relatively safe procedure with a high yield, and the finding of pauciimmune glomerulonephritis together with characteristic serology provides a relatively secure diagnosis. Characteristic histological features may be patchy in the lungs, and the yield from pulmonary biopsies may be low, especially with fine needle aspirations, but are better with transbronchial or open lung procedures. Frequent involvement of the upper respiratory tract in patients with WG (e.g., trachea, ears, nose, sinuses, and eyes) may offer sites for relatively noninvasive biopsy procedures; however, the yield from such sites is disappointingly low.[69] When the disease is isolated to these sites, definitive diagnosis may be difficult and may need to rely on nonspecific or incomplete histopathological confirmation, serological findings, and

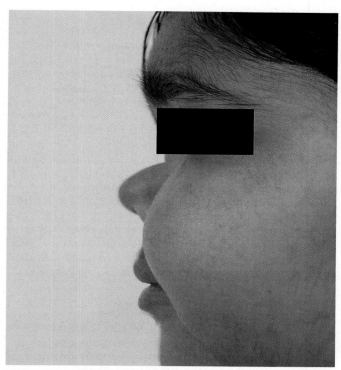

FIGURE 34–2 Saddle nose deformity in a girl with erosive sinusitis and Wegener granulomatosis.

the combined expertise of multiple disciplines, including the otorhinolaryngologist, ophthalmologist, pathologist, radiologist, and rheumatologist. The stringent need for tissue diagnosis in such cases may be influenced by disease severity, the need to embark upon toxic chemotherapy, and the need to exclude other diseases.

Laboratory Examination

White blood cell (WBC) counts may be particularly elevated in generalized disease, and may be associated with moderate eosinophilia, normochromic normocytic anemia, thrombocytosis, and markedly elevated erythrocyte sedimentation rate or C-reactive protein level.[65] In early disease, or disease limited to a single or few systems, these tests may be normal or only slightly abnormal. Abnormal urinalysis, characteristically with proteinuria, microscopic hematuria, and red blood cell casts, indicates glomerular disease.[65,70] Gross hematuria is uncommon.[20] Elevation of blood urea nitrogen and serum creatinine levels indicates the presence of significant renal disease.

Antinuclear antibodies of unknown specificity are uncommon in adults and are present in about 20% to 36% of children tested.[14,21] Rheumatoid factors are present in approximately 50% of adult and pediatric patients.[21,65] Serum levels of immunoglobulin (Ig) A may be increased.[5] Children with WG may be at risk for thrombosis because of antiphospholipid antibodies and factor V Leiden mutations.[71] Antiphospholipid antibodies were evident at presentation in 6 (18%) of 34 children without venous thrombosis tested in one series,[14] but 2 (22%) of nine children in another series had antibodies evident and had venous thromboses.[21]

ANCAs were present in 89% of 65 children with WG with cytoplasmic immunofluorescence staining pattern (cANCA) in 86%. By enzyme-linked immunosorbent assay (ELISA), 68% were positive for anti-PR3 (see Fig 34–1).[14] A perinuclear immunofluorescence staining pattern was present in 21%, and by ELISA anti-MPO antibodies were present in 14%. Similar frequencies of ANCA positivity were found in the pediatric series of Akikusa and colleagues[21] and relatively recent adult series.[4,72] While cANCA and antiPR3 are highly sensitive and specific for WG, they are also found in MPA and CSS. pANCA and anti-MPO although generally less characteristic of WG may be more frequent in so-called renal-limited WG,[73] in Chinese patients with multisystem WG,[74] and in patients with MPA and CSS. Although ANCAs are the unifying characteristic of these diseases collectively described as the AAV they have been demonstrated in inflammatory bowel diseases (usually pANCA), infection-associated vasculitis, and paraneoplastic syndromes (Table 34–3).[72,75-77]

Pathology

The full histological spectrum of WG includes necrotizing granulomas of the upper or lower respiratory tract, necrotizing or granulomatous vasculitis, predominantly of small arteries and veins (in the lungs and other organs), and focal, segmental necrotizing glomerulonephritis.[78] Granulomata most uniquely characterize the disease and show acute and chronic inflammation with central necrosis and histiocytes, lymphocytes, and giant cells; eosinophils may be present in small numbers (Fig. 34–3). The granulomas may be discreet, confluent, or poorly formed with scattered giant cells; at times, lung specimens will demonstrate nonspecific inflammation. The vasculitis is more often necrotizing than granulomatous. Leukocytoclastic vasculitis may involve small vessels as well.[79] Renal glomeruli are infiltrated with lymphocytes and histiocytes (Fig. 34–4). The earliest renal change may be glomerular thrombosis,[80] but the most commonly reported renal lesions are extracapillary proliferation (with or without fibrinoid necrosis) and crescent formation, found in a focal and segmental pattern, followed by necrotizing glomerulonephritis.[81,82] Glomerular sclerosis occurs quickly and is often seen on the initial biopsy, even with good renal function. Renal granulomata are rare.[83] Immunofluorescence microscopy is characteristic of a "pauciimmune" pattern with scanty deposition of Igs and complements.[5,81] Dense subendothelial deposits are visible on electron microscopy.[84]

Imaging

Approximately 45% of children with WG have abnormalities on chest radiographs, with nodules being twice as common as fixed infiltrates (Fig. 34–5).[14,21] Cavitations, pleural effusions, and pneumothoraces may also occur. While these gross abnormalities are readily detectable on conventional radiography,[85,86] high resolution computed tomography CT is more effective in detecting other characteristic changes, such as small nodules, linear opacities, focal low attenuation infiltrates,[87] and fluffy centrilobular, perivascular densities (Fig. 34–6).[88] Sinus radiographs or CT may demonstrate thickening of the sinus lining, opacification of the frontal or maxillary sinuses, or bony cavitation and destruction (Fig. 34–7). However, magnetic resonance imaging (MRI) is superior in defining highly active mucosal disease. MRI is also helpful in visualizing soft tissue changes involving the nose, orbits, mastoids, and upper airways (i.e., subglottic stenosis); characteristic patterns have been described.[89-91]

Treatment

Treatment of WG with a combination of glucocorticoids and oral cyclophosphamide (CYC) has been the standard of care and has induced remission in more than 90% of adult patients.[25,65] The disease was fatal in almost all children reported before such treatment.[92] CYC (2 mg/kg/day) and prednisone at a dose of 1 mg/kg/day for four weeks and then tapered to an alternate-day regimen induced remission in 97% of patients in one pediatric series.[20] This regimen continued for approximately

Table 34–3			
Common disease associations with Antibodies to neutrophil cytoplasmic antigens			
Antigen	ANCA Pattern	Disease Association	Frequency (%)
PR3	cANCA	Wegener granulomatosis	30 to 90
		Churg-Strauss	25 to 50
MPO	pANCA	Microscopic polyarteritis	25 to 75
		Ulcerative colitis	40 to 80
		Sclerosing cholangitis	65 to 85
		Crohn disease	10 to 40
BPI	ANCA	Cystic fibrosis	80 to 90
Actin	pANCA	Autoimmune hepatitis type 1	70 to 75

ANCA, Antibodies directed at neutrophil cytoplasmic antigen; BPI, Bactericidal permeability increasing protein; cANCA, cytoplasmic ANCA; pANCA, perinuclear ANCA.

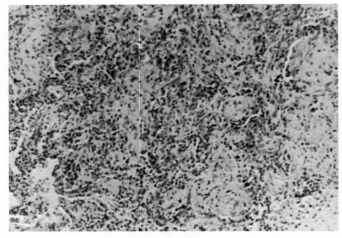

FIGURE 34–3 Lung biopsy specimen from a patient with Wegener granulomatosis. Necrotizing granulomata and fibrous tissue have obliterated the normal alveolar architecture. Hematoxylin and eosin stain, magnification X 480.

one year past remission, with CYC then tapered by 25 mg decrements every two months if there was no relapse, resulted in a median requirement for cytotoxic therapy of 28 months. As an alternative to oral therapy, dosing regimens modeled on the NIH protocol for treatment of severe SLE have been used, i.e., monthly pulses of CYC for six months followed by pulses at three monthly intervals for an additional period up to 18 months. In the only multicenter cohort of pediatric patients with WG, 83% of 65 patients were initially treated with CYC and corticosteroids, although there were several permutations of regimens, and routes of administration, and no followup data were reported.[14] The most common treatment alternative to CYC in this series[14] and other single center case series was methotrexate (MTX),[21,93] but efficacy relative to CYC was not reported.

Because of the significant toxicity risks of CYC (infections, bone marrow failure, infertility, hemorrhagic cystitis, and bladder cancer), newer strategies are evolving to reduce the cumulative CYC dose burden. One strategy is to administer CYC for three to six months to induce remission, and then to maintain remission with less aggressive drug therapy. Administration of CYC by intermittent intravenous (IV) pulses every three weeks (Table 34–4) as an alternative to the oral regimen will reduce the total CYC burden. Initial trials[94-96] comparing these two regimens were promising with respect to remission induction; however, they were inconclusive because of small numbers and because of the inclusion of patients with MPA and PAN. Relapse rates following pulse CYC therapy also seemed more frequent.[97] The results of the more recent CYCLOPS trial studying WG together with other AAVs demonstrated that patients receiving pulse CYC received 50% less CYC than those receiving oral therapy, that remission induction was as frequent, and

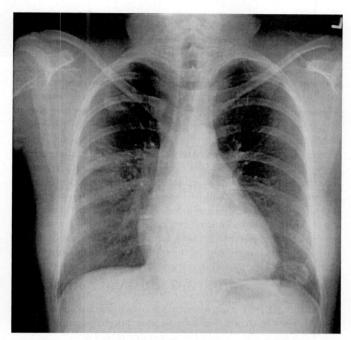

FIGURE 34–5   Patchy, lower lobe infiltrates and several well-defined granulomata (left, lower lobe; right, upper and middle lobes) are evident in the lung of an adolescent with Wegener granulomatosus.

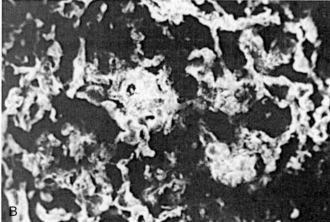

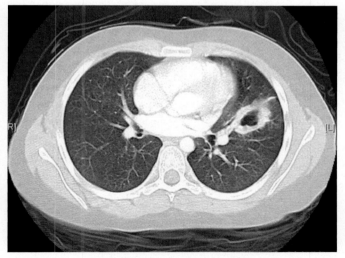

FIGURE 34–4   A, Renal biopsy specimen from a child with Wegener granulomatosis. The glomerulus on the right shows areas of hypercellularity and fibrinoid necrosis with interstitial inflammation. Hematoxylin and eosin stain, magnification × 480. B, Positive immunofluorescent stain for fibrin in a renal biopsy specimen from a patient with Wegener granulomatosis. Magnification × 480.

FIGURE 34–6   Cavitating lung disease and main bronchus stenosis in a child with Wegener granulomatosis.

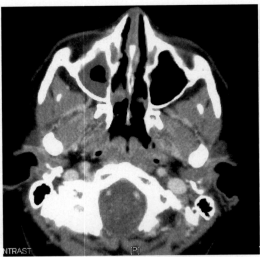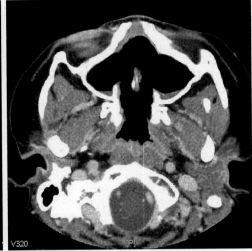

FIGURE 34–7 Erosive sinusitis in a 12-year-old girl with Wegener granulomatosis. Computed tomography of the sinuses in September 2008 **(A)** and October 2009 **(B)** of a patient with Wegener granulomatosis treated with immunosuppressive medication showing almost complete destruction of the medial walls of the maxillary sinuses bilaterally.

Table 34–4

Recommended Therapy of Wegener Granulomatosis (*Traditional Standard Therapy Italicized*)

Phase	Drug	Regimen
Induction (3 to 6 mo)	Prednisone	*1-2 mg/kg/day PO in two or three divided doses (max, 60 mg) for 2-4 weeks before tapering*
	PLUS	*(exceptionally ill patients initially receive methylprednisolone, 30 mg/kg/day [max, 1 g/day] for 1-3 d IV)*
	Cyclophosphamide	*2 mg/kg/day PO (exceptionally ill patients may receive initial doses as IV pulse, 0.50-0.75 g/m², for two doses two weeks apart; if limitations or contraindications to oral therapy, 0.5 - 1.0 g/m² monthly IV pulses)* or 15mg/kg (max, 1g) IV every 2 weeks for 3 doses and then 3 weekly
	OR Methotrexate	0.5 - 1mg /kg SC once weekly (max 30-40 mg) (for early systemic/localized disease without renal disease)
Maintenance (minimum 18 to 24 mo)	Prednisone *PLUS*	After 4 wk, prednisone is consolidated and tapered as long as the patient remains well.
	Cyclophosphamide *OR*	2 mg/kg/day PO (taper after 1 yr of disease control or remission)
	Azathioprine *OR*	2 mg/kg/day PO
	Methotrexate	0.3-1 mg/kg SC once each week (max, 30-40 mg)
Refractory	Infliximab or	5mg/kg IV twice monthly
	Rituximab or	375mg/m² /week for 4 weeks
	Intravenous or immunoglobulin	2g/kg monthly

that patients were less likely to have leukopenia as a side effect.[98] Relapse rates may have been more frequent in the patients receiving pulse therapy (17%) compared to those receiving oral therapy (8%); however, the study was not powered to determine if this was a significant difference. Prolonged maintenance therapy with other immunosuppressive agents was not used.

Glucocorticoids are the cornerstone of therapy for remission induction and maintenance of remission, but they also carry a toxicity burden. In critically ill patients, high dose IV methylprednisolone can be used initially.[99] Otherwise, for remission or induction prednisone should be started at a dose of 1 to 2 mg kg/day to a maximum of 60 mg in two or three divided doses to be given for a minimum of two weeks (see Table 34–4). Reduction in therapy to twice daily and/or to a single daily dose should take place over four to six weeks. Dose reductions of about 10% to 15% should be on a regular schedule every two to four weeks, as long as the patient remains well with no evidence of worsening disease activity, ultimately aiming to establish the patient on a prolonged low "maintenance" dose, for at least 12 months.[100] In one study where glucocorticoids were withdrawn rapidly,[101] and in another study when maintenance therapy of any kind was discontinued after 12 months,[102] relapse rates were high.

With the assumption that individuals with less severe disease need less aggressive therapy, clinical trials in adults have depended on subclassifying or "staging" patients according to disease severity (Table 34–5).[103,104] These disease subclassifications have not been evaluated in children, so severity-associated treatment strategies for children are being extrapolated from experience in adults. Several immunosuppressive therapies, other than CYC for remission induction or maintenance of remission, have been proposed. In the CYCAZAREM trial,[105] patients with ANCA-associated vasculitis who went into remission in three to six months with standard glucocorticoid and oral CYC therapy were randomized to continue either CYC or azathioprine as maintenance for 12 months, after which all patients were continued on azathioprine. Relapse rates in follow-up were similar in the group receiving long-term (13.7%) versus short-term (15.5%) CYC. There have been no trials to determine the role of azathioprine for induction of remission. MTX has been used for both remission induction and for maintenance therapy as an alternative to CYC. Studies evaluating the role of MTX for induction treatment have all been limited to patients with nonlife- or organ-threatening disease and minimal or no renal disease.[102,106-108] In the most recent of these trials,[102] remission rates for MTX (89.8%) and CYC (93.5%) were comparable, and with long-term follow-up,[107] renal outcome was not impaired. Both treatment arms were continued for 12 months, and then maintenance was discontinued in all patients. High relapse rates at six months for both MTX (69.5%) and CYC (46.5%) suggested the need for more prolonged maintenance therapy. Two trials investigating the use of MTX for maintenance of remission in WG following remission induction with oral CYC showed relapse rates of 36% and 52%; however, when compared to prolonged CYC therapy, adverse events from MTX in both trials were rare.[100,109] In a trial comparing MTX with azathioprine for maintenance therapy, the relapse rates and safety profiles of both drugs were similar.[110] Leflunomide has been used as an agent to maintain remission.[111] The risks and benefits have been compared with those of MTX;[112] the results were not conclusive, but leflunomide probably has some role as an alternative to azathioprine or MTX. Mycophenolate mofetil (MMF) has also been used for maintenance of remission following CYC induction, but the results in two studies[113,114] were at variance. The current IMPROVE trial will compare the use of MMF against azathioprine and might be more conclusive. Trimethoprim-sulfamethoxazole has been effective in reducing the rate of relapse of disease of the ear, nose, and throat, but should be considered only as adjunctive therapy in patients with upper respiratory tract disease.[115,116] As *Pneumocystis jiroveci* pneumonia has been reported as a major complication of immunosuppression in patients with WG,[117] the use of prophylactic trimethoprim-sulfamethoxazole (three times weekly dosing) has been recommended at least during the induction phase with CYC, when the risk factors for infection (high glucocorticoid doses and lymphopenia, specifically low CD4+ T cell counts) are highest.[118] The relative risks and benefits for such a strategy in children are not known.

TNF blockade has been used for the treatment of both refractory disease and as a potentially safer maintenance therapy. The WG etanercept trial demonstrated that etanercept used as maintenance therapy was no better than standard therapy in maintaining remission; however, six out of 91 (7%) patients developed solid tumors, compared to none receiving standard therapy.[101] As a result, etanercept as maintenance therapy for WG is contraindicated. Infliximab use for patients with WG refractory to standard therapy has been reported to be effective in some open-label clinical trials[119-121] and in additional case reports,[122] including one pediatric report.[123] Rituximab use for refractory disease has been reported in several single case reports and in some small series of no more than 11 patients, where it has induced complete or partial remission in all patients, with variable frequencies of relapse.[124-129] However, in two series, where a total of 10 patients had predominantly granulomatous disease, rather than vasculitis, rituximab was not effective.[46,130] It is difficult to interpret the best strategy for using rituximab, because of the wide variety of adjunctive therapies in these studies. It has also been successfully used as primary induction therapy for patients with limited disease[131] and in conjunction with CYC for induction in a small pediatric series as a CYC dose-limiting strategy.[132] The results of the RAVE trial comparing CYC and rituximab for primary induction therapy are still unknown. Deoxyspergualin, a synthetic analogue of a bacterial product, has been successfully used in some pilot studies to induce remission in patients' refractory to conventional therapy.[133-135] IVIG has led to some modest improvements in disease activity, particularly in patients without severe organ dysfunction, but the benefits were not sustained.[136]

For patients with pulmonary hemorrhage, intensive care unit management with ventilatory support and even extracorporeal membrane oxygenation may be required for initial life support.[14] For such patients, plasmapheresis may have a role, in addition to other aggressive immunosuppressive therapy.[137] Tracheal stenosis may be resistant to local or systemic immunosuppression because of fibrosis and may respond to intralesional glucocorticoid injections.[138] It may ultimately require tracheostomy or stent placement.[139] Endoscopic dilatation and laser surgery followed by a mitomycin-C application to reduce re-scarring may limit

Table 34–5

Classification schemes for staging (subclassifying) Wegener Granulomatosis

European Vasculitis Network (EUVAS) scheme[103]

Subgroup	Organ Involvement
Localized	Confined to upper and/or lower respiratory tract
Early systemic	Any organ system except renal, and no imminent vital organ failure
Generalized	Renal with serum creatinine level <500 μmol/L and/or other imminent vital organ failure
Severe renal	Renal with serum creatinine level >500 μmol/L
Refractory	Progressive disease despite standard therapy with glucocorticoids and cyclophosphamide

Vasculitis Clinical Research Consortium (VCRC) Scheme[280]

Subgroup	Definition
Limited	No red blood cell casts in urine. If hematuria is present, serum creatinine is ≤1.4mg/dL and creatinine rise no greater than 25% above baseline. If pulmonary involvement, PO_2 in room air >70 mm Hg and O_2 saturation >92%. Pulmonary hemorrhage may be included provided there is no evidence of progression. No other critical organ involvement requiring immediate institution of maximal therapy
Severe	Any patient whose disease is not classifiable as limited

the ultimate need for tracheostomy.[140,141] Current therapeutic recommendations are summarized in Table 34–4.

Course of the Disease and Prognosis

Prognosis arguably depends in part on the clinical state or stage of disease at diagnosis, which may be influenced by the interval from symptom onset to diagnosis. The one year mortality of adult patients with untreated WG was ~ 80%,[65,142] whereas more recent studies report five year mortality rates of treated patients of around 10% to 25%.[25,143,144] 22 children younger than 15 years old died of the disease in a 10-year period ending in 1988 in the U.S.[5] The cause of death of 28 adult patients with WG in a long-term follow-up of subjects used in development of the ACR classification criteria were infection in 29%, cardiac disease in 18%, renal failure in 18%, and malignancy in 14%.[145] In adults treated with prednisone and CYC, over 90% of patients responded completely or partially; however, over 50% relapsed within five years.[25,144] Similar rates of remission and relapse are reported in two pediatric series.[20,21] The pediatric series reported 23 and 25 patients who are followed for a mean of 8.7 years and a mean of 2.7 years respectively. In the former series reported by Rottem and associates, one patient died of severe lung disease and cor pulmonale, and one died of sepsis.[20] No patients died in the series reported by Akikusa and associates.[21] No patient developed malignancy in either series.[20,21] Approximately 25% of children with WG have at least one serious infection during the course of the illness.[20] Although subglottic stenosis was present in only 4% of patients at presentation, during follow-up 48% had this problem, and half of these required tracheostomy.[20] Such therapy might arguably be mitigated with current treatment strategies. Nonetheless, subglottic stenosis in this series was four times as common and nasal deformity twice as common in children as in adults. Persistent sinus pain and dysfunction, hearing loss, and pulmonary insufficiency may ensue. In one-third of children, irreversible renal insufficiency develops. Treatment-related morbidity included cystitis or infertility in 22%.[25] Glucocorticoid side effects included cataracts and glaucoma in 12%, steroid myopathy and symptomatic vertebral compression fractures in 4% each, and adverse growth effects were described as prominent.[21] Long-term multicenter follow-up of a cohort of contemporary similarly-treated patients is needed to appreciate the effects of the disease in childhood. As a corollary to this, pediatric modification and validation of standardized disease assessment tools, such as the Birmingham Vasculitis Activity Scale[146] and the Vasculitis Damage Index,[147] will be essential.

CHURG-STRAUSS SYNDROME (ALLERGIC GRANULOMATOSIS)

CSS or allergic granulomatosis and angiitis, a disorder found in patients with severe asthma or allergic rhinitis, is characterized by pulmonary and systemic small vessel vasculitis, extravascular granulomas, and eosinophilia. Because of the high frequency of associated ANCA, specifically anti- MPO-ANCA,[148] CSS has been classified as a distinct entity among the other ANCA associated vasculitides. Originally described by Churg and Strauss in 1951 and based on pathological findings found on autopsy, the disease was distinguished from PAN because it predominantly involved small vessels rather than medium-size arteries.[149]

Definition and Disease Classification

A patient meets the CHCC definition of CSS if they have asthma, peripheral eosinophilia, eosinophilic granulomatous inflammation of the respiratory tract, and necrotizing vasculitis of small to medium vessels.[12] The criteria proposed by Lanham and colleagues require a patient to have asthma, peripheral blood eosinophilia, and systemic vasculitis in two or more extrapulmonary sites.[150] The ACR classification criteria for CSS aim to distinguish this disease from the other vasculitides (Table 34–6). There are no specific criteria for the diagnosis of CSS in children.

Epidemiology

CSS is a rare disease with an estimated annual incidence of one to three cases per million, and, similar to WG, there may be an increasing frequency in higher latitudes and rural areas, suggesting environmental influences.[17,18,151,152] CSS characteristically occurs in middle-age[150] and is rare in children. In a report of 117 children with ANCA-associated vasculitis from 30 U.S. and Canadian centers, two children had CSS compared to 76 with WG and 17 with MPA.[14] Zwerina and colleagues, in a systematic review of the literature in 2008, identified 33 reported cases of childhood CSS in whom the mean age was 12 with a slight

---

Table 34–6

American College of Rheumatology criteria for classification of Churg-Strauss Syndrome

Criterion*	Description
Asthma	History of wheezing or diffuse high-pitched rales on expiration
Eosinophilia	Eosinophils >10% of white blood cell differential count
History of allergy	History of seasonal allergy (e.g., allergic rhinitis) or documented allergies, including food, contactants, and others (except for drug allergies)
Mononeuropathy or polyneuropathy	Mononeuropathy, multiple mononeuropathies, or polyneuropathy (i.e., glove/stocking distribution) attributable to a systemic vasculitis
Pulmonary infiltrates	Migratory or transitory pulmonary infiltrates on radiographs attributable to a systemic vasculitis
Paranasal sinus abnormality	History of acute or chronic paranasal sinus pain or tenderness or radiographic opacification of the paranasal sinuses
Extravascular eosinophils	Biopsy including artery, arteriole, or venule, showing accumulation of eosinophils in extravascular areas

*For classification purposes, a patient is said to have Churg-Strauss syndrome it at least four of these criteria are present. The presence of any four or more criteria has a sensitivity of 85% and a specificity of 99.7%.

preponderance of females.[153] The predominance of males versus females varies between different adult studies suggesting an adult sex ratio of 1:1.[150,154-156]

Pathogenesis

The etiology of CSS remains poorly understood, although there is likely some pathogenic role for both ANCA[157] and eosinophils.[158,159] ANCA is reported less frequently in CSS (38% to 73%) than in WG or MPA,[154,157,160] and among reported pediatric patients,[153] it was found in 25% of those tested. The clinicopathological differences described between ANCA positive and ANCA negative disease[155] suggest that CSS may represent more than one disease entity.[161] A report that cysteinyl leukotriene receptor antagonists (montelukast) given to asthmatic agents precipitated CSS were initially misinterpreted. The association was not that montelukast had a pathological role, but rather it was effective in reducing the corticosteroid requirements of the "asthmatics" and it thereby unmasked the underlying CSS or CSS-like syndrome.[162]

Clinical Manifestations

CSS usually has a very prolonged prodromal course of many years, consisting of asthma and other allergic manifestations, such as chronic allergic rhinitis and nasal polyposis.[150] An eosinophilic phase with eosinophilia and pulmonary infiltrates is then followed by vasculitis.[150] These three phases do not always occur sequentially, and asthma may occasionally follow the onset of vasculitis.[160,163] Among the 33 reported pediatric cases,[153] presenting features in order of frequency were asthma in 91%, pulmonary involvement with nonfixed infiltrates in 85%, sinusitis in 77%, skin involvement in 66%, cardiac disease in 55% (cardiomyopathy 42%, pericarditis 27%), gastrointestinal involvement in 40%, peripheral neuropathy (mononeuritis multiplex) in 39%, myalgia in 22%, and kidney disease in 16%. Other organs occasionally involved included joints (arthralgia), lymph nodes, orbits, salivary glands, mammary glands, testicles, and thymus. Although there was likely significant selection bias in this collection of case reports, the low disease prevalence precludes any other type of case series, and when the pediatric cases were compared in the same review [153] to 205 adult cases from two combined multicenter retrospective cohorts,[155,156] there were more similarities than differences. The significant differences in organ involvement were that compared to children, adults less frequently had pulmonary infiltrates (59%) and cardiac disease, (26%) but they more frequently had peripheral neuropathy (69%) and myalgia (54%).

Asthma is the hallmark of the disease in both adults and children, and it is usually steroid requiring, if not steroid dependent, with severity and frequency of attacks increasing prior to the onset of vasculitis.[154,164] The presence of skin manifestations in a majority of patients reflects involvement of small vessels, and the specific manifestations resemble those of the other small vessel vasculitides and include petechiae or palpable purpura, maculopapular rash, cutaneous nodules, livedo reticularis, ulcers,

and bullae.[165] Cardiac disease, predominantly because of cardiomyopathy, was an important cause of mortality in the pediatric[153] and adult series.[154] Renal disease is generally mild and rarely progresses,[150,163] although it may advance occasionally.[166] Hypertension, ocular involvement, and pseudotumor cerebri occur in some patients.[167] Peripheral neuropathy, usually mononeuritis multiplex but also polyneuropathy, is an important cause of morbidity.[168,169] The spectrum of gastrointestinal manifestations includes abdominal pain, nausea, vomiting, diarrhea, acute abdomen, and bleeding or perforation likely because of small vessel vasculitis involving the mesentery or small or large bowel.[154,170]

Pathology

The characteristic histopathological findings in specimens from any involved site are angiitis and extravascular necrotizing granulomas usually with eosinophilic infiltrates.[78] The angiitis may be granulomatous or nongranulomatous and involve arteries, veins, and pulmonary and systemic blood vessels.[78] The so-called "Churg Strauss granuloma," which describes the skin nodules and papules over the extensor surfaces of joints and the histological pattern of palisading granulomas with central necrosis, is not unique to CSS, but also occurs in WG, SLE, and other diseases.[171] Similarly, many of the skin manifestations and the associated histopathology of leukocytoclastic vasculitis with or without eosinophils are not unique to CSS.[165]

Diagnosis and Differential Diagnosis

Ultimately the diagnosis of CSS, like the other systemic vasculitides, is made on the basis of clinical and histopathological features. CSS should be considered in patients with chronic asthma, a fever, a deteriorating clinical course, and eosinophilia. There may also be features suggestive of vasculitis at other extrapulmonary sites[150] as described previously (see Table 34–6). Diagnosis should ideally be confirmed histopathologically with biopsy of renal, skin, or lung tissue showing eosinophilic infiltration of granulomas and vasculitis. The main differential diagnoses are the pulmonary eosinophilic syndromes and other vasculitides. When extrapulmonary features are not prominent, conditions in need of exclusion are parasitic infections, drug reactions, acute and chronic eosinophilic pneumonia, allergic bronchopulmonary aspergillosis, and idiopathic hypereosinophilic syndrome. This last disorder may also involve multiple organs. In the presence of ANCA, CSS needs to be distinguished from other chronic vasculitides, particularly WG and MPA.

Laboratory Examination

Elevation of acute phase reactants accompanies active disease. Peripheral blood eosinophilia (with eosinophils accounting for 10% or more of leukocytes) and elevation of serum levels of IgE are typical. Chest radiographs or computed tomography of the chest may reveal diffuse pulmonary infiltrates (Fig. 34–8), and pulmonary function tests demonstrate poor lung diffusing capacity and

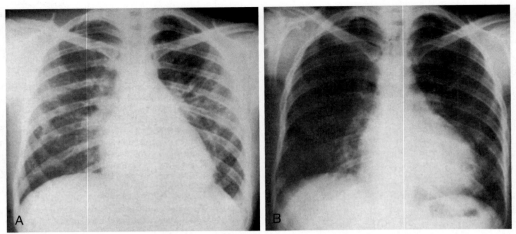

FIGURE 34–8   Chest radiographs of a young man with allergic granulomatosis. **A,** The initial film demonstrates an enlarged cardiac silhouette and relatively normal pulmonary fields. **B,** The film was taken during an acute episode of left- and right-sided heart failure. Notice the cardiac enlargement and disappearance of the normal pulmonary vascular markings, indicating acute pulmonary hypertension and cor pulmonale, which, in this case, is due to vasculitis.

low PO_2. ANCAs, most commonly anti-MPO, are found in fewer than 50% of patients.[153,154,157,160] Examination of bronchopulmonary lavage fluid may be useful to confirm the presence of eosinophilic inflammation[172,173] and to exclude infectious and other pathologies. Transbronchial biopsy is less invasive than transthoracic biopsy for obtaining lung specimens.[174]

Treatment

There are no clinical trials in adults or pediatrics to help guide therapy. The principles of treatment should be similar to that described for WG. Glucocorticoids, initially at high dose, are the mainstay of treatment.[153] The addition and choice of an additional immunosuppressive agent should be determined by the severity of the disease. The disease might be considered severe if it is life- or organ-threatening and in the presence of some defined prognostic risk factors (i.e., significant renal disease, cardiomyopathy, CNS, or gastrointestinal involvement)[175] when induction treatment with CYC may be warranted. Alternative immunosuppressants for less severe or steroid dependent disease include MTX, azathioprine, and MMF.[176-178] IFN-α[179] and rituximab[180] have been used in a few CSS patients with refractory disease.

Course of the Disease and Prognosis

When first described CSS seemed to be universally fatal.[149] More recent mortality rates have ranged from being no different than the general population,[160] to 40%.[154,163,181] Increasing mortality was related to increasing age[181] and the presence of risk factors described previously.[175] The most frequent cause of death in both adults and children is cardiac involvement.[150,153] In the literature review of 33 pediatric patients, the mortality was 18%. A majority of patients in long-term remission may require continuing treatment with corticosteroids (oral or inhaled) because of residual asthma.[154]

MICROSCOPIC POLYANGIITIS

MPA, originally described as a subset of PAN, became more clearly recognized as a distinct entity among the systemic vasculitides because of the presence of necrotizing glomerulonephritis.[182] Although some clinical features are similar to PAN, it is distinguished from that disease by the presence of small vessel disease, notably with involvement of the kidneys and lungs.[183] Because of the high frequency of associated ANCA, specifically anti-MPO-ANCA, it has been grouped together with the ANCA-associated vasculitides.

Definition and Disease Classification

MPA is described as a small vessel vasculitis by the CHCC[12] and in the EULAR/PReS proposal for classification of pediatric vasculitis.[13] It is defined as a necrotizing vasculitis, with few or no immune deposits, predominantly affecting small vessels (i.e., capillaries, venules, or arterioles), although arteritis of the small- and medium-sized arteries may be present.[12] Necrotizing glomerulonephritis and pulmonary capillaritis are common. Classification criteria for MPA were not described within the ACR 1990 criteria for classification of vasculitis[11] nor in the recent pediatric proposals. As a result, it is inevitable that patients defined as having MPA might also be concurrently classified as having WG[14] or PAN.[184] Watts and colleagues[185] criticized the poor performance of existing criteria[11,12,150] in classifying adult patients with PAN or any of the ANCA associated vasculitides in mutually exclusive categories, and they proposed an algorithm to address this issue. The concept of the algorithm is to apply the different criteria in a stepwise approach, firstly defining CSS patients where criteria are most specific and subsequently and sequentially applying elements of different criteria to the remaining patients to classify each into a single category for study purposes.

Epidemiology

Epidemiological data on MPA are limited because of its origins as a subset of PAN and because it is now frequently described collectively with the other ANCA associated vasculitides. Following the CHCC description of MPA, Watts and colleagues estimated a regional UK incidence of 3.6 per million compared to the incidence of PAN of 2.4 per million.[184] Mohamed and colleagues, using an algorithm to uniquely classify patients, described the following prevalence figures of primary systemic vasculitis in southern Sweden per million inhabitants in order of decreasing frequency: WG 160, MPA 94, PAN 31, and CSS 14.[186] By survey, pediatric rheumatologists in US and Canada recognize MPA among their patients equally frequently as PAN and about half as frequently as WG.[9] The average age of onset is around 50-years-old, and the male to female ratio ranges from 1.0 to 1.8:1.[183,186,187] In the limited pediatric cases series, the mean age of onset in children is from 9- to 12-years-old,[188-191] and over 80% of patients were female, with the exception of a Turkish study[190] where the sex ratio was equal.

Pathogenesis and the Role of Myeloperoxidase Antineutrophil Cytoplasmic Antibodies

MPA is described as one of the ANCA associated vasculitides, and 75% of patients have pANCA with specificity for MPO.[73,192] MPO-ANCA interacting with neutrophils likely has a direct pathogenic role as demonstrated both *in vitro* and in animal models. ANCA both activates TNF-α primed neutrophils and promotes neutrophil adhesion to endothelial cells and their lysis.[193-195] Immunization with MPO, or passive transfer of anti-MPO antibodies in both mouse[196] and rat models,[38] result in the development of systemic vasculitis (involving lung, spleen, and lymph nodes) and pauci-immune glomerulonephritis, closely resembling human disease. Two case reports of transplacental transfer of MPO-ANCA from mother to newborn causing neonatal MPA also support the concept that MPO-ANCA has a direct pathogenic role in MPA.[197,198]

Clinical Manifestations

Reports on clinical manifestations of MPA in both adults[183,187,192,199,200] and children[188-191] should be interpreted in the context that MPA is often described collectively with other types of vasculitis.[190] Additionally, MPA is not always defined by criteria mutually exclusive of diseases such as WG, CSS, or PAN.[185] Clinical manifestations of MPA in children are described in three retrospective case series of 21, 7, and 26 patients from Japan,[188] Serbia,[191] and Turkey respectively.[190] General features such as fever, weight loss, myalgias, and arthralgias described only in two series[188,191] were present in virtually all children except for three in the Japanese series,[188] where the disease was first identified through a routine urine screening program. Renal involvement, including hypertension, hematuria, proteinuria, and even

renal failure present in 33% of patients at time of diagnosis,[188] occurred in 100% of patients.[188,190,191] This frequency in series reported from departments of nephrology may represent a referral bias. Pulmonary involvement, not specifically characterized in all of the pediatric series, occurred in 17% to 62% of patients.[188,190,191] In the Japanese series, one-third of patients had hemoptysis as a presenting manifestation, and about one-half had pulmonary hemorrhage at some time.[188] In adult series, pulmonary involvement ranges from mildly bloody sputum or episodic cough, through dyspnea, to massive pulmonary hemorrhage, occurring in 25% to 72% of patients.[183,187,192,199,200] Pulmonary manifestations most frequently occur as part of a pulmonary-renal syndrome, but lung disease may rarely be present without kidney involvement. Skin manifestations, predominantly purpura but also ulcers, are present in 38% to 100% of pediatric patients. In adults, the predominant skin manifestation is purpura (often palpable),[183,187,192,199,200] but other lesions such as petechiae, livedo, ulcers, urticaria and erythema also occur.[201-204] Other less frequent manifestations include CNS disease (convulsions, severe headaches), gastrointestinal symptoms (abdominal pain and gastrointestinal bleeding), and ocular symptoms (episcleritis and conjunctivitis).[188,190,191] Peripheral neuropathy was not described in the series where PAN was actively excluded.[188,191]

Pathology

Pauci-immune necrotizing vasculitis predominantly affecting small vessels and necrotizing glomerulonephritis defines MPA (see previously).[12] Patients with ANCA-associated glomerulonephritis without other organ manifestations may have renal histopathology indistinguishable from patients with MPA. In the Japanese series of 31 patients, 21 had MPA and 10 had necrotizing crescentic glomerulonephritis. In 22 of 31 biopsies crescent were found in 75% of the glomeruli. Extraglomerular vasculitis was present in four cases.[188]

Diagnosis and Differential Diagnosis

Patients presenting with renal disease and ANCA-associated glomerulonephritis should be clinically assessed for extrarenal manifestations of MPA. One-third of patients with Goodpasture syndrome may have antiglomerular basement membrane antibodies and ANCA[205] and will be differentiated from MPA with immunofluorescence microscopy of a renal biopsy. WG may be distinguished from MPA by the presence of PR3-ANCA, granulomatous inflammation, upper respiratory tract involvement (specifically nasal septal perforation and/or saddle nose deformity), and chest imaging findings of nodules, nodular infiltrates, or cavitation representing granulomatous inflammation rather than capillaritis.[188] PAN may be distinguished by the absence of MPO-ANCA, rapidly progressive glomerulonephritis and lung hemorrhage, and the presence of microaneurysms and other abnormal angiographic findings.[183,206,207] Other small vessel vasculitides, such as Henoch-Schönlein purpura and cryoglobulinemic vasculitis, may present similarly but are distinguished by their clinical course and/or histopathology showing well-defined or prominent immune complex deposits and IgA in the case of Henoch-Schönlein purpura.

Laboratory Examination

As with the other AAVs, nonspecific measurements of inflammation (increased erythrocyte sedimentations rate and C-reactive protein, anemia, thrombocytosis, and hypoalbuminemia) and characterization of urinalysis and renal function are useful for following disease activity and course. The presence of pANCA in 75% of patients with MPA is useful diagnostically depending on the prior clinical probability of systemic vasculitis and on the MPO specificity.[208] During the course of the disease, the relationship of ANCA titers with disease activity, relapse, or mortality risk is not consistent.[188,209,210]

Treatment

There are no clinical trials in pediatrics to guide therapy for MPA, but treatment principles and practices are based on studies in adults and use regimens similar to those described for patients with the WG (see Table 34–4) with induction and maintenance therapy and strategies for treating refractory or relapsing disease. In the pediatric MPA series, most patients initially received glucocorticoids and/or CYC, intravenously or orally in various regimens. Plasmapheresis was used for some patients.[188,190,191] Patients receiving CYC seemed to do better than patients receiving corticosteroids alone,[190,192] but immunosuppressive other than CYC should be used in patients with a better prognosis. Poor prognostic factors (i.e., significant renal disease, cardiomyopathy, CNS, or gastrointestinal involvement) were established for patients with PAN, CSS,[175] and MPA.[211] Massive pulmonary hemorrhage is also a bad prognostic sign.

Course of the Disease and Prognosis

Of the 30 patients in the Japanese[188] and Serbian[191] series, only one patient died three months after diagnosis with cytomegalovirus infection. In the Turkish[190] series of 26 patients (including two patients with PAN) where only 13 patients received CYC, there were nine deaths: four due to renal failure, two from CNS disease, two from massive gastrointestinal hemorrhage, and one from cardiac failure. Follow-up in these series ranged from less than six months to 10 years. Of the 64 patients (including 10 with ANCA-associated necrotizing crescentic glomerulonephritis), 25 developed end-stage renal disease. A shorter interval between disease onset and treatment seemed to be associated with a better outcome. The renal lesions of patients treated early after disease onset in, showed focal segmental necrosis on kidney in biopsies, while those with later diagnosis and treatment had a predominance of circumferential fibrosis and/or crescents.[191] Among the 30 Japanese patients, the 10 diagnosed early through a school-based urine screening program for hematuria and proteinuria had a more favorable renal outcome than the other 20 patients.[188]

GIANT CELL ARTERITIS

The term *giant cell arteritis (GCA)* includes two phenotypically distinct vasculitides involving predominantly large vessels with the common histological hallmark of GCA.[212] In children and adolescents, Takayasu Arteritis (TA) describing a large vessel vasculitis affecting the aorta and its major branches is the most common form.[213] In adults, temporal (cranial) arteritis is the most common GCA,[214] and it is the most common vasculitis seen in adults. The incidence of temporal arteritis in the Caucasian population is estimated at 15 to 30/100,000 persons over 50-years-old.[215] In contrast, juvenile temporal arteritis is a rare, nonprogressive disease.[216] Temporal arteritis can be the initial presentation of PAN in children.[217]

TAKAYASU ARTERITIS

In 1908 the Japanese ophthalmologist Takayasu and his colleagues initially reported retinal vessel abnormalities and subsequently their association with absent wrist pulses.[218] TA is a rare chronic, relapsing large vessel vasculitis affecting the aorta and its major branches, and presenting manifestations include fatigue, weight loss, hypertension, headaches, strokes, and ischemic abdominal pain.[213,219] Absence of peripheral pulses has given it the name "pulseless disease."

Definition and Classification

The ACR criteria for the classification of TA include six features: bruits, decreased brachial artery pulses, claudication, blood pressure differences of more than 10mm Hg, patient younger than 40-years-old at onset, and angiographic evidence of aortic and/or primary aortic branches disease. A patient must meet three or more of the six criteria to fulfill the requirements for classification as having TA. The presence of any three or more criteria has a sensitivity of 90.5% and a specificity of 97.8% in adults.[220] In the proposed PReS/EULAR criteria for TA in children,[221] angiographic abnormalities of the aorta or its main branches is a mandatory criterion, and patients should have one of the four criteria shown in Table 34–7 for classification of TA. The PReS/EULAR criteria have not been prospectively validated.

Table 34–7

Proposed EULAR/PReS criteria for the classification of Takayasu Arteritis in children

Angiographic abnormalities (conventional, computed tomography, *or magnetic resonance angiography) of the aorta or its main branches* (mandatory criterion) plus at least one of the following four features:

- Decreased peripheral artery pulse(s) and/or claudication of extremities
- Blood pressure difference >10 mmHg
- Bruits over aorta and/or its major branches
- Hypertension (related to childhood normative data)

Epidemiology

Estimates of the incidence of TA in adults range from 0.8/1,000,000/year in Great Britain, to 2.6/1,000,000/year in North America, to 1 to 2.9/1,000,000/year in Europe.[222-224] Higher incidences are reported for Asia, Africa, and South America.[225-228] The mean prevalence of TA was 4.7/million.[229] Pediatric incidence data for TA are not available. TA usually occurs in adolescence rather than young childhood. Pediatric series reported from Chandigarh, India,[225] describing 20 year experience (1978 to 1998) of 24 pediatric patients (20 female, 4 male) with a median age of 14 years. A series from Leuven, Belgium[230] recounted a mixed cohort of 15 adults and children(14 female, 1 male) with a median age of 25 years (range 5 to 65 years). A South African series[227] included 31 children (18 female, 13 male) with a median age of 8 years old (range 2.4- to 14.5 years old). All series have a female predominance ranging from 14:1 to 1.4:1. Geographic variations remain unexplained.

Etiology and Genetic Factors

An association of mycobacterium tuberculosis exposure and TA has been suggested.[231-233] Tuberculosis exposure requiring therapy was present in from 29%[234] to 87%[227] of patients from developing countries. In an adult autopsy series, Kinare found active tuberculosis in 60% of patients with TA versus 10% in other adults in the same region of India.[235,236] An association between TA and the histocompatibility antigen HLA Bw52 has been reported from Japan[237] and Mexico.[238] A possible association with HLA-DR4 and HLA-DQ3 alleles in Caucasians has been noted.[239] Reports of markedly elevated serum interleukin (IL) 6 and IL18 levels in TA patients suggest a preferential use of a distinct proinflammatory pathway similar to TB infections.[240]

Clinical Manifestations

Patterns of blood vessel involvement in TA determine the clinical manifestations. The frequencies of symptoms described below are summarized from the larger pediatric or mixed series.[219,226-228,234,241-246] Supradiaphragmatic "aortic arch disease" is commonly associated with CNS manifestations, chest disease, blood pressure differences, claudication, and absent wrist pulses. Arterial ischemic strokes (AIS) are found in 16% to 35% of pediatric patients. Syncope is reported in 16% of children. Seizures can occur secondary to cerebrovascular disease or systemic hypertension. Chest pain, palpitations, and features of cardiac failure due to congestive heart disease, valvular disease or cardiomyopathy can be present in 10% to 57% of patients. Hemoptysis is uncommon. Supradiaphragmatic disease uncommonly occurs in isolation. In the authors' experience, less than 10% of children have isolated aortic arch disease in TA (unpublished data). The vast majority have both supra- and infradiaphragmatic TA.

Infradiaphragmatic "midaortic syndrome" disease is often present with hypertension, abdominal bruits, and abdominal pain. Renal artery involvement presenting as renal hypertension is the single most common TA symptom, occurring in 66% to 93% of children. Clinical manifestations of hypertension, such as encephalopathy, can occur. Hypertension may be detected in the absence of associated clinical symptoms or in association with bruits only. Mesenteric artery disease can present as bloody diarrhea and as intermittent severe abdominal pain. Combined supra- and infradiaphragmatic manifestations are seen in two-thirds of pediatric patients.

Systemic features of weight loss, fevers, and fatigue are found in 42% to 83% of children at diagnosis of active TA. Musculoskeletal disease, including arthritis, arthralgia, and myalgia, is present in 12% to 65% of children. Skin manifestations and lymphadenopathy are infrequently reported. TA-associated diseases include inflammatory bowel disease,[247-249] pyoderma gangrenosum,[250] ankylosing spondylitis,[247] and juvenile rheumatoid arthritis.[251] Uncommon manifestations include refractory abdominal pain,[252] posterior reversible encephalopathy syndrome,[253] keratouveitis,[254] bilateral ocular ischemic syndrome,[255] and relapsing polychondritis.[256]

Diagnosis

The diagnosis of TA in children is most commonly based on the angiographic demonstration of stenoses of the aorta and its major branches. Vessel imaging is commonly performed in children with hypertension, stroke, and symptoms of claudication. The differential diagnosis is limited. Proximal stenoses of the large vessels can be found in children with fibromuscular dysplasia (FMD).[257,258] Vessel wall imaging can determine TA characteristics of wall edema, concentric wall thickening, and contrast enhancement, which are not found in FMD.[259] Other differential diagnoses, such as infectious vasculitis, are rare in children.

Laboratory Investigations

Elevated inflammatory indices are found in the majority of patients with active disease; however, no TA-specific marker has been identified. Elevated ESR, CRP, WBC and platelet count, C3 complement levels, von Willebrand-Factor (vWF) antigen levels, and/or anemia may be detected.[219,226-228,234,241-245] The sensitivity of these markers is unknown. Autoantibodies are not present. Disease flares may be accompanied by raised inflammatory markers. One-third of patients have no elevation of inflammatory markers at presentation, possibly reflecting burnt-out disease.

Pathology

Histopathological studies of pediatric and adult TA patients are limited. The presence of intramural multinucleated giant cells in the walls of affected arteries is diagnostic. The histopathology of arterial lesions of TA and GCA is indistinguishable.[214,260] In an autopsy series of 10 young TA patients from India, mean age of 22.6+/-10.2 years, vascular lesions in the aorta comprised stenosis (eight patients), dilatation,[6] aneurysm,[2] and dissection of aorta involving its arch, thoracic, and abdominal segments.[1] The abdominal aorta was the most common site of involvement (9 out of 10 patients); renal arteries were involved in six patients. The inflammatory infiltrate leads to thickening of all layers of the vessel wall and is thought to be triggered by dendritic cell activation.[261] Active lesions histologically have acute exudative inflammation and granulomata. Fibrosis characterizes inactive lesions. Both may be present at the same time. Active lesions may be found in clinically quiescent patients.[262,263]

Radiological Examination

Vascular imaging is the cornerstone of diagnosis and monitoring in TA.[264,265] After establishing the diagnosis with an angiogram (Table 34–8) the most commonly used modality for monitoring is MRI and magnetic resonance angiography (MRA). The addition of gadolinium contrast may enhance the ability to determine the activity of vessel wall inflammation. Hoffman studied the imaging characteristics of adults with TA in detail.[266,267] Although MR provides a safe, noninvasive means of assessing changes in vascular anatomy, Hoffman emphasized the limitations of MRI in reflecting activity of wall inflammation.[268] Positron emission tomography (PET) appears to be a promising technique. However, in a recent study, Arnaud found no statistical association between the semiquantitative assessment of FDG uptake and the presence of vascular wall thickening, gadolinium uptake, acute phase reactants, or the presence of vascular wall edema.[269] Innovative fusion of PET and MRI images may be helpful in supporting the diagnosis of active TA, especially when the site of vascular involvement is atypical.[270]

In children, MRI/MRA is the preferred imaging modality. In a recent series of 26 children with TA, stenosis of the aorta was the most consistent finding with both fusiform and saccular aneurysms being encountered.[271] Noninvasive quantification of intimal media thickness and elastic properties of the aorta may help to assess aortic involvement and possibly help to follow disease activity and response to therapy.[272,273]

Treatment

The treatment of TA includes immunosuppression for active vessel wall inflammation, anticoagulation, and surgical or endovascular management, such as percutaneous transluminal angioplasty.

Immunosuppression in children follows the treatment protocols proposed for adult TA. Commonly used treatment options include corticosteroids, MTX and CYC. In a retrospective cohort of six children, patients with limited disease received oral corticosteroids and MTX, and patients with extensive disease received oral corticosteroids and oral CYC for remission induction followed by oral MTX for maintenance. In this study, one patient died of pulmonary vasculitis during the first month of therapy. All other children entered remission and subsequently had aortic or aortorenal bypass surgery, balloon dilatation, and unilateral nephrectomy performed. The authors concluded that CYC induction and corticosteroids followed by MTX was effective and safe treatment.[274] Filocamo reported that two of four children with refractory TA treated with TNF antagonists achieved remission, and two achieved a partial response.[275] Similar encouraging data have been published for refractory disease in adult TA.[276]

In children with inactive TA but with significant stenoses or aneurysms, surgical and endovascular procedures may be beneficial. McCulloch reported that from a cohort of 26 patients angioplasty was successful in all 8 patients in whom it was performed.[271] Lee reported the efficacy and safety of endovascular management of 24 adult and pediatric TA patients with 35 lesions in the chronic inactive stage.[277] Twenty-six lesions achieved excellent to good target lesion revascularization with no residual or only minimal residual stenosis; five had a moderate result. Thirty lesions achieved satisfactory hemodynamic correction. Restenosis was observed in eight lesions treated with angioplasty alone (n=18) and in three lesions treated with angioplasty and stenting (n=17). All recurrent stenoses underwent successful reintervention without significant complication. After 47 months of follow-up, the majority of patients had an excellent outcome. Kalangos reported that despite significant extent and severity of vascular lesions, children with TA could benefit from reconstructive surgery, with low mortality and morbidity and satisfactory long-term results.[278]

Course of Disease and Prognosis

TA is a relapsing, chronic disease with an overall survival of 70% to 93% at five years in adults.[279] The average duration of remission and frequency of flare in the pediatric population is unknown. Long-term observations of children with TA are rare. Maksimowicz-McKinnon stated that, despite improvement of symptoms in TA following immunosuppressive therapy, for adults with TA, relapses usually occur with dosage reduction. Attempts to restore vascular patency are often initially successful, but restenosis occurs frequently. Chronic morbidity and disability occur in most patients with TA.[266] Long-term morbidity and mortality information for children with TA is not available.

CHILDHOOD CENTRAL NERVOUS SYSTEM VASCULITIS

In 1922 Harbitz first described a patient with angiitis of the CNS.[281] Cravioto and Feigin first recognized noninfectious, granulomatous angiitis of the CNS as a unique class of vasculitis in 1959.[282] By 1979, 30 cases of "granulomatous vasculitis of the neuraxis" had been reported in patients ages 15- to 96-years-old. All but one

---

Table 34–8

Proposed 1994 angiographic classification of Takayasu Arteritis

Type	Vessel involvement
Type I	Branches from the aortic arch
Type IIa	Ascending aorta, aortic arch and its branches
Type IIb	Ascending aorta, aortic arch and its branches, thoracic descending aorta
Type III	Thoracic descending aorta, abdominal aorta, and/or renal arteries
Type IV	Abdominal aorta and/or renal arteries
Type V	Combined features of types IIb and IV

According to this classification system, involvement of the coronary or pulmonary arteries should be designated as C (+) or P (+), respectively.

of these patients died within three years of diagnosis. Calabrese and colleagues first systematically reviewed adult PACNS, proposed diagnostic criteria, and suggested a clinical approach.[283-285]

In 2001, Lanthier and colleagues described two children with CNS vasculitis and distinguished the entities of small and large vessel disease.[286] Gallagher and colleagues reported four children with angiography positive primary CNS vasculitis and their immunosuppressive treatment regimens.[287] In 2006, a cohort of 62 children with angiography-positive childhood primary CNS angiitis (cPACNS) was described at Toronto Hospital for Sick Children.[288] An additional four children with negative cerebral angiographies had small vessel cPACNS (SV-cPACNS) histopathologically demonstrated in elective brain biopsies.[289] Over the past five years, recognition of CNS vasculitis has increased, and mimics of childhood CNS vasculitis recognized within the wider spectrum of inflammatory brain diseases include antibody-mediated brain inflammation,[290-291] genetically defined systemic inflammatory diseases with predominant CNS manifestations,[292] and a metabolic disease presenting with associated inflammation of the CNS.[293-294]

Definition and Classification

CNS vasculitis of childhood is an inflammatory disease of blood vessels in the brain. It is, by definition, not associated with vasculitis in other organs. It may be primary or secondary; secondary forms are associated with infection, rheumatic or systemic inflammatory disease, malignancies, metabolic diseases,[295] and exogenous factors such as medications and radiation therapy (Table 34–9). Similar patterns of CNS vessel involvement are seen in primary and secondary disease.

The terminology of cPACNS remains challenging. The proposed classification is based on the size of the affected vessels: (1) SV-cPACNS (normal angiography) versus (2) large-medium cPACNS (abnormal angiography). Large-medium vessel cPACNS has been further characterized as being progressive or nonprogressive,[288] with progressive disease being defined when there is evidence of inflammatory vessel disease (vessel stenoses) in a new vascular segment or territory on repeat vascular imaging beyond three months of disease onset. Progression within an affected segment is commonly seen and does not support the classification of progressive cPACNS. Nonprogressive cPACNS is characterized by unilateral stenosis of the distal internal carotid artery, the proximal middle cerebral artery, and/or the proximal anterior cerebral artery. By definition, the stenoses are stable or improved in appearance on repeat imaging at three months without evidence of new vascular bed involvement.

The Toronto series demonstrated that the anterior CNS circulation is most commonly affected by cPACNS. About a third of children have both anterior and posterior vessel disease;[288] the very small subgroup of children with vasculitis solely affecting the posterior basilar system were found to have progressive disease. Patients with this pattern of involvement appear to be distinctly different from those with the previously described nonprogressive

posterior circulation vasculopathy predominantly affecting teenage boys.[296]

The diagnosis of cPACNS is commonly based on the Calabrese criteria proposed for adult PACNS.[285] These criteria have not been validated in children and do not capture those children, who may potentially present with predominant psychiatric features or development-related phenotypes, such as autism or attention deficit disorder. The proposed modified Calabrese criteria are shown in Table 34–10.

Epidemiology

No epidemiological data are available for SV-cPACNS and childhood inflammatory brain diseases in general. An estimated 40% to 60% of arterial ischemic strokes

---

Table 34–9

Differential Diagnosis of childhood inflammatory brain diseases

White Matter Disease
Demyelinating diseases
- Acute demyelinating encephalomyelitis (ADEM)
- Multiple sclerosis
Optic neuritis
- Idiopathic/primary
- Secondary/associated with demyelinating diseases, cPACNS, infections

Gray and White Matter Disease
Vasculitis
- Primary CNS angiitis of childhood (cPACNS)
  - Large- and medium-sized vessel vasculitis
    - Progressive cPACNS
    - Nonprogressive cPACNS
  - Small vessel CNS vasculitis
- Secondary CNS angiitis in children
- Infections, inflammatory or rheumatic diseases, metabolic diseases, other
Transverse myelitis
- Idiopathic/primary
- Associated with cPACNS, demyelinating diseases, infections, SLE, others

Other Inflammatory Brain Diseases
Postinfectious inflammatory brain disease
Neuromyelitis optica (NMO)
Opsoclonus-myoclonus syndrome OMS
NMDA-receptor encephalitis
Inflammatory movement disorders
- Idiopathic/primary
- Secondary infection, cPACNS, demyelinating diseases, SLE, APLS, others

---

Table 34–10

Proposed diagnostic criteria for childhood primary angiitis of the central nervous system (cPACNS)

Modified Calabrese Criteria
- A newly acquired neurological and/or psychiatric deficit **plus**
- Angiographic and/or histological evidence of CNS vasculitis *in the absence of* any systemic condition known to be associated with or mimic CNS vasculitis

(AIS) in children is thought to be related to CNS vasculitis.[297,298] The incidence of childhood AIS is estimated at 3.3-7.9/100 000 children/year[299-301] with a male predominance.[302] Boys are more commonly affected with large-medium vessel cPACNS consistent with the male predominance of childhood AIS in general.[288,302] In contrast, small vessel vasculitis is more commonly seen in females.[289]

Etiology and Genetic Factors

The trigger for inflammation targeting the cerebral vessels remains unknown. Viral studies have been uniformly uninformative. The histopathology of the affected tissue is nonspecific. Angiographic abnormalities in the nonprogressive, angiography-positive cPACNS are very similar to those in postvaricella angiopathy (PVA) that commonly result in a stroke. PVA is believed to occur when Varicella Zoster Virus (or other viruses) latent in the trigeminal ganglion are reactivated and trigger an inflammatory proximal cerebral vessel stenosis.[296] Predisposing immune dysregulations, such as complement deficiencies and T-cell killing defects (perforin deficiency), are shown to be associated with the development of inflammatory brain diseases.[292]

Clinical manifestations

The understanding of the clinical spectrum of children with CNS vasculitis and inflammatory brain diseases is rapidly expanding. Large-medium vessel cPACNS more commonly presents with focal deficits and headaches. Children may present with AIS, fine motor deficits, cranial neuropathy or movement disorder, and ischemic disease syndromes corresponding to stenosis of specific cerebral vessels and their vascular distributions.[288] SV-cPACNS patients classically present with significant diffuse neurological deficits and/or psychiatric features.[286,289,304] Seizures are the single most common presentation of SV-cPACNS. Some children with intractable seizures have been identified as having an inflammatory brain disease, most commonly SV-cPACNS.[305] The clinical spectrum includes new onset of nonspecific cognitive dysfunction, school difficulties, behavior or mood disorders, or atypical presentations of psychiatric diseases of childhood. Stroke features are less common in SV-cPACNS; however, in children who present with "behavior abnormality," it is critical to identify transient weakness and subtle focal deficits as these are important red flags that might suggest an underlying inflammatory vascular problem.

Children with SV-cPACNS may be diagnosed with other conditions, such as movement disorder or demyelinating disease/multiple sclerosis (MS). The presence of clinical features characteristic of MS, such as optic neuritis or spinal inflammatory disease, may be misleading, since they are not specific for demyelinating disease and are found in up to one-third of children with SV-cPACNS (personal experience of author). Atypical clinical MS features, such as severe headaches and meningeal enhancement on MRI, may be diagnostic clues for cPACNS.[306] The course of illness varies. Completely

healthy children may develop severe focal or diffuse deficits within a few days, and these may or may not persist. Clinical features can improve spontaneously or with medications given for treatment of raised intracranial pressure (i.e., acetazolamide), headaches, or seizures. Other children may have months or years of smoldering inflammatory illness before the diagnosis is considered. A high index of suspicion is required in children presenting with a new neurological and/or psychiatric abnormality (Table 34–11).

Differential Diagnosis

The differentiation of angiography-positive cPACNS from noninflammatory vasculopathies is limited by our ability to histologically demonstrate vessel wall inflammation; large vessel biopsies are contraindicated and parenchymal brain biopsies to examine small vessels are commonly inconclusive (personal observation of authors). Gadolinium enhancement of the vessel wall on MRI is a promising tool that requires further validation.[307,308] Vessel wall enhancement is absent in mimics of cPACNS, such as idiopathic moyamoya disease, FMD, and other noninflammatory vasculopathies.[308] Channelopathies, genetic diseases affecting the function of ion channels such as in the voltage-gated calcium channel gene family, have variable CNS phenotypes, including vascular stenoses and associated strokes.[309]

Calabrese proposed the term "benign CNS angiitis" to describe a group of patients in whom he subsequently recognized there might be a noninflammatory, vasospastic etiology. He has more recently proposed the revised term *reversible vasoconstrictive syndromes (RVS)* to describe these patients, and the syndrome definition requires complete resolution of the vascular stenosis on repeat imaging.[310] The syndrome has been reported in children,[311] and vasodilating agents have been successfully used in RVS in adults and children.

Laboratory Examination

Inflammatory markers differ between the subtypes of CNS vasculitis in children. In angiography-positive cPACNS elevated ESRs were found in 51% of those tested, raised CRP were found in 74%, and mildly elevated IgG were found in 35%.[288] Hematological abnormalities including anemia, platelet abnormalities, or raised WBC counts were present in only 20% of children. Cerebrospinal fluid (CSF) abnormalities, including pleocytosis and/or raised protein, were found in 39% of the children tested. Negative inflammatory markers therefore do not exclude large-medium cPACNS.

SV-cPACNS patients more commonly present with elevated or abnormal inflammatory markers.[289] Raised CRP, elevated ESR, elevated C3, neutrophilia, anemia, thrombocytosis and elevated vWF antigen levels are found in the majority of children.[312] CSF abnormalities (including pleocytosis or elevated protein) and/or elevated opening pressure on lumbar puncture are found in virtually all children with SV-cPACNS; however, the abnormal test elevations may be small, and serial tests may be required.

Table 34–11

Clinical characteristics at diagnosis of with primary childhood CNS vasculitis (cPACNS) at childhood CNS vasculitis clinic, Toronto

	Large vessel cPACNS (Angiography Positive) N=144	Small Vessel cPACNS (Angiography Negative, Biopsy Positive) N=58
Reduced level of consciousness	5%	38%
Focal deficit		
Hemiparesis	72%	14%
Focal gross motor deficit	88%	22%
Fine motor deficit	90%	54%
Gait abnormality	86%	62%
Hemisensory deficit	64%	18%
Language production	52%	78%
Cranial nerve deficit	64%	14%
Optic neuritis	-	10%
Movement abnormality (ataxia, chorea, dystonia)	24%	17%
Diffuse deficit		
Cognitive dysfunction	42%	69%
Memory deficit	32%	64%
Behavior abnormality	38%	66%
Concentration deficit	34%	64%
Seizures		
Focal seizures	10%	69%
Generalized seizures	4%	33%
Status epilepticus	-	24%

Oligoclonal banding is present in one-third of children with biopsy-confirmed SV-cPACNS.[312]

The investigation of children with suspected inflammatory brain diseases should include metabolic screening and targeted genetic testing, depending on the clinical phenotype. This may include assessments for POLG mutations in children with features of epilepsia partialis continua, status epilepticus, or vision loss.[313-314] Mitochondrial disease such as, Mitochondrial Encephalopathy, Lactic Acidosis, and Stroke-like episodes (MELAS) in children presenting with recurrent strokes,[294] and Rolandic Mitochondrial Encephalomyelopathy (ROME) in children with myoclonic seizures and mild delays should be considered.[315] A prothrombotic and an infectious evaluation including tuberculosis status, cultures, and serologies is mandatory in children with suspected cPACNS. Neuroimmunology testing is indicated in children with suspected inflammatory brain diseases presenting with a broad spectrum of acquired deficits, including movement disorders, encephalitis, psychosis, or seizures. These symptoms may be associated with N-Methyl-D-Aspartate Receptor (NMDA-R) antibodies in the serum and/or CSF, as seen in NMDA-R encephalitis.[291,316,317] Neuromyelitis optica is a severe, inflammatory brain disease in children characterized by optic neuritis, transverse myelitis, encephalopathy, eye muscle paresis, ataxia, seizures, intractable vomiting, or hiccups.[318] Evidence of autoantibodies targeting the CNS water channel aquaporin-4 (AQP4) confirms the diagnosis. A characteristic MRI pattern reflecting the CNS and spinal distribution of AQP4 is frequently found.[319]

Pathology

Brain biopsy is the confirmatory test of choice in suspected SV–cPACNS, and an adequate brain biopsy sample is crucial for diagnosis.[312] Optimal sampling for diagnostic assessment requires all three superficial layers of brain tissue, including leptomeninges, gray matter cortex, and subcortical white matter. Biopsies may be obtained from the lesion, if the site does not correspond to an eloquent region of the brain, or outside the lesion usually from the nondominant frontal cortex. Inflammatory infiltrate (predominantly lymphocytes and macrophages, with occasional plasma cells, neutrophils, and eosinophils) can be seen within the walls of arterioles, capillaries, or venules (Fig. 34–9). The majority of patients have evidence of vasculitis in all three layers of the brain. Granulomatous inflammation and multinucleate giant cells are rarely reported in children. Nonspecific perivascular inflammation with lymphocytes (both B and T cells) and macrophages can be found in patients with a prolonged disease course. Electron-microscopy may demonstrate swollen, reactive endothelial cells, and tubuloreticular inclusions.[305,312]

Histological studies of brain biopsies of children with angiography-negative cPACNS demonstrate a nongranulomatous vessel inflammation with a predominant

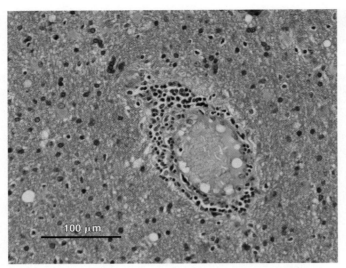

FIGURE 34–9   Lymphocytic vasculitis on brain biopsy of a child with primary central nervous system (CNS) vasculitis. Hematoxylin and eosin stain of a small muscular artery in the brain parenchyma of a patient with small vessel CNS vasculitis. Magnification x400.

lymphocytic cell infiltrate (see Fig. 34–9).[286,289,320] The histology of brain parenchyma in angiography-positive cPACNS is commonly nondiagnostic, since large vessel stenosis often leads to ischemia in the absence of specific vasculitis changes. Viral inclusion screening, cultures, and PCR studies for infectious agents have been consistently negative in SV-cPACNS.

Radiological Examinations

Conventional angiography is considered the gold standard for the diagnosis of cPACNS; however, it is an invasive method with limited use for follow-up assessments.[321] Computerized tomography (CT) angiography is an alternative; however, repeated studies over time expose the child to significant radiation. The sensitivity of CT scans for CNS inflammation is limited. In a recent series of patients with brain biopsy-confirmed SV-cPACNS patients, only 23% had an abnormal CT scan at diagnosis.[312,321-323] MRA, the most commonly used technique, has limitations in visualizing distal vessel segments, may underestimate the extent of disease, and may lead to misclassifications. MRI has a sensitivity of 98% for cPACNS (unpublished data). Most commonly, children have both MRA and conventional angiography at diagnosis, with MRA studies preferably used as the follow-up tool. Vessel wall imaging using gadolinium enhanced MRI sequences to detect inflammation is a promising imaging modality, but is not widely available.[308]

T2 and Fluid Attenuated Inversion Recovery sequences visualize inflammatory lesions, and gadolinium enhancement may be present. Both acute ischemic lesions and inflammatory lesions may be present in patients with large-medium vessel cPACNS. Diffusion restriction is the characteristic feature of brain ischemia and stroke and can be detected in diffusion weighted images (DWI). Children with inflammatory, nonischemic lesions have normal DWI imaging.

Treatment

Immunosuppressive therapy, including corticosteroids and CYC, is proposed to treat children with CNS vasculitis.[322,324] In angiography-positive, progressive cPACNS and angiography-negative SVcPACN remission induction therapy comprising IV CYC (500-750mg/m^2) monthly x 7 pulses together with high dose corticosteroids (2mg/kg, maximum of 60mg/day with a monthly taper to 50-40-30-25-20-17.5-15-12.5-10-7.5-5-2.5mg) for a total of 13 months, followed by maintenance therapy with a second-line agent such as MMF at a dose of 1000 to 1200 mg/m^2 /day was found to be effective in observational cohorts.[322] The treatment of nonprogressive angiography-positive cPACNS is controversial. Adjunctive corticosteroids with anticoagulation may decrease the restroke rate and improve the long-term neurological outcome.[325] Many centers treat children with Trimethoprim-sulfamethoxazole for pneumocystis prophylaxis during induction. Specific symptoms of CNS vasculitis, including seizures, psychosis, and movement abnormalities, require coordinated, targeted therapy. All patients require supportive care.

The evidence for anticoagulation and/or anti-platelet therapy is limited.[326] Commonly, children with angiography-positive cPACNS and stroke receive low-molecular weight or conventional heparin at the time of presentation. Many centers switch to antiplatelet therapy after two to six weeks. Children with SV-cPACNS are commonly given antiplatelet agents after a brain biopsy (acetylsalicylic acid at 3-5mg/day). These approaches need to be further evaluated.

Course of Disease and Prognosis

In the Toronto series, two-thirds of large-medium vessel cPACNS patients had monophasic, nonprogressive course.[288] Seventy-nine percent of patients were treated with anticoagulation/antiplatelet therapy without immunosuppression. Despite being nonprogressive, the neurological long-term outcome of this group is the least favorable. Inflammatory proximal stenoses of large vessels lead to extensive ischemic, largely irreversible lesions in the vascular distribution. The restroke rate in nonprogressive cPACNS patients is 40% to 60%.[288] Significant neurological deficits impacting function were found in 60% to 80% of children.[288] In small studies, the restroke rates in children with nonprogressive large vessel cPACNS treated with a short three-month course of immunosuppression appear significantly lower.[325]

Progressive large-medium vessel cPACNS and SV-cPACNS are largely treatable, and clinical features potentially reversible with immunosuppressive therapy. Ischemic lesions are less commonly found. The neurological outcome of patients with SV-cPACNS is reported to be excellent when they are treated with combination immunosuppression.[288] Flares are seen in one-third of SV-cPACNS patients and can occur as late as seven years after the first episode.[322] A minority of children is nonresponsive to the proposed cPACNS protocol and has progressive disease, despite high-dose corticosteroids and CYC. It may mandate other treatment options as described for adults with refractory vasculitis.[327] The cognitive burden of inflammatory brain diseases and therapy in children has yet to be studied.

INFLAMMATORY BRAIN DISEASES

The spectrum of childhood inflammatory brain diseases is expanding beyond the confines of childhood CNS vasculitis in part because of the increased sensitivity of neuroimaging techniques and advances in neuroimmunology research.[328] Rheumatologists may become involved in these inflammatory diseases as they are important mimics of SV-cPACNS and may ultimately require similar therapies.

Infection-Triggered Inflammatory Brain Diseases

Encephalitis is an inflammation of the brain characterized by altered mental status, seizures, or focal neurological signs. The annual incidence of encephalitis in the pediatric age group is 10.5 per 100,000 child-years.[329] Both infectious and noninfectious etiologies can lead to a similar encephalitic presentation. Previously healthy children can develop encephalopathy, seizures, and coma within days after the onset of a common childhood febrile infection, such as influenza A or parainfluenza. Other viruses such as enterovirus,[330] Ebstein-Barr virus,[331] varicella zoster, cytomegalovirus, and herpes simplex virus are proven infectious agents causing severe encephalitis.[332]

Mycoplasma-Associated Encephalitis

Mycoplasma is a ubiquitous pathogen found in the lungs in healthy individuals, but it also causes respiratory disease and, likely on an autoimmune basis, CNS and other extrapulmonary manifestations. In the California Encephalitis Project, evidence of acute *M. pneumonia* infection was found in approximately 5% of patients with encephalitis; three-quarters of these patients were children, and they had rapidly progressive disease.[333] Children with mycoplasma-associated encephalitis typically present with decreased level of consciousness, psychiatric features, and seizures following an upper respiratory tract infection.[334] Typical MRI finding are bilateral posterior thalamic lesions.[335] The confirmatory test is evidence of mycoplasma IgM in the serum and/or CSF.[336] The treatment includes antimicrobial therapy, IVIG, and/or corticosteroids.[337]

Neuromyelitis Optica

In 2008, McKeon reported 88 consecutive children, 4- to 18-years-old, found to be positive for a novel auto-antibody against the water channel aquaporin 4.[318,338] Clinically all children presented with attacks of optic neuritis (83%), transverse myelitis (78%), and/or other episodic cerebral symptoms (45% including encephalopathy, ataxia, seizures, and vomiting). Seventy-six percent had additional autoantibodies. MRI abnormalities in only 68% involved periventricular areas, medulla,

supra/infratentorial white matter, midbrain, cerebellum, thalamus, and hypothalamus. Ninety-three percent had recurrent attacks, and 90% residual disability. In the same year, in a retrospective study of 25 patients, including two children,[339] Jacob reported the efficacy of rituximab in reducing the frequency of attacks and improving the long-term deficits.

Opsoclonus-Myoclonus Syndrome

Previously healthy young children can present with a new onset of severe eye movement disturbance, myoclonia, ataxia, and cognitive dysfunction.[340] The incidence was recently calculated at 0.18 cases per million per year. The mean age at presentation was 18-months-old (range 3 to 42 months). A fraction of opsoclonus-myoclonus syndrome (OMS) cases are secondary to neuroblastoma.[341] IgG3 autoantibodies are suspected to be the result of an autoimmune response directed against crossreactive proteins of tumor and neuronal cells.[342] In the UK series, typical OMS features were present in 40% of children, including very delayed presentation of opsoclonus and dysphagia. Only 26% of cases were associated with neuroblastoma.[343] The treatment of OMS includes rituximab;[344,345] alternatively, CYC and dexamethasone may be used.[346] Pranzatelli reported that rituximab affords long-term protection against CSF B cell expansion in OMS.[344]

Mitochondrial Mutations and Inflammatory Brain Diseases

Mutations in the mitochondrial DNA (mtDNA) may cause respiratory chain deficiencies that will clinically manifest in tissues, such as the brain, where there is high energy expenditure.[347] MELAS[294,348] and ROME with associated MT-ND3 mutations[293] may both causes new neurological deficits and MRI lesions in children that can mimic cPACNS. Mutations in the POLG1 gene (partly encoding for an enzyme crucial for mtDNA repair and replication) are estimated to account for 25% of all adult onset mitochondrial disease. In children, POLG1 mutations have been reported to be responsible for a spectrum of phenotypes, including Alpers syndrome,[349] ataxia neuropathy spectrum disorders, childhood neurodegenerative myocerebrohepatopathy spectrum disorders, myoclonus epilepsy myopathy sensory ataxia,[350] and in association with intractable seizures.[314] CNS manifestations in the absence of liver and muscle disease are increasingly recognized and can present with an associated inflammatory brain disease targeting the small cerebral vessels and warrant immunosuppressive therapy.

Many of newly recognized inflammatory brain diseases continue to be labeled idiopathic including idiopathic transverse myelitis. Demyelinating diseases such as acute demyelinating encephalomyelitis and childhood MS are distinct white matter diseases in the spectrum of inflammatory brain diseases. The diagnoses of childhood CNS vasculitis, inflammatory brain diseases and their mimics, and differential diagnoses require an interdisciplinary team approach.

REFERENCES

5. M.F. Cotch, G.S. Hoffman, D.E. Yerg, et al., The epidemiology of Wegener's granulomatosis. Estimates of the five-year period prevalence, annual mortality, and geographic disease distribution from population-based data sources,, Arthritis Rheum. 39 (1996) 87–92.

7. J.M. Gardner-Medwin, P. Dolezalova, C. Cummins, et al., Incidence of Henoch-Schonlein purpura, Kawasaki disease, and rare vasculitides in children of different ethnic origins, Lancet 360 (2002) 1197–1202.

9. N.M. Wilkinson, J. Page, A.G. Uribe, et al., Establishment of a pilot pediatric registry for chronic vasculitis is both essential and feasible: a Childhood Arthritis and Rheumatology Alliance (CARRA) survey, J. Rheumatol. 34 (2007) 224–226.

10. V.M. Belostotsky, V. Shah, M.J. Dillon, Clinical features in 17 paediatric patients with Wegener granulomatosis, Pediatr. Nephrol. 17 (2002) 754–761.

11. J.F. Fries, G.G. Hunder, D.A. Bloch, et al., The American College of Rheumatology 1990 criteria for the classification of vasculitis. Summary, Arthritis Rheum. 33 (1990) 1135–1136.

12. J.C. Jennette, R.J. Falk, K. Andrassy, et al., Nomenclature of systemic vasculitides. Proposal of an international consensus conference, Arthritis Rheum. 37 (1994) 187–192.

13. S. Ozen, N. Ruperto, M.J. Dillon, et al., EULAR/PReS endorsed consensus criteria for the classification of childhood vasculitides, Ann. Rheum. Dis. 65 (2006) 936–941.

14. D.A. Cabral, A.G. Uribe, S.M. Benseler, et al., Classification, presentation and initial treatment of Wegener's Granulomatosis in childhood, Arthritis Rheum. 60 (2009) 3413–3424.

20. M. Rottem, A.S. Fauci, C.W. Hallahan, et al., Wegener granulomatosis in children and adolescents: clinical presentation and outcome, J. Pediatr. 122 (1993) 26–31.

21. J.D. Akikusa, R. Schneider, E.A. Harvey, et al., Clinical features and outcome of pediatric Wegener granulomatosis, Arthritis Rheum. 57 (2007) 837–844.

22. C.G. Kallenberg, Pathogenesis of PR3-ANCA associated vasculitis, J. Autoimmun. 30 (2008) 29–36.

25. G.S. Hoffman, G.S. Kerr, R.Y. Leavitt, et al., Wegener granulomatosis: an analysis of 158 patients, Ann. Intern. Med. 116 (1992) 488–498.

35. J.A. Savige, D.J. Davies, P.A. Gatenby, Anti-neutrophil cytoplasmic antibodies (ANCA): their detection and significance: report from workshops, Pathology. 26 (1994) 186–193.

37. J.C. Jennette, R.J. Falk, Small-vessel vasculitis, N. Engl. J. Med. 337 (1997) 1512–1523.

38. M.A. Little, C.L. Smyth, R. Yadav, et al., Antineutrophil cytoplasm antibodies directed against myeloperoxidase augment leukocyte-microvascular interactions in vivo, Blood 106 (2005) 2050–2058.

65. A.S. Fauci, B.F. Haynes, P. Katz, et al., Wegener's granulomatosis: prospective clinical and therapeutic experience with 85 patients for 21 years, Ann. Intern. Med. 98 (1983) 76–85.

70. R.Y. Leavitt, A.S. Fauci, D.A. Bloch, et al., The American College of Rheumatology 1990 criteria for the classification of Wegener's granulomatosis,, Arthritis Rheum. 33 (1990) 1101–1107.

78. J.T. Lie, Illustrated histopathologic classification criteria for selected vasculitis syndromes. American College of Rheumatology Subcommittee on Classification of Vasculitis, Arthritis Rheum. 33 (1990) 1074–1087.

85. M.B. McGregor, G. Sandler, Wegener's Granulomatosis. A clinical and radiological survey, Br. J. Radiol. 37 (1964) 430–439.

86. J.F. Cordier, D. Valeyre, L. Guillevin, et al., Pulmonary Wegener's granulomatosis. A clinical and imaging study of 77 cases, Chest. 97 (1990) 906–912.

92. A.V. Moorthy, R.W. Chesney, W.E. Segar, et al., Wegener granulomatosis in childhood: prolonged survival following cytotoxic therapy, J. Pediatr. 91 (1977) 616–618.

93. B.S. Gottlieb, L.C. Miller, N.T. Ilowite, Methotrexate treatment of Wegener granulomatosis in children, J. Pediatr. 129 (1996) 604–607.

95. L. Guillevin, J.F. Cordier, F. Lhote, et al., A prospective, multicenter, randomized trial comparing steroids and pulse cyclophosphamide versus steroids and oral cyclophosphamide in the treatment of generalized Wegener's granulomatosis, Arthritis Rheum. 40 (1997) 2187–2198.

98. G.K. de Groot, L. Harper, D.R. Jayne, et al., Pulse versus daily oral cyclophosphamide for induction of remission in antineutrophil cytoplasmic antibody-associated vasculitis: a randomized trial, Ann. Intern. Med. 150 (2009) 670–680.

100. E. Reinhold-Keller, C.O. Fink, K. Herlyn, et al., High rate of renal relapse in 71 patients with Wegener's granulomatosis under maintenance of remission with low-dose methotrexate, Arthritis Rheum. 47 (2002) 326–332.

101. WGET Research Group, Etanercept plus standard therapy for Wegener's granulomatosis, N. Engl. J. Med. 352 (2005) 351–361.

102. K. de Groot, N. Rasmussen, P.A. Bacon, et al., Randomized trial of cyclophosphamide versus methotrexate for induction of remission in early systemic antineutrophil cytoplasmic antibody-associated vasculitis, Arthritis Rheum. 52 (2005) 2461–2469.

105. D. Jayne, N. Rasmussen, K. Andrassy, et al., A randomized trial of maintenance therapy for vasculitis associated with antineutrophil cytoplasmic autoantibodies, N. Engl. J. Med. 349 (2003) 36–44.

109. C.A. Langford, C. Talar-Williams, K.S. Barron, et al., Use of a cyclophosphamide-induction methotrexate-maintenance regimen for the treatment of Wegener's granulomatosis: extended follow-up and rate of relapse, Am. J. Med. 114 (2003) 463–469.

110. C. Pagnoux, A. Mahr, M.A. Hamidou, et al., Azathioprine or methotrexate maintenance for ANCA-associated vasculitis, N. Engl. J. Med. 359 (2008) 2790–2803.

150. J.G. Lanham, K.B. Elkon, C.D. Pusey, et al., Systemic vasculitis with asthma and eosinophilia: a clinical approach to the Churg-Strauss syndrome, Medicine (Baltimore) 63 (1984) 65–81.

153. J. Zwerina, G. Eger, M. Englbrecht, et al., Churg-Strauss Syndrome in Childhood: A Systematic Literature Review and Clinical Comparison with Adult Patients,, Semin. Arthritis Rheum. 39 (2008) 108–115.

154. L. Guillevin, P. Cohen, M. Gayraud, et al., Churg-Strauss syndrome. Clinical study and long-term follow-up of 96 patients, Medicine (Baltimore) 78 (1999) 26–37. 1999.

164. L. Guillevin, T. Guittard, O. Bletry, et al., Systemic necrotizing angiitis with asthma: causes and precipitating factors in 43 cases, Lung 165 (1987) 165–172.

175. L. Guillevin, F. Lhote, M. Gayraud, et al., Prognostic factors in polyarteritis nodosa and Churg-Strauss syndrome. A prospective study in 342 patients, Medicine (Baltimore) 75 (1996) 17–28.

183. C.O. Savage, C.G. Winearls, D.J. Evans, et al., Microscopic polyarteritis: presentation, pathology and prognosis, Q. J. Med. 56 (1985) 467–483.

184. R.A. Watts, V.A. Jolliffe, D.M. Carruthers, et al., Effect of classification on the incidence of polyarteritis nodosa and microscopic polyangiitis, Arthritis Rheum. 39 (1996) 1208–1212.

188. M. Hattori, H. Kurayama, Y. Koitabashi, Antineutrophil cytoplasmic autoantibody-associated glomerulonephritis in children, J. Am. Soc. Nephrol. 12 (2001) 1493–1500.

190. N. Besbas, S. Ozen, U. Saatci, et al., Renal involvement in polyarteritis nodosa: evaluation of 26 Turkish children, Pediatr. Nephrol. 14 (2000) 325–327.

192. L. Guillevin, B. Durand-Gasselin, R. Cevallos, et al., Microscopic polyangiitis: clinical and laboratory findings in eighty-five patients, Arthritis Rheum. 42 (1999) 421–430.

196. H. Xiao, P. Heeringa, P. Hu, et al., Antineutrophil cytoplasmic autoantibodies specific for myeloperoxidase cause glomerulonephritis and vasculitis in mice, J. Clin. Invest. 110 (2002) 955–963.

206. A. Bakkaloglu, S. Ozen, E. Baskin, et al., The significance of antineutrophil cytoplasmic antibody in microscopic polyangitis and classic polyarteritis nodosa,, Arch. Dis. Child 85 (2001) 427–430.

211. M. Gayraud, L. Guillevin, P. le Toulemin, et al., Long-term followup of polyarteritis nodosa, microscopic polyangiitis, and Churg-Strauss syndrome: analysis of four prospective trials including 278 patients, Arthritis Rheum. 44 (2001) 666–675.

282. H. Cravioto, I. Feigin, Noninfectious granulomatous angiitis with predilection for the nervous system, Neurology 9 (1959) 599–609.

283. L.H. Calabrese, J.A. Mallek, Primary angiitis of the central nervous system: report of 8 new cases, review of the literature, and proposal for diagnostic criteria, Medicine 67 (1988) 20–39.

286. S. Lanthier, A. Lortie, J. Michaud, et al., Isolated angiitis of the CNS in children, Neurology 56 (2001) 837–842.

287. K.T. Gallagher, B. Shaham, A. Reiff, et al., Primary angiitis of the central nervous system in children: 5 cases, J. Rheumatol. 28 (2001) 616–623.

288. S.M. Benseler, E. Silverman, R.I. Aviv, et al., Primary central nervous system vasculitis in children, Arthritis Rheum. 54 (2006) 1291–1297.

289. S.M. Benseler, G. deVeber, C. Hawkins, et al., Angiography-negative primary central nervous system vasculitis in children: a newly recognized inflammatory central nervous system disease, Arthritis Rheum. 52 (2005) 2159–2167.

290. B. Banwell, S. Tenembaum, V.A. Lennon, et al., Neuromyelitis optica-IgG in childhood inflammatory demyelinating CNS disorders, Neurology 70 (2008) 344–352.

291. N.R. Florance, R.L. Davis, C. Lam, et al., Anti-N-methyl-D-aspartate receptor (NMDAR) encephalitis in children and adolescents, Ann. Neurol. 66 (2009) 11–18.

292. D. Moshous, O. Feyen, P. Lankisch, et al., Primary necrotizing lymphocytic central nervous system vasculitis due to perforin deficiency in a four-year-old girl, Arthritis Rheum. 56 (2007) 995–999.

293. K.G. Werner, C.F. Morel, A. Kirton, et al: RoME: Rolandic Mitochondrial Encephalomyelopathy with Epilepsia Partialis Continua and ND3 mutations, *Ped Neurol* accepted for publication, 2009.

295. J. Elbers, S.M. Benseler, Central nervous system vasculitis in children, Curr. Opin. Rheumatol. 20 (2008) 47–54.

296. V. Ganesan, W.K. Chong, T.C. Cox, et al., Posterior circulation stroke in childhood: risk factors and recurrence, Neurology 59 (2002) 1552–1556.

297. R. Askalan, S. Laughlin, S. Mayank, et al., Chickenpox and stroke in childhood: a study of frequency and causation, Stroke 32 (2001) 1257–1262.

302. M.R. Golomb, H.J. Fullerton, U. Nowak-Gottl, et al., Male predominance in childhood ischemic stroke: findings from the international pediatric stroke study, Stroke 40 (2009) 52–57.

305. S. Venkateswaran, C. Hawkins, E. Wassmer, Diagnostic yield of brain biopsies in children presenting to neurology, J. Child Neurol. 23 (2008) 253–258.

308. W. Kuker, S. Gaertner, T. Nagele, et al., Vessel wall contrast enhancement: a diagnostic sign of cerebral vasculitis, Cerebrovasc. Dis. 26 (2008) 23–29.

318. A. McKeon, V.A. Lennon, T. Lotze, et al., CNS aquaporin-4 autoimmunity in children, Neurology 71 (2008) 93–100.

321. R.I. Aviv, S.M. Benseler, E.D. Silverman, et al., MR imaging and angiography of primary CNS vasculitis of childhood, AJNR. 27 (2006) 192–199.

323. R.I. Aviv, S.M. Benseler, G. DeVeber, et al., Angiography of primary central nervous system angiitis of childhood: conventional angiography versus magnetic resonance angiography at presentation, AJNR. 28 (2007) 9–15.

328. R.C. Dale, F. Brilot, B. Banwell, Pediatric central nervous system inflammatory demyelination: acute disseminated encephalomyelitis, clinically isolated syndromes, neuromyelitis optica, and multiple sclerosis, Curr. Opin. Neurol. 22 (2009) 233–240.

339. A. Jacob, B.G. Weinshenker, I. Violich, et al., Treatment of neuromyelitis optica with rituximab: retrospective analysis of 25 patients, Arch. Neuro. 65 (2008) 1443–1448.

342. A. Kirsten, S. Beck, V. Fuhlhuber, et al., New autoantibodies in pediatric opsoclonus myoclonus syndrome, Ann. N. Y. Acad. Sci. 1110 (2007) 256–260.

Entire reference list is available online at www.expertconsult.com.

Chapter 35

PEDIATRIC SARCOIDOSIS

Carlos D. Rosé and Carine H. Wouters

Pediatric sarcoidosis encompasses a spectrum of childhood granulomatous inflammatory conditions with the hallmark being the presence of noncaseating epithelioid giant cell granulomas in a variety of tissues and organ systems. The finding in 2001 of a mutation in the nucleotide-binding oligomerization domain 2/caspase activation recruitment domain 15 (NOD2/CARD15) gene among patients with a history of familial granulomatous arthritis constituted a major advance and revealed the complexity and heterogeneity of the spectrum of pediatric sarcoidosis.[1]

Blau syndrome (BS) and Early Onset Sarcoidosis (EOS) constitute the familial and sporadic forms of a pediatric disease characterized by a triad of polyarthritis, uveitis and rash; and a unique association with mutations in or near the central NOD/NACHT domain of the NOD2 gene.[1–5] The term Pediatric Granulomatous Arthritis (PGA) proposed for both conditions[6,7] falls short in describing the systemic and visceral manifestations that have been documented in a number of patients with PGA.

Many children with sarcoidosis are NOD2 mutation negative and tend to exhibit systemic and visceral manifestations at presentation. Within this group, the authors recently identified a distinct entity, Infantile Onset Panniculitis, with uveitis and systemic granulomatosis.[8]

The form of sarcoidosis observed in adults, characterized mainly by interstitial pulmonary involvement and hilar adenopathy, is rarely seen in the pediatric age group and is limited to older children. Certain clinical symptom complexes of granulomatous inflammation, including Löfgren and Mikulicz syndromes, can occur in children. Granulomatous inflammation can be seen secondary to immunodeficiencies or in the context of certain drug therapies.

EPIDEMIOLOGY

Scarce data exist on the epidemiology of pediatric sarcoidosis. A Danish National Registry study included 48 children within a cohort of 5536 patients with sarcoidosis, resulting in a calculated overall incidence for childhood sarcoidosis of 0.29/100,000/year. The incidence ranged from 0.06/100,000/year for children below five years old to 1.02/100.000/year for children 14 to 15 years old.[9,10]

An earlier international registry reported on 53 pediatric patients of whom 14 had a family history yielding a ratio of 1:5 for familial to sporadic forms.[11] The International Registry of Pediatric Sarcoidosis established in 2005 shows no gender difference or geographic predominance; the majority of patients exhibiting the classic triad of arthritis, uveitis, and rash have disease onset before reaching five years old.[5]

ETIOPATHOGENESIS

The familial cases manifesting the classic clinical triad and an autosomal dominant transmission pattern have been termed BS.[12] Using linkage analysis of the original pedigree, the susceptibility locus for BS was mapped to a region of chromosome 16, which was found to contain a gene associated with Crohn's Disease (CD) called IBD1.[13,14] The IBD1 gene was later found to be NOD2.[15] In 2001, Miceli and colleagues identified mutations within the NOD/NACHT domain of the NOD2 gene in four French families with the Blau phenotype.[1] This seminal work revealed that NOD2 substitutions associated with BS were located in a different domain of the protein than those associated with CD. Wang and colleagues reported NOD2 mutations in 50% of 10 pedigrees with the BS phenotype.[16] Later, identical mutations were reported among patients with EOS, a sporadic disease with the same phenotype of granulomatous arthritis, uveitis, and rash.[4,5] Currently, BS and EOS are considered to be the same disease, and the term PGA (Pediatric Granulomatous Arthritis) has been proposed to refer to both.[7] Conversely, mutations in NOD2 are not found in variant forms of pediatric sarcoidosis displaying a more heterogeneous phenotype, nor are they found in adult sarcoidosis.[7,17,18]

The NOD2 gene encodes a 1,040 amino-acid protein composed of three main functional domains, two amino-terminal Caspase Recruitment Domains (CARDs), a central Nucleotide Binding Oligomerization Domain (NOD/NACHT), and carboxyterminal Leucine-Rich repeats (LRRs). To date, 14 mutations causing amino-acid substitutions in and near the NOD domain have been documented (Table 35–1). Substitutions R334W (Arginine to Glutamine in position 334) and R334Q (Arginine to Tryptophan) are by far the most common. Mutations associated with CD are concentrated in the carboxyterminal LRR region; although CD and EOS have very different phenotypes, they are both characterized by the presence of giant cell granulomas.

Table 35–1

NOD2 mutations (and amino-acid substitutions) associated with pediatric sarcoidosis (Familial forms [Blau syndrome] and sporadic forms [Early onset sarcoidosis] with their first publication

R334W (Arg334Trp)	Miceli-Richard et al., 2001
R334Q (Arg334Gln)	Miceli-Richard et al., 2001
D382E (Asp383Glu)	Kanazawa et al., 2005
E383K (Glu383Lys)	van Duist et al., 2005
L469F (Leu469Phe)	Miceli-Richard et al., 2001
H496L (His496Leu)	Kanazawa et al., 2005
M513T (Met513Thr)	Kanazawa et al., 2005
T605P (Thr605Pro)	Kanazawa et al., 2005
N670K (Asn670Lys)	Kanazawa et al., 2005
W490L (Try490Leu)	Gattorno et al., 2006
C495Y (Cys495Tyr)	Arostegui et al., 2007
R587C (Arg587Cys)	Arostegui et al., 2007
E383G (Glu383Gly)	Okafuji et al., 2009
T605N (Thr605Asn)	Milman et al., 2009

The NOD2 protein is a member of a growing family of NOD-like receptor cytosolic proteins comprising different functional domains and implicated in pathways of inflammation and apoptosis. The two amino-terminal CARD domains of NOD2 have an important role in the mediation of nuclear factor (NF)-κB activation and secretion of proinflammatory cytokines, resulting from CARD-CARD interactions between NOD2 and a pivotal downstream kinase protein receptor-interacting serine/threonine kinase [RICK] also known as RIP2 or CARDIAK. The centrally located NOD domain mediates self-oligomerization of NOD2 proteins and activation of downstream effector molecules. The LRR region is structurally related to the LRR regions of the Toll-like receptors, which are molecules of the innate immune system indispensable for the "sensing" of molecular motifs specific to pathogens, such as lipopolysaccharide. Studies have shown that the moiety recognized by NOD2 is actually muramyl dipeptide, a building block of peptidoglycan found in both Gram-positive and Gram-negative bacterial cell walls. NOD2 is expressed constitutively in monocytes, granulocytes, dendritic cells, and in Paneth cells in the villous crypts of the small intestine.[19,20]

The downstream effects of NOD2 mutations and their relationship with the clinical phenotype are largely unknown. The NOD2 mutations associated with PGA involve residues located in the NOD domain and reportedly act as constitutively active NOD2 mutants, which are gain-of-function variants consistent with the autosomal-dominant nature of the disease (Fig. 35–1). Using transfection systems, a constitutive NF-κB activation through an abnormal stabilization of the active conformation in the mutated NOD2 protein has been suggested, although these findings have not been replicated to date.[21,22] Conversely, experiments using patients' circulating mononuclear cells could not confirm the expected upregulation and release of interleukin (IL)-1 and other proinflammatory cytokines.[23]

The pathological hallmark of sarcoidosis is the presence of noncaseating epithelioid granulomas thought to result from an exaggerated immune-inflammatory response to a persistent unidentified antigen. The granulomas consist of a central cluster of monocytes/macrophages in various stages of activation, epithelioid cells aligned in a way reminiscent of epithelial cells, and multinucleated giant cells (Fig. 35–2). A corona of mostly CD4+ T lymphocytes, scattered CD8+ T lymphocytes, and plasma cells surrounds the central region. Immunohistochemistry studies in adult sarcoidosis have demonstrated the presence of T helper (Th)-1 type lymphokines (IL-2, interferon-γ) and proinflammatory cytokines (IL-1, tumor necrosis factor [TNF]-α, IL-6) in situ.[24] The relationship between the formation and persistence of inflammatory granulomas and the effect of NOD2 mutations on inflammatory and apoptosis pathways remains to be elucidated.

CLINICAL FEATURES

Sarcoidosis Associated with NOD2 Mutation

NOD2 mutation-associated sarcoidosis comprises patients with either BS or EOS manifesting a consistent clinical phenotype with polyarthritis, dermatitis and uveitis (Fig. 35–3). In recent years, because of the availability of genetic testing, a more protean clinical picture than initially conceived is being observed. That this form of sarcoidosis is different from the better-known adult form should not be forgotten.

The initial manifestations include the typical exanthema followed within months by a symmetrical polyarthritis. Ocular involvement tends to occur towards the second year. The median age at onset in the International PGA Registry was 26 months with two unusual cases with a debut at ages 2-months and 14-years.[7]

Cutaneous Involvement

The rash varies in color from pale pink with varied degrees of tan to intense erythema. The lesions appear on the trunk mainly dorsally and extend to the face and limbs with accentuation of the tan color on extensor surfaces, where it may become scaly brownish over time (see Fig. 35–3A). The lesions are tiny (5 to 7 millimeter), round, and barely palpable. At onset, the rash often shows a very fine desquamation, which may lead to confusion with atopic dermatitis. Over the course of years the rash waxes and wanes. With time, the desquamation predominates, and, in adolescence, it may mimic ichthyosis vulgaris.

Subcutaneous nodules, often located in the lower limbs, are the second most common dermatological manifestation and may be clinically indistinguishable from erythema nodosum.[7] The nodules are mildly tender and resolve without atrophy or pigmentation, even in patients with recurrent episodes. Erysipelas-like lesions have been observed as well, and in one case an urticarial rash showed typical histological features of leukocytoclastic vasculitis.[25]

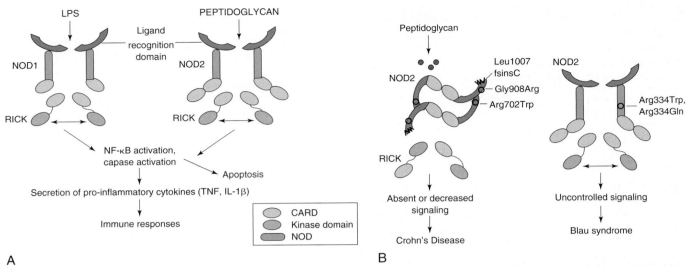

FIGURE 35–1   A, Nucleotide-binding oligomerization domain (NOD) 1 and NOD2 proteins recognition bacterial-derived LPS and peptidoglycan through their leucine-rich repeat (LRR) domains. Signaling through NOD1 and NOD2 is mediated through the receptor-interacting serine/threonine kinase (RICK), which interacts with NOD1 and NOD2 through caspase activation recruitment domain (CARD)-CARD interactions. RICK mediates nuclear factor (NF)-κB activation and promotes caspase activation that leads to the secretion of pr-inflammatory cytokines. **B,** NOD2 variants that are associated with Crohn's Disease (Leu1007fsinsC, Gly908Arg, Arg702Trp) are located in or near the LRRs. These variants are defective in their response to bacterial peptidoglycan, resulting in absent or decreased signaling. NOD2 mutations associated with Blau syndrome (Arg334Trp, Arg334Gln) are located in the NOD and are activating mutations that lead to uncontrolled signaling in the absence of a ligand.

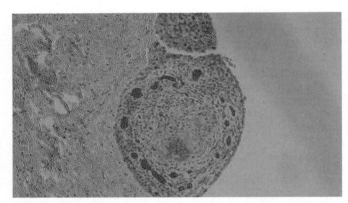

FIGURE 35–2   Synovial biopsy showing a typical noncaseating epithelioid cell granuloma with multinucleated giant cells.

Articular Disease

The majority of patients present with a polyarticular symmetrical, generalized, or additive arthritis, affecting large and small peripheral joints and tendon sheaths. A characteristic feature of both synovitis and tenosynovitis is the exuberance of the swelling. The distal flexor tendons of the digits, the extensor and peroneal compartments, and the flexor groups of the carpus can reach significant size. The anserine tendon sheath diameter can reach one centimeter in some cases. The synovial outpouching can acquire a cystic appearance in the dorsum of carpus and tarsus. Despite the prominent "boggy" synovitis, pain and morning stiffness appear to be moderate and are overall well tolerated. Except for the proximal interphalangeal joints, where a characteristic flexion contracture described as "camptodactyly" can be seen, the range of

motion is relatively well preserved, at least in childhood (see Fig. 35–3*B*). The course of the arthritis is variable, and erosive changes are mostly modest. However, limited joint mobility and joint contractures may develop with time; ulnar deviations, wrist subluxations, and joint space narrowing have been described.[12,26]

Ocular Disease

An insidious granulomatous iridocyclitis and posterior uveitis can evolve into a severe destructive panuveitis. Of the clinical triad elements, the ocular disease exhibits the most somber functional prognosis. It tends to start within the first two years of disease, and initially there is little to no redness or photophobia. Over time characteristic iris nodules, focal synechiae, cataract, increased intraocular pressure, and characteristic clumpy keratic precipitates at the limbus ensue. Nodules may also occur in the conjunctivae and, in this location, offer an early diagnostic clue and biopsy site. A description of the slit lamp appearance of sarcoid uveitis compared to juvenile idiopathic arthritis (JIA)-associated uveitis was published by Lindsley and Godfrey.[27] Posterior involvement includes vitritis, multifocal choroiditis, retinal vasculopathy, and optic nerve edema (see Fig. 35–3*C*). Significant visual loss is observed in 20% to 30% of the affected individuals.[7,11,12,26]

Visceral Involvement

As our understanding of the disease spectrum evolves, it has become apparent that the clinical phenotype is not restricted to the classic triad. Among patients with sarcoidosis and associated NOD2 mutations, a myriad of clinical manifestations including granulomatous and interstitial nephritis, chronic renal insufficiency, small

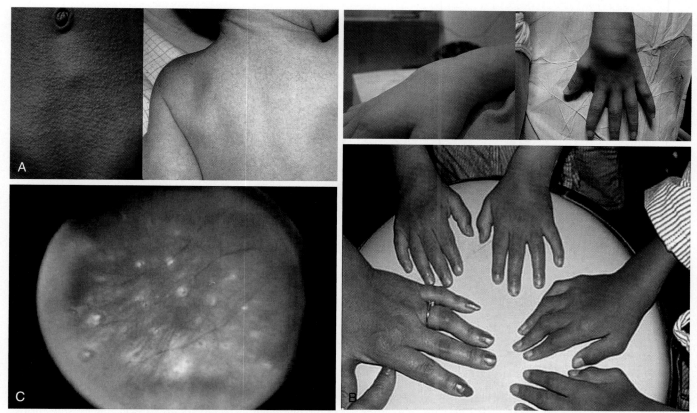

FIGURE 35–3   Clinical triad typical of *NOD2*-associated Pediatric Sarcoidosis. **A**, Cutaneous features with fine maculopapular erythematous/tan eruption with ichthyosiform appearance *(right)*. **B**, Typical "boggy" synovitis with preserved range of motion and cyst-like synovial swelling. *Below*, a family with *NOD2*-associated polyarthritis and PIP contractures causing camptodactyly. **C**, Multifocal choroiditis characteristic of granulomatous panuveitis.

vessel vasculitis, interstitial pneumonitis, peripheral and mediastinal (excluding hilar) lymphadenitis, pericarditis, cranial neuropathy (VII cranial nerve), and parotitis have been documented.[6,25,27] Visceral manifestations have been described in patients with BS before the NOD2 mutation was known.[28-31] Systemic manifestations including prolonged fever have been reported at the onset and may recur during first few years of the disease.[6,32] Large vessel vasculopathy has been reported in past studies,[33–35] and in one NOD2 mutated family studied by Wang,[16] but it was not confirmed in more recent series.[6,7,32] Severe arterial hypertension without demonstrable vascular involvement by digital imaging has been observed, suggesting renal vasculopathy of a diameter beyond imaging resolution.[32]

Until recently, no cases of asymptomatic mutation carrying have been observed; however, one family with a mutation E383K in four asymptomatic members has been reported.[32,36]

Sarcoidosis Without NOD2 Mutation

Sarcoidosis with wild-type *NOD2* constitutes a heterogeneous group of granulomatous inflammatory disorders with protean manifestations. Within this group, two distinct subsets have been identified, including infantile-onset panniculitis with systemic granulomatosis and pediatric-onset adult sarcoidosis.

Infantile-Onset Panniculitis with Uveitis and Systemic Granulomatosis

Five infants with a unique phenotype, including recurrent lobular nonlipophagic panniculitis, severe systemic involvement with persistent fever, hepatosplenomegaly, and granulomatous inflammation affecting joints, eyes, internal organs, and the central nervous system (CNS), have been described. The disease course is progressive, although a partial response to anti-TNF agents can be seen. This condition has been considered a new clinical and pathological entity.[8]

Pediatric-Onset Adult Sarcoidosis

Overall, this form of sarcoidosis is characterized primarily by systemic features: pulmonary and lymph node involvement, rather than articular disease. The incidence increases with age and tends to cluster in early adolescence. A review of published pediatric sarcoidosis cohorts reveals the presence of systemic features (malaise, fever, weight loss) at presentation in 60% to 98% of patients, lung involvement in 90% to 100%, hilar and peripheral lymphadenopathies in 40 to 67%, and 71 to 76% of patients respectively. Hepatomegaly and splenomegaly were seen in up to 43% of patients; mild elevation of liver enzymes is common, but severe sarcoid hepatitis rarely occurs. A liver biopsy may show granulomas but also cholestatic, necroinflammatory, and vascular changes.

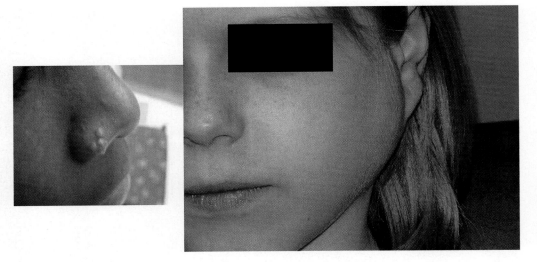

FIGURE 35–4 Clinical signs in sarcoidosis with wild-type *NOD2*. *Left,* Typical maculopapular lesion consisting of multiple noncaseating granulomas on nose. *Right,* Mikulicz syndrome with parotid and lacrimal gland involvement in a girl presenting with sicca symptoms.

Cutaneous manifestations including erythema nodosum, erythematous macules, papules, and plaques were observed in 25% to 42% (Fig. 35–4). Eye involvement was seen in 23% to 51%, and uveitis, the most common ocular manifestation, was observed in 25%. Neurological manifestations, mainly CNS involvement, was seen in 23%.[10,37,38]

Some particular presentations of adult sarcoidosis can rarely be observed in older children as well. Löfgren's syndrome is characterized by an acute onset of arthritis (mainly of the ankles), erythema nodosum, and hilar adenopathy, and occurs in 9% to 34% of adult sarcoidosis patients.[38,39] The authors have observed one case of Mikulicz syndrome (parotid and lacrimal gland enlargement) with granulomatous inflammation on a lacrimal gland biopsy in a child who later developed interstitial pneumonitis (see Fig. 35–4).

Particular Features of Organ Involvement in Pediatric-Onset Adult Sarcoidosis

Neurosarcoidosis in children presents differently than in adults. Seizures as the manifestation of sarcoid encephalopathy are common in prepubertal children, whereas cranial nerve palsy, the most common neurological complication among adults, is less frequent and only seen at an older age. A review of 29 pediatric cases of neurosarcoidosis by Baumann and colleagues showed that masslike lesions on imaging are more common than previously recognized; additional features were leptomeningeal enhancement and multifocal T2 hyperintense MRI lesions within cortical grey and subcortical white matter. Cerebrospinal fluid analysis characteristically reveals a mild lymphocytosis, mildly elevated protein, and increased immunoglobulins with oligoclonal banding. Evidence of hypothalamic dysfunction is also common with patients showing growth failure, diabetes insipidus, and failure of sexual maturation.[40]

Renal sarcoidosis deserves attention because of the risk of renal dysfunction and coexistent calcium metabolism abnormalities. In a review of 15 pediatric case series, the frequency of a decreased creatinine clearance was 26% to 45%. Mild to moderate proteinuria and sediment changes (especially leukocyturia) were noted in 31% of patients. Hypercalciuria was found in 47% and hypercalcemia in 21% of patients. Pathology most often showed interstitial and granulomatous nephritis; tubulopathy, glomerular, and vascular changes were rarely seen.[41] In fact, the same pattern of interstitial nephritis with renal failure was documented by Meiorin and colleagues in a child with proven *NOD2* mutation, suggesting that similar renal manifestations are seen in both *NOD2* mutation related and unrelated forms.[25]

Symptomatic sarcoid myositis is rare in children and adults, although asymptomatic granulomatous involvement has been detected in up to 80% of muscle biopsy specimens.[42] Three distinct clinical patterns reported in children comprise an acute inflammatory myositis with myalgia and increased muscle enzymes,[43] a long-lasting myopathy with progressive muscle weakness,[44] and a nodular myopathy with palpable muscle nodules.[45]

Similarly, although clinically recognized cardiac involvement in uncommon, autopsy studies demonstrate granulomatous infiltration of the myocardium in as many as 27% of adults. The most common clinical manifestations in adults include conduction and rhythm disturbances. Heart failure and sudden death are rare but have been described as well.[46] Death from multiorgan failure and chronic congestive heart failure 10 years after disease onset has been reported in a child; autopsy revealed sarcoid granulomas throughout the myocardium.[28]

The cumulative clinical manifestations in a cohort of 75 patients with sarcoidosis in the International PGA Registry are presented in Fig. 35–5. In *NOD2*-associated sarcoidosis, the majority of patients display a typical clinical triad of skin, joint, and eye involvement, but incomplete forms and extended manifestations are observed (see Fig. 35–5A). Conversely, a tremendous heterogeneity in clinical manifestations is seen in sarcoidosis with wild-type *NOD2*, although specific subgroups may be identified (see Fig. 35–5B).

Secondary Granulomatous Inflammatory Diseases

Children with primary immunodeficiency disorders can develop granulomatous inflammation without an identifiable infectious cause. These granulomas have been

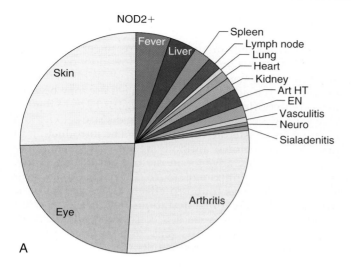

A

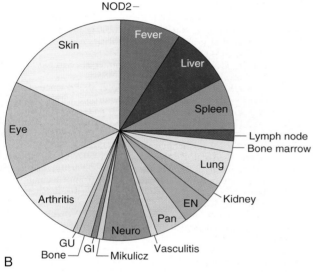

B

FIGURE 35–5 Cumulative clinical manifestations in 75 patients with pediatric sarcoidosis recruited through the International PGA Registry. **A,** The large majority of patients with *NOD2*-associated sarcoidosis display a clinical triad with skin, joint, and eye involvement, although incomplete forms and extended manifestations exist. **B,** A large heterogeneity of clinical manifestations is typical of sarcoidosis with wild-type *NOD2*.

described in association with ataxia telangiectasia, common variable immunodeficiency, Wiscott-Aldrich syndrome, chronic granulomatous disease, Ig-A deficiency, X-linked hypogammaglobulinemia, and severe combined immunodeficiency. The mechanism is unknown, and the extent of organ involvement varies, although lymphatic nodes, skin, lung, liver, and spleen are reportedly the main sites involved.[47,48] The etiology of granulomas in children with primary immunodeficiencies remains to be elucidated; immunohistochemical studies have documented a predominance of CD8+ T cells and a lower CD4+/CD8+ ratio in these granulomas as compared to the findings in sarcoidosis.[49]

A rare form of chronic granulomatous cheilitis in children with noncaseating giant cell granulomas in the inflammatory infiltrate is considered a monosymptomatic variant of the Melkersson-Rosenthal syndrome, a granulomatous disorder of unknown etiology comprising a triad of recurrent orofacial swelling, relapsing facial paralysis, and a fissured tongue.[50]

Granulomatous inflammation of the lungs, and less frequently lymph nodes, skin, and bone marrow, has been observed in patients receiving anti-TNF therapy for nongranulomatous inflammatory diseases. This is an emerging entity probably related to the anti-TNF agent, but is still poorly understood.[51,52]

DIAGNOSIS

Laboratory Parameters

There is no laboratory test diagnostic of sarcoidosis. The sedimentation rate and acute phase reactants reflect clinical disease activity. Peripheral blood cell counts are usually within normal limits, although mild anemia, leucopenia, or lymphopenia can be seen. Hypergammaglobulinemia is often present, but autoantibodies are absent. Elevation of angiotensin converting enzyme (ACE) is not consistent, and the value of serum ACE levels in diagnosing and managing sarcoidosis remains unclear. ACE levels are influenced by ACE-gene polymorphisms, and physiological values vary according to age with a higher normal range of serum values in children.[12] Hypercalciuria and hypercalcemia result from overproduction of 25-hydroxyvitamin D-1 α-hydroxylase, which converts 25-hydroxyvitamin D to 1,25 dihydroxyvitamin D, by sarcoid macrophages. Hypercalciuria can lead to nephrocalcinosis and nephrolithiasis.

Pathology

The diagnosis of sarcoidosis is confirmed by the finding of characteristic noncaseating epithelioid and giant cell granulomas, which can be documented in biopsies of skin, synovium, conjunctiva, lymph node, or any involved tissue. It has to be noted that asymptomatic granulomatous inflammation has been observed in various organs including liver, skeletal muscle, and myocardium.[29,42,46]

Genetic Testing

The published frequencies of *NOD2* mutation among patients exhibiting the clinical triad of dermatitis, arthritis, and uveitis vary between 50% in familial forms[16] and 90% in sporadic forms.[22] We found *NOD2* mutations in 98% of the patients of the International PGA Registry exhibiting the classic triad phenotype with either a sporadic or a familial form. The recent discovery of *NOD2* mutations in a few asymptomatic individuals of a large family, and the finding of extended clinical manifestations, suggest the interference of supplementary modulating genes in the clinical phenotype. The role for *NOD2* mutation analysis in the diagnosis of sarcoidosis in children remains to be established.

DIFFERENTIAL DIAGNOSIS

The diagnosis of sarcoidosis in a child with granulomatous inflammation requires a concerted effort to exclude chronic infections, notably mycobacteria and fungi, by appropriate staining and cultures. Various primary immunodeficiency disorders can present with granulomatous inflammation without an identifiable infectious cause, and should to be excluded by evaluation of neutrophil function and analysis of circulating lymphocyte subsets and serum levels of immunoglobulins.

Pediatric sarcoidosis needs to be differentiated from other systemic inflammatory disorders in children, such as CD, and necrotizing granulomatous vasculitides, notably Wegener granulomatosis, Churg-Strauss syndrome, and lymphomatoid granulomatosis. Wegener granulomatosis often is associated with granulomatous inflammation of the upper respiratory tract; careful examination of tissue will reveal signs of small-vessel vasculitis. CD can present with a wide array of extraintestinal manifestations seen in sarcoidosis, including erythema nodosum, uveitis, arthritis, and vasculitis.[53]

NOD2 mutation associated sarcoidosis bears resemblance to other causes of polyarthritis with uveitis in children, especially JIA and Behçet syndrome. The cutaneous rash in patients with the classical phenotype is commonly confused with atopic dermatitis or with ichthyosis vulgaris. The presence of fever and visceral involvement in *NOD2* associated sarcoidosis can evoke systemic onset JIA as well.[6]

PROGNOSIS

There are limited data on the outcome of *NOD2* mutation-associated sarcoidosis in children. EOS is reportedly not always a benign disease with possible dissemination and vital organ involvement occurring at a later stage.[28] Severe hypertension and visceral involvement, including glomerulonephritis with renal failure and interstitial pneumonitis, have been observed in patients from the International PGA Registry, indicating the necessity of careful surveillance throughout the disease course.[32] Ocular disease can be relentless and causes visual loss in more than one-third of patients. Uveitis severity is variable even among patients with the same *NOD2* substitution, suggesting the influence of additional genetic factors. Arthritis seems to be nondestructive, especially during the first years, but as the disease progresses, flexion deformities, camptodactyly, and erosions can be observed. The outcome of pediatric sarcoidosis with wild-type *NOD2* is very variable. The large majority of patients with adult-type sarcoidosis enter into remission within 2.2 (0.5 to 5.9) years after disease onset. On the other hand, chronic active inflammation and organ damage involving lung, eye, CNS, and/or kidney have been noted in up to one-fifth of patients. The outcome is worse in patients with severe lung/organ involvement at presentation, multiorgan involvement, CNS, or eye disease.[38]

Infantile-onset panniculitis with systemic granulomatosis is a separate entity with a potentially fatal course; two out of six affected children died before age 15 because of widespread visceral organ inflammation.[8]

TREATMENT

Evidence-based data on the optimal treatment of pediatric sarcoidosis are scarce. Moderate- to low-dose daily corticosteroid therapy is effective to control uveitis and joint disease, but the side effects of prolonged use may become unacceptable. Methotrexate at a dosage of 10 to 15 mg/m2 once weekly is effective in suppressing disease activity and allowing corticosteroid tapering.[54,55] The introduction of anti-TNF monoclonal antibody agents may constitute a major therapeutic advance in the treatment of pediatric sarcoidosis.[56,57] Infliximab (5 to 10 mg/kg every four to eight weeks) was found to effectively control chronic arthritis and visceral manifestations; however. the effect on uveitis activity may be less convincing.[7] The experience with IL-1 antagonists (e.g., Anakinra) is minimal and associated with variable results.[6,23]

REFERENCES

1. C. Miceli-Richard, S. Lesage, M. Rybojad, et al., CARD15 mutations in Blau syndrome, Nat. Genet. 29 (2001) 19–20.
2. E.B. Blau, Familial granulomatous arthritis, iritis, and rash, J. Pediatr. 107 (1985) 689–693.
3. A.F. North Jr., C.W. Fink, W.M. Gibson, et al., Sarcoid arthritis in children, Am. J. Med. 48 (1970) 449–455.
4. N. Kanazawa, S. Matsushima, N. Kambe, et al., Presence of a sporadic case of systemic granulomatosis syndrome with a CARD15 mutation, J. Invest. Dermatol. 122 (2004) 851–852.
5. C.D. Rosé, T.M. Doyle, G. McIlvain-Simpson, et al., Blau syndrome mutation of CARD15/NOD2 in sporadic early onset granulomatous arthritis, J. Rheumatol. 32 (2005) 373–375.
6. J.I. Aróstegui, C. Arnal, R. Merino, et al., NOD2 gene-associated pediatric granulomatous arthritis: clinical diversity, novel and recurrent mutations, and evidence of clinical improvement with interleukin-1 blockade in a Spanish cohort, Arthritis Rheum. 56 (2007) 3805–3813.
7. C.D. Rosé, C.H. Wouters, S. Meiorin, et al., Pediatric granulomatous arthritis: an international registry, Arthritis Rheum. 54 (2006) 3337–3344.
8. C.H. Wouters, T.M. Martin, D. Stichweh, et al., Infantile onset panniculitis with uveitis and systemic granulomatosis: a new clinicopathologic entity, J. Pediatr. 151 (2007) 707–709.
9. K.E. Byg, N. Milman, S. Hansen, Sarcoidosis in Denmark 1980-1994. A registry-based incidence study comprising 5536 patients, Sarcoidosis Vasc. Diffuse Lung Dis. 20 (2003) 46–52.
10. A.L. Hoffmann, N. Milman, K.E. Byg, Childhood sarcoidosis in Denmark 1979-1994: incidence, clinical features and laboratory results at presentation in 48 children, Acta. Pediatr. 93 (2004) 30–36.
11. C.B. Lindsley, R.E. Petty, Overview and report on international registry of sarcoid arthritis in childhood, Curr. Rheumatol. 2 (2000) 343–348.
12. C. Wouters, C. Rosé, A.M. Prieur, Rhumatologie pédiatrique, Flammarion Médecine-Sciences, Paris, 2009.
13. G. Tromp, H. Kuivaniemi, S. Raphael, et al., Genetic linkage of familial granulomatous inflammatory arthritis, skin rash, and uveitis to chromosome 16, Am. J. Hum. Genet. 59 (1996) 1097–1107.
14. J. Cavanaugh, International collaboration provides convincing linkage replication in complex disease through analysis of a large pooled data set: Crohn's Disease and chromosome 16, Am. J. Hum. Genet. 68 (2001) 1165–1171.
15. J.P. Hugot, M. Chamaillard, H. Zouali, et al., Association of NOD2 leucine-rich repeat variants with susceptibility to Crohn's disease, Nature 411 (2001) 599–603.
16. X. Wang, H. Kuivaniemi, G. Bonavita, et al., CARD15 mutations in familial granulomatosis syndromes: a study of the original Blau syndrome kindred and other families with large-vessel arteritis and cranial neuropathy, Arthritis Rheum. 46 (2002) 3041–3045.
17. B.A. Rybicki, M.J. Maliarik, C.H. Bock, et al., The Blau syndrome gene is not a major risk factor for sarcoidosis, Sarcoidosis Vasc. Diffuse Lung Dis. 16 (1999) 203–208.

18. M. Schürmann, R. Valentonyte, J. Hampe, et al., CARD15 gene mutations in sarcoidosis, Eur. Respir. J. 22 (2003) 748–754.

19. N. Inohara, G. Nunez, NODS: Intracellular Proteins involved in inflammation and apoptosis, Nature Reviews 3 (2003) 371–382.

20. N. Inohara, M. Chamaillard, C. McDonald, et al., NOD-LRR Proteins: Role in Host-microbial interactions and inflammatory disease, Annu. Rev. Biochem. 74 (2005) 355–383.

21. M. Chamaillard, D. Philpott, S.E. Girardin, et al., Gene-environment interaction modulated by allelic heterogeneity in inflammatory diseases, Proc. Natl. Acad. Sci. USA 100 (2003) 3455–3460.

22. N. Kanazawa, I. Okafuji, N. Kambe, et al., Early-onset sarcoidosis and CARD15 mutations with constitutive nuclear factor-kappaB activation: common genetic etiology with Blau syndrome, Blood 105 (2005) 1195–1197.

23. T.M. Martin, Z. Zhang, P. Kurz, et al., The NOD2 defect in Blau syndrome does not result in excess interleukin 1 activity, Arthritis Rheum. 60 (2009) 611–618.

24. C. Agostini, A. Meneghin, G. Semenzato, T lymphocytes and cytokines in sarcoidosis, Curr. Opin. Pulm. Med. 8 (2002) 435–440.

25. S.M. Meiorin, G. Espada, C.E. Costa, et al., Granulomatous nephritis associated with R334Q mutation in NOD2, J. Rheumatol. 34 (2007) 1945–1947.

26. C. Wouters, D. Rosé, Childhood sarcoidosis, in: R. Cimaz, T. Lehman (Eds.), Pediatrics in systemic autoimmune diseases, vol. 6, Handbook of systemic autoimmune diseases, Elsevier, Amsterdam, 2008.

26a. C.B. Lindsley, W.A. Godfrey, Childhood sarcoidosis manifesting as juvenile rheumatoid arthritis. Pediatrics 76 (1985) 765–768.

27. M.L. Becker, T.M. Martin, T.M. Doyle, et al., Interstitial pneumonitis in Blau syndrome with documented mutation in CARD 15, Arthritis Rheum. 56 (2007) 1292–1294.

28. C.W. Fink, R. Cimaz, Early onset sarcoidosis: not a benign disease, J. Rheumatol. 24 (1997) 174–177.

29. S.K. Saini, C.D. Rosé, Liver involvement in familial granulomatous arthritis (Blau syndrome), J. Rheumatol. 23 (1996) 396–399.

30. S.S. Ting, J. Ziegler, E. Fischer, Familial granulomatous arthritis (Blau syndrome) with granulomatous renal lesions, J. Pediatr. 133 (1998) 450–452.

31. D.A. Jabs, J.L. Houk, W.B. Bias, et al., Familial granulomatous synovitis, uveitis, and cranial neuropathies, Am. J. Med. 78 (1985) 801–804.

32. C.D. Rosé, J.I. Aróstegui, T.M. Martin, et al., NOD2-Associated Pediatric Granulomatous Arthritis (PGA): an Expanding Phenotype. A Study of an International Registry and a National Cohort, Arthritis Rheum. 60 (2009) 1797–1803.

33. D. Rotenstein, D.L. Gibbas, B. Majmudar, et al., Familial granulomatous arteritis with polyarthritis of juvenile onset, N. Engl. J. Med. 306 (1982) 86–90.

34. K.R. Gross, P.N. Malleson, G. Culham, et al., Vasculopathy with renal artery stenosis in a child with sarcoidosis, J. Pediatr. 108 (1986) 724–726.

35. A. Gedalia, A.K. Shetty, K. Ward, et al., Abdominal aortic aneurysm associated with childhood sarcoidosis, J. Rheumatol. 23 (1996) 757–759.

36. F. Saulsbury, C.H. Wouters, T. Martin, et al., Incomplete penetrance of the NOD2 E383K substitution among members of a Pediatric Granulomatous Arthritis pedigree, Arthritis Rheum. 60 (2009) 1804–1806.

37. E.N. Pattishall, E.L. Kendig, Sarcoidosis in children, Pediatr. Pulmonol. 22 (1996) 195–203.

38. N. Milman, A.L. Hoffmann, Childhood sarcoidosis: long-term follow up, Eur. Respir. J. 31 (2008) 592–598.

39. N. Thelier, C. Assous, Job-Deslandre, et al., Osteoarticular involvement in a series of 100 patients with sarcoidosis referred to rheumatology departments, J. Rheumatol. 35 (2008) 1622–1628.

40. R.J. Baumann, W.C. Robertson Jr., Neurosarcoid presents differently in children than in adults, Pediatr. 112 (2003) e480–e486.

41. R. Coutant, B. Leroy, P. Niaudet, et al., Renal granulomatous sarcoidosis in childhood: a report of 11 cases and a review of the literature, Eur. J. Pediatr. 158 (1999) 154–159.

42. F. Fayad, F. Liote, F. Berenbaum, et al., Muscle involvement in sarcoidosis: a retrospective and followup studies, J. Rheumatol. 33 (2006) 98–103.

43. M.M. Jamal, A.M. Cilursu, E.L. Hoffman, Sarcoidosis presenting as acute myositis. Report and review of the literature, J. Rheumatol. 15 (1988) 1868–1871.

44. G.A. Rossi, E. Battistini, M.E. Celle, et al., Long-lasting myopathy as a major clinical feature of sarcoidosis in a child: case report with a 7-year follow-up, Sarcoidosis Vasc. Diffuse Lung Dis. 18 (2001) 196–200.

45. E.N. Pattishall, G.L. Strope, S.M. Spinola, et al., Childhood sarcoidosis, J. Pediatr. 108 (1986) 169–177.

46. K.J. Silverman, G.M. Hutchins, B.H. Bulkley, Cardiac sarcoid: a clinicopathologic study of 84 unselected patients with systemic sarcoidosis, Circulation 58 (1978) 1204–1211.

47. L.J. Mechanic, S. Dikman, C. Cunningham-Rundles, Granulomatous disease in common variable immunodeficiency, Ann. Intern. Med. 127 (1997) 613–617.

48. D.F. Arnold, J. Wiggins, C. Cunningham-Rundles, et al., Granulomatous disease: distinguishing primary antibody disease from sarcoidosis, Clin. Immunol. 128 (2008) 18–22.

49. M. de Jager, W. Blokx, A. Warris, et al., Immunohistochemical features of cutaneous granulomas in primary immunodeficiency disorders: a comparison with cutaneous sarcoidosis, J. Cutan. Pathol. 35 (2008) 467–472.

50. M.R. Greene, R.S. Rogers III, Melkersson-Rosenthal syndrome, J. Am. Acad. Dermatol. 21 (1989) 1263–1270.

51. E. Toussirot, E. Pertuiset, B. Kantelip, et al., Sarcoidosis occuring during anti-TNF-alpha treatment for inflammatory rheumatic diseases: report of two cases, Clin. Exp. Rheumatol. 26 (2008) 471–475.

52. M. Ramos-Casals, P. Brito-Zerón, M.J. Soto, et al., Autoimmune diseases induced by TNF-targeted therapies, Best Pract. Res. Clin. Rheumatol. 22 (2008) 847–861.

53. C.D. Rosé, T.M. Martin: Caspase recruitment domain 15 mutations and rheumatic diseases, Curr. Opin. Rheumatol. 17 (2005) 579–585.

54. M.C. Ianuzzi, B.A. Rybicki, A.S. Teirstein, Sarcoidosis, NEJM 357 (2007) 2153–2165.

55. R.P. Baughman, D.B. Winget, E.E. Lower, Methotrexate is steroid sparing in acute sarcoidosis: results of a double blind, randomized trial, Sarcoidosis Vasc. Diffuse Lung Dis. 17 (2000) 60–66.

56. A.M. Brescia, G. McIlvain-Simpson, C.D. Rosé, Infliximab therapy for steroid-dependent early onset sarcoid arthritis and Blau syndrome, Arthritis Rheum. 46 (2002) S313.

57. N. Milman, C.B. Andersen, A. Hansen, et al., Favourable effect of TNF-alpha inhibitor (infliximab) on Blau syndrome in monozygotic twins with a de novo CARD15 mutation, APMIS 114 (2006) 912–919.

Chapter 36

BEHÇET DISEASE

Seza Ozen and Ross E. Petty

In 1937, the Turkish dermatologist Hulusi Behçet[1] described the vasculitis syndrome that bears his name: the triad of aphthous stomatitis, genital ulceration, and uveitis. Superficial thrombophlebitis was identified as the fourth criterion in 1946.[2] Matteson[3] identified even earlier reports of this condition, including those from Japan. The geographical distribution of disease prevalence retraces the historical route of the Silk Road from Japan to the eastern edge of the Mediterranean Sea and through areas of the Ottoman Empire.[4] However, Behçet disease (BD) is by no means confined to these areas and reflects emigration patterns in the 20th century. The history of BD has been reviewed by Kaklamani and colleagues.[5]

DEFINITION AND CLASSIFICATION

There is no unanimous agreement about the definition of this syndrome, and several sets of diagnostic criteria have been proposed. Those of the International Study Group (ISG)[6] (Table 36–1) are most widely used. If only one of the criteria is present along with oral ulcerations, the term *incomplete or partial Behçet disease* is applied. Criteria proposed by Mason and Barnes[7] (Table 36–2) emphasize the broader spectrum of disease. The ISG criteria have a specificity of 96% and sensitivity of 91%; the Mason and Barnes criteria have a specificity of 84% and sensitivity of 86%.[8] Both have been applied to the diagnosis of BD in children, although neither has been validated.

EPIDEMIOLOGY

Incidence and Prevalence

The frequency of BD varies widely from one geographical area and ethnic group to another. It is most common in Japan, Turkey, and other parts of the Middle East, where Ozen and coworkers[9] have proposed that the prevalence is less than 10 cases per 100,000 children. In contrast, the frequency of BD in French children younger than 15-years-old is approximately one case in 600,000.[10] It may be underrecognized, however, and a recent report from France showed that among adult vasculitides, BD was much more common than had previously been appreciated, occurring at a higher frequency than other rare vasculitides.[11]

Age at Onset and Sex Ratio

The age at onset of disease ranges widely (Table 36–3), and BD has been reported in neonates born to mothers with BD.[12-15] The mean age at onset in children in one large study was just over 12 years old. Several reviews document BD in childhood and adolescence.[10,16-25] There have also been series reported from Saudi Arabia,[19] Turkey,[20] Korea,[21] Italy,[22] Japan,[23] and Israel.[16, 24] Overall, 5.4% to 13% of all patients have onset of BD in childhood.[16,22,25]

In most series, boys and girls are affected with equal frequency,[10,16] and BD is reported to be more common in women in Japan but more common in men in the Middle East.[5]

GENETIC BACKGROUND

The higher frequency of BD in Japan and the countries of the Middle East and the high frequency of familial occurrence suggest that there may be a genetic or environmental component to the disease. A recent study reported that the rate of BD among North African immigrants in France was comparable with rates reported from North Africa and Asia. These results support a genetic basis for the disease.[11] A study of adult Turkish patients showed that the risk of the sibling of a patient with BD also having BD was 4.2%.[26] In an international study of BD in European children,[27] 15% had parents or siblings with the disease. An autosomal recessive mode of inheritance has been suggested in children.[28]

The strongest genetic marker in BD is the human leukocyte antigen (HLA) B*5101.[29] In healthy populations of most ethnic origins, the frequency of HLA B51 is around 20%; in BD, it is increased to 50% to 80%.[29] It is likely that B51 confers significant risk of BD (relative risk, 6.3 to 6.44), particularly in patients with a family history of the disease,[30] but only approximately 20% of the risk in siblings can be attributed to B51.[31] MHC class-I related chain (MHC-A) alleles[32] and another locus, DF6S285, may be important in explaining the occurrence of BD in HLA B51 negative subjects.[31] Karasneh and colleagues have reported many other putative susceptibility loci in a genome-wide linkage study.[33]

Table 36–1

Criteria of the International Study Group for the diagnosis of Behçet disease

Criterion	Description
Recurrent oral ulceration	Minor aphthous, major aphthous, or herpetiform ulceration recurring at least three times in one 12-month period, observed by physician or patient
Plus two of the following:	
Recurrent genital ulcers	Aphthous ulceration or scarring observed by physician or patient
Eye lesions	Anterior uveitis, posterior uveitis, cells in vitreous on slit-lamp examination, or retinal vasculitis observed by an ophthalmologist
Skin lesions	Erythema nodosum observed by physician or patient, pseudofolliculitis or papulopustular lesions, or acneiform nodules observed by physician in post-adolescent patient not on corticosteroid treatment
Pathergy	Skin reaction to a needleprick observed by physician at 24 to 48 hr

From International Study Group for Behçet's Disease: Criteria for diagnosis of Behçet's disease, *Lancet* 335:1070-1080, 1990.[6]

Table 36–2

Mason and Barnes criteria for a diagnosis of Behçet disease

Major Criteria*	Minor Criteria
Buccal ulceration	Cardiovascular lesions
Gastrointestinal lesions	Arthritis
Genital ulceration	Central nervous system lesions
Thrombophlebitis	Family history of Behçet disease
Eye lesions	
Skin lesions	

*Diagnosis requires the presence of at least three major criteria or two major plus two minor criteria.
From Mason RM, Barnes CG: Behçet's syndrome with arthritis, *Ann Rheum Dis* 28:95-103, 1969.[7]

Despite clinical similarities of BD to some of the autoinflammatory diseases, a search for genes associated with mevalonic kinase deficiency (MVK1 gene), PAPA syndrome (PSTP1P1 gene), and cryopyrin-associated periodic syndromes (CIAS1 gene) showed no increased frequency in patients with BD.[34] On the other hand, Touitou and colleagues have shown that mutations in the gene for Familial Mediterranean Fever (FMF) were more frequent among patients with BD, suggesting that they may act as additional susceptibility factors in BD.[35]

ETIOLOGY AND PATHOGENESIS

The cause of BD is unknown. Evidence for a microbial cause of BD is reviewed by Verity and colleagues.[36] It is speculated that a microbial agent (Herpes simplex Virus 1, Parvo B19, and streptococcus) is responsible for inducing an aberrant immune response in a genetically predisposed individual. The role of heat shock proteins has been recently reviewed.[37] The γ/δ T cells from patients with BD are highly responsive to four peptides from the human 60-kD heat-shock protein compared with healthy controls, patients with systemic illnesses, or patients with recurrent oral ulcers but no other manifestations of the disease.[38]

Neutrophils and the inflammation mediated by the innate immune system play a major role in BD. Hyperactive neutrophils are characteristic of BD and HLA B51 transgenic mice.[39] The involvement of the innate immune system, the absence of autoimmune features, and the episodic nature of the disease course has led to the classification of BD as an autoinflammatory disease of multifactorial origin.[40] That an antibody-mediated process may be responsible is suggested by the observation of transient neonatal BD in the offspring of mothers with the disorder.[12-15]

CLINICAL MANIFESTATIONS

The clinical manifestations of BD are varied and often emerge asynchronously over several years. In a study of 40 Korean children, the mean interval between the first and the second major manifestations was seven years.[21] The usual course of BD in any organ system is that of exacerbations and remissions, with the overall activity generally declining with time. The frequencies of the major and minor manifestations are given in Table 36–3.

Mucocutaneous Disease

Oral and Genital Ulcerations

Most children with BD (around 87%)[16] have oral ulcerations; it usually occurs at disease onset and may persist for much of the course of the disease.[10,16,23,24] Crops of extremely painful ulcers, usually indistinguishable from canker sores appear on the lips, tongue, palate, and elsewhere in the gastrointestinal tract (Fig. 36–1). They last for three to 10 days (sometimes longer), recur at various intervals, and usually heal without scarring. The exception to this is neonatal disease, in which extensive scarring may result.[12] Minor ulcers (<10 mm) are most common. Major aphthae (1 to 3 cm) are uncommon, but they may scar. Herpetiform ulcers are rare, very small, and multiple. Recurrent, painful ulcerations of the scrotum, and, less commonly, the glans penis, prepuce, and perianal area in the male and of the vulva and vagina in the female are more common after puberty, but much less common than oral ulcers. The ulcerations occurred in 6% in one large series.[16] These ulcers usually occur after oral ulcers and, unlike the oral ulcers, may scar with healing.

Skin Lesions

A variety of skin lesions occur in more than 90% of children with BD.[10,24] These include erythema nodosum, papulopustular (acneiform) lesions, folliculitis, purpura, and, rarely, ulcers.[24,25] Pathergy, an unusual cutaneous

Table 36–3

Behçet disease in childhood

Study	N	M:F	Onset (yr)	OU	GU	Skin	Uveitis Pathergy
Lang et al[17]	37	19:18	8.7	100	75	84*	30	?
Bahabri et al[19]	12	7:5	11.5	100	65	83*	92	57
Koné-Paut et al[10]	65	33:32	8.4	100	96	92*	45	80
Eldem et al[20]	20	15:5	15.1	100	65	35*	80	?
Kim et al[21]	40	16:24	10.6	100	82	72*	27	?
Pivetti-Pezzi et al[22]	16	9:7						
Fujikawa and Suemitsu[23]	31	14:17						
Uziel et al[24]	15	7:8	6.6*	100	33	100*	53	40
Karincaoglu et al[16]	83	38:45	12.3	100	82	**	35	37

*Includes pathergy
**Includes erythema nodosum (51%) and papulopustular lesions (50.5%)
GU, genital ulceration; M:F, sex ratio; OU, oral ulceration

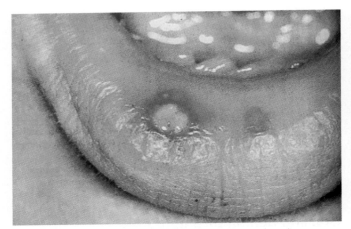

FIGURE 36–1 Oral aphthous lesion in a girl with Behçet disease.

pustular reaction occurring 24 to 48 hours after a sterile 20 gauge needle puncture of the dermis, is highly characteristic but not pathognomonic of the syndrome.[41] Pathergy test positivity varies considerably in frequency from one series to another and occurs most commonly (50% to 70%) in patients from the Middle East.[5]

Ocular Disease

Eye lesions occur in 30% to 61% of children with BD.[10,19-24] The most common ocular complication is uveitis: panuveitis in 54%, posterior uveitis in 29%, isolated anterior uveitis in 15%, and intermediate uveitis in 2%.[10,20,42-44] The disease is bilateral in 75%.[10,20,42-44] Uveitis occurs almost three times more frequently in boys than in girls.[10,20,42-44] The eye may be painful and red. The course tends to be characterized by frequent relapses. Hypopyon may occur, and severe uveitis may lead to blindness; however, currently most reports document improved visual outcome with treatment.[42,43] Complications of uveitis may include glaucoma and cataracts. Corneal ulceration, cystoid macular degeneration, retinal vasculitis, retinal detachment, and retrobulbar neuritis are rare events.

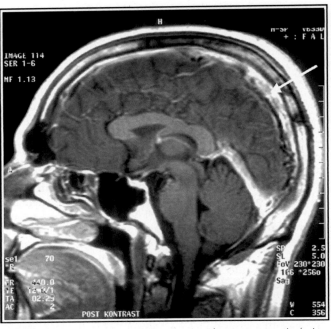

FIGURE 36–2 Magnetic resonance imaging demonstrates sagittal sinus thrombosis in a patient with Behçet disease. (Courtesy of Dr. A. Dinc.)

Central Nervous System Disease

The reported frequency of central nervous system (CNS) disease in children with BD varies from 5% to 15%.[10,16,23,24] It may be parenchymal or nonparenchymal (vascular).[45] Meningoencephalitis with headache, stiff neck, focal neurological abnormalities, and pleocytosis of the cerebrospinal fluid are common. However, the findings are diverse, and three other neurological syndromes are recognized in patients with BD[46]: encephalomyelitis (e.g., pyramidal, extrapyramidal, cerebellar, spinal cord abnormalities, seizures), benign intracranial hypertension (e.g., pseudotumor cerebri, papilledema, dural sinus thrombosis) (Fig. 36–2), and organic psychiatric disturbances (e.g., psychoses, depression, dementia). Several of these manifestations may occur simultaneously. The subject has been comprehensively reviewed by Al Araji and Kidd.[47]

Musculoskeletal Disease

Arthritis occurs in 50%[10] to 75%[24] of children with BD. It most commonly affects the knees, ankles, wrists, and elbows, but may occur in other joints as well.[10,24] The disease is usually oligoarticular, but polyarthritis is observed in at least one third of patients.[10] The disease does not usually result in erosions or joint destruction. There is probably no association of BD with sacroiliac arthritis, at least in childhood.[10,48]

Acute, localized myositis is uncommon, is rarely multifocal, and has been reported in only a few children.[17,24] It may be confused with vasculitis or venous thrombosis, especially when it affects the gastrocnemius muscle.[17,49] Generalized myositis may also occur, and both forms are reviewed by Sarui and associates.[50]

Vascular Disease

Adamantiades[2] recognized the importance of vasculitis in BD, which is the only vasculitis that involves both the arterial and venous systems. It is characteristically associated with arterial or venous thromboses and aneurysms or occlusions in arteries of any size. Superficial or deep-vein thromboses are common in adults, but occur only in 5% to 15% of children.[10] Most thromboses develop in veins, especially those of the lower extremities. A prothrombotic state has been demonstrated in BD.[51] Arteritis and arterial aneurysms may occur,[52-54] and involvement of the pulmonary artery and central retinal artery has been reported.[10] Pulmonary artery thrombosis is rare, but it is one of the most severe features of the disease and is associated with high morbidity and mortality rates.[55,56] Patients who develop superficial thrombophlebitis are more likely to develop major venous occlusions, and they must be carefully monitored. Although rare in childhood, vascular involvement is a major cause of morbidity and mortality.[57] Dilatation and dropout of periungual capillaries were reported in 75% of adults in one study.[58]

Uncommon Manifestations

Gastrointestinal Disease

Gastrointestinal manifestations (diarrhea, abdominal pain) are characterized by exacerbations and remissions. Ulceration of the ileum, cecum, and colon[10,23,24] is present. Gastrointestinal tract lesions may be indistinguishable from those of Crohn Disease or ulcerative colitis. Hepatic vein occlusion may result in Budd-Chiari syndrome.[59,60]

Renal Disease

Renal involvement is probably more common than was initially recognized. The most common manifestations are amyloidosis (occurring in patients as young as 13-years-old). In a survey of 253 adult patients with renal BD, 43% had amyloidosis, 35% glomerulonephritis, 13% renal artery aneurysms or stenosis, 12% microvascular or interstitial disease, and 5% renal vein thrombosis.[61]

Other Uncommon Manifestations

A number of cardiac complications (e.g., endocarditis, myocarditis, pericarditis, dysrhythmias) have been reported in adults but are rare in children. Dilatation of the proximal aorta, interatrial septal aneurysm, mitral valve prolapse, and mitral valve regurgitation were the most common abnormalities reported in one survey.[62] Pulmonary disease, most commonly thrombosis, has been reviewed by Erkan and colleagues.[63] Deafness has been reported in adults with BD.[64]

PATHOLOGY

The underlying pathological lesion of BD is an occlusive vasculitis in arterioles and veins. In the skin, the lesions may be necrotizing but do not exhibit fibrinoid degeneration.[6] Inflammation in the synovium is nonspecific with a predominantly neutrophil infiltration. Muscle biopsies have demonstrated a wide range of abnormalities from perivascular infiltrates and fibrosis[17] to muscle necrosis.[65]

There is some controversy regarding the histopathology of the pathergy reaction. A serial study of the lesion revealed a superficial and deep perivascular mixed inflammatory cell infiltrate, with neutrophils peaking at 24 hours.[66] True vasculitis was not present. However, leukocytoclastic vasculitis and a neutrophilic vascular reaction with endothelial swelling has also been reported.[47]

LABORATORY EXAMINATION

No laboratory findings are diagnostic of BD. There is a generalized increase in acute phase reactants with active disease. The frequencies of antinuclear antibodies, anticardiolipin antibodies, rheumatoid factors, and antibodies to neutrophil cytoplasmic antigens are probably not increased, but antibodies to ocular antigens[67] and *Saccharomyces cerevisiae*[68] have been observed.

There appears to be a procoagulant state in BD, although the question is not entirely resolved The often conflicting data are reviewed by Kiraz and colleagues[51] and suggest possible abnormalities in levels of coagulation factors and fibrinolysis coupled with endothelial cell damage. Elevated von Willebrand factor antigen levels and decreased thrombomodulin levels are associated with vasculitis and active disease. Increased serum levels of tumor necrosis factor (TNF) α[69] and soluble TNF-α receptors[70] may serve as markers of active disease. The pathogenic significance of elevated interleukins and the association of certain cytokine polymorphisms with BD requires further evaluation.

Neutrophils are prominent infiltrating cells in the skin, synovium, and eye lesions of BD, and inconsistent abnormalities of their function have been reported. Carletto and colleagues[71] studied neutrophil function in 15 adults and found that although superoxide production and adhesion were normal, migration was significantly increased in patients with active disease compared with those with inactive disease or with controls. Enhanced migration into inflammatory sites facilitates their participation in the leukocytoclastic vasculitis or neutrophilic vasculitis that may occur in BD and may be at least partly responsible for pathergy. In other studies,[72] levels of reactive oxygen species were increased. Synovial fluid analysis is characterized by a predominance of neutrophils in relatively low numbers (<15,000/mm^3 [<15 × 10^9/L]) and low glucose levels but no other distinguishing features.[73]

IMAGING STUDIES

CNS lesions are evaluated by angiography and magnetic resonance imaging (MRI) (see Fig. 36–2). MRI is less accurate for imaging smaller arteries.[74] In a study of 98 adult patients,[75] brainstem or basal ganglia lesions were demonstrated, especially during an attack. Similar findings were evident by single photon emission computed tomography.[76] MRI changes in muscle have been described.[49,50]

DIAGNOSIS

In general, aphthous stomatitis is the presenting sign of BD; other components of the syndrome may not appear for years. The diagnosis is principally clinical, with laboratory tests supplying only supporting evidence. The differential diagnosis includes inflammatory bowel disease, aphthous stomatitis, and erythema nodosum. Posterior uveitis is more common in BD than in inflammatory bowel disease.

TREATMENT

BD is difficult to treat, and therapy depends largely on the site and severity of involvement. There are no controlled studies evaluating treatment of BD in children, and physicians must therefore depend on the experience gained in treating adults. Yazici and colleagues[45] suggest that young men have the worst prognosis and should be treated most aggressively. Arthritis is usually treated with colchicine or low doses of prednisone. The recent European League Against Rheumatism (EULAR) guidelines for the management of BD[77] is a carefully prepared consensus based on evidence and expert opinion. The recommendations discussed later reflect these guidelines, although they were not specifically developed for the treatment of childhood BD.

Oral and Genital Ulcers

Topical sucralfate or corticosteroids should be the first line of treatment for oral or genital ulcers.[78] During the acute stage of ulceration, a short course of oral prednisone helps provide fast relief.[77] A double-blind study enrolling adults with BD showed that colchicine significantly reduced the frequency of genital ulcers, erythema nodosum, and arthritis among women, and of arthritis among men.[79]

For severe ulceration, including intestinal ulceration, thalidomide is very effective.[80,81] A number of regimens have been used. An initial dose of thalidomide of 50 mg/day for adolescents is reduced to 50 mg twice per week if the patient responds. Alternatively, the drug may be started in a dose up to 1 mg/kg/day and tapered to 1 mg/kg taken two or three days each week. Peripheral neuropathy may be a limiting side effect of this drug, and thalidomide is a potent teratogen that must not be used in women of childbearing age without contraception. Dapsone (100 mg/day) has been reported to benefit the mucocutaneous lesions.[82]

Ocular Inflammation

All patients with BD should be followed by an experienced ophthalmologist. The EULAR guidelines[77] note that topical corticosteroids are widely used during acute flares, but that strong evidence to support their efficacy is lacking. Azathioprine (2 mg/kg/d) has been beneficial in trials surveyed in the Cochrane Controlled Trials Register[83] and is the recommended initial treatment for uveitis in BD.[77] The EULAR guidelines recommend that patients with inflammatory eye disease affecting the posterior segment should be treated with a combination of azathioprine and systemic corticosteroids. In patients with severe loss of visual acuity, retinal vasculitis, or macular involvement, the addition of cyclosporine or infliximab is recommended.[77] The results of treatment with cyclosporine alone (3-5 mg/kg/day for two years) in 16 patients was generally favorable, and complete clinical remission was attained in 14 patients within six months.[84] In a study of adults with intractable uveitis complicating BD, all seven responded to infliximab (3 mg/kg) in from seven days to three weeks and achieved remission after three infusions.[85] Combination therapy with azathioprine and interferon-α or methotrexate have been successful for severe uveitis.[77,86]

Treatment of Central Nervous System Disease

Parenchymal disease is treated with systemic corticosteroids (intravenous methylprednisolone followed by a tapering dose of oral prednisone).[47] Unresponsive or relapsing parenchymal CNS disease has been shown to respond to various immunosuppressive drugs and infliximab. CNS manifestations may reflect venous sinus or other vascular thrombosis, although there is no consensus about the use of anticoagulants.[77] Low-dose methotrexate[87] may be of some benefit.

COURSE OF THE DISEASE AND PROGNOSIS

BD tends to run a very long, relapsing course. Young age at onset and male gender are both indicators of a prolonged disease course. The ocular and CNS manifestations in particular can be extremely incapacitating.[24] The young child who presents with only recurrent oral mucocutaneous lesions may develop genital ulcerations and gastrointestinal tract disease during adolescence. Potentially fatal lesions include occlusion or aneurysms of arteries supplying the CNS or heart, pulmonary hemorrhage, and bowel perforation.[88] In a series of 65 children and adolescents, the mortality rate was 3%.[10]

REFERENCES

1. H. Behçet, Über rezidivierende Aphthöse, durch ein Virus verusachte Geschwüre am Mund, am Auge und an den Genitalien, Dermatol. Wochenschr. 105 (1937) 1151–1157.
2. B. Adamantiades, Le thrombophlébite comme quatriéme symptome de l'iritis récidivante à hypopyon, Ann. Ocul. (Paris) 179 (1946) 143–148.
3. E.L. Matteson, Notes on the history of eponymic idiopathic vasculitis: the diseases of Henoch and Schönlein, Wegener, Churg and Strauss, Horton, Takayasu, Behçet, and Kawasaki, Arthritis Clin. Res. 13 (2000) 237–245.
4. N. Dilsen, History and development of Behçet's disease, Rev. Rhum. (Engl. Ed.) 63 (1996) 512–519.
5. V.G. Kaklamani, G. Vaiopoulos, P.G. Kaklamanis, Behçet's disease, Semin. Arthritis Rheum. 27 (1998) 197–217.
6. International Study Group for Behçet's Disease, Criteria for diagnosis of Behçet's disease, Lancet 335 (1990) 1070–1080.
7. R.M. Mason, C.G.L. Barnes, Behçet's syndrome with arthritis, Ann. Rheum. Dis. 28 (1969) 95–103.
8. A.S. Rigby, M.A. Chamberlain, B. Bhakta, Classification and assessment of rheumatic diseases. Part I. Behçet's disease, Baillieres Clin. Rheumatol. 9 (1995) 375–395.
9. S. Ozen, Y. Karaaslan, O. Ozdemir, et al., Prevalence of juvenile chronic arthritis and Familial Mediterranean Fever in Turkey. A field study, J. Rheumatol. 25 (1998) 2445–2449.
10. I. Koné-Paut, S. Yurdakul, S.A. Bahabri, et al., Epidemiological features of Behçet's syndrome in children: an international collaborative survey of 86 cases, J. Pediatr. 132 (1998) 721–725.
11. A. Mahr, L. Belarbi, B. Wechsler, et al., Population based prevalence study of Behçet's disease: Differences by Ethnic origin and low variation by age at immigration, Arthritis Rheum. 58 (2008) 3951–3959.
12. A.G. Fam, K.A. Siminovitch, S. Carette, et al., Neonatal Behçet's syndrome in an infant of a mother with the disease, Ann. Rheum. Dis. 40 (1981) 509–512.
13. M.A. Lewis, B.L. Priestly, Transient neonatal Behçet's disease, Arch. Dis. Child 61 (1986) 805–806.
14. A.C. Stark, B. Bhakta, M.A. Chamberlain, et al., Life-threatening transient neonatal Behçet's disease, Br. J. Rheumatol. 36 (1997) 700–702.
15. P.S. Wu, H.L. Chen, Y.M. Jeng, et al., Intestinal Behçet disease presenting as neonatal onset chronic diarrhea in an 11-month-old baby, Eur. J. Pediatr. 164 (2005) 523–525.
16. Y. Karincaoglu, M. Borlu, S. Toker, et al., Demographic and clinical properties of juvenile-onset Behçet's disease: a controlled multicenter study, J. Am. Acad. Dermatol. 58 (2008) 597–584.
17. B.A. Lang, R.M. Laxer, P. Thorner, et al., Pediatric onset of Behçet's syndrome with myositis: case report and literature review illustrating unusual features, Arthritis Rheum. 33 (1990) 418–425.
18. G. Vaiopoulos, V.G. Kaklamani, N. Markomichelakis, et al., Clinical features of juvenile Adamantiades-Behçet's disease in Greece, Clin. Exp. Rheumatol. 17 (1999) 256–259.
19. S.A. Bahabri, A. Al-Mazyed, S. Al-Balaa, et al., Juvenile Behçet's disease in Arab children, Clin. Exp. Rheumatol. 14 (1996) 331–335.
20. B. Eldem, C. Onur, S. Ozen, Clinical features of pediatric Behçet's disease, J. Pediatr. Ophthalmol. Strabismus 35 (1998) 159–161.
21. D.K. Kim, S.N. Chang, D. Bang, et al., Clinical analysis of 40 cases of childhood-onset Behçet's disease, Pediatr. Dermatol. 11 (1994) 95–101.
22. P. Pivetti-Pezzi, M. Accorinti, M.A. Abdulaziz, et al., Behçet's disease in children, Jpn. J. Ophthalmol. 39 (1995) 309–314.
23. S. Fujikawa, T. Suemitsu, Behçet disease in children: a nationwide retrospective survey in Japan, Acta Paediatr. Jpn. 39 (1997) 285–289.
24. Y. Uziel, R. Brik, S. Padeh, et al., Juvenile Behçet's disease in Israel, Clin. Exp. Rheumatol. 16 (1998) 502–505.
25. R. Sarica, G. Azizlerli, A. Kose, et al., Juvenile Behçet's disease among 1784 Turkish Behçet's patients, Int. J. Dermatol. 35 (1996) 109–111.
26. A. Gül, M. Insanü, L. Öcal, et al., Familial aggregation of Behçet's disease in Turkey, Ann. Rheum. Dis. 59 (2000) 622–625.
27. I. Koné-Paut, I. Geisler, B. Wechsler, et al., Familial aggregation in Behçet's disease, J. Pediatr. 135 (1999) 89–93.
28. N. Molinari, I. Kone-Paut, R. Manna, et al., Identification of an autosomal recessive mode of inheritance in paediatric Behçet's families by segregation analysis, Am. J. Med. Genet. A 122 (2001) 115–118.
29. K. Sano, K. Yabuki, Y. Imagawa, et al., The absence of disease-specific polymorphisms within the HLA-B51 gene that is the susceptible locus for Behçet's disease, Tissue Antigens 58 (2001) 77–82.
30. T. Chajek-Shaul, S. Pisanty, H. Knobler, et al., HLA-B51 may serve as an immunogenetic marker for a subgroup of patients with Behçet's syndrome, Am. J. Med. 83 (1987) 666–672.
31. A. Gul, A.H. Hajeer, J. Worthington, et al., Linkage mapping of a novel susceptibility locus for Behçet's disease to chromosome 6p22-23, Arthritis Rheum. 44 (2001) 2693–2696.
32. G.R. Wallace, D.H. Verity, L.J. Delamaine, et al., MHC-A allele profiles and HLA class I associations in Behçet's disease, Immunogenetics 49 (1999) 613–617.
33. J. Karasneh, A. Gul, W.E. Ollier, et al., Whole genome screening for susceptibility genes in multicase families with Behçet's disease, Arthritis Rheum. 52 (2005) 1836–1842.
34. I. Kone-Paut, E. Sanchez, A. LeQuellec, et al., Autoinflammatory gene mutations in Behçet's disease, Ann. Rheum. Dis. 66 (2007) 832–834.
35. I. Touitou, X. Magne, N. Molinari, et al., MEFV mutations in Behçet's disease, Hum. Mutat. 16 (2000) 271–272.
36. D.H. Verity, G.R. Wallace, R.W. Vaughan, et al., Behçet's disease: from Hippocrates to the third millennium, Br. J. Ophthalmol. 87 (2003) 1175–1183.
37. H. Direskeneli, G. Saruhan-Direskeneli, The role of heat shock proteins in Behçet's disease, Clin. Exp. Rheum. 21 (2003) S44–S48.
38. A. Hasan, F. Fortune, A. Wilson, et al., Role of gamma delta T cells in pathogenesis and diagnosis of Behçet's disease. Lancet 347 (1996) 1631–1632.
39. M. Takeno, A. Kariyone, N. Yamashita, et al., Excessive function of peripheral blood neutrophils from patients with Behçet's disease and from HLA-B51 transgenic mice, Arthritis Rheum. 38 (1995) 426–433.
40. S. Ozen, H.M. Hoffman, J. Frenkel, et al., Familial Mediterranean fever (FMF) and beyond: a new horizon, Ann. Rheum. Dis. 65 (2006) 961–964.
41. H. Yazici, Y. Tuzun, H. Pazarli, et al., The combined use of HLA-B5 and the pathergy test as diagnostic markers of Behçet's disease in Turkey, J. Rheumatol. 7 (1980) 206–210.
42. M. Kramer, R. Amer, M. Mukamel, et al., Uveitis in juvenile Behçet's disease: clinical course and visual outcome compared with adult patients, Eye (2009) 1–8 (e-publication).
43. R. Friling, M. Kramer, M. Snir, et al., Clinical course and outcome of uveitis in children, J. AAPOS 9 (2005) 379–382.
44. M.R. Kesen, D.A. Goldstein, H.H. Tessler, Uveitis associated with pediatric Behçet disease in the American Midwest, Am. J. Ophthalmol. 146 (2008) 819–827.
45. H. Yazici, S. Yurdakul, V. Hamuryudan, Behçet's syndrome, Curr. Opin. Rheumatol. 13 (2001) 18–22.
46. I. Koné-Paut, B. Chabrol, J.M. Riss, et al., Neurologic onset of Behçet's disease: a diagnostic enigma in childhood, J. Child Neurol. 12 (1997) 237–241.
47. A. Al-Araji, D.P. Kidd, Neuro-Behçet's disease: epidemiology, clinical characteristics and management, Lancet Neurol. 8 (2009) 192–203.
48. M.A. Chamberlain, R.J. Robertson, A controlled study of sacroiliitis in Behçet's disease, Br. J. Rheumatol. 32 (1993) 693–698.
49. G. Akansel, Y. Akgoz, E. Ciftci, et al., MRI findings of myositis in Behcet disease, Skeletal. Radiol. 33 (2004) 426–428.
50. H. Sarui, T. Maruyama, I. Ito, et al., Necrotising myositis in Behçet's disease: characteristic features on magnetic resonance imaging and a review of the literature, Ann. Rheum. Dis. 61 (2002) 751–752.

51. S. Kiraz, I. Ertenli, M.A. Ozturk, et al., Pathological haemostasis and "pro-thrombotic" state in Behcet's disease, Thrombosis Res. 105 (2002) 125–133.

52. V. Kutay, C. Yakut, H. Ekam, Rupture of the abdominal aorta in a 13-year-old girl secondary to Behçet disease. A case report, J. Vasc. Surg. 39 (2004) 901–902.

53. S.D. Cohl, T. Colby, Fatal hemoptysis from Behçet disease in a child, Cardiovasc. Pathol. 11 (2002) 296–299.

54. N. Besbas, E. Ozyurek, F. Balkanci, et al., Behçet disease with severe arterial involvement in a child, Clin. Rheumatol. 21 (2002) 176–179.

55. F. Erkan, Pulmonary involvement in Behçet disease, Curr. Opin. Pulm. Med. 5 (1999) 314–318.

56. R. Sarica, et al., Pulmonary artery involvement in Behçet's disease, Adv. Exp. Med. Biol. 528 (2003) 419–422.

57. H. Yazici, F. Esen, Mortality in Behçet's syndrome, Clin. Exp. Rheumatol. 26 (2008) S138–S140.

58. G. Vaiopoulos, N. Pangratis, M. Samarkos, et al., Nailfold capillary abnormalities in Behçet's disease, J. Rheumatol. 22 (1995) 1108–1111.

59. Y. Bayraktar, E. Ozaslan, D.H. van Thiel, Gastrointestinal manifestation of Behçet's disease, J. Clin. Gastroenterol. 30 (2000) 144–154.

60. I. Ben Ghorbel, R. Ennaifer, M. Lamloum, et al., Budd-Chiari syndrome associated with Behçet's disease, Gastroenterol. Clin. Biol. 32 (2008) 316–320.

61. T. Akpolat, M. Dilek, K. Aksu, et al., Renal Behçet's Disease: An update, Semin. Arthritis Rheum. 38 (2008) 241–248.

62. C. Gürgün, E. Ercan, C. Ceyhun, et al., Cardiovascular involvement in Behçet's disease, Jpn. Heart J. 43 (2002) 389–399.

63. F. Erkan, A. Gül, E. Tasali, Pulmonary manifestations of Behçet disease, Thorax 56 (2001) 572–578.

64. L. Pollak, L.M. Luxon, D.O. Haskard, Labyrinthine involvement in Behcet's syndrome, J. Laryngol. Otol. 115 (2001) 522–529.

65. C.R. Arkin, B.M. Rothschild, N.T. Florendo, et al., Behçet syndrome with myositis: a case report with pathologic findings, Arthritis Rheum. 23 (1980) 600–604.

66. T. Ergun, O. Gurbuz, J. Harvell, et al., The histopathology of pathergy: a chronologic study of skin hyperreactivity in Behçet's disease, Int. J. Dermatol. 37 (1998) 929–933.

67. Y. Okunuki, Y. Usui, M. Takeuchui, et al., Proteomic surveillance of autoimmunity in Behçet's disease with uveitis: selenium binding protein is a novel autoantigen in Behcet's disease, Exp. Eye Res. 84 (2007) 823–831.

68. I. Fresko, S. Ugurlu, F. Ozbakir, et al., Anti-Saccharomyces cerevisiae antibodies ASCA in Behçet's syndrome, Clin. Exp. Rheumatol. 23 (2005) S67–S70.

69. N. Sayinalp, O.I. Ozcebe, O. Ozdemir, et al., Cytokines in Behçet's disease, J. Rheumatol. 23 (1996) 321–322.

70. B. Turan, H. Gallati, H. Erdi, et al., Systemic levels of the T cell regulatory cytokines IL-10 and IL-12 in Behçet's disease; soluble TNFR-75 as a biological marker of disease activity, J. Rheumatol. 24 (1997) 128–132.

71. A. Carletto, M.L. Pacor, D. Biasi, et al., Changes of neutrophil migration without modification of in vitro metabolism and adhesion in Behçet's disease, J. Rheumatol. 24 (1997) 1332–1336.

72. M. Takeno, A. Kariyone, N. Yamashita, et al., Excessive function of peripheral blood neutrophils from patients with Behçet's disease and from HLA-B51 transgenic mice, Arthritis Rheum. 38 (1995) 426–433.

73. S. Yurdakul, H. Yazici, Y. Tuzun, et al., The arthritis of Behçet's disease: a prospective study, Ann. Rheum. Dis. 42 (1983) 505–515.

74. T. Akpolat, M. Danaci, U. Belet, et al., MR imaging and MR angiography in vascular Behçet's disease, Magn. Reson. Imaging 18 (2000) 1089–1096.

75. G. Akman-Demir, S. Bahar, O. Coban, et al., Cranial MRI in Behçet's disease: 134 examinations of 98 patients, Neuroradiology 45 (2003) 851–859.

76. F. Nobili, M. Cutolo, A. Sulli, et al., Brain functional involvement by perfusion SPECT in systemic sclerosis and Behçet's disease, Ann. NY Acad. Sci. 2966 (2002) 409–414.

77. G. Hatemi, A. Silman, D. Bang, EULAR recommendations for the management of Behçet disease, Ann. Rheum. Dis. 67 (2008) 1656–1662.

78. S. Ozen, The spectrum of vasculitis in children, Baillieres Best Pract. Res. Clin. Rheumatol. 16 (2002) 411–425.

79. S. Yurdakul, C. Mat, Y. Tüzün, et al., A double-blind trial of colchicine in Behçet's syndrome, Arthritis Rheum. 44 (2001) 2686–2692.

80. J.A. Kari, V. Shah, M.J. Dillon, Behçet's disease in UK children: clinical features and treatment including thalidomide, Rheumatology 40 (2001) 933–938.

81. K. Yasui, N. Uchida, Y. Akazawa, et al., Thalidomide for treatment of intestinal involvement of juvenile onset Behçet disease, Inflamm. Bowel Dis. 14 (2008) 396–400.

82. K.E. Sharquie, R.A. Najim, A.R. Abu-Raghif, Dapsone in Behçet's disease: a double blind placebo controlled cross over study, J. Dermatol. 29 (2002) 267–279.

83. A. Saenz, M. Ausejo, B. Shea, et al., Pharmacotherapy for Behçet's Syndrome, Cochrane Database Syst. Rev. 2 (2004) CD001084.

84. M.L. Pacor, D. Biasi, C. Lunardi, et al., Cyclosporin in Behçet's disease: results in 16 patients after 24 months of therapy, Clin. Rheumatol. 13 (1994) 224–227.

85. E.W. Lindstedt, G.S. Baarsma, R.W.A.M. Kuijpers, et al., Anti-TNF-a therapy for sight threatening uveitis, Br. J. Ophthalmol. 89 (2005) 533–536.

86. M. Schirmer, K.T. Calamia, H. Direskeneli, International conference on Behçet's disease. Seoul, Korea, 2000, J. Rheumatol. 28 (2000) 636–639.

87. N. Piptone, I. Olivieri, A. Padula, et al., Infliximab for the treatment of neuro-Behçet's disease: a case series and review of the literature, Arthritis Rheum. 59 (2008) 285–290.

88. H. Yazici, F. Essen, Mortality in Behçet's disease, Clin. Exp. Rheumatol. 26 (2008) S138–S140.

Chapter 37

INFECTIOUS ARTHRITIS AND OSTEOMYELITIS

Ronald M. Laxer and Carol B. Lindsley

The relation of infectious agents to arthritis is an area of great interest to the rheumatologist. Important discoveries have led to an understanding of the origin, pathogenesis, treatment, and cure of at least one infection-related arthritis—Lyme disease—and have given impetus to investigations of other possible arthrogenic infectious agents.

Arthritis related to infection can be regarded as septic, reactive, or postinfectious.[1] *Septic arthritis* occurs when a viable infectious agent is present or has been present in the synovial space. Although direct bacterial infection of the joint constitutes the most widely recognized form of septic arthritis, direct infection with viruses, spirochetes, or fungi also occurs. *Reactive arthritis* is a response to an infectious agent that is or has been present in some other part of the body, usually the upper airway, gastrointestinal tract, or genitourinary tract. By definition, viable infectious agents are not recoverable from the synovial space in patients with reactive arthritis, which may be regarded as an autoimmune disorder resulting from immunological crossreactivity between articular structures and infectious antigens. The reactive arthritis group merges pathogenically with diseases such as the spondylarthritides. *Postinfectious arthritis* may be considered a special type of reactive arthritis in which immune complexes containing nonviable components of an initiating infectious agent may be present in the inflamed joint. Lyme disease is discussed in Chapter 38, the reactive arthritides in Chapter 40, and poststreptococcal arthritis in Chapter 41.

The precise relation of infection to arthritis is complex and by no means completely understood. As techniques for the demonstration of infectious organisms improve, the frequency with which they are detected in synovial fluid or membrane is increasing, lending authority to the suspicion that some or many of the chronic arthritides of children are related to infectious diseases. Perhaps many of the so-called reactive arthritides will be found to represent diseases in which living pathogens are present in the joint and are, by definition, septic. In some of the viral arthritides that fit the concept of reactive arthritis (i.e., joint disease follows the onset of the acute illness by days or weeks), viral antigen or living virus can be isolated from synovial fluid lymphocytes or membrane when appropriate techniques are used. The same has been true for Lyme disease, in which early attempts to demonstrate *Borrelia* were unsuccessful, although the organisms have since been demonstrated by silver stain in several different laboratories. The lesson implicit in all of these observations is that in chronic arthritides, which we currently consider aseptic, concerted investigations for infectious agents using the most powerful techniques of molecular biology may yet demonstrate the causative agent in the joint space. Although study of infectious agents, such as viruses, as possible initiators of some forms of arthritis in children has attracted much attention, it is important to remember that intraarticular and systemic bacterial infections remain the most important curable causes of arthritis in childhood.

SEPTIC ARTHRITIS

Epidemiology

Septic arthritis of bacterial origin accounts for approximately 6.5% of all childhood arthritides.[2] It has been suggested that its frequency might be increasing,[3,4] although the retrospective reviews from Dallas[5] and Memphis[6] did not document an increase in incidence. In a 1997 report, 12.7% of 1158 patients with septic arthritis were children younger than 10 years old.[7]

Sex Ratio and Age at Onset

Septic arthritis is slightly less common in girls than in boys, who account for 55% to 62% of patients in reported series.[8-10] Septic arthritis is found most often in the very young[11] and the very old; it may occur in the neonate, is most common in children younger than 2-years-old, and diminishes in frequency throughout childhood.[5,12]

Familial and Geographical Clustering

There does not appear to be a genetic predisposition to septic arthritis. Typical cases of presumed septic arthritis in which no pathogen is identified tend to occur in the summer and fall,[4] but geographical clustering has not been reported. In spirochetal arthritis, such as Lyme disease, there are marked geographic and seasonal outbreaks.

Etiology and Pathogenesis

A wide range of microorganisms can cause septic arthritis in children; *Staphylococcus aureus* and nongroup A and B streptococci are most common overall.[7,12-14] However, different organisms are more common at some ages and in certain circumstances (Table 37–1). *Haemophilus influenzae* type B had been the most common infection identified in children younger than 2-years-old, but vaccination of infants for *H. influenzae* has significantly decreased the frequency of infection with this organism.[13,15-18] *Streptococcus pneumoniae* is a frequent cause of infection in children younger than 2 years old and is common in the older child.[19,20] After a child reaches 2 years old, *S. aureus* is the most frequently occurring organism.[13] Group A streptococci and enterococci account for a small proportion of all cases of septic arthritis in childhood and are most prevalent in the 6- to 10-year age group. *Salmonella* arthritis constitutes approximately 1% of all cases of septic arthritis, and it is commonly associated with sickle cell disease.[21] Infection with *Mycobacterium*

tuberculosis is an unusual cause of septic monarthritis in childhood. Other rare causes of infectious arthritis in children include *Streptobacillus moniliformis* (rat-bite fever), *Pseudomonas aeruginosa*, *Bacteroides* species, *Campylobacter fetus*, *Serratia* species, *Corynebacterium pyogenes*, *Neisseria meningitis*, *Pasteurella multocida*, and *Propionibacterium acnes*. *Kingella kingae* is emerging as an important pathogen in children with septic arthritis[22-24] and may account for a significant portion of culture negative cases.[25] Most infections with this organism occur in children younger than 5 years old, and 60% occur in children younger than 2 years old.[26] In the neonate, *S. aureus* (40% to 50%) or group B *Streptococcus* (20% to 25%) are the most common causative organisms.[5,9,27] Enterobacteriaceae, gonococcus, and *Candida* species are also significant pathogens in the neonate.

Septic arthritis usually results from hematogenous spread from a focus of infection elsewhere in the body.[28] Direct extension of an infection from overlying soft tissues (e.g., cellulitis, abscess) or bone (e.g., osteomyelitis)[29] or traumatic invasion of the joint accounts for only 15% to 20% of cases. In the hips, shoulders, ankles, and elbows, the joint capsule overlies a portion of the metaphysis. As a result, if a focus of underlying osteomyelitis breaks through the metaphysis, it may enter the joint and result in septic arthritis. Joint damage results from several mechanisms. Proliferation of bacteria in the synovial membrane results in accumulation of polymorphonuclear (PMN) leukocytes and the inflammatory effects outlined in Chapter 4. Synovial fluid contains high levels of proinflammatory cytokines (tumor necrosis factor-α, interleukin-1β)[30] that mediate cartilage damage by metalloproteinases.[31] The ensuing damage to cartilaginous surfaces of the bone and the supporting structures of the joint may be severe and permanent if treatment is not urgently initiated.

Although trauma or extraarticular infection preceding onset of septic arthritis is common in case histories, knowledge of the etiological significance of these factors is incomplete.[32] In one series, upper respiratory tract infections preceded septic arthritis in approximately 50% of patients, and approximately one-third had received antibiotics within one week of onset.[4] A history of a mild, nonpenetrating injury to the affected extremity was elicited in approximately one-third of patients. Intravenous (IV) drug users are at particular risk for septic arthritis of the sacroiliac and sternoclavicular joints, usually caused by gram-negative organisms.[33] Other recognized risk factors include prosthetic joints, diabetes, alcoholism, recent intraarticular steroids, and cutaneous ulcers.[34] Chronic inflammatory arthritis, such as juvenile idiopathic arthritis (JIA), may predispose to joint infection.[35]

Clinical Manifestations

Septic arthritis is usually accompanied by systemic signs of illness (e.g., fever, vomiting, headache)[36] and may be a component of a more generalized infection that might include meningitis, cellulitis, osteomyelitis, or pharyngitis.[37] Joint pain is usually severe, and the infected joint and periarticular tissues are swollen, hot, and sometimes erythematous. Passive and active motion

Table 37–1		
Common microorganisms involved in septic arthritis and osteomyelitis		
Age	**Organisms**	
Neonate	Group B *Streptococcus*	
	Staphylococcus aureus	
	Gram-negative bacilli	
Infant	*Staphylococcus aureus*	
	Streptococcus species	
	Haemophilus influenzae	
Child	*Staphylococcus aureus*	
	Streptococcus pneumoniae	
	Group A *Streptococcus*	
	Kingella kingae (some areas)	
Adolescent	*Staphylococcus aureus*	
	Streptococcus pneumoniae	
	Group A *Streptococcus*	
	Neisseria gonorrhoeae	

of the joint is severely, often completely, restricted (i.e., pseudoparalysis). Osteomyelitis frequently accompanies bacterial arthritis, and the presence of bone pain (as opposed to joint pain) should alert the examiner to this possibility. Other sites of hematogenous spread, although less common, are nonetheless important (Table 37–2).[4,8,9]

Affected Joints

The joints of the lower extremity are most commonly the sites of infection. Knees, hips, ankles, and elbows account for 90% of infected joints in children. Septic arthritis affecting the small joints of the hands or feet is rare (Table 37–3).[5,9,10] Pyogenic sacroiliac joint disease can occur.[38]

Multiple Infected Joints

Although septic arthritis is most often a monarthritis, two or more joints are infected simultaneously or during the course of the same illness in a few children. In the large clinical experience reported by Fink and Nelson,[5] septic arthritis was monarticular in 93.4% but affected two joints in 4.4%, three in 1.7%, and four in 0.5% of patients.

Geographical variation exists with up to 24% multisite involvement reported in some studies.[39] Certain immune deficiencies, such as chronic granulomatous disease or acquired immunodeficiency syndrome (AIDS), may predispose to septic arthritis in multiple joints.

Diagnosis

A recent systematic review concluded that in the absence of positive cultures in either the synovial fluid or the blood, the overall clinical judgment of an experienced clinician is superior to laboratory or radiological investigations for the diagnosis of septic arthritis.[40] Guidelines for the management of suspected septic arthritis have been published for adults and may be applicable to the older child as well.[41] It is essential that every child with acute unexplained monarthritis undergo aspiration of the affected joint immediately, because septic arthritis continues to be associated with considerable morbidity and mortality.[18,42,43] Synovial fluid examination is outlined in Table 37–4.

If an anaerobic organism or mycobacterium is suspected, enriched culture medium and special anaerobic culture conditions are necessary. Children in whom septic arthritis is considered should also have cultures of blood and of any potential source of infection (e.g., cellulitis, abscess, and cerebrospinal fluid) performed. Rapid antigen latex agglutination tests for *H. influenzae*, group B and C streptococci, *Neisseria meningitidis*, and *S. pneumoniae* are available in most clinics. The polymerase chain reaction (PCR) has proved useful in detecting evidence of infectious agents in synovial fluid,[44-47] and real-time PCR may be even more beneficial in the investigation of culture-negative septic arthritis.[23,48]

In a group of children with septic arthritis in whom the bacterial agent was identified,[5] Fink and Nelson reported that synovial fluid was culture positive in 307 (79%) of 389 patients (Table 37–5).[4,9,10] The remaining 21% had positive cultures from sites other than the joint: blood (10%), cerebrospinal fluid (3.8%), blood and cerebrospinal fluid (2.3%), and vagina (1.3%). One of five children with culture-positive septic arthritis had a negative synovial fluid culture but a positive culture from elsewhere, most often the blood. Initial inoculation of synovial fluid

Table 37–2

Extraarticular sites of infection in children with septic arthritis

Sites of Infection	Nelson and Koontz[8] n = 117 (%)	Welkon et al[4] n = 95 (%)	Speiser et al[9] n = 86 (%)
Osteomyelitis	12	12	26
Meningitis	4	4	11
Cellulitis, abscess	–	–	9
Respiratory tract	19	–	9
Middle ear	–	20	3
Urine	–	–	1
Genital tract	4	–	1
Pericardium	–	–	1
Pleura	–	–	1

Table 37–3

Frequency of infected joints in septic arthritis

Infected Joint	Fink and Nelson[5] n = 591 (%)	Welkon et al[4] n = 95 (%)	Speiser et al[9] n = 86 (%)	Wilson and DiPaola[10] n = 61 (%)	Overall n = 833 (%)
Knee	40	46	30	29	39
Hip	23	25	29	40	25
Ankle	13	15	17	21	14
Elbow	14	5	11	3	12
Shoulder	4	4	2	3	4
Wrist	4	-	1	1	3
PIP, MCP, MTP	1	-	10	-	2
Other	1	5	-	1	1

MCP, metacarpophalangeal; MTP, metatarsophalangeal; PIP, proximal interphalangeal.

into blood culture bottles may increase the yield of some organisms, especially *Kingella kingae*.[24] Although an organism can be identified in one-third to two-thirds or more of patients by the culturing of all appropriate sites, no causative organisms are ever identified in approximately one-third of children with pyogenic arthritis.[49] In these patients, the diagnosis of septic arthritis is based on a typical history and the demonstration of frank pus by arthrocentesis.

Synovial Fluid Analysis

The characteristics of the synovial fluid depend somewhat on the duration and severity of the disease and previous administration of antibiotics. Synovial fluid may appear normal, turbid, or grayish green with bloody streaks (see Table 37–4). The synovial fluid white blood cell (WBC) count is often markedly elevated, with 90% PMNs. Speiser and colleagues[9] reported that synovial WBC counts in septic arthritis were less than 50,000/mm^3 (50 × 10^9/L) in 15% of children, 50,000 to 100,000/mm^3 (50-100 × 10^9/L) in 34%, and more than 100,000/mm^3 (100 × 10^9/L) in 51%. Fink and Nelson[5] found a relatively low WBC count (less than 25,000/mm^3 or 25 × 10^9) in one-third of their patients.

The protein content is high (more than 2.5 g/dL), and the glucose concentration compared with plasma glucose is usually low in septic arthritis, although it may be normal. A Gram stain identifies the organism in one-half of untreated patients but in only one-fifth of those who have received antibiotics. A Gram stain provides rapid confirmation of bacterial infection and tentative identification of the organism (if the findings are positive), permitting rational antibiotic therapy. Special procedures such as counterimmunoelectrophoresis, latex agglutination, or evaluation by PCR may sometimes identify bacterial antigens in a culture-negative fluid (i.e., blood, urine, or cerebrospinal fluid). These techniques have the advantage of providing antigenic identification much more rapidly than cultures, but they do not provide antibiotic sensitivities.

Blood Studies

At least two blood cultures should always be performed for a child suspected of having septic arthritis. An elevated WBC count with a predominance of PMNs and bands and a markedly elevated erythrocyte sedimentation rate (ESR) or C-reactive protein (CRP) level—although of limited help in specific diagnosis—provide a baseline whereby the efficacy of subsequent treatment can be judged. CRP is a better predictor than ESR. If the CRP value is less than 1 mg/dL, the likelihood that the patient does not have septic arthritis is 87%.[50] Concentrations of other acute phase reactants are usually increased, but provide no additional useful information.

Radiological Examination

A number of imaging techniques may be helpful in evaluating a child with septic arthritis (Fig. 37–1).[51-55] Plain radiographs are not diagnostic but might be helpful in excluding other disorders. They may show an underlying osteomyelitis as the etiology of the septic arthritis and may demonstrate only increased soft tissue and capsular swelling. Juxtaarticular osteoporosis reflects inflammatory hyperemia and is evident within several days after onset of infection. Cartilage loss and narrowing of the joint space develop as the disease progresses. These changes are followed by marginal erosions and eventually by ankylosis (Fig. 37–2).[54] Computerized tomography (CT) and especially magnetic resonance imaging (MRI) are additional confirmatory techniques.

In the hip, accumulation of fluid within the joint displaces the gluteal fat lines laterally, or the obturator sign (i.e., displacement of the margins of this muscle medially) may be present. Traction applied to the leg during the radiographic procedure normally induces a radiolucent outline of the femoral head; this is referred to as the

---

Table 37–4

Synovial fluid examination in a child with suspected septic arthritis

Synovial fluid aspiration must be done under strictly aseptic conditions to minimize the risk of bacterial contamination.

Septic arthritis is strongly suggested if:
- Visual inspection finds cloudy, serosanguineous, or greenish fluid.
- Cell count reveals elevated numbers of neutrophils (50,000 to 300,000/mm^3) (50–300 × 10^9/L).
- Synovial fluid viscosity is low.
- Synovial fluid glucose is low (<30 mg/dL).
- Lactate dehydrogenase level is high (>500 IU).
- Gram stain is positive.
Culture is positive for about 70% of those tested.

Table 37–5

Laboratory confirmation of septic arthritis in children

Laboratory Confirmation	Fink and Nelson[5]	Welkon et al[5]	Speiser et al[9]	Wilson and DiPaola[10]
	n = 591 (%)	n = 95 (%)	n = 86 (%)	n = 61 (%)
Confirmed diagnosis (culture positive)	66	64	84	92
Positive synovial fluid Gram stain	33	–	19 to 54*	–
Positive synovial fluid culture	79	84	36 to 70*	71 to 80†
Positive blood culture	33	46	46	41

*Depends on prior administration of antibiotics.
†Depends on procedure (aspiration = 80, arthrotomy = 71).

"vacuum" phenomenon. This lucency does not occur in the presence of increased intraarticular fluid.[54]

Computerized tomography

As MRI is much better for the evaluation of soft tissues, the role of CT is limited, except for the evaluation of sacroiliac and sternoclavicular joints. It is also helpful to guide aspirations and biopsies.

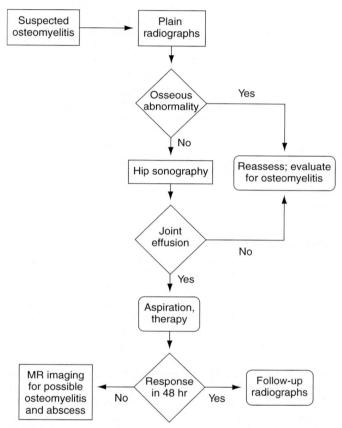

FIGURE 37–1 Flowchart of recommendations for evaluating septic arthritis in children. (Adapted from Jaramillo D, Treves ST, Kasser JR et al: Osteomyelitis and septic arthritis in children: appropriate use of imaging to guide treatment, *AJR Am J Roentgenol* 165:399-403, 1995.)

Ultrasonography

Detection of joint fluid by ultrasound helps guide fluid aspiration. The ultrasonic detection of an effusion in the hip of a child treated for osteomyelitis of the femur indicates the presence of septic arthritis of the joint.[54] Color Doppler may show increased capsular vascularity.

Radionuclide Scans

During the first few days of disease, when plain radiographs show only soft tissue changes, 99mTc-MDP scans reflect hyperemia of the infected area on blood flow studies and increased uptake of the isotope on both sides of the joint.[55] Occasionally, decreased uptake may occur if significant accumulation of intraarticular fluid impedes local blood flow. This technique is useful in the early detection of joint or bone inflammation or infection, but it does not differentiate the two with certainty and cannot differentiate septic arthritis from synovitis from other causes (e.g., JIA). It is helpful in differentiating septic arthritis from osteomyelitis and soft tissue infection and in the detection of multifocal joint infections.[56] Radionuclide scans with gallium 67 or the patient's indium 111-labeled granulocytes or monoclonal antibodies may be helpful but are not routinely needed. 2-deoxy-2 [^{13}F] fluoro-D-glucose (FDG)-positron emission tomography (PET)/CT may have an important role in the diagnosis of difficult cases owing to the fact that PET is a relatively fast, whole-body imaging modality and can be used to find infectious foci outside of the bone or joint.[56] It may be particularly helpful for infections of the vertebrae.

Magnetic Resonance Imaging

Delineation of soft tissue structures by MRI is superior to that provided by CT.[53,54] Changes may be seen as soon as 24 hours following infection. Synovial enhancement is detected in virtually all patients. Signal-intensity alterations in the bone marrow are characteristic but not diagnostic of septic arthritis (i.e., low intensity on fat-suppressed, gadolinium-enhanced, T1-weighted spin-echo images, and high signal intensity on fat-suppressed, T2-weighted, fast spin-echo images).[57] Articular cartilage and growth cartilage are depicted along with other

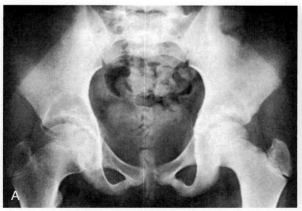
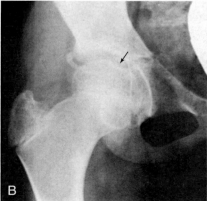

FIGURE 37–2   **A,** Questionable joint space widening of the right hip of a 10-year-old girl with fever and an irritable hip. **B,** Repeat x-ray film taken 20 days later demonstrated epiphyseal demineralization and erosion *(arrow).*

fibrous structures, muscle, blood vessels, and synovial fluid. An abnormal collection of fluid or debris, often displacing the joint capsule, eroding into other tissues, or in children, leading to subluxation, supports the possibility of septic arthritis. Fat suppressed, gadolinium-enhanced MRI is 100% sensitive and 79% specific for the diagnosis of septic arthritis in adults.[58]

Treatment

The child with septic arthritis requires hospitalization and consultation with an orthopaedic surgeon and specialist in infectious diseases. Nonsteroidal antiinflammatory drugs (NSAIDs) may be used to help minimize the effects of inflammation, to control fever, and to contribute to pain relief. IV dexamethasone was shown to reduce duration of symptoms and minimize joint damage in a randomized, double-blind study, but is rarely, if ever, used.[59] A clinical practice guideline for the management of septic arthritis in children has been proposed.[60] It was demonstrated that this approach was effective in minimizing bone scans, in minimizing the rate of joint drainage, in accelerating the change to oral antibiotic administration, and in shortening the duration of hospital stay. There were no differences in outcomes such as readmission to the hospital, recurrence of infection, or the development of residual joint damage.

Antibiotics

In a child with septic arthritis, IV antibiotics should be administered as promptly as possible. The choice of antibiotic depends on the presence of predisposing factors, the age of the child, and the organisms suspected because of the Gram stain or rapid antigen detection tests (although it is hazardous to narrow initial treatment based solely on these results because either can be wrong). If the Gram stain and results of rapid antigen detection are negative or not available, an approach based on age outlined in Table 37–6 is suggested.[38] The demonstration of an organism or antigen may support or contradict the generalizations outlined in this table and should influence the physician in selection of the initial antibiotic treatment.[42,61]

It is prudent to monitor intravenous antibiotic efficacy with serum bactericidal titer determinations at frequent intervals initially and at follow-up for compliance, especially if home therapy is instituted. After satisfactory control of the infectious process with IV antibiotic

administration is achieved (including resolution of fever, significant decrease in pain, improvement in range of motion, and falling laboratory measures of inflammation), treatment by the oral route in the hospital or on an outpatient basis may be appropriate.[62-64] Home IV antibiotic programs may also be effective in reducing the hospital stay. Such programs should be undertaken only after careful consideration and consultation with an expert in pediatric infectious disease.

If the cultures are negative, IV antibiotics should be continued for a minimum of 21 days.[1] If the child's clinical state is improving (i.e., temperature returning to normal, pain diminishing, range of motion improving) and the WBC count and ESR are falling, the initial antibiotics should be maintained. If the patient does not appear to be responding, additional IV antibiotic coverage should be instituted. Because of various patterns of antibiotic susceptibility and resistance, guidelines regarding antibiotic choice and duration of treatment are constantly changing, and the physician is urged to review the most current recommendations. This is especially important with the rise in the incidence of community-acquired *Methicillin-resistant Staphylococcus aureus* (CA-MRSA), which requires specific antibiotic management.

Aspiration and Drainage

The usefulness of repeated aspiration and drainage of an infected joint has been hotly debated. There is no dispute that an initial diagnostic arthrocentesis must be performed. Any joint that appears to be under pressure from an effusion can probably benefit from aspiration, if only for pain relief. Studies of the importance of repeated aspirations under other circumstances, however, have failed to show a consistent benefit. Similarly, open drainage is worse than closed needle aspiration (except for specific joints such as the hip and shoulder) and is attended by significantly increased morbidity. Irrigation of the joint at the time of aspiration has no demonstrated additional benefit. Occasionally, arthroscopic examination is indicated. Intraarticular administration of antibiotic is unnecessary because therapeutic synovial fluid antibiotic levels are readily achieved,[65] and it may induce chemical synovitis in the infected joint.

Special Cases

Neonatal Septic Arthritis

In addition to *S. aureus*, group B *Streptococcus* and gram-negative bacteria can be the offending organisms in the neonate.[66] They are rare but potentially very serious infections in this age group, may have a subtle presentation, and can occasionally be bilateral. They are much more likely to occur in association with osteomyelitis than in older children. Most affected newborns show no fever, toxemia, or leukocytosis.[67,68] Any infant who has swelling in the region of the thigh or holds the leg flexed, abducted, or externally rotated must be investigated promptly. Problems in early recognition of disease undoubtedly contribute to the often disastrous outcome of this involvement.[69]

Table 37–6	
Recommended empirical antibiotic therapy by age	
Age	**Recommended Empirical Antibiotic Therapy**
Neonate	Cloxacillin + gentamicin OR cloxacillin + cefotaxime
Infant	Cefotaxime + cloxacillin OR cefuroxime
Child	Cefazolin OR cloxacillin OR clindamycin
Adolescent	Ceftriaxone OR cefixime + azithromycin

Alternatives appropriate to local epidemiology and patient comorbidities (e.g., immunocompromise) may be needed. Vancomycin should be included in patients with high risk for MRSA.

Septic Hip Joint

Septic arthritis of the hip is such an important problem that it merits special attention.[70,71] Because the risks of missing this diagnosis are so high, there must a very low threshold for hip aspiration to establish the diagnosis.[72] The femoral head is intracapsular, and the arterial supply passes through the ligamentum teres through the intracapsular space. Increased intracapsular pressure can therefore interrupt the blood supply to the femoral head, with disastrous consequences to its viability and to the subsequent development of avascular necrosis.[73] Metaphyseal osteomyelitis readily leads to septic arthritis of the hip joint in the infant because nutrient blood vessels pass from the metaphysis through the epiphyseal growth plate and terminate in the distal ossification center.

Septic arthritis of the hip joint is most common in infants and very young children; 70% of patients are 4-years-old or younger.[74] The typical clinical picture is that of an infant or young child who may have an unexplained fever; is irritable; and refuses to move an extremity, bear weight, or walk. Any movement of the hip is extremely painful; and the affected leg is held in a position of partial flexion, abduction, and external rotation at the hip. Occasionally, the child has lower abdominal pain or tenderness, sometimes with paralytic ileus.

In very young or premature infants, a number of risk factors predispose to septic hip joint arthritis.[75] In a study of septic arthritis of the hip of 16 infants younger than 4 weeks old, 11 were premature, 7 had an umbilical catheter, and 12 had septicemia. In contrast, of 13 children with septic arthritis between the ages of 1 month and 3 years, none was premature or had an umbilical catheter, and only five were septicemic. A high frequency of preceding or accompanying osteomyelitis of the femur or pelvis has been observed. The association of septic arthritis of the hip and femoral venipuncture has been recorded[76] and may account in part for the high frequency of arthritis of this site in the premature neonate.

Management of septic arthritis of the hip requires open drainage to minimize intraarticular pressure.[77,78] Traction and immobilization for the first two to three days of treatment provide pain relief, but should be followed by passive and then active physiotherapy to prevent loss of range of motion. Prognosis is guarded even with the best treatment, especially in the neonate. The anatomy of the shoulder joint is not unlike that of the hip with respect to vascular supply. Septic arthritis of this joint, although rare, should be treated similarly.[79]

Gonococcal Arthritis

In reported series of septic arthritis in children and adolescents, disease caused by *N. gonorrhoeae* appears to be uncommon. When it occurs, it is most common in the adolescent, although it occasionally occurs in the neonate in association with disseminated infection.[80] It is more common in girls than in boys and is particularly likely just after menstruation or with pregnancy.[81] Gonococcal arthritis usually develops in patients with primary asymptomatic genitourinary gonorrhea or with a gonococcal infection of the throat or rectum. The patient presents with a systemic illness characterized by fever and chills.[82] A vesiculopustular rash, sparsely distributed on the extremities, commonly yields organisms on culture or Gram stain of the smear. Gonococcal arthritis may have an initial migratory phase and may be accompanied by tenosynovitis. In contrast to most patients with septic arthritis, those with gonococcal arthritis may present with a purulent arthritis of several joints. For a patient with suspected gonococcal arthritis, it is important to culture samples from the genital tract, throat, rectum, and any vesicles in addition to the affected joint. Special culture media with chocolate agar will help in isolating the organism. The possibility of sexual abuse should be considered and appropriately investigated.

Tuberculous Arthritis

Tuberculous arthritis is seldom encountered in North America or Europe, although its frequency may be increasing because of immunosuppressive therapy, drug-resistant strains of tuberculosis, and the human immunodeficiency virus (HIV) epidemic.[83-85] Tuberculous arthritis is by no means rare in other parts of the world. Typically, arthritis arises on a background of pulmonary tuberculosis as indolent, chronic monarthritis, often of the knee or wrist, that eventually results in extreme destruction of the joint and surrounding bones. Rarely, it manifests as acute arthritis.[86] Al Matar and colleagues[87] have observed two young children with tuberculous monarthritis that mimicked oligoarticular JIA. They were unresponsive to NSAIDs and intraarticular corticosteroids. One had a history of exposure, but the other child had no identifiable contact with tuberculosis.

Joint infection occurs by hematogenous dissemination of the organism from adjoining osteomyelitis. Pott disease is a consequence of vertebral osteomyelitis (Fig. 37–3). Tuberculous dactylitis may occur with cystic expansion and destruction of bone (i.e., spina ventosa) (Fig. 37–4).[88] A family or environmental history of pulmonary tuberculosis and a positive purified protein derivative (Mantoux) skin test result suggest the possibility of tuberculous arthritis. Although synovial fluid cultures are positive in approximately three-fourths of patients, synovial membrane biopsy and culture are preferred and confirm the diagnosis in almost all patients (Fig. 37–5). The synovial WBC count is classically less than $50,000/mm^3$ ($50 \times 10^9/L$), with a high proportion of mononuclear cells. Genus-specific PCR is invaluable in the diagnosis.[46] Rarely, a polyarthritis accompanies tuberculosis (i.e., Poncet disease); it probably represents a reactive arthritis because culture of the inflamed joints fails to demonstrate tubercle bacilli.[89,90]

Leprosy can result in articular changes and inflammatory disease, including polyarthritis and subcutaneous nodules.[91] Clinical differentiation from JIA may be difficult, especially if the possibility of leprosy is not considered in a nonendemic area.[92] *Mycobacterium leprae* is not always easily identified in synovial biopsies.[93,94]

Arthritis Associated with Brucellosis

Human *Brucella* infections are reported primarily from European,[95,96] Israeli,[97] and South American[98,99] clinicians with a substantial number of patients having arthritis. Cases in North America are more likely to have

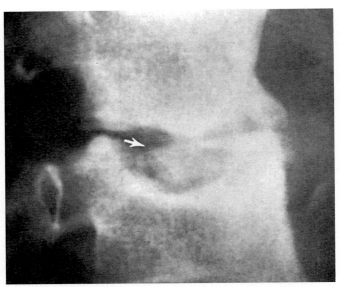

FIGURE 37–3 Pott disease of the vertebral column in an adolescent boy with pulmonary tuberculosis produced destruction of the disk space and vertebral end-plate erosion *(arrow)*.

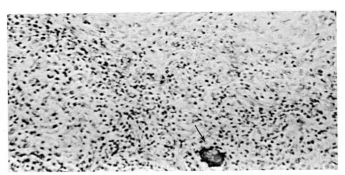

FIGURE 37–5 Synovial biopsy specimen of chronic inflammation in tuberculous joint disease in which a giant cell *(arrow)* is indicated.

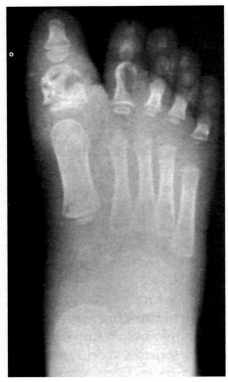

FIGURE 37–4 Advanced osseous destruction occurred in the foot of a child with tuberculous dactylitis (i.e., spinal ventosa).

been acquired elsewhere.[100] The species most frequently implicated are *Brucella melitensis*[96,98,99] and, less commonly, *Brucella canis*.[101] Unpasteurized milk is a source of infection.

The systemic illness is often mild in children but is usually characterized by undulant fever, gastrointestinal complaints, lymphadenopathy, and sometimes dermatitis.

In 88 children from Israel,[97] the classic triad of fever (91%), arthralgia or arthritis (83%), and hepatosplenomegaly (63%) was characteristic of most patients. In a large series of cases from Peru,[98] almost one-third were children, and one third had arthritis. In the birth to 15-year-old age group, peripheral arthritis of a hip or knee was most common. Spondylitis and sacroiliac arthritis became predominant after children reached 15 years old. Gomez-Reino and colleagues[96] found that periarthritis without effusion was most common and that small joints and the spine were not affected. Whether this reflects differences in the infecting organism or in ascertainment is not known. No association with HLA-B27 has been demonstrated.[95] Synovial fluid WBC counts are only modestly elevated with a slight predominance of mononuclear cells.[98,102] Joint fluid culture is positive for the organism in some patients. Tetracyclines, aminoglycosides, rifampin, and trimethoprim-sulfamethoxazole, often in combination, provide effective treatment of the acute infection, although permanent sequelae may result.[96,99]

Mycoplasma and Arthritis

Myalgia and arthralgia are common during pulmonary infection with *Mycoplasma pneumoniae*. Objective oligoarticular, polyarticular, or migratory arthritis has also been described.[103] Sensitive screening tests may uncover *Mycoplasma* as a cause of arthritis even in the absence of pneumonia.[104,105]

Bartonella Infection and Arthritis

There have been rare reports of *Bartonella henselae* infection causing arthritis in children (i.e., cat-scratch disease).[106-108] In two children, the disease mimicked systemic JIA[107,108]; a third child had polyarthritis and subcutaneous nodules.[106] Arthropathy occurred in 3% of patients in an Israeli registry. It was characterized by large- and medium-sized mono-, oligo-, or polyarthritis (most commonly symmetric oligoarthritis), which was debilitating. Despite cat-scratch disease being a disease of children and adolescents, in this series no patient under 20 years old had joint involvement. The arthropathy usually occurred concurrent with the lymphadenopathy. Erythema nodosum was more common in those with than without arthropathy.[109,110]

Arthritis in Immunocompromised Patients

Chronic inflammatory arthritis in patients with a primary immunodeficiency is discussed in Chapter 42. Typical septic arthritis has been reported infrequently in immunodeficient children.[111] *Mycoplasma* is the most common cause of severe chronic erosive arthritis in patients with congenital immunodeficiency syndromes[112] and has been recovered from joints of patients with AIDS.[113] *Ureaplasma urealyticum* has been identified in patients with agammaglobulinemia.[114] *Candida albicans* is occasionally responsible for arthritis in immunosuppressed patients.[114,115]

Course of the Disease and Prognosis

The outcome in septic arthritis is somewhat guarded because, even with early and appropriate antibiotic treatment, permanent damage is common. The child usually recovers from the acute illness, but with the passage of time, reduction in range of motion, pain, and eventually degeneration of the surfaces of the affected joint may require surgical intervention. It is estimated that residual dysfunction occurs in 10% to 25% of children, although the changes (e.g., limited joint mobility, joint instability of chronic subluxation) may not be apparent until years later.[4] Recently, a simplified radiographic classification system has been developed to determine prognosis and to guide surgical management of the sequelae of septic arthritis of the hip.[116]

OSTEOMYELITIS

Although osteomyelitis, like septic arthritis, is most often encountered and treated by specialists in orthopaedics and infectious diseases, its frequent association with septic arthritis and the diagnostic problems that it presents require that it be included in this discussion.[3,63,117-122]

Definition and Classification

Osteomyelitis is an intraosseous infection with bacteria or, rarely, fungi. It is classified as acute, subacute, or chronic. *Acute osteomyelitis* is of recent onset and short duration. It is most often hematogenous in origin but may result from trauma such as a compound fracture or puncture wound. It can be metaphyseal, epiphyseal, or diaphyseal in location. *Subacute osteomyelitis* is of longer duration and is usually caused by less virulent organisms. *Chronic osteomyelitis* results from ineffective treatment of acute osteomyelitis and is characterized by necrosis and sequestration of bone.

Epidemiology

Acute osteomyelitis is somewhat less common than acute septic arthritis. An incidence of 16.7 cases per year was reported from an institution at which acute septic arthritis occurred at a rate of 28.4 cases per year.[5] However, it may be more common than septic arthritis in developing countries of the world.[123] Although its incidence may be

declining in many parts of the world, that is not necessarily the case everywhere.[124] It occurs twice as often in boys as in girls[5,123] and is more common in younger children. It can occur in the neonate.[66]

Etiology and Pathogenesis

S. aureus (50% to 80%) and the group A streptococci (5% to 10%) are the predominant organisms at all ages.[5,125] Recently, CA-MRSA has emerged as an important pathogen.[6,126,127] Up to 15% of children with CA-MRSA that carry the genes encoding Panton-Valentin leukocidin (*pvl*) have multiple sites of infection.[128] These organisms are also associated with chronic osteomyelitis. Even before specific immunization, *H. influenzae* seldom caused osteomyelitis (2% to 10%) and should now be even less common.[16,129] In certain circumstances, specific or unusual organisms (15%) are found. For example, infection of the calcaneus or other bone in the foot associated with a puncture wound through athletic footwear is likely caused by *P. aeruginosa*.[28,32,130,131] Osteomyelitis caused by *S. pneumoniae*[19,132] usually occurs in children with associated diseases such as sickle cell anemia,[133-135] asplenia,[119,136] or hypogammaglobulinemia,[120,137] although it has been observed in young infants without underlying disease.[138] *Salmonella* osteomyelitis is a complication of sickle cell anemia but also occurs in normal children.[139] In the neonate, group B streptococci,[140,141] gram-negative organisms,[142-144] and *Candida* in addition to *S. aureus* are all potential causes of osteomyelitis. *B. melitensis* uncommonly results in osteomyelitis, but when it does, it has a predilection for the vertebral bodies.[101] Tuberculous osteomyelitis may take various forms and may mimic chronic pyogenic disease, Brodie abscess, tumor, or other types of granuloma.[145-147] *B. henselae* (the organism of cat-scratch disease) has been identified as the causative agent in a few patients with osteomyelitis.[148-150]

Clinical Manifestations

Fever, severe bone pain, and tenderness with or without local swelling should suggest the possibility of acute osteomyelitis. Although a history of prior trauma is elicited in approximately one-third of young patients, its significance is uncertain. In the infant, fever may be minimal, and localization of the pain may be difficult on physical examination.[151] Pseudoparalysis of a limb is often evident. The examiner may find clinical evidence of a preceding systemic infection. The site of the bone infection is usually metaphyseal, and bony tenderness is elicited by pressure near or over the infected area. There may also be an area of overlying cellulitis, especially in the infant, in whom the thin cortex allows pus to erode into the periosteal structures. The presence of a joint effusion adjacent to the site of bone infection may reflect septic arthritis or a sterile noninflammatory "sympathetic" effusion.[152]

Osteomyelitis in children has a predilection for the metaphysis of rapidly growing bone. Many explanations have been suggested for this tendency. The anatomical differences in vasculature in this area in children and its easily compromised blood supply may in part explain the clinical observation (see Chapter 2). In one anatomical model,

Table 37–7

Affected sites in septic osteomyelitis

Bone	Osteomyelitis* (%)
Tibia	25
Clavicle	<1
Fibula	6
Spine	1
Femur	27
Metatarsus, metacarpus, phalanx	4
Radius	4
Pelvis	6
Humerus	11
Ulna	2
Sternum	<1
Mandible	<1
Scapula	<1
Rib	<1
Talus	1
Calcaneus	6

*Data from Fink CW, Nelson JD: Septic arthritis and osteomyelitis in children, *Clin Rheum Dis* 12:423, 1986, and from Cole WG, Dalziel RE, Leitl S: Treatment of acute osteomyelitis in childhood, *J Bone Joint Surg Br* 64: 218, 1982.

Table 37–8

Brodie abscess

Characteristic	Findings or Procedures
Symptoms	Pain may be severe; child awakens at night.
Signs	Evidence of a penetrating injury of hematogenous spread First week: soft tissue swelling Second week: metaphyseal osteolytic lesion with surrounding sclerosis
Investigations	Sterile joint effusion; curettage samples and cultures may be negative.
Treatment	Immobilization, nonsteroidal antiinflammatory drugs, antibiotics

bacteremia and, in some cases, preceding microtrauma were sufficient to initiate disease.[153] The bones of the lower extremity are affected in two-thirds of patients; those of the upper extremity account for approximately 25%, but those of the skull, face, spine, and pelvis are the sites of infection in fewer than 10% (Table 37–7).[5,123,154-156] Less than 10% of children have two or more simultaneously infected bones; in some cases, five or more bones are involved as part of a severe septicemic illness, usually caused by staphylococci. This type of involvement must be distinguished from chronic recurrent multifocal osteomyelitis (see Chapter 44).

Acute osteomyelitis can be associated with the development of deep-vein thromboses (DVT).[157] In a series of 35 patients from Dallas who had osteomyelitis involving the proximal humerus, femur, proximal tibia or fibula, pelvis, or vertebrae, 10 had evidence of DVT based on imaging studies, although it was only symptomatic in one patient. In two patients, the DVT was related to a central catheter placed for long-term antibiotic therapy, where as in the remaining eight, the DVT occurred in veins adjacent to the site of infection. The authors attributed the DVTs to the inflammatory response leading to localized endothelial damage and activation of the coagulation cascade. Compounding factors include the local edema, venous compression and immobility in patients with lower extremity involvement. Organisms with the *pvl* gene were more likely to be associated with DVTs.[158]

Subacute Osteomyelitis

Compared with acute osteomyelitis, patients with subacute osteomyelitis usually have a longer duration of illness (more than two weeks), experience less pain, often have no fever, and have frequently taken a trial of antibiotics.

Laboratory changes are less common, but radiographs are usually abnormal and may be confused with Ewing sarcoma or osteoid osteoma.[124] Brodie abscess, a unique form of subacute osteomyelitis, is usually of staphylococcal origin and may develop after a penetrating injury or by hematogenous spread of an infection to the metaphysis. It is characterized clinically by localized soft tissue swelling and tenderness with marked pain that may awaken the child at night (Table 37–8). Radiographs demonstrate only soft tissue swelling in the first week, but metaphyseal osteolytic lesions are evident by the second week of the illness. They are most common in the proximal or distal ends of the tibia (Fig. 37–6).[159,160] Culture of the abscess may be negative. Treatment includes IV antibiotics, an NSAID, and immobilization.

Chronic Osteomyelitis

Chronic osteomyelitis take places when symptoms occur for longer than three months and develops in states of impaired host or antibiotic resistance. Reduced blood flow leads to the formation of a sequestrum, which may be surrounded by a sleeve of periosteal new bone (involucrum) and represents inadequate treatment. This in turn requires surgical excision. Complications of chronic osteomyelitis include growth plate arrest or stimulation, avascular necrosis, pathological fracture, septicemia, and amyloidosis.[124]

Neonatal Osteomyelitis

Neonatal osteomyelitis merits special consideration.[67] Up until a child reaches the age of approximately 18-months-old, metaphyseal blood vessels can cross over the open physis into the epiphysis, permitting infection to move across the growth plate. The thin cortical bone of newborns allows infection to spread rapidly into the subperiosteal region, and the relative immune deficient state of the newborn allows for rapid spread. The lack of a systemic inflammatory response often leads to a delay in diagnosis, and involvement of more than one site is common. Although *S. aureus* remains the most common organism responsible for neonatal osteomyelitis, especially in newborns with central lines, group B streptococci, gram-negative bacteria, and *Candida albicans* may also be responsible.

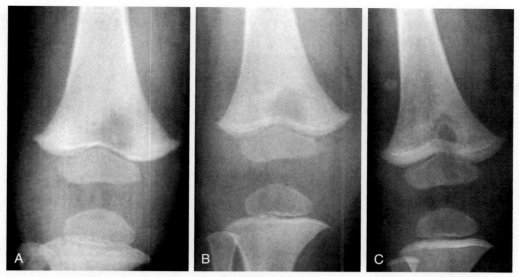

FIGURE 37–6   Brodie abscess is revealed in radiographs of the knee of a 16-month-old boy with acute hematogenous osteomyelitis inadequately treated one month earlier. **A,** Central sequestration with a surrounding, ill-defined lytic margin. The patient was appropriately treated with antibiotics at this stage. **B,** One month later, the sequestrum has been removed by osteoclasts. **C,** One month later, the radiograph shows a well-defined lesion with sclerotic borders. (**A** to **C,** courtesy of Dr. B. Wood.)

Diagnosis

As in septic arthritis, it is essential that every reasonable attempt be made to identify the organism and determine its antibiotic susceptibility.[119] A high index of suspicion for this diagnosis must be maintained in any child with unexplained pain, fever, or lack of use of an extremity. Aspiration of subperiosteal pus is the diagnostic procedure of choice and, together with cultures of the blood, synovial fluid, or an infected wound, should yield an organism in approximately 70% to 80% of cases. Blood cultures alone are positive in 30% to 50% of infants and children.[161] A bone biopsy may be desirable or necessary if other sites of culture prove negative. The elevated WBC count and ESR are nonspecific and provide little help with diagnosis; they are useful in assessing effectiveness of therapy.

Radiographic evaluation may delineate soft tissue swelling very early, but osteoporosis is not evident until days 10 to 14, and diagnostic findings may not be clear until days 10 to 21 (Fig. 37–7).[52] Radionuclide scanning (i.e., technetium 99m polyphosphonate or diphosphonate) provides a sensitive if nonspecific method for the early detection of increased blood flow and uptake in the infected bone (see Fig. 37–7C).[28,55,162] A bone scan is particularly helpful in localizing osteomyelitis in the neonate or infection of the axial skeleton and in searching for subclinical areas of infection in multifocal osteomyelitis. A positive result is not necessarily diagnostic of osteomyelitis, but a negative scan is unlikely for a child with bacterial osteomyelitis, except in the very early stages of the illness.

MRI is superior to other modalities in identifying changes in the marrow (see Fig. 37–7D).[38,163-165] T1- or T2-weighted MR images, fat suppression, and gadolinium enhancement can confirm a focal area of increased inflammatory exudate (i.e., protons or water). A major advantage of MRI in early disease over plain radiographs, ultrasonography,[166-168] or CT is the delineation of soft tissue or subperiosteal pus (Fig. 37–8).[169]

Treatment

In the absence of specific indications to the contrary,[64] the initial antibiotic choices in the treatment of acute osteomyelitis should be effective against MRSA (see Table 37–6). Screening of *S. aureus* for inducible clindamycin resistance with the D-test helps determine whether the patient should be treated with clindamycin or vancomycin.[170] Linezolid may become an important oral agent in the initial treatment and in the treatment of clindamycin-resistant MRSA, although studies to date are limited.[171] IV antibiotics for four to six weeks have been traditionally recommended with subsequent oral coverage if appropriate. Because of the complications that may occur from central venous catheters required to maintain IV access[174] recent recommendations have included a shortened course of IV treatment.[169,172,173] Surgical treatment, which should be kept to a minimum,[175] includes drainage of subperiosteal and soft tissue abscesses and débridement of associated lesions. Surgery is often needed for subacute and chronic osteomyelitis. Immobilization of the extremity for relief of pain is often necessary; otherwise, weight-bearing may be permitted as tolerated by the patient.

Course of the Disease and Prognosis

The most dreaded complications of acute osteomyelitis are chronic osteomyelitis and impaired bone growth.[175] Chronic osteomyelitis should be suspected in a child whose systemic symptoms have responded slowly or incompletely to antibiotics or in whom there is a late recurrence of pain at the affected site.

Differential Diagnosis and Related Disorders

Both chronic recurrent multifocal osteomyelitis and synovitis, acne, pustulosis, hyperostosis, and osteomyelitis syndrome are discussed extensively in Chapter 44.

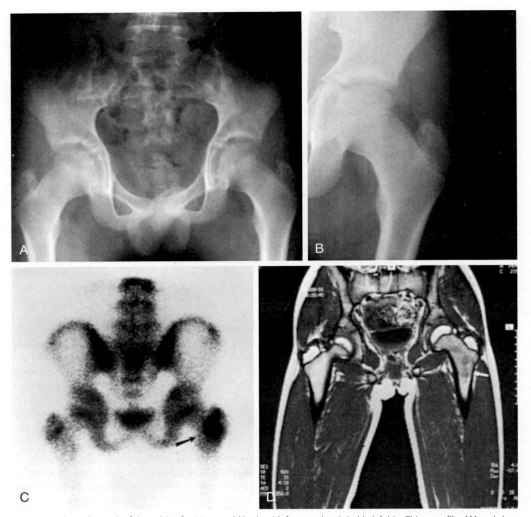

FIGURE 37–7 **A,** Anteroposterior radiograph of the pelvis of a 14-year-old body with fever and an irritable left hip. This x-ray film **(A)** and close-up film of the left hip **(B)** are normal. **C,** Bone scan documents increased uptake of technetium 99m in the area of the left proximal femur *(arrow).* **D,** Magnetic resonance imaging demonstrates an increased marrow signal in the same area of the left hip *(arrow),* which indicates acute osteomyelitis.

Arthritis Associated with Acne

The association between arthritis and acne has been noted for decades. Most patients are male and have onset of musculoskeletal complications during adolescence. The syndrome includes severe truncal acne followed in several months by fever and arthralgia or arthritis, most often involving hips, knees, and shoulders. Myopathy may also accompany the disorder (see Chapter 24).[176] It is possible that this syndrome is another example of reactive arthritis, or it may even be part of the autoinflammatory group of diseases. Although arthritis lasts for only a few months in some patients, recurrences over many years have been documented.[177,178] Treatment with NSAIDs and with antibiotics for control of the acne is indicated. Treatments for acne may also be associated with arthritis, such as minocycline-induced autoimmune phenomena[179] and isotretinoin causing an acute arthritis.[180-183] Infliximab for the treatment of arthritis has been reported to cause acne.[184]

Diskitis

There is considerable dispute about whether diskitis is an infectious process. Infection of an intervertebral disk space from osteomyelitis of an adjoining vertebral body is rare.[185] However, acute diskitis unassociated with vertebral osteomyelitis is a self-limited inflammation of an intervertebral disk that may be caused by pathogens of low virulence, although bacteria or viruses are seldom recovered by aspiration. *S. aureus* and Enterobacteriaceae or *Kingella* organisms are responsible in some patients. Diskitis occurs throughout childhood, but one-half of the cases manifest before the patient reaches 4 years old (peak age, 1- to 3-years-old).[186,187] The sex ratio is approximately equal, although one review observed that diskitis occurred more frequently in girls.[188]

Clinical signs may be subtle. Diskitis is characterized by vague back pain and stiffness, often resulting in a characteristic tripod position during sitting or other unusual posturing.[189] The child, who usually has a low-grade fever, often refuses to walk, stand, or bend over; and may complain of abdominal pain. Palpation of the spine produces well-localized tenderness, usually in the lower lumbar region. The ESR is usually moderately elevated.

Plain radiographs of the affected area often appear normal until late in the disease (Fig. 37–9). A technetium 99m bone scan is valuable diagnostically (Fig. 37–10). The L4-L5 interspace is most often affected (44%), followed by L3-L4 (37%), L2-L3 (7%), and L5-S1 (6%).[186-191] The cervical spine may also be involved. In one study, disk space narrowing occurred in 82% of children, and a bone scan was positive in 72%.[192] MRI may be valuable in differentiating infection from other conditions, including idiopathic disk calcification (Fig. 37–11).[193-195] Aspiration of the disk space or disk biopsy should not be routinely necessary. Immobilization provides symptomatic relief. If bacterial infection is suspected, IV antibiotics should be instituted until results of blood cultures are available.

Whipple Disease

Whipple disease, first described in 1907,[196] is rare in childhood; approximately five afflicted children younger than 15 years old have been reported.[197] It is caused by the bacterium *Tropheryma whipplei,* a ubiquitous organism present in the environment, and is characterized by abdominal pain, weight loss, diarrhea, and, in 65% to 90% of patients, arthralgias or arthritis.[198-200] Whipple disease occurs 10 times more frequently in males than in females and is most common in middle age, although it has been identified in a 3 month old boy[201] and a 7 year old boy.[202] There is also one report of central nervous system disease in a young boy.[197] Migratory, peripheral joint pain and inflammation lasting hours to months occur over a period of many years, often in association with fatigue, weight loss, and anemia. Joint swelling with increased synovial fluid and restriction of range of motion may occur,[203] although residual deformity does not.[204] The joints most frequently affected are the ankles, knees, shoulders, and wrists,[203] and spondylitis has been reported in 20%.[204] Occasionally, arthritis or spondylodiscitis may be present in the absence of gastrointestinal symptoms, and Whipple disease should be considered in patients who are resistant to antirheumatic treatment.[205] A small percentage of the population, especially those who work with soil or in sewage plants, may be asymptomatic carriers. Periodic acid-Schiff-positive material and bacteria are detectable in macrophages infiltrating the upper small intestine and abdominal lymph nodes. Other diagnostic tools include PCR and immunohistochemistry. Because it takes several months to culture the organism, cultures

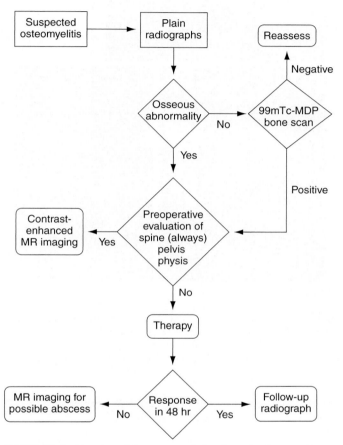

FIGURE 37–8 Flowchart of the recommendations for evaluating acute hematogenous osteomyelitis in children. (Adapted from Jaramillo D, Treves ST, Kasser JR et al: Osteomyelitis and septic arthritis in children: appropriate use of imaging to guide treatment, *AJR Am J Roentgenol* 165:399-403, 1995.)

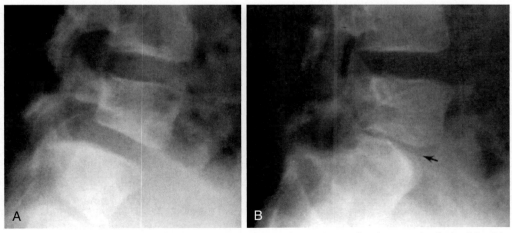

FIGURE 37–9 **A,** Normal disk space is demonstrated on a lateral view of the lumbar spine. **B,** Diskitis has caused collapse of the disk space *(arrow).*

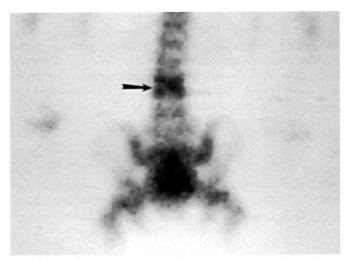

FIGURE 37–10 Technetium 99m bone scan of a 2.5-year-old girl with back pain demonstrates increased uptake of the isotope in the inferior end plate of L2 and superior end plate of L3 *(arrow)*, which is characteristic of diskitis. (courtesy of Dr. H. Y. Nadel.)

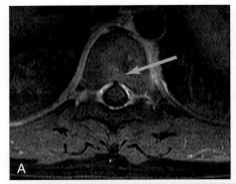
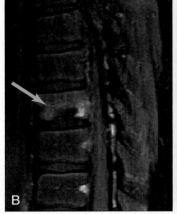
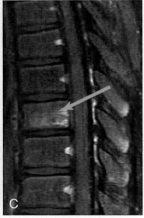

FIGURE 37–11 A 10 year old male with back pain and diskitis. **A,** Axial T1 weighted fat-suppressed MR image postcontrast showing bone enhancement. **B,** Sagittal T1-weighted fat-suppressed MR image following contrast administration with increased signal on the inferior aspect of the vertebral body surrounding an area of decreased enhancement. **C,** Sagittal T2 weighted MR image showing increased signal intensity within the T7 vertebral body and narrowing of the adjacent inferior disk (courtesy by Dr. P. Babyn).

are not recommended as a diagnostic tool, A genetic predisposition has been suggested based on the ubiquitous nature of the organism, but causative genes have not been identified. Antimicrobial therapy (e.g., ceftriaxone, penicillin, doxycycline, cotrimoxazole, streptomycin) has greatly improved the outcome in this disease.

ARTHRITIS CAUSED BY VIRUSES

A classification of viruses known to be associated with arthritis in humans is shown in Table 37–9.[206] The togaviruses account for most of the viral arthritides. In general, viral arthritides occur much more often in adults than in children.[207] Arthralgia is more common than objective arthritis, and both are usually migratory and of short duration (one to two weeks), disappearing without residual joint disease. There are a number of potential mechanisms by which viruses may lead to arthritis, including targeting the cells of innate immunity and adaptive immunity, inducing the production of autoantibodies and T cell mediated autoimmunity, or directly infecting synovial cells.[208] As arthritis is seldom the main symptom of viral disease, clues as to the etiology should be sought in the history, including travel to areas where alphaviruses and Human T-cell leukemia virus type-1 (HTLV-1) may be common, a history of blood transfusions, IV drug abuse, recent vaccinations, or ongoing epidemics or exposures.

Small joints are most often affected by rubella, hepatitis B, and members of the alphavirus group (e.g., Ross River, chikungunya), whereas one or two large joints (usually the knees) are most often affected by mumps, varicella, and other viruses. In some viral arthritides, virus (e.g., rubella, varicella, herpes simplex, cytomegalovirus) can be isolated from the joint space; in others, only virus-containing immune complexes (e.g., hepatitis B, adenovirus 7) are found; and in still others, neither virus nor viral antigen can be recovered from the joint.[209] Whether this represents limitations of recovery and culture techniques

or the fact that culture-negative viral arthritis is "reactive" rather than "septic" is unknown.

Rubella Virus

Rubella-associated arthropathy was recognized by Osler[210] and was one of the most commonly identified virus-associated arthritides in North America. Musculoskeletal symptoms after natural rubella infection are relatively common in young women. These symptoms are unusual in preadolescent children and in males, however, and are much less frequent after rubella immunization than after natural infection. Arthritis is more common after natural infection, and it is more severe and lasts longer.[211]

Arthralgia usually begins within seven days of the appearance of the rash or 10 to 28 days after immunization. The joints of the fingers and, later, the knees are most frequently affected. Joint pain may be accompanied by warmth, erythema, and effusion, and tenosynovitis is common. Carpal tunnel syndrome has also been reported. These findings usually disappear within three to four weeks but occasionally persist for months or even years.

In a study of natural rubella infection in 37 teenage students, 52% of girls and 8% of boys developed objective arthritis,[211] and an additional 13% and 48%, respectively, experienced arthralgia. In a group of young

Table 37–9

Viruses that cause arthritis in humans

Virus	Comment
Togaviruses	
Rubivirus	
Rubella	Global; most reports from North America and Europe
Alphaviruses	
Ross River	Australasia
Chikungunya	Africa, Asia
O'nyong-nyong	Africa
Mayaro	South America
Sindbis	Africa, Asia, Australia
Ockelbo	Sweden
Pogosta	Finland
Parvoviruses	B19 associated with fifth disease, aplastic crises
Hepadnaviruses	
Hepatitis B	Global
Hepatitis C	Global
Adenoviruses	
Adenovirus 7	Rare
Herpesviruses	
Epstein-Barr	Rare; suggested role in rheumatoid arthritis
Cytomegalovirus	Rare
Varicella-zoster	Rare
Herpes-simplex	Rare
Paramyxoviruses	
Mumps	Rare
Enteroviruses	
Echovirus	Rare
Coxsackievirus B	Rare
Orthopoxvirus	
Variola virus (smallpox)	Nonexistent today
Vaccinia virus	Rare

Adapted from Petty RE, Tingle AJ: Arthritis and viral infection, *J Pediatr* 113:948, 1998.

women who received RA 27/3 rubella vaccine, 14% developed an acute polyarthritis. Arthralgia and arthritis are most common in adults, although approximately 25% of prepubertal females develop arthralgia, and 10% arthritis.[212,213] Chronic arthritis in adult women has been reported after vaccination in 5% to 11%.[214,215] It has been suggested that reinfection contributes to arthritis in susceptible hosts.[216,217] Rubella virus has been recovered from the synovial fluid of patients with rubella arthritis in many[218,219] but not all instances.[207,220] The virus was isolated from synovial or peripheral blood mononuclear cells in seven of 19 children with juvenile rheumatoid arthritis but from no control subjects.[221] Other investigations have shown no association.[222]

Parvovirus

Parvoviruses are the latest candidates in the list of viruses putatively involved in the cause of rheumatoid arthritis in adults.[223,224] Parvovirus RA-1 has been isolated from the synovial membrane of one patient with classic rheumatoid arthritis.[225] A second parvovirus, B19, is the agent responsible for erythema infectiosum (i.e., fifth disease or slapped cheek syndrome).[226,227] This illness is sometimes accompanied by an arthritis not unlike that of rubella infection.[227-230]

Arthralgia, symmetrical joint swelling, and morning stiffness have been described in adults, especially women, after parvovirus B19 infection.[230] Carpal tunnel syndrome, hepatitis, and angioedema have been described. This syndrome may be more widespread than previously thought and may be considerably underdiagnosed. In some patients, symptoms have persisted for years. An early study of erythema infectiosum in 364 patients indicated that joint pain, most often affecting knees and wrists, was present during the first week in 77% of adults and 8% of patients younger than 20-years-old.[231] Subsequently, it was determined that arthritis was most common in patients who were HLA-DR4 positive.[232] Whether or not a chronic arthritis results from parvovirus B19 infection is still controversial.[209,233]

Parvovirus infection is common and widespread. Parvovirus B19 genome consists of a linear, 5.6-kD, single-stranded deoxyribonucleic acid (DNA). There is only one serotype of parvovirus B19. Human parvovirus B19 has been implicated as the causative agent in erythema infectiosum, aplastic crises, some cases of hemophagocytic syndrome, and hydrops fetalis.[234] Erythema infectiosum, is a common exanthem of older children that lasts for a few days to a week and presents with a low-grade fever, an erythematous facial rash ("slapped cheeks"), and a lacy, reticular rash on the extremities. These manifestations often recur with malaise, irritability, and arthralgia.

Only a few cases of children with documented B19-associated arthritis have been reported.[228,235-237] Joint symptoms tend to be mild and transient. In the children reported by Reid and coworkers,[238] there was symmetrical involvement of the small joints of the hands and feet. In one child, the arthritis preceded development of the rash. In another, arthritis persisted for three months. Antinuclear antibodies and rheumatoid factors (RFs) were absent in all of the patients in this series. Rivier and colleagues[236] described a 5-year-old boy with arthritis of one knee that lasted for six weeks after typical erythema infectiosum. Nocton and associates[235] described acute arthritis in 20 children with parvovirus B19 infections. The arthritis was associated with constitutional symptoms in one-half of the children and was of brief duration (less than four months) in 14. Six children had persistent arthritis lasting up to 13 months; criteria for a diagnosis of JIA would have been met in this group. Laboratory results were generally normal, except for serological evidence of the B19 infection. Usually, NSAID treatment will suffice, but for patients with persistent symptoms, intravenous immunoglobulin (IVIG) may be a treatment option.[239] A recent study on seroprevalence of parvovirus B19 did not show an increase in patients with JIA compared with diseased or healthy controls.[240]

The precise relation of the viral infection to arthritis has not been clarified. The virus has not been grown from synovial fluid or blood from patients with joint symptoms, although B19-specific DNA has been identified by hybridization in the synovial fluid of adults[238] and by PCR amplification in synovial tissue.[241] However, Soderlund and colleagues[242] demonstrated genomic B19 DNA in the synovium of joints that had suffered trauma even more frequently than in those of children with chronic arthritis. Inflammatory synovitis may not be identifiable by arthroscopy. Although infection gives rise first to IgM antibodies[243] and then to IgG antibodies, there is no evidence that the arthropathy represents an immune complex disease. Demonstration of IgM antibodies, however, is essential to diagnosis. The prevalence of IgG antibodies in the general population is too high to be diagnostically helpful, unless a fourfold increase concurrent with the clinical symptoms is demonstrated.[244-246]

Hepatitis B Arthritis–Dermatitis Syndrome

In adults, up to 20% of infections with hepatitis B virus are characterized by a period of rash and arthritis that resembles serum sickness.[247] The arthritis is often explosive in onset and often occurs in the preicteric phase of hepatitis B infections. In a review of reported cases of arthritis associated with hepatitis B infection,[248] the age of the patients ranged from 14 to 56 years, and the male-to-female ratio was 1.5:1. The dermatitis is characterized by a maculopapular rash, sometimes with petechiae, or urticaria, and is most prominent on the lower extremities. The arthritis usually begins abruptly and symmetrically and affects the interphalangeal joints in 82%, knees in 30%, and ankles in 24% of patients. Although erythema and warmth are present, synovial effusions are uncommon. Joint symptoms last for four weeks on average, respond well to NSAIDs, and disappear without sequelae. The ESR is usually normal, although serum and synovial fluid complement levels are low in the early stages of the illness.[249] Synovial fluid has been reported to show a mononuclear cell predominance.[250] Electron microscopic evidence of hepatitis antigen in the synovial membrane has been reported.[251]

Hepatitis C

Hepatitis C virus is lymphotrophic and is associated with rheumatic symptoms resulting from mixed cryoglobulinemia[207] and producing an intermittent monoarticular or oligoarticular nondestructive arthritis affecting large- and medium-sized joints.[252] A rheumatoid arthritis-like picture may also occur.[253] As many of these patients may be rheumatoid factor positive, the presence of anti-CCP has been proposed as a useful tool in diagnosing true RA in the hepatitis-C infected individual.[254]

Alphaviruses

Epidemic polyarthritis caused by infection with one of the alphaviruses is the most common virus-associated arthritis in Australia, the islands of the South Pacific, Africa,

and Asia.[255] These viruses are transmitted by arthropods, usually the mosquito, and incite an illness characterized by arthritis and a rash that may be macular, papular, vesicular, or purpuric. Although there are some virus-specific differences in these illnesses, they usually are mild in children and occur with equal frequency in males and in females.

In Ross River virus disease, the wrist is most commonly affected and is often accompanied by tenosynovitis and enthesitis at the insertion of the plantar fascia into the calcaneus.[255,256] The synovial fluid is said to be highly characteristic, with a predominance of vacuolated macrophages and very few PMNs. In chikungunya, the knee is the most commonly involved joint, and back pain and myalgia are prominent. The arthritis lasts one to two weeks and is followed by complete recovery. Diagnosis rests on the clinical presentation and an elevated level of antibodies to the specific virus. Viral antigen has not been recovered from synovial fluid.

Herpesviruses

Four of the herpesviruses have been associated with arthritis. Herpes simplex virus type 1 has been isolated from the synovial fluid of one patient with arthritis and disseminated herpes simplex infection.[257] Epstein-Barr virus has long been thought by some investigators to have a primary role in the cause or pathogenesis of rheumatoid arthritis, although direct evidence is lacking.[258-260] Arthritis is a rare complication of infectious mononucleosis.[261-263] Cytomegalovirus is occasionally associated with arthritis and has been isolated from synovial fluid in one instance.[257]

Varicella-zoster infection is uncommonly complicated by arthritis.[264-271] However, there have been instances of bacterial septic arthritis complicating chickenpox.[269,272,273] In one instance, varicella-zoster virus was grown from synovial fluid of an 8-year-old girl with acute, painless monarthritis occurring three days after the onset of chickenpox.[264] The synovial fluid cells were predominantly lymphocytes.[264,271,274] Occasionally, chickenpox is associated with the emergence of psoriatic arthritis.[275] Acute monarthritis has been reported in association with herpes zoster in two adults.[276,277]

Mumps Virus

The paramyxovirus (mumps) rarely causes arthritis. In a 1984 review,[278] only 32 cases were well documented. Since then, two additional patients have been reported.[279,280] The male-to-female ratio is 3.6:1, and the peak age of occurrence is 21- to 30-years-old. Four patients younger than 11 years old and seven between the ages of 11 and 20 years have been described. Arthritis occasionally preceded parotitis but usually followed by one to three weeks. In children, the arthritis was mild, affected few joints, and lasted one to two weeks. In postadolescent males, arthritis was often accompanied by orchitis and pancreatitis.[278] It is reported that the arthritis responds to ibuprofen or prednisone but not to aspirin.[278] The pathogenesis is unknown, and no attempts at recovery of mumps virus from synovium or synovial fluid have been reported. Arthritis has not occurred after mumps immunization.

Human Immunodeficiency Virus

The spectrum of rheumatic diseases that can accompany HIV infection is extremely large and has changed with the introduction of highly active antiretroviral (HAART) treatment. AIDS resulting from HIV infection may be complicated by septic arthritis, although this is now considered rare.[281] Virtually any organism can be responsible; *S. aureus* and Streptococcus species are the most common. Although the precise nature of rheumatic syndromes associated with HIV infection remains controversial, a number of stereotypical presentations have been documented in adults.[282] These include reactive arthritis, psoriasiform arthritis, and an undifferentiated spondyloarthropathy,[283-287] often more severe than in patients without HIV infection. A similar picture has been observed in children infected with HIV.[287a] Arthralgias occur initially with viremia; lower extremity oligoarthritis or persistent polyarthritis can supervene later. A study of 270 patients concluded that the most frequent pattern of joint involvement was one of an acute onset, short duration, few if any recurrences, and no erosive sequelae.[288] The authors have observed chronic oligoarthritis in two young children with HIV infection (one transplacental and one related to blood products). Osteomyelitis may also occur; tuberculosis infection is a relatively common cause.[289] In the post-HAART era, there has been a decline in reactive, psoriatic, and infectious causes of musculoskeletal syndromes, but disorders such as osteoporosis, osteomalacia, and osteonecrosis have become more prevalent.[281]

Other Viruses

There are reports of arthritis associated with adenovirus type 7 infections, although the virus was not isolated from the synovial fluid, and diagnosis was confirmed only on clinical and serological grounds.[288,290,291] Echoviruses[292-294] and coxsackie B viruses[291,295] have been rarely implicated as the cause of arthritis. Smallpox (variola virus infection), now eradicated from the world, was often accompanied by arthritis, especially in children younger than 10 years old. Arthritis also followed cowpox vaccination.[296] Human T cell leukemia virus type 1 HTLV-1 has been associated with a number of rheumatic disorders in adults, including arthritis and Sjögren's syndrome.[297] A 1998 report[298] outlined an outbreak of Sindbis virus-induced Pogosta disease (e.g., fever, rash, joint symptoms) in Finland.

Syndromes Presumably Related to Viral Infection

Transient or toxic synovitis of the hip is an idiopathic disorder often preceded by a nonspecific upper respiratory tract infection. It occurs most commonly in boys (70%) between 3- and 10-years-old.[299] Pain in the hip, thigh, or knee may be of sudden or gradual onset and lasts for an average of six days. Bilateral involvement occurs in approximately 4% of cases. There is loss of internal rotation of the hip, and the hip may be held in the flexed, abducted position. The ESR and WBC count are usually normal.[299,300] Radiographs often appear normal or may document widening of the joint space with lateral displacement of the femoral head because of effusion. These findings can be confirmed by CT or ultrasound studies.[299] Radionuclide scanning may demonstrate a transient decrease in uptake of technetium 99m phosphate. Signal intensity is normal with MRI and differentiates toxic synovitis of the hip from a septic process,[57] which is often the principal differential diagnosis.[301]

After a diagnostic ultrasound scan to confirm the presence of fluid, the hip joint should be aspirated to exclude bacterial sepsis.[302] The synovial fluid has a normal or minimally increased cell count but may be under high pressure.[299] After aspiration, the pain and range of motion are dramatically improved, at least temporarily. Treatment includes the use of analgesics or NSAIDs, bed rest, and skin traction with the hip in 45 degrees of flexion to minimize intracapsular pressure.[299] Long-term sequelae include Legg-Calvé-Perthes disease in about 1.5% of cases,[303,304] coxa magna, and osteoarthritis. Recurrences are often accompanied by low-grade fever.

ARTHRITIS ASSOCIATED WITH OTHER INFECTIONS

Fungal Arthritis

Arthritis caused by fungal infection is rare[305] and is almost unknown in children beyond the neonatal period. Fungi that have been reported as causing arthritis or osteomyelitis are *C. albicans*,[306] *Sporothrix schencii*,[307,308] *Actinomyces israelii*,[309] *Aspergillus fumigatus*,[310] *Histoplasma capsulatum*,[311] *Cryptococcus neoformans*,[311] *Blastomyces dermatitidis*,[312] *Coccidioides immitis*,[313] *Paracoccidioides brasiliensis*,[314] *Nocardia asteroides*,[315] and *Pseudallescheria boydii*.[316] Candidal arthritis,[306] often with accompanying osteomyelitis, is a recognized entity in the newborn[317,318] and occurs occasionally in immunocompromised patients[319,320] and in patients with prosthetic joints.[321]

Sporotrichosis and Plant Thorn Synovitis

Infection with *Sporothrix schenckii* is a rare but significant occupational hazard of gardeners, night-crawler farmers, and field workers.[307,308] Monarthritis or, less commonly, polyarthritis resembling rheumatoid arthritis, has been reported (Fig. 37–12). Synovial biopsy is often necessary to make the diagnosis (Fig. 37–13). Other fungal infections are even less common causes of bone or joint infection in children. The interested reader is referred to the review by Goldenberg and Cohen[308] and to other select references.[310-316,318,321]

Synovitis caused by the penetration of a plant thorn into the joint space or surrounding structures is probably a reaction to the foreign material rather than an

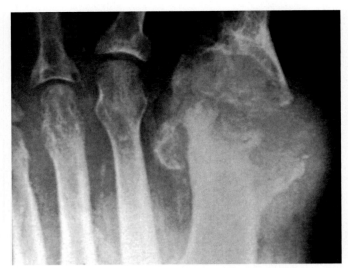

FIGURE 37–12   Destruction of the first metatarsophalangeal joint was caused by sporotrichosis.

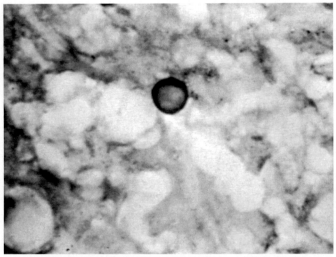

FIGURE 37–13   *Sporothrix schenckii* is identified in a Gram-stained preparation of the synovial fluid aspirate.

outright infection, although the circumstances of the injury may suggest the latter. The synovial effusion is inflammatory, and culture occasionally yields a relatively nonvirulent organism. In the case of rose thorn penetration, *S. schenckii* is the probable cause. More commonly, the thorn of the palm tree or blackthorn is implicated. There are signs of local inflammation, and radiographs demonstrate periosteal new bone formation, a radiolucent defect in bone, or the presence of radiopaque foreign material. CT is indicated if plain radiographic results are negative. Because this disorder may develop months after the initial injury, foreign-body synovitis may be ignored as a diagnostic possibility. Treatment should be directed at appropriate surgical exploration and removal of the foreign material.[322]

Arthritis Caused by Spirochetes

Lyme Disease

The geographical and temporal clustering of cases of what was thought to be juvenile rheumatoid arthritis in Old Lyme, Connecticut, led to the discovery and description of the cause, pathogenesis, and cure of Lyme disease. This epidemiological work is one of the most important developments of the past three decades in rheumatology and provides a model for approaching the question of the infectious cause of other chronic arthritides of childhood. Unfortunately, work on the development of a safe and effective vaccine has stalled.[323] Chapter 38 provides a complete discussion of classic Lyme disease.

Other Spirochetes and Arthritis

Arthritis rarely complicates leptospirosis *(Leptospira icterohemorrhagica)*[324] and syphilis *(Treponema pallidum)*[325,326] Congenital syphilis causes juxtaepiphyseal osteochondritis and periarthritis in infancy and syphilitic dactylitis in early childhood (Fig. 37–14). Clutton joints—relatively painless, recurrent, nonprogressive, symmetrical synovitis of the knees—develop later.[327]

Parasites and Arthritis

There have been case reports of arthritis accompanying a wide range of parasitic infestations,[328] including *Giardia intestinalis (lamblia)*,[329] *Endolimax nana*,[330] *Toxocara canis*,[331] schistosomiasis,[332] and others.[333] In general, the joint disease is presumably reactive or postinfectious rather than septic and pursues a benign course with a good prognosis.

Musculoskeletal Manifestations of Systemic Bacterial Infections

Bacterial infection of ventricular shunts for the management of hydrocephalus may result in arthritis and nephritis.[334] RFs may be demonstrable in the sera of these patients. Meningococcemia is complicated by arthritis in up to 10% of cases.[335] It is usually oligoarticular and occurs most often during the recovery phase, when immune complexes can be demonstrated in the synovium.[336] It can also be complicated by acute septic arthritis in the early stage of the disease. *H. influenzae* type B meningitis may lead to a sterile arthritis.[337]

Infective endocarditis frequently causes arthralgia or arthritis[338,339] and signs suggesting vasculitis (e.g., Osler nodes, Janeway lesions, Roth spots). The musculoskeletal signs and symptoms (e.g., arthralgia, arthritis, myalgia, low back pain) may precede other manifestations of infective endocarditis by weeks.[339] The arthritis is characteristically polyarticular and symmetrical, affecting both large and small joints. An immune complex-mediated pathogenesis is thought to be responsible, and the presence of hypocomplementemia,[340] circulating immune complexes,[313] and sometimes RFs[340] support this theory. Specificity of the RFs is directed to the patient's IgG in combination with the infecting organism.

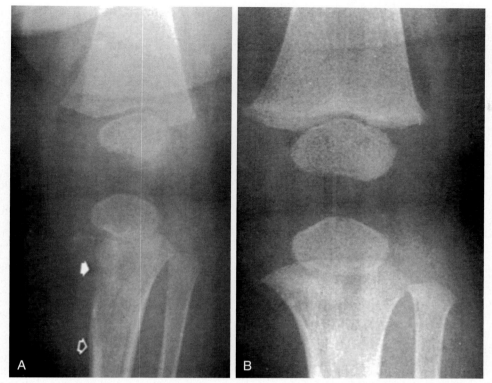

FIGURE 37–14 Lesions of congenital syphilis were identified in a 6-month-old girl brought to the child abuse clinic because of multiple fractures that occurred during the previous 10 days. Her rapid plasma reagin test result was 1:256. **A,** Bilateral, symmetrical, destructive metaphysitis lesions of the proximal ends of the tibiae (Wimberger sign) *(solid arrow)* and periosteal new bone apposition *(open arrow)* can be seen. **B,** With penicillin therapy, the lesions have almost healed two months later.

REFERENCES

3. P. Christiansen, B. Frederiksen, J. Glazowski, et al., Epidemiologic, bacteriologic, and long-term follow-up data of children with acute hematogenous osteomyelitis and septic arthritis: a ten-year review, J. Pediatr. Orthop. B 8 (1999) 302–305.
5. C.W. Fink, J.D. Nelson, Septic arthritis and osteomyelitis in children, Clin. Rheum. Dis. 12 (1986) 423–435.
16. A.W. Howard, D. Viskontas, C. Sabbagh, Reduction in osteomyelitis and septic arthritis related to Haemophilus influenzae type B vaccination, J. Pediatr. Orthop. 19 (1999) 705–709.
23. S. Chometon, Y. Benito, M. Chaker, et al., Specific real-time polymerase chain reaction places Kingella kingae as the most common cause of osteoarticular infections in young children, Pediatr. Infect. Dis. J. 26 (2007) 377–381.
24. P. Yagupsky, Kingella kingae: from medical rarity to an emerging paediatric pathogen, Lancet Infect. Dis. 4 (2004) 358–367.
25. K.M. Kiang, F. Ogunmodede, B.A. Juni, et al., Outbreak of osteomyelitis/septic arthritis caused by Kingella kingae among child care center attendees, Pediatrics 116 (2005) e206–e213.
34. C.J. Mathews, G. Coakley, Septic arthritis: current diagnostic and therapeutic algorithm, Curr. Opin. Rheumatol. 20 (2008) 457–462.
39. T.R. Nunn, W.Y. Cheung, P.D. Rollinson, A prospective study of pyogenic sepsis of the hip in childhood, J. Bone Joint Surg. Br. 89 (2007) 100–106.
40. C.J. Mathews, G. Kingsley, M. Field, et al., Management of septic arthritis: a systematic review, Ann. Rheum. Dis. 66 (2007) 440–445.
46. I.M. van der Heijden, B. Wilbrink, L.M. Schouls, et al., Detection of mycobacteria in joint samples from patients with arthritis using a genus-specific polymerase chain reaction and sequence analysis, Rheumatology (Oxford) 38 (1999) 547–553.
49. R.M. Lyon, J.D. Evanich, Culture-negative septic arthritis in children, J. Pediatr. Orthop. 19 (1999) 655–659.
51. R.F. Buchmann, D. Jaramillo, Imaging of articular disorders in children, Radiol. Clin. North Am. 42 (2004) 151–168. vii.
52. D. Jaramillo, S.T. Treves, J.R. Kasser, et al., Osteomyelitis and septic arthritis in children: appropriate use of imaging to guide treatment, AJR 165 (1995) 399–403.
56. K.D. Stumpe, K. Strobel, Osteomyelitis and arthritis, Semin. Nucl. Med. 39 (2009) 27–35.
58. M. Karchevsky, M.E. Schweitzer, W.B. Morrison, et al., MRI findings of septic arthritis and associated osteomyelitis in adults, AJR 182 (2004) 119–122.
60. M.S. Kocher, R. Mandiga, J.M. Murphy, et al., A clinical practice guideline for treatment of septic arthritis in children: efficacy in improving process of care and effect on outcome of septic arthritis of the hip, J. Bone Joint Surg. Am. 85-A (2003) 994–999.
62. P.O. Newton, R.T. Ballock, J.S. Bradley, Oral antibiotic therapy of bacterial arthritis, Pediatr. Infect. Dis. J. 18 (1999) 1102–1103.
68. A.C. Offiah, Acute osteomyelitis, septic arthritis and discitis: differences between neonates and older children, Eur. J. Radiol. 60 (2006) 221–232.
69. R.R. Betz, D.R. Cooperman, J.M. Wopperer, et al., Late sequelae of septic arthritis of the hip in infancy and childhood, J. Pediatr. Orthop. 10 (1990) 365–372.
72. M.S. Kocher, How do you best diagnose septic arthritis of the hip? in: J.G. Wright (Ed.), Evidence-based orthopedics, Saunders, Philadelphia, 2009.
81. S.P. Brogadir, B.M. Schimmer, A.R. Myers, Spectrum of the gonococcal arthritis-dermatitis syndrome, Semin. Arthritis Rheum. 8 (1979) 177–183.
100. M.W. Shen, Diagnostic and therapeutic challenges of childhood brucellosis in a nonendemic country, Pediatrics 121 (2008) e1178–e1183.
110. E. Maman, J. Bickels, M. Ephros, et al., Musculoskeletal manifestations of cat scratch disease, Clin. Infect. Dis. 45 (2007) 1535–1540.
113. M.S. Gilbert, L.M. Aledort, S. Seremetis, et al., Long term evaluation of septic arthritis in hemophilic patients, Clin. Orthop. Relat. Res. (1996) 54–59.

114. B.I. Asmar, J. Andresen, W.J. Brown, Ureaplasma urealyticum arthritis and bacteremia in agammaglobulinemia, Pediatr. Infect. Dis. J. 17 (1998) 73–76.
116. E. Forlin, C. Milani, Sequelae of septic arthritis of the hip in children: a new classification and a review of 41 hips, J. Pediatr. Orthop. 28 (2008) 524–528.
121. R.J. Scott, M.R. Christofersen, W.W. Robertson Jr., et al., Acute osteomyelitis in children: a review of 116 cases, J. Pediatr. Orthop. 10 (1990) 649–652.
126. R.J. Gorwitz, A review of community-associated methicillin-resistant Staphylococcus aureus skin and soft tissue infections, Pediatr. Infect. Dis. J. 27 (2008) 1–7.
127. J. Saavedra-Lozano, A. Mejias, N. Ahmad, et al., Changing trends in acute osteomyelitis in children: impact of methicillin-resistant Staphylococcus aureus infections, J. Pediatr. Orthop. 28 (2008) 569–575.
143. L.T. Gutman, Acute, subacute, and chronic osteomyelitis and pyogenic arthritis in children, Curr. Probl. Pediatr. 15 (1985) 1–72.
147. M.N. Wang, W.M. Chen, K.S. Lee, et al., Tuberculous osteomyelitis in young children, J. Pediatr. Orthop. 19 (1999) 151–155.
152. M.H. Perlman, M.J. Patzakis, P.J. Kumar, et al., The incidence of joint involvement with adjacent osteomyelitis in pediatric patients,, J. Pediatr. Orthop. 20 (2000) 40–43.
156. P.N. Tyrrell, V.N. Cassar-Pullicino, S.M. Eisenstein, et al., Back pain in childhood, Ann. Rheum. Dis. 55 (1996) 789–793.
160. N.E. Green, R.D. Beauchamp, P.P. Griffin, Primary subacute epiphyseal osteomyelitis, J. Bone Joint Surg. Am. 63 (1981) 107–114.
161. J.J. McCarthy, J.P. Dormans, S.H. Kozin, et al., Musculoskeletal infections in children. Basic treatment principles and recent advancements, J. Bone Joint Surg. Am. 86-A (2004) 850–863.
164. G.A. Mandell, Imaging in the diagnosis of musculoskeletal infections in children, Curr. Probl. Pediatr. 26 (1996) 218–237.
172. A. Karwowska, H.D. Davies, T. Jadavji, Epidemiology and outcome of osteomyelitis in the era of sequential intravenous-oral therapy, Pediatr. Infect. Dis. J. 17 (1998) 1021–1026.
174. R. Ruebner, R. Keren, S. Coffin, et al., Complications of central venous catheters used for the treatment of acute hematogenous osteomyelitis, Pediatrics 117 (2006) 1210–1215.
185. F.L. Sapico, J.Z. Montgomerie, Pyogenic vertebral osteomyelitis: report of nine cases and review of the literature, Rev. Infect. Dis. 1 (1979) 754–776.
193. M. Fernandez, C.L. Carrol, C.J. Baker, Discitis and vertebral osteomyelitis in children: an 18-year review, Pediatrics 105 (2000) 1299–1304.
205. T. Schneider, V. Moos, C. Loddenkemper, et al., Whipple's disease: new aspects of pathogenesis and treatment, Lancet Infect. Dis. 8 (2008) 179–190.
206. R.E. Petty, A.J. Tingle, Arthritis and viral infection, J. Pediatr. 113 (1988) 948–949.
208. R. Franssila, K. Hedman, Infection and musculoskeletal conditions: Viral causes of arthritis, Best Pract. Res. Clin. Rheumatol. 20 (2006) 1139–1157.
235. J.J. Nocton, L.C. Miller, L.B. Tucker, et al., Human parvovirus B19-associated arthritis in children, J. Pediatr. 122 (1993) 186–190.
248. R.D. Inman, Rheumatic manifestations of hepatitis B virus infection, Semin. Arthritis Rheum. 11 (1982) 406–420.
253. I. Rosner, M. Rozenbaum, E. Toubi, et al., The case for hepatitis C arthritis, Semin. Arthritis Rheum. 33 (2004) 375–387.
269. P. Schreck, P. Schreck, J. Bradley, et al., Musculoskeletal complications of varicella, J. Bone Joint Surg. Am. 78 (1996) 1713–1719.
281. N. Patel, N. Patel, L.R. Espinoza, HIV infection and rheumatic diseases: the changing spectrum of clinical enigma, Rheum. Dis. Clin. North Am. 35 (2009) 139–161.
299. H. Wingstrand, Transient synovitis of the hip in the child, Acta. Orthop. Scand. (Suppl.) 219 (1986) 1–61.
301. M.S. Kocher, D. Zurakowski, J.R. Kasser, Differentiating between septic arthritis and transient synovitis of the hip in children: an evidence-based clinical prediction algorithm, J. Bone Joint Surg. Am. 81 (1999) 1662–1670.

Entire reference list is available online at www.expertconsult.com.

Chapter 38

LYME DISEASE

Hans-Iko Huppertz and Frank Dressler

Lyme arthritis was first described in 1977 by Steere and colleagues[1] in a cluster of children thought to have juvenile rheumatoid arthritis. They lived in and around Old Lyme, Connecticut. Subsequent studies documented that the disease was caused by the spirochete *Borrelia burgdorferi*[2,3] and that arthritis was only one of many possible manifestations of this infection, now known as *Lyme borreliosis* or *Lyme disease*.[4-6]

Clinical case descriptions of various manifestations of this disease date back more than a century. Acrodermatitis chronica atrophicans was described in Germany in 1883.[7] Erythema migrans, the early skin manifestation of Lyme borreliosis, was reported in Sweden in 1909.[8] The first case of neuroborreliosis and its association with a tick bite was reported in France in 1922.[9] Among the cases of lymphocytic meningitis and inflammatory polyneuritis studied by Bannwarth[10] in Germany in 1941, several patients described had "rheumatism," probably the first report of what is now called Lyme arthritis. Successful treatment with penicillin was described in 1946.[11] Erythema migrans was transferred by skin biopsy to healthy human volunteers in 1955.[12] These observations suggested an infectious cause.

DEFINITION AND CLASSIFICATION

Lyme disease is a complex disease with cutaneous, articular, neurological, and other systemic manifestations that results from infection with the spirochete *B. burgdorferi* transmitted by the bite of a tick of the genus *Ixodes*. Various components of the disease (e.g., erythema migrans, arthritis, neuroborreliosis) may occur in isolation. The term *Lyme borreliosis* is often used in Europe; *Lyme disease* is the most frequent term used in North America.

EPIDEMIOLOGY

Geographical Distribution

Lyme disease has been documented only in the temperate zones of the northern hemisphere.[4,13] In North America, the disease is recognized most commonly in the northeastern, mid-Atlantic and north-central United States; it occurs less commonly on the West Coast and in southern Canada.[14] Lyme borreliosis is rare or absent in the other parts of the United States and Canada. In Europe, the disease is most common in central Europe but occurs endemically from southern Sweden to the northern Mediterranean and from Portugal to Russia. Although sporadic cases of Lyme disease have been reported in eastern Russia, China, Korea, and Japan, it appears to be much less common in Asia than in the endemic areas of North America or Europe.

Incidence and Prevalence

The Centers for Disease Control and Prevention have reported a rapid increase in the frequency of Lyme disease in the United States since 1982. Between 1992 and 2002, the incidence more than doubled, and 23,763 cases were reported in 2002.[14] Case numbers were slightly smaller for the years 2003 to 2006, the last year for which a detailed analysis has been published. Between 1992 and 2006, the highest average incidence was 73.6 cases per 100,000 of the general population in Connecticut. Throughout this period, the highest local incidence shifted from the island of Nantucket, Massachusetts, to Columbia County, New York, with a peak incidence of 962 per 100,000 during the years 2002 to 2006.[14] Data from the Slovenian National Registry document annual incidences of Lyme disease of 176 to 223 cases per 100,000 between 2003 and 2007[15] with a further increase to 258 in 2008 (F. Strle, personal communication, 2009). A study in southern Sweden reported an incidence of 69 cases per 100,000; Lyme arthritis was present in 7% of all cases.[16] In a population-based study in Würzburg, Germany, the incidence was 111 per 100,000, with higher rates among children younger than 16-years-old.[17]

In a community-based Connecticut cohort study of 201 consecutive cases in children in whom Lyme disease had been newly diagnosed, 13 (6%) had arthritis, and 5% had facial palsy.[18] In Europe, Lyme arthritis and neuroborreliosis have been reported in similar frequencies, and in the Würzburg study, arthritis was more common.[17] Compared with adults, children more frequently had manifestations other than isolated erythema migrans.[17]

Early onset of cutaneous disease and neural involvement are closely related to tick activity in the spring to autumn; there is no seasonal pattern for late manifestations, such as Lyme arthritis.[4,5,17,19]

Sex Ratio and Age at Onset

Both sexes are affected equally. Cases have been reported among all age groups, with peaks occurring in school-age children and people between 40- and 74-years-old.[16,17]

GENETIC BACKGROUND

Although Lyme disease may affect several members of the same family, genetic factors appear to have a limited influence on its occurrence. Nonetheless, host factors influence the course of the disease. In American patients, the development of chronic Lyme arthritis and antibiotic unresponsiveness has been associated with the presence of human leukocyte antigen (HLA)-DR4. HLA-DR2 is an additional risk factor, especially in patients who are HLA-DR4 negative.[20] These results have not been confirmed in European patients. Recently a DR4-positive mouse model has been established.[21]

ETIOLOGY AND PATHOGENESIS

Etiology

Lyme disease is the most common vector-borne infection in North America and Europe and is transmitted by hard-bodied ticks of the genus *Ixodes*[4,22] (Fig. 38–1). Transmission by other ticks or flying hematophagous insects has been suggested but has not been proven. Ticks of the genus *Ixodes* include *Ixodes ricinus* in central Europe, *Ixodes persulcatus* in Eastern Europe and Asia, *Ixodes scapularis* in the northeastern and north-central United States and Ontario, Canada and *Ixodes pacificus* in the western United States.[4]

To become active, ticks require a warm and humid environment and are affected by climatic variability.[23] Infection is acquired in tick habitats, including forests, shaded valleys, gardens, lawns, and inner-city parks. After gaining access to unprotected skin, ticks crawl to the preferred feeding locations in the popliteal region, thighs, groins, breasts, axillae, neck, or head. *Ixodes* ticks feed only once during each of the three stages of their life cycle. Most human infections occur after the painless bite of nymphs (Fig. 38–2). *Ixodes* ticks also transmit tick-borne encephalitis virus, *Ehrlichia*, *Anaplasma phagocytophila*, and *Babesia* organisms. Coinfection of these organisms with *B. burgdorferi* has been reported in rare cases.[24-26]

Microbiology

Lyme disease is caused by infection with one of several species of *B. burgdorferi sensu lato*. These spirochetes have a protoplasmic cylinder surrounded by a cell membrane, a periplasmic flagellum, and an outer membrane.[27]

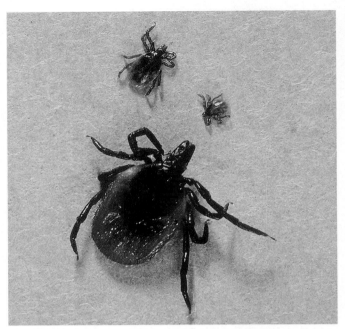

FIGURE 38–1   *Ixodes scapularis*, a member of the *Ixodes ricinus* complex. Clockwise, beginning upper left: nymph, larva, and adult female.

They are microaerophilic and grow best at 33° C in a special liquid medium. They grow slowly, with doubling times between 12 and 24 hours. *B. burgdorferi sensu lato* has been subdivided into several species, of which only *B. burgdorferi sensu stricto* has been found to cause human disease in North America; *Borrelia garinii* and *Borrelia afzelii* also have been identified regularly in patients in Europe.[4,5] A fourth species, *Borrelia spielmanii*, has been isolated in Europe and associated with cases of erythema migrans.[28,29] Up to now, this species has not yet been demonstrated in cases of Lyme arthritis, but this will likely change with time. Recently, *Borrelia lusitaniae* was isolated from a 13-year-old girl with a vasculitis-like syndrome in Portugal.[30] This was the second human isolate and the pathological potential of this species remains to be defined. In general, diversity in *B. burgdorferi* organisms has been greater in Europe and Asia than in North America. Concurrent infection with more than one species of *B. burgdorferi* was described in a patient with acrodermatitis and erythema migrans,[31] as was culture-confirmed reinfection in patients with several episodes of erythema migrans.[32]

B. burgdorferi species differ genomically. Even within a species, different strains express proteins of different molecular weights as identified on gel electrophoresis. The major proteins identified in sonicates of *B. burgdorferi* are the 41-kD flagellar antigen; the 60-kD GroEL heat-shock protein; the three major outer surface proteins (Osp) OspA (30- to 32-kD), OspB (34- to 36-kD), and OspC (21- to 25-kD); the vlsE lipoprotein, the 39-kD BmpA protein; and the 83- to 100-kD antigen. Two membrane glycolipids of *B. burgdorferi* have recently been shown to lead to strong IgG responses in patients with Lyme arthritis.[33] The linear chromosome and 11 plasmids of *B. burgdorferi sensu stricto* strain B31 have been sequenced.[34]

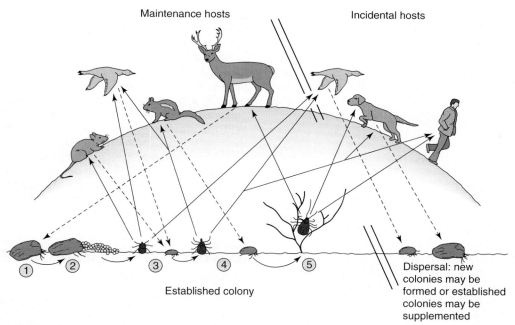

Maintenance hosts   Incidental hosts

Established colony

Dispersal: new
colonies may be
formed or established
colonies may be
supplemented

FIGURE 38–2 Life cycle of *Ixodes scapularis*. **1,** Engorged adult female; **2,** adult female laying eggs; **3,** questing and engorged larva; **4,** questing and engorged nymph; **5,** questing adult. A questing tick successfully finds a host *(solid arrows)*. The tick engorges and drops from the host *(dashed arrows)*. The tick develops to the next stage *(curved arrows)*. (Redrawn from Anderson JF, Magnarelli LA: Avian and mammalian hosts for spirochete-infected ticks and insects in a Lyme disease focus in Connecticut. In Steere AC, Malawista AC, Craft JE et al, editors: First International Symposium on Lyme Disease, New Haven, CT. *Yale J Biol Med* 57:638, 1984.)

The natural reservoirs of *B. burgdorferi* are mice and voles, although hedgehogs and birds may also serve this function. The life cycle of *Ixodes* ticks lasts two years (see Fig. 38–2).[35] The eggs hatch and larvae develop in the spring of the first year. The larvae feed once that summer on their preferred host (i.e., mice and voles) and so become infected with *B. burgdorferi*. The next spring, the larvae molt into nymphs, which feed on the preferred host before becoming mature ticks, at which time larger animals (e.g., deer) act as hosts. Mating occurs while the female tick feeds. The female then detaches and lays her eggs on the ground.

Pathogenesis

Lyme arthritis provides a fascinating model for other arthritides because the causative organism and the clinical picture are well known. However, knowledge of the pathogenesis of this disease remains fragmented. *B. burgdorferi* excreted through tick salivary glands spread locally in the skin and can frequently be found at the advancing edge of erythema migrans. They attach to human cells by binding to various integrins, such as the fibronectin and vitronectin receptors.[36] Binding of the organism to platelets may play a role in its hematogenous spread.[37] Recently, some of the molecular mechanisms involved in vascular interactions of *B. burgdorferi* have been described in a living mouse model.[38] *B. burgdorferi* organisms are presumed to reach the synovium through the bloodstream. It is probable that their presence in synovium is required at the onset of arthritis.

Survival of *B. burgdorferi* for decades in the lesions of acrodermatitis chronica atrophicans indicates that the spirochetes are able to evade the host immune response.

There is also evidence that *B. burgdorferi* may survive intracellularly in endothelial cells, fibroblasts, and synovial cells.[39-41] *B. burgdorferi* uses the mechanism of sequential variation of their outer surface proteins to attempt to evade the host immune response. This contributes to the survival of the organisms in spite of a strong antibody response. Arthritis appears to be largely due to the host inflammatory response.[42] *B. burgdorferi* has stimulatory effects on B cells,[43] and a dominant T-helper (Th)-1 cell response has been found in synovial fluid of patients with Lyme arthritis.[44,45] A *B. burgdorferi*-specific CD8+ cytotoxic T-cell response has also been reported for patients with Lyme arthritis.[46] These cells were found only after the disappearance of arthritis.[46] *B. burgdorferi* also stimulate synovial γ/δ T cells from patients with Lyme arthritis, leading to high and prolonged expression of Fas ligand associated with cytolytic activity.[47,48] A number of cytokines are induced, including interleukin (IL)-1 and IL-6,[49,50] tumor necrosis factor,[51] CXCR3, CCR5, CXCL9,[52] and interferon (IFN) γ and IL-10.[53]

Molecular mimicry may also play a role in the pathogenesis of some of the manifestations of Lyme disease. Sequence homologies have been identified between *B. burgdorferi* flagellin and human myelin basic protein, as well as cross-reactivity between flagellin and a human axonal protein.[54,55] In America, antibody reactivity to OspA and OspB occurred late in the course of infection in patients with chronic Lyme arthritis.[56] Th cells from patients with treatment-resistant Lyme arthritis demonstrated dominant recognition of an OspA peptide of *B. burgdorferi*,[57] and high levels of CXCL9 and IFN-γ were found in synovial fluid and tissue.[52] Human homologues of the borrelial T-cell epitope were found, but reactivity with the self-peptides was lower implying that molecular mimicry is unlikely to be the critical mechanism.[58] The human leukocyte function-associated antigen-1 (LFA-1) was implicated as a candidate autoantigen in treatment-resistant Lyme arthritis.[59] However, later work from the same group cast doubt that LFA-1 is a relevant autoantigen.[60] It has recently been suggested that IL17 and Th17 lymphocytes have an additional role in Lyme arthritis.[61,62] This still needs to be confirmed.

CLINICAL MANIFESTATIONS

Many persons infected with *B. burgdorferi* are asymptomatic. Very often, a tick bite is not recalled. In symptomatic patients, the cutaneous, nervous, and musculoskeletal systems are most frequently involved.[4,5] Symptoms of Lyme disease can be divided into early and late manifestations (Table 38–1). Early signs of infection become evident within weeks or a few months of the tick bite, whereas late organ involvement begins several months or even years later. Early symptoms are usually self-limiting, whereas late manifestations may become chronic and occasionally lead to irreversible damage of involved organs. Most patients present with disease that affects only one organ system.

Cutaneous Disease

The earliest and most common skin manifestation, *erythema migrans*, typically occurs days to several weeks after infection as an enlarging, warm, but usually painless erythematous rash at the site of the bite, and it lasts for days or weeks (Fig. 38–3).[4,5,63] In its classic form, this lesion begins as a red macule or papule and expands peripherally with partial central clearing occurring later. Sometimes, this clearing does not appear; in other cases, the clearing is so complete that erythema migrans becomes a mere curved red streak. In children, the neck and head are the most frequently affected sites. It is also common in the groin, axilla, or thigh and may become quite large (up to 30 cm). Secondary lesions can occur at sites distant from the tick bite. Erythema migrans may be accompanied by flu-like symptoms of fever, chills,

arthralgia, musculoskeletal pain, headaches, malaise, and fatigue. Lyme disease may also begin as a flu-like illness in the absence of erythema migrans.[64]

Weeks to months after infection, *borrelial lymphocytoma*, also known as *lymphadenosis cutis benigna* (i.e., a purple swelling most commonly at an earlobe, the scrotum, or a nipple), is occasionally reported in European patients.[65] *Acrodermatitis chronica atrophicans*, a late skin manifestation, rarely affects European children and then only years after infection.[63,66] In the early phase of acrodermatitis, the affected limb develops inflammatory changes with a red or bluish discoloration. Later, cutaneous atrophy becomes apparent. A peripheral neuropathy can accompany the skin lesion. Lymphocytoma and acrodermatitis are extremely uncommon in North America.

Nervous System Disease: Neuroborreliosis

Early neuroborreliosis most frequently presents as lymphocytic meningitis or a cranial nerve palsy weeks to months after infection.[67,68] It may be accompanied by fever, headache, nausea, vomiting, radicular paresthesias, or pain. Unilateral or bilateral facial nerve palsy is the most common focal neurological manifestation, but cranial nerves III, IV, VI, and VIII may also be affected. Signs of meningitis may be mild or absent in spite of increased protein and lymphocytes in the cerebrospinal fluid. A painful meningoradiculoneuritis is the most common neurological manifestation in European adults but is relatively uncommon in children. Months to years after infection, a small number of patients develop progressive encephalomyelitis or an encephalopathy.[68,69] Other rare neurological manifestations include the Guillain-Barré

Table 38–1		
Major clinical manifestations of Lyme Disease in children and adolescents		
Organ System	**Early Lyme Disease**	**Late Lyme Disease**
Skin	Erythema migrans	Acrodermatitis chronica atrophicans*
	Borrelial lymphocytoma*	
Nervous system	Cranial nerve palsy	Chronic encephalomyelitis*
	Lymphocytic meningitis	
Musculoskeletal system	Arthralgia	Arthritis
Other	Carditis*	

*Rare in childhood.

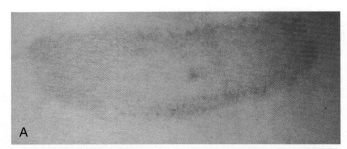
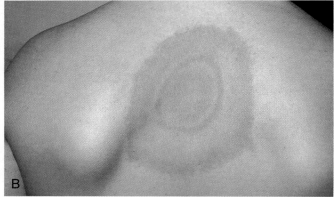

FIGURE 38–3 Erythema migrans. **A,** The site of the tick bite is visible near the center of the lesion. **B,** Typical "bull's eye" lesion.

syndrome,[70,71] pseudotumor cerebri,[72] optic neuritis,[73] cerebral vasculitis,[74,75] and neurogenic bladder.[76]

Musculoskeletal Disease

After erythema migrans, arthritis is the most common manifestation of Lyme borreliosis in many series of pediatric patients and is perhaps slightly more common in North America than in Europe.[4,5,22,77-79] There is little evidence that the musculoskeletal symptoms of Lyme borreliosis otherwise differ between Europe and North America. Myalgia and myositis occur less often, and enthesitis is not a common feature, although *B. burgdorferi* have been identified in a few patients with enthesitis or nodular fasciitis.[80-82] Arthralgia and myalgia develop as early as days to weeks after infection, sometimes concurrent with erythema migrans or flu-like symptoms. However, arthritis appears typically months to years after infection.[83]

The two largest series of pediatric patients with Lyme arthritis include 90 children from Connecticut[79] and 109 from Germany,[83] 62 of whom have been described in detail.[19] Monarthritis of a knee occurred in approximately two-thirds of all children.[19,79] Both knees or other large joints may also be affected.[19,79,83] Polyarticular involvement of small joints was rare. At onset, the arthritis was usually episodic, with relatively painless swelling lasting only a few days and disappearing without therapy. Recurrent episodes of arthritis may become prolonged, and chronic arthritis (duration of more than three months) has been reported in up to 18% of patients.[19] Among 109 German children with Lyme arthritis, 70 had monoarthritis, 32 oligoarthritis, and 7 polyarthritis.[83] The pattern of oligoarticular involvement differed from that found in patients with early-onset oligoarticular juvenile idiopathic arthritis or juvenile rheumatoid arthritis. Ocular involvement with keratitis and anterior and intermediate uveitis may occur in children with Lyme arthritis.[84] In a recent study of acute monoarthritis, fever was a negative predictor for Lyme arthritis versus septic arthritis, and knee involvement was a positive predictor.[85]

Lyme arthritis was reported in a woman after autologous chondrocyte transplantation.[86] The investigators hypothesize that *B. burgdorferi* was asymptomatically present in the patient's joint before the chondrocyte transplant procedure. Myositis has only rarely been described in adult patients,[80] and only myalgia has been reported in children.[87] A dermatomyositis-like picture has also occurred in an adult patient.[88] *B. burgdorferi* was isolated from a child with subacute multifocal osteomyelitis.[89] Fibromyalgia may follow Lyme borreliosis and does not respond to antibiotic therapy.[90]

Other Manifestations

Involvement of other organ systems is much more uncommon. Carditis is rare in children and most commonly manifests as a reversible atrioventricular block.[91] Ocular involvement, including conjunctivitis, keratitis, iridocyclitis, intermediate uveitis, choroiditis, or optic neuritis, has been described in children with Lyme arthritis.[84,92,93] Even more uncommonly, patients may develop hepatitis.[94] There have been anecdotal reports of transplacental transmission of *B. burgdorferi*,[95] but this has not been confirmed in controlled studies.[96] The offspring of five of 19 pregnant women who had Lyme disease during pregnancy had one or more of the following abnormal outcomes: prematurity, syndactyly, rash, cortical blindness, developmental delay, or intrauterine fetal death.[97,98] Whether any of these complications is attributable to infection with *B. burgdorferi* or with other spirochetes (more probably with *Treponema pallidum*) is not certain. There is no evidence that maternal infection presents a significant risk to the fetus.

PATHOLOGY

The synovitis of Lyme arthritis resembles that of juvenile idiopathic arthritis or juvenile rheumatoid arthritis, with villous hypertrophy, synovial cell hyperplasia, and infiltration of lymphocytes and plasma cells.[99] Lymphoid follicles may also be present. Endarteritis is a characteristic finding in patients with Lyme synovitis. In one study, spirochetes were detected in two of 17 synovia, mainly in a perivascular distribution.[99] Other studies using special silver stains have also identified *B. burgdorferi* in synovium or synovial fluid.[100,101] The organism has been recovered from the margins of the erythema migrans lesion and cardiac tissue.[102-104] Although cardiomyopathy may result from the initial myocarditis, valvular endocarditis does not develop. Myositis may in part account for the myalgia and fatigue that occur in this disease, and DNA from *B. burgdorferi* has been identified in the muscle of such patients.[105]

LABORATORY EXAMINATION

Nonspecific Abnormalities

The erythrocyte sedimentation rate is elevated in one-half of the patients, especially during the early phase of Lyme arthritis. Meningoencephalitis causes mild cerebrospinal fluid lymphocytic pleocytosis.[106] The mean synovial fluid white blood cell count ranges from less than 1000/mm^3 to greater than 50,000/mm^3, with a predominance of neutrophils in samples with high cell counts.[19]

Confirmation of Infection with *Borrelia burgdorferi*

Laboratory methods to document infection with *B. burgdorferi* include direct tests, such as culture or the polymerase chain reaction (PCR) to detect borrelial sequences, and indirect tests, such as serology (Table 38–2).[107] The latter tests are most frequently used and universally available. In spite of the standardization of the laboratory evaluation in North America, the approach suggested by the American College of Physicians[108,109] has not been widely adopted for European patients. Common problems with standardization of test procedures for the diagnosis of Lyme disease have been reviewed.[110]

Table 38–2

Laboratory diagnosis of Lyme arthritis

Method	Assessment
Culture of *Borrelia burgdorferi*	Requires weeks; rarely successful
Histochemistry using silver stain or monoclonal antibodies	Rarely successful in synovial tissue
Polymerase chain reaction for borrelial DNA	Efficiency varies widely: Urine, 5% to 30% Synovium, 6% to 90% (higher in membrane than in fluid)
Enzyme immunoassay or immunofluorescence assay using serum	High sensitivity, low specificity, rarely false negative, >10% false positive
Immunoblot using serum	Confirmatory test with high specificity; healthy blood donors <3% positive
Lymphocyte-proliferation assay with borrelial antigens	Sensitivity and specificity <80% Limited availability

All diagnostic tests bear the risk of false-negative or false-positive results. No test is of value in a patient with low pretest probability of having Lyme arthritis.

Adapted from Huppertz HI: Lyme arthritis. In Wahn U, Seger R, Wahn V et al, editors: *Paediatrische Allergologie und Immunologie*, ed 4, Elsevier, 2005, Munich.

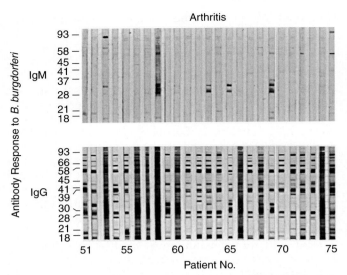

FIGURE 38–4 Western blots of immunoglobulin M (IgM) and IgG antibody responses of 25 patients with Lyme arthritis to a sonicated whole-cell lysate of *Borrelia burgdorferi sensu stricto* strain G39/40. Molecular masses (in kilodaltons) are indicated on the left side. Characteristic of Lyme arthritis, strong IgG responses against many antigens are demonstrated. In North America, the criteria for a positive IgG blot are the detection of at least five of the following 10 bands: 18 kD, 21-kD Osp C, 28 kD, 30 kD, 39-kD BmpA, 41-kD flagellin, 45 kD, 58 kD, 66 kD, and 93 kD. All patients met these criteria. A minority of patients also have IgM responses to a smaller number of antigens. Molecular masses depend on the strain used for testing. (Adapted from Dressler F, Whalen JA, Reinhardt BN et al: Western blotting in the serodiagnosis of Lyme disease, *J Infect Dis* 167:392, 1993.)

Direct Methods to Detect Infection

Culture of *B. burgdorferi* usually takes two weeks to a few months, requires immediate suspension of the test material in special medium, and has high rates of recovery only from skin biopsies of patients with dermatological manifestations of the disease.[102] Culture of the organism from blood and synovial fluid has been relatively unsuccessful. The possibility of obtaining positive cultures is somewhat better from the cerebrospinal fluid of patients with early neuroborreliosis.[111] Methods such as silver staining of spirochetes in tissue specimens or staining with monoclonal antibodies are not routinely performed and are prone to artefacts.

The PCR can demonstrate DNA of *B. burgdorferi* in tissues or body fluids, including synovial fluid.[112-118] In a large North American study of synovial fluid from patients with Lyme arthritis,[112] PCR results were positive for 96% of patients not previously treated with antibiotics and 37% of those who had been treated. In a later study from the same group, borrelial sequences were undetectable in synovial specimens from patients with chronic Lyme arthritis after appropriate antibiotic therapy.[113]

Other groups have found a smaller percentage of positive PCR results in synovial fluid of patients with Lyme arthritis. The precise role of PCR in routine diagnosis remains unclear. False-positive or false-negative results may occur. Optimization of PCR includes using more than one primer pair, targeting genes situated on the bacterial chromosome and the plasmids, performing nested PCR, and analyzing synovial fluid and urine.[114] There is evidence that PCR of synovial tissue may have a higher positivity rate than in synovial fluid[117] and may remain positive in patients with ongoing arthritis whose synovial fluid is negative by PCR after antibiotic treatment.[118] PCR results for urine may be positive in healthy humans whose sera contain *B. burgdorferi*-specific antibodies.[119]

Indirect Methods to Detect Infection

Specific antibodies can be demonstrated after *B. burgdorferi* infection by a variety of tests including enzyme-immunoassay (EIA), immunofluorescence, hemagglutination, and Western blotting[120] (Fig. 38–4). It is recommended that a sensitive EIA be used as a screening test and that all results in the indeterminate or positive ranges be confirmed by Western blotting; this has been called two-tier testing.[121]

Typical IgM and IgG responses of patients with Lyme arthritis and the North American criteria for a positive IgG blot are shown in Fig. 38–4.[121,122] In early Lyme borreliosis, IgM blots are considered positive if at least two of the following three bands are present: 21-kD OspC, 39-kD BmpA, and 41-kD flagellin.[121,123] Antigens from different strains of *B. burgdorferi* have different molecular weights, and, for this reason, North American criteria cannot easily be applied in Europe or Asia, where there is greater strain diversity. Even so, a two-test approach is the best available method for diagnosis of Lyme disease in European children.[19] In a German pediatric Lyme arthritis study,[19] at least six specific bands were required for a positive IgG Western blot, similar to the American criteria. Commonly, patients with Lyme disease have 10 or more IgG bands (see Fig. 38–4), including the ones mentioned earlier. Specific blot-positivity criteria have been established for each of the three pathogenic species in Europe, with different positivity criteria for each strain.[124,125] A North American study found that kinetic EIAs detecting IgG responses to recombinant *B. burgdorferi* antigen vlsE1 or to a conserved internal sequence of vlsE1 were equally sensitive and specific in assessing patients with Lyme arthritis and more sensitive in assessing patients with early skin or neurological manifestations of Lyme borreliosis.[126] European studies have also shown the usefulness of EIAs or Western blots using recombinant vlsE1 peptide antigen in children with Lyme arthritis[127] or adults with neuroborreliosis.[128] In the most recent North American study comparing two-tier testing with ELISA and Western blot with a vlsE C6 peptide ELISA, both methods had similar sensitivity, but two-tier testing had slightly better specificity.[129] Within the first weeks after infection, all serological results may be negative because specific IgM antibodies usually do not appear until three to four weeks after infection, and IgG antibodies cannot be detected until four to eight weeks after infection. Frequently, EIA may give false-positive results related to crossreactive antibodies such as rheumatoid factors or after infection with Epstein-Barr virus[130] or other spirochetes, including *Treponema pallidum*, *Treponema denticola*, *Borrelia hermsii*, and leptospirosis.[131] Antibodies to *B. burgdorferi* occasionally are found in children with juvenile rheumatoid arthritis,[132,133] systemic lupus erythematosus,[134] and other illnesses (e.g., bacterial endocarditis, mumps, Rocky Mountain spotted fever, and other rickettsial diseases).

Serological tests cannot distinguish patients with active infection from those with a previous infection who have responded to therapy. In particular, about 10% of patients with late manifestations of Lyme disease continue to demonstrate an IgM response in addition to the IgG response. Because IgG titers tend to remain elevated for years,[135] serology cannot be used to monitor treatment success or failure. Contrary to claims that the rate of decline of antibodies to the conserved internal sequence of vlsE1 could be useful to monitor treatment efficacy, this was not true in German children with Lyme arthritis.[127] In an endemic area, serological tests should be performed only in patients with clinical signs suggestive of the disease because a positive result in a patient with a low pretest probability of Lyme disease is much more likely to represent a false-positive rather than a true-positive result.[110,136] Given these restrictions, serology is useful diagnostically in patients with suspected Lyme arthritis because almost all patients are clearly IgG seropositive.[19,79] Table 38–3 provides a simplified overview of the laboratory evaluation.

Seronegative Lyme arthritis has been described[137-140] but must be considered so uncommon that vigorous attempts must be undertaken by centers with special experience with this disease to rule out another diagnosis. In these cases, the cellular immune response induced by *B. burgdorferi* can be evaluated,[137-141] and this is the route that is recommended when clinical symptoms and serological results are discordant.[139] However, lymphoproliferative assays are not well standardized and have high rates of false positivity and false negativity.[137-139]

Table 38–3

Assessment of patients with suspected Lyme arthritis

Patient living in or having visited an endemic area
Presence of arthritis documented
No other obvious cause of arthritis
Serology positive (enzyme immunoassay [EIA] and Western blot for IgG antibodies to *B. burgdorferi*):
  No further laboratory test needed:
  Start therapy
Serology negative (EIA and Western blot):
  Rule out other diagnosis
  Refer for specialized evaluation

DIAGNOSIS

Clinical characteristics of patients with arthritis that suggest a diagnosis of Lyme arthritis include residence in or travel to an endemic area, a preceding tick bite, episodic oligoarthritis involving the knee joint, the absence of arthralgias preceding the onset of arthritis, and an adolescent age at onset. Specific criteria have been combined to form a clinical diagnostic score that would confirm or exclude Lyme arthritis in two-thirds of children with arthritis[142] (Table 38–4). For a diagnosis of Lyme arthritis, arthritis (i.e., swelling and effusion or painful limitation of motion in the absence of trauma) must be observed by a physician. Arthralgias alone or reports by the patient or the parents that the joint was swollen are not objective signs of arthritis in this context.

Frequently, however, the clinical presentation of Lyme arthritis may be indistinguishable from that of other rheumatic diseases of childhood with arthritis as a principal manifestation, making laboratory tests mandatory in all patients with arthritis living in or having traveled to an endemic area.[110]

The Centers for Disease Control and Prevention established the following criteria for the diagnosis of Lyme disease:[143]

The presence of erythema migrans larger than 5 cm in diameter,

or

At least one clinical sign (i.e., arthritis, meningitis, radiculoneuritis, mononeuritis, or carditis) and the presence of specific antibodies to *B. burgdorferi*

These criteria were developed for epidemiological research and may not always be applicable in the clinical setting. For example, borrelial lymphocytoma may initially occur in the absence of specific antibodies. Moreover, the mere combination of an objective sign with specific antibodies may include chance associations between two frequent events: arthritis of some kind may affect one in 1000 children, and in endemic areas, 3% or more of healthy blood donors may be positive for specific antibodies to *B. burgdorferi*.[144] Serology can provide evidence of current or prior infection but cannot absolutely confirm a pathogenic link between the infection and the clinical manifestation. The child may have been infected with *B. burgdorferi* as documented by serology; however, arthritis may result from other known or unknown causes. Overdiagnosis of Lyme disease in children has also been reported.[145]

Table 38-4

Diagnosis of Lyme arthritis using a clinical score

Criterion	Score*
Episodic arthritis	+4
Arthralgia before onset of arthritis	−3
Age at onset of arthritis	+0.3 × age (yr)
Initial arthritis in knee joint	+2
History of tick bite	+2
Number of joints involved	−0.4 × number of large joints affected

Scoring example: A 10-year-old boy without prior arthralgia or history of a tick bite developed arthritis in a knee. The arthritis resolved after 10 days but recurred after a 3-month interval. †

Episodic arthritis present	+4
No initial arthralgias	+0
Age at onset × 0.3	+3
Initial arthritis in knee	+2
No history of tick bite	+0
1 large joint affected	−0.4
Total score	+8.6

*If a criterion is recognized, its indicated value is added to or subtracted from the total score for the patient. If it is not identified, the item is scored as 0. Values of 6 or greater indicate the presence of Lyme arthritis, and values of 2.5 or less exclude the diagnosis.

†The patient's serum was later shown to contain IgG antibodies to *Borrelia burgdorferi* by enzyme immunoassay and immunoblot. He was treated with ceftriaxone for 2 weeks. Arthritis disappeared during therapy and did not recur in the subsequent 2 years of follow-up.

Adapted from Huppertz HI, Bentas W, Haubitz I et al: Diagnosis of pediatric Lyme arthritis using a clinical score, *Eur J Pediatr* 157:304, 1998.

Synovial fluid analysis is of little help in establishing a diagnosis of Lyme arthritis because the white blood cell count and type of cells vary greatly.[116,146] However, synovial fluid analysis can exclude septic arthritis and other infection-associated arthritides, yields material for testing by PCR, and confirms the presence of inflammation. Although a positive PCR result from an experienced laboratory indicates a persistent infection, a negative result does not exclude the diagnosis. Synovial tissue may be more suitable than synovial fluid for PCR testing, especially after antibiotic treatment has failed to produce a remission of symptoms.[117,118]

A lumbar puncture should be performed in patients with suspected neuroborreliosis, including those with facial palsy. Lymphocytic pleocytosis and elevated cerebrospinal fluid protein levels are characteristic.[67,68] The reliable standard in diagnosing neuroborreliosis in European patients remains detection of intrathecal antibody production.[67,68,147] However, specific antibody production frequently occurs only after several weeks to months of infection and has been less commonly demonstrable in American patients.

TREATMENT

Antibiotic Regimens

Recommendations by the Infectious Diseases Society of America (IDSA) for the treatment of Lyme disease (Table 38–5) have been published and vary according to disease

manifestations.[148] In the treatment of patients with erythema migrans or neuroborreliosis, amoxicillin is as effective as doxycycline.[149] Cephalosporins were only marginally better than penicillin G.[149-154] Cefuroxime axetil was equally efficacious as doxycycline in adults or as amoxicillin in children with erythema migrans.[155,156] Whereas doxycycline and ceftriaxone have been equally effective,[156] macrolide antibiotics are inferior to other antibiotics.[157-160] It is not known whether these results are applicable to patients with Lyme arthritis, for whom a variety of antibiotics have been recommended, including parenteral penicillin G, oral penicillins, amoxicillin with or without probenecid, ceftriaxone, cefotaxime, cefuroxime, erythromycin, roxithromycin (plus cotrimoxazole), azithromycin, tetracycline, doxycycline, and others.[19,161] For Lyme arthritis, oral antibiotic therapy for four weeks with amoxicillin in young children or with doxycycline in adolescents has been recommended by the IDSA; however, controlled trials of oral versus intravenous antibiotics have not been performed. Oral treatment may be more convenient for the patient and more cost-effective but involves administration of up to 84 doses of amoxicillin. Intravenous treatment with ceftriaxone once daily for 14 days can be performed as an outpatient and may be more convenient for other patients. Before the physician assumes failure of antibiotic therapy, at least two courses of sufficient duration and well-documented compliance are required. When confronted with failure of a treatment program with appropriate antibiotics, the correctness of a diagnosis of Lyme arthritis should be questioned and reconfirmed.

Among 51 German patients followed for at least 12 months after initiation of antibiotic treatment, eight patients still had arthritis, and four had arthralgias.[162] Risk factors for a prolonged course of disease were female gender, age over 10 years, and intra-articular steroids before antibiotic treatment.

Duration of therapy is a matter of debate. Because *B. burgdorferi* is a slow-growing organism, treatment should be continued for at least 10 days. In adults with erythema migrans, extension of treatment with doxycycline from 10 days to 20 days provided no additional benefit.[163] In a retrospective study of Swedish children with early neuroborreliosis, antibiotic treatment for 10 days was considered sufficient.[164] There is also no proof that treatment extending beyond one month is of any additional benefit. The success of antibiotic treatment must be determined clinically because serological results remain positive for a long time after resolution of all manifestations.[135,165]

An approach to treatment is shown in Table 38–5. In young children, erythema migrans is treated with amoxicillin (50 mg/kg/day) in three doses for 10 days to three weeks. In children 9-years-old or older, doxycycline (200 mg/day) is given once daily for 10 days to three weeks. If erythema migrans resolves within a week, 10 days of treatment may be long enough; otherwise a longer duration up to three weeks is recommended. In neuroborreliosis or Lyme carditis, ceftriaxone (50 mg/kg/day) is administered intravenously for 14 days. Because only one 20-minute infusion is required per day, treatment can be provided in an outpatient setting using an indwelling

Table 38–5

Treatment recommendations for lyme disease in children and adolescents

Manifestation	Drugs*	Dose*	Duration
Erythema migrans	Amoxicillin	50 mg/kg/day in 3-4 doses	10-21 days‡
	Doxycycline†	200 mg/day in 1-2 doses	10-21 days‡
Neuroborreliosis and Lyme carditis	Ceftriaxone	50-100 mg/kg/day in 1 dose	2-4 wk
	Cefotaxime	150 mg/kg/day in 3 doses	2-4 wk
Lyme arthritis	Ceftriaxone	50 mg/kg/day in 1 dose	2-4 wk
	Amoxicillin	50 mg/kg/day in 3-4 doses	4 wk
	Doxycycline†	200 mg/day in 1-2 doses	4 wk
	Cefuroxime	30 mg/kg/day in 2 doses	4 wk
	Roxithromycin	5 mg/kg/day plus cotrimoxazole, 6 mg/kg/day in 2 doses each	4 wk

*Ceftriaxone and cefotaxime are administered intravenously; amoxicillin and doxycycline are taken orally.
Maximum daily dose of amoxicillin = 2 g; doxycycline = 200 mg; ceftriaxone = 2 g; cefotaxime = 6 g.
†Doxycycline should not be administered to patients younger than 10-years-old.
‡Continue treatment for another 10 days if erythema migrans is still present at the end of 10 days.

venous access line. Patients with Lyme arthritis also benefit from intravenous therapy, but have been treated successfully with oral antibiotics, including amoxicillin or doxycycline, for four weeks. The latter approach to treatment is more convenient for most patients and more cost-effective than intravenous regimens, but it should not be used in patients with a Baker cyst, neuroborreliosis, or carditis.[166] There is growing evidence that oral doxycycline is as effective as intravenous ceftriaxone for the treatment of European adults with neuroborreliosis.[167] In case of allergy to penicillin, amoxicillin, or cephalosporins, macrolide antibiotics are recommended in children younger than 9 years, although these drugs are less effective than the β-lactam antibiotics. [157,169] This disadvantage may be overcome by a combination of roxithromycin and cotrimoxazole.[168] Infection during pregnancy should be treated with antibiotics not posing a risk to the fetus (i.e., amoxicillin, intravenous penicillin G, or cephalosporins).

During antibiotic treatment, up to 10% of patients with arthritis develop a Jarisch-Herxheimer reaction, with fever, a nonpruritic, nonpalpable rash, and severe pain. This complication usually develops after the first few doses of antibiotics but may occur up to 10 days after beginning treatment. It must be distinguished from allergic reactions to the administered drug.[19] In the authors' experience, most reactions thought to be allergic are Jarisch-Herxheimer reactions. Whereas an allergic response to the antibiotic requires immediate interruption of administration of the drug, a Jarisch-Herxheimer reaction is a favorable, self-limited sign, and treatment can be continued.

Although nonsteroidal anti-inflammatory agents are frequently given to patients with Lyme arthritis, often before the correct diagnosis is made, their efficacy has not been established; however, nonsteroidal anti-inflammatory agents can be used as analgesics or used after antibiotics have failed. Treatment failures in patients with Lyme arthritis or late neuroborreliosis are often associated with prior administration of glucocorticoids.[150] In

such instances, repetition of antibiotic treatment with the same or another antibiotic is recommended. Intra-articular steroids, sulfasalazine, methotrexate, or arthroscopic synovectomy[169] with a further course of antibiotics (in that order) are treatment options. In addition, Steere has given hydroxychloroquine or infliximab in adult patients.[170] The total duration of arthritis was shortened in those patients with ongoing arthritis after antibiotic therapy in comparison to patients that were not treated with antibiotics.[170]

Prevention

Recommendations for the prevention of Lyme disease have been published by the American Academy of Pediatrics,[171] and the subject has been reviewed in detail.[172]

Avoidance of Tick Bites

Avoiding tick bites in endemic areas is difficult. Reduction of tick numbers on residential properties and gardens can be achieved through landscaping measures that create a drying barrier between forest and lawn, the use of acaricides, and the removal of deer from specified areas.[172] Appropriate clothing with light-colored long trousers tucked into socks makes it more difficult for ticks to attach to a human host. Tick repellents containing N,N-diethylmeta-toluamide (DEET), or permethrin applied to clothing can reduce tick attachment for several hours.[22] DEET may also be applied directly to skin, but the use of repellents on skin should be limited because toxic side effects can occur. In Europe, icaridin is usually used instead of DEET. Ticks should be removed promptly because *B. burgdorferi* resides in the tick's midgut, and proliferation starts only after the host's blood has entered the tick's gut. Thereafter, *B. burgdorferi* organisms spread by the acarial hemolymph to the tick's salivary glands. Because this takes 24 to 36 hours, a daily search for and removal of ticks is helpful in endemic areas.[22] There is evidence that *B. afzelii* may be transmitted more quickly than *B. burgdorferi sensu stricto*.[173] Ticks should be grasped with tweezers or fingernails as close to their point of attachment as possible and pulled steadily away from the skin to allow the tick to detach its mouth parts.[22] Mouth parts that remain in the skin do not pose a risk for further transmission of *B. burgdorferi* but may lead to a superficial bacterial infection. The site of the tick bite should be disinfected after the tick is removed. The use of prophylactic antibiotics after a tick bite is controversial. A single dose of 200 mg of doxycycline after *I. scapularis* bites was found to reduce the occurrence of erythema migrans.[174] However, most tick bites remain unnoticed, and in most geographical areas, the frequency of antibiotic side effects exceeds the estimate of preventable disease manifestations. Failures of prophylactic treatment also have been described.[175,176] Prompt antibiotic treatment of the early manifestations of Lyme disease usually prevents late manifestations such as arthritis.

Immunization

Two human vaccines have been developed with a recombinant fragment of OspA of *B. burgdorferi sensu stricto*. These vaccines were first evaluated in North American adults and were found to be safe. After three injections, vaccine efficacy in adults was 76% to 92%.[176,177] One of these vaccines was safe and efficacious in North American children,[178] and recommendations for the use of the vaccine were published.[179] However, these vaccines were never intended for use in Europe or Asia because of the greater strain variation on these continents. The only licensed vaccine was withdrawn from the American market due to economic reasons in 2002. A study of patients with a new onset of arthritis following Lyme disease vaccination found no evidence for an unusual OspA response or more common occurrence of HLA-alleles associated with treatment-resistant Lyme arthritis compared with vaccinated and healthy controls.[180] While efforts to develop new vaccines are ongoing, none of them is close to broader use.

COURSE OF THE DISEASE AND PROGNOSIS

The prognosis for children with erythema migrans or early neuroborreliosis is excellent when the disease has been promptly treated with appropriate antibiotics.[164,181-183] Even in children with Lyme arthritis who have not been treated, manifestations usually diminish and eventually disappear over time.[93] Among 90 children with Lyme arthritis treated with appropriate antibiotics, four had ongoing musculoskeletal complaints seven years later.[79] Of 51 German children with Lyme arthritis examined one year after initiation of antibiotic treatment, eight patients had chronic arthritis, and four had persistent arthralgias in joints previously affected by arthritis.[162] In rare cases, flares of arthritis in a previously affected joint have been observed several years after antibiotic treatment and the initial disappearance of arthritis. Among 94 children with Lyme arthritis, 39% had resolution of arthritis longer than six months after onset of antibiotic therapy, and 13% had resolution after more than 12 months.[184] No clinical or laboratory feature could be identified to distinguish antibiotic responsive patients from those with longer disease duration.

Erosion of cartilage is rare in children. Arthralgia in joints previously affected by arthritis may persist for several months, but children generally do not fulfill diagnostic criteria for fibromyalgia, and arthralgias usually do not restrict the physical or educational performance of adolescents. Late neurological complications have been described in untreated children with Lyme arthritis[93] but have not been observed after appropriate treatment.[185] However, transient neurocognitive abnormalities may occur.[69] Late development of keratitis has occurred in treated and in untreated children.[93] Lyme disease is not fatal and rarely results in significant persistent organ damage, but co-infection with tick-borne encephalitis virus or with *Ehrlichia* or *Babesia* organisms may lead to a more severe disease course.[24-26]

A follow-up study of American adult patients found more musculoskeletal disease and verbal memory impairment in patients than in controls.[186] Poor prognosis of Lyme arthritis in American adults has been associated with the DRB1*0401 and DRB1*0101 alleles[59,60] and the presence of antibodies to OspA. The risk of treatment failure seems to increase with increasing age and when intra-articular steroids were given before antibiotics.[150,162]

In adult patients with medically unexplained symptoms, including diffuse pain and the belief of suffering from chronic Lyme disease, an increased rate of psychiatric problems including depression, negative affect and catastrophizing were found.[187] The authors recommend a multidisciplinary treatment protocol rather than prolonged antibiotic treatment and perpetuation of the role of the chronically ill patient.

Szer and colleagues[93] studied 46 American children (25 boys) with chronic Lyme arthritis with onset of disease between 1976 and 1979. None had been treated with antibiotics for the first four years of the disease. Almost all (98%) had arthralgias during the early phase, with a median time from disease onset to development of arthritis of three months (range, two to 24 months). The number of children with recurrent episodes declined each year. Older children tended to have arthritis of longer duration. At the end of the study, 12 children (31%) still had occasional brief episodes of joint pain. One child had marked fatigue, and two developed keratitis. All 46 children had persistently positive IgG antibody responses. IgM responses were more frequent, and IgG titers were higher in children with recurrent symptoms than in those who became asymptomatic.

REFERENCES

1. A.C. Steere, S.E. Malawista, D.R. Snydman, et al., Lyme arthritis. An epidemic of oligoarticular arthritis in children and adults in three Connecticut communities, Arthritis Rheum. 20 (1977) 7–17.
2. W. Burgdorfer, A.G. Barbour, S.F. Hayes, et al., Lyme disease-a tick-borne spirochetosis? Science 216 (1982) 1317–1319.
3. A.C. Steere, R.L. Grodzicki, A.N. Kornblatt, et al., The spirochetal etiology of Lyme disease, N. Engl. J. Med. 308 (1983) 733–740.
4. G. Stanek, F. Strle, Lyme borreliosis, Lancet. 362 (2003) 1639–1647.
5. A.C. Steere, Lyme disease, N. Engl. J. Med. 345 (2001) 115–125.
6. F. Dressler P. Irigoyen, N. Ilowite, et al., Lyme arthritis, in: S.K. Sood (Ed.), Lyme borreliosis in Europe and North America, 2010, John Wiley, in print.
7. A. Buchwald, Ein Fall von diffuser idiopathischer Hautatrophie, Arch. Dermatol. Syph. 10 (1883) 553.

17. H.I. Huppertz, M. Böhme, S.M. Standaert, et al., Incidence of Lyme borreliosis in the Würzburg region of Germany, Eur. J. Clin. Microbiol. Infect. Dis. 18 (1999) 697–703.

19. H.I. Huppertz, H. Karch, H.J. Suschke, et al., Lyme arthritis in European children and adolescents, Arthritis Rheum. 38 (1995) 361–368.

27. A.G. Barbour, S.F. Hayes, Biology of Borrelia species, Microbiol. Rev. 50 (1986) 381–400.

29. V. Fingerle, U.C. Schulte-Spechtel, E. Ruzic-Sabljic, et al., Epidemiological aspects and molecular characterization of Borrelia burgdorferi s.l. from southern Germany with special respect to the new species Borrelia spielmanii sp. nov, Int. J. Med. Microbiol. 298 (2008) 279–290.

38. M.U. Norman, T.J. Moriarty, A.R. Dresser, et al., Molecular mechanisms involved in vascular interactions of the Lyme disease pathogen in a living host, PLoS. Pathog. 4 (2008) e1000169.

41. H.J. Girschick, H.I. Huppertz, H. Rüssmann, et al., Intracellular persistence of Borrelia burgdorferi in human synovial cells, Rheumatol. Int. 16 (1996) 125–132.

42. A.C. Steere, L. Glickstein, Elucidation of Lyme arthritis, Nat. Rev. Immunol. 4 (2004) 143.

45. D.M. Gross, A.C. Steere, B.T. Huber, T helper 1 response is dominant and localized to the synovial fluid in patients with Lyme arthritis, J. Immunol. 160 (1998) 1022–1028.

46. D.H. Busch, C. Jassoy, U. Brinckmann, et al., Detection of Borrelia burgdorferi-specific CD8+ cytotoxic T-cells in patients with Lyme arthritis, J. Immunol. 157 (1996) 3534–3541.

61. G. Codolo, A. Amedei, A.C. Steere, et al., Borrelia burgdorferi NapA-driven Th17 cell inflammation in Lyme arthritis, Arthritis Rheum. 58 (2008) 3609–3617.

62. D.T. Nardelli, S.M. Callister, R.F. Schell, Lyme arthritis: Current concepts and a change in paradigm, Clin. Vaccine Immunol. 15 (2008) 21.

64. H.M. Feder, M.A. Gerber, P.J. Krause, et al., Early Lyme disease: a flu-like illness without erythema migrans, Pediatrics 91 (1993) 456–459.

67. H.J. Christen, F. Hanefeld, H. Eiffert, et al., Epidemiology and clinical manifestations of Lyme borreliosis in childhood. A prospective multicentre study with special regard to neuroborreliosis, Acta. Paediatr. 82 (1993) 1–75.

79. M.A. Gerber, L.S. Zemel, E.D. Shapiro, Lyme arthritis in children: clinical epidemiology and long-term outcomes, Pediatrics 102 (1998) 905–908.

83. H.I. Huppertz, H. Michels, Pattern of joint involvement in children with Lyme arthritis, Br. J. Rheumatol. 35 (1996) 1016–1018.

84. H.I. Huppertz, D. Münchmeier, W. Lieb, Ocular manifestations in children and adolescents with Lyme arthritis, Br. J. Ophthalmol. 83 (1999) 1149–1152.

85. A. Thompson, R. Mannix, R. Bachur, Acute pediatric monoarticular arthritis: Distinguishing Lyme arthritis from other etiologies, Pediatrics 123 (2009) 959.

90. L.H. Sigal, S.J. Patella, Lyme arthritis as the incorrect diagnosis in pediatric and adolescent fibromyalgia, Pediatrics 90 (1992) 523–528.

93. I.S. Szer, E. Taylor, A.C. Steere, The long-term course of Lyme arthritis in children, N. Engl. J. Med. 325 (1991) 159–163.

98. D. Nadal, U.A. Hunziker, H.U. Bucher, et al., Infants born to mothers with antibodies against Borrelia burgdorferi at delivery, Eur. J. Pediatr. 148 (1989) 426–427.

107. M. Golightly, Laboratory considerations in the diagnosis and management of Lyme borreliosis, Am. J. Clin. Pathol. 99 (1993) 168–174.

108. American College of Physicians, Guidelines for laboratory evaluation in the diagnosis of Lyme disease. Clinical guideline, part 1, Ann. Intern. Med. 127 (1997) 1106–1108.

109. P. Tugwell, D.T. Dennis, A. Weinstein, et al., Laboratory evaluation in the diagnosis of Lyme disease. Clinical guideline, part 2, Ann. Intern. Med. 127 (1997) 1109–1123.

110. L.H. Sigal, Pitfalls in the diagnosis and management of Lyme disease, Arthritis Rheum. 41 (1998) 195–204.

112. J.J. Nocton, F. Dressler, B.J. Rutledge, et al., Detection of Borrelia burgdorferi DNA by polymerase chain reaction in synovial fluid from patients with Lyme arthritis, N. Engl. J. Med. 330 (1994) 229–234.

121. Centers for Disease Control and Prevention (CDC), Recommendations for test performance and interpretation from the Second National Conference on Serologic Diagnosis of Lyme Disease, MMWR. Morb. Mortal. Wkly. Rep. 44 (1995) 590–591.

122. F. Dressler, J.A. Whalen, B.N. Reinhardt, et al., Western blotting in the serodiagnosis of Lyme disease, J. Infect. Dis. 167 (1993) 392–400.

123. S.M. Engstrom, E. Shoop, R.C. Johnson, Immunoblot interpretation criteria for serodiagnosis of early Lyme disease, J. Clin. Microbiol. 33 (1995) 419–427.

124. U. Hauser, G. Lehnert, R. Lobentanzer, et al., Interpretation criteria for standardized Western blots for three European species of Borrelia burgdorferi sensu lato, J. Clin. Microbiol. 35 (1997) 1433–1444.

127. T. Heikkilä, H.I. Huppertz, I. Seppälä, et al., Recombinant or peptide antigens in the serology of Lyme arthritis in children, J. Infect. Dis. 187 (2003) 1888–1894.

129. A.C. Steere, G. McHugh, N. Damle, et al., Prospective study of serologic tests for lyme disease, Clin. Infect. Dis. 47 (2008) 188–195.

136. G. Nichol, D.T. Dennis, A.C. Steere, et al., Test-treatment strategies for patients suspected of having Lyme disease: a cost-effectiveness analysis, Ann. Intern. Med. 128 (1998) 37–48.

137. F. Dressler, N.H. Yoshinari, A.C. Steere, The T-cell proliferative assay in the diagnosis of Lyme disease, Ann. Intern. Med. 15 (1991) 533–539.

139. H.I. Huppertz, S. Mösbauer, D.H. Busch, et al., Lymphoproliferative responses to Borrelia burgdorferi in the diagnosis of Lyme arthritis in children and adolescents, Eur. J. Pediatr. 155 (1996) 297–302.

142. H.I. Huppertz, W. Bentas, I. Haubitz, et al., Diagnosis of pediatric Lyme arthritis using a clinical score, Eur. J. Pediatr. 157 (1998) 304–308.

143. M. Wharton, T.L. Chorba, R.L. Vogt, et al., Case definitions for public health surveillance, MMWR. Morb. Mortal. Wkly. Rep. 39 (1990) 19.

145. M. Zahid Qureshi, D. New, N.J. Zulqarni, et al., Overdiagnosis and overtreatment of Lyme disease in children, Pediatr. Infect. Dis. J. 21 (2002) 12–14.

148. G.P. Wormser, R.J. Dattwyler, E.D. Shapiro, et al., The clinical assessment, treatment, and prevention of Lyme disease, human granulocytic anaplasmosis, and babesioisis: clinical practice guidelines by the Infectious Diseases Society of America, Clin. Infect. Dis. 43 (2006) 1089–1134.

161. A.C. Steere, R.E. Levin, P.J. Molloy, et al., Treatment of Lyme arthritis, Arthritis Rheum. 37 (1994) 878–888.

162. W. Bentas, H. Karch, H.I. Huppertz, Lyme arthritis in children and adolescents: outcome 12 months after initiation of antibiotic therapy, J. Rheumatol. 27 (2000) 2025–2030.

163. G.P. Wormser, R. Ramanathan, J. Nowakowski, et al., Duration of antibiotic therapy for early Lyme disease, Ann. Intern. Med. 138 (2003) 697–704.

165. P. Kannian, G. McHugh, B.J.B. Johnson, et al., Antibody responses to Borrelia burgdorferi in patients with antibiotic-refectory, antibiotic-responsive, or non-antibiotic-treated Lyme arthritis, Arthritis Rheum. 56 (2007) 4216–4225.

166. M.H. Eckman, A.C. Steere, R.A. Kalish, et al., Cost effectiveness of oral as compared with intravenous antibiotic therapy for patients with early Lyme disease or Lyme arthritis, N. Engl. J. Med. 337 (1997) 357–363.

170. A.C. Steere, S.M. Angelis, Therapy for Lyme arthritis—strategies for the treatment of antibiotic-refractory arthritis, Arthritis Rheum. 54 (2006) 3079–3086.

171. American Academy of Pediatrics, Committee on Infectious Diseases: Prevention of Lyme disease, Pediatrics 105 (2000) 142–147.

172. E.B. Hayes, J. Piesman, How can we prevent Lyme disease? N. Engl. J. Med. 348 (2003) 2424–2430.

175. S. Warshafsky, J. Nowakowski, R.B. Nadelman, et al., Efficacy of antibiotic prophylaxis for prevention of Lyme disease, J. Gen. Intern. Med. 11 (1996) 329–333.

181. W.V. Adams, C.D. Rose, S.C. Eppes, et al., Cognitive effects of Lyme disease in children: a 4 year followup study, J. Rheumatol. 26 (1999) 1190–1194.

182. J.C. Salazar, M.A. Gerber, C.W. Goff, Long-term outcome of Lyme disease in children given early treatment, J. Pediatr. 122 (1993) 591–593.

183. E.G. Seltzer, M.A. Gerber, M. Cartter, et al., Long-term outcomes of persons with Lyme disease, JAMA. 283 (2000) 609–616.

184. A.C. Brescia, C.D. Rose, P.T. Fawcett, Prolonged synovitis in pediatric Lyme arthritis cannot be predicted by clinical or laboratory parameters, Clin. Rheumatol. 28 (2009) 591–593.

186. N.A. Shadick, C.B. Phillips, E.L. Logigian, et al., The long-term clinical outcomes of Lyme disease. A population-based retrospective cohort study, Ann. Intern. Med. 121 (1994) 560–567.

187. A.L. Hassett, D.C. Radvanski, S. Buyske, et al., Role of psychiatric comorbidity in chronic Lyme disease, Arthritis Rheum. 59 (2008) 1742–1749.

Entire reference list is available online at www.expertconsult.com.

Chapter 39

REACTIVE ARTHRITIS

Rubén Burgos-Vargas and Janitzia Vázquez-Mellado

The reactive arthritides, among the most common rheumatic diseases of childhood, constitute a group of diverse inflammatory arthropathies in which the joint and extra-articular manifestations are preceded by an extra-articular infection with specific organisms. This chapter reviews arthritis related to enteric or genitourinary bacterial infections.

DEFINITION AND CLASSIFICATION

In this chapter, use of the term *reactive arthritis* (ReA) is restricted to the arthritides triggered by enteric and genital bacterial infections, and often associated with human leukocyte antigen (HLA) B27. ReA is a nonseptic arthritis developing after an extraarticular infection with one of the so-called arthritogenic bacteria, particularly *Chlamydia, Yersinia, Salmonella, Shigella,* or *Campylobacter.*[1-3]

Reiter syndrome is a presentation of ReA defined by the triad of arthritis, conjunctivitis, and urethritis (or cervicitis). The term has been frequently used in the pediatric rheumatology literature in the past.

CLASSIFICATION AND DIAGNOSTIC CRITERIA

The diagnosis of ReA is a clinical challenge. The criteria currently used most commonly to make a diagnosis of ReA are those of the 1995 Berlin Third International Workshop on ReA[4] (Table 39–1), which require the presence of a predominantly lower limb, asymmetrical oligoarthritis, and clinical or laboratory evidence of a preceding infection (Table 39–2). The problem of definition and classification of ReA has been reviewed by Pacheco-Tena and colleagues.[5] In general, the value of diagnostic tests depends on the pretest probability of the diagnosis.[6]

EPIDEMIOLOGY

The frequency of ReA is related to the prevalence of HLA-B27 and probably to the rate of infections by arthritogenic bacteria in the general population.[7] However, ReA may occur in HLA-B27 negative patients and in recent series of *Salmonella*- and *Yersinia*-triggered arthritis a minority of patients has HLA-B27. Reports of *Yersinia*-triggered ReA in children have usually come from countries in which infection with *Yersinia* is common. *Mycoplasma pneumoniae* has been linked to ReA.[8]

In studies summarized by Keat,[3] ReA was estimated to occur in 1% of patients with sexually acquired infections, 2.4% of those with either *Shigella* or *Campylobacter* infections, 3.2% with *Salmonella* infections, and up to 33% of adult patients with yersiniosis. ReA develops in 5% to 10% of children with yersiniosis.[9,10] In a *Salmonella* outbreak in Germany,[11] no cases of ReA occurred among 286 infected children, although six children had brief arthralgia. In contrast, 20% of 207 children reported joint, eye, or mucocutaneous symptoms after an outbreak of *Salmonella typhimurium* phage type 135a in Australia.[12] ReA occurred in 43% of adults infected; and the role of HLA-B27 was considered to be of minor relevance.

The relative frequency of ReA among patients in pediatric rheumatology clinics in the United States,[13,14] United Kingdom,[15] and Canada[16] ranged between 4.1% and 8.6%. This wide variation is consistent with differences in the stringency of diagnostic and classification criteria used in each study. Reports from other sources suggest that clinical recognition of ReA may be increasing.[17-23] Most cases of ReA occur in boys between the ages of 8 and 12 years, but sex and age distribution vary according to the causative organism. In an Italian study of children with *Yersinia*-triggered ReA, most cases occurred between the ages of 3 and 7 years, and there was a slight predominance of females.[22] Enteric infections are responsible for ReA at all ages, but ReA following genital infections with *Chlamydia* occurs more frequently during adolescence.

GENETIC BACKGROUND

Although the susceptibility to the primary infection is not related to any genetic marker, ReA most frequently occurs in HLA-B27 individuals. In fact, the frequency and severity of joint pain after intestinal infections by *Salmonella, Shigella,* and *Yersinia* is associated with the presence of HLA-B27.[24] The frequency of HLA-B27 in children with

Table 39–1

The Berlin diagnostic criteria for reactive arthritis

Typical Peripheral Arthritis
(Predominantly lower limb, asymmetric oligoarthritis)
plus

Evidence of Preceding Infection
If there is a clear history of diarrhea or urethritis within the preceding 4 weeks, laboratory confirmation is desirable but not essential.
Where no clear clinical infection is identified, laboratory confirmation of infection is essential.

Exclusion Criteria
Patients with other known causes of monarthritis or oligoarthritis (such as other defined spondyloarthropathies, septic arthritis, crystal arthritis, Lyme disease, and streptococcal Reactive arthritis) should be excluded.

Modified from Kingsley G, Sieper J: Third International Workshop on Reactive Arthritis: an overview, *Ann Rheum Dis* 55:564-570, 1996, with permission from the BMJ Publishing Group.

Table 39–2

Laboratory tests for documenting preceding infection in reactive arthritis

Routine
  Culture of stool and urethra
  Serology: antibodies against specific arthritogenic bacteria
Research Studies
  Urethral swab for detection of Chlamydial DNA by polymerase chain reaction (PCR)*
  Synovial fluid or synovial membrane biopsy for detection of bacterial DNA by PCR*
  Immunofluorescence microscopy for detection of bacteria in synovial biopsy specimen**
  Stimulation of synovial fluid lymphocytes with antigens from arthritogenic bacteria**

*A potential diagnostic test.
**Research tools, not suitable for routine diagnostic use.
Modified from Kingsley G, Sieper J: Third International Workshop on Reactive Arthritis: an overview, *Ann Rheum Dis* 55:564-570, 1996, with permission from the BMJ Publishing Group.

ReA varies widely; in children with mild forms of *Yersinia*-, *Campylobacter*-, and *Chlamydia*-related ReA, the frequency of B27 is similar to that of the population.[8,9,25] In others, the prevalence may reach 60%.

Other associations have been reported in specific populations. An association with the tumor necrosis factor c1 allele independent of B27 was reported in a predominantly adult Finnish population with ReA.[26] In a similar population, TAP2J, a polymorphism of transporters associated with antigen processing (TAP2), was more frequent in B27 positive patients with ReA.[27] An association between the toll-like receptor 2 and ReA has been described after an outbreak of *S. enteritidis* in Canada.[28] Single nucleotide polymorphisms in the interferon gamma (IFNγ) gene (rs2430561 and rs1861493) appear to predispose to ReA in the Dutch population,[29] and solute carrier family 11 member A1 gene polymorphisms are increased in the Chinese.[30]

ETIOLOGY AND PATHOGENESIS

Arthritogenic Bacteria

Several bacteria are involved in the etiology of ReA. In preadolescent patients, *Salmonella*, *Shigella*, *Yersinia*, or *Campylobacter* enteric infections precede the onset of arthritis in 80% of instances. *Shigella flexneri*,[31-35] *Yersinia enterocolitica*,[35] *Salmonella enteritidis*,[36] *Salmonella oranienburg*,[37] and *Salmonella typhimurium*[38] have all been isolated from children with the post-dysenteric ReA conjunctivitis and urethritis triad. In at least two youths and three children, *Chlamydia trachomatis*[38] has been identified in synovial fluid. Respiratory tract infection with *Mycoplasma pneumoniae*[39] or *Chlamydia pneumoniae*[40] has preceded the development of ReA in a few children, and the latter agent was responsible for approximately 10% of cases of ReA in a Finnish study.[40] HLA-B27 ReA has also been associated with *Clostridium difficile*.[41,42]

Role of HLA-B27

The role of HLA-B27 in the pathogenesis of ReA is still unknown.[43-47] The arthritogenic peptide hypothesis[48-51] postulates that the HLA-B27 molecule is able to bind a unique bacterial or self antigenic peptide (not yet identified, but supposedly present in the joints), which is then presented to an HLA-B27-restricted cytotoxic (CD8+) T cell.[52] CD8+ T cells crossreaction with bacterial epitopes may then lead to inflammation and tissue damage.[53] Several bacterial amino acid sequences homologous to HLA-B27 amino acid sequences have been described.[54,55,56] These sequences include, among others, that of a primase derived from *Chlamydia trachomatis*[57,58] and even the Epstein-Barr virus LMP2 epitope.[59]

Equally relevant is the B27 misfolding hypothesis,[60,61] which refers to the accumulation of misfolded heavy chains of HLA-B27 in the endoplasmic reticulum, leading to the activation of nuclear factor-κB and proinflammatory cytokines.[60-63] Instability of the HLA-B27 molecule leads to the formation of HLA-B27 homodimers, which are likely to act as receptors for humoral or cell-mediated autoimmune responses mediated by class I HLA molecules or as proinflammatory targets that consequently lead to excessive cytokine production.[64,65] The same process seems to be responsible for the deposition of β2 microglobulin in the synovium and perhaps other tissues, leading to inflammation.[66]

HLA-B27 modulates the production of cytokines and influences both bacterial invasion of cells and killing of bacteria.[67,68] As a result, intracellular survival of arthritogenic bacteria is prolonged. Arthritogenic bacteria invade the gut mucosa and replicate within polymorphonuclear cells and macrophages.[69-71] Studies in murine fibroblasts transfected with B27, not replicated in human cells, indicated that the expression of this antigen inhibited cell invasion by arthritogenic bacteria.[72-76] Persistence of the organism within B27 cells was prolonged.[77] Various bacterial components (including lipopolysaccharide, DNA, and RNA) have been identified in both synovial fluid cells and synovial membranes of patients with ReA.[78-87]

The antibody response against arthritogenic bacteria in ReA lasts longer than in infected patients who do not develop arthritis. Nevertheless, the role of antibodies in the pathogenesis of ReA is probably minimal. Additional findings suggest a role for heat-shock proteins[88] and bacterial peptidoglycan in the pathogenesis or ReA.[89]

CLINICAL MANIFESTATIONS

The course and severity of ReA vary considerably. Symptoms of infection usually precede the onset of arthritis, enthesitis, or extraarticular disease by one to four weeks. After an active period of weeks to months, the arthritis subsides and the patient then enter a sustained remission or a phase of recurrent disease activity, which may evolve into enthesitis related arthritis or ankylosing spondylitis.

Characteristics of the Primary Infection

An appreciation of the characteristics of the enteric or genitourinary infections which trigger ReA could possibly aid in the identification of the bacteria involved in the pathogenesis of the disease.

Shigella Enteritis

A period of high fever, with or without watery diarrhea, and cramping abdominal pain lasting 48 to 72 hours, may be followed in seven to 21 days by the sudden onset of non-migratory oligoarthritis (knees and ankles) lasting from several weeks to three or four months. Diagnosis requires a history, the presence of agglutinins to *Shigella flexneri* serotype 2 or 2a,[33-35] and an attempt to isolate the organism from the stool. Because of the long interval between the diarrhea and the joint complaints, blood cultures are positive in fewer than 4% of patients.

Salmonella Infection

The acute onset of oligoarthritis, mostly in the knees and ankles, may follow an enteric infection with *Salmonella typhimurium* or *Salmonella enteritidis* by one to three weeks.[90,91] The enteric infection may be mild, but the onset of arthritis is usually accompanied by low-grade fever. Because *Salmonella* infection can also result in osteomyelitis and septic arthritis, it is important to make certain that the synovial fluid is sterile. The erythrocyte sedimentation rate (ESR) is usually elevated, and the leukopenia that may accompany the acute infection is generally followed by leukocytosis. Stool cultures are usually positive, even late in the disease course, but seroconversion to *Salmonella* H and O antigens occurs in only 50% of patients.

Yersinia Infection

ReA triggered by *Yersinia* may affect some children.[22,35,92] The interval between infection and onset of arthritis in 18 children with *Yersinia*-triggered ReA[22] was seven to 30 days. The diarrhea preceding ReA was notably very mild, much more so than in the usual *Yersinia* enterocolitis. Contact with the organism is through infected drinking water or milk. *Yersinia enterocolitica* causes gastroenteritis in young children and a syndrome of abdominal pain similar to that of appendicitis in older children. In a study of children hospitalized because of *Yersinia* infection, 35% had arthritis lasting three to 22 months (average, 6.5 months).[9] Of those with arthritis, 85% had HLA-B27. *Yersinia* can occasionally cause septic arthritis.

Campylobacter Infection

In an epidemic of *Campylobacter jejuni* enteritis in Finland, 2.6% of patients—all adults—developed oligoarthritis or polyarthritis four days to four weeks after infection. Synovial fluid cultures were negative, and 33% of the patients with arthritis were positive for HLA-B27.[93]

Chlamydia Infection

Genitourinary tract infection with *Chlamydia trachomatis* is often asymptomatic but may cause dysuria, frequency, and a urethral or vaginal discharge. ReA may also be related to upper respiratory tract infections with *Chlamydia pneumoniae*.[40] Artamonov and colleagues[94] found evidence of nasopharyngeal infection in 45 of 52 children with ReA. Although the prevalence of HLA-B27 was higher than that in the control population (relative risk, 2.5), it was much lower than that in those who developed ReA after intestinal infection.

Musculoskeletal Disease

Acute arthritis with marked pain and sometimes erythema over the affected joints is characteristic of ReA, but some children present with only slight to moderate joint pain and swelling over several weeks.[9,22,38,35,90-98] Enthesitis may occur alone or with arthritis, tenosynovitis, or bursitis (Figs. 39–1 and 39–2). In other children, arthralgias antedate the onset of arthritis for a variable amount of time. The initial episode of arthritis usually affects the knees or ankles. The pattern of arthritis in the metatarsophalangeal (MTP) joints and the proximal and distal interphalangeal (IP) joints of the feet may be that of a dactylitis and may involve two or three joints in one or more digits in combination with tenosynovitis and bursitis. Arthritis of the small joints of the hands has also been described in ReA caused by *Yersinia* and *Salmonella*.[9,22,35,90-92]

The synovial fluid effusion is usually marked, but proliferative synovitis is uncommon. In addition to involvement of peripheral joints and entheses, there may be inflammation of joints of the axial skeleton resulting in spinal and sacroiliac pain, stiffness, and reduced mobility of the lumbar and cervical spine.

In a study of 11 children with ReA followed for 0.9 to 6.7 years, Hussein[95] observed recurrent episodes of arthritis in most patients: four children had severe arthritis, five had sacroiliitis, but none had significant disability. Cuttica and colleagues[96] found that, at a mean follow-up of 28.6 months, 18 of 26 children with the triad of arthritis, conjunctivitis, and urethritis developed oligoarthritis, seven polyarthritis, and one monarthritis, with axial symptoms in six. Five patients followed for a mean of 83.5 months developed radiographic sacroiliitis. Symptoms remitted in most patients, but some had either a sustained or a fluctuating course. In a group of nine

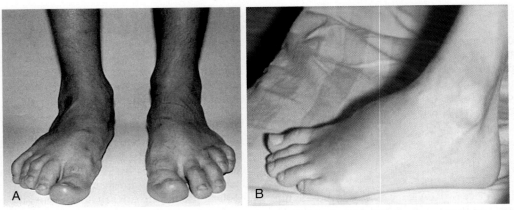

FIGURE 39–1   A, There is slight swelling of the midfoot and dactylitis involving the second right toe and the fourth and fifth left toes in an adolescent with *Salmonella*-triggered reactive arthritis of six months' duration. **B,** The foot of a teenage girl with post-*Yersinia* reactive arthritis showing swelling and erythema of the dorsum of the foot.

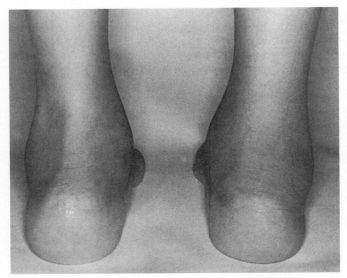

FIGURE 39–2   Achilles tendinitis and swelling of the retrocalcaneal bursa of the right foot of a patient with ReA.

Greek children with *Salmonella*-triggered ReA, disease was active at four to 13 months, and there were one to four recurrences in four patients during 48 to 78 months but no axial symptoms.[91]

Constitutional Signs and Symptoms

Apart from the infection itself, children with ReA may continue to have fever, weight loss, fatigue, and muscle weakness during active periods of disease. Polyarthralgia, muscle pain, and joint stiffness affecting peripheral joints and the axial skeleton sometimes accompany these symptoms. Myocarditis and pericarditis have been described during the active phase of the disease in children with *Salmonella enteritidis*-triggered ReA.[99]

Mucocutaneous and Ocular Disease

Painless, shallow ulcers of the oral mucosa and palate are common and often asymptomatic. Aphthous stomatitis occurs in some patients. Urethritis and cervicitis are rare

manifestations, occurring more frequently in adolescents with sexually acquired ReA caused by *Chlamydia*.[38] These conditions are often mild, and girls tend to have no symptoms; they are detected only because of the presence of sterile pyuria. Diarrhea occurs in association with bacterial infection but may also be part of a generalized episode of mucositis.

Skin lesions in ReA include erythema nodosum in some children with *Yersinia*-triggered ReA, circinate balanitis, (Fig. 39–3) and keratoderma blennorrhagicum (Fig. 39–4), with or without conjunctivitis or urethritis.[11,38,100] Keratoderma may be clinically and histologically indistinguishable from psoriasis. Mucocutaneous involvement in ReA tends to parallel disease activity in the peripheral joints.

Conjunctivitis occurs in about two thirds of children at onset. In *Yersinia*-triggered ReA, conjunctivitis may be purulent and severe.[101] Acute iridocyclitis in these cases is characterized by flare and cells in the anterior chamber, small keratic precipitates, cells in the vitreous, and occasionally fibrinous exudates, posterior synechiae, and macular edema in a unilateral or bilateral pattern. Acute anterior uveitis has also been described in ReA triggered by *Salmonella typhimurium*.[102] Although there are few studies of the visual prognosis in children with ReA, the frequency of patients with permanent ocular sequelae appears to be low.

LABORATORY EXAMINATION

In the early inflammatory phase, there may be a slight decrease of hemoglobin, hematocrit, mild leukocytosis, and neutrophilia. The platelet count and serum levels of immunoglobulins (Ig) M, G, and occasionally A may be elevated. The ESR and C-reactive protein (CRP) correlate with disease activity. In patients with severe disease—particularly in those with polyarthritis and polyenthesitis, fever, weight loss, fatigue, mucositis, or dermatitis—these laboratory abnormalities may be extreme. In particular, the hemoglobin concentration may fall to 8 to 10 g/dL, and the platelet count rise well above 400,000 mm³. The ESR and CRP values may remain elevated for a

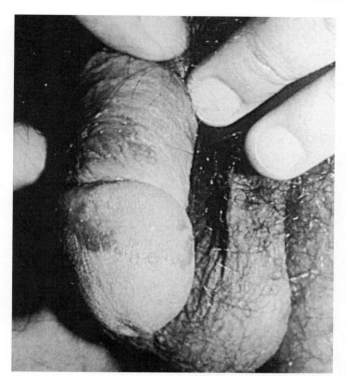

FIGURE 39–3 Circinate balanitis in an adolescent with *Chlamydia*-triggered reactive arthritis. The shallow ulcers on the glans penis are usually painless.

protracted period. Autoantibodies (e.g., rheumatoid factor, antinuclear antibodies) are usually absent. Synovial fluid analysis and culture helps to distinguish between ReA and septic arthritis.[103]

With the exception of epidemics and some isolated reports, the clinical and laboratory confirmations of infection as a trigger in children with ReA are seldom made. When available, cultures obtained at the time of the infection may be helpful: *Salmonella*, *Yersinia*, *Shigella*, and *Campylobacter* may be isolated from the gut during an episode of diarrhea, or *Chlamydia* may be cultured from the urethra, but negative results do not exclude the diagnosis of infection-related arthritis. Because *Salmonella* and *Chlamydia* may also be present in asymptomatic carriers, these organisms can occasionally be cultured from patients who have arthritis not directly related to these organisms.

More frequently, ReA is diagnosed in the appropriate clinical setting because of the presence of high titers of serum antibodies against arthritogenic bacterial antigens.[4,5] Hemagglutination tests are useful in documenting recent infections with *Salmonella* or *Yersinia*.[7,22,35,38,90-92] Both the sensitivity and the specificity of circulating IgA and IgM antibodies to *Salmonella*, *Yersinia*, and *Campylobacter* detected by enzyme-linked immunoassay are acceptable, but results must be compared with those in the control population. IgG antibodies are useful if levels change significantly; a rising titer of IgA antibodies may be noted.

Lymphoproliferation assays performed on cells from peripheral blood or synovial fluids also have some use as diagnostic tools.[4,5] Unfortunately, these tests are not easy to perform and often demonstrate nonspecific responses to several antigens.

Yersinia or *Chlamydia* antigens may be detected in intestinal or genital smears or biopsies. By using electron and immunofluorescence microscopy and immunohistochemistry, it has been possible to identify intraarticular chlamydial elemental bodies,[38,78,79] *Yersinia* 60 kD heat-shock proteins and the urease β subunit,[79,80] and *Salmonella* lipopolysaccharide.[81] Likewise, bacterial DNA or RNA from several bacterial species, including *Chlamydia* sp, *Salmonella* sp, *Shigella* sp, and *Campylobacter* sp has been identified in synovial fluid cells or the synovial membrane by polymerase chain reaction.[82-87] The role of these tests as diagnostic tools is restricted at present.

RADIOLOGICAL EXAMINATION

Radiographic abnormalities early in the disease consist only of nonspecific soft tissue swelling, juxta-articular osteopenia, and (less frequently) slight periosteal irregularities at tendon attachments.[104] The occurrence of subchondral cysts, erosions, and sometimes extensive destruction of joints, such as the hips, proximal and distal IPs of the hands and feet, and less commonly, joints of the wrist, indicate the severity of the synovitis that can occur in ReA. Ultrasonographic studies may delineate synovial sheath and tendon thickening and the accumulation of synovial fluid within the tendon sheath and bursae. Hyperintense signals on magnetic resonance imaging (MRI) result from edema associated inflammation that may be seen in the bone, synovial membrane, and joint space with T2 fat suppressed and short tau inversion recovery sequences, with and without gadolinium. In certain areas, particularly the foot, osteopenia may be extensive and may affect entire bones. Various entheses, especially those at the attachment of the plantar fascia to the calcaneus, develop erosions and marked bony proliferation and spur formation. These abnormalities may also be apparent in the navicular bone, greater trochanter, and ischium. Unilateral or bilateral subchondral cysts and bony erosions of the hip, metacarpophalangeal, MTP, and proximal IP joints of the hands and feet characterize more extensive and unremitting disease. An association between joint erosions and occult inflammation of the gut has been described in patients with ReA.[105]

Symptomatic and radiographic involvement of the sacroiliac joint and spine are rare in children with ReA, but MRI of the sacroiliac joints may revealed acute and chronic changes in up to one-half.

DIFFERENTIAL DIAGNOSIS

Differentiation of ReA from other types of arthritis is often difficult (Table 39–3). Reactive and infectious arthritides not associated with HLA-B27 have similar symptoms, although the primary site of infection is usually the upper airway. ReA is usually more painful and is associated with erythema of the overlying skin, a feature rarely seen in juvenile idiopathic arthritis (JIA). Specific clinical features, such as rash, subcutaneous nodule, and lymphadenopathy,

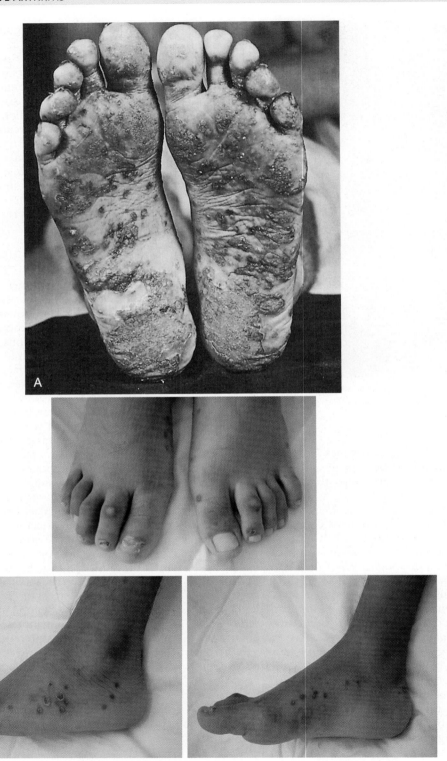

FIGURE 39–4   Keratoderma blennorrhagicum. **A,** This scaly eruption on the soles of the feet of an 18-year-old youth with reactive arthritis is difficult to distinguish from psoriasis. **B,** Dorsal, lateral, and medial aspects of the feet of a 16-year-old patient with chronic reactive arthritis. *Dorsal view,* While the third digit on the right foot shows some diffuse swelling and hyperpigmentation, the first toe looks more atrophic than its counterpart on the left foot. *Lateral view,* Midfoot and ankle swelling. *All views.* There is nail dystrophy of the first three digits in the right foot (clearly seen on the first toe) and multiple keratoderma blennorrhagic lesions. This patient had recurrent episodes of severe arthritis and enthesitis involving both feet but only recently skin lesions.

Table 39-3

Differential diagnosis of reactive arthritis

Arthritis Related to Infection

Presumed viral arthritis (including transient synovitis of the hip)

Poststreptococcal arthritis (including rheumatic fever)

Lyme disease

Septic arthritis, tuberculosis, gonococcal arthropathy

Idiopathic Inflammatory Diseases

Juvenile idiopathic arthritis

Arthritis associated with Crohn's Disease and ulcerative colitis

Synovitis, acne, pustulosis, hyperostosis, and osteomyelitis (SAPHO) syndrome

Behçet disease

Kawasaki disease

Orthopedic and Amplification Pain Syndromes

Legg-Calvé-Perthes, Osgood-Schlatter disease

"Growing pains"

Idiopathic pain syndromes (fibromyalgia, reflex sympathetic dystrophy)

help differentiate diseases such as Kawasaki disease[107] and Lyme disease from ReA. Early juvenile idiopathic arthritis (JIA) and the arthritis of inflammatory bowel disease must also be considered. Laboratory test abnormalities, such as a positive synovial fluid culture or elevated antistreptolysin O titers suggest septic arthritis or rheumatic fever. The presence of elevated inflammatory indices helps exclude orthopaedic conditions.

TREATMENT

Disease activity, functional status, and quality of life should be evaluated in children with ReA. Although no specific instruments have been developed for this disease, the use of validated measures of health status designed for other chronic arthritides of childhood is appropriate (Chapters 7 and 8).[108,109]

There are no special nutritional recommendations for children with ReA. Any measure taken to avoid bacterial contamination of food, from slaughtering of the animals to refrigeration, cooking, and serving, is essential to avoid enteric infections. ReA is not only an epidemic disease but is also endemic to some areas of the world. Programs that improve the sanitary conditions of the community to prevent the spread of infectious diseases are required. Counseling of the family about the risk of recurrences in case of enteric infections is advisable. This applies to adolescents with regard to sexual activities and the risk of sexually transmitted diseases.

Pharmacologic Therapy

The inflammatory manifestations of ReA require the administration of nonsteroidal antiinflammatory drugs (NSAIDs) in nearly all patients and glucocorticoids in some. The requirement for NSAIDs tends to be intermittent rather than constant. However, in patients in whom ReA becomes chronic, medications including, sometimes, sulfasalazine, should be maintained for long periods Except for the use of antibiotics in selected cases, there is no clear evidence that any drug alters the course of the disease.

Recommended doses and therapeutic regimens of NSAIDs in children with ReA are similar to those used in other forms of childhood arthritis. Because episodes of ReA tend to be self-limiting, lasting from three to six months, NSAIDs may be discontinued in many children with onset of a remission. Glucocorticoids may be required for children with severe and disabling polyarthritis and polyenthesitis. Enthesitis responds poorly and may require higher doses and longer courses of drug therapy than usual. Fever, fatigue, and anemia tend to disappear, and CRP and ESR levels tend to fall after several weeks of treatment. Glucocorticoid dose reduction and withdrawal in children with ReA are usually easily achieved.

The required doses of prednisone or prednisolone vary between 5 and 10 mg/day, and of deflazacort between 6 and 24 mg/day. To minimize the risk of adverse events, it is advisable to administer the drug as a single dose very early in the morning and to start reducing the dose after two to three weeks. In patients with slight or mild synovitis, the intra-articular administration of triamcinolone hexacetonide or analogues of methylprednisolone or hydrocortisone, produces rapid and sustained relief. There is no reported experience regarding the injection of synovial sheaths, bursae, or entheses in children with ReA. Injection of entheses may result in postinjection pain and local soft tissue calcification or atrophy.

Because of the possible occult nonspecific inflammation of the gut in patients with HLA-B27 associated arthritis, including ReA,[110,111] and their responsiveness to sulfasalazine,[112,113] this drug is often recommended in the management of resistant arthritis and enthesitis. The administration of sulfasalazine (30 to 50 mg/kg/day; maximum 1.5 to 2.0 g/day in adolescents) may reduce the number of painful and swollen joints, pain intensity, and ESR. The response to sulfasalazine is moderate; some patients enter remission after three to six months of therapy, but this also may occur spontaneously. This time corresponds to the natural history of the disease, and in many trials, the six month placebo response equals that of sulfasalazine. It is advisable to continue the drug for an additional period of three to six months after remission has been achieved in order to avoid a flare. The frequency of adverse events with sulfasalazine ranges from 10% to 20% (see Chapter 6). Some beneficial effect of the drug has also been observed in patients with uveitis and skin manifestations, such as *keratoderma blennorrhagicum*. Because of limited response of SpA to methotrexate, this drug is not recommended for ReA. In contrast, its effects on iritis and *keratoderma blennorrhagicum* in children may be satisfactory. Uveitis usually responds to topical or systemic glucocorticoids, but severe, resistant ocular inflammation occasionally requires other immunosuppressive drugs (see Chapter 20).

No antibiotic regimen has been clearly efficacious in ReA. Double-blind and open trials of various tetracycline derivatives (except for one using lymecycline) or ciprofloxacin have noted no significant differences when compared with placebo in the short- and long-term. Compared with placebo, lymecycline[114] reduced the time to recover from arthritis in patients with *Chlamydia* but not in those with enteritis-related ReA. Antibiotic treatment, however, did not change the natural history of ReA.[115] In children, it has been suggested that amoxicillin alone or in combination with clavulanic acid may be useful.[116]

The use of TNF alpha blockers, specifically infliximab, has been reported to be of benefit in adults with ReA,[117-119] although no data are yet available in children.

Physical Therapy and Rehabilitation

In the acute inflammatory phase, treatment of ReA is similar to that for other forms of chronic arthritis (Chapter 12). Rest, ice, hot packs, and ambulation aids may be useful. Custom-made insoles relieve pain caused by enthesitis at the heel and metatarsal heads and help preserve the longitudinal arch of the foot. The use of night resting splints helps avoid joint contractures associated with tendonitis or tenosynovitis. Both active and passive stretching of joints and muscle strengthening should be prescribed when inflammation is being controlled and pain permits. Children with chronic and recurrent ReA tend to develop fibrous ankylosis first, followed by bone ankylosis of the midtarsal joints and subluxation of the MTP joints, and therefore require special attention to insoles and shoes. Knee, hip, and axial disease benefits from activities such as biking and swimming.

Orthopaedic Surgery

Arthroscopic synovectomy is potentially beneficial for children with recurrent synovitis of the knee or small joints of the hands and feet, although is seldom necessary. Early soft tissue release of contractures at the hip, knee, MTP, and IP joints increases functional capacity and may reduce the risk of severe impairment thereafter. Adolescents with severe hip or knee disease may require joint replacements in the long term.

COURSE OF THE DISEASE AND PROGNOSIS

The course of arthritis in children with ReA varies. Most children have only a single episode of monarthritis or oligoarthritis. This is typical of ReA triggered by *Yersinia*[13,38,96] or *Campylobacter*.[27] Others have recurrent episodes of oligoarthritis or an extended form of disease affecting multiple joints and entheses that may account for most of those attending specialized clinics. Although remission may still occur in these patients, many others evolve into ERA or ankylosing spondylitis with sacroiliac arthritis.

There are no reports of long-term outcome of ReA in children. Children with ReA who have HLA-B27 have more severe involvement.[31,41,92] Extra-articular disease, including iridocyclitis and the triad of arthritis, conjunctivitis, and urethritis, also occurs more frequently among children with ReA who are B27 positive. In one report, three of five HLA B27 positive children with *Salmonella*-triggered ReA developed psoriasis.[92] The number of joints involved at onset, the presence of fever or anemia, and the number and duration of episodes of disease activity influence the outcome.

The prognosis of *Chlamydia*- or *Yersinia*-triggered ReA is less severe than that described after *Shigella* or *Salmonella* infection. Whether this is a direct influence of the infectious agent or represents different frequencies of association with HLA-B27 is uncertain.

REFERENCES

1. K. Aho, M. Leirisalo-Repo, H. Repo, Reactive arthritis, Clin. Rheum. Dis. 11 (1985) 25–40.
3. A. Keat, Reiter's syndrome and reactive arthritis in perspective, N. Engl. J. Med. 309 (1983) 1606–1615.
4. G. Kingsley, J. Sieper, Third international workshop on reactive arthritis. An overview, Ann. Rheum. Dis. 55 (1996) 564–584.
5. C. Pacheco-Tena, R. Burgos-Vargas, J. Vázquez-Mellado, et al., A proposal for the classification of patients for clinical and experimental studies on reactive arthritis, J. Rheumatol. 26 (1999) 1338–1346.
6. J. Sieper, M. Rudwaleit, J. Braun, et al., Diagnosing reactive arthritis: role of clinical setting in the value of serologic and microbiologic assays, Arthritis Rheum. 46 (2002) 319–327.
8. M. Harjacek, J. Ostojic, O. Djakovic Rode, Juvenile spondyloarthropathies associated with Mycoplasma pneumoniae infection, Clin. Rheumatol. 25 (2006) 470–475.
9. R. Leino, A.L. Mäkelä, A. Tiilikainen, et al., *Yersinia* arthritis in children, Scand. J. Rheumatol. 9 (1980) 245–249.
10. J.A. Hoogkamp-Korstanje, V.M. Stolk-Engelaar, *Yersinia enterocolitica* infection in children, Pediatr. Infect. Dis. J. 14 (1995) 771–775.
11. M. Rudwaleit, S. Richter, J. Braun, et al., Low incidence of reactive arthritis in children following a salmonella outbreak, Ann. Rheum. Dis. 60 (2001) 1055–1057.
12. A.T. Lee, R.G. Hall, K.D. Pile, Reactive joint symptoms following an outbreak of Salmonella typhimurium phage type 135a, J. Rheumatol. 32 (2005) 524–527.
13. B.A. Denardo, L.B. Tucker, L.C. Miller, et al., Demography of a regional pediatric rheumatology patient population, J. Rheumatol. 21 (1994) 1553,–1561.
14. S. Bowyer, P. Roettcher, and the members of the Pediatric Rheumatology Database Research Group: Pediatric Rheumatology Clinic populations in the United States: results of a 3 year survey, J. Rheumatol. 23 (1996) 1968–1974.
15. D.P.M. Symmons, M. Jones, J. Osborne, et al., Pediatric rheumatology in the United Kingdom: data from the British Pediatric Rheumatology Group National Diagnostic Register, J. Rheumatol. 23 (1996) 1975–1980.
16. P.N. Malleson, M.Y. Fung, A.M. Rosenberg, for the Canadian Pediatric Rheumatology Association, The incidence of pediatric rheumatic diseases: results from the Canadian Pediatric Rheumatology Association Disease Registry, J. Rheumatol. 23 (1996) 1981–1987.
19. K.G. Oen, M. Cheang, Epidemiology of chronic arthritis in childhood, Semin. Arthritis Rheum. 26 (1996) 575–591.
22. G. Taccetti, S. Trapani, M. Ermini, et al., Reactive arthritis triggered by *Yersinia enterocolitica*: a review of 18 pediatric cases, Clin. Exp. Rheumatol. 12 (1994) 681–684.
25. K. Johnsen, M. Ostensen, A.C. Melbye, et al., HLA-B27-negative arthritis related to *Campylobacter jejuni* enteritis in three children and two adults, Acta. Med. Scand. 214 (1983) 165–168.
32. A.L. Florman, H.M. Goldstein, Arthritis, conjunctivitis and urethritis (so-called Reiter's syndrome) in a 4-year-old boy, J. Pediatr. 33 (1948) 172–177.
34. B.H. Singsen, B.H. Bernstein, K.G. Koster-King, et al., Reiter's syndrome in childhood, Arthritis Rheum. 20 (1977) 402–407.
35. A.S. Russell, Reiter's syndrome in children following infection with *Yersinia enterocolitica* and shigella, Arthritis Rheum. 20 (1977) 471–472.

36. J.M.I. Iveson, B.S. Nanda, J.A.H. Hancock, et al., Reiter's disease in three boys, Ann. Rheum. Dis. 34 (1975) 364–368.

37. A.G. Jacobs, A case of Reiter's syndrome in childhood, Br. Med. J. 2 (1961) 155.

38. A.M. Rosenberg, R.E. Petty, Reiter's disease in children, Am. J. Dis. Child 133 (1979) 394–398.

41. R.Q. Cron, P.V. Gordon, Reactive arthritis to *Clostridium difficile* in a child, West. J. Med. 166 (1997) 419–421.

69. M.A. Penttinen, K.M. Heiskanen, R. Mohapatra, et al., Enhanced intracellular replication of Salmonella enteritidis in HLA-B27-expressing human monocytic cells: dependency on glutamic acid at position 45 in the B pocket of HLA-B27, Arthritis Rheum. 50 (2004) 2255–2263.

70. S. Vähämiko, M.A. Penttinen, K. Granfors, Aetiology and pathogenesis of reactive arthritis: role of non-antigen-presenting effects of HLA-B27, Arthritis Res. Ther. 7 (2005) 136–141.

72. K. Kapasi, R.D. Inman, HLA B27 expression modulates gram-negative bacterial invasion into transfected L cells, J. Immunol. 148 (1992) 3554–3559.

74. O. Ortiz-Alvarez, D.T. Yu, R.E. Petty, et al., HLA-B27 does not affect invasion of arthritogenic bacteria into human cells, J. Rheumatol. 25 (1998) 1765–1771.

79. K. Granfors, S. Jalkanen, R. von Essen, et al., *Yersinia* antigens in synovial fluid cells from patients with reactive arthritis, N. Engl. J. Med. 320 (1989) 216–221.

81. K. Granfors, S. Jalkanen, A.A. Lindberg, et al., *Salmonella* lipopolysaccharide in the synovial cells from patients with reactive arthritis, Lancet 335 (1990) 685–688.

82. D. Taylor-Robinson, C.B. Gilroy, B.J. Thomas, et al., Detection of *Chlamydia trachomatis* DNA in joints of reactive arthritis patients by polymerase chain reaction, Lancet 340 (1992) 81–82.

85. C. Pacheco-Tena, C. Alvarado de la Barrera, Y. López-Vidal, et al., Bacterial DNA in synovial fluid cells of patients with juvenile onset spondyloarthropathies, Rheumatology 40 (2001) 920–927.

88. P. Life, A. Hassell, K. Williams, et al., Responses to gram negative enteric bacterial antigens by synovial T cells from patients with juvenile chronic arthritis: recognition of heat shock protein HSP60, J. Rheumatol. 20 (1993) 1388–1396.

90. W.L. Carroll, W.F. Balistreri, R. Brilli, et al., Spectrum of *Salmonella*-associated arthritis, Pediatrics 68 (1981) 717–720.

92. C. Jezequel, J.Y. Prigent, M.N. Loiseau-Corvez, et al., Reactive arthritis caused by *Yersinia* in children. Report of 4 cases, Ann. Pediatr. (Paris) 38 (1991) 318–322.

94. V.A. Artamonov, S. Akhmadi, I.S. Polianskaia, The clinical and immunogenetic characteristics of reactive arthritis in children, Ter. Arkh. 63 (1991) 22.

95. A. Hussein, Spectrum of post-enteric reactive arthritis in childhood, Monatsschr. Kinderheilkd. 135 (1987) 93–98.

96. R.J. Cuttica, E.J. Scheines, S.M. Garay, et al., Juvenile onset Reiter's syndrome—a retrospective study of 26 patients, Clin. Exp. Rheumatol. 10 (1992) 285–288.

97. G.N. Lockie, G.G. Hunder, Reiter's syndrome in children: a case report and review, Arthritis Rheum. 14 (1971) 767–772.

98. J. Fris, Reiter's disease with childhood onset having special reference to HLA B27, Scand. J. Rheumatol. 9 (1980) 250–252.

100. D. Zivony, J. Nocton, D. Wortmann, et al., Juvenile Reiter's syndrome: a report of four cases, J. Am. Acad. Dermatol. 38, 1998. 32–32.

101. K.M. Saari, M. Mäki, T. Päivönsalo, et al., Acute anterior uveitis and conjunctivitis following *Yersinia* infection in children, Int. Ophthalmol. 9 (1986) 237–241.

102. J.D. Fischel, J. Lipton, Acute anterior uveitis in juvenile Reiter's syndrome, Clin. Rheumatol. 15 (1996) 83–85.

103. H.I. Huppertz, H. Karch, J. Heesemann, Diagnostic value of synovial fluid analysis in children with reactive arthritis, Rheumatol. Int. 15 (1995) 167–170.

107. C. Bauman, R.Q. Cron, D.D. Sherry, et al., Reiter syndrome initially misdiagnosed as Kawasaki disease, J. Pediatr. 128 (1996) 366–369.

109. E. Müller-Godeffroy, H. Lehmann, R.M. Küster, et al., [Quality of life and psychosocial adaptation in children and adolescents with juvenile idiopathic arthritis and reactive arthritis], Z. Rheumatol. 64 (2005) 177–187.

113. H.J. Suschke, Treatment of juvenile spondyloarthritis and reactive arthritis with sulfasalazine, Monatsschr. Kinderheilkd. 140 (1992) 658–660.

114. A. Lauhio, M. Leirisalo-Repo, J. Lahdevirta, et al., Double-blind, placebo-controlled study of three-month treatment with lymecycline in reactive arthritis, with special reference to *Chlamydia* arthritis, Arthritis Rheum. 34 (1991) 6–14.

115. K. Laasila, L. Laasonen, M. Leirisalo-Repo, Antibiotic treatment and long term prognosis of reactive arthritis, Ann. Rheum. Dis. 62 (2003) 655–658.

116. D. Astrauskiene, Efficacy of empirically prescribed amoxicillin and amoxicillin + clavulanic acid in children's reactive arthritis: a randomised trial, Clin. Exp. Rheumatol. 21 (2003) 515–521.

Entire reference list is available online at www.expertconsult.com.

Chapter 40

ACUTE RHEUMATIC FEVER AND POSTSTREPTOCOCCAL REACTIVE ARTHRITIS

Khaled Alsaeid and James T. Cassidy

ACUTE RHEUMATIC FEVER

Definition and Classification

Acute rheumatic fever (ARF) is a disease characterized by an inflammatory process that affects several organs of the body. It is one of the few rheumatic diseases for which the cause has been identified—tonsillopharyngitis due to the group A β-hemolytic *Streptococcus pyogenes*. The streptococcal infection and the onset of the clinical manifestations of ARF are separated by a period of latency of two to three weeks. During this time, the patient is asymptomatic. The clinical presentations include arthritis, carditis, chorea, a characteristic rash, and subcutaneous nodules. Arthritis is the most common but least specific of these manifestations, whereas carditis is the most specific and serious. The pathological process underlying the inflammatory reaction in the various organs is a vasculitis mediated by an immune reaction to the streptococcal infection. This nonpurulent complication of group A streptococcal disease can be prevented by appropriate treatment of the streptococcal pharyngitis.

Epidemiology

Incidence and Prevalence

ARF was prevalent worldwide until the middle part of the 20th century. The advent of industrialization and improved public hygiene in Western Europe and North America was associated with a sharp decline in the incidence of this disease. During the early part of the 20th century, incidence rates of 100 to 200 cases per 100,000 members of the general population were documented in the United States.[1] Although this rate still prevails in developing countries,[2] current estimates of the incidence of ARF in children in the United States document a markedly lower incidence rate of 0.5 to 3 cases per 100,000 children.[3] Between 1985 and 1990, a marked resurgence of the disease occurred in several areas of the United States.[4-13] This dramatic reappearance of what had been an increasingly rare disease was followed by a persistently higher rate in the incidence of ARF in these geographical areas.[14-16] However, the focal nature of these episodes has not significantly affected the overall prevalence of the disease in the United States.

Age at Onset and Sex Ratio

The age-related incidence of ARF follows that of group A streptococcal pharyngitis and peaks between the ages of 6- and 15-years-old. ARF is rarely encountered in the United States in children younger than 5-years-old.[17-19] Among adults at high risk for streptococcal pharyngitis, such as military recruits and persons working in crowded settings, the incidence of the disease is higher. There is no difference in the incidence of ARF between males and females.

Geographical and Racial Distribution

ARF used to be considered a disease of temperate climates but is now more common in countries with tropical climates, particularly in developing countries. In the United States, the highest seasonal incidence is in the spring, following the peak season of streptococcal pharyngitis in the winter. In other countries, a season of peak frequency is less well defined.

Despite the decline of ARF in industrialized countries, its prevalence in developing areas of the world remains very high. Incidence rates per 100,000 population range from 23 in Kuwait, 35 in Iran, to 51 in India. It has been estimated that 95% of the nearly 20 million cases of RHD in the world each year occur in developing countries.[20,21] Factors invoked in explaining the decreased incidence of the disease in the United States include less crowding in homes and schools and the increased availability of health care to children.[22,23] Observations during the recent resurgence of ARF suggest that these factors may not be important because this disease is now occurring primarily in children from middle- to high-income families with ready access to medical care.[4]

Differences in the incidence of ARF among racial and ethnic groups have been described. In New Zealand, the disease is more common among the Maori population compared with local non-Maoris of similar socioeconomic status.[24] ARF in the United States is more prevalent among African Americans and Hispanics than among whites.[3] Although genetic factors can account for these racial and ethnic differences, environmental factors may also be instrumental in explaining these observations.[2]

Etiology and Pathogenesis

ARF is a complication of a group A streptococcal tonsillopharyngitis in a predisposed human host; streptococcal pyoderma does not lead to this nonpurulent complication.[25] There is no experimental model for this disease. Specific factors that influence its evolution include the characteristics of the etiological organism, the site of the streptococcal infection, and a genetic predisposition of the host (Fig. 40–1). Less than 2% to 3% of previously healthy persons who acquire streptococcal pharyngitis develop ARF. This complication can be prevented by prompt identification and treatment of the streptococcal infection.

Etiological Agent

β-Hemolytic streptococci have been divided into 20 serogroups (A to H and K to V) by Lancefield[26] based on immunochemical differences in their cell-wall polysaccharide. The group A *Streptococcus* is the most common bacterial pathogen associated with tonsillopharyngitis and is the only member that can initiate ARF. Several cellular components and extracellular products produced by this streptococcus *in vivo* and *in vitro* have been identified.

The streptococcal bacterium consists of a cytoplasm enclosed in a membrane composed predominantly of lipoproteins. This structure is surrounded by a rigid cell wall made up of three components. The primary component is a peptidoglycan that imparts rigidity to the cell wall. A complex of this component and the cell-wall polysaccharide elicits arthritis and a recurrent nodular reaction when injected into the skin of experimental animals.[27-29] Integrated into the peptidoglycan is the cell-wall polysaccharide or group-specific carbohydrate whose immunochemical structure determines the serogroup specificity. This polysaccharide has been reported to share antigenic determinants with a glycopeptide present in mitral valve tissue.[30] Traversing through and extending outside the cell wall as hairlike fimbriae is the M protein, part of a mosaic that also includes the R and T proteins. The M protein is a coiled protein with an α-helical structure consisting of a free, distal, hypervariable aminoterminus and a proximal carboxylterminus anchored to the cell wall.[31] This protein is the type-specific antigen of the group A *Streptococcus*.

About 100 M proteins have been identified by differences in immunochemical composition of the variable aminoterminus. A major biological property of the M protein resides in its capacity to inhibit phagocytosis of the streptococcus, which is neutralized by antibody to its aminoterminal region. Immunity to group A streptococcal infections is therefore type specific, predicated on formation of antibodies to the various M proteins. Additional attributes include the association of certain serotypes with potential pathogenicity and virulence. Data procured during a resurgence of ARF confirmed that serotypes 3 and 18, particularly strains that produced mucoid colonies when cultured on blood agar, were primarily associated with the disease.[32,33] These two serotypes and the M1 serotype were also associated with severe, invasive group A streptococcal disease, including the streptococcal toxic shock syndrome.[34] Studies have indicated that bacterial strains that have conserved parts of the carboxylterminal portion of the M-protein molecule exposed on their cell surface (class I strains) were associated with ARF, whereas strains that did not have this characteristic (class II) were not.[35] It was reported that phages and phagelike elements were the sources for variation in the genome of an M18 isolate, recovered from a patient with ARF, and an M1 strain.[36]

The pathogenetic importance of the M proteins is supported by data indicating that several epitopes of the M-protein molecule crossreact antigenically with human myocardium, myosin, and brain tissue, ostensibly leading to tissue inflammation.[37,38] M protein also functions as a "superantigen."[39] These findings indicate that this streptococcal molecule can induce an inflammatory response in certain tissues by eliciting "autoimmune" antibodies and tissue inflammation by nonspecific stimulation of cell-mediated immunity as a superantigen.

The cellular component of the group A streptococci that has been implicated in the pathogenesis of arthritis is the hyaluronate capsule. Like the M protein, this moiety appears to carry epitopes that elicit antibodies that crossreact with human cartilage and synovial hyaluronate.[40] Some studies have documented that components of the M3 and M18 epitopes aggregate type IV collagen, a component of the human basement membrane. This reaction is affected in M3 strains by the production of a collagen-binding factor. M18 strains bind collagen through the hyaluronic acid capsule. Patients with ARF have higher

PATHOGENESIS OF RHEUMATIC FEVER

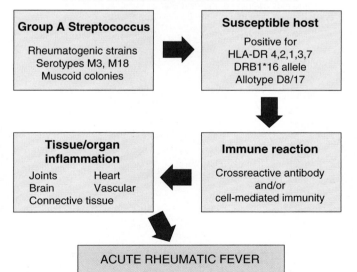

FIGURE 40–1 Interactions between the group A *Streptococcus* and the human host that lead to acute rheumatic fever. HLA, human leukocyte antigen. (Adapted from Ayoub EM: Acute rheumatic fever. In Emmanouilides GC, Riemenschneider TA, Allen HD et al, editors: *Moss and Adams' heart disease in infants, children, and adolescents, including the fetus and young adult*, vol II, ed 5, Baltimore, 1995, Williams & Wilkins.)

levels of anticollagen intravenous (IV) antibodies than controls;[41] mice immunized with recombinant M3 protein produce anticollagen antibodies.

In addition to the cellular components, extracellular products of the group A streptococci have important biological activities and are of practical value in the diagnosis of group A streptococcal infections and their nonpurulent complications. Most of these products are proteins with enzymatic properties, and they possess specific biological and antigenic activity. The streptococcal pyrogenic exotoxins (SPEs) A, B, C, and F (i.e., the mitogenic factor) and Streptococcus supre antigen (SSA) are of particular interest because they act as superantigens that induce proliferation of T lymphocytes *in vitro* and the synthesis and release of several lymphokines *in vivo*.[37-43] This biological activity reflects the ability of SPEs to bind simultaneously to class II major histocompatibility antigens (HLA) of antigen-presenting cells and to the Vβ region of the T-cell receptor. Production of these exotoxins is associated *in vivo* with a febrile response, alteration of membrane permeability, and enhancement of susceptibility to endotoxin-induced lethal shock.[44] Selective activation of lymphocytes has been ascribed to different SPEs. SPE A activates T cells bearing T-cell receptor β-chain segments Vβ8, Vβ12, and Vβ14, whereas SPE B activates T cells bearing segments Vβ2 and Vβ8.[45] SPE B has been identified as a cysteine protease that inhibits phagocytosis and enhances dissemination of the organism *in vivo*. It also induces apoptosis of phagocytic cells.[46]

The frequencies of the *spe* genes and their expression vary among group A streptococci; *speA* is found in 45% of strains, *speB* in almost all strains, and *speC* in 30% of strains. SPE A is expressed by 43% and SPE B by 76% of strains.[34,47,48] The frequencies of the *speA* genes and their products are similar among M1 and M3 serotypes.[47] The association of certain serotypes with various clinical manifestations of streptococcal infections, such as toxic shock syndrome, has been ascribed to the capacity of the infecting strain to produce one of the SPEs.[34,45,47] However, the ubiquity of the production of these toxins makes confirmation of the specificity of these associations questionable.[48]

Streptococcal Antibody Tests

The specific antigenicity of most of the streptococcal extracellular products led to the establishment of antibody tests for these products. These tests are used to confirm evidence of a group A streptococcal infection, primarily in patients with ARF and glomerulonephritis. The first and still most universally used is the antistreptolysin O (ASO) test, which was designed by Todd[49] to measure neutralizing antibodies to purified streptolysin O in patients with scarlet fever and ARF. This test proved helpful in providing evidence for antecedent group A streptococcal infection, particularly when throat cultures were negative. Subsequently, tests were developed to assay for antibodies to other streptococcal antigens (Table 40–1). The anti-DNAse B test, which assays for antibodies to the most ubiquitous of four deoxyribonuclease isozymes produced by the group A streptococcus (A, B, C, and D), proved to be as reliable and reproducible as the ASO test. The other tests, which are no longer readily available, and the streptozyme test, which was widely used at one time, lacked standardization and reproducibility and should not be relied on for evidence of antecedent group A streptococcal infection.[50]

The pattern of the antibody response to the streptococcal antigens is illustrated in Figure 40–2. Antibodies peak approximately three weeks after the acute infection. Because of the period of latency between the infection and the onset of the clinical manifestations of ARF, serum obtained at the time of clinical presentation should document the necessary evidence for antecedent group A streptococcal infection. However, as outlined in Table 40–2, only about 83% of patients with ARF mount an ASO response. Another streptococcal antibody test, such as anti-DNAse B, can provide evidence for an antecedent streptococcal infection in patients in whom an ASO response has not been diagnostic.

Table 40–1

Group A streptococcal antigens and corresponding antibody tests

Streptococcal Antigen	Antibody Test
Extracellular Product	
Streptolysin O	ASO
Streptokinase	Antistreptokinase
Hyaluronidase	Antihyaluronidase
DNAse B	Anti-DNAse B
NADase	Anti-NADase
Multiple antigens	Streptozyme
Cellular Component	
M protein	Type-specific antibody
Group-specific polysaccharide	Anti-A-carbohydrate

ASO, Antistreptolysin O; DNAse B, deoxyribonuclease B; NADase, nicotinamide adenine dinucleotidase.
Adapted from Ayoub EM: Streptococcal antibody tests in rheumatic fever, *Clin Immunol Newsletter* 3:107-111, 1982.

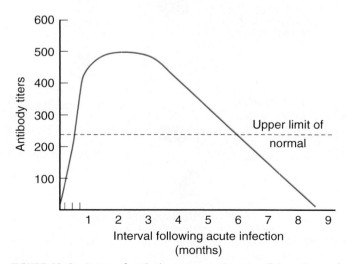

FIGURE 40–2 Pattern of antibody response to the extracellular antigens of the group A *Streptococcus* after tonsillopharyngeal infection in humans. (From Ayoub EM: Streptococcal antibody tests in rheumatic fever, *Clin Immunol Newsletter* 3:107-111, 1982.)

Tests for antibodies to the cell-wall components of group A streptococci are available but not widely used. Determination of type-specific antibody to the different M proteins is employed in epidemiological studies to determine previous exposure or immunity to specific M serotypes. Testing for antibody to the group-specific carbohydrate is available in some laboratories. Because this antibody tends to persist for prolonged periods in patients with rheumatic valvular disease, it may help to confirm the rheumatic cause of mitral valve disease in a patient without a history of ARF.[51-54]

Mechanism of Tissue Injury

Initial suggestions that tissue injury in ARF was caused by direct invasion by the streptococcus or the effect of its extracellular toxins were subsequently replaced by the theory that an immune mechanism was responsible for the inflammatory response in the affected organs. The potential role of an immunological process as the cause of tissue injury was predicated on the observation that the clinical manifestations of ARF occurred after a period of latency of about three weeks from the inciting group

A streptococcal infection. Evidence for involvement of an immune mechanism in pathogenesis was first advanced by Kaplan and coworkers.[55,56] These investigators and others described the presence of common antigenic determinants among the cellular components of the group A streptococci and myocardial tissues. Structures that share crossreactive antigenic determinants included components of the M protein and myocardial sarcolemma,[55-60] cell-wall carbohydrate, and valvular glycoprotein,[30] streptococcal protoplast membrane, and neuronal tissue of the subthalamic and caudate nuclei,[61,62] and the hyaluronate capsule, and articular cartilage.[40] Based on these studies, it was concluded that antibodies formed against the streptococcal antigens crossreacted with the corresponding tissues and ostensibly led to inflammation in the heart, joints, and brain (Fig. 40–3).[37,38]

As attractive as the process of "antigenic mimicry" is in explaining the inflammatory reaction in ARF, there are several flaws in this hypothesis. The most compelling of these arguments is the presence of high levels of crossreactive antibodies in the sera of patients who do not have any manifestations of acute carditis or arthritis. An alternative explanation was provided by subsequent studies that documented a potential role for cell-mediated immunity in inducing tissue damage. These studies confirmed that peripheral blood lymphocytes from patients with acute rheumatic carditis were cytotoxic to human myocardial cells in tissue culture.[63] Addition of plasma from the same patients abrogated this cytotoxic effect. The latter observation suggested that the crossreactive antibodies elicited by group A streptococci had a protective rather than a detrimental effect on the host. Based on these arguments, the prevalent hypothesis for explaining tissue injury in this disease is that an immunological mechanism involving the humoral or the cellular immune system may be responsible for tissue inflammation in ARF.

Genetic Background

Early postulates regarding the epidemiology of rheumatic fever suggested that persons who acquired this disease had a peculiar susceptibility to it. This postulate was based on the observation that 30% to 80% of patients who

Table 40–2			
Frequency of patients with acute rheumatic fever with elevated titers of antistreptolysin O or antideoxyribonuclease B			
Group	ASO	Anti-DNAse B	ASO and anti-DNAse B
Normal controls	19%	19%	30%
Acute rheumatic fever	83%	82%	92%
Sydenham chorea (isolated)	67%	40%	80%

ASO, Antistreptolysin O; DNAse B, deoxyribonuclease B.
Adapted from Ayoub EM, Wannamaker LW: Evaluation of the streptococcal deoxyribonuclease B and diphosphopyridine nucleotidase antibody tests in acute rheumatic fever and acute glomerulonephritis, *Pediatrics* 29:527-538, 1962, and from Ayoub EM, Wannamaker LW: Streptococcal antibody titers in Sydenham's chorea, *Pediatrics* 38: 946-956, 1966.

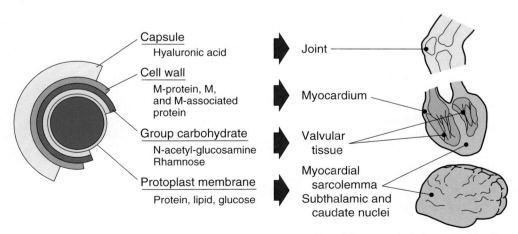

FIGURE 40–3   Group A streptococcal components and corresponding human tissues reported to exhibit immunological crossreactivity. (From Ayoub EM, Schiebler GL: Acute rheumatic fever. In Kelley VC, editor: *Practice of pediatrics,* vol 8, New York, 1987, Harper & Row.)

had had ARF developed a recurrence of the disease after subsequent group A streptococcal pharyngitis, whereas only about 2% of normal persons would develop ARF after such an infection.[64] Studies by several investigators documented the familial occurrence of the disease.[65-67] Citing their studies, these investigators concluded that susceptibility to ARF is inherited as a single recessive gene.

More substantial evidence for a genetic association was provided by Khanna and associates,[68] who reported that a B-cell alloantigen, designated D8/17, was present in 99% of patients with ARF but in only 14% of normal controls, data that have been confirmed in subsequent studies.[69] Further support for the role of genetic factors in susceptibility was provided by studies on the association of this disease with inheritance of the major HLAs .[70-78] The results of these investigations, summarized in Table 40–3, document a significant association of susceptibility with class II HLA antigens. These associations with rheumatic heart disease are more evident and consistent among clinically homogeneous patients.[79] Studies have also documented an association with ARF and HLA class II alleles, such as with DRB1*16[80] and DRB1*07.[81]

Early investigators proposed that susceptibility to ARF was related to a state of hyperreactivity to streptococcal antigens. Studies of hyperresponsiveness to a number of streptococcal and nonstreptococcal antigens suggested a hyperimmune response to streptococcal extracellular products, particularly streptolysin O, although subsequent reports did not confirm these findings.[82,83] Later studies on the immune response to the group A streptococcal group-specific carbohydrate documented an unusual pattern of hyperimmune response to this antigen in patients with rheumatic valvular disease.[51-54,84] This response was associated with inheritance of HLA-DR2 and HLA-DR4 antigens.[70] This finding is relevant in view of data that indicate that the immune response to streptococcal cell-wall antigen is under genetic control in experimental animals and humans.[85-87]

Clinical Manifestations

Arthritis, carditis, Sydenham chorea (SC), erythema marginatum, and subcutaneous nodules constitute the *major* clinical manifestations of ARF (Fig. 40–4). A patient may present with only one, two, or more of these manifestations and with varying degrees of severity of each. Although the severity and frequency of these manifestations vary considerably from patient to patient, their overall frequencies in various populations are similar (Table 40–4). Minor manifestations of ARF include fever, arthralgia, abnormal acute phase reactants, and a prolonged PR interval.

Arthritis

Arthritis occurs in about 70% of patients. Although it is the most common of the major manifestations, it is relatively less specific than the other major criteria are because it is encountered in such a large number of other rheumatic diseases. As such, it is the most common cause of a misdiagnosis of ARF. Despite its lower specificity, the arthritis of ARF has characteristics that can help in its differentiation from that due to other causes. The arthritis primarily affects large joints, particularly the knees, ankles, wrists, and elbows. Small peripheral joints are only occasionally involved, and axial disease occurs rarely, if ever. The arthritis of ARF is characteristically migratory and additive; it is usually initially a monarthritis but can be polyarticular.[88] Symptoms in an affected joint may resolve spontaneously within hours of onset, only to reappear in a different joint. The affected joint manifests the cardinal signs of inflammation with swelling, erythema, warmth, and pain. The latter symptom is the most prominent. It occurs at rest and is accentuated by passive or active movement of the joints. The severity of pain induces guarding of the joints, which may lead to pseudoparalysis.

Table 40–3

Reported associations of histocompatibility antigens-DR antigens and alleles with rheumatic fever

Study	Location	No. of Patients	Ethnicity	HLA-DR Antigen/Allele	Percent Positive Controls	Percent Positive Patients
Ayoub et al[70]	Florida, USA	24	White	DRB1*16	32	63
		48	African American	DR2	23	54
Anastasiou-Nana et al[71]	Utah, USA	33	White	DR4	32	52
Jhinghan et al[72]	New Delhi, India	134	Indian	DR3	26	50
Rajapakse et al[73]	Riyadh, Saudi Arabia	40	Arab	DR4	12	65
Maharaj et al[74]	Durban, South Africa	120	African American	DR1	3	13
Taneja et al[75]	New Delhi, India	54	Indian	DQw2	32	63
Guilherme et al[76]	San Paulo, Brazil	40	Brazilian (mulatto)	DR7	26	58
Ozkan et al[77]	Istanbul, Turkey	107	Turkish	DR3	23	49
				DR7	33	57
Weidebach et al[78]	Sao Paulo, Brazil	24	Brazilian (mulatto)	DR16 DRw53	34	83
Ahmed et al[80]	Florida, USA	18	White	DRB1*16	4	15

HLA-DR, Histocompatibility antigens DR.
Adapted from Ayoub EM: Rheumatic fever. In Rich RR, Fleisher TA, Schwartz BD et al, editors: *Clinical Immunology: Principles and Practice*, St. Louis, 1996, Mosby-Year Book.

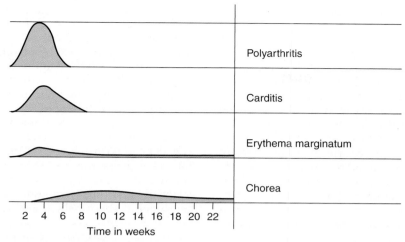

FIGURE 40–4 Major manifestations of acute rheumatic fever. This diagram illustrates the expected occurrence of each manifestation. The relative duration in weeks is indicated on the abscissa. The maximum clinical activity of each finding is represented by the *peak of the shaded area*. The expected frequency of each clinical manifestation is represented by the *relative height of each shaded area*. Polyarthritis and carditis usually are manifestations of acute disease. Chorea, although it may be an early manifestation, usually occurs about three months after the inciting episode of pharyngitis. It may be unaccompanied by other manifestations of the disease. Erythema marginatum is present for a longer period during and after the initial acute attack. This manifestation, although it is often associated with severe disease, is relatively uncommon in children.

Table 40–4

Frequency of major manifestations of acute rheumatic fever in patients in U.S. and non-U.S. patients

	U.S. Patients			Non-U.S. Patients
Manifestation	1958-1962	1962-1980	1985-1989	1960-1980
Arthritis	75%	53%	65%	30-79%
Carditis	48%	78%	59%	41-93%
Sydenham chorea	16%	5%	20%	1-12%
Erythema marginatum	6%	2%	6%	0-16%
Subcutaneous nodules	7%	5%	5%	1-9%

Adapted from Ayoub EM: Resurgence of rheumatic fever in the United States: the changing pictures of a preventable disease, *Postgrad. Med.* 92: 133-142, 1992.

Carditis

Cardiac inflammation develops in about 50% of the patients. The high frequency of this manifestation reported from developing countries probably reflects a bias toward hospitalization of patients with severe heart disease. Carditis is the most common cause of morbidity and mortality. As with other manifestations, the severity of the carditis is highly variable.[89] In some patients, such as those with SC, signs of carditis may be subtle, and cardiac involvement may be missed unless its diagnosis is pursued vigorously with echocardiographic examination.[90] Other patients may present with acute pancarditis and severe, life threatening congestive heart failure. Carditis usually occurs in tandem with other major manifestations, such as arthritis. If it is not present initially, carditis may follow arthritis within one week; the onset of carditis beyond this interval is rare.

Inflammation of the heart in ARF usually involves the myocardium and endocardium. Pericarditis is a sign of pancarditis: involvement of all cardiac layers in the inflammatory process. It is an ominous development associated with a high mortality rate. Unlike its occurrence in other rheumatic diseases, isolated pericarditis is rare in patients with ARF.

Myocarditis occurs during the initial stage of cardiac involvement; it is recognized clinically by the presence of tachycardia at rest in an afebrile patient and obliteration of the normal respiratory variation in heart rate. Myocarditis may be associated with heart block,[91] cardiac dysrhythmias, and a prolonged PR interval on electrocardiography.

Endocarditis affects principally valvular tissue and leads to the hallmark lesion of rheumatic carditis, valvular insufficiency. The mitral valve is affected alone or in conjunction with other valves in 94% of patients. Isolated mitral valve disease occurs in 65% to 70% of patients, isolated aortic disease in 6% to 13%, and simultaneous involvement of both valves in 29% to 97% of patients. The pulmonic and tricuspid valves are only occasionally affected.

Mitral insufficiency or regurgitation is identified clinically by the presence on auscultation of a high-frequency, smooth, holosystolic, apical murmur. This murmur radiates to the left axilla and is best heard with the patient in a left lateral decubitus position. A mid- to late-diastolic flow murmur of relative mitral stenosis (i.e., Carey-Coombs murmur) may be heard in patients with severe mitral insufficiency.

The murmur of aortic insufficiency is a high-frequency, diastolic murmur that starts with the aortic component of the second heart sound. It is best heard with the diaphragm of the stethoscope over the third left intercostal space with the patient in the upright position and leaning forward. The murmur of mild aortic insufficiency is faint and often difficult to hear. Murmurs of severe insufficiency are loud and accompanied by a diastolic thrill. In these patients, an increased pulse pressure due to aortic runoff is associated with bounding peripheral pulses (i.e., Corrigan pulse). Mitral and aortic valve stenoses result from valvular scarring and develop during the chronic stages of the disease.

Acute heart failure due to severe myocarditis or valvular insufficiency occurs in about 5% of children with ARF. The clinical manifestations vary greatly and include cough, chest pain, dyspnea, orthopnea, and anorexia. Tachycardia, cardiomegaly, and hepatomegaly with tenderness of the liver are present on physical examination.

Sydenham Chorea

Also known as *St. Vitus' dance,* this manifestation of inflammatory involvement of the basal ganglia and caudate nucleus of the central nervous system occurs in about 15% of patients. A higher frequency of SC was documented by several centers during the recent resurgence of ARF in the United States.[60] The latency period between the inciting streptococcal pharyngitis and the onset of clinical signs of chorea is longer than that of the other major manifestations of the disease, averaging two to four months, and sometimes extending to as long as 12 months.

A patient with SC presents with persistent involuntary and purposeless movements of the extremities usually symmetric and with muscular incoordination.[92] These movements are jerky and most prominent in the face, trunk, and distal extremities. These symptoms disappear during sleep. On examination, the patient grimaces and fidgets constantly. The protruded tongue darts in and out and resembles a bag of worms (i.e., wormian tongue). Speech is halting and explosive, and a steady tone cannot be maintained for even a short time. Extension of the arms above the head leads to pronation of the hands (i.e., pronator sign); extension of the arms anteriorly results in hyperextension of the fingers (i.e., spoon or dishing sign). When the patient is asked to squeeze the examiner's fingers, the examiner feels irregular contractions of the hand muscles (i.e., milkmaid's grip or milking sign). Handwriting, particularly drawing vertical straight lines, is clumsy and irregular because of the loss of fine muscle coordination. The patient has difficulty putting on clothes or buttoning a shirt. Such attempts lead to easy frustration and emotional upsets. Parents and teachers often complain about the child's clumsiness, inability to concentrate on tasks, or emotional lability. These symptoms usually resolve spontaneously in two to three weeks, but in severe cases they may persist for several months and sometimes for years.

A condition akin to SC, at least in pathophysiology, is Pediatric Autoimmune Neuropsychiatric Disorders Associated with Streptococcus infections (PANDAS). This condition represents a subset of childhood obsessive-compulsive disorders (OCD) and tick disorders (TD) triggered by group A beta-hemolytic streptococcus infections. Physicians have long noted that up to 70% of these patients would present with symptoms indistinguishable from classic OCD. In 1998, the National Institute of Mental Health characterized a group of children with a subset of OCD and TD and termed it PANDAS.[91] The clinical characteristics that define the PANDAS group are the presence of an OCD or a TD, prepubertal age at onset, abrupt onset relapsing-remitting symptom course, association with neurological abnormalities during exacerbations (adventitious movements or motoric hyperactivity), and temporal association between symptoms exacerbation and Group A streptococcus (GAS) infection. In a systematic clinical evaluation of 50 children who met the diagnostic criteria for PANDAS, Swedo found that patients with PANDAS typically had a young age at illness onset and an abrupt onset of neuropsychiatric symptoms. Group A beta hemolytic streptococcus infection preceded 45 (31%) of 114 exacerbations of TD or OCD.[91] Antibrain and antibasal ganglia antibodies have been documented in children with PANDAS, further supporting this hypothesis.[92] Prophylaxis with oral penicillin or azithromycin effectively reduced streptococcal infections and neuropsychiatric exacerbations among children with PANDAS. In contrast to SC where carditis is highly prevalent, 70% in some studies, carditis is not associated with PANDAS.[93] In fact, the discovery of a carditis in a child with suspected PANDAS indicate SC, rather than PANDAS, as a diagnosis.

Erythema Marginatum

Erythema marginatum is characteristic of rheumatic fever and occurs in about 5% of patients. This rash is nonpruritic and macular with a serpiginous erythematous border (Fig. 40–5). The individual lesions are about 0.4 cm in diameter and are usually located on the trunk and proximal inner aspects of the limbs, particularly where they join the trunk. The rash is rare on the face or other exposed areas. It is accentuated by warmth, such as the application of warm towels or a bath. Erythema marginatum is difficult to detect in patients with dark skin.

Subcutaneous Nodules

The subcutaneous nodules of ARF that were most common in patients who developed chronic rheumatic heart disease and were a sign of severe involvement are now rare. They are usually located on the extensor surfaces of the joints, particularly the elbows, knees, ankles, and knuckles, and occasionally on the occiput and spine. The overlying skin is not discolored. Their size varies from 0.5 to 2 cm, and they are freely movable. In many respects, they clinically and histologically resemble benign rheumatoid nodules.

Minor Manifestations of the Disease

The minor manifestations of fever, arthralgia, and elevated acute phase reactants are nonspecific and encountered in a number of other rheumatic diseases. The severity and

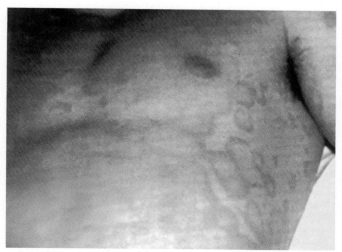

FIGURE 40–5   Rash of erythema marginatum in an adolescent boy with acute rheumatic fever occurred with its characteristic serpiginous and erythematous margins.

duration of fever vary; the patient may have a temperature of 38.5°C=101°F to 40°C=104°F during the acute phase of the disease. Arthralgia (i.e., pain without objective changes in the joint) should be differentiated from arthritis. Abnormally elevated acute phase reactants are indicators of tissue inflammation and are present during the acute stage of the disease. A prolonged PR interval on the electrocardiogram is another nonspecific finding. It occurs frequently in ARF but does not alone constitute an adequate criterion for carditis; PR prolongation also does not correlate with the ultimate development of chronic rheumatic heart disease.

Pathology

The inflammation that occurs in ARF is the result of a diffuse vasculitis. The organs most commonly affected are the joints, heart, brain, and peripheral vascular system. The vasculitis affects the smaller vessels and is characterized by proliferation of endothelial cells. This vasculitic process is reflected in the rash of ARF; inflammation of collagen occurs primarily in arthritis, valvulitis, and pericarditis. The synovitis of ARF is typified by a mononuclear cell infiltrate with fibrinoid degeneration. Joint cartilage is usually not involved.[93,94]

Inflammation of the heart, the most serious complication of the disease, usually involves the myocardium and endocardium. Unlike other rheumatic diseases, such as systemic lupus erythematosus (SLE) or juvenile rheumatoid arthritis (JRA), sole involvement of the pericardium is distinctly uncommon in ARF. Valvular endocarditis is the more common and characteristic inflammatory process and the principal cause of chronic cardiac disease. Acute inflammation leads to valvular insufficiency, and persistence of the inflammation results in scarring and stenosis (Fig. 40–6). The mitral valve is the most commonly involved, and mitral insufficiency is the hallmark of rheumatic carditis. A review of the cardiac pathology by Roberts[95] indicated that isolated mitral valve disease was of rheumatic origin in 76% of cases, whereas aortic valve disease was ascribable to ARF in only 13% of cases.

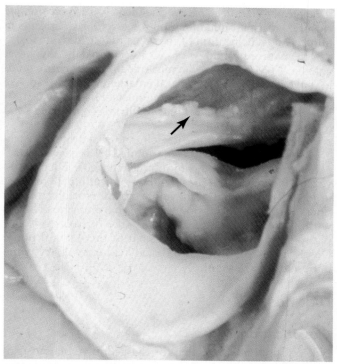

FIGURE 40–6   Chronic rheumatic valvular heart disease. Verrucal endocardial thickening was present along the line of closure of the valve leaflets (*arrow*).

The simultaneous presence of mitral and aortic disease was related to a rheumatic cause in 97% of cases. Serum cardiac troponin I, a sensitive and specific marker of myocardial injury, is not elevated in cases of ARF with cardiac involvement, indicating that congestive heart failure in ARF is related to valvar insufficiency rather than specific myocardial inflammation.[96]

The histological changes in acute rheumatic carditis are not specific, and the degree of abnormality does not necessarily correlate with the severity of carditis.[93,94] In the early stage, when dilatation of the myocardium is present, histological changes can be minimal. Despite this, cardiac function may be severely impaired and associated with a high rate of mortality. Progression of the inflammation leads to an exudative and proliferative reaction in the myocardium characterized by edematous changes followed by a cellular infiltrate of lymphocytes and plasma cells with few granulocytes. CD4- cells predominate in the lymphocytic infiltrate[97] Degenerating collagen fibers are visible throughout the tissue as eosinophilic, granular deposits consisting of a mixture of fibrin, globulin, and other substances. This stage is followed by the formation of the *Aschoff body*.[98,99] This lesion consists of a perivascular infiltrate of large cells with polymorphous nuclei and basophilic cytoplasm arranged in a rosette around an avascular center of fibrinoid. The Aschoff body is pathognomonic of rheumatic carditis and occurs most commonly in patients with subacute or chronic carditis. It may develop in any area of the myocardium but is not present in other tissues.

Tissue edema and cellular infiltrates characterize the inflammation of valvular tissue. This inflammatory process also involves the chordae tendineae. Verrucae may form at the edge of the leaflets, preventing the valves from complete closure. Persistent inflammation for several years results in fibrosis and calcification of the valve that lead to stenosis.

The pathophysiology of SC is centered in the basal ganglia.[100] Magnetic resonance imaging volumetric studies have indicated focal striatal enlargement and response of the chorea to dopamine antagonists. Histological studies have documented cellular infiltration and neuronal loss in the basal ganglia.[101,102]

Subcutaneous nodules are characterized by a central area of fibrinoid necrosis surrounded by loosely demarcated zones of scattered mononuclear cells. Edema and vascular islands are present, but palisading of epithelioid cells is not well developed. Interstitial collagen fibers and scar formation occupy the outermost layers without formation of a capsule. The histology is not pathognomonic but resembles that of the Aschoff body. Descriptions of the pathological features of erythema marginatum are scant.

Diagnosis

Classification Criteria

No specific test is available for the definitive diagnosis of ARF. The diagnosis continues to be based on guidelines of clinical and laboratory criteria initially promulgated by T. Duckett Jones and subsequently revised by several committees of the American Heart Association. The latest modification of the Jones Criteria is outlined in Table 40–5.[103] The purpose of these guidelines is to assist in the diagnosis of an initial attack of rheumatic fever and to minimize overdiagnosis. As stated under these guidelines, the presence of two major manifestations or one major plus two minor manifestations provides the basis for the diagnosis of ARF—if supported by evidence of antecedent group A streptococcal infection. The latter is a *sine qua non* for establishing the diagnosis.

A positive throat culture or rapid antigen test can confirm an antecedent group A streptococcal pharyngitis. However, the period of latency between the inciting pharyngitis and the onset of ARF reduces the frequency of positive cultures to less than one third of patients.[104]

More reliable evidence can be obtained by the use of the streptococcal antibody tests listed in Table 40–1. Because of the latency period, serum obtained at the time of the initial evaluation of the patient coincides with the peak of the antibody response (see Fig. 40–2). An elevated ASO or anti-DNAse B level is expected in about 85% of patients (see Table 40–2). When both tests are performed (considered by many to be a reasonable and conservative approach to diagnostic specificity), more than 90% of patients have an elevated titer for one of these tests. If the result of the ASO test is negative, a DNAse B titer should be performed. A fourfold (two-tube) increase or decrease in titers should be demonstrated over time because normal children in many geographical areas may have elevated titers.[105] Results of these antibody tests may be normal for most patients with chronic rheumatic heart disease, and a high proportion of patients with SC may have normal ASO or anti-DNAse B titers (see Table 40–2). Neither the ASO nor the other streptococcal antibody tests are

diagnostic of ARF; they provide supportive evidence for antecedent streptococcal infection.

The three acute phase reactants most commonly used in diagnosis are the peripheral blood leukocyte count, the erythrocyte sedimentation rate (ESR), and the C-reactive protein (CRP) level. The leukocyte count is the most variable and least dependable. It is normal in about one half of the patients with ARF. The ESR is markedly elevated in patients with acute disease but may be normal even with severe congestive failure.[106] The CRP level is also elevated in patients with acute disease,[107] and unlike the ESR, its concentration is not affected by congestive heart failure. These tests are most useful in following the course of the disease and its response to treatment. Serum cardiac troponin 1 levels, known to be associated with myocardial injury, are not elevated in active rheumatic carditis.[89,96,108]

The role of echocardiography is controversial to date. According to the modified Jones criteria, echocardiographic abnormalities without concomitant clinical findings are not considered in the diagnosis of rheumatic carditis. In certain regions of the world where populations are at increased risk of rheumatic fever, such as the Maori and Pacific people in New Zealand and the aboriginal Australians, echocardiography has a central role in the diagnosis of rheumatic carditis. Australian criteria and the New Zealand guidelines for rheumatic fever diagnosis suggest that subclinical carditis, namely echocardiographic valvulitis without clinical findings, should be accepted as carditis for the diagnosis of rheumatic fever.[109] Other studies useful in diagnosis include chest radiography and electrocardiography. A chest radiograph can detect cardiac enlargement or pericardial fluid. These findings are best confirmed by echocardiographic studies, which can also define the presence of

Table 40–5

Guidelines for the diagnosis of an initial attack of rheumatic fever (Modified Jones Criteria, 1992)

Major Manifestations*	Minor Manifestations*
Carditis	Clinical
Polyarthritis	Fever
Sydenham chorea	Arthralgia
Erythema marginatum	Laboratory
Subcutaneous nodules	Elevated acute phase reactants:
	Erythrocyte sedimentation rate
	C-reactive protein level
	Prolonged PR interval

Supporting Evidence of Antecedent Group A Streptococcal Infection
Elevated or rising streptococcal antibody titers
Positive throat culture or rapid streptococcal antigen tests

*The presence of two major manifestations or of one major and two minor manifestations indicates a high probability of acute rheumatic fever if supported by evidence of preceding group A streptococcal infection.
Adapted from Dajani AS, Ayoub EM, Bierman FZ et al: Guidelines for the diagnosis of rheumatic fever: Jones Criteria, updated 1992, *JAMA* 87:302-307, 1992.

myocarditis by assessing myocardial contractility and the nature and extent of valvular lesions. Electrocardiography is most useful in confirming abnormalities in conduction and rhythm during acute myocardial inflammation.

Differential Diagnosis

Other rheumatic diseases account for most of the disorders misdiagnosed as ARF. JRA can be confused with ARF without carditis (see Chapters 14 to 17). Characteristics indicating a diagnosis of JRA rather than ARF include an onset of oligoarticular arthritis in a child before the age of 5-years-old; absence of erythema of the joint; a protracted, recurrent course with an incomplete response to nonsteroidal antiinflammatory drug (NSAID) therapy; and particularly the absence of evidence for antecedent group A streptococcal infection.

Poststreptococcal reactive arthritis (PSRA) poses some difficulty in differentiation from ARF. Clinical findings that should assist in the diagnosis of this disorder are discussed later in this chapter. Other conditions in which joint involvement is common include SLE, Kawasaki disease, mixed connective tissue disease, other reactive arthritides, and serum sickness.[110] Infectious arthritis, particularly gonococcal arthritis, and brucellosis in endemic areas, may present a problem in differential diagnosis. Leukemia and hemoglobinopathy with bone infarcts can be mistaken for ARF.

Patients with carditis and pericarditis may develop secondary infections by a variety of bacterial, viral, rickettsial, or mycoplasmal agents. Endocardial involvement occurs in patients with bacterial endocarditis and in patients with SLE and Libman-Sacks endocarditis. A murmur and systolic clicks are present in patients with mitral valve prolapse. Some children with Kawasaki disease develop clinically obvious myocarditis and valvular disease during the early stages of illness. In these patients, the lack of evidence for antecedent group A streptococcal infection allows an initial differentiation from ARF.

Differentiation of SC from other neurological disorders requires careful evaluation.[111] Imaging studies of the central nervous system are usually normal for patients with SC. Other neurological conditions that may be confused with SC include congenital or acquired "habitual" TDs, attention-deficit disorders, and obsessive-compulsive behavior.[112] ASO and anti-DNAse B tests should provide evidence for antecedent streptococcal infection in more than 80% of children with SC. Chorea is also a characteristic symptom in children with the antiphospholipid antibody syndrome (see Chapter 23).

Treatment

The initial treatment of ARF should address the eradication of streptococci that initiated this complication and the inflammatory process that has affected the various organs. Patients with ARF should be promptly evaluated for cardiac involvement. Subsequent management includes prophylaxis to prevent recurrence of streptococcal infections and treatment of residual cardiac disease when present.

Eradication of Streptococci

Patients should receive a streptococcal eradicating regimen of antimicrobials even if their throat culture or rapid antigen test is negative (Table 40–6).[113] Penicillin is the primary agent of choice administered intramuscularly as a single dose or orally for 10 days. The intramuscular route is preferable in children with cardiac involvement because of its greater dependability and efficacy. Patients allergic to penicillin should receive one of the following: a narrow spectrum cephalosporin, clindamycin, azithromycin, or clarithromycin.

Treatment of Clinical Manifestations

CARDITIS

Acute carditis requires immediate attention.[114] For mild to moderate carditis, aspirin is administered in a dose of 80 to 100 mg/kg/day in four divided doses. This schedule is maintained for four to eight weeks, depending on clinical response, and then is reduced gradually and discontinued during the next four weeks. Other NSAIDs may be as effective as aspirin,[115,116] but have not yet been recommended by the expert committee of the American Heart Association.

Glucocorticoid therapy is reserved for patients with severe carditis and congestive heart failure, particularly those with pancarditis, in whom it may be life saving. The use of glucocorticoids, rather than aspirin in patients with heart failure, is also justified to avoid solute overload from aspirin. It should be emphasized that neither form of therapy has been demonstrated to influence the subsequent evolution of valvular disease.[117-119] Unlike most rheumatic diseases, the use of IV methylprednisone as a single antiinflammatory agent is inferior to conventional treatment with oral prednisone in the control of severe rheumatic carditis.[120-122] Prednisone is given orally in a dose of 2 mg/kg once daily. The duration of daily steroid therapy should rarely exceed two weeks, and the drug should be tapered and withdrawn during the next two to three weeks. One week before termination of therapy, aspirin should be instituted (following the regimen described earlier) to avoid the rebound of symptoms and acute phase reactants that occurs when steroid therapy is abruptly terminated.

The ESR and CRP levels are essential in monitoring the response to antiinflammatory therapy. In patients with heart failure and a falsely low ESR, a rise in this reactant may occur with recovery; the CRP level is more reliable in monitoring the response in these patients. Ancillary therapy for cardiac failure includes the judicious use of drugs such as digitalis; inotropic agents such as dobutamine, dopamine, or amrinone; vasodilators (captopril or enalapril); and diuretics.

General aspects of initial management include bedrest for patients with acute carditis. This recommendation, overly emphasized in the past, led to prolonged confinement in bed and cardiac neurosis and should be discouraged. Gradual resumption of normal activity should be allowed after the acute carditis subsides. Echocardiographic follow-up is predicated on the type

Table 40–6

Antibiotic regimens for primary prevention (streptococcal eradication) and secondary prevention of rheumatic fever

Antibiotic	Dose	Route	Duration
Primary Prevention			
Benzathine penicillin G	600,000 U for patients <27 kg 1,200,000 U for patients > 27 kg	Intramuscular	Single dose
Penicillin V	<27 kg 250 mg 2 to 3 times daily > 27 kg 500 mg 2 to 3 times daily	Oral	10 days
For individuals allergic to penicillin Narrow-spectrum cephalosporins	Variable	Oral or	10 days
Clindamycin	20 mg/kg/day 3 times daily	Oral or	10 days
Azithromycin	12 mg/kg once daily	Oral or	5 days
Clarithromycin	15 mg/kg/day twice daily	Oral	10 days
Secondary Prevention			
Benzathine penicillin G	600,000 U for patients <27 kg 1,200,000 U for patients >27kg	Intramuscular	Every 4 weeks*
Penicillin V	250 mg twice daily	Oral	
Sulfadiazine	0.5 g once daily <27 kg 1.0 gm daily >27 kg	Oral	
For individuals allergic to penicillin and sulfadiazine Macrolide or azalide	Variable	Oral	

*May be given every 3 weeks in high-risk situation.
Adapted from Gerber MA, Baltimore RS, Eaton CB et al: Prevention of rheumatic fever and diagnosis and treatment of acute streptococcal pharyngitis: a scientific statement from the American Heart Association Rheumatic Fever, Endocarditis, and Kawasaki Disease Committee of the Council on Cardiovascular Disease in the Young, the Interdisciplinary Council on Functional Genomics and Transitional Biology, and the Interdisciplinary Council on Quality of Care and Outcomes Research, *Circulation* 119:1541-1551, 2009.

and severity of the initial carditis and its response to therapy.[121]

ARTHRITIS

The arthritis characteristically pursues a self-limiting course, rarely lasting more than one week in any one joint. A hallmark of the arthritis in this disease is its exquisite sensitivity to salicylates. A dose of aspirin of 50 to 75 mg/kg/day given in three to four divided doses is usually effective. This therapy continues for no more than two weeks and is thereafter gradually withdrawn. A rapid resolution of the fever and a decline in the ESR usually parallel resolution of the arthritis. A lack of improvement of the arthritis within about five days of salicylate therapy should prompt a reconsideration of the correctness of the diagnosis. No data are available regarding the efficacy of other NSAIDs in the treatment of ARF. Steroids should not be used in patients with isolated arthritis.

CHOREA

Mild manifestations of SC require only bedrest and avoidance of physical and emotional stress. Although anticonvulsant drugs may help control severe symptoms, the response to these agents is unpredictable. Phenobarbital, haloperidol, carbamazepine, and valproate have been used with varying success. Antiinflammatory agents are not needed for the treatment of chorea.

Prophylaxis of Rheumatic Heart Disease

Medical management after the acute stage of the disease centers on prevention of recurrences of rheumatic fever and continued treatment of residual heart disease, including prevention of bacterial endocarditis. Antimicrobial prophylaxis against streptococcal pharyngitis has proved highly effective in reducing recurrences of rheumatic fever and in preventing cumulative heart damage.

Regimens for streptococcal prophylaxis recommended by the American Heart Association are outlined in Table 40–6. Because recurrences of rheumatic fever are most common during the five years after the initial attack,[17,37,93] intramuscular benzathine penicillin prophylaxis is preferable and should be given once monthly in areas of low incidence of rheumatic fever and every three weeks in areas endemic to this disease. Oral prophylaxis is acceptable for patients without cardiac involvement. Although sulfonamides are ineffective in eradicating streptococcal infections, these agents are as effective, if not more effective, than oral penicillin for prophylaxis against recurrent streptococcal infections.

The American Heart Association has recently revised recommendations on rheumatic fever prophylaxis. Current protocols are based on the risk of reinfection and the development of streptococcal pharyngitis.[122] This risk is highest in school-aged children, in persons working in crowded conditions, military recruits, and those in close contact with children, such as parents, teachers, and health providers. Therefore, patients with carditis should receive prophylaxis well into adulthood, preferably for life, whereas it may be discontinued at the age of 21-years-old in those with no cardiac involvement (although all such patients should receive prophylaxis for a minimum of five years regardless of age).[123] Prophylaxis should be continued after surgical valve repair.

Endocarditis Prophylaxis

Supplemental doses of antibiotic should be prescribed for surgical or dental procedures in children with known rheumatic heart disease. Specific recommendations vary, depending on the procedure and age of the patient.

Course of the Disease and Prognosis

Major morbidity in rheumatic fever is associated exclusively with the degree of cardiac damage. Severe carditis, which leads to chronic residual valvular disease (see Fig. 40–6), primarily occurs in children in developing countries. The availability of cardiac surgery has alleviated to a considerable extent the crippling effect of this complication. Mortality is rare and occurs predominantly in patients with pancarditis. A better understanding of the relationship of streptococcal infection to the occurrence of initial attacks and recurrences of rheumatic fever has led to the institution of prophylactic regimens that have prevented subsequent attacks of the disease and reduced the cumulative heart damage produced by these exacerbations.[124] The study by Tompkins and colleagues[125] emphasizes the singular value of prophylaxis by confirming that signs of rheumatic valvular disease resolve in about 80% of patients who receive continuous, long-term prophylaxis. This information is of particular importance in encouraging patients with rheumatic heart disease to adhere to the prescribed regimen of prophylaxis.

Rheumatic arthritis is self-limited. A rare form of nonerosive but deforming arthropathy ascribed to rheumatic fever (i.e., Jaccoud arthritis) has been reported in adults but does not occur in children.[126] It is more commonly associated with SLE. SC and erythema marginatum are also self-limited with no permanent residua. Patients who escape severe heart disease can be assured of a benign course and a good prognosis.

POSTSTREPTOCOCCAL REACTIVE ARTHRITIS

Definition and Classification

The occurrence of arthritis after group A streptococcal infection in children who did not fulfill criteria for the diagnosis of ARF was described first by Crea and Mortimer in 1959.[127] Subsequently, a number of other studies reported on this entity which was designated *poststreptococcal reactive arthritis* (PSRA).[80,128-135] In contrast to the arthritis of ARF, arthritis observed in these patients was nonmigratory, protracted in course, and responded poorly to aspirin or other NSAIDs. Despite these clinical differences, several investigators have maintained that PSRA is an extension of the spectrum of ARF.[129,136] Some studies, however, suggest that this syndrome differs significantly in pathogenesis and clinical characteristics from the arthritis of rheumatic fever.[137]

Epidemiology

Although it is difficult to assess accurately, the incidence of this disease in North-Central Florida is estimated to be one to two cases per 100,000 children at risk per year; 17 of 455 patients with rheumatic diseases encountered over a period of two years had PSRA.[80,138] This incidence was twice that for ARF during the same period. The age of the patients varied from 5- to 16-years-old with a mean of 9.7-years-old. A slightly but not significantly higher incidence of the disease occurred in males (56% versus 44%). There was no ethnic preponderance.

Etiology and Pathogenesis

Evidence for group A streptococcal infection should be documented in all patients. In contrast to ARF, in which throat cultures or rapid antigen tests are positive in one third of patients, results are positive in about 75% of patients with PSRA. This difference can be ascribed to the shorter latency (less than 10 days) for this disease.[130,131,134] Streptococcal pharyngitis is associated with an ASO and an anti-DNAse B response in most patients.[80] Skin infection does not elicit an ASO response. The high frequency of elevated ASO titers in patients with PSRA suggests that streptococcal pharyngitis is the primary inciting cause of the disease.[139]

Genetic Background

Studies of the relationship of PSRA with HLA-B27 failed to document a significant association;[80] only three of 18 (16.7%) white American patients were positive. This frequency contrasts with reactive arthritis in children, in which 93% are HLA-B27 positive.[140] Further studies, however, documented a significant association of PSRA with HLA class II alleles. Compared with normal controls and patients with ARF, these patients had a significant increase in the frequency of DRB1*01.[80] In ARF, there is an increased frequency of the DRB1*16 allele. These associations with DRB1 alleles suggest a common pathogenetic mechanism for PSRA and ARF.

Clinical Manifestations

In addition to a pharyngitis present in 66% of patients,[80,138] approximately 30% report the occurrence of low-grade fever, and a similar number describe a nonscarlatinal rash that precedes onset of the arthritis. About one half of the children complain of morning stiffness of varying duration.

Most patients present with arthritis involving one or more joints. About 10% complain only of arthralgia. The frequency of joint involvement is illustrated in Fig. 40–7. The arthritis is asymmetric and nonmigratory in

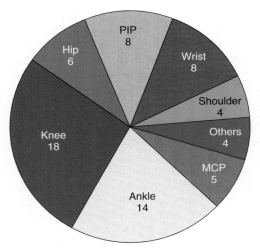

FIGURE 40–7 Frequency of joint involvement in patients with poststreptococcal reactive arthritis. Values represent the number of patients with involvement of that joint. MCP, metacarpopharyngeal; PIP, proximal interphalangeal. (From Ahmed S, Ayoub EM, Scornik JC et al: Poststreptococcal reactive arthritis: clinical characteristics and association with HLA-DR alleles, *Arthritis Rheum* 41: 1096-1102, 1998. Copyright © 1998 John Wiley & Sons, Inc. Reprinted with permission of Wiley-Liss, Inc., a subsidiary of John Wiley & Sons, Inc.)

70% to 80% and involves joints of the lower extremities in almost all patients. One half of the patients also have arthritis involving the upper extremities.[80] Axial disease occurs in 25%; in our experience, these patients account for any possible association with HLA-B27.

Cardiac disease was present in 5.8% of 86 patients described in the literature.[80] In almost all cases, valvular disease was only detected, if at all, several months after onset. Most of these patients had not been placed on penicillin prophylaxis. The delay in onset of cardiac abnormalities should be contrasted with the carditis associated with ARF, in which cardiac involvement usually occurs during the acute stage of the disease and in tandem with the arthritis. Some investigators have described patients who presented with "silent carditis," indicating that this complication was not clinically detectable and required echocardiographic studies for confirmation.[131] This suggests that the frequency of carditis in this disease may be higher than that reported to date.

Extraarticular manifestations include vasculitis, tenosynovitis, and glomerulonephritis.[141] Acquired Brown syndrome, the inability to elevate the affected eye in full adduction resulting from inflammatory tenosynovitis of the superior oblique tendon, has been reported in one child.[142]

Diagnosis and Differential Diagnosis

Proposed criteria for the diagnosis of PSRA are in Table 40–7.[138] The differential diagnosis includes most of the same arthritides outlined for ARF. The similarity in cause, and in some of the clinical manifestations of both diseases, poses unresolved difficulty in differentiating these two entities. However, as outlined in Table 40–8, clinical and laboratory differences should permit the separation of this entity from ARF and other reactive arthritides in most children.

Table 40–7

Proposed criteria for the diagnosis of poststreptococcal reactive arthritis

A. Characteristics of the arthritis
  1. Acute-onset arthritis, symmetrical or asymmetrical, usually nonmigratory, can affect any joint
  2. Persistent or recurrent
  3. Poorly responsive to aspirin or nonsteroidal antiinflammatory drugs
B. Evidence of antecedent group A streptococcal infection
C. Does not fulfill the modified Jones Criteria for the diagnosis of acute rheumatic fever

Adapted from Ayoub EM, Ahmed S: Update on complications of Group A streptococcal infections, *Curr Probl Pediatr* 27:90-101, 1997.

Table 40–8

Clinical and laboratory characteristics of poststreptococcal reactive arthritis and acute rheumatic fever

Characteristics	PSRA	ARF
Antecedent group A streptococcal infection	Yes	Yes
Onset of arthritis after infection	<2 weeks	2 to 3 weeks
Migratory arthritis	No	Yes
Axial arthritis	Yes	No
Heart involvement	6%	50%
Response to ASA	Not dramatic	Dramatic
Association with HLA-B27	No	No
Association with HLA-DRβ alleles	DRB1*01	DRB1*16

ARF, acute rheumatic fever; ASA, 5-aminosalicylic acid; HLA, histocompatibility antigens; PSRA, poststreptococcal reactive arthritis.
Adapted from Ahmed S, Ayoub EM, Scornik JC et al: Poststreptococcal reactive arthritis: clinical characteristics and association with HLA-DR alleles. *Arthritis Rheum* 41: 1096-1102, 1998. Copyright © 1998 John Wiley & Sons, Inc. Reprinted with permission of Wiley-Liss, Inc., a subsidiary of John Wiley & Sons, Inc.

Laboratory Examination

The leukocyte count is normal in the majority of patients. However, the ESR is elevated in 75%. As in ARF, this test is helpful in assessing the course of the arthritis. Streptococcal antibody tests are more dependable than in ARF for documenting evidence for an antecedent group A streptococcal infection. The ASO level is elevated in 88% and the anti-DNAse B in 80% of patients. At least one of these antibodies should be elevated in almost all patients at the time of presentation or shortly thereafter.[80] Because of the shorter period of latency between the streptococcal infection and the onset of arthritis, these patients have a higher frequency of positive throat cultures or rapid antigen tests for group A streptococci than patients with ARF.

Treatment

NSAIDs (e.g., naproxen, ibuprofen, and tolmetin) are the principal drugs used in treatment. Aspirin probably offers no particular advantage. The value of disease-modifying drugs, such as methotrexate, has not been assessed. Physical therapy should be instituted for relief of joint pain and stiffness.

As recommended for patients with group A streptococcal pharyngitis and its complications, antimicrobial therapy should be prescribed at the time of initial diagnosis to eradicate streptococci from the tonsillopharyngeal tissue (see Table 40–6). Antimicrobial prophylaxis to prevent recurrences, and possibly subsequent cardiac disease, has been recommended by some investigators, but this issue is controversial.[143] Because carditis can occur in this disease, albeit probably at a lower rate than in patients with rheumatic fever, the American Heart Association has suggested prophylaxis for one year.[122] If carditis is not detected by then, prophylaxis is discontinued. If carditis occurs during this interval, the patient is considered to have had ARF and should continue to receive prophylaxis in accordance with previously stated recommendations. However, discontinuing prophylaxis after only one year potentially leaves the patient at risk for the development of carditis. Our preference is to institute a prophylactic regimen similar to that proposed by the American Heart Association for patients with ARF who have arthritis but no carditis—that is, to continue prophylaxis until the patient reaches the age of 21-years-old and for a minimum of at least five years.[122] All patients should be reevaluated for evidence of carditis for a period extending over five years.

Course of the Disease and Prognosis

Unlike the arthritis of ARF, the course of the arthritis in PSRA is often protracted, lasting five days to eight months, with a mean duration of 66 days from onset to resolution.[80] Some patients continue to have arthralgia for several months after remission of the arthritis. This prolonged course is not altered significantly by the administration of NSAIDs or antimicrobials.

Acknowledgment

This chapter is dedicated to the memory of Elia Ayoub, MD.

REFERENCES

1. G.H. Stollerman, Rheumatogenic group A streptococci and the return of rheumatic fever, Adv. Intern. Med. 35 (1990) 1–25.
2. A.C. Steer, J.R. Carapetis, T.M. Nolan, et al., Systematic review of rheumatic heart disease prevalence in children in developing countries: the role of environmental factors, J. Paediatr. Child Health 38 (2002) 229–234.
3. M. Markowitz, The decline of rheumatic fever: role of medical intervention, Lewis W. Wannamaker Memorial Lecture, J. Pediatr. 106 (1985) 545–550.
4. L.G. Veasy, S.E. Wiedmeier, G.S. Orsmond, et al., Resurgence of acute rheumatic fever in the intermountain area of the United States, N. Engl. J. Med. 316 (1987) 421–427.
8. S.P. Griffiths, W.M. Gersony, Acute rheumatic fever in New York City (1969 to 1988): a comparative study of two decades, J. Pediatr. 116 (1990) 882–887.
16. L.G. Veasy, L.Y. Tani, H.R. Hill, Persistence of acute rheumatic fever in the intermountain area of the United States, J. Pediatr. 124 (1994) 9–16.
20. K.B. Tibazarwa, J.A. Volmink, B.M. Mayosi, Incidence of acute rheumatic fever in the world: a systematic review of population-based studies, Heart 84 (2008) 1534–1540.
21. J.R. Carapetis, A.C. Steer, E.K. Mulholland, et al., The global burden of group A streptococcal diseases, Lancet. Infect. Dis. 5 (2005) 685–694.
23. L. Gordis, The virtual disappearance of rheumatic fever in the United States: lessons in the rise and fall of disease. T. Duckett Jones memorial lecture, Circulation 72 (1985) 1155–1162.
25. L.W. Wannamaker, Differences between streptococcal infections of the throat and of the skin (second of two parts), N. Engl. J. Med. 282 (1970) 78–85.
30. I. Goldstein, B. Halpern, L. Robert, Immunologic relation between *Streptococcus* A polysaccharide and the structural glycoproteins of heart valve, Nature 213 (1967) 44–47.
31. V.A. Fischetti, Streptococcal M protein, Sci. Am. 264 (1991) 58–65.
33. J.C. Smoot, E.K. Korgenski, J.A. Daly, et al., Molecular analysis of group A *Streptococcus* type emm18 isolates temporally associated with acute rheumatic fever outbreaks in Salt Lake City, Utah, J. Clin. Microbiol. 40 (2002) 1805–1810.
35. D. Bessen, K.F. Jones, V.A. Fischetti, Evidence for two distinct classes of streptococcal M protein and their relationship to rheumatic fever, J. Exp. Med. 169 (1989) 269–283.
36. J.C. Smoot, K.D. Barbian, J.J. Van Gompel, et al., Genome sequence and comparative microarray analysis of serotype M18 group A *Streptococcus* strains associated with acute rheumatic fever outbreaks, Proc. Natl. Acad. Sci. U. S. A. 99 (2002) 4668–4673.
38. E.M. Ayoub, E. Kaplan, Host-parasite interaction in the pathogenesis of rheumatic fever, J. Rheumatol. (Suppl. 30) (1991) 6–13.
40. J. Sandson, D. Hamerman, R. Janis, et al., Immunologic and chemical similarities between the streptococcus and human connective tissue, Trans. Assoc. Am. Physicians 81 (1968) 249–257.
44. D.L. Stevens, Streptococcal toxic-shock syndrome: spectrum of disease, pathogenesis, and new concepts in treatment, Emerg. Infect. Dis. 1 (1995) 69–78.
51. B.A. Dudding, E.M. Ayoub, Persistence of streptococcal group A antibody in patients with rheumatic valvular disease, J. Exp. Med. 128 (1968) 1081–1098.
52. E.M. Ayoub, S.T. Shulman, Pattern of antibody response to the streptococcal group A carbohydrate in rheumatic patients with or without carditis, in: S.E. Read, J.B. Zabriskie (Eds.), Streptococcal disease and the immune response, Academic Press, New York, 1980.
54. E.M. Ayoub, Immune response to group A streptococcal infections, Pediatr. Infect. Dis. J. 10 (1991) S15–S19.
55. M.H. Kaplan, M. Meyeserian, An immunological cross-reaction between group-A streptococcal cells and human heart tissue, Lancet 1 (1962) 706–710.
61. G. Husby, I. van de Rign, J.B. Zabriskie, et al., Antibodies reacting with cytoplasm of subthalamic and caudate nuclei neurons in chorea and acute rheumatic fever, J. Exp. Med. 144 (1976) 1094–1110.
69. L. Harel, A. Zeharia, Y. Kodman, et al., Presence of the d8/17 B-cell marker in children with rheumatic fever in Israel, Clin. Genet. 61 (2002) 293–298.
78. W. Weidebach, A.C. Goldberg, J.M. Chiarella, et al., HLA class II antigens in rheumatic fever, Analysis of the DR locus by restriction fragment-length polymorphism and oligotyping, Hum. Immunol. 40 (1994) 253–258.
79. Y. Guedez, A. Kotby, M. El Demellawy, et al., HLA class II associations with rheumatic heart disease are more evident and consistent among clinically homogeneous patients, Circulation 99 (1999) 2784–2790.
80. S. Ahmed, E.M. Ayoub, J.C. Scornik, et al., Poststreptococcal reactive arthritis: clinical characteristics and association with HLA-DR alleles, Arthritis Rheum. 41 (1998) 1096–1102.
88. J.R. Carapetis, B.J. Currie, Rheumatic fever in a high incidence population: the importance of monoarthritis and low grade fever, Arch. Dis. Child. 85 (2001) 223–227.
89. R.V. Williams, L.L. Minich, R.E. Shaddy, et al., Evidence for lack of myocardial injury in children with acute rheumatic carditis, Cardiol. Young 12 (2002) 519–523.
91. S.E. Swedo, H.L. Leonard, M. Garvey, et al., Pediatric autoimmune Neuropsychiatric disorders associated with streptococcal infections: clinical description of the first 50 cases, Am. J. Psychiatry 155 (1998) 264–271.
92. P. Pavone, R. Bianchini, E. Parano, et al., Anti-brain antibodies in Pandas versus uncomplicated streptococcal infection, Pediatr. Neurol. 30 (2004) 107–110.

93. L.A. Snider, V. Sachdev, J.E. MaCkaronis, et al., Echocardiographic findings in the PANDAS subgroup, Pediatrics 114 (2004) e748–e751.

96. M. Gupta, R.W. Lent, E.L. Kaplan, et al., Serum cardiac troponin I in acute rheumatic fever, Am. J. Cardiol. 89 (2002) 779–782.

100. P.C. Faustino, M.T. Terreri, A.J. da Rocha, et al., Clinical, laboratory, psychiatric and magnetic resonance findings in patients with Sydenham chorea, Neuroradiology 45 (2003) 456–462.

105. S. Sethi, K. Kaushik, K. Mohandas, et al., Anti-streptolysin O titers in normal healthy children of 5-15 years, Indian Pediatr. 40 (2003) 1068–1071.

107. Z. Golbasi, O. Ucar, T. Keles, et al., Increased levels of high sensitive C-reactive protein in patients with chronic rheumatic valve disease: evidence of ongoing inflammation, Eur. J. Heart Fail. 4 (2002) 593–595.

108. B. Oran, H. Coban, S. Karaaslan, et al., Serum cardiac troponin-I in active rheumatic carditis, Indian. J. Pediatr. 68 (2001) 943–944.

109. J.R. Carapetis, A. Brown, N.J. Wilson, K.N. Edwards, on behalf of the Rheumatic Fever Guidelines Writing Group: An Australian guideline for rheumatic fever and rheumatic heart disease: an abridged outline, MJA. 186 (2007) 581–586.

110. H.M. Sondheimer, A. Lorts, Cardiac involvement in inflammatory disease: systemic lupus erythematosus, rheumatic fever, and Kawasaki disease, Adolesc. Med. 12 (2001) 69–78.

113. S.T. Shulman, Acute streptococcal pharyngitis in pediatric medicine: current issues in diagnosis and management, Paediatr. Drugs 5 (2003) 13–23.

115. S. Karademir, D. Oguz, F. Senocak, et al., Tolmetin and salicylate therapy in acute rheumatic fever: Comparison of clinical efficacy and side-effects, Pediatr. Int. 45 (2003) 676–679.

116. P.J. Hashkes, T. Tauber, E. Somekh, et al., Naproxen as an alternative to aspirin for the treatment of arthritis of rheumatic fever: a randomized trial, J. Pediatr. 143 (2003) 399–401.

117. United Kingdom and United States Joint Report, The treatment of acute rheumatic fever in children: a cooperative clinical trial of ACTH, cortisone and aspirin, Circulation 11 (1955) 343–371.

118. United Kingdom and United States Joint Report, The evolution of rheumatic heart disease in children: five year report of a cooperative clinical trial of ACTH, cortisone and aspirin, Circulation 22 (1960) 503–515.

119. United Kingdom and United States Joint Report, The natural history of rheumatic fever and rheumatic heart disease. Ten-year report of a cooperative clinical trial of ACTH, cortisone, and aspirin, Circulation 32 (1965) 457–476.

121. F.E. Figueroa, M.S. Fernandez, P. Valdes, et al., Prospective comparison of clinical and echocardiographic diagnosis of rheumatic carditis: long term follow up of patients with subclinical disease, Heart 85 (2001) 407–410.

122. M.A. Gerber, R.S. Baltimore, C.B. Eaton, et al., Prevention of rheumatic fever and diagnosis and treatment of acute streptococcal pharyngitis: a scientific statement from the American Heart Association Rheumatic Fever, Endocarditis, and Kawasaki Disease Committee of the Council on Cardiovascular Disease in the Young, the Interdisciplinary Council on Functional Genomics and Transitional Biology, and the Interdisciplinary Council on Quality of Care and Outcomes Research, Circulation 119 (2009) 1541–1551.

124. Committee on Infectious Diseases American Academy of Pediatrics, Red Book 2006 Report of the Committee on Infectious Diseases, ed 27, AAP, Elk Grove Village, IL, 2006.

125. D.G. Tompkins, B. Boxerbaum, J. Liebman, Long-term prognosis of rheumatic fever patients receiving regular intramuscular benzathine penicillin, Circulation 45 (1972) 543–551.

135. E.M. Ayoub, H.A. Majeed, Poststreptococcal reactive arthritis, Curr. Opin. Rheumatol. 12 (2000) 306–310.

137. E. Tutar, S. Atalay, E. Yilmaz, et al., Poststreptococcal reactive arthritis in children: is it really a different entity from rheumatic fever? Rheumatol. Int. 22 (2002) 80–83.

138. E.M. Ayoub, S. Ahmed, Update on complications of group A streptococcal infections, Curr. Probl. Pediatr. 27 (1997) 90–101.

141. A. Iglesias-Gamarra, E.A. Mendez, M.L. Cuellar, et al., Poststreptococcal reactive arthritis in adults: long-term follow-up, Am. J. Med. Sci. 321 (2001) 173–177.

Entire reference list is available online at www.expertconsult.com.

Chapter 41

MUSCULOSKELETAL MANIFESTATIONS OF SYSTEMIC DISEASE

James T. Cassidy and Ross E. Petty

Many nonrheumatic systemic disorders cause musculoskeletal signs or symptoms, most commonly arthralgia, arthritis, myalgia or bone pain. Sometimes these are trivial; occasionally, they are the presentations of the underlying disease. This chapter outlines some systemic disorders that may present in the guise of rheumatic disease. It is not our intent to describe comprehensively the clinical and laboratory manifestations or management of such disorders, which can be found in standard textbooks dealing with the specific diseases.

DISORDERS RELATED TO NUTRITION

A number of disorders in which there is a nutritional deficiency or excess result in signs or symptoms suggesting a rheumatic disease.[1]

Rickets

Rickets a term introduced into the English literature around 1650, includes several diseases associated with defective ossification of bone matrix (Table 41–1).[2] The affected child presents with joint pain and tenderness over the bones. Bowing of the long bones and splaying of the rib cage are characteristic features. Proximal muscle weakness, particularly of the lower extremities, is occasionally prominent. Defective bone growth results from suppression of calcification and maturation of epiphyseal cartilage. The result is a wide, frayed, irregular zone of uncalcified osteoid at the epiphyseal line—the rachitic metaphysis (Fig. 41–1).

Most cases of rickets worldwide result from exclusion from the sun for social or cultural reasons or from insufficient dietary intake of vitamin D.[3,4] Vitamin D–deficiency rickets is seldom encountered in developed countries but may occur in infantile and adolescent forms in the rest of the world.[1,5] It may also develop in the presence of sufficient dietary vitamin, when there is impaired absorption because of celiac disease, inflammatory bowel disease, scleroderma, or liver disease. It can result from deficiency of the active form of vitamin D (1,25-dihydroxyvitamin D_3), from a deficiency of phosphate, or rarely, from a lack of calcium. Some types (i.e., hypophosphatemic rickets and rickets associated with hypophosphatasia) are associated with defective mineralization and are classified as osteochondrodysplasias, as discussed in Chapter 50. Disorders such as cystinosis that result in renal tubular acidosis may present as rickets with pain in the joints and metaphyseal enlargement (Fig. 41–2). Administration of anticonvulsant medications in children deprived of sunlight may also be a cause.

The normal source of vitamin D_3 in humans is the skin in which ultraviolet rays of sunlight convert 7-dehydrocholesterol into the vitamin prohormone.[6] This compound is subsequently transformed to the 25-hydroxy form in the liver and then to active 1,25-dihydroxyvitamin in the kidney (Fig. 41–3). A deficiency of 1,25-dihydroxyvitamin D_3 may result from a nutritional deficiency, from hepatic failure to convert vitamin D to 25-hydroxyvitamin D, or from failure of the kidney to convert 25-hydroxyvitamin D to 1,25-dihydroxyvitamin D_3.

Hypophosphatemic vitamin D–resistant rickets, when expressed in infancy, leads to short stature, bowing of

Table 41–1

Causes of Rickets

Type	Cause or Biochemical Abnormality
Vitamin D deficiency	Exclusion from light or insufficient dietary vitamin D
Calcium deficiency	Impaired calcium absorption in celiac disease, inflammatory bowel disease, scleroderma, or liver disease
Vitamin D resistance	Impaired parathormone-dependent proximal renal tubular reabsorption of phosphate
Vitamin D dependence	
Type 1	Defect in renal 1-α-hydroxylase
Type 2	End-organ unresponsiveness to 1, 25-dihydroxyvitamin D_3
Hypophosphatasia	Decreased serum alkaline phosphatase

the legs, and ectopic calcification.[2,7] This disorder is inherited as an X-linked recessive or autosomal dominant trait, although sporadic cases occur. The basic defect is impaired parathormone-dependent proximal renal tubular reabsorption of phosphate. A low serum phosphate concentration with a normal calcium level is characteristic.

Type I vitamin D–dependent rickets is an autosomal recessive defect in renal 1-α–hydroxylase that results in failure of hydroxylation of 25-hydroxyvitamin D to 1,25-dihydroxyvitamin D_3. The onset of typical features of rickets occurs before the age of 2 years. Type II vitamin D–dependent rickets is rare and characterized by defective intracellular interaction between 1,25-dihydroxyvitamin D_3 and its receptor. Symptoms of rickets begin in early infancy. Alopecia and absence of eyelashes occur frequently in this disorder.[8]

Hypophosphatasia, a rare autosomal recessive disorder caused by a mutation in the gene for tissue-nonspecific alkaline phosphatase (TNSALP),[9] has onset in infancy as severe rickets and fractures.[2,9] Band keratopathy, proptosis and papilledema develop. There may be early loss of teeth. Chondrocalcinosis and pseudogout may be associated features. There is a marked depression in the concentration of serum alkaline phosphatase. Treatment with nonsteroidal anti-inflammatory drugs may lead to

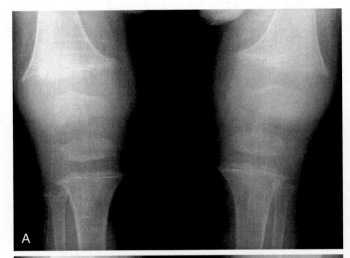

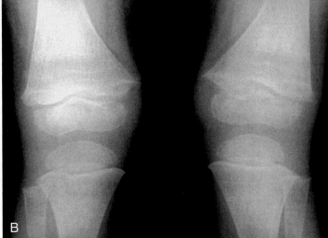

FIGURE 41–1 Vitamin D–deficient rickets in a toddler. *A*, Radiographs of knees demonstrate rachitic metaphyseal changes, indistinct cortices, and poorly defined trabeculation. The zone of provisional calcification is almost absent, the axial height of the epiphyseal plate is markedly increased, and cupping is evident. *B*, X-ray films taken 6 months later demonstrate progressive healing with replacement of vitamin D.

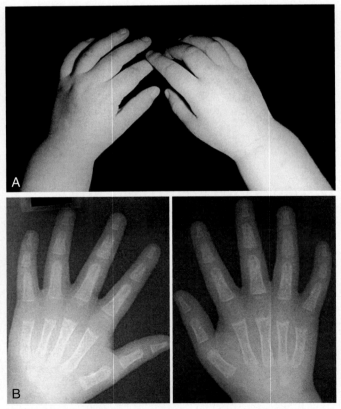

FIGURE 41–2 Cystinosis. An 18-month-old girl presented with joint pain primarily involving the large joints and profound muscle weakness due to cystinosis. *A*, Hands demonstrate swelling predominantly in the metaphyseal area of the radius and ulna, but not in the wrist joint proper. *B*, Radiographs document metaphyseal resorption that is typical of rickets.

symptomatic improvement.[10] Recent reports have noted an association between hypophosphatasia and chronic recurrent multifocal osteomyelitis (chronic non-bacterial osteomyelitis) in at least 4 children.[11,12]

Scurvy

Ascorbic acid (vitamin C) is required for the formation of normal collagen and chondroitin sulfate.[13] Vitamin C is neither synthesized nor stored in the body and in the malnourished child, a deficiency of dietary vitamin C may lead to scurvy with poor collagen synthesis and intradermal, gingival and subperiosteal hemorrhage.[14] Subperiosteal hemorrhage results in severe bone pain in arms and legs; the child, usually an infant, assumes the flexed posture of pseudoparalysis and is irritable when picked up. Hemarthroses may also occur. In severe cases "scorbutic beads," resulting from subluxation of the sternum at the costochondral junctions, may be visible on physical examination. Radiographs demonstrate subperiosteal new-bone apposition. Treatment with oral or parenteral vitamin C results in definite improvement within 2 weeks.[13-15]

Hypervitaminosis A

A large number of physiologic functions, organogenesis, and embryogenesis are affected by vitamin A and the derivative retinoids.[16] Excess intake of vitamin A or retinoids causes pain in the extremities, irritability, apathy, alopecia, and delayed growth.[17] Cortical hyperostosis (e.g., metatarsal bones, ulnas, spine) is a typical radiographic finding. Abnormal epiphyseal growth and periosteal new-bone apposition occur occasionally.

Disorders Related to Environmental Factors

Kashin-Beck Disease

An endemic progressive osteoarthropathy affecting millions of individuals occurs in certain regions of northwestern China, northeastern Russia, and North Korea. It is unassociated with systemic or visceral manifestations. It may result from mycotoxins in fungus-infected grain or from selenium or iodine deficiency.[18–26] There is depletion of aggregating proteoglycan (aggrecan),[27] which results in an epiphyseal dysplasia from a zonal necrosis of chondrocytes of the epiphyses and metaphyses.[28] These abnormalities increase in severity as long as the child lives in the endemic area and eats foods made with the contaminated grain. Excessive amounts of iron in the water and diet may contribute further to the polyarthritis. Experimental animals fed grain infected with Fusarium species develop a similar form of epiphyseal dysplasia.[21] A genetic influence has been proposed in humans[29] and in a murine model.[30] Differences in gene expression by osteoarthritis cartilage and cartilage from adults with Kashin-Beck disease imply different pathogenic mechanisms.[31]

Kashin-Beck disease causes symmetric polyarthritis and progressive enlargement and limitation of motion involving multiple joints (i.e.,elbows, interphalangeal joints, wrists, knees, and ankles).[32,33] In the school-age child, morning stiffness, aching, and muscle weakness are the initial symptoms. Joint effusions and laboratory indices of inflammation are absent early in the disease. The eventual dwarfing, epiphyseal deformity, and short digits resemble those encountered in the lysosomal storage diseases. Radiographic findings include irregular erosions of the small bones of the hands and feet. Treatment with selenium may be beneficial[34] although iodine supplementation may be more important.[35]

Mseleni Joint Disease

A chronic polyarthritis affects a large proportion of the Tsonga population of the Mseleni area of northern Zululand on the eastern seaboard of South Africa.[36–38] Onset of joint pain in childhood or adolescence is the first symptom of the disease. Restriction of movement and limitation of mobility develop at a variable rate. Mild stunting of growth is common, and a few patients develop severe dwarfing (Table 41–2). The life span is not shortened. Characteristic radiographic abnormalities include irregularity of the surface, density, and shape of the epiphyses that progresses to a secondary osteoarthritis; in the hips, which bear the brunt of the disease, protrusio acetabuli

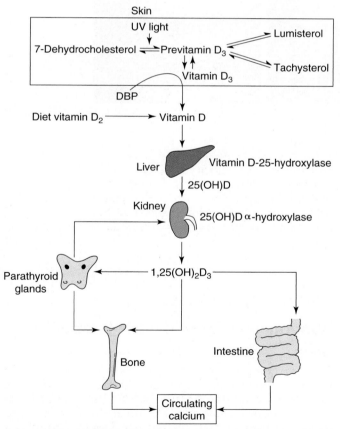

FIGURE 41–3 Metabolism of vitamin D. Previtamin D_3 is formed in the skin and isomerizes to vitamin D_3 or other biologically inert isomers. Vitamin D binding protein (DBP) has an affinity only for vitamin D_3, which is translocated to the circulation. Vitamin D is then hydroxylated in the liver and kidney to the active metabolite, $1,25(OH)_2D_3$. (From Bhalla AK: Osteoporosis and osteomalacia. *In* Maddison PJ, Isenberg DA, Woo P, Glass DN [eds]: Oxford Textbook of Rheumatology. Oxford, England, Oxford University Press, 1993, p 1005.)

Table 41–2

Mseleni Joint Disease and Kashin-Beck Disease

Characteristic	Mseleni Joint Disease	Kashin-Beck Disease
First noted	6 yr adult	6-10 yr
Inherited	Probably not	Probably not
Sex ratio	More females	More males
Stunting of growth	Slight to severe	Moderate
Posture	Lumbar lordosis, genu valgum	Lumbar lordosis, neck extended, knees flexed
Precocious osteoarthritis	Yes	Yes
Radiology	Fragmented epiphyses, flared metaphyses, brachymetacarpia, protrusio acetabuli, platyspondyly	Dysplastic interphalangeal, wrist, knee, ankle joints intra-articular loose bodies

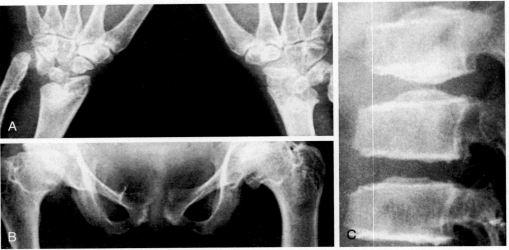

FIGURE 41–4 Mseleni joint disease. *A,* Irregularity and deformity of the distal ends of the ulnar and radius with distraction of the radius from the ulna. *B,* Marked deformation of the femoral heads. *C,* Platyspondyly. (Courtesy of Dr. G. Lockitch.)

occurs in females (Fig. 41–4). Short metacarpals, ulna, and radius, and a deformity of the distal end of the ulna, are also present. The diagnosis is usually obvious in the geographic and racial context, but the clinical presentation may suggest cretinism, brucellosis, hemochromatosis, alkaptonuria, and Legg-Calvé-Perthes disease at different stages of its development. Hips, knees, and ankles are the predominant sites of involvement in 66% of the women, 25% of the men, 7% of the girls, and 4% of the boys. Hands, wrists, shoulders, and elbows are less commonly affected. Neither a genetic nor an environmental cause has been identified. Handigodu, an idiopathic familial arthropathy found in a small area of southern India, closely resembles Mseleni Joint disease both clinically and radiographically.[38]

Fluorosis

Fluorosis is endemic in certain areas of the world, particularly Asia and Africa, and results in chronic rheumatic symptoms in children.[39] High levels of fluoride may occur naturally in the water supply or may result from pollution. Radiologically identified skeletal fluorosis was reported in 8% of children living in households with indoor coal-burning stoves in southern China.[40] Dental fluorosis is

an early sign of toxicity.[41] Knee pain is often an early symptom, followed by limb, hand, or spinal abnormalities that suggest a chronic inflammatory arthropathy. Radiographs demonstrate increased bone density and later show calcification of the spinal ligaments, intervertebral disks, and entheses.[42] Cord compression can result from narrowing of the spinal canal.

METABOLIC DISEASES

Abnormalities of Uric Acid Metabolism

Gout

The term gout refers to a group of disorders characterized by hyperuricemia and deposition of monosodium urate monohydrate crystals in tissues.[43-45] Its major clinical manifestations include an acute monarthritis, most commonly in the first metatarsophalangeal joint; chronic erosive arthritis associated with subcutaneous periarticular deposits of urate (tophi); and nephrolithiasis, often leading to chronic renal failure.

Serum urate levels increase normally at puberty, particularly in males, from approximately 3.5 mg/dL (0.21 mmol/L) in childhood to an upper limit of 7 mg/dL

Table 41–3
Causes of Hyperuricemia and Gout

Increased Uric Acid Production
Primary
    Lesch-Nyhan syndrome
    Becker's syndrome (phosphoribosyl pyrophosphate synthetase superactivity)
Secondary
    Glycogenosis type I (glucose-6-phosphate dehydrogenase deficiency)
    Myeloproliferative disorders
    Lymphoproliferative disorders
    Severe psoriasis
    Gaucher's disease
    Cytotoxic drugs
    Hypoxia
    Chronic hemolysis
    Secondary polycythemia

Decreased Uric Acid Excretion
Reduced glomerular filtration rate
Reduced fractional urate excretion
    Down syndrome
    Lead nephropathy
    Analgesic nephropathy
    Amyloidosis
    Sickle cell anemia
    Sarcoidosis
    Hypothyroidism
    Hyperparathyroidism
Increased levels of organic acids
    Type I glycogen storage disease
    Maple syrup urine disease
Drugs
    Diuretics
    Salicylates (low dose)
    Levodopa

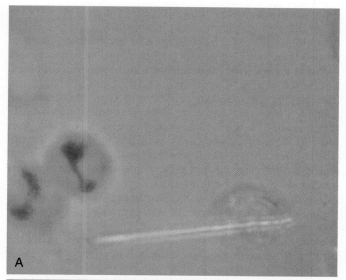

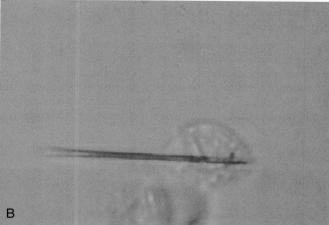

FIGURE 41-5 Urate crystals visualized with a polarizing microscope. A bright needle-shaped crystal of sodium urate monohydrate (A) shows negative birefringence (B) when viewed with a compensated polarized light microscope.

(0.42 mmol/L) in adult males, and 6 mg/dL (0.36 mmol/L) in adult females. Above these concentrations, the serum becomes saturated with urate.

Gout may result from increased production or decreased excretion of uric acid (Table 41–3). Diagnosis is confirmed by demonstration with compensated polarized light microscopy of negatively birefringent, needle-shaped monosodium urate crystals in synovial fluid (Fig. 41-5). Treatment of the acute attack with nonsteroidal anti-inflammatory drugs (NSAIDs) such as indomethacin, or with colchicine, is usually effective. After the acute episode has subsided, allopurinol is the drug of choice for prevention of recurrences.[46]

Gouty arthropathy is rare in children. Treadwell identified 66 patients younger than 20 years who were reported between 1769 and 1960 and added two additional cases.[47] In many early publications, the exact diagnosis is in doubt. The onset of gouty arthritis in a 14-year-old boy as a result of chronic compensated hemolysis of unknown cause has been described.[48] Yarom and colleagues[49] reported two children with marked hyperuricemia, mild renal failure, and acute, episodic, painful swelling of one

joint, often the first metatarsophalangeal joint, knee, ankle, elbow, or a proximal interphalangeal joint of the hand. The authors have seen two unrelated boys with gout presenting as polyarthritis. Gout has also been reported in children with glycogen storage disease,[50,51] malignancy,[52] and renal failure.[53-55] Typical radiographic changes in a teen-age boy are shown in Fig 41-6.

An exceptionally large group of children and youth with juvenile gout has been reported from Taiwan.[56] Juvenile gout accounted for 543 patients, 1.9% of all patients with the disease, and occurred in children as young as 8 years of age; 97% were male. Although greater than one-half of the patients had a paternal history of gout, there is as yet no genetic explanation for this disease or for the uniquely high prevalence of gout in this age group in Taiwan.

Lesch-Nyhan Syndrome

The Lesch-Nyhan syndrome, first described in 1967 as an X-linked recessive disorder of uric acid metabolism and central nervous system dysfunction, results from a deficiency of the enzyme hypoxanthine-guanine phosphoribosyltransferase (HPRT) (Table 41–4).[57-60] There is a range of clinical phenotypes, the most severe of which is characterized by the childhood onset of choreoathetosis, spasticity, mental retardation, severe growth retardation, self-mutilation, hyperuricemia with increased uric acid synthesis, and uric acid crystalluria. Severity of the disorder is determined by the degree of HPRT deficiency resulting from unique mutations in each family.[60] With rare exceptions,[61,62] affected boys do not develop acute gouty arthritis, at least not until the adolescent or adult years. Treatment with allopurinol effectively prevents the rheumatic complaints but does not alter the central nervous system disease, for which there is no effective therapy. An incomplete hereditary deficiency of the enzyme *(Kelley-Seegmiller syndrome)* may occur in adolescent or adult males as severe gouty arthritis with renal calculi, but it lacks the dramatic neurologic and mutilating characteristics of the complete enzyme deficiency.

Phosphoribosyl Pyrophosphate Synthetase Superactivity

An X-linked mutation resulting in excessive activity of phosphoribosyl pyrophosphate synthetase (PPRPS), the enzyme that converts ribose-5-phosphate to PP-ribose-phosphate, results in increased purine production and gout in children and young adults, sometimes with neurologic deficits and sensorineural deafness.[63,64] Allopurinol effectively controls this disorder.

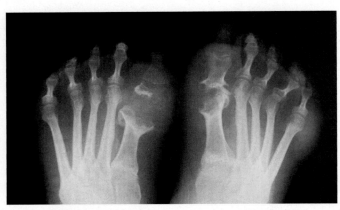

FIGURE 41-6 Radiograph of the fore-feet of an adolescent boy with gout. Note destructive changes in the first metatarsophalangeal joints. Soft tissue swellings adjacent to these joints and the right fifth metatarsophalangeal joint are sites of tophi. (Photograph courtesy of Dr Jorge Jaimes).

Table 41–4	
Lesch-Nyhan Syndrome	
Clinical characteristics	Progressive development of choreo-athetosis, spasticity, and mental retardation with self-mutilation
Genetics	X-linked recessive
Biochemical defect	Deficiency of hypoxanthine-guanine phosphoribosyltransferase
Laboratory findings	Hyperuricemia and uric acid crystalluria

Glucose-6-Phosphatase Deficiency

Glycogen storage disease type I (von Gierke's disease) may be associated with the onset of gouty arthritis[65,66] or tendinitis[51] in childhood. Children with this disorder are stunted and have marked hepatosplenomegaly, progressive mental retardation, abnormalities of platelet function, and hypoglycemia. Hyperuricemia results from increased catabolism of adenosine triphosphate and decreased urate excretion. Other types of glycogen storage disease and other metabolic disorders may have musculoskeletal manifestations, especially myopathy.[67-69]

Calcium Pyrophosphate Deposition Disease

Crystals of calcium pyrophosphate dihydrate (CPPD) in synovial fluid and joint structures are associated with a chronic inflammatory and degenerative joint disease *(pseudogout)*.[70] The wrists, knees, shoulders, and ankles are most commonly affected. Synovial fluid CPPD crystals are positively birefringent when viewed through a compensated polarized light microscope and are shorter than urate crystals.

Chondrocalcinosis, the deposition of CPPD crystals in hyaline cartilage and fibrocartilage, is primarily a disorder of the adult. Radiographs demonstrate linear calcifications in the menisci of the knee and in other cartilaginous structures such as the triangular cartilage of the wrist.[71] In descriptions of familial chondrocalcinosis, however, there have been rare reports of adolescents in whom the disorder presented as an acute, self-limited polyarthritis, often precipitated by exercise or trauma.[72] The characteristics of the clinical disease have varied, however, depending on the kindred, age at onset, severity, and the presence of an associated osteoarthritis or chondrodysplasia.

Ochronosis

Ochronosis (alkaptonuria) is an autosomal recessive defect in homogentisic acid oxidase resulting in the accumulation of homogentisic acid in tissues, and pigmentation of cartilage (e.g., ears, sclerae, heart valves), calcification and ossification of the intervertebral disks, accelerated osteoporosis and osteoarthritis, and vascular disease.[73,74] Black urine or staining of the diapers is often the sign that prompts referral of the child with this metabolic defect. Arthritis has not been reported in children.

Hyperlipoproteinemia

Defects in lipoprotein metabolism are associated with a high risk of premature atherosclerosis, coronary artery disease, and musculoskeletal abnormalities.[75] Articular and tendinous swelling accompany essential familial hypercholesterolemia and hypertriglyceridemia; both of these conditions are autosomal dominant traits.[75-77] In *type II hyperlipoproteinemia (familial hypercholesterolemia)*, the Achilles, patellar, and extensor tendons of the hands are the principal locations of xanthomata.[78,79] These lesions are associated with recurrent episodes of an acute migratory polyarthritis. In type IV hyperlipoproteinemia *(hypertri-glyceridemia)*, the hands, knees, and ankles are primarily affected by mild chronic or migratory oligoarthritis.[80] The onset is often acute, and fever and an elevated white blood cell count may occur. The arthritis is self-limited but may be misdiagnosed as acute rheumatic fever, especially if the tendon xanthomata are mistaken for nodules.

Xanthomata of the tendons also occur in *sitosterolemia*, a syndrome resulting from accumulation of sterols derived from vegetable sources. The xanthomata initially appear in childhood and usually involve the extensor tendons of the hands and, later, the patellar, Achilles, and plantar tendons. Plasma sterol levels are elevated, and cholesterol levels may be increased.[81,82]

SPHINGOLIPIDOSES

In the sphingolipidoses, lipid accumulates in cells as a result of specific enzyme deficiencies.[83] Of the many different sphingolipidoses, three have prominent musculoskeletal signs and symptoms (Table 41–5). *Farber's lipogranulomatosis* is an autosomal recessive disorder marked in the neonatal period by a hoarse cry and irritability.[84,85] Painful red masses develop along tendon sheaths and over pressure points, as well as around the joints, especially the wrists, small joints of the hands and feet, elbows, knees, and ankles.[86] Nodules have also been described in conjunctivae, ears, and nares. Epiglottal and laryngeal swelling results in repeated pulmonary infections, leading to death by about 2 years of age. Delayed motor development and mental retardation are prominent. The basic process underlying this disease is the cytoplasmic accumulation of a glycolipid ceramide in fibroblasts, histiocytes, macrophages, and neurons, attributable to a deficiency of lysosomal acid ceramidase. The central nervous system, retina, respiratory tract, heart, liver, spleen, lymph nodes, synovium, and bone are all affected to various degrees. Radiographic changes in the skeleton consist of osteoporosis, juxta-articular erosions, and disruption of the normal trabecular pattern.

In *Gaucher's disease*, an autosomal recessive disorder, glucocerebroside accumulates in the reticuloendothelial cells of the bone marrow, spleen, liver, lymph nodes, and viscera as a result of deficiency of glucocerebrosidase. Hepatosplenomegaly and pathologic fractures of the femur or vertebrae suggest the diagnosis. Premature

osteoarthritis of weight-bearing joints is an important feature of the juvenile form of this disease.[86,87] One of the diagnostic hallmarks of Gaucher's disease is widening of the distal femur. Characteristic areas of rarefaction and osteoporosis are visible in the peripheral and axial skeleton, including the skull.

Fabry's disease is characterized by the progressive accumulation of birefringent deposits of triglycosylceramide in the endothelial, perithelial, and smooth muscle cells of blood vessels, and in ganglion and perineural cells of the autonomic nervous system.[2] The disease results from an X-linked recessive deficiency of ceramide trihexosidase. Affected boys in late childhood or adolescence have recurrent attacks of fever and severe arthritis and a characteristic burning, tingling pain in the extremities that is aggravated by hot weather or exercise. The fingers, elbows, and knees may become swollen, and a characteristic deformity limiting extension of the fingers develops.[88] Other bones may also be involved, and secondary effects of osteonecrosis become increasingly important, especially in weight-bearing joints such as the hips. A typical rash consisting of purple papules, *angiokeratoma corporis diffusum universale*, accompanies the other features of Fabry's disease. Enzyme activity may be assayed in skin fibroblasts and leukocytes. Female heterozygotes may develop milder forms of this disorder. Renal, cardiac, or cerebral disease leads to death in the mid-adult years in untreated patients. Recombinant α-galactosidase enzyme replacement therapy and renal allograft transplantation, if renal failure has developed, correct the metabolic defect.[89]

A number of other rare disorders present in a manner similar to that of the diseases discussed earlier, but they have not been clearly identified as involving a lysosomal degradative enzyme. One such entity, *multicentric reticulohistiocytosis*, or lipoid dermatoarthritis, is a rare, mutilating, symmetric polyarthritis.[90,91] An important diagnostic clue is the presence of clear histiocytic cutaneous nodules (Fig. 41–7). Stiffness and contractures appear

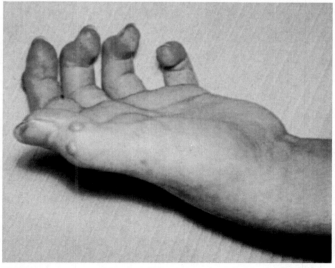

FIGURE 41–7   Multicentric reticulohistiocytosis in a 14-year-old boy. There is marked swelling and subluxation of the wrist and swelling of the distal interphalangeal joints of the fingers and the interphalangeal joint of the thumb. Cutaneous nodules are visible over the thumb.

Table 41-5		
Sphingolipidoses		
Disorder	**Genetics**	**Musculoskeletal Abnormalities**
Farber's disease	AR	Painful red masses along tendons at wrists, elbows, knees, and ankles
Gaucher's disease	AR	Osteoporosis with pathologic fractures of femur and vertebrae
Fabry's disease	XR	Recurrent fever and severe distal arthritis with burning pain; rash

AR, autosomal recessive; XR, X-linked recessive.

early, and the joints (with a predilection for the interphalangeal and metacarpophalangeal joints) are swollen and tender. Biopsy of the lesions of the skin, mucous membranes, or synovium demonstrates lipid-laden histiocytes and foamy multinucleated giant cells. Most described cases have been in adults and are not familial.

HEMATOLOGIC DISORDERS

Hemoglobinopathies

Homozygous *sickle cell disease*[92] and *β-thalassemia*[93-95] cause severe musculoskeletal manifestations as a result of skeletal changes that accompany hematopoietic expansion of the bone marrow and repeated episodes of avascular necrosis.[96] Sickle cell anemia is an autosomal dominant trait and occurs almost exclusively in black children. Acute arthritis and long bone pain may be severe and incapacitating during sickle cell crises. In the infant, dactylitis and periostitis of the small bones of the hands may cause painful swollen extremities and the hand-foot syndrome.[97] Each acute episode lasts 1 to 3 weeks and is characterized by diffuse, symmetric, painful swelling of the hands or feet. In a 1997 review, dactylitis was reported to occur before 1 year of age in 41 (10%) of 392 children and was a predictor of severe disease in later life.[98] Osteonecrosis may occur in any bone and leads to marked abnormalities of growth and deformity. The hip is particularly vulnerable and is the usual site of the septic arthritis caused by Salmonella or other species to which these children are unduly susceptible. Differentiation of sickle cell bone infarction from osteomyelitis is sometimes difficult and is aided by scintigraphy, ultrasonography, and magnetic resonance imaging.[99]

The thalassemias are a group of heterogeneous syndromes of inherited hypochromic anemias of differing severity. Thalassemia minor is characterized by anemia, hepatosplenomegaly, and recurrent brief episodes of joint pain, swelling, and effusion, especially in the ankles.[100] Bone pain was frequently reported in patients with β thalassemia.[101] Deferiprone, an iron chelating agent used to treat patients with thalassemia has been associated with arthritis.[102]

Hemophilia

Recurrent intra-articular hemorrhage is a hallmark of classic hemophilia A (i.e. factor VIII deficiency) and is one of the most important causes of morbidity in this X-linked recessive coagulopathy.[103] The frequency of episodes of hemarthrosis is related to the plasma concentration of factor VIII; hemarthroses almost invariably occur in children with levels below 5% of normal.[104] A similar association is found in *von Willebrand's disease*.[105] The presence of inhibitors is associated with greater risk for hemarthroses.[106] Iron deposition within the synovium is central to the pathogenesis of the proliferative synovitis that characterizes hemophilic arthropathy.[107]

Hemarthrosis can occur even before the child starts walking, and the frequency of episodes increases during the early childhood years. The joints most commonly affected are the knees, elbows, and ankles.[108] Bleeding into the small joints of the hands, feet, or spine is unusual. Hemorrhage into soft tissues, especially muscle, may mimic hemarthrosis.[109,110] Acute hemarthrosis is signaled by onset over a few minutes to an hour of increasing pain, a feeling of fullness in the joints, and loss of range of motion. The joint is warm and distended. Resorption of the hemarthrosis takes place over several days with effective factor VIII replacement. Intra-articular bleeds, however, tend to be recurrent, and lead to secondary proliferation of synovium with hemosiderosis that produces a diffuse increase in the density of the soft tissues on radiographs and characteristic MRI findings that are highly suggestive of the diagnosis. These debilitating changes may develop in as little as 1 to 2 years. Radiographic abnormalities range from changes in the density of soft tissues to epiphyseal overgrowth, widening of the femoral intercondylar notch, osteoporosis, subchondral cyst formation and bony sclerosis, squaring of the patella, narrowing of the joint space, and eventually, osteoarthritis (Fig. 41–8).[111,112] Intensive physical therapy with strengthening of the muscles around affected joints helps to prevent hemarthroses.[113] Management of the acute bleed consists of factor VIII replacement,[108,114] application of ice to the affected joint, splinting, and rest. Agents that affect coagulation (e.g., NSAIDs) should be avoided. Joint aspiration has only a limited therapeutic role and must be preceded by factor VIII administration.[111] Arthrocentesis accompanied by intra-articular glucocorticoid is sometimes dramatically effective in reducing the severity and frequency of hemarthroses,[115] as is prophylactic administration of factor VIII. Surgical synovectomy with or without a sclerosing agent (radioactive or chemical) has a place in treating the older child with early destructive changes.[116,117]

DISORDERS OF ENDOCRINE AND EXOCRINE GLANDS

Diabetes Mellitus

With the exception of diabetes mellitus, musculoskeletal disease is rarely associated with endocrinopathies in childhood. Grgic and others[118] described a syndrome of juvenile-onset insulin-dependent diabetes mellitus, short stature, and contractures of the finger joints: *diabetic cheiroarthropathy* or stiff-hand syndrome (Fig. 41–9). In a survey of 229 diabetics aged 7 to 18 years, 29% had flexion contractures of one or more joints of the fingers, most often the proximal interphalangeal joints of the fifth or fourth fingers.[118] In a few children, flexion contractures occurred in other joints (e.g., wrists, elbows, ankles, toes, knees), and spinal motion was decreased. In most instances, the child was unaware of any joint limitations and had no pain. Functional disability was uncommon. The prevalence of joint contractures increased from less than 10% in those with diabetes for less than 1 year to close to 50% in children with disease for longer than 9 years.[118] However, there did not appear to be a correlation with the severity of the diabetes or adequacy of its control. Tightening of the skin over the distal phalanges mimicked the acrosclerosis of scleroderma.[119] The precise

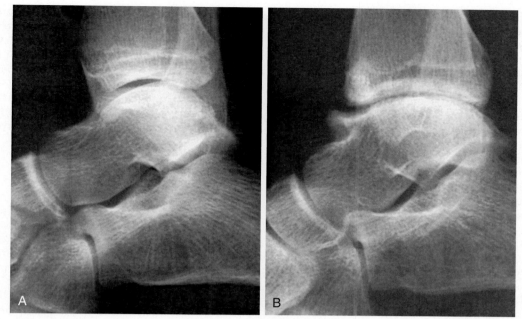

FIGURE 41-8   Hemophilic arthropathy. *A*, Normal ankle. *B*, Recurrent hemarthroses resulted in arthritis characterized by a loss of joint space and development of a talar osteophyte. (Courtesy of Dr. R. Cairns.)

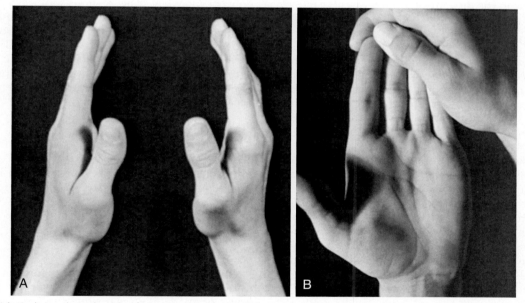

FIGURE 41-9   Diabetic cheiroarthropathy with soft tissue contractures that limit extension of the metacarpophalangeal and interphalangeal joints of the hands *(A)* and flexor tendon contractures in the palm *(B)*. In this 16-year-old boy, multiple flexion contractures without evidence of intra-articular or muscle inflammation had failed to respond to physical therapy over a 2-year period. A diagnosis of insulin-dependent diabetes mellitus was made, and 2 months after institution of insulin therapy, flexion contractures were considerably improved.

relation of diabetes mellitus to contractures is unknown. Studies have demonstrated increased glucosylation of collagen in this syndrome.[119] Perhaps increased cross-linking of collagen leads to the contractures. Magnetic resonance imaging demonstrates thickening of the tendon sheaths.[120] NSAIDs have no beneficial effect on this disorder. The frequency of inflammatory arthritis may be increased in children with diabetes mellitus.[121]

Occasionally, hemochromatosis occurs with diabetes mellitus and leads to an arthropathy that results in a characteristic bony enlargement of the second and third metacarpophalangeal joints; other joints are affected less commonly.[122] This disorder has not been documented in childhood. *Juvenile hemochromatosis*, unrelated to diabetes, is a rare autosomal recessive disorder (1q21) that results in iron overload lending to hypogonadism and cardiomyopathy.[123,124] *Diabetic osteopathy* is characterized by pain and osteoporosis of the distal metatarsal heads that may progress to erosion or even complete resorption of the ends of the bones. The cause of this phenomenon is unknown, and the disorder has not been recorded in childhood. These and other musculoskeletal complications of diabetes mellitus have been recently reviewed.[125]

Pancreatitis with Arthritis

Acute or chronic pancreatitis or pseudocyst formation from trauma to the pancreas may be accompanied by disseminated fat necrosis, leading to the development of subcutaneous nodules and osteolytic lesions resembling multicentric osteomyelitis or arthritis.[126-130] The nodules are tender, erythematous, widely disseminated, and similar to those of erythema nodosum. They are often accompanied by systemic illness and fever. Joint pains and effusions may develop 2 to 3 weeks later. The arthropathy is usually self-limited and remits spontaneously. Soft tissue swelling is evident on radiographs, which show multiple sites of periosteal new-bone apposition and diaphyseal lytic lesions. Because the bony lesions are delayed in appearance by a few months, the initiating abdominal trauma may have been forgotten. Diagnosis is confirmed during the acute illness by elevation of the serum lipase and amylase concentrations. A bone scan may demonstrate increased uptake of isotope in the metaphyses or diaphyses because of the infarctions that have resulted from the disseminated intravascular fat.

Disorders of other Endocrine Glands

Hyperparathyroidism is rare in children; in adults, it may be characterized by fever, abdominal pain, musculoskeletal pain, osteoporosis,[131] mental disturbances, and headaches. Elevation of serum parathormone levels confirms the diagnosis.[132] Pseudohypoparathyroidism and pseudopseudohypoparathyroidism are classified as forms of acromelic dysplasia.

Hyperthyroidism and hypothyroidism can be associated with diffuse musculoskeletal pain and muscle weakness, although these disorders and their complications appear to be rare in childhood. *Hashimoto's thyroiditis* can complicate systemic lupus erythematosus,[133] and autoimmune hyperthyroidism (i.e., Graves' disease) is occasionally associated with JRA. *Thyroid acropachy* is a rare form of hyperostosis of the phalanges, metacarpals, and metatarsals that is associated with hyperthyroidism, pretibial myxedema, exophthalmos, and clubbing.[134]

CYSTIC FIBROSIS

Musculoskeletal disease occurs in a small proportion of children with cystic fibrosis.[135,136] Cystic fibrosis associated arthropathy is estimated to occur in from 2 to 8.5% of patients with cystic fibrosis.[135,137] The cystic fibrosis associated arthropathy described by Newman and Ansell,[138] was an episodic arthritis lasting 1 – 10 days and recurring at intervals of weeks to months in 3 boys and 2 girls, aged 2 to 20 years. One or more joints were affected during each episode. A pruritic nodular rash occurred in all 5 children. Results of serologic studies for rheumatoid factors and antinuclear antibodies were negative, and radiographs demonstrated no abnormalities.

The cause and pathogenesis of this self-limited arthropathy are unknown, but it may be a reaction to chronic bacterial infection in the lung. Management usually requires non-steroidal anti-inflammatory drugs, but in patients in whom the arthritis becomes chronic, disease modifying agents may be indicated.[136]

Secondary hypertrophic osteoarthropathy occurs in approximately 5% of children with cystic fibrosis.[139,140] The occurrence rheumatoid factor–positive JIA[141] and sarcoidosis[142] has been reported.

CELIAC DISEASE

Musculoskeletal complications of celiac disease are quite common in adults. Lubrano et al[143] described arthritis in 26% of patients compared to 7.5% of controls, and noted that this complication was more common in patients on a regular diet, than in those on a gluten-free diet. Arthritis occurred in peripheral joints in 19 patients, in joints of the axial skeleton in 15, and in both in 18 patients. It is usually non-erosive and non-deforming. Stagi and colleagues[144] reported the incidence of IgA anti-tissue transglutaminase antibodies in 10 of 151 children (6.6%). Seven children had oligoarticular JIA, 3 had polyarticular JIA. The diagnosis of celiac disease was confirmed by intestinal biopsy. Neuhausen et al[145] noted an increased incidence of JIA in first degree relatives of patients with celiac disease. Alpigiani et al[146] also noted an increased prevalence of celiac disease in 108 children with JIA studied over a 13 year period. Improvement in joint disease following institution of a gluten-free diet has been described in at least two patients.[144,146]

HYPEROSTOSIS

Hyperostosis, the abnormal subperiosteal or endochondral deposition of bone, may be primary or secondary.

Primary Hyperostosis

Pachydermoperiostosis

Pachydermoperiostosis is a rare autosomal dominant disorder characterized by onset (usually in adolescent boys) of spade-like enlargement of the hands and feet, sometimes accompanied by pain along the distal long bones.[147-149] In addition to the cylindrical enlargement of the digits, forearms and lower legs, there may be minimal joint effusions, coarsening of the facial features, excessive oiliness of the skin, and occasionally gynecomastia, female hair distribution, striae, and acne. It is caused by a mutation in the gene encoding the major enzyme for the degradation of prostaglandins.[150]

Familial infantile cortical hyperostosis (Caffey disease)

This rare disorder presents before 4 months of age with fever, irritability, abnormal acute phase indices, and swelling, tenderness, erythema or altered contour of the mandible, shoulder girdles, and long bones.[151] A more severe, sometimes lethal form of the disease with pre-natal onset has been reported.[152] Bone involvement tends to be asymmetric. The calvarium is never affected. The ribs and clavicles are often involved by marked cortical thickening with altered bone shape. The cause is unknown, although the condition appears to be inflammatory and may be triggered by an infection. It usually has a self-limited course of weeks to months, after which it subsides without sequelae. Short-term treatment with glucocorticoids may be considered for the infant with severe disease and marked systemic symptoms. There appears to be a familial but non-genetic basis.

The *Goldbloom syndrome* is a form of idiopathic, periosteal new-bone formation associated with fever, constitutional symptoms, severe pain in the extremities, elevated serum immunoglobulin levels, and an increased erythrocyte sedimentation rate.[153,154] Radiographs demonstrate typical periosteal new-bone apposition along the long bones. The child may develop limited motion in contiguous joints and refuse to walk if the lower extremities are involved. The disorder runs a chronic course over several months; a spontaneous recovery is expected. NSAIDs are sometimes useful for symptomatic control. There is no known cause, but the disorder may follow an infectious disease or viral syndrome.

Secondary Hyperostosis

Hypertrophic osteoarthropathy (Secondary hyperostosis) is characterized by clubbing of the fingers and toes, painful subperiosteal apposition of new bone along the shafts of the long bones, and occasionally, arthritis. In children, it most commonly complicates suppurative lung disease, primary or secondary tumors of the lung, pleura, or mediastinum, and may occur in inflammatory bowel disease, or thyroid disease. Radiographs are characterized by a distinctive apposition of periosteal new-bone along the shafts of long bones, soft tissue swelling, and joint effusions. Bone scintigraphy demonstrates increased isotope uptake in the areas of new-bone formation. Asymptomatic, isolated clubbing can occur in children with cyanotic congenital heart disease. Familial clubbing can develop without associated systemic disease and is usually asymptomatic. Secondary hyperostosis is seen in several unrelated disorders (Table 41–6).

Table 41–6

Causes of Secondary Hypertrophic Osteoarthropathy

Malignant metastases to chest (lungs, pleura, mediastinum)
  Osteosarcoma
  Neuroblastoma
  Lymphoma
Chronic suppurative pulmonary disease
  Cystic fibrosis
Cyanotic congenital heart disease
Gastrointestinal disease
  Inflammatory bowel disease
  Biliary cirrhosis or ductal atresia
  Thyroid acropathy

REFERENCES

3. S.A. Abrams, Nutritional rickets: an old disease returns, Nutr. Rev. 60 (2002) 111–115.
4. B. Wharton, N. Bishop, Rickets, Lancet 362 (2003) 1389–1400.
12. M.P. Whyte, D. Wenkert, W.H. McAlister, et al., Chronic recurrent multifocal osteomyelitis mimicked in childhood hypophosphatasia, J. Bone Miner. Res. 24 (2009) 1493–1505.
13. O. Fain, Musculoskeletal manifestations of scurvy, Joint Bone Spine 72 (2005) 124–128.
16. S. Perrotta, B. Nobili, F. Rossi, et al., Vitamin A and infancy. Biochemical, functional, and clinical aspects, Vitam. Horm. 66 (2003) 457–591.
24. W.H. Zhang, J. Neve, J.P. Xu, et al., Selenium, iodine and fungal contamination in Yulin District (People's Republic of China) endemic for Kashin-Beck disease, Int. Orthop. 25 (2001) 188–190.
27. J. Cao, S. Li, Z. Shi, et al., Articular cartilage metabolism in patients with Kashin-Beck disease. An endemic osteoarthropathy in China, Osteoarthritis Cartilage 16 (2008) 680–688.
29. X.W. Shi, X. Guo, F.L. Ren, et al., The effect of short tandem repeat loci and low selenium levels on endemic osteoarthritis in China, J. Bone Joint Surg. Am. 92 (2010) 72–78.
31. C. Duan, X. Guo, X.-D. Zhang, et al., Comparative analysis of gene expression profiles between primary knee osteoarthritis and an osteoarthritis endemic to northwestern China, Kashin-Beck disease, Arthritis Rheum. 62 (2010) 771–780.
34. K. Zou, G. Liu, T. Wu, L. Du, Selenium for preventing Kashin-Beck osteoarthropathy in children – a meta-analysis, Osteoarthritis Cartilage 17 (2009) 144–1512.
35. R. Moreno-Reyes, F. Mathieu, M. Boelaert, Selenium and iodine supplements of rural Tibetan children affected by Kashin-Beck osteoarthropathy, Am. J. Clin. Nutr. 78 (2003) 137–144.
38. S.S. Agarwal, S.R. Phadke, V. Fredlund, et al., Mseleni and Handigodu familial osteoarthropathies: syndrome identity? Am. J. Med. Genet. 72 (1997) 435–439.
40. X. Qin, S. Wang, M. Yu, et al., Child skeletal fluorosis from indoor burning of coal in southwestern China, J. Environ. Pub. Health 2009. Article ID 969764.
46. N. Schlesinger, management of acute and chronic gouty arthritis, Drugs 64 (2004) 2399–2416.
50. C.B. Hoyningen-Huene, Gout and glycogen storage disease in preadolescent brothers, Arch. Intern. Med. 118 (1966) 471–477.
51. C. Carves, A. Duquenoy, F. Toutain, et al., Gouty tendinitis revealing glycogen storage disease type Ia in two adolescents, Joint Bone Spine 70 (2003) 149–153.
57. M. Lesch, W.L. Nyhan, A familial disorder of uric acid metabolism and central nervous system function, Am. J. Med. 36 (1964) 561–570.
61. A. Zamora, R.O. Escarcega, R. Vazquez, et al., HPRT deficiency in a two-month-old child presenting acute renal failure and gout with a new deletion of two bases in exon 3 of the HPRT gene, Arch. Med. Res. 38 (2007) 460–462.
62. H.K. Ea, T. Bardin, H.A. Jinnah, et al., Severe gouty arthritis and mild neurologic symptoms due to F199C, a newly identified variant of the hypoxanthine guanine phosphoribosyltransferase, Arthritis Rheum. 60 (2009) 2201–2204.
63. M.A. Becker, J.G. Puig, F.A. Mateos, et al., Inherited superactivity of phosphoribosylpyrophosphate synthetase: association of uric acid overproduction and sensorineural deafness, Am. J. Med. 85 (1988) 383–390.
67. W. Zhang, C. Bao, Y. Gu, S. Ye, Glycogen storage disease manifested as gout and myopathy: three case reports and review of the literature, Clin. Rheumatol. 27 (2008) 671–674.
70. A.K. Rosenthal, Calcium crystal-associated arthritides, Curr. Opin. Rheumatol. 10 (1998) 273–277.
80. R.B. Buckingham, G.G. Bole, D.R. Bassett, Polyarthritis associated with type IV hyperlipoproteinemia, Arch. Intern. Med. 135 (1975) 286–290.
85. C. Sana, E. Larbi, A. Samir, et al., Farber disease in a newborn, Pediatr. Dermatol. 26 (2009) 44–46.
86. K.F. Lutsky, N.C. Tejwani, Orthopaedic manifestations of Gaucher disease 65 (2007) 37–42.
87. G.M. Pastores, Musculoskeletal complications encountered in the lysosomal storage disorders, Best Pract. Res. Clin. Rheumatol. 22 (2008) 937–947.

88. R. Cimaz, S. Guillaume, M.J. Hilz, et al., Awareness of Fabry Disease among rheumatologists- Current status and perspectives, Clin. Rheumatol. 2010 April 15. EPub.

91. M. Uhl, J. Gutfleisch, E. Rother, et al., Multicentric reticulohistiocytosis. A report of 3 cases and review of literature, Bildgebung 63 (1996) 126–129.

92. J. Fixler, L. Styles, Sickle cell disease, Pediatr. Clin. North Am. 49 (2002) 1193–1210. vi.

94. M.I. Arman, B. Butun, A. Doseyen, et al., Frequency and features of rheumatic findings in thalassaemia minor: a blind controlled study, Br. J. Rheumatol. 31 (1992) 197–199.

97. V.C. Ejindu, A.L. Hine, M. Mashayekhi, et al., Musculoskeletal manifestations of sickle cell disease, Radiographics 27 (2007) 1005–1021.

101. M.G. Vogiatzi, E.A. Macklin, E.B. Fung, et al., Bone disease in thalassemia: a frequent and still unresolved problem, J. Bone Min. Res. 24 (2009) 543–557.

104. W.D. Arnold, M.W. Hilgartner, Hemophilic arthropathy. Current concepts of pathogenesis and management, J. Bone Joint Surg. Am. 59 (1977) 287–305.

105. A. Ahlberg, J. Silwer, Arthropathy in von Willebrand's disease, Acta. Orthop. Scand. 41 (1970) 539–544.

106. W.K. Hoots, Arthropathy in inhibitor patients: differences in the joint status, Semin. Hematol. 45 (2008) S42–49.

107. W.K. Hoots, Pathogenesis of hemophilic arthropathy, Semin. Hematol. 43 (2006) S18–S22.

110. E.C. Rodriguez-Merchan, Management of musculoskeletal complications of hemophilia, Semin. Thromb. Hemost. 29 (2003) 87–96.

112. A. Jelbert, S. Vaidya, N. Fotiadis, Imaging and staging of hemophilic arthropathy, Clin. Radiol. 64 (2009) 1119–1128.

116. M.W. Hilgartner, Current treatment of hemophilic arthropathy, Curr. Opin. Pediatr. 14 (2002) 46–49.

118. A. Grgic, A.L. Rosenbloom, F.T. Weber, et al., Joint contracture—common manifestation of childhood diabetes mellitus, J. Pediatr. 88 (1976) 584–588.

119. B.A. Buckingham, J. Uitto, C. Sandborg, et al., Scleroderma-like syndrome and the non-enzymatic glucosylation of collagen in children with poorly controlled insulin dependent diabetes, Pediatr. Res. 15 (1981) 626.

123. M. De Gobbi, A. Roetto, A. Piperno, et al., Natural history of juvenile haemochromatosis, Br. J. Haematol. 117 (2002) 973–979.

124. C. Camaschella, A. Roetto, M. De Gobbi, Juvenile hemochromatosis, Semin. Hematol. 39 (2002) 242–248.

125. A. Del Rosso, M. Cerenic, F. De Giorgio, et al., Rheumatological manifestations in diabetes mellitus, Curr. Diabet. Rev. 2 (2006) 455–466.

126. P.G. Shackelford, Osseous lesions and pancreatitis, Am. J. Dis. Child 131 (1977) 731–732.

130. J. Narvaez, M. Bianchi, P. Santo, et al., Pancreatitis, Panniculitis and Polyarthritis, Semin. Arthritis Rheum. 39 (2010) 417–423.

132. A.K. Bhalla, Musculoskeletal manifestations of primary hyperparathyroidism, Clin. Rheum. Dis. 12 (1986) 691–705.

133. B.A. Eberhard, R.M. Laxer, A.A. Eddy, et al., Presence of thyroid abnormalities in children with systemic lupus erythematosus, J. Pediatr. 119 (1991) 277–279.

134. R.A. Kinsella Jr., D.K. Back, Thyroid acropachy, Med. Clin. North Am. 52 (1968) 393–398.

135. E. Botton, A. Saraux, H. Laselve, et al., Musculoskeletal manifestations in cystic fibrosis, Joint Bone Spine 70 (2003) 327–335.

138. A.J. Newman, B.M. Ansell, Episodic arthritis in children with cystic fibrosis, J. Pediatr. 94 (1979) 594–596.

143. E. Lubrano, C. Ciacci, P.R.J. Ames, et al., The arthritis of celiac disease: prevalence and pattern in 200 adult patients, Br. J. Rheumatol. 35 (1996) 1314–1318.

144. S. Stagi, T. Giani, G. Simonini, F. Falcini, Thyroid function, autoimmune thyroiditis and coeliac disease in juvenile idiopathic arthritis, Rheumatology 44 (2005) 517–520.

145. S.I. Neuhausen, L. Steele, S. Ryan, et al., Co-occurrence of celiac disease and other autoimmune disease in celiacs and their first degree relatives, J. Autoimmunity 31 (2008) 160–165.

146. M.G. Alpigiani, R. Haupt, S. Parodi, et al., Coeliac disease in 108 patients with juvenile idiopathic arthritis: a thirteen- year follow-up study, Clin. Exp. Rheumatol. 26 (2008) 162.

147. M. Castori, L. Sinibaldi, R. MIngarelli, et al., Pachydermoperiostosis: an update, Clin. Genet. 68 (2005) 477–486.

150. S. Uppal, C.P. Diggle, I.M. Carr, et al., Mutations in 15 hydroxy prostaglandin dehydrogenase cause primary hypertrophic osteoarthropathy, Nature Genet. 40 (2008) 789–793.

151. A. Kamoun-Goldrat, M. le Merrer, Infantile cortical hyperostosis (Caffey Disease): a review, J. Oral Maxillofac. Surg. 66 (2008) 2145–2150.

153. R.B. Goldbloom, P.B. Stein, A. Eisen, et al., Idiopathic periosteal hyperostosis with dysproteinemia. A new clinical entity, N. Engl. J. Med. 28 (1966) 873–878.

Entire reference list is available online at www.expertconsult.com.

Chapter 42

IMMUNODEFICIENCIES AND THE RHEUMATIC DISEASES

Nico M. Wulffraat, Joris van Montfrans, and Wietse Kuis

Genetic disorders of the immune system enable the study of the relationship between the clinical expression of immunodeficiencies and the underlying immune defect. Although infections are the most common, and early clinical expressions of primary immunodeficiencies, autoimmune diseases (as well as malignancies) often occur in immunodeficient patients. This association can provide new understanding of the mechanisms of tolerance and the pathophysiology of autoimmunity. In recent years, knowledge of the genetic basis of immunodeficiencies has increased, and the molecular abnormalities of these diseases have started to unravel. An increasing number of associated genetic defects have been identified by a variety of techniques, such as positional cloning and complementation. Monogenic primary immunodeficiencies provide information on genes that can be involved in the mechanisms of immune tolerance.

Better understanding of the molecular basis of immunodeficiencies will provide insight into why autoimmune diseases develop under these circumstances. This knowledge permits the linking of observations in immunodeficient patients with autoimmune diseases and a known gene defect, to patients with comparable autoimmune diseases in whom there is no clear understanding of pathogenesis. In this paradigm, autoimmune diseases are regarded as subtle immunodeficiencies. The expectation is that this approach will help clarify the pathogenesis of many autoimmune diseases. This chapter focuses on genetically determined primary immunodeficiencies in which autoimmune disorders may occur (Table 42–1).

DISORDERS OF INNATE IMMUNITY ASSOCIATED WITH RHEUMATIC DISEASES

Defective Control of Lymphocyte Survival

Apoptosis (or *programmed cell death*) is one of most essential physiological mechanisms to regulate embryonic development, cell differentiation, and tissue turnover.

Of the several mechanisms leading to apoptosis, that best studied is the death pathway initiated by the interaction of CD95 (Fas/APO-1) and its ligand.[1,2] Recently, the molecular pathway of this process was unraveled. After binding of Fas-ligand to the extracellular part of the Fas molecule, the so-called "death domain" of this molecules associates with Fas-associated death domain and pro-caspases 8 and 10.[3-5] This complex of molecules, called the death inducing signaling complex, induces activation of caspase 8/10 and cell death.

MRL-lpr/lpr mice have mutations in the Fas-encoding gene leading to faulty Fas (CD95) expression on T cells.[6] This mutation results in a syndrome characterized by lymphoproliferation of CD4-CD8- T cells, associated with autoimmune manifestations. The severity of the disease depends not only on mutations on the Fas-encoding gene but also on the genetic background of the mice. Mutations of the Fas-ligand gene (gld mutation) also result in lymphoproliferation.[6]

The human counterpart of this murine abnormality is called the autoimmune lymphoproliferative syndrome (ALPS), which is a lymphoproliferative disorder with accumulation of CD4-CD8- T cells and B cells and variable autoimmunity.[7,8] Subtypes of ALPS (type Ia, Ib, I-mosaic, II, III, and IV) result from defects in different parts of the Fas pathway.[7,9,10] Type 1a results from a mutation in the death domain of the Fas receptor *TNFRSF6 (CD95)*; more than 60 mutations are described. Transmission is autosomal dominant. Homozygous mutations are rare and associated with a severe phenotype. Type 1b results from a mutation in the Fas ligand *(TNFSF6)*, and only three patients with this subtype have been described. Type Im (mosaic) shows heterozygous CD95 mutations on select cell lines only, such as double negative T cells; 10 patients have been described. Type 2 results from a mutation in caspase-10 *(CASP10)*, reducing its activity. The clinical phenotype is similar to type I. In type III ALPS, no genetic defect has been found. Type IV ALPS was described as an intrinsic defect of apoptosis. Note that expansion of double negative (DN) cells is absent in yet another ALPS variant named Dianzani autoimmune lymphoproliferative disease.[11]

In homozygous Fas deficiency, lymphoproliferation is already present at birth. Stimulated lymphocytes do not

Table 42–1

Classification of immunodeficiency disorders

Disorders of Innate Immunity
Abnormalities of Fas-mediated apoptosis
Phagocytic abnormalities
Complement abnormalities
Disorders of Adaptive Immunity
Abnormalities of T and B lymphocytes
Abnormalities of T lymphocytes
Abnormalities of B lymphocytes

express Fas and are insensitive to treatment by an agonist anti-Fas antibody.[8,12] Apoptotic lymphocytes can be detected in the peripheral blood and in the spleen, indicating that other death pathways are operating. Some ALPS patients (two type Ia patients and five type III patients) were successfully treated with the antimalarial drug pyrimethamine; however, treatment failures have also been reported.[13,14] For the more severe cases, allogeneic bone marrow transplantation can be performed.[8,15,16]

Heterozygous Fas gene mutations are more common.[12,17,18] The majority of these mutations reside in the Fas (TNFRSF6) gene and in the genes encoding the Fas ligand and caspase-8 and caspase-10, all involved in Fas mediated signalling.[17] These patients are characterized by lymphadenopathy at an early age, autoimmune hemolytic anemia, and thrombocytopenia. Less frequently, glomerulonephritis, the Guillain-Barré syndrome, and urticaria are also described. Variable heterozygous Fas mutations are present, leading to defective Fas-mediated apoptosis. Parents of affected children have Fas mutations without clinical symptoms of lymphoproliferation or autoimmunity. This important observation indicates that for the disease to be expressed, the single-allele Fas mutation must be combined with another gene defect (digenic disease).[8]

Mutations in the Fas-ligand gene can also result in lymphoproliferative diseases associated with autoimmunity. Mutations have been detected in a patient with systemic lupus erythematosus (SLE).[19,20] Molecular cloning and sequencing indicated that the genomic DNA of this patient contained an 84-bp deletion within exon 4 of the Fas-ligand gene, resulting in a predicted 28-amino acid in-frame deletion.[20]

Knowledge of the basic mechanisms controlling cell survival or death and the identification of genetic defects in death pathways have led to new concepts of the pathogenesis of autoimmune disease. In addition to Fas-induced apoptosis, a rapidly increasing number of other death pathways are being discovered. Future research will evaluate their role in preventing autoimmune disease and recognize defects leading to disease.

INNATE IMMUNITY INTERACTING WITH ADAPTIVE IMMUNITY

The interaction between innate and adaptive immunity determines the course of many autoimmune diseases, such as rheumatoid arthritis (RA). Studies in animal models of arthritis show evidence for this interaction involving circulating immune complexes, cytokine-induced Receptor Activator for Nuclear Factor κ B Ligand (RANKL), direct osteoclast activation, T cell factors such as interferon (IFN) γ and interleukin (IL) 17, and granulocytes. Spontaneous T cell-dependent arthritis in IL1Ra-/- mice is absent under germ-free conditions: in sterile conditions, in absence of micro-organisms, and markedly suppressed in Toll-like receptor (TLR) 4-deficient mice. Moreover, TLR4 blocking with a receptor antagonist suppresses erosive arthritis.[21]

Innate immunity can be triggered by recognizing invading microorganisms through pathogen-associated molecular patterns (PAMPs) and by reacting to tissue damage signals called damage-associated molecular patterns (DAMPs).[22] DAMP molecules, including alarmins, high mobility group box 1 protein, (HMGB-1), heat-shock proteins (HSPs), uric acid, altered matrix proteins, and S100 proteins, represent important danger signals that mediate inflammatory responses through the receptor for advanced glycation end-products (RAGE) and TLRs. A prototypical DAMP molecule, the nuclear protein HMGB-1, is either passively released by necrotic cells or actively secreted with delay by activated cells. To function as an alarmin, HMGB1 translocates from the nucleus of the cell to the extracellular milieu, a process that can take place with cell activation and cell death. HMGB1 can interact with receptors that include RAGE and TLR-2 and TLR-4 and function in a synergistic fashion with other proinflammatory mediators to induce responses.

The calprotectins S100A8, S100A9, and S100A12 are calcium-binding proteins expressed in the cytoplasm of phagocytes. They are rapidly secreted by activated monocytes or neutrophils, which are abundant in inflamed synovial tissue. The S100 A molecules can bind TLR-4. They are elevated in RA but specifically in systemic onset juvenile idiopathic arthritis (JIA).[23-26] HSPs are involved in the crosstalk between innate and adaptive immune systems, and primarily mediate immune regulatory functions. Multiple positive feedback loops between DAMPs and PAMPs and their receptors exist and represent the molecular basis for the observation that infections and nonspecific stress factors can trigger flares in rheumatic diseases.

Rheumatic Diseases Associated with Disorders of Phagocytes

There is an increasing awareness of the association of rheumatic diseases with abnormalities of phagocytic cell function and the complement pathways (Table 42–2).

Chronic Granulomatous Disease

Chronic granulomatous disease (CGD) is a rare (one in 250,000), inherited primary immunodeficiency of phagocytic leukocytes characterized by recurrent, life-threatening bacterial, fungal, and yeast infections of the subcutaneous tissues, airways, lymph nodes, liver, and bones.[27] The disorder results from absence or malfunction of the reduced form of the nicotinamide adenine dinucleotide phosphate (NADPH) oxidase enzyme system that produces superoxide in the professional phagocytic

Table 42–2

Classification of deficiencies of Innate Immunity associated with Rheumatic Disease

Disorders of Innate Immunity	Rheumatic Disease Association
Phagocytic Defects	
Chronic granulomatous disease	DLE, SLE
Familial lipochrome histiocytosis	Arthritis
Chédiak-Higashi disease	SLE-like disease in animals
Streaking leukocyte syndrome	Polyarthritis
Complement Deficiencies	
Deficiency of C1q	SLE-like GTN, RTS
Deficiency of C1r	SLE, DLE, GTN
Deficiency of C1s	SLE, DLE
Deficiency of C1 INH	SLE, DLE
Deficiency of C4	SLE, Sjögren's syndrome
Deficiency of C2	SLE, DLE, PM, HSP, vasculitis, GTN, Hodgkin disease, JIA, RA
Deficiency of C3	SLE, vasculitis, GTN, arthralgias, SLE
Deficiency of C5	SLE
Deficiency of C6	SLE, DLE
Deficiency of C7	SLE, sclerodactyly, RA, vasculitis
Deficiency of C8	SLE, JRA

DLE, Discoid lupus erythematosus; GTN, glomerulotubulonephritis; HSP, Henoch-Schönlein purpura; JIA, juvenile idiopathic arthritis; PM, polymyositis; RA, rheumatoid arthritis; RTS, Rothmund-Thomson syndrome (congenital poikiloderma); SLE, systemic lupus erythematosus.
Adapted from Ruddy S: Complement deficiencies and rheumatic diseases. In Kelley WN, Harris ED Jr, Ruddy S et al, editors: *Textbook of Rheumatology*, ed 4, Philadelphia, 1993, Saunders.

cells (neutrophils, monocytes, macrophages, and eosinophils). Deficiency of this oxidase (which is required for the production of microbicidal oxygen metabolites) renders the phagocytes unable to kill ingested microorganisms. NADPH oxidase consists of several subunits, each encoded by a separate gene.[27] Treatment consists of antimicrobial prophylaxis and recombinant human IFN-γ treatment.[27-29] In the more severe cases, stem cell transplantations can be performed.[29]

The majority of patients (70%) suffer from the X-linked form of the disease, which is caused by mutations in *CYBB*, the gene that encodes the beta-subunit of cytochrome b558, also called gp91phox. Mutations in three other subunits cause autosomally inherited forms of CGD. This concerns the α-subunit of cytochrome b558 (p22phox) needed for stabilization of the cytochrome in the plasma membrane of phagocytes, and the cytoplasmic proteins p47phox and p67phox that translocate to the cytochrome during cell activation, a process needed for induction of the bactericidal enzymatic activity after phagocytosis of microorganisms.[30] The molecular basis of CGD has been extensively reviewed.[31] Clinical variability in CGD is considerable and is mainly associated with the degree of residual respiratory burst activity.

A mucocutaneous syndrome characterized by discoid lupus erythematosus (DLE), photosensitive dermatitis,

and recurrent aphthous stomatitis occurs in up to one-third of carriers of the CGD gene.[32-34] Occasionally, other rheumatic complaints are noted, and some mothers of patients with CGD have autoantibodies to nuclear antigens. Few cases are described of children with CGD who developed convincing clinical, serological, and pathological evidence of SLE; other children have features of discoid lupus and photosensitivity.[34-37] However, the frequency of defects in neutrophil function among patients with discoid lupus erythematosus (DLE) who lack a family history of CGD appears to be very low.[36] The pathogenesis of these cutaneous lesions of lupus in patients with CGD or carriers is unknown. It has been proposed that a partial defect in bactericidal ability leads to chronic antigen persistence and immune activation, possibly provoking autoantibody formation. Ultraviolet irradiation seems to be an environmental trigger.

A girl of Chinese ancestry with autosomal recessive CGD (p47phox) was described as having polyarthritis since the age of 4 years, involving the large joints (wrists, ankles, knees, and hips) and the small joints (metacarpophalangeal and metatarsophalangeal joints).[38] There was early-morning stiffness and joint swelling with synovial thickening, stiffness, and tenderness. Infections were excluded. Serological markers included several autoantibodies, such as rheumatoid factor (RF), antinuclear antibodies (ANAs), and anti-dsDNA antibodies. Serum complement factors were not depressed. The patient did not develop SLE-like symptoms in the 22-month period of follow-up,[38] although such symptoms occurred later. Bland peripheral arthritis and bursitis in two boys with CGD and erosive polyarthritis in a young girl with the disease have been reported. However, apart from susceptibility to septic arthritis and osteomyelitis, children with CGD have only rarely developed a rheumatic disease.[39]

Suppurative and granulomatous infections in CGD patients are established soon after birth, first at body surfaces normally in contact with bacteria and fungi (e.g., the skin, the airways, and the gut).[27] From these areas, infectious organisms may be carried to lymph nodes and internal organs such as the liver. Failure to contain the infection may result in bacteremia that enables further infectious foci to develop. The major clinical manifestations of CGD are thus pyoderma, pneumonia, gastrointestinal involvement, lymphadenitis, liver abscesses, and osteomyelitis.[27,39,40] In contrast with normal children, in whom osteomyelitis usually involves the metaphyseal areas of long bones, patients with CGD more often develop infections of the small bones of the hands and feet.[27,40] Multiple sites are often infected. Aspiration of pus is mandatory for identification of the pathogenic microorganism.

A variety of bacterial pathogens has been isolated from the lesions of CGD.[27] *Staphylococcus aureus*, *Staphylococcus epidermidis*, and enterobacteria predominate. Common gram-negative organisms include *Escherichia coli*, *Salmonella*, *Pseudomonas aeruginosa* and *cepacia*, *Klebsiella-Aerobacter*, *Proteus*, *Serratia marcescens*, *Arizona*, and *Legionella*. Infections with *Nocardia* species and *Mycobacteria* (BCG strain) are of special importance. Fungal pathogens isolated most commonly in CGD are *Aspergillus* species and, to a lesser extent,

Candida albicans. The response to viral pathogens is normal, and parasitic infections, except for *Pneumocystis carinii*, are rare.

Patients with CGD may be considerably shorter than expected based on parental height.[41] This phenomenon is not fully explained. Infections often suppress growth temporarily, but catch-up growth is normal. Protein-calorie malnutrition does not seem to explain the shorter stature. Patients have a normal pubertal growth spurt.

Chédiak-Higashi syndrome

The rare Chédiak-Higashi syndrome is characterized by susceptibility to bacterial infection beginning in early childhood and associated with the presence of large cytoplasmic granules in neutrophils. The hemophagocytic lymphohistiocytosis syndrome, which characterized the evolution of the Chédiak-Higashi syndrome results from defects affecting intracellular trafficking.[42,43]

Arthritis, Pyoderma Gangrenosum, and Streaking Leukocyte Factor

A 2-year-old boy developed massive monarticular joint effusions and later severe pyoderma gangrenosum after minor trauma.[44] The sterile pyoarthritic episodes, leading to the repetitive erroneous diagnosis of septic arthritis, were ultimately self-limited or could be controlled by prednisone. The pyoderma responded to FK 506. A second case has been reported by Jacobs.[45] Pyoderma gangrenosum can also be seen in inflammatory bowel disease.[46] The mechanism of this disorder remains unknown, although the pattern of episodes of arthritis in response to minor trauma is quite similar to the PAPA syndrome, an autoinflammatory syndrome associated with a mutation of the PSTPIP1-gene.[47]

Rheumatic Diseases Associated with Complement Deficiencies

Primary genetic deficiencies of complement are inherited as autosomal recessive traits with the exception of C1 inhibitor deficiency (causing hereditary angioneurotic edema [HANE], an autosomal dominant disease, and properdin deficiency, an X-linked disorder). The heterozygous state can usually be detected by measuring the complement protein in serum.

The clinical manifestations of complement deficiencies vary.[48-55] Some patients are asymptomatic, but most suffer from rheumatic diseases, particularly a syndrome resembling SLE.[56,57] The clinical findings include early onset of skin lesions resembling discoid lupus, alopecia, photosensitivity, and mild renal and pleuropericardial involvement. The two other main clinical presentations are increased susceptibility to infection (repeated bacterial infections with pathogens such as *Streptococcus pneumoniae* and *Neisseria meningitidis* and viral infections),[58,59] and angioedema in the case of HANE. Frequent infections are the predominant manifestations of deficiencies of C3 and factors I and H, the absence of which leads to consumption of C3. Primary or secondary C3 deficiency leads to infections with encapsulated bacteria such as *S. pneumoniae*, underlining the importance

of C3 as a mediator of opsonization. Deficiencies of components of the membrane attack complex C5-C8 particularly predispose to recurrent infections with *Neisseria* species.[53,60,61]

SLE-like rheumatic disorders are the major clinical manifestations of classic pathway complement deficiencies.[49,51,53,56,62] The frequency and severity of disease vary with each deficiency. SLE was observed in 28 of 30 C1q-deficient persons, 12 of 16 with C4 deficiency, approximately 40% with C2 deficiency, but in only four of 24 patients with C3 deficiency.[57] These observations imply a physiological protective activity of the early activation of the classic complement pathway against the development of the immune complex-mediated syndrome SLE.

Binding of C1 to immune complexes activates the classic complement pathway, resulting in the cleavage of C4 and C3 to C4b and C3b, which bind covalently to immune complexes, thus leading to two important effects.[53,63] First, binding of C3b (and, to a lesser extent, of C4b) promotes the solubility of immune complexes. Second, immune complexes are bound via C3b and C4b to CR1 receptors on peripheral blood cells, mainly erythrocytes, and transported to the liver and spleen; there immune complexes are transferred to fixed macrophages, after which the erythrocytes return to the circulation.[64,65] The observation that erythrocytes transport immune complexes in lupus is demonstrated by the depression of CR1 numbers in active disease. This defect is also found in other diseases that are accompanied by complement fixation on red blood cells, whether by immune complexes or directly by red blood cell antibodies.[64,65]

It has been proposed that failure of the mononuclear phagocytic system to effectively remove immune complexes from the circulation and tissues allows a cycle to develop in which immune complexes deposit in tissue, causing inflammation and release of autoantigens, which in turn stimulate the production of autoantibodies and the production of more immune complexes. Thus autoantibody synthesis in lupus may be primarily antigen-driven rather than due to polyclonal activation of B cells. The specific autoantibodies are formed against defined antigens such as DNA, histones, and non-histone proteins in the DNA nucleoprotein particle.[49,53] There is a less frequent disease association with C2 deficiency than with deficiencies of C1 and C4; this is because in C2-deficient subjects, complement fixation proceeds as far as C4, which (albeit to a lesser degree) subserves functions otherwise carried out by fixed C3.

Lesser degrees of defective complement function, either genetic or acquired, may also predispose to lupus.[66,67] In the case of the relatively common heterozygous C4 deficiency, the increase in SLE is associated with deficiency of C4A (C4AQ0 allele) (relative risk, 2 to 5) but not the C4B allele. C4A is the isotype of C4 that is more effective in inhibiting immunoprecipitation and, compared with C4B, binds much more effectively to CR1.[64]

The hypothesis that the complement component deficiency per se is not responsible for the increased incidence of SLE but is merely a marker for a true susceptibility gene seems unlikely, because C1q encoded on chromosome 1, C1r and C1s on chromosome 12, and C4 and C2 in the major histocompatibility complex (MHC) on chromosome 6 are all associated with the same disease. Even for the MHC-linked complement loci, the marker gene role seems to be excluded, because Caucasian C2 deficiency is nearly always found as part of one particular haplotype (A10, B18, C4A2B4, DR2), whereas the complete C4 deficiency haplotypes are variable and quite different. Finally, C1 inhibitor deficiency, which results in a secondary subtotal deficiency of C2 and C4, is also associated with an increased incidence of autoimmune immune-complex disease.[50,53,64,68]

The frequency of complement deficiencies in the general population is probably very low. C2 deficiency is still the most frequently recognized component deficiency.[56,57] Heterozygous deficiency for C2 is estimated to be 1%. In patients with SLE, homozygous complement component deficiency is also low (estimated to be about one in 2000 for women in the United Kingdom). Nevertheless, particularly in children with early-onset (preschool age) SLE-like disease and, in instances of familial SLE, hereditary primary deficiencies of complement should be considered (Table 42-2).

C1 Deficiency

The absence of C1q is the most common abnormality of the first component of complement.[65] About 30 patients with homozygous C1q deficiency have been reported in the literature.[69] Of these, 28 subjects suffered from SLE, one had discoid lupus alone, and a 38-year-old male was healthy. A number of characteristic clinical features of SLE are associated with C1q deficiency.[69] Disease onset tends to be early, with a median age at onset of 7 years (range, 6-months- to 42 years). Skin rash was present in 25 cases. The SLE may be severe; six patients had central nervous system disease (five of six with grand mal seizures), and 11 had glomerulonephritis. Seventeen of 23 patients had ANA, and autoantibodies to extractable nuclear antigens were reported in 10 patients (anti-RNP in six, anti-Sm in six, and anti-Ro in four). Anti-dsDNA antibodies are unusual in the context of C1q deficiency. Therapy with hydroxychloroquine and oral corticosteroids may relieve some symptoms. Thalidomide corticosteroids therapy may benefit the skin lesions.[70]

Case Report

The authors treated a C1q-deficient girl with homozygous nonfunctional C1q with weekly infusions of fresh-frozen plasma for seven years. She was born of healthy non-consanguinous Caucasian parents. She began having recurrent otitis and tonsillitis, recurrent fever, and arthralgia at the age of 3 years. At 5 years, she had aseptic meningitis, and a few months later developed nephrotic syndrome. A kidney biopsy revealed mesangioproliferative glomerulonephritis with granular deposits of immunoglobulin (Ig) M, IgG, C3, and C5—but not C1q—along the basement membrane. Apart from a malar rash after sun exposure, the patient had no other lupus-like symptoms. The nephrotic syndrome responded rapidly to prednisone.

However, in the following years, despite therapy with prednisone and hydroxychloroquine, she developed a severe malar rash even after the mildest sun exposure; alopecia; oral ulcerations; Raynaud phenomenon; livedo reticularis; and severe vasculitis of the palms and fingers, soles, and toes, making it impossible to write, walk, or wear shoes. Recurrent respiratory tract infections provoked exacerbations of vasculitis, arthralgias, headaches, and depression. Intravenous immunoglobulin (IVIG) every three weeks prevented recurrent infections and SLE exacerbations but failed to achieve clinical remission. The girl developed anemia, leukopenia with lymphopenia, and thrombocytopenia. She had ANAs, and tests for anti-dsDNA, anti-Sm, and anti-RNP were positive. RFs were present, and slightly raised levels of anticardiolipin antibodies were detected. Hemolysis of sensitized sheep erythrocytes was defective (CH50 <5 %), but the functional activity of the alternative complement pathway was intact. Levels of complement factors C3 and C4 were increased even during active disease; C2 was normal. Family investigation confirmed the patient to be homozygous for a gene that resulted in the production of low-molecular-weight C1q unable to activate the classic complement pathway.[71] Both parents were heterozygous for the abnormality and asymptomatic.

Fresh-frozen plasma infusions (initially, 2 L every 3 weeks; later, 800 mL once a week) resulted in clinical remission and normalization of hemoglobin, white blood cell count, and platelet count until the onset of menarche, when severe headaches, vasculitis of the hands and feet, malar rash, alopecia, and arthralgias required reinstitution of prednisone and transient treatment with thalidomide, 100 mg/day. In 2008, the patient was still on this regimen. During the entire illness, results of tests for ANA and other autoantibodies have remained positive, despite clinical remission. Antibodies to C1q have not been observed.

Inherited deficiency of C1r, often with a concomitant deficiency of C1s, has been reported in eight children, five of whom had SLE, and many of whom also had multiple episodes of upper respiratory tract infections, skin infections, meningitis, unexplained fevers, and glomerulonephritis.[65,72]

HANE, caused by a deficiency in C1q esterase inhibitor, has no known human leukocyte antigen (HLA) association but is associated with a Sjögren's syndrome or lupus-like disease in some families.[48,72,73] The authors observed a girl with familial C1q esterase deficiency who developed classical DLE with anti-Ro and La antibodies in the absence of ANA or dsDNA antibodies.

C2 Deficiency

Lack of the second component of complement is the most common genetic deficiency of complement.[74-76] Heterozygous C2 deficiency may occur in approximately 1% of the normal population, 1.4% of adults with RA, 3.7% of children with juvenile idiopathic arthritis (JIA), and 6% of patients with SLE.[75] About 60% of homozygous and 13% of heterozygous C2-deficient persons have been found to have associated autoimmune disease, most commonly SLE. These patients usually exhibit a restricted set of clinical manifestations, including sun-sensitive skin lesions, alopecia, febrile episodes, arthritis, and renal disease. The lupus-like disease, particularly in association with heterozygous C2 deficiency, tends to be somewhat milder than one would otherwise expect, with less clinically significant nephritis but more florid cutaneous lesions.[58,72] Steinsson and colleagues successfully treated a 43-year-old woman with homozygous C2 deficiency and SLE with infusions of fresh-frozen plasma and were able to discontinue previously required medications (prednisone and azathioprine).[77]

C3 Deficiency

Almost all reported patients with homozygous C3 deficiency have been infants or young children with severe bacterial infections (meningitis, pneumonitis, peritonitis, or osteomyelitis).[72,78,79] Other associations described in children have included SLE, vasculitis, arthralgia, and glomerulonephritis. Successful renal transplantation in a C3-deficient patient with glomerulonephritis has been reported.

C4 Deficiency

At least seven homozygous C4-deficient children have been recorded.[53,67,72,80] Five had SLE, one had glomerulonephritis, and three had serious infections. SLE is associated with an extended HLA haplotype that includes the C4A null allele.[67,80]

Deficiency of Late Complement Components

Deficiency of C5, although unusual, is more common in adults and older children.[50] Both of the reported C5-deficient adolescents had *Neisseria meningitidis* meningitis, but neither had rheumatic complaints. Absence of C6 has been reported in six children younger than 18-years-old, most of whom had *N. meningitidis* meningitis.[81] Although no child with C6, C7, or C8 deficiency and a rheumatic disease has been reported, adults with these deficiencies have developed DLE, Sjögren's syndrome, or SLE.[82] The authors reported a 13-year-old boy who presented with a 6-month history of recurrent fever; an exanthem involving the trunk and extremities, and arthritis of the wrists, knees, and the metacarpophalangeal and proximal interphalangeal joint of both hands.[83] The patient was found to have deficiency of the β-subunit of C8. Infection, particularly meningococcal infection, was excluded. Deficiencies of C9 and of components of the alternate complement pathway are very rare.[72,82]

Mannose Binding Lectins

Mannose binding lectin (MBL) is a serum protein with a specific role in innate immunity.[84,85] MBL has structural similarities to C1q, binds to mannose structures present in the cell surface of bacteria and yeasts, thus facilitating opsonisation by phagocytes, and initiates complement activation through the classical pathway. This happens by activation of the mannan-binding lectin-associated serine protease 2 (MASP-2), which then cleaves complement factors C4 and C2, generating the C3 convertase C4bC2b. Activation of C3 initiates the alternative pathway and the formation of the membrane-attack complex. An inherited MASP-2 deficiency has been described in a man with ulcerative colitis since the age of 13 years, SLE since the age of 29 years, and severe pneumococcal pneumonias.[86]

The human MBL2 gene on chromosome 10 has three variant alleles. Mutations in these alleles may cause low serum MBL values. Low serum values are associated with an increased risk of infections, although individuals with MBL deficiency may be asymptomatic.[87,88] Because Kawasaki disease is an acute vasculitis with a possible infectious cause, a possible role of the MBL gene in Caucasian patients with Kawasaki disease was investigated.[89,90] In a group of 90 children with Kawasaki disease, there was a higher frequency of MBL gene mutations compared to healthy children. Similar studies of MBL gene polymorphisms in SLE, Sjögren's syndrome, and sarcoidosis reported contrasting results.[91-96]

DISORDERS OF ADAPTIVE IMMUNITY ASSOCIATED WITH RHEUMATIC DISEASES

Adaptive immunity is mediated by lymphocytes and their products. Deficiencies are classified according to abnormalities of T and/or B lymphocytes.[97] Acquired abnormalities of adaptive immunity are common in children with rheumatic diseases. It is thought that these laboratory abnormalities (e.g., hypergammaglobulinemia and altered lymphocyte numbers) reflect a response to the disease rather than a primary abnormality, although the validity of this conclusion is uncertain. Rare but instructive examples of the association of primary immunodeficiencies and rheumatic diseases are discussed in the following paragraphs (Table 42–3). The association of immunodeficiency and rheumatic disease has been reviewed by several authors.[54,55,98-100]

Primary Abnormalities of T and B Lymphocytes

This part of the chapter discusses diseases characterized clinically and immunologically by defects in both T and B lymphocytes (Tables 42–4 and 42–5).[8,97,98,101,102]

Table 42–3

Disorders of Adaptive Immunity associated with Rheumatic Disease

Disorders of Adaptive Immunity	Rheumatic Disease Associations
Combined Immunodeficiencies	
Wiskott-Aldrich syndrome	Chronic arthritis, vasculitis
Immunodeficiency with thymoma (Good syndrome)	Chronic arthritis
Nezelof syndrome	Chronic arthritis, SLE
Humoral Immunodeficiencies	
Selective IgA deficiency	JIA, SLE, RA, others
Hypogammaglobulinemia	Chronic arthritis, SLE
IgG subclass deficiencies	JIA, SLE

Ig, immunoglobulin; JIA, juvenile idiopathic arthritis; RA, rheumatoid arthritis; SLE, systemic lupus erythematosus.

Genetic defects have been identified in a substantial number of these disorders.

Severe Combined Immunodeficiency

Severe combined immunodeficiency (SCID) is a rare disorder characterized by severe congenital defects in cellular and humoral immunity.[8,98,101,103] The incidence is approximately one in 75,000 births. Because of absent T cell-mediated immunity, affected children develop severe lung infections with *Pneumocystis carinii*, chronic candidiasis, persistent diarrhea, and failure to thrive, usually within the first year of life. There is lymphoid aplasia, and the thymus usually cannot be detected radiographically. Laboratory tests confirm the presence of agammaglobulinemia (although some maternal IgG can be detected in the first months of life) and T cell lymphopenia with absent *in vitro* responses to mitogens.

In the X-linked form of SCID, which accounts for 50% to 60% of cases, B lymphocytes are present but natural killer (NK) cells are absent. In these patients (T⁻B⁺ SCID), the agammaglobulinemia is a direct consequence of deficient T cell help. The X-linked form results from a gene defect located at Xq12-13.1.[104,105] This gene encodes the common γ chain, present in the IL receptors IL-2R, IL-4R, IL-7R, IL-9R, and IL-15R. In the autosomal recessive form of SCID, B cells are lacking, and NK cells may be present (T⁻B⁻ SCID). In *adenosine deaminase (ADA) deficiency*, a variety of ADA gene mutations have been described. A lack of ADA in precursor lymphocytes results in a maturation arrest by accumulation of deoxyadenosine tri

phosphate (ATP), which inhibits cell division.[8,9,99,106] The clinical course is fatal within the first two years of life. Janus Kinase-3 (JAK-3) deficiency causes autosomal recessive SCID, as a result of a mutation in the JAK-3 kinase gene.[8] This enzyme mediates post-IL-2R signaling. Another form of autosomal recessive SCID is Zeta chain-associated protein kinase-70 deficiency, a key signal transduction molecule in T cells.[8] ZAP-70 is involved in T cell receptor down-modulation, thus rendering a T cell anergic.[107] A spontaneous point mutation of the gene encoding Src homology 2 domain (SH2) of ZAP-70, causes chronic autoimmune arthritis in mice that resembles human rheumatoid arthritis in many aspects.[107] However, arthritis has not yet been described in its human counterpart, and naturally acquired immunological self-tolerance is not entirely accounted for by this T cell-anergy. The T cell-repertoire of healthy individuals harbors self-reactive lymphocytes with a potential to cause autoimmune disease, and these lymphocytes are under dominant control by a unique subpopulation of CD4+ T cells now called regulatory T cells (Tregs).[108]

The only curative treatment for SCID is allogeneic hemopoietic stem cell transplantation. As in patients with adenosine deaminase deficiency, patients with the X-linked IL-2R deficiency may benefit from gene therapy.[109,110] This approach has been initially very successful but is associated with an increased risk of acute lymphatic leukemia.[111]

There are no reports of rheumatic diseases in children with SCID.[112] This may be because they usually die before the age of 2 years unless they undergo transplantation, but it may also illustrate the essential role of T cells in the initiation of an autoimmune disorder. In SCID due to *Purine nucleoside phosphorylase* deficiency, autoimmune thyroiditis, idiopathic thrombopenia, SLE, and cerebral vasculitis were described before stem cell transplantation was performed.[17] After stem cell transplantation, autoimmune hematologic phenomena have been described in patients with graft-versus-host disease (GVHD), a positive Coombs test result, and autoimmune hemolytic anemia. Chronic GVHD of the skin leads to skin changes that resemble those that occur in systemic scleroderma. Patients with ADA deficiency frequently have cupping deformities of the ribs and flat iliae without joint problems.

Table 42–4		
Primary immunodeficiencies of T and B lymphocytes		
	Inheritance	Gene
Disease	**Pattern**	**Product**
SCID	XL	γ chain
SCID	AR	JAK3, RAG1, RAG2, DNA-PK
Adenosine deaminase deficiency	AR	Adenosine deaminase
Purine nucleoside phosphorylase deficiency	AR	Purine nucleoside phosphorylase
MHC class II deficiency	AR	CIITA (also called MHC2TA), RFX5
Wiskott-Aldrich syndrome	XL	WASP (also called WAS)
Reticular dysgenesis	AR	?
Ataxia telangiectasia	AR	ATM
Omenn syndrome	AR	RAG1, RAG2
CD3γ and CD3ε deficiency	AR	?
CD8 deficiency	AR	ZAP70 (zeta chain-associated protein kinase 70 kD)
DiGeorge syndrome	AR	Candidate gene exists
Cartilage-hair hypoplasia	AR	Candidate gene exists

AR, autosomal recessive; MHC, major histocompatibility complex; SCID, severe combined immune deficiency; XL, X-linked.

Table 42–5
Primary humoral immunodeficiencies
X- linked agammaglobulinemia (Bruton agammaglobulinemia)
X-linked hypogammaglobulinemia with growth hormone deficiency
X-linked Hyper-IgM
Autosomal recessive Hyper-IgM
IgG subclass deficiencies
Selective IgA deficiency
κ light chain deficiency
Antibody deficiency with normal immunoglobulins (Nezelof syndrome)
Common variable immunodeficiency
Hyper-IgD syndrome
Hyper-IgE syndrome

Combined Immunodeficiency

The term *combined immunodeficiency* is applied to a group of disorders of variable clinical severity associated with defects in both cellular and humoral immunity.[98,113] The *Wiskott-Aldrich syndrome* (WAS) is characterized by a progressive abnormality in both T and B lymphocyte function.[114] It is thought to be caused by defects in immunoregulatory peptides involved in cell-cell interactions. There is a low expression of sialophorin (CD43), and the syndrome is associated with mutations of the gene located at Xp11.23.[115] The precise function of the protein (the WAS protein) that this gene encodes is uncertain. A female WAS patient has been described in whom the gene mutation was discovered to be present on one of the X chromosomes. That she was nevertheless affected was explained by a nonrandom inactivation of the X chromosomes. Discovery of the gene mutation has also led to the identification of related male adults with only thrombocytopenia.

Children with the WAS have persistent eczema, thrombocytopenia with a low platelet volume, and recurrent ear, nose, and throat infections. They often have chronic cytomegalovirus infection, and laboratory abnormalities vary widely. The characteristic Ig pattern includes normal IgG and elevated IgA and IgE levels, with absence of antibodies to polysaccharide antigens (such as pneumococcal capsular antigen) and absent blood group isohemagglutinins. There is a high incidence of Coombspositive hemolytic anemia, vasculitis, and (mostly transient) arthritis.[115-118] The syndrome is a premalignant condition with a high frequency of thymomas and sarcomas later in life, although the precise incidence of these malignancies is unknown, because persons with the WAS gene mutation may be asymptomatic. In a survey of the long-term outcome following hematopoietic stem-cell transplantation in WAS, a striking result was the observation of host autoimmunity in 20% of patients strongly associated with a persistent mixed/split chimerism status after stem cell transplantation.[117]

T Cell Immunodeficiencies

In the T cell immunodeficiencies, T lymphocytes are, in contrast with SCID, present in the peripheral blood, although in reduced numbers. This is a heterogeneous and often poorly defined group of disorders. Various functional and genetic defects have been described (see Table 42–4). Clinically, these children do not have life-threatening infections in the first months of life but show a more gradually developing immunodeficiency. An imbalance between T and B lymphocytes may explain the high incidence of autoimmune disorders, infections, allergies, and malignancies. Severe and chronic autoimmune manifestations, mostly involving blood cells, develop between the ages of 1 and 12 years.[113] In addition, vasculitis, autoimmune hepatitis, and thyroiditis have been described. In younger patients, without severe ongoing infections, bone marrow transplantation may be performed. The Di George syndrome (DGS) is a T cell disorder of variable severity and is caused by mutations in the 22q11 region. Several case reports describe an increased incidence of (polyarticular) JIA in DGS.[119-122]

In a cohort of 80 patients with DGS and a proven chromosome 22q11.2 deletion, three patients were found to have polyarticular JIA.[122]

Cartilage-hair hypoplasia (CHH) consists of bony dysplasia, short-limbed dwarfism, fine sparse hair, short fingernails, and various immune defects, including neutropenia, combined immunodeficiency, or mild humoral deficiency.[123,124] The disease-causing gene has been identified as the RNA component of mitochondrial RNA processing endoribonuclease (RMRP) gene on the short arm of chromosome 9. Affected infants have generalized hypermobility. However, inflammatory rheumatic diseases have not been reported. In addition, four children were described with a similar syndrome of short stature due to spondylometaphyseal dysplasia and severe infections because of a combined humoral and cellular immune deficiency.[125] They all had a normal RMRP gene expression, thus excluding CHH. ADA activity was normal. There were several autoimmune diseases present (idiopathic thrombocytopenia 3/4; hypothyroidism 3/4; vitiligo 2/4; oligoarticular JIA 1/4 and Crohn disease 1/4).[125] The immunological abnormalities were comparable with those seen in CHH.[124] One patient died of encephalitis of unknown cause.

Disorders of Regulation by T Cells and Natural Killer T Cells

CD4+CD25+ Tregs play a critical role in immune tolerance.[126] Tregs exert immune surveillance activities by modifying the function of antigen presenting cells (APCs). Tregs can induce apoptosis of APCs or inhibit their activation and function. These actions of Tregs are mediated by both soluble factors (IL-10, transforming growth factor-β, perforins, and granzymes) and cell-associated molecules such as cytotoxic T lymphocyte antigen 4 (CTLA4). However, in autoimmunity, chronically activated APCs under the influence of intracellular signaling pathways, such as phosphatidyl inositol 3 kinase, JAK-STAT, MAPK, and nuclear factor-κB pathways, can escape surveillance by Tregs, leading to the activation of T cells refractory to suppression by Tregs. Moreover, APCs and APC-derived inflammatory cytokines, such as tumor necrosis factor (TNF), IL-6, IL-1β, and IL-23 can render Tregs defective and can also reciprocally enhance the activity of the IL-17-producing pathogenic T-helper (Th)17 T cell subset. Th17 is a recently defined subset of CD4+ T cells distinct from the traditional subsets of Th1, Th2, and Treg cells. Emerging data on recall responses seen in vaccine studies and in pathogenesis of autoimmune diseases have suggested that Th17 plays an essential role in the host defense against extracellular bacteria and fungi. Designated Th17 cells selectively produce proinflammatory cytokines including IL-17, IL-21, and IL-22. In human cells, IL-1β, IL-6, and IL-23 promote human Th17 differentiation.

Deficiencies in Tregs development, functions, numbers, and T cell receptor repertoire are among the main factors contributing to autoimmunity pathogenesis in many (if not all) primary immunodeficiencies most frequently manifesting with autoimmune features.[23]

The immunodysregulation, polyendocrinopathy, enteropathy, X-linked (IPEX) syndrome is a rare disease, characterized by absence of Tregs and is due to a mutation in the Foxp-3 gene, resulting in the defective development of CD4+ CD25+ Tregs.[127] Disease manifestations are characterized by autoimmune enteritis, type 1 diabetes mellitus occurring during the first months of life, eczema, hypothyroidism, autoimmune hemolytic anemia, membranous nephropathy and recurrent infections. Patients presenting with IPEX syndrome usually die before the age of 2 years, unless allogeneic stem cell transplantation is performed.[128]

Autoimmune polyendocrinopathy-candidiasis-ectodermal dystrophy (APECED) syndrome is a recessive autosomal disease defined by at least two of the following symptoms: chronic cutaneo-mucous candidiasis, hypoparathyroidism, and Addison disease.[129] Candidiasis is usually the first clinical manifestation of the disease, occurring around the age of 5 years, followed in most cases by hypoparathyroidism before the age of 10 years and adrenocortical failure before the age of 15 years. Other organ-specific autoimmune manifestations encountered in this condition include hypothyroidism, hypogonadism, type 1 diabetes mellitus, autoimmune hepatitis, pernicious anemia, vitiligo, alopecia, primary biliary cirrhosis, and ectodermal dysplasia. APECED syndrome results from a defect in the autoimmune regulator (AIRE) gene. AIRE is involved in the expression of a variety of peripheral tissue antigens in medullary epithelial cells of the thymus.[130] In healthy individuals, AIRE increases the transcription of these antigens and allows the negative selection of self-reactive T cells leading to their deletion. Mice deficient in AIRE also show evidence of spontaneous organ-specific autoimmunity.

Natural Killer T Cells

NKT cells express a highly restricted repertoire of T cell receptors that recognize glycolipid antigens bound with the antigen-presenting molecule CD1d. NKT cells produce high amounts of immunomodulatory cytokines upon antigenic stimulation, which endows these cells with potent immunoregulatory properties giving protection against autoimmunity.[131-133] Consequently, NKT cells have been implicated in regulating a wide variety of immune responses, including immune responses against autoantigens. In patients and mice with a variety of autoimmune diseases, numbers and functions of NKT cells are disturbed.[134] Also, in some mouse models of autoimmunity such as collagen-induced-arthritis, NKT cell-deficiency exacerbates disease.[133]

Primary Humoral Immunodeficiencies

These antibody deficiency syndromes result from either impaired intrinsic B cell development or ineffective B cell responses to T cell-derived signals. The association of primary humoral immunodeficiencies and rheumatic disease is a well-known phenomenon.

Selective IgA Deficiency

Selective IgA deficiency (sIgA-D) is the most common primary immunodeficiency. In Western countries, the prevalence ranges between one in 330 and one in 2200 persons.[135-137] It is characterized by serum IgA levels of less than 0.01 to 0.05 g/L.[137] IgA is also absent in secretions, although the secretory component of IgA is normally present in saliva. Patients with sIgA-D identified by routine immunodiffusion assays have trace amounts of circulating IgA detectable by the more sensitive radioimmunoassay.[135] Although the term *sIgA-D* denotes an isolated deficiency of IgA, this Ig is also deficient in 20% of patients with IgG subclass deficiency and in 40% of patients with a defective antipolysaccharide antibody response. Antibodies of the IgM or the IgG class directed against IgA are commonly found in sera from patients with sIgA-D.[138]

The etiology of sIgA-D is largely unknown. Anti-IgA autoantibodies may play a role in the induction of IgA deficiency. This is supported by the observation that IgA deficiency is more common in children of affected mothers than in children of affected fathers.[139] Transplacental passage of maternal anti-IgA antibodies might interfere with the developing IgA system. That plasma cells producing anti-IgA could not be detected locally along the mucosal linings has led to the hypothesis that sIgA-D results from systemic exposure to endogenous anti-IgA. sIgA-D with anti-IgA antibodies could thus be regarded as an autoimmune disorder.[140] Moreover, such antibodies are more common in IgA-deficient patients with autoimmune and rheumatic diseases than in asymptomatic IgA-deficient patients. In the majority of patients, B cells expressing IgA on their surface and in the cytoplasm are still present in the blood, albeit in low numbers.[141] Exposure to an oral vaccine induces a normal mucosal immune response by B cells that secrete antigen-specific IgG or IgM. Nevertheless, a B cell maturation defect may be present because, in contrast with B cells of normal persons, B cells from IgA-deficient persons also express surface IgM and IgD.

Comparable with common variable immunodeficiency (CVID), T cellular proliferative responses to mitogens are decreased in a proportion of patients with IgA deficiency.[141] Both defective Th cell function and suppressor T cells inhibiting IgA production have been described. sIgA-D can be familial, and in some families an autosomal dominant inheritance pattern is found. The mother and three siblings of an IgA-deficient girl with JIA lacked serum IgA. The mother had very high levels of anti-IgA antibodies detected by a hemagglutination assay. The incidence of sIgA-D is increased in families of patients with CVID or hypogammaglobulinemia. sIgA-D may also precede CVID. As in CVID, a putative gene defect resides on chromosome 6 between the HLA-B and the HLA-DQ regions (see later), and an increased incidence in the TNFSR13B gene, encoding Transmembrane activator and CAML interactor (TACI), has been reported.[142,143]

sIgA-D is usually congenital and permanent, although transient cases have been described.[141] In some patients with JIA and sIgA-D, the IgA deficiency developed before antirheumatic drugs were prescribed.[144,145] Drug-induced IgA deficiency is well known, however. In particular, nonsteroidal antiinflammatory drugs such as diclofenac and sulfasalazine, parenteral gold, and D-penicillamine are associated with IgA deficiency that is sometimes reversible on discontinuation of the drug.[146,147]

DISEASE ASSOCIATIONS

The clinical spectrum varies from asymptomatic healthy persons to those with recurrent respiratory and gastrointestinal infections. The heterogeneity of this disorder

Table 42–6

Selective IgA Deficiency in patients with Rheumatic Diseases

Rheumatic Disease	Author	IgA deficient*	(%)
JIA-like arthritis	Cassidy[144,150]	18/477	(3.8)
	Panush et al[a]	3/176	(1.7)
	Pelkonen et al[b]	11/300	(3.7)
	Barkley et al[c]	2/582	(0.34)
	Salmi et al[d]	5/115	(4.3)
SLE	Cassidy et al[144]	10/50	(20.0)
Dermatomyositis	Cassidy et al[144]	3 patients	
Systemic scleroderma	Cassidy[e]	1/15	(6.7)
Ankylosing spondylitis	Cassidy et al[e]	2 patients	
MCTD	Cassidy et al[144]	1 patient	

*Number of IgA deficient patients/number of patients with specific rheumatic disease.
[a]Panush et al., Clin Exp Immunol 10 (1972) 103-115
[b]Pelkonen et al., Scand J Rheumatol 8 Suppl 1 (1975) 4
[c]Barkley et al., J Rheumatol 6 (1979)219-224
[d]Salmi et al., Ann Clin Res 5 (1973) 395-397
[e]Cassidy, in Moore TD., Arthritis in Childhood. Ross Conference 1981 p 82

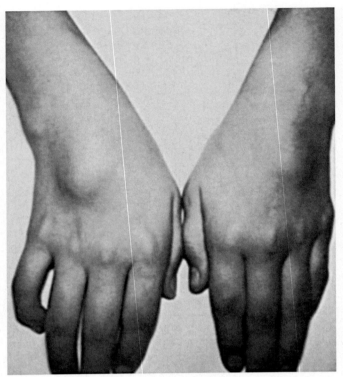

FIGURE 42–1 Hands of an 11-year-old girl with chronic arthritis, tenosynovitis, and selective immunoglobulin A deficiency. Hand and wrist involvement gradually returned to normal, but a minimally symptomatic effusion of her right knee persisted.

is further illustrated by a variety of associated diseases. Organ-specific autoimmune diseases are more frequent in patients with sIgA-D, in addition to those rheumatic diseases. The frequency of autoimmune disease as reported in large studies of IgA-deficient individuals ranges between 7% and 36%.[146-148] It has been established that among the rheumatic diseases JIA, SLE, and RA are most frequent (Table 42–6). In general, rheumatic diseases in these patients respond to conventional anti-rheumatic therapy.

Chronic Arthritis. The prevalence of sIgA-D in JIA varies from 2% to 4%.[142,148,149] In general, the clinical picture, sex ratio, and age at onset of arthritis do not differ from those in children with JIA and normal or elevated levels of IgA. The distribution of onset types is also similar: oligoarticular onset in 64%, polyarticular onset in 32%, and systemic onset in 4% (Figs. 42–1 to 42–3).[141,144] In the majority of patients, the course of the disease is mild and remains oligoarticular with little or no functional limitations. Erosive arthritis, however, has been described in up to 28%.[150] Patients with sIgA-D associated with oligoarticular JIA may be more prone to chronic uveitis and they have ANAs more frequently,[144] although this could not be confirmed in a study by Pelkonen and colleagues.[141]

Systemic Lupus Erythematosus. The prevalence of sIgA-D in patients with SLE is 1% to 4%, which is 20 to 30 times higher than that in the normal population.[136,148,151] In general, the clinical manifestations of SLE and the response to therapy do not differ between patients with or without sIgA-D, although in a series of 10 children with sIgA-D and SLE, there were more neuropsychiatric diseases but nephritis was absent.[152] Resolution of the sIgA-D has been described under intensive immunosuppressive

therapy, similar to low IgG-associated SLE and sIgA-D-associated JIA.[153]

Other Rheumatic Diseases. sIgA-D has been described sporadically in other systemic rheumatic diseases such as dermatomyositis, sarcoidosis, scleroderma, and ankylosing spondylitis.[148,154,155] However, these associations may merely reflect an ascertainment bias.

Hypogammaglobulinemia

The term *hypogammaglobulinemia* is applied to a number of disorders characterized by decreased levels of serum IgG and the inability to produce specific antibodies when exposed to an antigen. Unlike SCID and combined immunodeficiency, there are no severe T cell abnormalities although multiple abnormalities in the laboratory evaluations of T cells have been reported in patients with hypogammaglobulinemia. Among the primary hypogammaglobulinemias are X-linked agammaglobulinemia (Bruton agammaglobulinemia), CVID (also called *late-onset hypogammaglobulinemia*), and the hyper-IgM syndrome (Table 42–7). Clinical manifestations of hypogammaglobulinemia are recurrent pyogenic infections, often involving the respiratory tract, and an increased incidence of parasitic gastrointestinal infections. Non-infectious complications described are autoimmune manifestations, polyclonal lymphoid infiltration, enteropathy, and malignancies. Drug-induced hypogammaglobulinemia has been reported in patients exposed to various anti-convulsants and anti-rheumatic drugs.

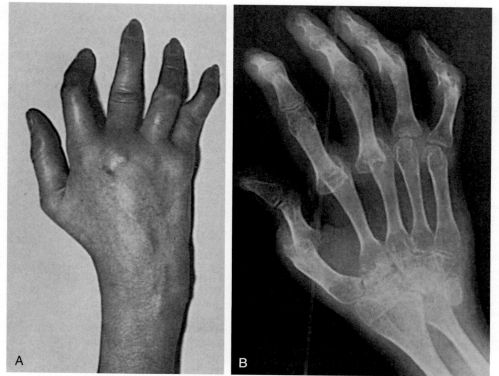

FIGURE 42–2   A, Hand of T. P. when 27-years-old. A chronic, deforming, erosive arthritis of the wrists and small joints of the hands was slowly progressive from the onset. These deformities and subluxation of metacarpophalangeal (MCP) joints are evident. The second proximal interphalangeal (PIP) joint had been surgically fused in a functional position. **B,** Hand of an 18-year-old girl with selective immunoglobulin A deficiency and systemic lupus erythematosus, with onset of arthritis at the age of 7-years-old. Destruction of joints is already far advanced, with subluxations of ulnar side of wrist, MCP joints 1 to 3, and PIP joints 4 and 5. Erosions, destruction of articulating surfaces, microfractures and bony collapse, and extreme juxtaarticular osteoporosis have occurred.

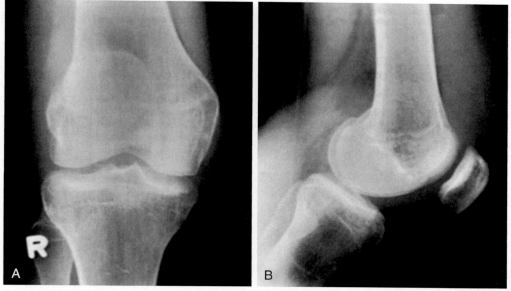

FIGURE 42–3   Radiographs of the knee of a patient with selective immunoglobulin A deficiency at 25-years-old. **A,** Anteroposterior view. **B,** Lateral view. Coarsening of the trabecular architecture and slight osteoporosis are evident, along with a moderate decrease in the cartilaginous space. There is sharpening of the tibial tubercles and the posterior aspect of the lateral femoral condyle. Erosions are not present despite 16 years of continuous joint effusion.

X-LINKED AGAMMAGLOBULINEMIA

X-linked agammaglobulinemia is characterized by recurrent severe bacterial infections from the age of 6 to 12 months onward.[156] Only males are affected with recurrent otitis media, pneumonia, meningitis, and septic arthritis mainly from extracellular encapsulated organisms such *as Streptococcus pneumoniae* and *Haemophilus influenzae*. The defective gene resides at Xq21.3-22 and causes defective production of Bruton tyronase kinase,

Table 42–7

Characteristics of hypogammaglobulinemia

Characteristic	X-linked	Common Variable
Sex	Males	Equal sex distribution
Genetics	X-linked recessive (Xq21.3-22)	Variable (? 6p21.3)
Age at onset of symptoms	6 mo to 2 yr	2 yr to adulthood
B lymphocytes	pre-B cell	B cell
Peripheral lymphoid tissue	Hypoplastic	Normal to enlarged
Plasma cells in nodes	Rare	Decreased or none
Surface immunoglobulins on B cells	Absent	Present
Serum IgG	<1 g/L	<5 g/L
Serum IgA, IgM	Very low	Variable
Natural antibodies	Very low	Variable
Specific antibodies	Absent	Variable (autoantibodies)
T lymphocytes	Numbers increased, subsets normal	Variable number and function
Clinical Characteristics		
Severe bacterial infections	Yes	Sometimes; less severe
Viral infections	Yes	Yes
Malabsorption	Sometimes	Frequent
Autoimmune diseases	No	Frequent
JIA-like arthritis	30%	Infrequent; frequency unknown
Control with Ig replacement	Partial	Partial

which leads to a block in B cell differentiation at the pre-B cell stage.[157] B cells are therefore absent. Serum IgG is usually less than 2 g/L; IgM, IgA, and IgE are absent. Patients should be treated with life-long Ig replacement therapy and should be treated vigorously with antibiotics for infections.

COMMON VARIABLE IMMUNODEFICIENCY

CVID is a heterogeneous primary immunodeficiency characterized by hypogammaglobulinemia and recurrent infections, predominantly by bacterial agents. Recurrent sinopulmonary infections often cause bronchiectasis, and an increased incidence of parasitic gut infections is observed. Apart from recurrent infections and their sequelae, CVID patients suffer from other disease-related complications in up to 45% of the cases. With respect to disease-related complications: CVID was recently divided into five distinct phenotypes, autoimmunity, enteropathy, polyclonal lymphoid infiltration, malignancies, or no complications.[158,159] Up to 87% of patients in this large patient cohort could be grouped into one of these groups. Autoimmunity is described in more detail later. Enteropathy includes different clinical entities; the majority of patients have polyclonal lymphocytic infiltration of the gut but increased incidences of sprue-like disease, inflammatory bowel disease, and several other entities have also been reported.[160] Patients with CVID have an increased risk (up to 10%) of malignancies of the lymphoid system or the gastrointestinal tract.[161,162] The category polyclonal infiltration includes granulomatous disease and may affect the spleen (resulting in splenomegaly), lungs, gastrointestinal tract, skin, and kidneys. The incidence of CVID is about five per 100,000. The age at onset varies from 1- to 71-years-old,[152-154] the majority of patients being between 30 and 45 years old at the onset of their disease. About 25% have onset before the age of 15 years.

Numerous immunological defects have been reported in CVID patients. The number of B lymphocytes in the peripheral blood of patients with CVID may be normal or decreased. Defects in early and late B cell differentiation, impaired upregulation of CD70 and CD86, impaired somatic hypermutation, and impaired antibody affinity maturation are among the defects described. When T cells from patients with CVID were co-cultured with normal B cells, normal Ig secretion was generally not depressed. Studies using B cell mitogens or soluble T cell factors confirmed that most B cells from patients with CVID could synthesize at least some Ig in the presence of an appropriate *in vitro* stimulus. Although this disease is regarded as an intrinsic B cell defect, distinct T cell abnormalities, including a decreased number of CD4+ T cells and decreased *in vitro* T lymphocyte proliferative responses to mitogens, have been reported.[161,163]

Several genetic defects have been described among CVID patients involving inducible costimulator (ICOS), CD19, CD21, CD81, transmembrane activator and calcium-modulator and cyclophilin ligand interactor (TACI), or B cell activating factor of the TNF family receptor (BAFF-R).[164-167] Except for ICOS, which is expressed on T cells and is involved in co-stimulation of B cells, all these gene the defects affect B cell surface receptors involved in activation and proliferation of B cells. Although defects in TACI have clearly been related to CVID, its role in the pathogenesis of CVID is unclear. Homozygous and compound heterozygous mutations have so far only been reported in affected patients; however, heterozygous TACI mutations have been reported in both affected and unaffected individuals. Mutations in TACI predispose to autoimmunity and other types of immune dysregulation; however, this relation is also likely to be influenced by other factors.[143] The current view is that heterozygous TACI mutations relate to increased susceptibility to CVID and to autoimmune diseases in CVID patients.

In the majority of patients (more than 85%), the precise B cell defect is still unknown, and the hypogammaglobulinemia may also result from a lack of appropriate T cell-derived stimulation necessary for normal B cell maturation, as is shown by the example of ICOS gene mutations.[168] Such a T cell abnormality may account for the observed predisposition of patients with CVID to malignancies and autoimmune disorders. A decreased number of T cells have been found in up to 30% of CVID patients.[163] In addition, an accelerated decline of thymic output with age has also been described, as shown by a more rapid decline of T cell receptor rearrangement excision circles (TRECS) and reduced numbers of CD31 positive recent thymic emigrants. Specifically, patient CD4+ cells produce less IL-2, possibly because of a selective defect in the ability to activate the IL-2 gene normally.[169] In addition, some patients with CVID have expanded activated (i.e., CD57+ and DR+) CD8+ populations, a pattern comparable with that in patients infected with cytomegalovirus, Epstein-Barr virus, or human immunodeficiency virus. It was thus speculated that a chronic viral infection in a genetically predisposed person could induce CVID (see later). A similar pathogenesis is thought to apply to the X-linked lymphoproliferative syndrome.

Autoimmune Disease. Autoimmune disease occurs in 20% to 30% of patients with CVID,[160,161] whereas there are only a few reports of autoimmune disease in X-linked agammaglobulinemia.[170] Thrombocytopenia and hemolytic anemia are most common.[171] The association of antibody-mediated autoimmunity and hypogammaglobulinemic states might seem contradictory but could be explained by defects in the anti-idiotypic network, which normally regulates expression of naturally occurring autoantibodies. The prevalence of arthritis in hypogammaglobulinemia ranges from 10% to 30%. It is divided into septic and aseptic forms.

Septic Arthritis. Septic arthritis, both with common and with rare microorganisms, occurs relatively frequently in patients with hypogammaglobulinemia.[169,172] Causative microorganisms are *Staphylococcus aureus*, *Streptococcus pneumoniae*, *Haemophilus influenzae*, *Mycobacteria* species, and *Mycoplasma* species (including *Ureaplasma*). *Mycoplasma* species are difficult to culture. Improved detection techniques (such as specific culture fluids, electron microscopy, polymerase chain reactions) may identify the presence of these microorganisms in a substantial number of cases that have heretofore been regarded as aseptic.[172,173]

Aseptic Arthritis. The association of rheumatic diseases and CVID or X-linked agammaglobulinemia is firmly established, with reported frequencies varying between 7% and 42% (see Table 42–7). In a large series of 103 patients with CVID, three were reported as having chronic arthritis similar to JIA, affecting one to four large peripheral joints.[161] Onset of arthritis is between ages 3 and 15 years, is often subtle, and is characterized by small to moderate effusions, soft tissue thickening, and limitation of motion (Figs. 42–4 and 42–5).[152] In about

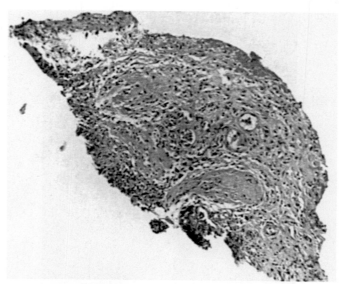

FIGURE 42–4   Needle biopsy of the synovium of R. B., who developed chronic synovitis of the left knee and was found to have common variable immunodeficiency. There is marked hypertrophy of the subsynovial layers with hyperplasia of vascular endothelium and compaction of collagen. A nonspecific infiltrate of mononuclear cells is visible, but there are no aggregations of round cells. Plasma cells are absent. Fibrin is present on the synovial surface. (From Petty RE, Cassidy JT, Tubergen DG: Association of arthritis with hypogammaglobulinemia, *Arthritis Rheum* 20: 441, 1977.)

50% of patients, arthritis is the presenting symptom.[174] In the remainder, arthritis is preceded by several years of infectious complications. Uluhan described a patient with a systemic-onset JIA and CVID.[175] This patient later developed neutropenia (found in up to 10% of patients with CVID and X-linked agammaglobulinemia), autoimmune hemolytic anemia, and a cellular immune deficiency. Despite Ig infusions, the patient died at the age of 22-years-old from infection.

Other Rheumatic Diseases. Whereas the prevalence of sIgA-D in patients with SLE is 20 to 30 times higher than that in the normal population, there is no marked association of hypogammaglobulinemia and SLE. To date, only nine cases of SLE with persistent hypogammaglobulinemia have been described.[176-178] After a 24 year disease history of SLE, one patient developed fatal extrapulmonary tuberculosis.[176,179] Cronin reported on 18 patients who developed low Ig G levels following the diagnosis of SLE.[153] There was no significant proteinuria that could account for a loss of Ig. The low IgG was transient in 10 patients and related to cytotoxic drugs in eight. Only four had recurrent infections. This low number suggests that the association of SLE and CVID may be coincidental. It is also difficult to understand an association of an autoimmune disease such as SLE, where B cell activation, elevated serum IgG, and circulating immune complexes are prominent, with another disorder characterized by deficient antibody production.

Dermatomyositis-Like Syndrome. There is considerable doubt that the dermatomyositis-like syndrome that sometimes complicates hypogammaglobulinemia has

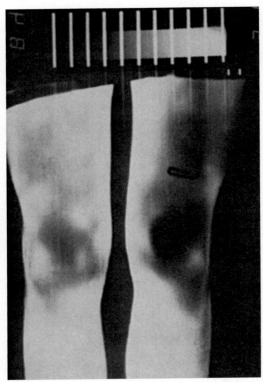

FIGURE 42–5 Thermograph of the knees of R. B. at 20-years–old show increased heat production on the left knee, the site of the inflammatory arthritis. (The paper clip on the left leg is used for standardization in thermography.)

the same pathogenesis as idiopathic dermatomyositis of childhood. It is characterized by subcutaneous edema, myalgia, muscle wasting, and sometimes polyarthritis followed by contractures of large joints. It is not clear whether the myopathy is proximal, distal, or diffuse in most instances. Cutaneous manifestations include heliotrope discoloration of the eyelids, rash on the extensor surfaces of the metacarpophalangeal and proximal interphalangeal joints, and sometimes a nonspecific rash. Electromyographic evidence of a myopathy was documented in one patient, and abnormalities on muscle biopsy consistent with a diagnosis of dermatomyositis were present in seven. Central nervous system disease and deafness frequently accompanied the myositis, and a fatal outcome was common. Other associations have also been described, including leukemia and lymphoma. Viral isolations (e.g., echovirus, adenovirus) from the cerebrospinal fluid and sometimes from muscle and other sites raise the question of a viral etiology of this syndrome and support a role for persistent latent viral infection in its pathogenesis.[155] A direct relation to idiopathic dermatomyositis remains unproven, however, in spite of speculations on its viral cause. One patient was successfully treated with IVIG.

IgG SUBCLASS DEFICIENCIES AND RHEUMATIC DISEASES

The availability of specific antisera for the IgG subclasses has enabled the detection of subclass deficiencies in a wide variety of normal and abnormal conditions.[180,181]

A 10-year-old boy with JRA and Hodgkin disease had low concentrations of IgA (0.19 g/L) and IgG2 (0.02 g/L). Another 10-year-old boy had SLE, undetectable IgA, and an IgG2 concentration of 0.02 g/L. Heiner and colleagues found low IgG4 levels (<30 mg/L) in 12 of 112 patients with "disseminated collagen vascular disease" but provided no further details.[182] Aucouturier and associates reported 450 patients with subclass deficiencies.[183] IgG2 deficiency was associated most frequently with vasculitis and cytopenias.[183,184] Another study found an increased frequency of Henoch-Schönlein purpura and glomerulonephritis.[174]

Hyper-IgE syndrome

Hyper-IgE syndrome is a primary immunodeficiency with recurrent pneumonia with pneumatocele formation, eczema, elevated Ig E, eosinophilia, vasculitis, erythema nodosum, and central nervous system symptoms.[102,185,186] Rarely, autoimmune manifestations are described.[187] It must be differentiated from the Omenn syndrome, which is associated with very high IgE levels and a severe T cell deficiency.

REFERENCES

7. F. Rieux-Laucat, F. Le Deist, C. Hivroz, et al., Mutations in Fas associated with human lymphoproliferative syndrome and autoimmunity, Science 268 (1995) 1347–1349.
8. A. Fischer, M. Cavazzana-Calvo, B.G. De Saint, et al., Naturally occurring primary deficiencies of the immune system, Annu. Rev. Immunol. 15 (1997) 93–124.
10. J.B. Oliveira, S. Gupta, Disorders of apoptosis: Mechanisms for autoimmunity in primary immunodeficiency diseases, J. Clin. Immunol. 28 (2008) S20–S28.
11. U. Dianzani, A. Chiocchetti, U. Ramenghi, Role of inherited defects decreasing Fas function in autoimmunity, Life Sci. 72 (2003) 2803–2824.
21. M.F. Roelofs, S. Abdollahi-Roodsaz, L.A.B. Joosten, et al., The orchestra of toll-like receptors and their potential role in frequently occurring rheumatic conditions, Arthritis Rheum. 58 (2008) 338–348.
22. D. Foell, H. Wittkowski, J. Roth, Mechanisms of Disease: a 'DAMP' view of inflammatory arthritis, Nat. Clin. Pract. Rheumatol. 3 (2007) 382–390.
23. T.M. Brusko, A.L. Putnam, J.A. Bluestone, Human regulatory T cells: role in autoimmune disease and therapeutic opportunities, Immunol. Rev. 223 (2008) 371–390.
25. H. Wittkowski, M. Frosch, N. Wulffraat, et al., S100A12 is a novel molecular marker differentiating systemic-onset juvenile idiopathic arthritis from other causes of fever of unknown origin, Arthritis Rheum. 58 (2008) 3924–3931.
26. D. Foell, H. Wittkowski, I. Hammerschmidt, et al., Monitoring neutrophil activation in juvenile rheumatoid arthritis by S100A12 serum concentrations, Arthritis Rheum. 50 (2004) 1286–1295.
30. D. Roos, X-CGDbase: a database of X-CGD-causing mutations, Immunol. Today 17 (1996) 517–521.
39. S.S. De Ravin, N. Naumann, E.W. Cowen, et al., Chronic granulomatous disease as a risk factor for autoimmune disease, J. Allergy. Clin. Immunol. 122 (2008) 1097–1103.
53. M.J. Walport, Complement and systemic lupus erythematosus, Arthritis Res. 43 (2002) S279–S293.
54. G. Bussone, L. Mouthon, Autoimmune manifestations in primary immune deficiencies, Autoimmun. Rev. 8 (2009) 332–336.
55. A. Coutinho, M. Carneiro-Sampaio, Primary immunodeficiencies unravel critical aspects of the pathophysiology of autoimmunity and of the genetics of autoimmune disease, J. Clin. Immunol. 28 (2008) S4–S10.
82. M. Carneiro-Sampaio, B.L. Liphaus, A.A. Jesus, et al., Understanding systemic lupus erythematosus physiopathology in the light of primary immunodeficiencies, J. Clin. Immunol. 28 (2008) S34–S41.

97. R.S. Geha, L.D. Notarangelo, J.L. Casanova, et al., Primary immunodeficiency diseases: An update from the International Union of Immunological Societies Primary Immunodeficiency Diseases Classification Committee, J. Allergy Clin. Immunol. 120 (2007) 776–794.

98. R.H. Buckley, Primary immunodeficiency diseases due to defects in lymphocytes, N. Engl. J. Med. 343 (2000) 1313–1324.

99. J.W. Sleasman, The association between immunodeficiency and the development of autoimmune disease, Adv. Dent. Res. 10 (1996) 57–61.

103. A. Fischer, Human primary immunodeficiency diseases: a perspective, Nat. Immunol. 5 (2004) 23–30.

107. N. Sakaguchi, T. Takahashi, H. Hata, et al., Altered thymic T-cell selection due to a mutation of the ZAP-70 gene causes autoimmune arthritis in mice, Nature 426 (2003) 454–460.

108. S. Hori, T. Takahashi, S. Sakaguchi, Control of autoimmunity by naturally arising regulatory CD4+ T cells, Adv. Immunol. 81 (2003) 331–371.

117. H. Ozsahin, M. Cavazzana-Calvo, L.D. Notarangelo, et al., Long-term outcome following hematopoietic stem-cell transplantation in Wiskott-Aldrich syndrome: collaborative study of the European Society for Immunodeficiencies and European Group for Blood and Marrow Transplantation, Blood 111 (2008) 439–445.

120. P. Pelkonen, P. Lahdenne, R. Lantto, et al., Chronic arthritis associated with chromosome deletion 22q11.2 syndrome, J. Rheumatol. 29 (2002) 2648–2650.

126. S. Andre, D.F. Tough, S. Lacroix-Desmazes, et al., Surveillance of antigen-presenting cells by CD4+CD25+regulatory T cells in autoimmunity immunopathogenesis and therapeutic implications, Am. J. Pathol. 174 (2009) 1575–1587.

127. T.R. Torgerson, H.D. Ochs, Immune dysregulation, polyendocrinopathy, enteropathy, X-linked: Forkhead box protein 3 mutations and lack of regulatory T cells, J. Allergy Clin. Immunol. 120 (2007) 744–750.

129. E. Lindh, S.M. Lind, E. Lindmark, et al., AIRE regulates T-cell-independent B-cell responses through BAFF, Proc. Natl. Acad. Sci. U.S.A. 105 (2008) 18466–18471.

131. L. Wu, L. Van Kaer, Natural killer T Cells and autoimmune disease, Curr. Mol. Med. 9 (2009) 4–14.

135. J.T. Cassidy, G. Oldham, T.A. Platts-Mills, Functional assessment of a B cell defect in patients with selective IgA deficiency, Clin. Exp. Immunol. 35 (1979) 296–305.

141. P. Pelkonen, E. Savilahti, A.L. Makela, Persistent and transient IgA deficiency in juvenile rheumatoid arthritis, Scand. J. Rheumatol. 12 (1983) 273–279.

148. C.M.A. Jacob, A.C. Pastorino, K. Fahl, et al., Autoimmunity in IgA deficiency: Revisiting the role of IgA as a silent housekeeper, J. Clin. Immunol. 28 (2008) S56–S61.

152. R.E. Petty, J.T. Cassidy, D.G. Tubergen, Association of arthritis with hypogammaglobulinemia, Arthritis Rheum. 20 (1977) 441–445.

160. C. Cunningham-Rundles, Autoimmune manifestations in common variable immunodeficiency, J. Clin. Immunol. 28 (2008) S42–S45.

161. C. Cunningham-Rundles, Clinical and immunologic analyses of 103 patients with common variable immunodeficiency, J. Clin. Immunol. 9 (1989) 22–33.

166. M.C. van Zelm, I. Reisli, M. van der Burg, et al., An antibody-deficiency syndrome due to mutations in the CD19 gene, N. Engl. J. Med. 354 (2006) 1901–1912.

171. C. Cunningham-Rundles, Hematologic complications of primary immune deficiencies, Blood Rev. 16 (2002) 61–64.

172. S. Itescu, Adult immunodeficiency and rheumatic disease, Rheum. Dis. Clin. North Am. 22 (1996) 53–73.

173. A.H. Lee, A.I. Levinson, H.R. Schumacher Jr., Hypogammaglobulinemia and rheumatic disease, Semin. Arthritis Rheum. 22 (1993) 252–264.

177. M. Fernandez-Castro, S. Mellor-Pita, M.J. Citores, et al., Common variable immunodeficiency in systemic lupus erythematosus, Semin. Arthritis Rheum. 36 (2007) 238–245.

Entire reference list is available online at www.expertconsult.com.

Chapter 43

PERIODIC FEVER SYNDROMES AND OTHER INHERITED AUTOINFLAMMATORY DISEASES

Karyl Barron, Balu Athreya, and Daniel Kastner

Fever is one of the most common signs of illness in children. Most episodes are acute, of short duration, and usually caused by upper respiratory infections. When febrile episodes are prolonged beyond two to three weeks, infection is still the most common etiological factor. However, after acute infectious causes and conditions such as chronic infections have been excluded, rheumatic illnesses and malignancy enter the differential diagnosis.

Repeated febrile episodes lasting for a few days to a few weeks are common in young children attending day care centers and kindergarten. Such episodes are often caused by repeated viral infections, although parents frequently worry about immune system defects. Infections in immunodeficient children are often caused by unusual or opportunistic pathogens. Immunocompromised children often develop failure to thrive and other clinical signs of underlying pathology. Frequent localization of infections to the same organ system should raise the suspicion of anatomical defects.

If repeated infections due to immunodeficiency or organ malformations can be excluded, unexplained bouts of fever with a characteristic frequency and constellation of symptoms fall under the term *recurrent* or *periodic fever syndrome*. Such disorders are defined as three or more episodes of unexplained fever in a six-month period, occurring at least seven days apart.[1] These conditions may demonstrate strict periodicity or recur with varying intervals between attacks. Specific genetic mutations have been linked to some syndromes, although the etiology of others remains obscure. With increasing understanding of the genetics and pathophysiology of innate immunity and inflammation, the clinical concepts of periodic fever syndromes may change.

HEREDITARY AUTOINFLAMMATORY SYNDROMES

The term *autoinflammatory* has been used to describe a group of illnesses characterized by attacks of seemingly unprovoked inflammation without significant levels of either autoantibodies or antigen-specific T cells more characteristic of autoimmune disease.[2-8] The hereditary periodic fever syndromes, a group of Mendelian disorders manifesting with recurrent fever and inflammation, were the first illnesses to be classified as autoinflammatory, but there are now several other Mendelian autoinflammatory diseases. A key insight has been the recognition that the autoinflammatory syndromes represent disorders of the innate immune system. In contrast to adaptive immunity, which is based upon lymphocytes and receptors that rearrange and mutate somatically, the innate immune system is phylogenetically more ancient, based on myeloid cells and hard-wired receptors for pathogen-associated molecular patterns. In general, the more classically recognized autoimmune diseases, such as systemic lupus erythematosus, are disorders of adaptive immunity, although the Mendelian autoinflammatory diseases are inborn errors of innate immunity. Advances in our understanding of the autoinflammatory diseases have sometimes come hand-in-hand with advances in immunomodulatory therapy and have given an added stimulus to research in this area. The recent identification of a deficiency in interleukin-1 (IL-1) receptor antagonist (DIRA) is a case in point.[9,10]

The range of autoinflammatory diseases has expanded to include several other diseases, such as gout, systemic onset juvenile idiopathic arthritis, and Behçet's disease, which are currently not considered simple Mendelian hereditary syndromes, but may in fact prove to have a polygenic origin.[8] Discussed in this chapter are nine distinct disorders grouped among the hereditary auto-inflammatory syndromes, based on clinical findings and Mendelian patterns of inheritance (Table 43–1). Several of these have been termed *hereditary periodic fevers*, but Table 43–2 reclassifies these syndromes based on the current understanding of innate immunity and the inflammasome, a protein complex containing caspases involved in the proteolytic cleavage of IL-1 precursors to produce active forms of IL-1.[11]

Familial Mediterranean Fever

Genetics and Pathogenesis

Familial Mediterranean Fever (FMF) is the most common Mendelian autoinflammatory syndrome, resulting from autosomal recessive mutations in the *MEFV*

(MEditerranean FeVer) locus.[12,13] This disorder occurs most frequently among Sephardi and Ashkenazi Jewish, Arab, Armenian, Italian, and Turkish populations, with carrier frequencies as high as 1:3 to 1:5 in population-based surveys.[14-19] FMF occurs at lower frequencies in other populations and ethnicities.[14,15,20-26]

MEFV is comprised of 10 exons encoding a 781 amino acid protein called pyrin (after the Greek for fever) or marenostrin (after the Latin for the Mediterranean Sea), expressed primarily in the innate immune system, including granulocytes, cytokine-activated monocytes, dendritic cells, and serosal and synovial fibroblasts.[27] The N-terminal domain of pyrin defines a motif, called the pyrin domain (PYD), which is similar to the structure of the death domain (DD), death effector domains (DEDs), and the caspase recruitment domains (CARDs).[28-32] Through homotypical domain interactions, pyrin binds the apoptosis-associated speck-like protein with a CARD (ASC)[4,33-37] and participates in at least three important cellular processes: apoptosis, recruitment, and activation of procaspase-1 (also known as IL-1β converting enzyme),[34,38-41] with associated processing and secretion of IL-1 and IL-18; and activation of the nuclear factor-κB transcription factor.[4,33-36,42,43] Depending on experimental conditions, wild-type pyrin has been found either to inhibit or accentuate caspase-1 activity through the interaction of its N-terminal PYD with ASC, a key molecule in the inflammasome. Pyrin also inhibits caspase-1 activation through a second interaction involving the binding of its C-terminal B30.2 domain to the catalytic domains of caspase-1.[44] The net effect of pyrin, and the molecular mechanisms of FMF-associated mutations, remains controversial.[8] Until recently, the recessive inheritance of FMF, combined with data from animal models and biochemical studies,[34] seemed to support a model in which FMF is caused by loss-of-function mutations in an antiinflammatory molecule. Recent genetic data on FMF patients with only a single demonstrable mutation,[45] taken together with newer data on animal models, suggest that FMF may actually result from gain-of-function mutations in a proinflammatory molecule.[8] In either case, mutations

Table 43–1
Inheritance patterns of the hereditary autoinflammatory syndromes
Autosomal Dominant Pattern
Tumor necrosis factor receptor-associated periodic syndrome (TRAPS)
Familial cold autoinflammatory syndrome (FCAS)
Muckle-Wells syndrome (MWS)
Neonatal onset multisystem inflammatory disease (NOMID), also called chronic infantile neurological cutaneous and articular syndrome (CINCA)
Cyclic hematopoiesis (CH), also called cyclical neutropenia (CN)
Pyogenic arthritis, pyoderma gangrenosum, and acne syndrome (PAPA)
Autosomal Recessive Pattern
Familial Mediterranean fever (FMF)
Hyperimmunoglobulinemia D with periodic fever syndrome (HIDS)
Deficiency of interleukin-1 receptor antagonist (DIRA)

Table 43–2		
Classification of the hereditary periodic fever syndromes[a]		
Disease	**Gene (chromosome)**	**Protein (synonyms)**
IL-1β Activation Disorders (inflammasomopathies)		
Familial Mediterranean fever (FMF)	*MEFV* (16p13.3)	Pyrin (marenostrin)
Hyperimmunoglobulin D with periodic fever syndrome (HIDS)	*MVK* (12q24)	Mevalonate kinase
Familial cold autoinflammatory syndrome (FCAS), Muckle-Wells syndrome (MWS) Neonatal-onset multisystem inflammatory disease (NOMID)/Chronic infantile neurological cutaneous and articular syndrome (CINCA)	*NLRP3/CIAS1* (1q44)	Nucleotide-binding domain, leucine-rich repeat, and pyrin domain containing protein (NALP3, Cryopyrin, PYPAF1)
Pyogenic arthritis, pyoderma gangrenosum, and acne (PAPA)	*PSTPIP1* (15q24-25.1)	Proline serine threonine phosphatase-interacting protein (PSTPIP1); CD2-binding protein (CD2BP1)
Deficiency of the interleukin-1 receptor antagonist (DIRA)	*IL1RN* (2q14.2)	IL-1Ra
Protein Folding Disorders of the Innate Immune System		
TNF receptor-associated periodic syndrome (TRAPS)	*TNFRSF1A* (12p13)	TNF receptor superfamily 1A (TNFRSF1A, TNFR1, p55, CD120a)

[a]Adapted from reference 8.

appear to result in increased IL-1β activation and accentuated innate immune activation, and in fact there are anecdotal reports of favorable responses to IL-1 inhibition in FMF patients who cannot tolerate or do not respond to conventional therapy.[44,46]

Clinical Manifestations

The first clinical episode usually occurs during childhood or adolescence, with 90% of patients having had onset by age 20-years-old (Table 43–3).[26,47-50] There is often a modest male predominance.[47,48,51] FMF attacks last between 12 and 72 hours and consist of inflammation involving the peritoneum, pleura, joints, or skin, sometimes in combination. Between episodes, patients usually feel completely well and remain so for a few days to a few months. In children, fever may be the only sign of FMF, although other symptoms generally develop progressively with time.[49] The attacks vary not only between patients but also between episodes in a given affected individual.[52] The exact mechanism of triggering periodic attacks in FMF is unclear, with patients often noting menstruation or stress associated with the onset of an attack.

Abdominal symptoms often accompany the fever and range from mild discomfort and distention to severe pain with rigidity.[14,47,50] Constipation is more common than diarrhea, and in extreme cases, peristalsis may cease and result in paralytic ileus. Pain can be generalized or focused in a quadrant, sometimes mimicking acute appendicitis. Pleural pain is generally unilateral, occurring with decreased breath sounds. Less commonly, a small effusion, friction rub, or atelectasis may be present.[53]

Joint manifestations are common and are sometimes the first sign of the disease in children.[54] Arthralgia occurs more frequently than arthritis. Arthritis in adults usually is monoarticular, although children may have involvement of several joints, symmetrically or asymmetrically, with pain and large effusions.[14,50,55] Synovial aspirates from joints are sterile but may demonstrate leukocyte counts as high as 100,000/mm.[3] Rarely, in the precolchicine era, arthritis in the knees and hip may have had a protracted course.[56] In these cases, radiographical changes may have included severe juxtaarticular osteoporosis, erosions, and osteonecrosis. Muscle pain is a classical manifestation of FMF and occurs in about 20% of patients.[57] Usually the pain is not severe, appears in the lower extremities after physical exertion, mostly in the evenings, lasts from a few hours to two to three days, and subsides with rest. Treatment with nonsteroidal antiinflammatory drugs (NSAIDs) may be needed. Protracted febrile myalgia is an uncommon dramatic manifestation of FMF and requires treatment with corticosteroids.[57,58] It is important to differentiate colchicine-induced myopathy, a rare side effect, from an attack of prolonged febrile myalgia, an even rarer disease manifestation. Fever, high erythrocyte sedimentation rate (ESR), normal creatine kinase (CPK) levels, and the evidence of inflammatory myopathy on electromyogram (EMG) should help rule out colchicine as a likely causative factor.[57]

Cutaneous findings are less common than serosal or synovial involvement. Most commonly, there is an erysipeloid erythematous rash on the dorsum of the foot, ankle, or lower leg.[14,50,59,60] The rash may occur alone or in conjunction with other manifestations. Biopsies of the rash are characterized by a prominent mixed cellular infiltrate.[60]

Findings less commonly associated with FMF include episodes of unilateral acute scrotal pain in prepubescent boys[50,61,62] and diverse cutaneous manifestations including Henoch-Schönlein purpura.[47,50,63,64] Rarely, pericarditis is observed.[65] Behçet's disease,[66-68] polyarteritis nodosa,[69,70] microscopic polyarteritis,[71] and glomerulonephritis[72,73] may occur more frequently in FMF patients than in the general population. Although headache and febrile seizures may occur in pediatric patients, other neurological symptoms are rare. There may also be a higher than expected frequency of inflammatory bowel disorders among FMF patients.[74,75]

Laboratory Investigations

During attacks, concentrations of acute phase reactants such as C-reactive protein (CRP), serum amyloid A (SAA), and complement increase. Leukocytosis and an increased ESR are commonly observed.[14]

The continuous elevation of these acute phase serum proteins during and even between attacks[76-78] predisposes to the development of AA systemic amyloidosis, the most serious sequela of FMF (Fig. 43–1). SAA deposition occurs in several organs, including the gastrointestinal tract, spleen, kidneys, adrenals, thyroid, and lungs, but usually not the tongue, peripheral nerves, or heart.[47] Renal failure occurred by the age of 40 in many patients before effective treatment was available. The risk of amyloidosis increases with a positive family history of this complication, male sex, the α/α genotype at the SAA1 locus, and poor compliance with colchicine therapy.[79-82] In most studies, homozygosity for the M694V mutation also predisposes patients to amyloidosis, to arthritis, and to erysipeloid erythema,[54,80,83-85] although the M694V association with amyloidosis has not been observed universally.[86] For reasons not clear, the country of origin influences the phenotype of FMF and is a key risk factor for amyloidosis in FMF,[87,88] with a decreased incidence of amyloidosis in patients living in the United States. An early indicator of impaired renal function is microalbuminuria, and periodic urinalyses are an important part of continuing care for FMF patients. After proteinuria occurs, amyloidosis can be confirmed by biopsy of the kidney or rectum. Although kidney biopsy is more sensitive, rectal biopsy is preferred because it is safer, less invasive, and still has a sensitivity of 75%.[89]

Diagnosis

The clinical diagnosis of FMF is based on the presence of short (12 to 72 hours), recurrent (three or more) febrile episodes, with abdominal, chest, joint, or skin manifestations and no discernible infectious cause.[90,91] Appropriate ethnicity, positive family history, onset before the age of 20-years-old and a favorable response to colchicine also support the diagnosis.

Because physicians in the Western Hemisphere are not as familiar with FMF as clinicians in regions with a higher prevalence, genetic testing has become a valuable adjunct to clinical diagnosis, especially in North America and Europe. More than 70 mutations have been described in MEFV[12-13] (http://fmf.igh.cnrs.fr/infevers/),

Table 43-3

Clinical, demographical, and genetic features of Mendelian autoinflammatory diseases

	FMF	TRAPS	HIDS	FCAS	MWS	NOMID/CINCA	PAPA	DIRA
Inheritance	Autosomal recessive	Autosomal dominant	Autosomal recessive	Autosomal dominant	Autosomal dominant	Autosomal dominant or de novo	Autosomal dominant	Autosomal recessive
Ethnicity	Jewish, Arab, Turkish, Armenian, Italian	Any ethnic group	Dutch, French, other European	Mostly European	Northern European	Any ethnic group	Any ethnic group	Newfoundland, Puerto Rico, Netherlands, Lebanon
Chromosome	16p13	12p13	12q24	1q44	1q44	1q44	15q24	2q14.2
Gene	MEFV	TNFRSF1A	MVK	CIAS1	CIAS1	CIAS1	PSTPIP1/CD2BP1	IL1RN
Protein	Pyrin/marenostrin	TNFRSF1A	Mevalonate kinase	Cryopyrin	Cryopyrin	Cryopyrin	CD2-binding protein 2	Interleukin-1-receptor antagonist
Duration of episode	1-3 days	often >7 days	3-7 days	Usually <24 hours	2-3 days	Almost continuous, with exacerbations	Variable	Almost continuous
Cutaneous	Erysipeloid erythema	Migratory rash, underlying myalgia	Nonmigratory maculopapular rash; vasculitis	Cold-induced urticaria-like rash	Urticaria-like rash	Urticaria-like rash	Cystic acne; pyoderma gangrenosum	Pustulosis, pathergy
Abdominal	Peritonitis, constipation > diarrhea	Peritonitis, diarrhea or constipation	Severe pain, vomiting, diarrhea >constipation, rarely peritonitis	Nausea	Sometimes abdominal pain	Uncommon	None	Not reported
Serositis	Frequent	Frequent	Rare	Not seen	Rare	Rare	Not seen	Not seen
Joints	Monoarthritis, occasionally protracted in knees or hip	Arthralgia, arthritis in large joints	Arthralgia, polyarthritis	Polyarthralgia	Polyarthralgia, oligoarthritis	Epiphysial overgrowth, contractures, intermittent or chronic arthritis	Pyogenic, sterile arthritis	Neonatal onset sterile multifocal osteomyelitis, periostitis
Ocular	Uncommon	Conjunctivitis, periorbital edema	Uncommon	Conjunctivitis	Conjunctivitis, episcleritis	Conjunctivitis, uveitis, optic disc changes, vision loss	Not reported	Conjunctival injection reported
Distinctive features	Monoarthritis, peritonitis, erysipelas-like rash	Migratory myalgia and erythema and periorbital edema	Cervical adenopathy and aphthous ulcers	Cold-induced urticaria-like rash	Sensorineural hearing loss	Aseptic meningitis and arthropathy	Scarring cystic acne, PG, and pyogenic sterile arthritis	Multifocal osteomyelitis, periostitis, pustulosis
Vasculitis	HSP, polyarteritis nodosa	HSP, lymphocytic vasculitis	Cutaneous vasculitis, rarely HSP	Not seen	Not seen	Occasional	Not seen	Uncommon
Amyloidosis	Variable risk depending on MEFV, SAA genotypes, family history, gender, residence, compliance	Occurs in 10%	Rare	Uncommon	Occurs in 25%	May develop in portion of patients	Not reported	Not reported

FMF, familial Mediterranean fever; TRAPS, tumor necrosis factor receptor-associated periodic syndrome; HIDS, hyperimmunoglobulineia D with periodic fever syndrome; FCAS, familial cold autoinflammatory syndrome; MWS, Muckle-Wells syndrome; NOMID/CINCA, neonatal onset multisystem inflammatory disease, also called chronic infantile neurologic cutaneous and articular syndrome; PAPA, pyogenic arthritis with pyoderma gangrenosum and acne; HSP, Henoch-Schönlein Purpura DIRA, deficiency of the interleukin-1-receptor antagonist.

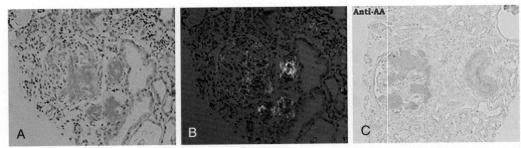

FIGURE 43–1 Amyloidosis in the kidney of an FMF patient. **A,** Stained with Congo red, viewed under nonpolarized light. **B,** The same field as in A, but viewed under polarizing light. **C,** Stained with a monoclonal antibody to serum amyloid A. (Courtesy of Dr. James E. Balow)

with the majority of mutations being missense changes and more than one half clustering in exons 2 and 10.[92] A subset of *MEFV* mutations (usually E148Q in exon 2 and M680I, M694V, and V726A in exon 10) may account for as many as 80% of FMF cases in classically affected populations.[21] Based on an autosomal recessive mode of inheritance, patients with FMF were expected to be homozygous for a single mutation or heterozygous for two different mutations. However, the reality is not always that simple. Certain mutations, most notably the substitution of alanine for valine at residue 726 (V726A) and the substitution of glutamine for glutamic acid at position 148 (E148Q), are sometimes found in cis in so-called complex alleles,[15,21] and it is possible for some patients to have three or even four demonstrable mutations. E148Q, P369S, and R408Q, which may also be inherited in Cis, are found at 1% or greater allele frequency in certain populations and may therefore represent functional polymorphisms.[8] Depending on the laboratory, DNA samples are often screened only for the most common mutations, and patients with rare mutations therefore may appear to have no mutations or only one. Even complete sequencing of *MEFV* exon 10 (where most mutations lie) will fail to diagnose patients with mutations in other regions of the gene. Sequencing of the entire *MEFV* coding sequence fails to identify any abnormalities in a small number of patients who respond well to colchicine and exhibit FMF symptoms, suggesting that there may be more than one gene causing FMF.[93,94] To further complicate the issue, some rare mutations appear inherited in a dominant fashion,[95] and approximately 30% of patients with clinical signs of FMF have only one demonstrable mutation,[15,83,94-98] despite complete sequencing of the coding region of *MEFV*.[45] A diagnosis of FMF should never be excluded based solely on the results of genetic testing. However, the clinical and ethnic spectra of FMF have definitely expanded with the availability of genetic testing,[14] suggesting that a combination of clinical evaluation with genetic testing for selected patients is the most sensible diagnostic approach.

Treatment

Colchicine therapy is highly effective for most patients in preventing febrile episodes and systemic amyloidosis.[50,99-101] Approximately 95% of patients demonstrate a marked improvement in symptoms, whereas almost 75% have a near-complete remission. Continuous therapy is generally more effective in controlling the attacks of FMF than intermittent treatment at the time of attacks, and daily therapy has the important added benefit of reducing the subclinical inflammation between episodes that potentially leads to amyloidosis.[76-78,102] Colchicine may have a number of beneficial actions in FMF, including its well-documented effects on the expression of adhesion molecules and on leukocyte migration.

Colchicine is generally safe in children, although colchicine pharmacokinetics may differ in younger patients, and doses adjusted for body weight may be greater in children than those used in adults may. The recommended adult colchicine dose is 1.2 to 1.8 mg/day given by mouth. Dosage should be started as low as possible (one half of a 0.6-mg tablet once daily in children) and slowly increased, titrating to maximize efficacy and minimize side effects, but usually not exceeding 1.8 mg/day in single or divided doses.[103,104] A gradual increase in dose often prevents or lessens diarrhea, the most common adverse effect. Some patients develop lactose intolerance due to colchicine, and a lactose-free diet may help to control gastrointestinal symptoms. In children with FMF, development of myopathy with progressive proximal muscle weakness and generalized myalgia is rarely observed on regular dosage.[101] Bone marrow alterations (hemolytic or aplastic anemia, pancytopenia, neutropenia, and thrombocytopenia) have been reported in cases of acute intoxication but are rarely observed in the usual doses given orally. Toxicity is more common with intravenous therapy and when given together with other drugs that are metabolized by CYP3A4 such as erythromycin and cimetidine.[105,106] There are no established alternatives in patients who are unresponsive to or cannot tolerate therapeutic doses of colchicine, although the role of pyrin, the FMF protein, in cytokine regulation suggests a possible future role for IL-1 inhibitors.[44,46]

Outcome and Prognosis

Among FMF patients with end-stage renal amyloidosis, the survival rate on hemodialysis is lower than among age-matched dialysis patients perhaps because of poor vascular access and hemodynamic instability.[107-109] Studies have confirmed little difference in patient and graft survival between FMF and control kidney transplant recipients.[110] Transplantation (with oral colchicine administration to prevent amyloidosis in the transplanted kidney) is the preferred treatment for renal failure.

Tumor Necrosis Factor Receptor-Associated Periodic Syndrome

One of the first clinical descriptions of tumor necrosis factor receptor-associated periodic syndrome (TRAPS) was that of a large family of Irish/Scottish ancestry, with an illness denoted as familial Hibernian fever.[111] With the discovery of mutations in the *TNFRSF1A* gene,[5] located in chromosome 12p13, which encodes the 55-kDa tumor necrosis factor (TNF) receptor in this family and in several other families of non-Irish ancestry, the current TRAPS nomenclature was proposed.

Genetics and Pathogenesis

TRAPS is inherited as an autosomal dominant trait, although in some cases, a clear pattern of inheritance cannot be discerned because of reduced penetrance in mutation-positive relatives or, rarely, because of de novo mutation. TRAPS has been reported in patients of many ethnicities. It is the second most common hereditary periodic fever disorder, with more than 50 known mutations in *TNFRSF1A*[5,112-128] (http://fmf.igh.cnrs.fr/infevers/).

The 55 kDa TNF receptor is widely expressed on cell membranes and mediates a number of proinflammatory effects. To date, all TRAPS-associated *TNFRSF1A* mutations lead to single amino acid substitutions in the extracellular domain of the receptor and many involve cysteine residues thereby disrupting highly conserved disulfide bonds. When the first of these mutations was discovered,[5] there were additional data supporting the hypothesis that mutations impair metalloprotease-mediated cleavage of receptors from the cell surface, the most common way of inactivating TNFRSF1A. Impaired receptor shedding might then lead to repeated signaling and prolongation of the immune response. Impaired receptor shedding has been observed by flow cytometry in patients with some but not all mutations.[5,114,120,121,129,130] Moreover, impaired cleavage does not seem to correlate with disease severity, suggesting that there must be other mechanisms by which *TNFRSF1A* mutations cause autoinflammatory disease.[131,132] Those include: reduced cell surface expression of mutant receptors,[133] an abnormal oligomerization or misfolding with retention in the endoplasmic reticulum (ER),[134-136] decreased binding of mutant forms of receptor to TNF,[137] ligand-independent signaling,[137,138] and a reduction in TNF-induced apoptosis.[130,139] The accumulation of misfolded proteins within the ER may induce stress responses prompting the release of proinflammatory cytokines.[135,140] This process is independent of TNF-TNFR1 interactions and is therefore "ligand-independent." In addition, mutant TNFR1 may accumulate within the cytoplasm forming oligomers triggering a range of DD-mediated signaling cascades. These processes, although ligand independent, require an intact DD to trigger an inflammatory response.

Clinical Manifestations

The clinical manifestations of TRAPS are similar to those of FMF and differ from those of the cryopyrinopathies (see Table 43–3). TRAPS causes episodic fever and inflammation with serosal, synovial, and cutaneous manifestations. Distinguishing characteristics of TRAPS include longer attacks (one to four weeks or more) and conspicuous eye and skin symptoms.[141-143] TRAPS attacks may be precipitated by minor trauma or infection or by stress and physical exertion. During attacks, patients exhibit vigorous acute phase responses that sometimes persist into the intercritical period, albeit at lower intensity.[142]

Cutaneous symptoms associated with TRAPS are often distinctive, consisting of macular areas of erythema that occur on the torso or on an extremity (Fig. 43–2).[141,142] These cutaneous lesions are warm and tender, may resemble cellulitis or bruises, and consist of superficial and deep perivascular infiltrates of mononuclear cells. When lesions occur on the limbs, they often migrate distally. There may be associated myalgia due to inflammation of the underlying fascia.[144] Magnetic resonance imaging (MRI) of affected muscle groups reveals focal areas of edema in discrete muscular compartments and intramuscular septa (see Fig. 43–2).[142] Other types of rash may also occur, including annular patches and generalized serpiginous plaques.[141,142]

Clinical attacks may include peritoneal inflammation or pleurisy, or both. Abdominal pain with tenderness is often a major feature resembling an acute abdomen. Recurrent pericarditis has also been reported. Ocular inflammation with periorbital edema or conjunctivitis is common (see Fig. 43–2).[142] Arthralgia is more prominent than arthritis, and it generally involves single joints, especially the hip, knees, and ankles. Scrotal inflammation may occur. Amyloidosis, although less common than in untreated FMF, affects about 10% of patients and can lead to renal failure.[20,114-116,142,145] The risk of amyloidosis appears to be greater among patients with cysteine mutations.[114] A positive family history of amyloidosis may increase the risk for other relatives.

Laboratory Investigations

Levels of SAA, CRP, and serum complement components are increased during flares, and most patients exhibit leukocytosis and thrombocytosis, with an accelerated ESR. Acute phase reactants may remain elevated in between clinical attacks, suggesting an elevated level of baseline inflammatory activity.

Diagnosis

The specific diagnosis is defined by mutations in *TNFRSF1A*. The majority are single nucleotide missense mutations in exons 2-4 encoding the first or second cysteine-rich extracellular domains (CRD1 and CRD2).[5,92] The binding site for TNF is formed by CRD2 and CRD3 of TNFRSF1A, whereas CRD1, also known as the pre-ligand assembly binding domain, is thought to mediate the TNFRSF1A self assembly. Genotype-phenotype studies showed that mutations at cysteine residues are associated with more severe phenotype and a higher incidence of amyloidosis.[114,142] Although most TRAPS associated mutations are fully penetrant, 2 TNFRSF1A variants, P46L and R92Q, have also been identified in asymptomatic family members and at low frequency in healthy populations.[124,131] Recent experience suggests

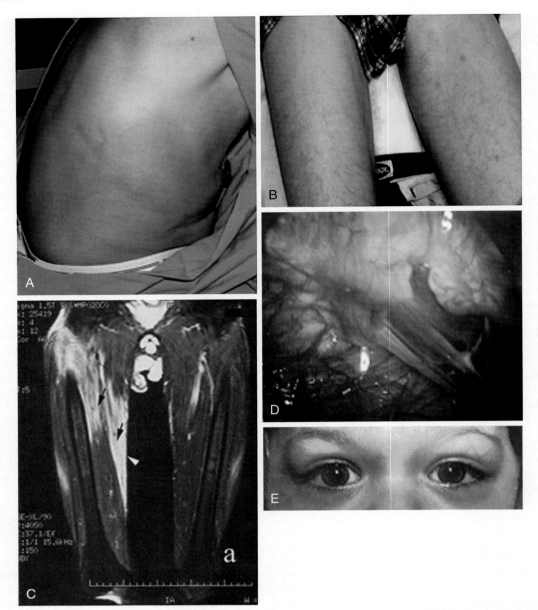

FIGURE 43–2 Cutaneous symptoms associated with TRAPS may consist of macular areas of erythema on the torso **(A)**[142] or on an extremity **(B)**.[144] **C,** Sagittal views of the proximal thighs of a TRAPS patient demonstrating edematous changes within muscle compartments *(black arrows),* here and extending to the skin *(white arrows).*[142] **D,** Peritoneal inflammation can lead to adhesions.[306] **E,** Periorbital edema is commonly observed in TRAPS patients during a flare.[142]

that patients with R92Q variant tend to have more frequent attacks of shorter duration and less frequent elevation of inflammatory markers. The clinical features of these patients may resemble those of PFAPA. In addition, they do not seem to respond as well to anti-TNF therapy.

Treatment

Treatment depends on the severity of the underlying disease. For some patients with relatively infrequent episodes, tapering doses of prednisone at the time of attacks may be effective and relatively safe.[142] For patients with more severe disease, etanercept (the recombinant TNF receptor antagonist), given weekly (once or twice a week) is effective in preventing attacks in some patients.[6,135,142,146-149]

Experience with infliximab (anti-TNF monoclonal antibodies) is limited. Treatment with this agent has led to exacerbation of the disease in some cases,[148-151] possibly due to the failure to shed infliximab-bound TNF/TNFR1 from the cell surface leading to an increase in cytokine secretion and an increased proinflammatory response.[152] Anakinra (IL-1 receptor antagonist) has also been shown to be effective in controlling the clinical and laboratory manifestations in some patients with TRAPS.[153-155] Colchicine usually has no effect on symptoms or the development of amyloidosis.[142,145] In patients with demonstrated amyloidosis, the goal should be to maintain the SAA levels at <10 mg/L. The prognosis depends on the development of amyloidosis. More aggressive therapy may be indicated in patients with a positive family history of amyloidosis or mutation at cysteine residues to suppress subclinical inflammation.

Hyperimmunoglobulinemia D with Periodic Fever Syndrome

Hyperimmunoglobulinemia D with periodic fever syndrome (HIDS) is an autosomal recessive disease[156] that was initially described in several patients of Dutch heritage.[157] HIDS is caused by mutations in the *MVK* gene, on chromosome 12, which encodes mevalonate kinase.[158-160] It occurs mainly in patients of northern European ancestry, and approximately 50% of patients are of Dutch ancestry.[143,161-165]

Genetics and Pathogenesis

Mevalonate kinase is the first enzyme to follow 3-hydroxy-3-methyl-glutaryl-CoA reductase (HMG-CoA reductase) in the mevalonate pathway and converts mevalonic acid to 5-phosphomevalonic acid. The mevalonate pathway produces cholesterol, a structural component of cellular membranes and precursor for bile acids and steroid hormones. In addition, the mevalonate pathway produces nonsterol isoprene compounds (Fig. 43–3).[160,166,167] Isoprenes are involved in a variety of cellular functions, including electron transport, protein glycosylation and synthesis, and prenylation of proteins involved in cell proliferation and differentiation. Mutations associated with HIDS lead to markedly reduced mevalonate kinase enzymatic activity,[158,159] whereas the mutations in the clinically more severe mevalonic aciduria result in the absence of enzymatic activity.[168] Although excessive production of proinflammatory cytokines by HIDS mononuclear cells may result from excessive accumulation of mevalonic acid substrate, recent data support an alternative hypothesis related to deficiencies in nonsterol isoprenoids synthesized through the mevalonate pathway.[169] If the latter possibility is correct, a shortage of geranylgeranylated proteins may be the link between the mevalonate pathway, increased IL-1β production, and the febrile attacks of HIDS.[170]

Clinical Manifestations

HIDS manifests in early childhood, often by the age of 6-months-old (see Table 43–3). Attacks last about three to seven days, usually separated by one- to two-month, symptom-free intervals. Episodes are often heralded by chills and headache, a rising fever, abdominal pain, nausea, and vomiting, sometimes precipitated by immunizations, surgery, trauma, and mild infections.[161,171] The mevalonate kinase enzyme in patients with HIDS-associated mutations loses activity at supraphysiological temperatures, perhaps explaining the association of immunizations, upper respiratory infections, and other inflammatory provocations with attacks.[172] Some patients develop a nondestructive arthritis, usually in the large joints, associated with attacks.[161,173,174] This arthritis is often polyarticular, unlike that associated with FMF. Protracted joint manifestations are rare.

During attacks, widespread erythematous macules that are sometimes painful develop.[161,175] The rash is usually not migratory, differentiating it from the rash associated with TRAPS, and it has no predilection for the lower legs, unlike that of FMF. The HIDS rash may be a diffuse maculopapular eruption (Fig. 43–4) extending to the palms and soles, or it can be nodular, urticarial, or morbilliform. Skin biopsies show perivascular inflammatory cells and deposits of antibody or complement component C3, or both. Oral and vaginal aphthous ulcers may be present. Henoch-Schönlein purpura[176] and erythema elevatum diutinum (a benign type of necrotizing vasculitis)[163] have been reported. Cervical lymphadenopathy is a common manifestation of HIDS, as are severe headache and splenomegaly.[161] Pleurisy is uncommon.

Patients with mevalonic aciduria have complete deficiency of mevalonic kinase and have developmental delays of varying severity, dysmorphic features, and hepatosplenomegaly. These patients have been known to develop periodic crises characterized by fever, rash, and arthralgia. HIDS is one end of the clinical spectrum of deficiency of mevalonate kinase.[168]

Laboratory Investigations

Most patients have elevated serum immunoglobulin (Ig) D levels, but how this observation contributes to the clinical disease is poorly understood. In a recent report, 22% of HIDS patients had normal levels of IgD,[161] suggesting that an elevated IgD concentration may be an epiphenomenon.[159,166,177] Levels of IgA may also be elevated.[178] Patients also exhibit an accelerated ESR, leukocytosis, and elevated levels of CRP[143,161,166,179] during and, less commonly, between attacks. Elevated levels of mevalonic acid may be detected in urine during attacks.[158,159,180,181]

Diagnosis

A diagnosis may require several lines of inquiry, including clinical observation, genetic testing, serum IgD measurement, and assay of mevalonate in urine. Modest elevations in IgD should be interpreted with caution, because this phenomenon is common in several other conditions, including chronic infections, acquired immunodeficiency syndrome, Hodgkin disease, and other periodic fever syndromes.[171,182-184] Most laboratories perform HIDS screenings for only the most common V377I and I268T mutations.[165,180,185,186] However, even with complete sequencing of the coding region of *MVK*, genetic testing may be inconclusive. Among patients with recurrent fevers and typical associated findings, up to 25% may be mutation negative.[161] The genetic and biochemical basis of disease in such patients remains to be elucidated.

Treatment

Various treatments have been proposed. A few patients may respond to colchicine. Glucocorticoids, intravenous immune globulin, and cyclosporine have all been tried with varying success rates. Small studies demonstrated improvement with etanercept[161,187] and simvastatin.[188] Consistent with the involvement of IL-1β in this disease, early studies suggest the efficacy of anakinra; however, larger confirmatory studies are needed. HIDS is not generally associated with a shortened lifespan. Although very rare, HIDS-associated amyloidosis has been reported.[189-192]

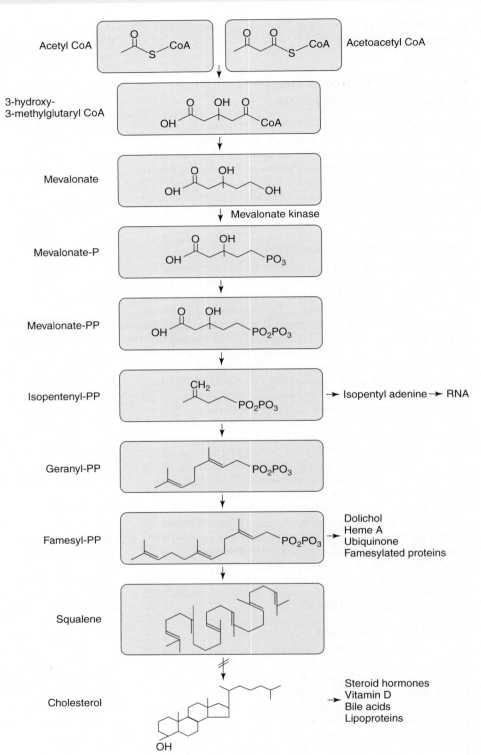

Acetyl CoA

Acetoacetyl CoA

3-hydroxy-
3-methylglutaryl CoA

Mevalonate

Mevalonate-P — Mevalonate kinase

Mevalonate-PP

Isopentenyl-PP → Isopentyl adenine → RNA

Geranyl-PP

Famesyl-PP → Dolichol / Heme A / Ubiquinone / Famesylated proteins

Squalene

Cholesterol → Steroid hormones / Vitamin D / Bile acids / Lipoproteins

FIGURE 43–3 Patients with the hyperimmu-noglobulinemia D with periodic fever syndrome have mutations in mevalonate kinase that result in enzyme activity markedly diminished but not absent. Patients with clinically more severe meva-lonic aciduria have mutations leading to an almost total loss of enzyme activity.

Cryopyrin-Associated Periodic Fever Syndromes

Among the episodic or periodic fever syndromes are three clinically distinguishable disorders caused by domi-nantly inherited abnormalities in cryopyrin (NLRP3), which results from missense mutations in the cold autoinflammatory syndrome 1 gene (*CIAS1*), also known as *NLRP3* or *NALP3* (discussed later in this chapter). These three disorders include: familial cold autoinflam-matory syndrome (FCAS), Muckle-Wells syndrome (MWS), and neonatal-onset multisystem inflammatory disease (NOMID), also called chronic infantile neurologi-cal cutaneous and articular syndrome (CINCA). These

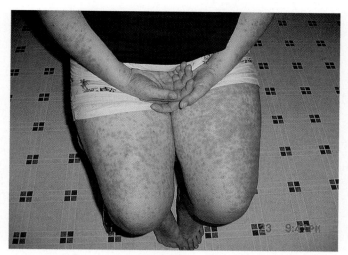

FIGURE 43–4 The rash of HIDS may be a diffuse maculopapular eruption, often extending to the palms and soles.

diseases were originally described as distinct clinical entities, but all phenotypes have some overlapping clinical symptoms; patients often present with fever, neutrophilic urticaria-like skin rash, and joint involvement of varying severity associated with neutrophil-mediated inflammation and an intense acute phase response. In reality, these three syndromes exist on a continuum of severity;[193] however, the clinical description is important regarding disease prognosis. While patients with FCAS have normal lifespans, the mortality rate is around 20% in children with NOMID before they reach adulthood.[194,195]

The skin rash—a key feature of all three diseases—is usually the first notable manifestation and develops shortly after birth or in early infancy. This rash exhibits the same clinical and histological characteristics regardless of syndrome: it is migratory, maculopapular, urticaria-like, and usually nonpruritic. A few patients report a burning sensation. The intensity of the skin rash can vary from patient to patient and with disease activity. Microscopic examination of lesional skin reveals a predominant perivascular neutrophilic infiltrate, dermal edema, and dilated blood vessels, without the presence of vasculitis, mast cells or mast cell degranulation.[52,196-198] These histological findings are in contrast with the typical lymphocytic and eosinophilic infiltration seen in classical urticaria. For this reason, the rash associated with FCAS, MWS, and NOMID is sometimes called pseudourticaria.[193,198,199]

FCAS

FCAS was first described in 1940.[200] This autosomal-dominant syndrome is characterized by recurrent short and self-limited episodes of fever, rash, and arthralgia precipitated by generalized exposure to cold (see Table 43–3).[196,199] The cold sensitivity in FCAS is unlike that in other cold-related disorders such as cryoglobulinemia; it is not only induced by a cool absolute ambient temperature but also by a rapid decrease in temperature. Air conditioning may be very problematic for patients with FCAS in hot climates and provides a clear example of an environmental influence on a genetic disease.[196,201]

Conjunctivitis is also frequently observed. Other commonly reported symptoms are muscle pain, profuse sweating, drowsiness, headache, extreme thirst, and nausea. Early onset of the disease, at birth or within the first six months of life, is characteristic. Typically, FCAS patients report the development of symptoms beginning one to two hours after generalized exposure to cold temperatures or to a considerable drop in temperature, and the duration of attacks is usually short (<24 hours). Predictably, attacks are more frequent in winter, on damp and windy days, and following exposure to air conditioning. Most patients describe a correlation between the severity of the crisis and the intensity of cold exposure. Many patients with FCAS also show evidence of chronic inflammation between attacks, particularly a daily pattern of rash developing in the afternoon that can be associated with headache, myalgia, and fatigue by the evening. The typical urticarial rash in FCAS does not necessarily occur on exposed areas of skin, unlike the classic urticarial rash in the more common acquired cold urticaria, in which direct contact with cold objects causes pruritic hives at the site of exposure.[197] The ice cube test is negative, in contrast to what is observed in acquired cold urticaria.[202] Amyloidosis is rarely reported,[202-206] in contradistinction to MWS and NOMID. Leukocytosis and increased acute phase reactants accompany episodes of inflammation.

Hoffman and colleagues[196] proposed a set of diagnostic criteria: (1) recurrent intermittent episodes of fever and rash that primarily follow natural, experimental, or both types of generalized cold exposure; (2) autosomal dominant pattern of disease inheritance; (3) age of onset <6-months-old; (4) duration of most attacks <24 hours; (5) presence of conjunctivitis associated with attacks; (6) absence of deafness, periorbital edema, lymphadenopathy, and serositis.

Muckle-Wells Syndrome

MWS was described in 1962 by Muckle and Wells as a perplexing syndrome of fever, urticarial rash, and limb pain that eventually led to progressive hearing loss and amyloidosis.[207] This disease is usually inherited as an autosomal dominant trait, but apparent sporadic cases also occur.[201,208] MWS is characterized by recurrent episodes of fever and rash associated with joint and eye manifestations, although fever is not always present (see Table 43–3).[193,208,209] Urticarial rash is the most common skin manifestation (Fig. 43–5). In contrast to FCAS, the rash of MWS and its other manifestations are not necessarily triggered by changes in temperature and last longer or can even be continuously present at varying intensity. Precipitating factors cannot usually be identified. The course of the disease varies between individuals from the typical recurrent attacks of inflammation to more persistent symptoms. Joint manifestations can be mild with brief episodes of arthralgia, but recurrent episodes of joint swelling affecting predominantly large joints can be observed.[193,210] Conjunctivitis is common, and episcleritis and iridocyclitis have been reported.[193] Sensorineural hearing loss is seen in approximately 70% of cases[193,203] and usually begins in late childhood or early adulthood. Abdominal pain and headache may occur in some cases.

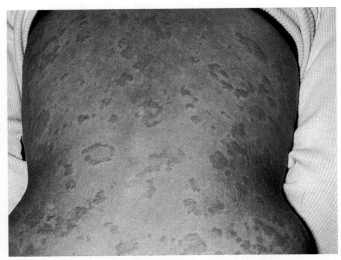

FIGURE 43–5 Urticarial rash is the most common skin manifestation seen in Muckle-Wells syndrome.[307]

AA amyloidosis, due to chronic inflammation, is the primary complication[198,201,211,212] and occurs in approximately one fourth of patients with MWS, reflecting the very intense and prolonged acute-phase response in this particular disorder. It usually manifests as proteinuria, followed by impaired renal function. AA amyloid fibrils are derived from the circulating acute-phase protein SAA. Other evidence of acute phase response includes elevation of the ESR and leukocytosis,[193,210] and may be observed during episodes of inflammation or nearly constant in severely affected individuals. Clinical manifestations of mild forms of MWS resemble those of FCAS, and more severe phenotypes overlap with NOMID/CINCA.[213,214]

NOMID/CINCA

NOMID/CINCA is associated with the most severe phenotype in the cryopyrin spectrum of diseases, although the clinical manifestations vary in severity (see Table 43–3). This syndrome was first described by both Prieur and Goldsmith in the early 1980s[195,215,216] as a chronic inflammatory disease with rash, articular involvement, and chronic aseptic meningitis. Most cases of NOMID appear sporadic, with a few reports of autosomal dominant transmission.[52] With increased quality of life afforded by currently available treatment, more patients with NOMID will reach childbearing potential, and as a result, more patients with autosomal dominant transmission may be recognized.

First symptoms occur at birth or in early infancy. Fever can be intermittent, very mild, or in some cases absent. An urticaria-like rash is usually present at birth or during the first months of life. The rash is nonpruritic and papular (Fig. 43–6). It varies in intensity from patient to patient, with time, and with disease activity. Bone and joint inflammation also vary in severity: in approximately two thirds of patients, joint manifestations are limited to arthralgia and transient swelling without effusion, and occur during flare-ups. In one third of patients,

joint abnormalities are severe and usually begin within the first year of life. The metaphyses and epiphyses of the long bones are affected, and bony overgrowth can result in gross deformity of the joints, articular and bone pain, and loss of range of motion (Fig. 43–7).[217] Joint involvement is most commonly asymmetrical and chiefly involves the knees; however, the condition can be symmetrical and affect other joints, including the ankles, wrists, and elbows.[217] Radiological manifestations, when present, are distinctive (see Fig. 43–7).[217,218] The first recognizable finding is swelling of the periarticular soft tissues, often with visible enlargement of the nonossified portion of the epiphyses. Fraying and cupping of irregular metaphyses follow. The hallmark of this disease is a bizarre enlargement of the ossified portions of the epiphyses of the involved joints. These epiphyses demonstrate erratically ossified, markedly coarsened trabeculae arranged in a random reticular pattern. The borders of the ossified portions of the epiphyses are spiculated and uneven. Eventually, long bones develop bowing of the ends and shortening of the diaphysis. Other radiographical findings include osteoporosis and prominent periosteal new bone formation along the diaphyses and metaphyses of affected long bones. Bone biopsy may show poorly organized cartilaginous columns on hematoxylin and eosin staining, nonhomogeneous spread of chondrocytes with staining for proteoglycans with Alcian blue, and a complementary pattern of calcification seen on von Kossa staining for calcium.[217]

Prematurity and dysmaturity are characteristic of one third of patients. Umbilical cord anomalies were observed in a few children.[195,218,219] Neurological manifestations, including chronic aseptic meningitis, cerebral ventricular dilation, cerebral atrophy, uveitis, optic disc edema, and high-frequency hearing loss are present in various subsets of patients.[193,195,220] High frequency progressive hearing loss is caused by chronic cochlear inflammation that can be seen on gadolinium enhanced images on MRI (Fig. 43–8).[221] Ocular manifestations can progress to blindness, and 25% of patients have a significant ocular disability.[195,209,219,222] Chronic headache, vomiting and papilledema are frequently observed consequences of chronic increased intracranial pressure (see Fig. 43–8.). Spastic diplegia and epilepsy may develop. Progressive cognitive impairment occurs in severely affected patients. Closure of the anterior fontanelle may be delayed, and macrocrania, frontal bossing, and saddle nose appearance are frequently observed due to increased intracranial pressure and the resulting macrocephaly. Cerebral spinal fluid (CSF) examination demonstrates variable hypercellularity with increased polymorphonuclear leukocytes, elevated protein levels, and an increased opening pressure. Computed tomography or MRI can be normal or document mild ventricular dilatation and enlarged subdural fluid spaces, suggesting mild cerebral atrophy.[193] Some patients develop progressive calcifications of the falx cerebri and dura mater. Leptomeningeal enhancement can be observed on MRI after gadolinium injection.[221] Amyloid A amyloidosis develops with increasing age in some patients. Severe disabilities are frequent, and premature death is possible in severely affected patients.[195,220]

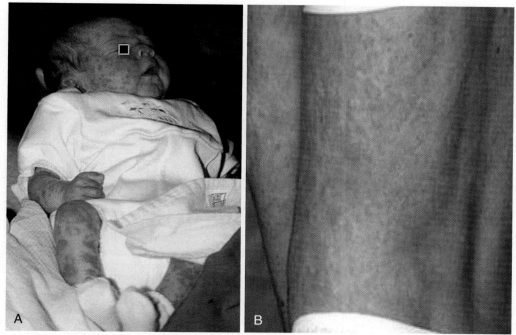

FIGURE 43–6   **A,** An urticaria-like rash is usually present at birth or during the first months of life. **B,** The rash is nonpruritic and papular. (Courtesy of Dr. Raphaela Goldbach-Mansky.)

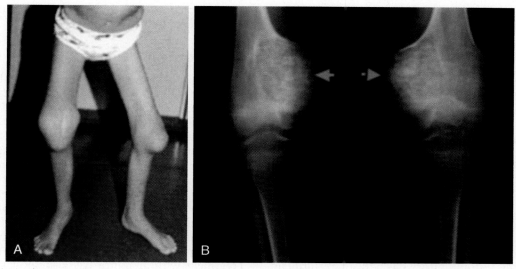

FIGURE 43–7   Joint involvement in NOMID is most commonly asymmetrical and chiefly involves the knees. **A,** The arthropathy can cause gross deformity of the joints with contractures. **B,** A hallmark of NOMID is a bizarre enlargement of the ossified portions of the epiphyses of the involved joints. (Courtesy of Dr. Raphaela Goldbach-Mansky)

Findings suggestive of an ongoing inflammatory process include lymphadenopathy, splenomegaly, a prolonged ESR, CRP, leukocytosis, eosinophilia, and hyperglobulinemia, but autoantibodies are generally not present.[195]

GENETICS OF CRYOPYRIN-ASSOCIATED PERIODIC SYNDROMES

Cryopyrin-associated periodic syndromes (CAPS) are associated with missense mutations of the *CIAS1 (NLRP3)* gene and are inherited in an autosomal dominant manner, although there are sporadic cases, and in some patients with clinical features of CAPS, no detectable *CIAS1* mutations can be detected.[201,203,209,220,223,224] This gene encodes the cryopyrin protein, also called NLRP3 or NALP3,[203] which is a member of the nucleotide-binding domain and leucine-rich repeat containing (NLR) family intimately involved in the innate immune system. Cryopyrin contains an N-terminal PYD, a nucleotide binding (NBS/NACHT) domain, and a C-terminal leucine-rich repeat (LRR) domain.[203,223] More than 90 mutations have been reported (http://fmf.igh.cnrs.fr/infevers/), and almost all are located in the region encoding the NACHT

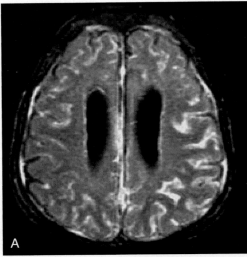
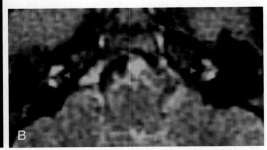

FIGURE 43–8 **A,** Leptomeningeal enhancement and ventriculomegaly seen on MRI of a patient with NOMID.[221] **B,** Cochlear inflammation seen on gadolinium enhanced MR images. (Courtesy of Dr. Raphaela Goldbach-Mansky)

domain and its flanking structures (i.e., in exon 3).[193] In the past five years, a small number of mutations have been identified in exons 4 and 6, within the region that encodes the LRR.[193,225-227] *CIAS1* mosaicism has been proposed to play a role in some mutation negative patients.[228,229] While some mutations are specific for a given disorder, particular *CIAS1* mutations may be involved in more than one disease.[52,201,224,230] These findings strongly suggest that additional modifier genes or environmental factors play a role in determining the disease phenotype.[220]

Cryopyrin/NLRP3 is a component of the macromolecular complex, the inflammasome, that senses various microbial products and endogenous "danger signals" and is involved in activation of IL-1β.[8] NLRP3 interacts with ASC by means of homotypical interaction between its PYD and the PYD of ASC.[231] This interaction mediates procaspase-1 activation, and caspase-1 activates pro- IL-1β to its proinflammatory active form, IL-1β. Current evidence suggests that the wild-type NLRP3 is kept in an inactive state through autoinhibition likely mediated by the interaction between the LRR domains with the NACHT domain of the protein. Mutations in the NACHT domain or some regions of the LRR domain might disrupt this autoinhibitory mechanism, resulting in increased inflammasome activation and subsequent IL-1β release.[11] *Nlrp3* knockout mice have been described and have established the requirement of NLRP3 for macrophage IL-1β production in response to Toll-like receptor agonists, plus adenosine triphosphate, to Gram-positive bacteria such as *Staphylococcus aureus* or *Listeria monocytogenes,* to bacterial RNA, to dsRNA and viral RNA, and to uric acid crystals.[232-235] Although NLRP3 is required to produce IL-1β in response to these many and varied insults, the disease-causing mutations in this protein do not seem to render CAPS patients clinically over responsive when faced with these challenges in nature, although some patients anecdotally report increased resistance to common viral infections.[8]

Cryopyrin is expressed on immune cells and chondrocytes.[203,223] Cryopyrin mutations are gain-of-function

mutations that lead to constitutive activation of the inflammasome,[11] generating the inappropriate release of IL-1β and leading to the excessive multisystem inflammation responsible for the symptoms associated with CAPS.[236] Consistent with this hypothesis is the finding of oversecretion of IL-1β by peripheral blood leukocytes from patients with CAPS.[11,220,237-240]

Treatment

Elucidation of the pathway involved in IL-1 action has allowed for the development of IL-1 targeted therapies. Targeting the IL-1 pathway has led to new treatment options for patients with CAPS. The use of an IL-1 receptor antagonist (IL-1RA; anakinra), a soluble IL-1 decoy receptor (IL-1 Trap; rilonacept), and an anti-IL-1β monoclonal antibody (canakinumab) have proven to be efficacious in treating mutation positive and mutation negative CAPS patients.[194,208,221,227,236,241-246] In addition to alleviating the fever, rash, conjunctivitis, joint pain, and evidence of systemic inflammation, there are reports of reversal of hearing loss associated with MWS,[238,247,248] and of improvement in the ESR, CRP and SAA levels.[208,249] Treatment with anakinra has also shown to resolve the meningitis, and the ocular and cochlear inflammation of NOMID.[221] Prior to the use of biological agents to treat these cryopyrin-associated autoinflammatory syndromes, there was no established treatment. NSAIDs and prednisone may offer temporary clinical relief. Colchicine is ineffective.

Periodic Fever with Aphthous Stomatitis, Pharyngitis, and Adenitis

Periodic fever with aphthous stomatitis, pharyngitis, and adenitis (PFAPA) syndrome (i.e., Marshall syndrome) was described in 1987.[250] It is a relatively common condition that has a benign prognosis.[251,252] The precise etiology is unknown; however, it has been suggested that there is a dysregulation of the immune response in patients with PFAPA that may contribute to the etiology.[253] No genetic mutations or ethnic factors have been associated with PFAPA, and although most cases occur sporadically, there have been reports of siblings and parents with similar presentations.[254,255]

Clinical Manifestations

The onset of PFAPA is usually before the age of 5-years-old. In an American series,[256] febrile episodes occurred approximately every 28 days and lasted for a mean of five days. Some say that it is the most clocklike of the periodic fevers in children. Children are healthy between episodes and grow normally.

Malaise, chills, fatigue, and oral lesions may herald the onset of a cycle. Fever may appear suddenly and reach a maximum of 40°C to 41°C and then resolve over a 24-to 48-hour period. In the largest series reported,[256] 70% of patients had aphthous stomatitis, characterized by shallow ulcers in the buccal mucosa and pharynx that lasted for three to five days and healed without scarring. Seventy-two percent had pharyngitis,[256] consisting of erythematous, enlarged tonsils.[257] Although cervical adenitis is a major feature of the disease in 88% of patients, generalized lymphadenopathy or noteworthy hepatosplenomegaly suggests a diagnosis other than PFAPA. Arthralgia and abdominal pain may be associated with the fever and are usually mild. Children may also complain of headache with the episodes.

Laboratory Investigations

During episodes, there is an increase in the total white blood cell count and elevation of acute phase reactants. Levels of CRP are substantially increased during the febrile episodes with higher values on days two to four compared to day one of fever.[258] Neutropenia usually is not present, but mild elevations in serum IgG, IgM, and IgA may occur. Elevated levels of IgD were reported in one study[252] but not in another.[256] Increased serum levels of interferon-γ, TNF, IL-1β, and IL-6 have been observed with fevers,[253,259] suggesting that perturbations in the cytokine network contribute to the disease phenotype.

Diagnosis

In order to encourage recognition and facilitate uniform reporting, diagnostic criteria for PFAPA have been established (Table 43–4).[260]

Treatment

Treatment of PFAPA is still a matter of debate. While NSAIDs may alleviate the fever in some patients, antibiotics and colchicine have not been effective in alleviating the spectrum of symptoms observed. The use of prednisone 0.6 mg/kg to 2 mg/kg given orally, as a single dose at the onset of symptoms, on day one and if necessary on day two causes a dramatic resolution of febrile episodes, although it does not prevent their recurrence and may actually shorten the interval between episodes.[250,252,256,261] Cimetidine may be effective at preventing recurrences.[262-264] Some investigators have reported that tonsillectomy and adenoidectomy may

Table 43–4

Clinical features of the syndrome of periodic fever with aphthous stomatitis, pharyngitis, and cervical adenopathy

- Onset of disease in early childhood, generally prior to the age of 5-years-old
- Regularly recurring abrupt episodes of fever lasting approximately 5 days, associated with constitutional symptoms, and both of the following:
  - Aphthous stomatitis and/or pharyngitis (with or without cervical adenitis) in the absence of other signs of respiratory tract infection
  - Acute inflammatory markers such as leukocytosis or elevated erythrocyte sedimentation rate
- Completely asymptomatic interval periods (generally lasting less than 10 weeks), benign long term course, normal growth parameters, and the distinct absence of sequelae
- Exclusion of cyclic neutropenia by serial neutrophil counts, before, during, and after symptomatic episodes
- Exclusion of other episodic syndromes (familial Mediterranean fever, hyper-IgD syndrome, TRAPS, Behçet disease) by family history and the absence of typical clinical features and laboratory markers
- Absence of clinical and laboratory evidence for immunodeficiency, autoimmune disease or chronic infection

From Marshall GS, Edwards KM, Lawton AR: PFAPA syndrome. *Pediatr Infect Dis J* 8:658-659, 1989.

eliminate attacks.[264-270] Two recent randomized studies on tonsillectomy or adenotonsillectomy have demonstrated that these surgical interventions may induce a remission of fever episodes compared with the control group.[266,269] While this is certainly promising news to those who care for these children, other nonsurgical interventions should also be considered.

Outcome and Prognosis

Prognosis seems to be excellent. In a 10-year registry,[256] cyclic episodes ceased after a mean of 4.5 years from the onset; approximately one third of patients stopped having episodes. In other patients, the symptoms became less intense and less frequent with the passage of time.[271]

Periodic Fever due to Cyclic Hematopoiesis

Cyclic hematopoiesis (CH), or cyclic neutropenia, is a rare disorder consisting of febrile episodes due to periodic neutropenia, interspersed between intervals of relatively normal neutrophil counts. CH may occur as a sporadic congenital disorder, an autosomal dominant inherited disease, or an acquired condition.[272-275] Cyclic neutropenia is a more common term for this condition, although cyclic hematopoiesis is more descriptive, because other formed elements of blood in addition to neutrophils also demonstrate cyclic variations in numbers.[274] Although the fevers associated with CH are sometimes caused by infectious agents, patients with CH may develop fevers in the absence of apparent infection, perhaps due to the large-scale apoptotic death of bone marrow precursors that underlies the variation in circulating mature forms.[275]

Genetics and Pathogenesis

The clinical features of autosomal dominant familial CH are indistinguishable from those of the sporadic form, suggesting that the sporadic variety may represent unrecognized familial cases or de novo mutations in CH genes. Inherited CH is caused by mutations in the neutrophil elastase-2 gene (ELA2),[276-278] which encodes neutrophil elastase (NE), a serine protease of neutrophil and monocyte granules. Mutations in the growth factor independent-1 gene (GFI1),[279] which encodes a transcription factor that controls expression of NE, cause severe congenital neutropenia, a noncyclical disorder. In dogs, CH has also been related to mutations in an adaptor protein (AP3B1) bound to NE.[278,280] The equivalent mutation is the cause of the Hermansky-Pudlak syndrome type 2 (HPS2) in humans caused by the absence of AP3B1, and is associated with intermittent neutropenia.[281,282]

There are several hypotheses to account for the periodicity of cyclic neutropenia. One hypothesis is that mutations in ELA2 lead to altered NE activity, thereby affecting digestion of a number of proteins regulating hematopoiesis, including granulocyte-CSF (G-CSF) and the G-CSF receptor, and most mutations reduce NE activity.[283] Other hypotheses are that CH is a mistrafficking/mislocalization disorder of NE[283] or that CH is caused by low level activation of the unfolded protein response. A more recent hypothesis is that the periodicity of cyclic neutropenia can be explained through a disturbance of a feedback circuit, in which mature neutrophils inhibit cell proliferation, thereby homeostatically regulating progenitor populations.[284]

Clinical Manifestations

Clinical manifestations of CH start in early childhood, with the earliest reported case occurring in the first few weeks of life (Table 43–5).[274] The cycle length is typically 21 days (range, 14 to 36 days), and each febrile cycle lasts three to 10 days.[274] In older persons, the cycles may not be evident. During attacks, the absolute neutrophil count (ANC) is less than 200/µL and may be zero. While patients are neutropenic, they are highly susceptible to infections from normal flora, resulting in recurrent oral ulcers, gingivitis, fever, and lymphadenopathy. Although these infections are usually mild to moderate in severity, severe infections due to *Clostridium* or *Escherichia coli*, with abdominal pain and vomiting rapidly progressing to necrotizing enterocolitis, may occur.[274] *Clostridium septicum* infection has caused enterocolitis, myonecrosis, and death.[285,286] Other symptoms include bone pain, fatigue, malaise, diarrhea, and headache. Symptoms improve rapidly as neutrophils counts recover. Children are well between attacks, with ANCs in the low normal to mildly neutropenic range.

Blood monocyte counts cycle in opposite fashion, so that the peak monocyte count coincides with the nadir of the ANC.[287] Reticulocytes, platelets, and eosinophils also may oscillate with neutrophils.[274,276,288] An acute phase response may be observed during the neutropenic

Table 43–5

Clinical features of cyclic hematopoiesis

1. Typical cycles recur approximately every 21 days.
2. Absolute neutrophil count is less than 0.2×10^9/L.
3. Absolute neutrophil count is low normal to mildly neutropenic between cycles.

episodes. Results of bone marrow examination are characterized by intramedullary destruction of promyelocytes and defects in granulopoiesis[289] due to accelerated apoptosis.[290] Adult-onset CH may be a benign neoplasm with clonal proliferation of large granular lymphocytes.[287,291,292]

Diagnosis

Based on extensive family studies,[274] the diagnosis of autosomal dominant CH can be established with reasonable accuracy based on the following criteria: regular, cyclic fluctuations in peripheral blood neutrophil counts, with a periodicity ranging from 19 to 21 days, and documentation of neutrophil counts less than 200/µL during periods of neutropenia. Complete blood counts should be determined two or three times each week for at least six weeks.[274] Genetic testing may play an adjunctive role, especially in families in which formes fruste are suspected or when there is no family history but there is a suspicion of de novo mutation.

Treatment

Treatment with granulocyte colony-stimulating factor (G-CSF)[293,294] or granulocyte-macrophage (GM-CSF) may be effective. The recommendation is to administer G-CSF subcutaneously at doses of 1-5 mc/kg/day. Symptoms are controlled by this treatment, and the cycles are shortened, with an increase in the nadir ANC.[294]

Infections must be treated promptly and aggressively. *E. coli* and *Clostridium* species precipitate serious and often fatal illness. Appropriate cultures should be obtained, particularly if a child develops abdominal pain with diarrhea and vomiting. Typhlitis (i.e., inflammation of the cecum) and perforating enterocolitis should always be considered.

Outcome and Prognosis

Prognosis appears to be good, except for the increased mortality rate associated with infection.[274] With age, the cycles are less prominent, and symptoms improve. Sinusitis and bone pain become more common, whereas fever, lymphadenopathy, and skin infections become rare. Early loss of permanent teeth associated with chronic gingivitis is common to all forms of neutropenia. No association with malignancy has been observed.

Pyogenic Arthritis, Pyoderma Gangrenosum, and Acne Syndrome

Pyogenic arthritis, pyoderma gangrenosum, and acne (PAPA) syndrome is a rare autosomal dominant auto-inflammatory syndrome characterized by early onset of

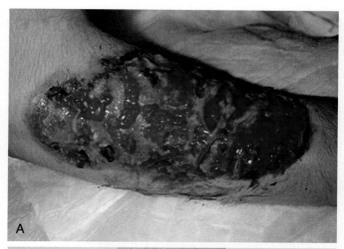

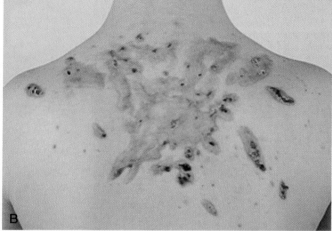

FIGURE 43–9 A, Aggressive ulcerative skin lesions indistinguishable from pyoderma gangrenosum seen in a patient with PAPA. **B,** Cystic acne in PAPA begins in adolescence and persists into adulthood.[302]

recurrent episodes of destructive inflammation of joints and skin (see Table 43–3).[295] PAPA syndrome manifests typically with recurrent episodes of sterile, erosive arthritis in early childhood, occurring spontaneously or after minor trauma, occasionally resulting in significant joint destruction.[295-297] Radiographic findings include periosteal proliferation of involved bones and in some cases ankylosis.[295] The arthritis may respond to corticosteroid therapy; however, the associated adverse effects often limit their use. As patients progress to puberty, cutaneous involvement may predominate. Dermatological manifestations are also episodic and recurrent, and are characterized by debilitating aggressive ulcerative skin lesions, often of the lower extremities, indistinguishable from pyoderma gangrenosum (Fig. 43–9).[297,298] While the synovial fluid and skin lesions may have the appearance of an infectious process, culture of skin and joints are sterile. The other component of this triad is cystic acne, which begins in adolescence and persists into adulthood (see Fig. 43–9).[296] Other possible manifestations of the PAPA syndrome include pathergy (the formation of sterile abscesses at injection sites), sporadic episodes of irritable bowel syndrome, aphthous stomatitis and, in one family, pancytopenia after administration of sulfa-containing medications.[295,296]

PAPA is caused by mutations in the proline serine threonine phosphatase-interacting protein [PSTPIP1, or CD2 binding protein 1 (CD2BP1)] on chromosome 15[297] that link PEST-type phosphatases to their substrates.[299] The encoded cytoplasmic protein modulates T cell activation,[300] cytoskeletal organization,[301] and IL-1β release.[302] To date, four missense mutations have been described in an online database of mutations (http://fmf.igh.cnrs.fr/in fevers/).

PSTPIP1 interacts with pyrin, and PAPA-associated PSTPIP1 mutations increase the strength of this interaction. Increased PSTPIP1-pyrin interaction, in turn, appears to cause increased IL-1β activation. Two possible mechanisms have been proposed. The first assumes an inhibitory role for pyrin, with PSTPIP1 mutations leading to sequestration of pyrin.[302] Alternatively, increased avidity of PSTPIP1 for pyrin may lead to the formation of macromolecular complexes denoted pyroptosomes, leading to cell death and inflammatory cytokine release.[303]

Consistent with this proposed pathogenesis, increased IL-1β levels have been noted,[302] and increased levels may contribute to TNF production,[304] raising the possibility that treatment with biological agents may be helpful. There are reports of successful treatment with anakinra,[302,305] etanercept,[304] and infliximab[298] in some patients; however, there is no consistently successful treatment for this syndrome suggesting that *PSTPIP1* mutations may have pathophysiological effects beyond IL-1 activation. There is anecdotal evidence that IL-1 inhibition may be more beneficial for joint manifestations and TNF inhibition for pyoderma gangrenosum.

Deficiency of the Interleukin-1 Receptor Antagonist

DIRA is a rare autosomal recessive autoinflammatory disease caused by mutations affecting the gene *IL1RN* encoding the endogenous IL-1 receptor antagonist.[9,10] There are founder mutations in Puerto Rico, Newfoundland, the Netherlands, and the Lebanese Israel border.[9] Children with DIRA present with strikingly similar clinical features including systemic inflammation in the perinatal period, bone pain, characteristic radiographical findings of multifocal sterile osteolytic bone lesions, widening of multiple anterior ribs, periostitis, and pustular skin lesions (Fig. 43–10). The skin manifestations range from groupings of small pustules to a generalized pustulosis. *IL1RN* mutations result in a prematurely truncated protein that is not secreted, resulting in to patient cells being hyperresponsive to IL-1 stimulation and increased production of proinflammatory cytokines and chemokines. Patients treated with anakinra, an IL-1 receptor antagonist, exhibited rapid clinical and immunological responses (see Chapter 44).[9,10]

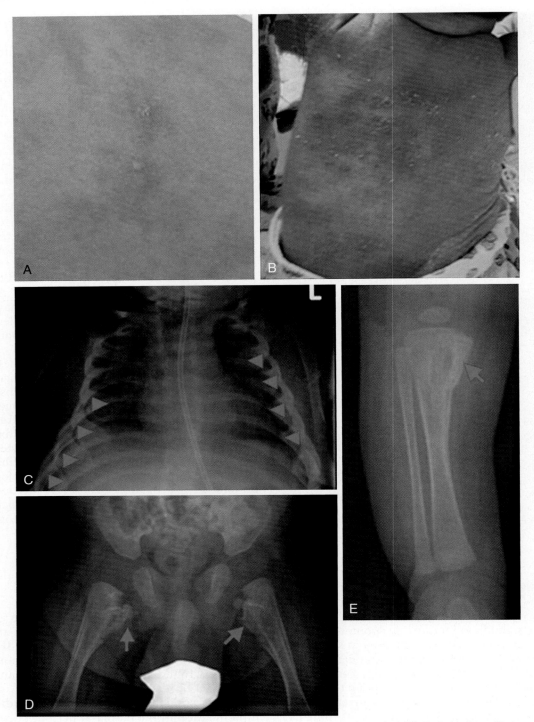

FIGURE 43–10   The skin manifestations range from groupings of small pustules **(A)** to a generalized pustulosis **(B)**. Typical radiographical manifestations include widening of multiple ribs (with affected ribs indicated with arrowheads) **(C)**, heterotopic ossification or periosteal cloaking of the proximal femoral metaphysis **(D,** *arrows*),[9] and an osteolytic lesion with a sclerotic rim **(E,** *arrow*). (Courtesy of Dr. Raphaela Goldbach-Mansky)

REFERENCES

1. C.C. John, J.R. Gilsdorf, Recurrent fever in children, Pediatr. Infect. Dis. J. 21 (2002) 1071–1077.
5. M.F. McDermott, I. Aksentijevich, J. Galon, et al., Germline mutations in the extracellular domains of the 55 kDa TNF receptor, TNFR1, define a family of dominantly inherited autoinflammatory syndromes, Cell 97 (1999) 133–144.
6. J. Galon, I. Aksentijevich, M.F. McDermott, TNFRSF1A mutations and autoinflammatory syndromes, Curr. Opin. Immunol. 12 (2000) 479–486.
8. S.L. Masters, A. Simon, I. Aksentijevich, et al., Horror autoinflammaticus: the molecular pathophysiology of autoinflammatory disease, Annu. Rev. Immunol. 27 (2009) 621–668.

9. I. Aksentijevich, S.L. Masters, P.J. Ferguson, et al., An autoinflammatory disease with deficiency of the interleukin-1-receptor antagonist, N. Engl. J. Med. 360 (2009) 2426–2437.

10. S. Reddy, S. Jia, R. Geoffrey, et al., An autoinflammatory disease due to homozygous deletion of the IL1RN locus, N. Engl. J. Med. 360 (2009) 2438–2444.

12. F.M.F. International, Consortium: Ancient missense mutations in a new member of the RoRet gene family are likely to cause familial Mediterranean fever, Cell 90 (1997) 797–807.

13. F.M.F. French, Consortium: a candidate gene for familial Mediterranean fever, Nat. Genet. 17 (1997) 25–31.

15. I. Aksentijevich, Y. Torosyan, J. Samuels, et al., Mutation and haplotype studies of familial Mediterranean fever reveal new ancestral relationships and evidence for a high carrier frequency with reduced penetrance in the Ashkenazi Jewish population, Am. J. Hum. Genet. 64 (1999) 949–962.

44. J.J. Chae, G. Wood, S.L. Masters, et al., The B30.2 domain of pyrin, the familial Mediterranean fever protein, interacts directly with caspase-1 to modulate IL-1beta production, Proc. Natl. Acad. Sci. U.S.A. 103 (2006) 9982–9987.

45. M.G. Booty, J.J. Chae, S.L. Masters, et al., Familial Mediterranean fever with a single MEFV mutation: where is the second hit? Arthritis Rheum. 60 (2009) 1851–1861.

47. E. Sohar, J. Gafni, M. Pras, et al., Familial Mediterranean fever. a survey of 470 cases and review of the literature, Am. J. Med. 43 (1967) 227–253.

48. A.D. Schwabe, R.S. Peters, Familial Mediterranean Fever in Armenians, Analysis of 100 cases, Medicine (Baltimore) 53 (1974) 453–462.

49. H.A. Majeed, M. Rawashdeh, H. el-Shanti, et al., Familial Mediterranean fever in children: the expanded clinical profile, Q. J. Med. 92 (1999) 309–318.

88. I. Touitou, T. Sarkisian, M. Medlej-Hashim, et al., Country as the primary risk factor for renal amyloidosis in familial Mediterranean fever, Arthritis Rheum. 56 (2007) 1706–1712.

92. I. Touitou, S. Lesage, M. McDermott, et al., Infevers: an evolving mutation database for auto-inflammatory syndromes, Hum. Mutat. 24 (2004) 194–198.

111. L.M. Williamson, D. Hull, R. Mehta, et al., Familial Hibernian fever, Q. J. Med. 51 (1982) 469–480.

114. I. Aksentijevich, J. Galon, M. Soares, et al., The tumor-necrosis-factor receptor-associated periodic syndrome: new mutations in TNFRSF1A, ancestral origins, genotype-phenotype studies, and evidence for further genetic heterogeneity of periodic fevers, Am. J. Hum. Genet. 69 (2001) 301–314.

135. F.C. Kimberley, A.A. Lobito, R.M. Siegel, et al., Falling into TRAPS—receptor misfolding in the TNF receptor 1-associated periodic fever syndrome, Arthritis Res. Ther. 9 (2007) 217.

136. S.L. Rebelo, S.E. Bainbridge, M.R. Amel-Kashipaz, et al., Modeling of tumor necrosis factor receptor superfamily 1A mutants associated with tumor necrosis factor receptor-associated periodic syndrome indicates misfolding consistent with abnormal function, Arthritis Rheum. 54 (2006) 2674–2687.

142. K.M. Hull, E. Drewe, I. Aksentijevich, et al., The TNF receptor-associated periodic syndrome (TRAPS): emerging concepts of an autoinflammatory disorder, Medicine (Baltimore) 81 (2002) 349–368.

149. E. Drewe, E.M. McDermott, P.T. Powell, et al., Prospective study of anti-tumour necrosis factor receptor superfamily 1B fusion protein, and case study of anti-tumour necrosis factor receptor superfamily 1A fusion protein, in tumour necrosis factor associated periodic syndrome (TRAPS): clinical and laboratory findings in a series of seven patients, Rheumatology (Oxford) 42 (2003) 235–239.

153. M. Gattorno, M.A. Pelagatti, A. Meini, et al., Persistent efficacy of anakinra in patients with tumor necrosis factor receptor-associated periodic syndrome, Arthritis Rheum. 58 (2008) 1516–1520.

157. J.W. van der Meer, J.M. Vossen, J. Radl, et al., Hyperimmunoglobulinaemia D and periodic fever: a new syndrome, Lancet 1 (1984) 1087–1090.

158. J.P. Drenth, L. Cuisset, G. Grateau, et al., Mutations in the gene encoding mevalonate kinase cause hyper-IgD and periodic fever syndrome. International Hyper-IgD Study Group, Nat. Genet. 22 (1999) 178–181.

159. S.M. Houten, W. Kuis, M. Duran, et al., Mutations in MVK, encoding mevalonate kinase, cause hyperimmunoglobulinaemia D and periodic fever syndrome, Nat. Genet. 22 (1999) 175–177.

161. J.C. van der Hilst, E.J. Bodar, K.S. Barron, et al., Long-term follow-up, clinical features, and quality of life in a series of 103 patients with hyperimmunoglobulinemia D syndrome, Medicine (Baltimore) 87 (2008) 301–310.

195. A.M. Prieur, C. Griscelli, F. Lampert, et al., A chronic, infantile, neurological, cutaneous and articular (CINCA) syndrome, A specific entity analysed in 30 patients, Scand. J. Rheumatol. 66 (Suppl.) (1987) 57–68.

196. H.M. Hoffman, A.A. Wanderer, D.H. Broide, Familial cold autoinflammatory syndrome: phenotype and genotype of an autosomal dominant periodic fever, J. Allergy Clin. Immunol. 108 (2001) 615–620.

200. R.I. Kyle, RH: A case of cold urticaria with unusual family history, JAMA 114 (1940) 1067.

203. H.M. Hoffman, J.L. Mueller, D.H. Broide, et al., Mutation of a new gene encoding a putative pyrin-like protein causes familial cold autoinflammatory syndrome and Muckle-Wells syndrome, Nat. Genet. 29 (2001) 301–305.

207. T.J. Muckle, Wellsm: Urticaria, deafness, and amyloidosis: a new heredo-familial syndrome, Q. J. Med. 31 (1962) 235–248.

209. I. Aksentijevich, C DP, E.F. Remmers, et al., The clinical continuum of cryopyrinopathies: novel CIAS1 mutations in North American patients and a new cryopyrin model, Arthritis Rheum. 56 (2007) 1273–1285.

213. B. Neven, I. Callebaut, A.M. Prieur, et al., Molecular basis of the spectral expression of CIAS1 mutations associated with phagocytic cell-mediated autoinflammatory disorders CINCA/NOMID, MWS, and FCU, Blood 103 (2004) 2809–2815.

215. A.M. Prieur, C. Griscelli, Arthropathy with rash, chronic meningitis, eye lesions, and mental retardation, J. Pediatr. 99 (1981) 79–83.

216. S.G. Hassink, D.P. Goldsmith, Neonatal onset multisystem inflammatory disease, Arthritis Rheum. 26 (1983) 668–673.

220. I. Aksentijevich, M. Nowak, M. Mallah, et al., De novo CIAS1 mutations, cytokine activation, and evidence for genetic heterogeneity in patients with neonatal-onset multisystem inflammatory disease (NOMID): a new member of the expanding family of pyrin-associated autoinflammatory diseases, Arthritis Rheum. 46 (2002) 3340–3348.

221. R. Goldbach-Mansky, N.J. Dailey, S.W. Canna, et al., Neonatal-onset multisystem inflammatory disease responsive to interleukin-1beta inhibition, N. Engl. J. Med. 355 (2006) 581–592.

223. J. Feldmann, A.M. Prieur, P. Quartier, et al., Chronic infantile neurological cutaneous and articular syndrome is caused by mutations in CIAS1, a gene highly expressed in polymorphonuclear cells and chondrocytes, Am. J. Hum. Genet. 71 (2002) 198–203.

236. H.M. Hoffman, M.L. Throne, N.J. Amar, et al., Efficacy and safety of rilonacept (interleukin-1 Trap) in patients with cryopyrin-associated periodic syndromes: results from two sequential placebo-controlled studies, Arthritis Rheum. 58 (2008) 2443–2452.

246. H.J. Lachmann, I. Kone-Paut, J.B. Kuemmerle-Deschner, et al., Use of canakinumab in the cryopyrin-associated periodic syndrome, N. Engl. J. Med. 360 (2009) 2416–2425.

249. P.N. Hawkins, H.J. Lachmann, M.F. McDermott, Interleukin-1-receptor antagonist in the Muckle-Wells syndrome, N. Engl. J. Med. 348 (2003) 2583–2584.

250. G.S. Marshall, K.M. Edwards, J. Butler, et al., Syndrome of periodic fever, pharyngitis, and aphthous stomatitis, J. Pediatr. 110 (1987) 43–46.

256. K.T. Thomas, H.M. Feder Jr., A.R. Lawton, et al., Periodic fever syndrome in children, J. Pediatr. 135 (1999) 15–21.

261. H.M. Feder, Jr., Periodic fever, aphthous stomatitis, pharyngitis, adenitis: a clinical review of a new syndrome, Curr. Opin. Pediatr. 12 (2000) 253–256.

266. M. Renko, E. Salo, A. Putto-Laurila, et al., A randomized, controlled trial of tonsillectomy in periodic fever, aphthous stomatitis, pharyngitis, and adenitis syndrome, J. Pediatr. 151 (2007) 289–292.

269. W. Garavello, M. Romagnoli, R.M. Gaini, Effectiveness of adenotonsillectomy in PFAPA syndrome: a randomized study, J. Pediatr. 155 (2009) 250–253.

273. D.C. Dale, A.A. Bolyard, W.P. Hammond, Cyclic neutropenia: natural history and effects of long-term treatment with recombinant human granulocyte colony-stimulating factor, Cancer Invest. 11 (1993) 219–223.

277. D.C. Dale, R.E. Person, A.A. Bolyard, et al., Mutations in the gene encoding neutrophil elastase in congenital and cyclic neutropenia, Blood 96 (2000) 2317–2322.

302. N.G. Shoham, M. Centola, E. Mansfield, et al., Pyrin binds the PSTPIP1/CD2BP1 protein, defining familial Mediterranean fever and PAPA syndrome as disorders in the same pathway, Proc. Natl. Acad. Sci. U.S.A. 100 (2003) 13501–13506.

Entire reference list is available online at www.expertconsult.com.

Chapter 44

AUTOINFLAMMATORY BONE DISORDERS

Polly J. Ferguson and Ronald M. Laxer

Autoinflammatory disorders, discussed extensively in Chapter 43, result from aberrant activation of the innate immune system.[1] They occur in the absence of high titer autoantibodies or autoreactive lymphocytes, distinguishing them from the classic autoimmune disorders.[1,2] The concept of autoinflammatory disorders was proposed in 1999, following the identification of the genetic basis of the prototypic periodic fever syndromes, familial Mediterranean fever, and TNF receptor–associated periodic syndrome.[1,3-5] There are now more than 30 disorders thought to be autoinflammatory, most of which affect children; included are a group of disorders that have bone inflammation as a main phenotypic feature including chronic recurrent multifocal osteomyelitis (CRMO); synovitis, acne, pustulosis, hyperostosis, osteitis (SAPHO) syndrome; Majeed syndrome; deficiency of interleukin-1 receptor antagonist (DIRA); and cherubism.[1,6]

CHRONIC RECURRENT MULTIFOCAL OSTEOMYELITIS

Overview

In 1972, Giedion recognized what is now commonly referred to as CRMO as a distinct clinical entity when he described four children who presented with subacute and chronic symmetrical osteomyelitis.[7] The term CRMO was coined by Probst, Bjorksten, and Gustavson to describe the recurrent nature of the illness.[8,9] Since then CRMO has been commonly used for this clinical entity, despite the disease being neither always multifocal nor recurrent. The co-occurrence of CRMO with pustulosis palmoplantaris (PPP) was reported in 1967 in a child with bilateral clavicular osteitis, but Bjorksten and colleagues firmly established the association with CRMO and PPP.[9,10] The correlation between CRMO and PPP has been confirmed by others, and descriptions of additional dermatological connections with CRMO, including psoriasis vulgaris, severe acne, generalized pustulosis (GP), and Sweet syndrome, followed shortly afterward.[11-20] Subsequently, reports of the co-occurrence of CRMO and inflammatory bowel disease (IBD) emerged, and the observation that CRMO may evolve into spondyloarthropathy over time in some patients suggested that CRMO might best fit in

spondyloarthropathy family of disorders.[21-34] Recently, the identification of the genetic basis for a subgroup of early onset CRMO cases and for murine models of disease has defined CRMO as an autoinflammatory syndrome.[6,35-41]

Nomenclature

It is difficult to review the CRMO literature because of the many terms used to describe similar clinical entities. Names used to describe cases of sterile inflammatory bone disorders that occur in the presence or absence of skin or intestinal inflammation are listed in Table 44–1.[33,42-55] The most common terms used in the literature are CRMO and SAPHO syndrome. SAPHO is an acronym proposed in 1987 by Chamot and colleagues as a broad umbrella term to denote a clinical syndrome characterized by inflammation of the bone, joint, and skin.[56,57] The SAPHO syndrome encompasses bone inflammation in the form of sterile osteomyelitis or as hyperostosis; inflammation of the skin including acne or pustulosis and inflammation of the joint in the form of synovitis. SAPHO syndrome is the term most frequently employed by adult rheumatologists, whereas the pediatric community has primarily applied the term CRMO.[31,43,58-61] SAPHO syndrome and CRMO may well be the same disorder presenting in different age groups, (CRMO in childhood and SAPHO in adults).

Another problem with the term CRMO is that sometimes the disease process is unifocal or is multifocal without recurrence, limiting the accuracy of the diagnostic term for many patients' clinical courses. In a German cohort of 89 patients with at least one noninfectious inflammatory bone lesion, approximately 20% had bone inflammation in one location with disease duration less than six months without recurrence (unifocal nonrecurrent), nearly 45% of patients had classic CRMO with multiple bone lesions with recurrent flares with remissions (recurrent multifocal), and the remaining 35% had persistent multifocal bone inflammation for longer than six months without remissions (persistent multifocal).[62] In addition, some children present with unifocal disease, yet over time go onto develop classic multifocal recurrent disease.[62] Similarly, in a cohort of 30 pediatric patients with sterile osteitis reported by Girschick and colleagues, 30% had unifocal nonrecurrent disease, 10% had unifocal recurrent disease,

Table 44–1

Alternative diagnostic labels

- Chronic recurrent multifocal osteomyelitis
- Chronic sclerosing osteitis
- Pustulotic arthrosteitis
- Chronic multifocal cleidometaphyseal osteomyelitis
- Chronic symmetrical osteomyelitis
- Chronic multifocal symmetrical osteomyelitis
- Sternocostoclavicular hyperostosis
- Sternoclavicular pustulotic osteitis
- Diffuse sclerosing osteomyelitis
- Multifocal recurrent periostitis
- Bone lesions of acne fulminans
- Clavicular hyperostosis and acne arthritis
- Chronic nonbacterial osteomyelitis

30% had multifocal nonrecurrent disease, and 30% had classic CRMO.[63] As a result, several authors have proposed other names, including chronic nonbacterial osteomyelitis (CNO) and chronic nonbacterial osteitis.[62,63] In this chapter, we will use the term CRMO.

Incidence, Geographic, and Racial Distribution

CRMO is a rare disorder. Several hundred cases have been reported in the literature, but the incidence of the disease is unknown. Early reports of CRMO were predominantly from Scandinavia; however, review of the literature suggests a worldwide distribution of disease affecting multiple ethnicities and races.[10,11,62,64]

Age at Onset and Sex Ratio

CRMO is primarily a disease of young girls with peak onset between the ages of 7 to 12 years.[62,65] Females are affected at a rate of two to four times that of males.[32,62,63,65-68] The majority of cases occur in childhood, but adults can be affected and are more likely to be reported as SAPHO syndrome.[58,67,69] Onset of CRMO prior to the age of 2 years is unusual and should prompt an evaluation for a syndromic form of CRMO including DIRA and Majeed syndrome.[35-37,39]

Etiology and Pathogenesis

CRMO best fits into the category of autoinflammatory disorders, a group of innate immune system disorders in which there are seemingly unprovoked episodes of inflammation.[1,2,70] In most cases of CRMO (and SAPHO), bone inflammation occurs in the absence of an identifiable trigger. Cultures of the bone are typically sterile, antibiotic therapy is rarely accompanied by clinical improvement, and antiinflammatory medications improve the condition.[62,65-68,71-76] Despite the inability to culture an organism in the vast majority of cases, many investigators have postulated that the osteitis is driven or triggered by exposure to a microbial agent. There are a few reports of bone cultures growing organisms, including *Propionibacterium acnes*, *Mycoplasma*, various *Staphylococcus*

species.[24,25,65,72,73,76-83] However, in many cases it is unclear if it is a contaminated specimen or a true infection.[76] In a cohort of adults with inflammatory osseous anterior chest wall lesions, most of whom also had PPP, *Propionibacterium acnes* was cultured in bone biopsy samples from 7 of the 15 patients, suggesting that for this population of adult patients infection may have played a role in pathogenesis.[81] However, in children with CRMO and for most adults with SAPHO syndrome the vast majority of cultures of pustules and bone are negative.[65,74,75]

Girshick and colleagues looked for evidence of microbial infection in 25 patients with CNO, all of whom had a bone biopsy performed as part of their diagnostic evaluation.[63] All biopsies were sent for aerobic and anaerobic bacterial, mycobacterial, and fungal organisms. Eubacterial polymerase chain reaction was performed on 12 of the 25 bone biopsy samples, but no bacterial ribosomal DNA was detected.[63] Serological testing for evidence of *Borrelia burgdorferi*, *Salmonella*, *Yersinia enterocolitica*, *Campylobacter jejuni*, and *Streptococcus pyogenes* showed no evidence of acute or chronic infection with any of these microbes.[63] Supporting the lack of an active infection as an etiology in CRMO or SAPHO syndrome, prolonged antimicrobial therapy rarely results in clinical improvement.[65,66,84,85] However, Schilling and colleagues reported that seven of 13 patients with CRMO treated with azithromycin had rapid clinical and radiological improvement.[82,86] However, azithromycin has a known antiinflammatory effect, so a response to azithromycin does not necessarily support the presence of an active infection in CRMO.[87,88] Bjorksten and colleagues and Jurik and coworkers reported that approximately 25% of CRMO patients presented with trauma preceding the development of chronic bone inflammation,[9,69] suggesting tissue damage as another possible trigger, although this has not been found in most series.

The immunological basis of CRMO remains unknown. There is no evidence of immune deficiency, and the lack of high titer autoantibodies suggests that it does not have an autoimmune basis.[65,73] Although in a German cohort antinuclear antibodies ≥1:120 were present in approximately one-third of cases, this hasn't been found other cohorts.[62] There is no significant association with human leukocyte antigen-(HLA) B27 positivity.[62,65,73] There are reports of neutrophil dysfunction in CRMO; however, the role of neutrophils in these disorders has not been fully elucidated.[9,69,89] Mouse models of CRMO have demonstrated that the adaptive immune system is not needed for disease development.[38,40,90] In addition, the discovery that some cases of infantile-onset noninfectious multifocal osteitis associated with GP are due to interleukin (IL)-1 pathway dysregulation lends additional support to the notion that CRMO, SAPHO and related disorders are autoinflammatory.[36,37]

Many authors have noted the tendency for CRMO or SAPHO syndrome to evolve into a picture consistent with spondyloarthropathy over time.[25,43,60,68,91] Rohekar and Inman point out that SAPHO syndrome has many features that fit into the spondyloarthropathy family and that suggest it lies in the spectrum of disease between ankylosing spondylitis and psoriatic arthritis (Fig. 44–1).[31,34] The connection between CRMO and IBD also supports the contention that CRMO is part of the spondyloarthropathy spectrum of disease. Crohn's Disease and ulcerative colitis have both been reported in conjunction with CRMO and SAPHO syndrome.[22-24,26-30,34] When IBD is associated with CRMO, pyoderma gangrenosum may accompany the inflammatory gut and bone disease.[19,30,92] The link between gut inflammation and spondyloarthropathies is well established with endoscopic gastrointestinal inflammation detectable in less than 40% of spondyloarthropathy patients.[93,94] In three CRMO cohorts, 13% of affected individuals had a first or second degree relative with Crohn's Disease, further supporting the link between IBD and autoinflammatory bone disease.[6,62,66]

Role of Genetics in CRMO Pathogenesis

Evidence that genetics play a prominent role in susceptibility to CRMO comes from reports of affected siblings, concordant monozygotic twins (with unaffected parents), and parent/child duos.[13,45,55,62,89,95] First-degree relatives with CRMO in one member and PPP or psoriasis in at least one other member have also been described.[6,62,69,95,96] Golla and colleagues performed an association study in CRMO and found evidence for a susceptibility locus on chromosome 18q21.3-22.[95] In addition, there are a spontaneous mutant mouse (cmo mouse) and a mouse made by chemical mutagenesis (lupo mouse) that developed chronic multifocal osteomyelitis with recessive inheritance.[38,40,41] Up to one-half of the first and second degree relatives of individuals with CRMO have another inflammatory disorder, most often some form of psoriasis (PPP or psoriasis vulgaris) or IBD.[6,62] Definitive proof that CRMO can be genetically determined came when *LPIN2* was identified as the causative gene for Majeed syndrome, followed by the identification of mutations in *pstpip2* in two murine models of disease (Fig. 44–2) and recently by the identification of mutations in *IL1RN* in infants with DIRA.[35-38,40] Identification of the genes involved in some forms of CRMO has resulted in a better understanding of disease pathogenesis.

Clinical Manifestations of CRMO

The typical clinical presentation of CRMO is local bone pain with or without fever.[9,25,65,68] Onset is usually insidious, although some people present with acute pain.[9,25,72] Tenderness, swelling, or warmth are often present overlying the involved bone but may also be absent.[9,25,32,65,72-74,97] At any one time, the number of osteomyelitis lesions can vary from one to 18.[65] The course typically waxes and wanes over many months to as many as 20 years.[65,66,98] However, many individuals have chronic unremitting symptoms that may vary in severity.[66] The disease may affect virtually any bone of the body, but the metaphyseal regions of the long bones, clavicle, vertebral bodies, and pelvis are the most commonly affected sites.[25,62,63,65,66] There is symmetrical bone involvement in 25% to 40% of individuals.[62,65]

The local swelling involving the soft tissues adjacent to the inflamed bone may mimic arthritis when the lesions affect the metaphyseal regions of the long bones.[25] Clavicular lesions often present with marked swelling and tenderness, most often involving the medial third of the

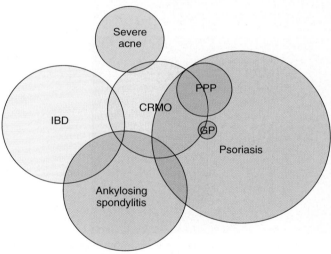

FIGURE 44–1   Overlapping features of the main inflammatory disorders associated with chronic recurrent multifocal osteomyelitis. CRMO, chronic recurrent multifocal osteomyelitis; GP, generalized pustular psoriasis; IBD, inflammatory bowel disease; PPP, palmoplantar pustulosis.

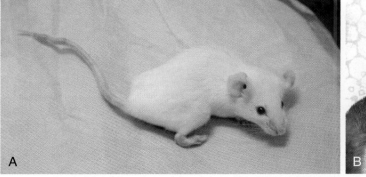
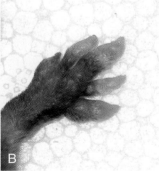

FIGURE 44–2   Tail kinks and hindfoot deformities in the cmo mouse model of CRMO. **A,** A cmo mouse with segmental swelling of the tail, swollen hindfoot, and increased erythema of the left ear. **B,** Swelling and deformity in the hindfoot and digits accompanied by thickening and discoloration of the nails in a cmo mouse. The swelling of the digits resembles dactylitis.

bone (Fig. 44–3).[9,68,69,99] When the pelvis or vertebrae are involved, pain is usually the only symptom.[68] Synovitis may accompany the bone lesions and can occur distant from the sites of bone involvement.[62,63] In one study, 80% of patients had been diagnosed with arthritis in joints adjacent to the lesion; a subset of these children had synovial biopsies that revealed histological evidence of synovitis.[63] Fever accompanies the bone pain at presentation in 33% of patients.[65] Most often the affected individuals appear well, although many complain of malaise and fatigue.[68,69] Twenty-five percent of CRMO patients present with an extraosseous manifestation; most

commonly a pustular rash on the palms and soles (Fig. 44–4).[25,63,65]

Laboratory Investigation

The majority of affected individuals have modest elevations of the erythrocyte sedimentation rate (ESR) and C-reactive protein (CRP).[62,65,69,76] White blood cell counts are typically normal or only mildly elevated.[25,62,65] High titer autoantibodies are typically absent and there is no strong association with HLA-B27 positivity.[32,63,65,72] Tumor necrosis factor (TNF) α was found to be elevated in the majority of

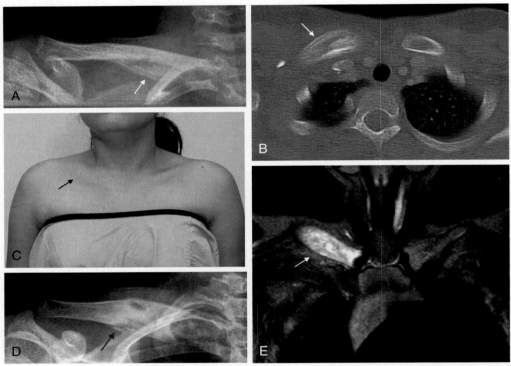

FIGURE 44–3 Clavicular involvement in CRMO. Adolescent female with unilateral clavicular involvement. **A,** Plain radiograph of the right clavicle at presentation reveals widening of the medial (⅔) clavicle with associated periosteal reaction. **B,** Corresponding computerized tomography scan of the right clavicle demonstrates expansion of the medial right clavicle, with areas of increased sclerosis accompanied by a surrounding periosteal reaction *(arrow)*. **C,** Flare of disease 18 months later showing further clavicular enlargement *(arrow)*. **D,** Plain radiograph of the right clavicle at that time demonstrates marked interval sclerosis and thickening. **E,** Magnetic resonance imaging at the same time shows increased signal intensity on fat suppressed contrast-enhanced T1 weighted MR images of the right medial clavicle consistent with continued inflammation. (Images courtesy of Dr. P. Babyn.)

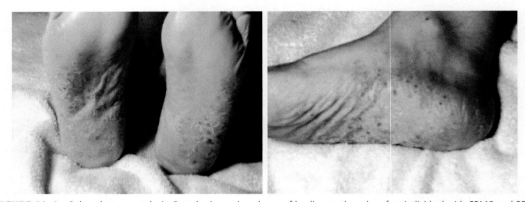

FIGURE 44–4 Palmoplantar pustulosis. Pustules in varying phases of healing on the soles of an individual with CRMO and PPP.

patients in one large study,[62] suggesting a role for TNF-α mediated inflammation in the pathogenesis of the disease.

Radiographic Studies

Very early in the disease, plain radiographs may be normal or may only show osteopenia; however, increased uptake on technetium bone scan or evidence of marrow edema on magnetic resonance imaging (MRI) can be seen at this stage. Mixed osteolytic and sclerotic lesions, with a predilection for the metaphyses of the long bones, are the most common radiological findings (Fig. 44–5).[8,68,98,100,101] Periosteal reaction may be present;[8,76] involvement of the small tubular bones is more likely to be accompanied by a significant periosteal reaction than is typically seen in the long bones.[76,101] Cortical thickening or progressive sclerosis of the lesions occurs later in the course of the disease, followed by gradual normalization of the radiographic appearance over several years.[8,62,66,68,76,98,101] Epiphyseal involvement is unusual but may occur and, when present, may lead to premature epiphyseal fusion.[76,101] Likewise, diaphyseal involvement is unusual but is typically adjacent to involved metaphyseal regions.[68]

Clavicular lesions are typically located in the medial clavicle and may have a lytic destructive appearance with periosteal new bone formation when the disease is active.[68,99,102] With time, the clavicle becomes increasingly sclerotic in appearance as the lesions heal.[68,99] Repeated periods of remission and active disease often result in progressive clavicular sclerosis and hyperostosis.[51,68] Vertebral lesions typically display erosion of vertebral plates sometimes accompanied by reduced intervertebral space, which can mimic infectious spondylodiscitis.[8,9,68,103,104] Alternatively, a destructive lytic lesion involving a vertebral body may occur, which may precede collapse of the affected vertebral body.[68,105] Vertebra plana may be seen.[34,75,106] Involvement of the bones of the pelvis may occur at joint surfaces or synchondroses and often has a sclerotic appearance (Fig. 44–6).[68] Sacroiliitis may also occur as part of the osseous pelvic lesions (Fig. 44–7).[25,32,66,68,101]

Asymptomatic lesions are common and can be detected by bone scan.[68,75,76,100] MRI is very useful for gauging activity and extent of the bone lesions.[68,101,107] In addition, it provides information about the extent of soft tissue involvement.[68,101] An active lesion typically has high signal intensity on T2-weighted MR images and on short tau inversion recovery (STIR) images accompanied by decreased signal intensity on T1-weighted images.[68] The ability to more clearly discern the extent of soft tissue involvement makes STIR images extremely useful.[68,101] Whole body STIR images can be performed at some institutions and offer an alternative to bone scan for detecting asymptomatic lesions.[101,108-110] The advantage of MRI over bone scan is that the lesions of CRMO often

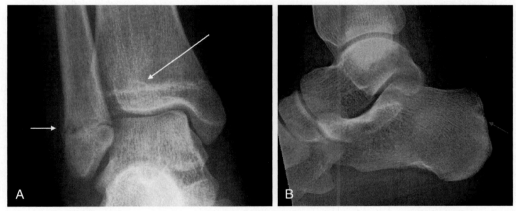

FIGURE 44–5 Typical lesions of CRMO. **A,** Osteolytic lesion with surrounding sclerosis in the metaphyseal area of the distal fibula *(short arrow)* and the distal tibia *(long arrow).* **B,** Osteolytic lesion with surrounding sclerosis in the calcaneus *(arrow).*

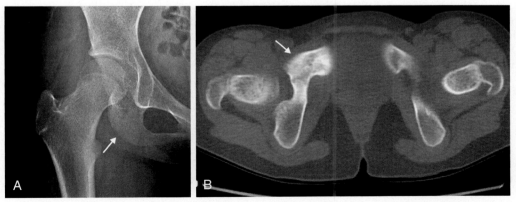

FIGURE 44–6 Pelvic involvement in CRMO. **A,** Plain film of the right pelvis demonstrates expansion of the ischium without visible osteolytic lesions. **B,** Computerized tomography of the region demonstrates expansion of the ischium with sclerosis and osteolytic lesions on the right.

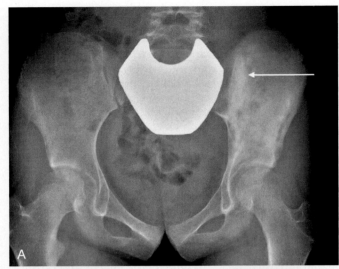

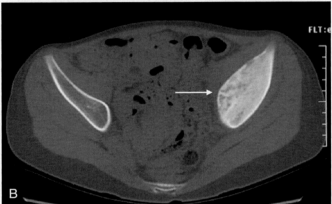

FIGURE 44–7 Involvement of the pelvis with sacroiliitis and osteomyelitis of the ilium. **A,** Unilateral sacroiliitis is present with sclerosis of the SI joint that is most prominent on the iliac side of the joint *(arrow)*. There is associated increased sclerosis of the left ilium with multiple moth eaten lesions scattered throughout the left side of the pelvis. **B,** Computerized tomography scan shows marked expansion of the left ilium with multiple small osteolytic lesions with surrounding sclerosis on the left *(arrow)*.

occur in the metaphyseal regions of the long bones and are often symmetrical. In a growing child, symmetrical inflammatory lesions in the metaphyses may be read as normal increased uptake due to metabolic activity in the open growth plate.

A reasonable radiographic approach in a child with suspected CRMO would be to start with plain radiographs of symptomatic regions, perform a bone scan or whole body MRI to detect asymptomatic lesions, obtain plain radiographs of the additional lesions, and use site-specific MRI to further delineate extent of disease as needed.

Histology

Histological findings in the bone vary depending on the age of the lesion, with neutrophils prominent in early lesions and a mixed inflammatory infiltrate consisting primarily of lymphocytes and plasma cells with varying degrees of sclerosis and fibrosis present later.[9,65,67,69,72,73]

Abscess formation surrounded by lymphocytes and increased osteoclasts with signs of bone resorption also can be seen early.[67] Later, a predominance of lymphocytes, accompanied by plasma cells, histocytes, and a few neutrophils, are seen.[65,67,69,73] Noncaseating granulomas have been reported in some biopsies.[9,67] Multinucleated giant cells, necrotic bone, areas of new bone formation, and fibrosis can also be seen in late lesions.[65,67,69,73] The histopathological picture may vary within the same sample; it is important to evaluate multiple sections from each biopsy specimen.[73]

Associated Inflammatory Conditions

There is a firm association of CRMO with inflammatory disorders of the skin and gut. These include PPP,[9,10,13,20,21] psoriasis vulgaris,[11,21] GP,[111] Sweet syndrome,[16-19] severe acne,[12,15] and pyoderma gangrenosum.[30,66,92] An association also exists with IBD, most often Crohn's Disease, but also with ulcerative colitis and celiac disease.[22-24,26-30,62,66] Peripheral arthritis has been reported with CRMO often adjacent to active bone lesions but can involve joints distant to the osteitis;[33,62,63,66] sacroiliac joint disease has also been reported.[25] Other disorders that have been reported in individuals with CRMO include Takayasu arteritis,[32,112,113] Wegener granulomatosus,[66,71] sclerosing cholangitis,[24,66] Ollier disease,[66] and parenchymal lung disease.[114,115]

Differential Diagnosis

There are no validated diagnostic criteria and no diagnostic tests for CRMO. Jansson and colleagues developed a clinical score to aid in differentiating nonbacterial osteitis from other bone lesions. They found that a normal complete blood count; symmetrical bone lesions; lesions with marginal sclerosis; absence of fever; lesion in a vertebra, clavicle, or sternum; the presence of a radiographical proven lesion, and CRP level ≥1 mg/dL were all diagnostically helpful. A clinical score can then be calculated that ranges from 0 to 63, with a score of ≥39 generating a positive predictive value of 97% and a sensitivity of 68% in their cohort.[62] The differential diagnosis includes infectious osteomyelitis; malignant bone tumors including primary intraosseous lymphoma, osteosarcoma, Ewing sarcoma, leukemia, and neuroblastoma; benign bone lesions including osteoid osteoma and osteoblastoma; Langerhans cell histiocytosis; Rosai-Dorfman disease; psoriatic arthritis or spondyloarthropathy; and hypophosphatasia.[8,86,108,116-120] Biopsy is often needed to exclude an infectious etiology and to exclude the possibility of malignancy. It is difficult to definitively rule out malignancy based on clinical picture and imaging. MRI of the affected region is helpful to guide the site to biopsy.[68] The best site to biopsy is the site felt to give the best diagnostic information with the lowest chance for functional or cosmetic consequences.[108] In some cases, a biopsy may not be needed. This occurs when a child has classic radiographical findings of CRMO (particularly if the clavicle is one of the bones involved) and has a comorbid condition such as Crohn's Disease or psoriasis.

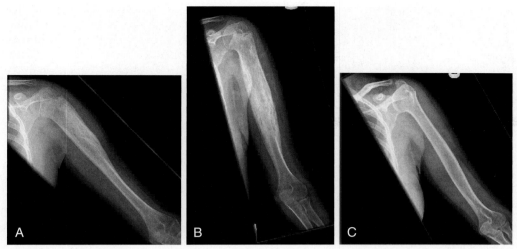

FIGURE 44–8   Plain radiographs of the left humerus. 10-year-old girl with noninfectious osteomyelitis of the left tibia diagnosed 7 months previously presents with a several month history of left arm pain. **A,** Initial radiograph shows marked proximal expansion with lateral cortical thickening extending down the proximal half of the humerus. She improves clinically on naproxen. **B,** 18 months later, she has a recurrence of pain with significant radiological progression, showing areas of lucency and sclerosis with extensive medullary expansion now involving almost the entire humerus. **C,** Plain radiograph taken one-year after a one-year course of intravenous pamidronate shows significant healing of the humerus lesion. (Courtesy of Dr. Paul Babyn.)

Treatment

Nonsteroidal antiinflammatory agents (NSAIDs) are used as a first line treatment strategy in CRMO, providing some degree of symptomatic relief in up to 80% of patients.[32,62,63,65,99,121] Indomethacin may be more effective than other NSAIDs.[122] However, many children continue to have symptoms despite NSAIDs.[32,62,63] The decision to escalate medical therapy must take into consideration the fact that most lesions resolve without significant sequelae.[63,66] Indications for escalation include persistent pain that affects normal activities, frequent recurrences, and functional limitations. Second line treatment agents used include corticosteroids, methotrexate, sulfasalazine, and azathioprine.[24,32,62,66,123] Most individuals obtain symptomatic relief with corticosteroids, but side-effects limit their usefulness in long term disease management.[32,63] There are reports of improvement in patients with CRMO or SAPHO treated with methotrexate, sulfasalazine, colchicine, hyperbaric oxygen, calcitonin, or azithromycin; however, the number of individuals treated was small, and there were also reports of treatment failures with several of these agents.[25,32,66,76,82,121,124] For NSAID resistant disease, there are case reports of marked improvement following treatment with TNF-α blocking agents,[27,62,125] interferon (INF)-α,[126] and INF-γ.[127] The data are strongest regarding the use of bisphosphonates in recalcitrant bone lesions. There is now information in the literature on more than 30 individuals with CRMO, CNO of the jaw, or SAPHO treated with various bisphosphonates, with a positive response to initial treatment reported in most of the individuals treated (Fig. 44–8).[62,128-137] In Miettunen and colleagues' series of 9 patients with CRMO, all nine were treated with pamidronate with a mean time to resolution of MRI abnormalities of six months. Four of the nine subsequently flared, but all responded to retreatment.[128] There are also reports of failure to respond to bisphosphonates and

failure to respond to TNF inhibitors.[62,129,134,137] Surgical approaches to treatment have included curettage or partial resection of the involved bone; however, surgical intervention is usually limited to obtaining tissue for cultures and histology. The optimal treatment strategy for CRMO remains unknown, and safety questions continue, with the long term use of both TNF inhibitors and with bisphosphonates in children. The use of IL-1 inhibitors to treat CRMO remains largely unexplored but could prove useful given the unequivocal role of IL-1 in the phenotype seen in patient with DIRA. All children should remain physically active despite ongoing inflammation. Referral to a physical therapist may be needed to regain strength and range of motion lost due to inactivity and guarding the extremity, especially for those with a delay in diagnosis and treatment.

Long-Term Outcome

For most affected individuals, the disease waxes and wanes with periods of exacerbations and remissions but with resolution of the disease process after several years, reportedly leaving most with no long-term sequelae (Fig. 44-9).[63,65] However, several long-term follow-up studies suggest that CRMO might be more persistent, lasting well over a decade in some[66,67,98] and might not be as benign as previously reported. The percentage of individuals with continued disease activity at follow-up ranges from 0% in a German cohort (mean follow-up 5.6 years) to18% in an Australian cohort (mean follow-up 7.5 years),[63] 25% in a Finnish cohort (mean follow-up 7.5 years),[71] 26% in a Canadian/Australian cohort (mean follow-up 12.4 years),[66] 57% in a French cohort (mean follow-up 5.3 years),[32] and 100% in a Dutch cohort (mean follow-up 5.5 years).[69] Pathological fractures, most often of a vertebral body, occurred in 49% of a German cohort.[62] Long-term skeletal deformities, particularly leg-length

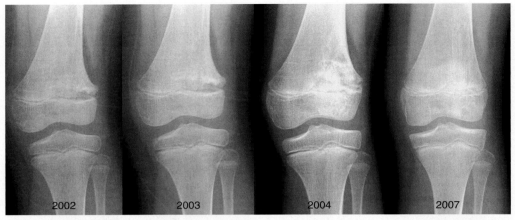

FIGURE 44–9   Radiographical resolution of distal femur lesion in a girl with CRMO over a 5-year time span. In 2002, there is an osteolytic lesion with surrounding sclerosis adjacent to the growth plate in the left distal femoral metaphysis. Minimal change is seen in the lesion one year later (2003). In 2004, the lesion begins to heal with significant sclerosis. In 2007, the lesion is almost healed, and the bone mineral density is nearly normal.

discrepancy, have been reported in up to 58% in one study.[76,98] Other long-term musculoskeletal abnormalities include residual hyperostosis and sclerosis of the bones, difficulty with mastication (following mandibular involvement), valgus deformity of the knee, vertebral collapse, persistent muscle atrophy, thoracic outlet syndrome, persistent arthritis, and evolution into spondyloarthropathy.[62,63,65,66,71,98,138] Disease recurrence may occur as long as six years after the last episode of osteitis.[8,98] Difficulty with employment, educational achievement, and participating in recreational sporting activities has been reported in a few cases.[66,98]

DISTINCT GENETIC AUTOINFLAMMATORY BONE SYNDROMES

Majeed Syndrome

The classic clinical triad in Majeed syndrome (OMIM reference # 609628) includes early onset CRMO, congenital dyserythropoietic anemia, and a neutrophilic dermatosis (consistent with Sweet syndrome) (Fig. 44–10).[17] This is a rare syndrome with only three unrelated Arabic families identified to date.[17,39,64] Affected individuals from all three families have homozygous mutations in the gene *LPIN2*.[35,39] Onset of the inflammatory bone disease is prior to the second birthday.[39,64] Bone pain with or without fever is the typical presenting feature. The histological and radiographical findings are identical to those of CRMO.[17,39,64] Cultures are negative, and there is no improvement with antibiotic therapy.[17,64]

Individuals with Majeed syndrome have varying degrees of anemia, ranging from mild to transfusion-dependent.[17,39,64] The red cells are typically microcytic.[17,139] Bone marrow biopsy reveals evidence of dyserythropoiesis with bi- and trinucleated normoblasts(see Fig. 44–10).[39,64] No other cell lines appear to be affected. Other laboratory abnormalities include leukocytosis, thrombocytosis, and a raised

ESR.[17,39,64] Despite the evidence that the protein Lipin2 is involved in fat metabolism, no lipid abnormalities have been reported in children with Majeed syndrome.[39] Cutaneous manifestations include a neutrophilic dermatosis consistent with Sweet syndrome in homozygous affected individuals.[17] Several of the carrier parents have psoriasis, which suggests that Lipin2 may play a role in the susceptibility to psoriasis.[6]

Treatment with corticosteroids results in clinical improvement in the inflammatory bone and skin disease; anemia is less responsive to treatment. However, undesirable long-term steroid induced side effects limits their long-term usefulness.[17,39] NSAIDs provide some degree of pain relief but do not produce disease control.[64] Colchicine was tried in three individuals without significant clinical improvement.[17] There are no published reports of using other disease modifying antirheumatic medications or biologicals in Majeed syndrome. Permanent joint contractures and growth disturbance have been reported after years of chronic inflammation (see Fig. 44–10).[64]

The role of Lipin-2 in inflammation of the bone and skin remains ill-defined. It is clear that Lipin-2 plays a role in fat metabolism and likely acts as a key phosphatidate phosphatase in the liver, but to date, there is no established link between the role of Lipin-2 in lipid metabolism and the inflammation seen in the bone and skin in Majeed syndrome.[140-142] However, hyper-immunoglobulin D syndrome, a hereditary periodic fever syndrome, is due to mutations in *MVK* that encodes for mevalonate kinase, an enzyme also involved in fat metabolism; yet how aberrant function in these lipid pathways genes causes autoinflammatory disease also remains unknown.[143] Lipin-2 may play a role in responses to oxidative stress as it is highly upregulated in animal models of tissue damage, including paraquat-induced pulmonary injury and 2,3,7,8-tetrachlorodibenzo-p-dioxin induced liver injury.[144,145] *Ned1* is an LPIN ortholog that, when mutated in yeast *Schizosaccharomyces pombe*, results in aberrantly shaped nuclei.[146] This suggests that Lipin-2 may be involved in mitosis as there are frequent bi- and trinucleated pronormoblasts in the bone marrow of children with Majeed syndrome.[147]

Table 44-2

Autoinflammatory bone disorders

	CRMO	Majeed Syndrome	DIRA	Cherubism	cmo and lupo Mice
Ethnicity	Worldwide, but mostly European	Arabic	European, Puerto Rican, Arabic	Worldwide	Occurs in various backgrounds
Fever	Uncommon	Common	Uncommon	No	Not assessed
Sites of osseous involvement	Metaphyses of long bones >vertebrae, clavicle, sternum, pelvis, others	Similar to CRMO	Anterior rib ends, metaphyses of long bones, vertebrae, others	Mandible > maxilla Rarely ribs	Vertebrae hind > forefeet
Extraosseous manifestations	PPP, psoriasis, IBD, others	Dyserythropoietic anemia, Sweet syndrome, HSM, growth failure	Generalized pustulosis, nail changes, lung disease, vasculitis	Cervical lymphadenopathy	Dermatitis, extramedullary hematopoiesis, splenomegaly
Family history of inflammatory disorders	Psoriasis, PPP, arthritis, IBD, others	Psoriasis in some obligate carriers	No known associations	No known associations	Heterozygotes normal
Inheritance	Not clear	Autosomal recessive	Autosomal recessive	Autosomal dominant; incomplete penetrance	Autosomal recessive
Gene defect	Unknown	*LPIN2*	*IL1RN*	*SH3BP2 >> PTPN11*	*Pstpip2*
Protein name	?	Lipin2	IL-1Ra	SH3BP2	PSTPIP2 (a.k.a. MAYP)
Protein function	?	Fat metabolism: (PAP enzyme activity), ↑ message to oxidative stress, ? role in mitosis	Antagonist of IL-1 receptor	↑myeloid cell response to M-CSF and RANKL, ↑TNF-α expression in macrophages	Macrophage proliferation, macrophage recruitment to sites of inflammation, cytoskeletal function
Cytokine abnormalities	↑ serum TNF-α	Not tested	↑IL-1α, IL-1β, MIP-1α, TNF-α, IL-8, IL-6 ex vivo monocyte assay; skin reveals IL-17 staining	↑ serum TNF-α in mouse model	cmo: ↑serum IL-6, MIP-1α, TNF-α, CSF-1, IP-10 Lupo: ↑serum MIP-1α, IL-4, RANTES, TGF-β

CRMO, chronic recurrent multifocal osteomyelitis; CSF, colony stimulating factor; DIRA, deficiency of interleukin-1 receptor antagonist; HSM, hepatosplenomegaly; IBD, inflammatory bowel disease; IL, interleukin; IL-1Ra, interleukin-1 receptor antagonist; IP-10, interferon-inducible protein-10; M-CSF, macrophage-colony stimulating factor; MIP-1α, macrophage inflammatory protein-1 alpha; PAP, phosphatidate phosphatase; PPP, palmer-plantar pustulosis; PSTPIP2, proline-serine-threonine phosphatase interacting protein; RANKL, receptor activator of nuclear factor-κB ligand; RANTES, regulated upon activation, normal T-cell expressed and secreted; SH3BP2, SH3 binding protein 2; TGF, transforming growth factor;TNF-α, tumor necrosis factor alpha.

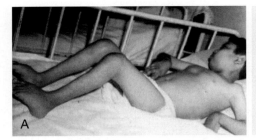
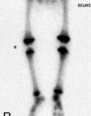
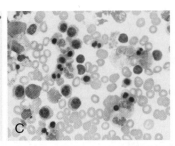

FIGURE 44–10 CRMO and dyserythropoietic anemia in Majeed syndrome. **A,** Affected male with contractures and failure to thrive. **B,** Tc99 bone scan from a girl with Majeed syndrome demonstrating increased radiotracer uptake in the metaphyses of the long bones of the lower extremities consistent with osteomyelitis. **C,** Dyserythropoiesis with multiple binucleated erythrocyte precursors in the bone marrow from a child with Majeed syndrome. (**A** from Majeed et al., Eur J Pediatr 160:705, 2001. **B** and **C** from Al-Mosawi et al., Arthritis Rheum 56:960, 2007.)

DIRA (Deficiency of the Interleukin-1 Receptor Antagonist)

DIRA (OMIM reference #612852) is an autosomal recessive autoinflammatory disorder caused by mutations in *IL1RN*, resulting in deficiency of the IL-1 receptor antagonist.[36,37] DIRA presents in infancy (usually within the first few weeks of life) with pustular rash, sterile osteitis, and periostitis, typically in the absence of fever.[36,37] Five of the 10 infants reported to date have been born near-term premature (33 to 36 weeks).[3 6,37] Respiratory problems were present in four of the 10 infants shortly after birth: either respiratory distress, apnea, or aspiration pneumonia.[36,37] Hepatomegaly was reported in five of the nine infants in one study.[36] All infants had elevated inflammatory markers including white blood cell counts in the 20,000 to 40,000 cells/mm³ range, ESRs up to 80 mm/hr, thrombocytosis ranging from 500,000 to 1,000,000 platelets/mm³, and CRP levels up to 30 mg/dL.[36,37] All but one of the 10 affected infants received prolonged courses of antibiotics for presumed sepsis without clinical improvement.[36,37] Clinical improvement was noted in all when treated with sizeable doses of corticosteroids.[36,37]

Inflammation of the skin has been present in 90% of the affected infants but can vary in severity from a few clusters of pustules to severe wide-spread GP, to ichthyosiform lesions.[36,37] Histologically, involved skin displays a neutrophilic infiltration of the epidermis and dermis, acanthosis, hyperkeratosis, and pustule formation along hair follicles.[36,37] Cultures of the skin lesions are generally negative; however, one infant had methicillin-resistant *Staphylococcus aureus* cultured from a pustular lesion on one occasion.[37] Other reported cutaneous manifestations included pathergy, oral ulcers, and pyoderma gangrenosum.[36] Nail abnormalities reminiscent of those seen in psoriasis have been reported in four of the children and range from nail pits to onychomadesis.[36]

There may be no objective evidence of osteitis on exam, but the infant may appear to be in pain with movement; only three infants had objective joint swelling. Yet, all had marked radiological abnormalities including multifocal osteolytic lesions, marked periostitis, widening of the medial clavicle, and flaring of the anterior rib ends (Fig. 44–11).[36,37] Nine of 10 infants had multifocal osteolytic lesions often involving the long bones.[36,37] Involvement of the vertebral bodies occurred in four children

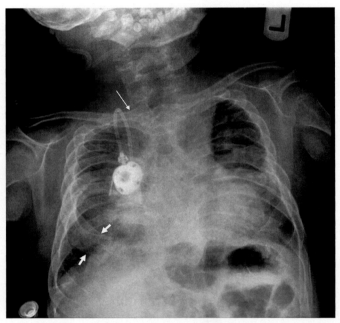

FIGURE 44–11 Chest radiograph in a patient with DIRA. Male infant with multiple bony abnormalities including expansion of the medial clavicles R>L *(long arrow)* and widening of the anterior rib ends *(shown by small thick arrows)*. Patchy opacifications are seen in the lung fields. This child developed interstitial lung disease. (Courtesy of Dr. P. Babyn.)

resulting in vertebral collapse in one and vertebral fusion in others.[36] Bone biopsies reveal neutrophilic infiltration with bone destruction, fibrosis, sclerosis, reactive new bone formation, and scattered osteoclasts.[36,37] Cultures of the bone were negative for anaerobes, aerobes, fungi, and acid-fast bacilli in all biopsies tested.[36,37]

Pulmonary involvement occurred in five of the 10 infants reported to date. Two of the five developed interstitial lung disease with pulmonary fibrosis found at autopsy in one and classic computed tomography findings of ground-glass opacities in another.[36,37] Central nervous system inflammation occurred in one infant, consisting of progressive inflammatory changes in the cortex ultimately leading to frank encephalomalacia of one of the involved gyri.[36] Histological evidence of vasculitis was found in the connective tissue seen in a bone biopsy from one of the affected children. The involved vessels had extensive neutrophilic infiltration with destruction of the vessel wall.[36] One infant developed multiple venous thromboses successfully treated with heparin.[37] Laboratory evaluations for genetic and immunological causes of clotting were negative in that infant. Other features include conjunctival injection, hypotonia, developmental delay, and failure to thrive.[36]

Antibiotics are ineffective in DIRA but all children improved when treated with high doses (2 mg/kg/day) of corticosteroids.[36,37] Prior to the discovery that children with DIRA were deficient in the IL-1 receptor antagonist, several steroid-sparing agents were used unsuccessfully including NSAIDs, intravenous gamma globulin, methotrexate, cyclosporine, azathioprine, etanercept, thalidomide, and INF-γ.[36] An empirical trial of anakinra in one child led to dramatic and rapid disease improvement, and this observation led investigators to sequence IL1 pathway genes and to the discovery of gene defect.[36] Mononuclear cells from DIRA patients produce high levels of inflammatory cytokines (including macrophage inflammatory protein-1α, TNF-α, IL-8 and IL-6) in vitro.[36,37] Left untreated, the unopposed action of IL-1 results in life-threatening systemic inflammation that predominately affects the skin and the bone.[36] Treatment with anakinra results in prompt and dramatic improvement within days of the initiation of treatment.[36] Once anakinra treatment was initiated, five of six infants were able to be weaned off corticosteroids.[36]

There is limited information about long-term outcomes in this condition given that it was unrecognized as a distinct clinical entity until its description in 2009. The disease is potentially fatal, with a 30% mortality rate in the first 10 patients described. Two deaths occurred in the first two years of life and were attributed to multisystem failure due to systemic inflammatory response syndrome.[36] One child lived until he was 9.5-years-old; he was treated with corticosteroids, methotrexate, and cyclosporin, but ultimately died of respiratory failure secondary to chronic interstitial lung disease.[36] Permanent skeletal deformities and failure to thrive occurred in several of the children prior to initiation of anakinra.[36] Allergic reaction to anakinra may occur in those that have complete deficiency of the protein, and desensitization therapy may allow continued treatment; alternatively, other IL-1 blocking agents may be used. Outcomes should improve significantly with early recognition accompanied by prompt initiation of appropriate treatment. Once the diagnosis of DIRA is made, genetic counseling should be offered to each family, so that they understand the recurrence risk. When genetic testing for IL1RN mutations is commercially available, determination of carrier status and prenatal diagnosis (if desired) would be options for family members of affected individuals.

Cherubism

Cherubism is an autosomal dominant autoinflammatory disorder (OMIM reference #118400) almost exclusively confined to the jaw.[148-151] The disorder was described by Jones in 1933 as a familial multilocular disease. Most children present between the ages of 2 and 7 years with symmetrical, progressive, nontender bony enlargement of the jaw without associated systemic symptoms.[148,150-153]

The expansion of the mandible and maxilla causes a chubby cheeked appearance and an upward gaze, features that Jones thought to be reminiscent of paintings of cherubs in Renaissance art.[153,154] The jaw hypertrophy is disfiguring and associated with significant dental problems, including malocclusion and loss of dentition with secondary difficulty with mastication in severely affected individuals.[153,154] Jaw enlargement begins to regress following puberty.[153] Regression may be accompanied by marked sclerosis, which may never fully resolve. Lymphadenopathy may be present during the active phase of the disease.[153] Extragnathic bone involvement is rare, but there are reports of lesions in the ribs, humerus, femur, and tibia.[153,155,156]

Radiographs reveal large multilocular, cystic-appearing lesions predominately affecting the mandible with less severe involvement of the maxilla. The lesions may appear osteolytic or radio-opaque with a coarse trabecular pattern associated with thinning of the cortices. Computerized tomography reveals osseous expansile remodeling and cortical thinning, dental derangement; many also show secondary maxillary sinus disease. MRI examination reveals extensive homogeneous isointense (to skeletal muscle) lesions on T1 MR images and hypointense on fast spin-echo T2-weighted MR images with fat suppression. Histologically, there are abundant osteoclasts interspersed throughout dense fibrostromal connective tissue without accompanying features of osteomyelitis. There have been no effective medical or surgical treatments.

A gene defect leading to cherubism was identified in 2001, when heterozygous mutations in the SH3 binding protein-2 (SH3BP2) were discovered in affected individuals from 12 families, with cherubism.[148] Mutations in SH3BP2 account for the vast majority of gene defects found in individuals with cherubism; however, mutations in *PTPN11* can also result in a cherubism phenotype.[157] To further understand the pathophysiology of cherubism, Ueki and colleagues created a murine cherubism model by knocking-in the most common human *SH3BP2* mutation.[158] One copy of the knock-in allele resulted in a surprisingly normal mouse.[158] However, mice homozygous for the knock-in allele (double knock-in) had widespread bone disease with osteoclast-rich inflammatory jaw lesions, systemic myeloid inflammation, and extensive trabecular bone loss throughout the remainder of the skeleton.[158] The inflammatory phenotype in cherubism mice occurs independent of a functioning adaptive immune system, is dependent on the presence of TNF-α, and is mediated by hematopoietically derived myeloid cells,[158] thus fulfilling criteria for an autoinflammatory bone disorder.[6] This finding that cherubism is an autoinflammatory disorder and is dependent on TNF-α offers hope that TNF-α inhibition may prove an effective therapy for this disfiguring disease.[159]

SUMMARY

Sterile bone inflammation is the cardinal feature of the autoinflammatory bone disorders. Many affected individuals also have a chronic inflammatory condition of the skin or intestinal tract, suggesting common immunological pathways are involved in CRMO, psoriasis, and IBD. A genetic defect has been found in two syndromic forms of CRMO and in a mouse model of the disease. The information learned from these single gene disorders implicates the innate immune system dysfunction in the pathogenesis of CRMO and related disorders.

REFERENCES

1. S.L. Masters, A. Simon, I. Aksentijevich, et al., Horror autoinflammaticus: the molecular pathophysiology of autoinflammatory disease (*), Annu. Rev. Immunol. 27 (2009) 621–668.
2. D. McGonagle, M.F. McDermott, A proposed classification of the immunological diseases, PLoS. Med. 3 (2006) e297.
6. P.J. Ferguson, H.I. El-Shanti, Autoinflammatory bone disorders, Curr. Opin. Rheumatol. 19 (2007) 492–498.
7. A. Giedion, W. Holthusen, L.F. Masel, et al., Subacute and chronic "symmetrical" osteomyelitis, Ann. Radiol. (Paris). 15 (1972) 329–342.
8. F.P. Probst, B. Bjorksten, K.H. Gustavson, Radiological aspect of chronic recurrent multifocal osteomyelitis, Ann. Radiol. (Paris) 21 (1978) 115–125.
9. B. Bjorksten, K.H. Gustavson, B. Eriksson, et al., Chronic recurrent multifocal osteomyelitis and pustulosis palmoplantaris, J. Pediatr. 93 (1978) 227–231.
11. R.M. Laxer, A.D. Shore, D. Manson, et al., Chronic recurrent multifocal osteomyelitis and psoriasis: a report of a new association and review of related disorders, Semin. Arthritis Rheum. 17 (1988) 260–270.
17. H.A. Majeed, M. Kalaawi, D. Mohanty, et al., Congenital dyserythropoietic anemia and chronic recurrent multifocal osteomyelitis in three related children and the association with Sweet syndrome in two siblings, J. Pediatr. 115 (1989) 730–734.
21. K. Bergdahl, B. Bjorksten, K.H. Gustavson, et al., Pustulosis palmoplantaris and its relation to chronic recurrent multifocal osteomyelitis, Dermatologica. 159 (1979) 37–45.
24. A. Bousvaros, M. Marcon, W. Treem, et al., Chronic recurrent multifocal osteomyelitis associated with chronic inflammatory bowel disease in children, Dig. Dis. Sci. 44 (1999) 2500–2507.
25. O. Vittecoq, L.A. Said, C. Michot, et al., Evolution of chronic recurrent multifocal osteitis toward spondylarthropathy over the long term, Arthritis Rheum. 43 (2000) 109–119.
31. G. Rohekar, R.D. Inman, Conundrums in nosology: synovitis, acne, pustulosis, hyperostosis, and osteitis syndrome and spondylarthritis, Arthritis Rheum. 55 (2006) 665–669.
32. C. Job-Deslandre, S. Krebs, A. Kahan, Chronic recurrent multifocal osteomyelitis: five-year outcomes in 14 pediatric cases, Joint Bone Spine 68 (2001) 245–251.
35. P.J. Ferguson, S. Chen, M.K. Tayeh, et al., Homozygous mutations in LPIN2 are responsible for the syndrome of chronic recurrent multifocal osteomyelitis and congenital dyserythropoietic anaemia (Majeed syndrome), J. Med. Genet. 42 (2005) 551–557.
36. I. Aksentijevich, S.L. Masters, P.J. Ferguson, et al., An autoinflammatory disease with deficiency of the interleukin-1-receptor antagonist, N. Engl. J. Med. 360 (2009) 2426–2437. 2009.
37. S. Reddy, S. Jia, R. Geoffrey, et al., An autoinflammatory disease due to homozygous deletion of the IL1RN locus, N. Engl. J. Med. 360 (2009) 2438–2444.
38. P.J. Ferguson, X. Bing, M.A. Vasef, et al., A missense mutation in pstpip2 is associated with the murine autoinflammatory disorder chronic multifocal osteomyelitis, Bone 38 (2006) 41–47.
39. Z.S. Al-Mosawi, K.K. Al-Saad, R. Ijadi-Maghsoodi, et al., A splice site mutation confirms the role of LPIN2 in Majeed syndrome, Arthritis Rheum. 56 (2007) 960–964.
40. J. Grosse, V. Chitu, A. Marquardt, et al., Mutation of mouse Mayp/Pstpip2 causes a macrophage autoinflammatory disease, Blood 107 (2006) 3350–3358.
56. A.M. Chamot, C.L. Benhamou, M.F. Kahn, et al., Acne-pustulosis-hyperostosis-osteitis syndrome, results of a national survey. 85 cases, Rev. Rhum. Mal. Osteoartic 54 (1987) 187–196.
57. C.L. Benhamou, A.M. Chamot, M.F. Kahn, Synovitis-acne-pustulosis hyperostosis-osteomyelitis syndrome (SAPHO), a new syndrome among the spondyloarthropathies? Clin. Exp. Rheumatol. 6 (1988) 109–112.
58. G. Hayem, A. Bouchaud-Chabot, K. Benali, et al., SAPHO syndrome: a long-term follow-up study of 120 cases, Semin. Arthritis Rheum. 29 (1999) 159–171.
61. M.F. Kahn, A.M. Chamot, SAPHO syndrome, Rheum. Dis. Clin. North Am. 18 (1992) 225–246.
62. A. Jansson, E.D. Renner, J. Ramser, et al., Classification of nonbacterial osteitis: retrospective study of clinical, immunological and genetic aspects in 89 patients, Rheumatology (Oxford) 46 (2007) 154–160.
63. H.J. Girschick, P. Raab, S. Surbaum, et al., Chronic non-bacterial osteomyelitis in children, Ann. Rheum. Dis. 64 (2005) 279–285.
65. C. Schultz, P.M. Holterhus, A. Seidel, et al., Chronic recurrent multifocal osteomyelitis in children, Pediatr. Infect. Dis. J. 18 (1999) 1008–1013.
66. A.M. Huber, P.Y. Lam, C.M. Duffy, et al., Chronic recurrent multifocal osteomyelitis: clinical outcomes after more than five years of follow-up, J. Pediatr. 141 (2002) 198–203.
67. B. Bjorksten, L. Boquist, Histopathological aspects of chronic recurrent multifocal osteomyelitis, J. Bone Joint Surg. (Br). 62 (1980) 376–380.
68. A.G. Jurik, Chronic recurrent multifocal osteomyelitis, Semin. Musculoskelet. Radiol. 8 (2004) 243–253.
82. F. Schilling, A.D. Wagner, Azithromycin: an anti-inflammatory effect in chronic recurrent multifocal osteomyelitis? A preliminary report, Z. Rheumatol. 59 (2000) 352–353.
83. M. Colina, A. Lo Monaco, M. Khodeir, et al., Propionibacterium acnes and SAPHO syndrome: a case report and literature review, Clin. Exp. Rheumatol. 25 (2007) 457–460.
95. A. Golla, A. Jansson, J. Ramser, et al., Chronic recurrent multifocal osteomyelitis (CRMO): evidence for a susceptibility gene located on chromosome 18q21.3-18q22, Eur J. Hum. Genet. 10 (2002) 217–221.
98. C.M. Duffy, P.Y. Lam, M. Ditchfield, et al., Chronic recurrent multifocal osteomyelitis: review of orthopaedic complications at maturity, J. Pediatr. Orthop. 22 (2002) 501–505.
99. H.J. Girschick, R. Krauspe, A. Tschammler, et al., Chronic recurrent osteomyelitis with clavicular involvement in children: diagnostic value of different imaging techniques and therapy with non-steroidal anti-inflammatory drugs, Eur. J. Pediatr. 157 (1998) 28–33.
101. G. Khanna, T.S. Sato, P. Ferguson, Imaging of chronic recurrent multifocal osteomyelitis, Radiographics 29 (2009) 1159–1177.
108. H.J. Girschick, C. Zimmer, G. Klaus, et al., Chronic recurrent multifocal osteomyelitis: what is it and how should it be treated?, Nat. Clin. Pract. Rheumatol. 3 (2007) 733–738.
125. A. Deutschmann, C.J. Mache, K. Bodo, et al., Successful treatment of chronic recurrent multifocal osteomyelitis with tumor necrosis factor-alpha blockage, Pediatrics 116 (2005) 1231–1233.
128. P.M. Miettunen, X. Wei, D. Kaura, et al., Dramatic pain relief and resolution of bone inflammation following pamidronate in 9 pediatric patients with persistent chronic recurrent multifocal osteomyelitis (CRMO), Pediatr. Rheumatol. Online J. 7(2) (2009).
129. P.J. Simm, R.C. Allen, M.R. Zacharin, Bisphosphonate treatment in chronic recurrent multifocal osteomyelitis, J. Pediatr. 152 (2008) 571–575.
130. H. Gleeson, E. Wiltshire, J. Briody, et al., Childhood chronic recurrent multifocal osteomyelitis: pamidronate therapy decreases pain and improves vertebral shape, J. Rheumatol. 35 (2008) 707–712.
131. H. Amital, Y.H. Applbaum, S. Aamar, et al., SAPHO syndrome treated with pamidronate: an open-label study of 10 patients, Rheumatology (Oxford) 43 (2004) 658–661.
132. S. Compeyrot-Lacassagne, A.M. Rosenberg, et al., Pamidronate treatment of chronic noninfectious inflammatory lesions of the mandible in children, J. Rheumatol. 34 (2007) 1585–1589.
140. K. Reue, The lipin family: mutations and metabolism, Curr. Opin. Lipidol. 20 (2009) 165–170.
147. H.I. El-Shanti, P.J. Ferguson, Chronic recurrent multifocal osteomyelitis: a concise review and genetic update, Clin. Orthop. Relat. Res. 462 (2007) 11–19.
148. Y. Ueki, V. Tiziani, C. Santanna, et al., Mutations in the gene encoding c-Abl-binding protein SH3BP2 cause cherubism, Nat Genet. 28 (2001) 125–126.
150. W.A. Jones, J. Gerrie, J. Pritchard, Cherubism: familial fibrous dysplasia of the jaws, J. Bone Joint Surg. Br. 32-B (1950) 334–347.

152. J. Southgate, U. Sarma, J.V. Townend, et al., Study of the cell biology and biochemistry of cherubism, J. Clin. Pathol. 51 (1998) 831–837.
154. X.M. Meng, S.F. Yu, G.Y. Yu, Clinicopathologic study of 24 cases of cherubism, Int. J. Oral. Maxillofac. Surg. 34 (2005) 350–356.
158. Y. Ueki, C.Y. Lin, M. Senoo, et al., Increased myeloid cell responses to M-CSF and RANKL cause bone loss and inflammation in SH3BP2 "cherubism" mice, Cell 128 (2007) 71–83.

Entire reference list is available online at www.expertconsult.com.

Chapter 45

MACROPHAGE ACTIVATION SYNDROME

Alexei A. Grom

DEFINITIONS

Macrophage Activation Syndrome (MAS) is a severe, potentially fatal condition associated with excessive activation and expansion of macrophages and T cells, leading to an overwhelming inflammatory reaction. The main manifestations of MAS include fever, hepatosplenomegaly, lymphadenopathy, severe cytopenias, serious liver disease, and coagulopathy consistent with disseminated intravascular coagulation.[1-6] Numerous, well-differentiated macrophages phagocytosing hematopoietic elements, the pathognomonic features of MAS, are often found in bone marrow (Fig. 45–1). Such cells can infiltrate almost any organ in the body and may account for many of the systemic features of this syndrome, including cytopenias, liver dysfunction, and coagulopathy. Although MAS has been reported to occur with almost all other rheumatic diseases, it is most common in the systemic form of Juvenile Idiopathic Arthritis (JIA). Systemic Lupus Erythematosus (SLE) and Kawasaki disease are also conditions in which MAS appears to occur more frequently than in other rheumatological diseases.[6-7]

It is now recognized that MAS bears a close resemblance to a group of histiocytic disorders known as *Hemophagocytic Lymphohistiocytosis (HLH)*,[4,8,9] a term that describes a spectrum of disease processes characterized by accumulations of well-differentiated mononuclear cells with a macrophage phenotype.[10,11] Since the macrophages represent a subset of histiocytes distinct from Langerhans cells, this entity should be distinguished from Langerhans cell histiocytosis and other dendritic cell disorders. In the contemporary classification of histiocytic disorders, HLH is further subdivided into primary or Familial HLH and secondary or Reactive HLH.[10,11] Clinically, however, it may be difficult to distinguish one from the other. Familial HLH is a constellation of rare autosomal recessive immune disorders. Its clinical symptoms usually become evident within the first two months of life, although initial presentation as late as the age of 22-years has been reported.[12] Reactive HLH tends to occur in older children and is more often associated with an identifiable infectious episode, most notably Epstein-Barr virus (EBV) or, cytomegalovirus infection. The group of secondary hemophagocytic

disorders also includes malignancy-associated HLH. As with MAS, the clinical course for the most typical form of HLH is characterized by persistent fever and hepatosplenomegaly.[11] Neurological symptoms can complicate and sometimes dominate the clinical course. Hemorrhagic rash and lymphadenopathy are observed less frequently. The laboratory findings—cytopenias (particularly thrombocytopenia), elevated liver enzymes, hypertriglyceridemia, hyperferritinemia, and hypofibrinogenemia—also overlap with MAS. As with MAS, hemophagocytosis in bone marrow is a hallmark of HLH. Despite all these clinical similarities, the exact pathophysiological relationship between MAS and HLH is unclear.

Epidemiology

The epidemiological studies of MAS have been complicated by the lack of well-defined diagnostic criteria. In one review originating from a tertiary level pediatric rheumatology unit, seven of 103 patients diagnosed with systemic JIA between 1980 and 2000 (approximately 7%) developed MAS at some point during the course of their illness.[5] The authors admitted, however, that the true incidence of MAS was likely much higher since relatively mild cases of MAS often remained unrecognized. Despite the lack of diagnostic criteria, increasing awareness of MAS has meant that it is recognized more frequently than previously. Increasing evidence suggest that mild subclinical MAS occurs in as many as one third of patients with active systemic disease.

Based on the authors' own experience and review of the literature, MAS occurs with equal frequency in boys and girls. There appears to be no racial predilection, and it may occur at almost any age. The youngest MAS patient reported to date was 12-months-old.[1] Although most patients develop this syndrome sometime during the course of their primary rheumatic disease, MAS occurring at the initial presentation of a rheumatic illness has been described as well.[1,13,14] The vast majority of patients have an active primary rheumatic disease prior to developing MAS. One report, however, described a patient whose polyarticular JIA was not active at the time of MAS presentation.[15]

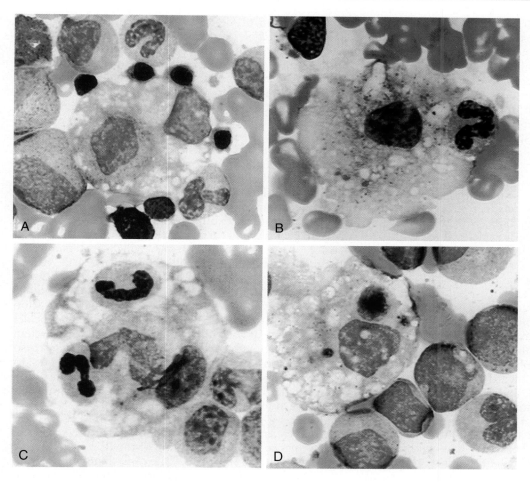

FIGURE 45–1 Activated macrophages phagocytosing hematopoietic elements in the bone marrow of a systemic JIA patient with MAS. Bone marrow aspirate specimen revealing activated macrophages (H&E stain, original magnification ×1000). **A,** Myelocyte within activated macrophage. There are also multiple adherent red blood cell and myeloid precursors. **B,** Activated macrophage engulfing a neutrophilic band form **C,** Neutrophilic band forms and metamyelocyte within an activated macrophage. Nuclei of band forms appear condensed, a result of destruction. **D,** Activated macrophage with hemosiderin deposits and a degenerating phagocytosed nucleated cell. (Redrawn from Prahalad et al. J Rheumatol 2001;28:2122.)[79]

TRIGGERS

A triggering event, such as infection or modification in the drug therapy, can be identified in about half of MAS episodes. It is now evident that development of MAS can be precipitated by virtually any infectious agent: viral, bacterial, fungal, and even parasitic. Viral illnesses, particularly EBV and other members of the Herpes family, appear to be the most commonly reported.[3,6,15] In several reports, the triggering of MAS coincided with the modifications in the drug therapy, most notably administration of gold preparations,[3,16] methotrexate,[17-19] and sulfasalazine.[20] These associations, however, should be interpreted cautiously, since many of the described patients had very active underlying rheumatic disease and might have been developing MAS as the drugs were started. In most patients, MAS appears to be triggered by a flare of the underlying rheumatic disease.

GENETIC BACKGROUND

The pathological mechanisms of MAS are not fully understood. In clinically similar HLH, there is uncontrolled proliferation of T cells and macrophages linked to decreased natural killer (NK) cell and cytotoxic T cell function,[21,22] often due to mutations in the gene encoding perforin.[23]

Perforin is a protein that cytolytic cells use to induce apoptosis of target cells, such as tumor cells or cells infected by viruses. More recently, mutations in another gene, MUNC13-4, have been implicated in the development of HLH in about 10% to 30% of patients with inherited HLH.[24] The protein encoded by the MUNC13-4 gene is an important player in the intracellular transport of perforin. More specifically the MUNC13-4 protein is involved in the process of fusing the perforin-containing granule with the plasma membrane of the cytolytic cells. Although the cytolytic cells of patients with Familial HLH caused by MUNC13-4 mutations produce sufficient amounts of perforin, the inability to deliver adequate perforin to the surface of the cells leads to profoundly decreased cytolytic activity against target cells. Defects in the granule-dependant cytotoxic functions of lymphocytes have also been implicated in three other genetic diseases associated with the hemophagocytic syndrome. Mutations in the gene-encoding Rab27a, one of the MUNC13-4 effector molecules, have been linked to the development of Griscelli syndrome type 2,[25] mutations in the Lyst gene have been identified as a cause of Chediak-Higashi syndrome,[26] and mutations in the gene encoding SH2D1A, an adaptor protein critical for lymphocyte activation, including granule-mediated cytotoxicity, have been associated with X-linked lymphoproliferative disease.[27] Recent observations suggest that as in HLH, MAS patients have profoundly depressed NK cell function, often associated with abnormal perforin expression,[28-30] and these abnormalities are associated with specific MUNC13-4[31,32] and perforin[33] gene polymorphisms. The presence of defects in the granule-dependant cytotoxic activity of lymphocytes in several diseases associated with hemophagocytic syndromes highlights the importance of this function in restoring the immune system to a state of equilibrium during some inflammatory responses.[34-35]

PATHOPHYSIOLOGY

The exact mechanisms to link deficient NK cell and cytolytic T lymphocyte (CTL) functions with the expansion of activated macrophages are not clear. Two explanations have been suggested in the literature. One is related to the fact that HLH/MAS patients appear to have a diminished ability to control some infections.[36,37] More specifically, NK cells and CTL fail to kill infected cells and to thus remove the source of antigenic stimulation. Such persistent antigen stimulation leads, in turn, to persistent antigen-driven activation and proliferation of T cells associated with escalating production of cytokines that stimulate macrophages. However, in many cases of MAS, attempts to identify an infectious trigger have not been successful, and some episodes appear to be triggered by modifications in drug therapy, rather than infection. Furthermore, the importance of NK cells and perforin-based systems in the downregulation of cellular immune responses has been demonstrated in experimental animal systems, where immune responses were elicited by anti-CD3 antibodies or staphylococcal toxins instead of viruses.[38] Some authors have hypothesized that abnormal cytotoxic cells may fail to provide the appropriate apoptotic signals for the removal of activated macrophages and T cells during the contraction stage of the immune response.[38,39] One intriguing possibility is that such perforin-dependant apoptotic signals may be delivered by the regulatory T cells.[40] Whatever the exact mechanism might be, the failure to deliver apoptotic signals leads to persistent expansion of T cells and macrophages secreting proinflammatory cytokines.[41] The clinical findings during the acute phase of HLH can largely be explained because of the prolonged production of cytokines and chemokines originating from activated macrophages and T cells.[11,42] Hemophagocytosis, the pathognomonic feature of the syndrome, is a hallmark of cytokine-driven excess activation of macrophages.[11]

A recent study of liver biopsies in MAS patients demonstrated massive infiltration of the liver by interferon (IFN) γ-producing CD8+ T lymphocytes and hemophagocytic macrophages producing tumor necrosis factor (TNF) α and IL-6.[43] Studies in perforin-deficient mice, an animal model of HLH, suggest that these cytotoxic CD8+ cells producing IFN-γ are particularly important in the pathogenesis of excessive macrophage activation.[44] Perforin-deficient mice manifest many features of MAS/HLH after infection with lymphocytic choriomeningitis virus. However, the MAS-like symptoms in these animals can be almost completely prevented

by elimination of CD8+ T cells or by neutralization of IFN-γ. Since IFN-γ is a well-known macrophage activator, it has been suggested to be critical to the expansion of macrophages in these animals. Consistent with the animal data, the increase in serum IFN-γ levels in MAS patients, compared to those in patients with active systemic JIA, is dramatically higher than the increase in the levels of any other cytokine.[4] Combined, these observations suggest that, similar to the animal models, massive activation and expansion of cytotoxic CD8+ T cells in MAS patients are associated with the production of IFN-γ and other macrophage-activating cytokines, such as GM-CSF (Fig. 45–2). This leads to subsequent activation and expansion of macrophages. The activated macrophages, in turn, exhibit hemophagocytic activity and secrete proinflammatory cytokines, including interleukin (IL) 1, TNF-α, IL-6, and IL-18, which are responsible for many of the clinical manifestations of MAS. Excess of circulating IL-1β, TNF-α, IL-6, IL-18, and IFN-γ is likely to contribute to the early and persistent findings of fevers, hyperlipidemia, and endothelial activation responsible in part for coagulopathy and later sequelae, including hepatic triaditis and central nervous system (CNS) demyelination.[11] The activated macrophages also secrete hemostatic tissue factor, which contributes to the development of the coagulopathy reminiscent of the disseminated intravascular coagulation (DIC) like syndrome seen in sepsis.

The hemophagocytic macrophages in MAS express the scavenger receptor CD163,[13,45,] a feature that provides clues to the understanding of the origin of extreme hyperferritinemia in MAS. The only known function of CD163 is related to its ability to bind hemoglobin-haptoglobin complexes and to initiate pathways important for the adaptation to oxidative stress induced by free heme and iron.[46] Since the sequestration of free iron by ferritin is an important component of these pathways, increased uptake of hemoglobin-haptoglobin complexes by CD163+ macrophages leads to increased synthesis of ferritin (Fig. 45–3). Therefore, increased release of free hemoglobin associated with increased erythrophagocytosis would require more production of ferritin to sequestrate excessive amount of free iron.

Two recent studies have suggested that expansion of CD163+ macrophages occurs in a substantial proportion of patients with systemic JIA without apparent MAS, and this phenomenon is highly specific to this disease.[47-49] It has been proposed that such expansion may represent early stages of MAS.[47-49] As shown in Fig.45–2, the expansion of overly activated T cells and macrophages is associated with shedding off some of their receptors including sIL2Rα and sCD163. The emerging consensus in the HLH literature is that serum levels of sIL2Rα and sCD163 reflect the degree of activation and expansion of T cells and phagocytic macrophages, respectively,[50,51] and, thus, serve as useful diagnostic markers. Limited experience in pediatric rheumatology suggests that assessment of serum levels of sIL2Rα and sCD163 may not only help diagnose MAS in patients with systemic JIA at the early stages, but may also provide a new way to monitor response to treatment.[47]

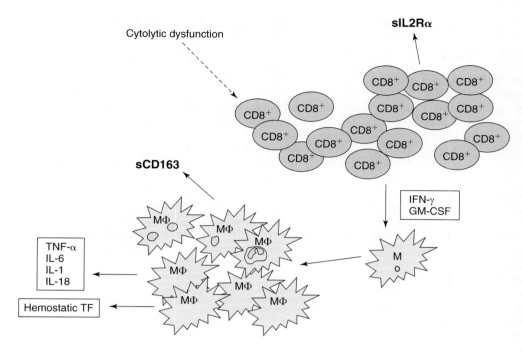

FIGURE 45–2 Pathogenesis of macrophage activation in hemophagocytic syndromes. The underlying cytolytic dysfunction leads to uncontrolled expansion and survival of activated cytotoxic CD8+ T cells. They continue to secrete proinflammatory cytokines, including IFN-γ and GM-CSF. Prolonged stimulation of monocytes with cytokines leads to their excessive activation and differentiation into macrophages with hemophagocytic activity. This is also associated with increased production of proinflammatory cytokines, such as TNF-α, IL-1, and IL-6. Hemophagocytosis of blood elements in the bone marrow leads to peripheral cytopenias. Production of procoagulant tissue factor (TF) combined with the TNF-α effects on vascular endothelial cells contribute to the development of coagulopathy.

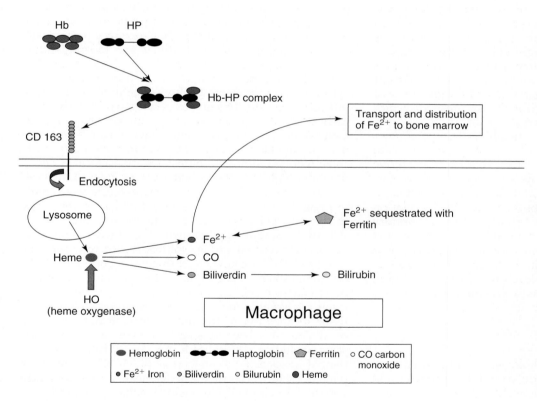

FIGURE 45–3 Role of the hemoglobin-haptoglobin scavenger receptor CD163, heme oxygenase (HO), and ferritin in adaptation to oxidative stress induced by free heme and iron. Free heme is a source of redox-active iron. To prevent cell damage caused by iron-derived reactive oxygen species, haptoglobin forms a complex with free hemoglobin. The haptoglobin-hemoglobin (Hp-Hb) complexes then bind to CD163 and are internalized by the macrophage. Endocytosis of Hp-Hb complexes leads to upregulation of HO enzymatic activity. HO degrades the heme subunit of Hb into biliverdin, which is subsequently converted to bilirubin, carbon monoxide, and free iron. The free iron is either sequestered with ferritin in the cell or transported and distributed to red blood cell precursors in the bone marrow. Increased uptake of Hp-Hb complexes by macrophages leads to increased synthesis of ferritin. Highly elevated levels of serum ferritin are an important diagnostic feature of both MAS and HLH.[50]

CLINICAL FEATURES

The clinical findings in overt MAS are dramatic.[1-6] Typically, patients with a chronic condition become acutely ill with persistent fever, mental status changes, lymphadenopathy, hepatosplenomegaly, liver dysfunction, easy bruising, and mucosal bleeding. These clinical symptoms are associated with precipitous fall in at least two of three blood cell lines (leukocytes, erythrocytes, and platelets).

The fall in platelet count is usually an early finding. Since bone marrow aspiration typically reveals significant hypercellularity and normal megakaryocytes, such cytopenias do not seem to be secondary to inadequate production of cells. Increased destruction of the cells by phagocytosis and consumption at the inflammatory sites are more likely explanations. Precipitous fall in erythrocyte sedimentation rate (ESR) is another characteristic laboratory feature, which probably reflects the degree of hypofibrinogenemia secondary to fibrinogen consumption and liver dysfunction.[2-6] Liver involvement is common in MAS, and significant hepatomegaly is frequently present. Some patients develop mild jaundice. Liver function tests often reveal high serum transaminases activity and mildly elevated levels of serum bilirubin, and moderate hypoalbuminemia has been reported. Serum ammonia levels are typically normal or only mildly elevated.

Encephalopathy is another frequently reported clinical feature of MAS. Mental status changes, seizures, and coma are the most common manifestations of CNS disease.[1-6] Cerebrospinal fluid pleiocytosis with mildly elevated protein has been noted in some studies.[2] Significant deterioration in renal function has also been noted in several series and was associated with particularly high mortality in one report.[5] Pulmonary infiltrates have been mentioned in several reports, and hemophagocytic macrophages can be found in bronchoalveolar lavage.

Additional laboratory findings in MAS include highly elevated serum levels of triglycerides, LDH, and ferritin. The elevation of serum ferritin is particularly marked (often above 10,000 ng/mL)[52] and appears to parallel the degree of macrophages activation. In normal physiological conditions, serum ferritin is usually 60% to 80% glycosylated while intracellular ferritin is not glycosylated. It is not clear what factors determine the balance between the glycosylated versus nonglycosylated forms, but it has been shown that the percentage of glycosylated ferritin in the serum of patients with hemophagocytic syndromes is very low (below 20%).[53] Based on these observations, it has been proposed that the assessment of the glycosylated ferritin may be a useful tool for the diagnosis of hemophagocytic syndromes.

A hemorrhagic syndrome resembling DIC is another striking abnormality in MAS.[1-6,54-55] Hemorrhagic skin rashes from mild petechiae to extensive ecchymotic lesions, epistaxis, hematemesis secondary to upper gastrointestinal bleeding, and rectal bleeding are most commonly described clinical symptoms caused by coagulation abnormalities observed in MAS. Further laboratory evaluation reveals prolonged prothrombin and partial thromboplastin times, marked hypofibrinogenemia, and moderate deficiency of vitamin K-dependant clotting factors. A decrease in Factor V levels is usually mild. Fibrin degradation products are present as well.

TISSUE HISTOLOGY

The most common histopathological finding in patients with MAS is tissue infiltration with T lymphocytes and cytologically benign yet actively phagocytic macrophages (see Fig. 45–1). Although the demonstration of macrophages phagocytosing hematopoietic elements in the bone marrow or lymph nodes is virtually diagnostic, negative reports may occur due to sampling difficulties or timing of the procedure. The hemophagocytic macrophages may also be found in tissues other than bone marrow. Thus, postmortem evaluation of one patient with MAS revealed extensive macrophagic infiltration of the heart, adrenal glands, liver, pancreas, and meninges.[3] In addition to sinusoidal and periportal infiltration with

macrophages, histological evaluation of the liver often reveals severe diffuse fatty changes.[54,55] The development of fatty changes in the liver may be related to the metabolic effects of TNF-α. TNF-α has been shown to stimulate hepatic lipogenesis and to inhibit synthesis of lipoprotein lipase, an enzyme needed to release fatty acids from circulating lipoproteins, so that they can be used by the tissues. The same mechanism also appears to be responsible for high triglyceridemia seen in MAS patients.

The most common cutaneous manifestations of MAS are panniculitis and purpura.[54-57] Most skin biopsy specimens show edema and hemorrhage associated with mononuclear cell infiltration with numerous macrophages occasionally showing hemophagocytosis. Two recent reports described systemic JIA/MAS patients who also had necrotizing histiocytic lymphadenopathy consistent with Kikuchi syndrome.[29,58] Given the rarity of both conditions, this association may not be random.

DIAGNOSIS

There are no validated diagnostic criteria for MAS, and early diagnosis is often difficult. Thus, in a patient with persistently active underlying rheumatological disease, a fall in the ESR and platelet count, particularly in a combination with persistently high C-reactive protein and increasing levels of serum D-dimer and ferritin, should raise a suspicion of impeding MAS. The diagnosis of MAS is usually confirmed by the demonstration of hemophagocytosis in the bone marrow. However, this method may be difficult to use due to sampling errors, particularly at the early stages of the syndrome. In addition, many reports have demonstrated that hemophagocytic macrophages may accumulate in tissues other than bone marrow. In some reports, additional biopsies were performed due to the initial failure to detect hemophagocytosis in the bone marrow, and hemophagocytic macrophages were found in organs, such as the liver, lymph nodes, or the lungs. In these patients, assessment of the levels of sIL2Rα and sCD163 in serum may help with the timely diagnosis of MAS. As discussed earlier, soluble IL2Rα receptors and soluble CD163 are now increasingly recognized as important biomarkers of MAS. Since they shed off the surface of activated T cells and macrophages respectively, their levels are likely to increase in the serum regardless of the tissue localization of the cells. Although mild elevation of sIL2Rα has been reported in many rheumatic diseases, including JIA and SLE,[58] a several fold increase in these diseases is highly suggestive of MAS.[47,59] One must remember, however, that other clinical entities associated with high levels of sIL2Rα include malignancies and some viral infections, including viral hepatitis, and these conditions should be considered in the differential diagnosis.

In contrast to MAS, the diagnosis of HLH is usually established based on the validated diagnostic criteria developed by the International Histiocyte Society[60] (Table 45–1). However, the application of the HLH diagnostic criteria to systemic JIA patients with suspected MAS is problematic. Some of the HLH markers, such as lymphadenopathy, splenomegaly, and hyperferritinemia, are common features of active systemic JIA itself and

Table 45-1

HLH-2004: Revised diagnostic guidelines for HLH[61]

The diagnosis HLH can be established if one of either (1) or (2) below is fulfilled:

(1) A molecular diagnosis consistent with HLH (i.e., reported mutations found in either PRF1 or MUNC13-4)

(2) Diagnostic criteria for HLH fulfilled (i.e., at least five of the eight criteria listed below are present):

- Persistent fever
- Splenomegaly
- Cytopenias (affecting ≥2 of 3 lineages in the peripheral blood):
  - Hemoglobin <90 g/L (in infants <4 weeks: <100g/L)
  - Platelets <100x10⁹/L
  - Neutrophils <1.0x10⁹/L
- Hypertriglyceremia and/or hypofibrinogenemia:
  - Fasting triglycerides ≥3.0 mmol/L (i.e., ≥265 mg/dL)
  - Fibrinogen ≤1.5 g/L
- Hemophagocytosis in bone marrow, spleen, or lymph nodes; no evidence of malignancy
- Serum ferritin ≥500 mcg/L (i.e., 500 ng/mL)
- Low or absent NK cell activity (according to local laboratory reference)
- Increased serum sIL2Rα (according to local laboratory reference)

If hemophagocytic activity is not proven at the time of presentation, further search for hemophagocytic activity is encouraged. If the bone marrow specimen is not conclusive, material may be obtained from other organs.

therefore do not distinguish MAS from a conventional systemic JIA flare. Other HLH criteria, such as cytopenias and hypofibrinogenemia, become evident only at the late stages. This is because systemic JIA patients often have increased white blood cell and platelet counts and serum levels of fibrinogen as a part of the inflammatory response seen in this disease. Therefore, when patients develop MAS, they reach the degree of cytopenias and hypofibrinogenemia seen in HLH only at the late stages of the syndrome when their management becomes challenging. This is even more problematic for the diagnosis of MAS in patients with SLE in whom autoimmune cytopenias are common and difficult to distinguish from those caused by MAS. In these patients, the presence of extreme hyperferritinemia and LDH elevation should raise suspicion for MAS.[61] Attempts to modify the HLH criteria to increase their sensitivity and specificity for the diagnosis of MAS in rheumatic conditions have been initiated.[62]

DIFFERENTIAL DIAGNOSIS

In addition to distinguishing MAS from a flare of an underlying rheumatological disease, one must consider other clinical entities associated with hepatic dysfunction, coagulopathy, cytopenias, or encephalopathy. In some MAS patients, the combination of hepatic dysfunction with encephalopathy may be reminiscent of Reye syndrome. The diagnosis of Reye syndrome, however, is based of viral prodrome, unexplained vomiting, behavioral changes, and a distinctive chemical profile characterized by rapid coordinated increase in serum aminotransferase levels, blood ammonia, and prothrombin time with relatively minimal changes in serum bilirubin. The DIC-like coagulopathy seen in MAS is not a feature of Reye syndrome. Conversely, sharp increase in blood ammonia levels, an important feature of Reye syndrome, is usually very mild in MAS.

The hemorrhagic syndrome seen in MAS may resemble thrombotic thrombocytopenic purpura. However, microangiopathic anemia with the emergence of fragmented red blood cells in peripheral circulation, a central feature of thrombotic thrombocytopenic purpura, is usually not seen in MAS.

It is also important to differentiate MAS from malignancy associated HLH and malignant histiocytic disorders. Some other important differential diagnoses include sepsis, drug reactions, and thorough infectious work up is necessary for the majority of these patients.

TREATMENT

MAS is a life-threatening condition still associated with high mortality rates. Therefore, early recognition of this syndrome and immediate therapeutic intervention to produce a rapid response are critical. Prompt administration of more aggressive treatment in these patients may, prevent a development of a full blown syndrome. To achieve rapid reversal of coagulation abnormalities and cytopenias, most clinicians start with intravenous methylprednisolone pulse therapy (30 mg/kg for three consecutive days) followed by 2-3 mg/kg/day divided in four doses. After normalization of hematological abnormalities and resolution of coagulopathy, steroids are tapered slowly to avoid relapses of MAS. However, MAS sometimes appears to be corticosteroid resistant with deaths being reported even among patients treated with massive doses of steroids.

Parental administration of cyclosporine A has been shown to be highly effective in patients with corticosteroid-resistant MAS.[63-65] From the primary effect of cyclosporine A, largely, but not entirely confined to T cells, a wide variety of other effects are mediated leading to profound and therapeutically useful immunosuppression.[66] In many patients, parental administration of cyclosporine A (2-7 mg/kg/day) not only provides rapid control of the symptoms, but also allows for avoiding of excessive use of steroids.

Patients in whom MAS remains active despite the use of corticosteroids and cyclosporine A present a formidable challenge. In these patients, one might consider using etoposide (or VP16), a podophyllatoxin derivative that inhibits DNA synthesis by forming a complex with topoisomerase II and DNA. The combination of steroids, cyclosporine A, and etoposide is the main component of the HLH-2004 treatment protocol developed by the International Histiocyte Society.[60] This protocol includes a combination of etoposide and CNS-penetrating dexamethasone (with or without methotrexate), followed by a maintenance dose of cyclosporine A and less frequent pulses of etoposide once clinical remission has been established. In accordance with the protocol, patients with Familial HLH and patients who experience a relapse after initially responding to HLH 2004 should proceed to definitive therapy with allogeneic hematopoietic stem cell transplantation.

Although successful use etoposide in MAS has been reported,[67] potential toxicity of the drug is a major concern, particularly in patients with hepatic impairment. Etoposide is metabolized by the liver, and then both the unchanged drug and its metabolites are excreted through the kidneys. Since patients who may require the use of etoposide are very likely to have hepatic and renal involvement, caution should be exercised to properly adjust the dosage and thus limit the extent of the potential side effects, such as severe bone marrow suppression, that may be detrimental. Reports describing deaths caused by severe bone marrow suppression and overwhelming infection have been published.

Recently, it has been suggested that antithymocyte globulin (ATG) might be a safer alternative to etoposide in patients unresponsive to the combination of steroids and cyclosporine A, particularly in those with renal and hepatic impairment. ATG depletes both CD4+ and CD8+ T cells through complement-dependant cell lysis. Mild depletion of monocytes is noted in some patients as well. Although in the reported cases, this treatment was tolerated well by patients,[43,59] one must remember infusion reactions, including anaphylaxis, are frequently reported with the use of ATG, and adequate laboratory and supportive medical resources must be readily available if this treatment is used.

The effectiveness of biological drugs in MAS treatment remains unclear. Although, TNF-inhibiting agents have been reported to be effective in occasional MAS patients,[68-71] other reports describe patients in whom MAS occurred while they were on the agents.[72-74]

Since MAS episodes are often triggered by the disease flare, at least in systemic JIA, biological drugs that neutralize IL-1, a cytokine that plays a pivotal role in systemic JIA pathogenesis, have been tried by some authors. As with TNF-inhibiting agents, the results, however, have been conflicting. Successful use of kineret in MAS complicating systemic JIA has been occasionally reported,[75] but in larger series, describing experience with this treatment in systemic JIA in general, several patients developed MAS while being treated with kineret.[76]

Based on some success with intravenous immunoglobulin administration in virus-associated Reactive HLH,[77] this treatment might be effective in MAS triggered by viral infection. If MAS, however, is driven by EBV infection, one might also consider Rituximab, a monoclonal antibody that depletes B lymphocytes, which are the main type of cells harboring EBV virus.[78] This approach has been successfully used in EBV-induced lymphoproliferative disease.

PROGNOSIS

MAS is a life-threatening condition, and the reported mortality rates reach 20%. Due to increasing awareness of this syndrome, MAS is now diagnosed relatively early, and the outcome is improving. A substantial proportion of MAS patients experience recurrent episodes, and these patients may require closer monitoring.

REFERENCES

1. E.D. Silverman, J.J. Miller, B. Bernstein, et al., Consumption coagulopathy associated with systemic juvenile rheumatoid arthritis, J. Pediatr. 103 (1983) 872–876.
2. M. Hadchouel, A.M. Prieur, C. Griscelli, Acute hemorrhagic, hepatic, and neurologic manifestations in juvenile rheumatoid arthritis: possible relationship to drugs or infection, J. Pediatr. 106 (1985) 561–566.
3. J.L. Stephan, J. Zeller, P. Hubert, et al., Macrophage activation syndrome and rheumatic disease in childhood: a report of four new cases, Clin. Exp. Rheumatol. 11 (1993) 451–456.
4. A.A. Grom, NK dysfunction: a common pathway in systemic onset juvenile rheumatoid arthritis, macrophage activation syndrome, and hemophagocytic lymphohistiocytosis, Arthritis Rheum. 50 (2004) 689–698.
5. S. Sawhney, P. Woo, K.J. Murray, Macrophage activation syndrome: A potentially fatal complication of rheumatic disorders, Arch. Dis. Child 85 (2001) 421–426.
6. J.L. Stephan, I. Kone-Paut, C. Galambrun, et al., Reactive Haemophagocytic syndrome in children with inflammatory disorders. A retrospective study of 24 patients, Rheumatology (Oxford) 40 (2001) 1285–1292.
7. A. Muise, S.E. Tallett, E.D. Silverman, Are children with Kawasaki disease and prolonged fever at risk for macrophage activation syndrome? Pediatrics 112 (2003) e495–e497.
8. B.H. Athreya, Is macrophage activation syndrome a new entity? Clin. Exper. Rheumatol. 20 (2002) 121–123.
9. A.V. Ramanan, E.M. Baildam, Macrophage activation syndrome is hemophagocytic lymphohistiocytosis—need for the right terminology, J. Rheumatol. 29 (2002) 1105.
10. B.E. Favara, A.C. Feller, M. Pauli, et al., Contemporary classification of histiocytic disorders. The WHO Committee On Histiocytic/Reticulum Cell Proliferations. Reclassification Working Group of the Histiocyte Society, Med. Pediatr. Oncol. 29 (1997) 157–166.
11. H.A. Filipovich, Hemophagocytic lymphohistiocytosis, Immunol. Allergy Clin. N. Am. 22 (2002) 281–300.
13. T. Avcin, S.M.L. Tse, R. Schneider, et al., Macrophage activation syndrome as the presenting manifestation of rheumatic diseases in childhood, J. Pediatr. 148 (2006) 683–686.
22. K.E. Sullivan, C.A. Delaat, S.D. Douglas, et al., Defective natural killer cell function in patients with hemophagocytic lymphohistiocytosis and first degree relatives, Pediatr. Res. 44 (1998) 465–468.
23. S.E. Stepp, R. Dufourcq-Lagelouse, F. Le Deist, et al., Perforin gene defects in familial hemophagocytic lymphohistiocytosis, Science 286 (1999) 1957–1959.
24. J. Feldmann, I. Callebaut, G. Raposo, et al., MUNC13-4 is essential for cytolytic granules fusion and is mutated in a form of familial hemophagocytic lymphohistiocytosis (FHL3), Cell 115 (2003) 461–473.
25. G. Menasche, E. Pastural, J. Feldman, et al., Mutations in Rab27a cause Griscelli syndrome associated with haemophagocytic syndrome, Nat. Genet. 25 (2000) 173–176.
26. M.D. Barbosa, Q.A. Nguyen, V.T. Tchernev, et al., Identification of the homologous beige and Chediak-Higashi syndrome genes (LYST), Nature 382 (1996) 262–265.
27. A.J. Coffey, R.A. Brooksbank, O. Brandau, et al., Host response to EBV infection in X-linked lymphoproliferative disease results from mutations in an SH2-domain encoding gene, Nat. Genet. 20 (1998) 129.
28. A.A. Grom, J. Villanueva, S. Lee, et al., Natural killer cell dysfunction in patients with systemic-onset juvenile rheumatoid arthritis and macrophage activation syndrome, J. Peds. 142 (2003) 292–296.
29. J. Villanueva, S. Lee, E.H. Giannini, et al., Natural killer cell dysfunction is a distinguishing feature of systemic onset juvenile rheumatoid arthritis and macrophage activation syndrome, Arthritis Res. Ther. 7 (2005) R30–R37.
30. N.M. Wulffraat, G.T. Rijkers, E. Elst, et al., Reduced perforin expression in systemic onset juvenile idiopathic arthritis is restored by autologous stem cell transplantation, Rheumatology (Oxford) 42 (2003) 375–379.
31. M.M. Hazen, A.L. Woodward, I. Hofman, et al., Mutations of the hemophagocytosis-associated gene UNC13D in a patient with systemic juvenile idiopathic arthritis, Arthritis Rheum. 58 (2008) 567–570.

32. K. Zhang, J. Biroscak, D.N. Glass, et al., Macrophage activation syndrome in systemic juvenile idiopathic arthritis is associated with MUNC13D gene polymorphisms, Arthritis Rheum. 58 (2008) 2892–2896.

38. D. Kagi, B. Odermatt, T.W. Mak, Homeostatic regulation of CD8+ T cells by perforin, Eur. J. Immunol. 29 (1999) 3262–3272.

40. J.W. Verbsky, W.J. Grossman, Hemophagocytic lymphohistiocytosis: diagnosis, pathophysiology, treatment, and future perspectives, Ann. Med. 38 (2006) 20–31.

41. G. Menasche, J. Feldmann, A. Fischer, et al., Primary hemophagocytic syndromes point to a direct link between lymphocyte cytotoxicity and homeostasis, Immunol. Rev. 203 (2005) 165–179.

43. A.D. Billiau, T. Roskams, T. Van Damme-Lombaerts, et al., Macrophage activation syndrome: characteristic findings on liver biopsy illustrating the key role of activated, IFN-γ-producing lymphocytes and IL-6 and TNF-α-producing macrophages, Blood 105 (2005) 1648–1651.

44. M.B. Jordan, D. Hildeman, J. Kappler, et al., An animal model of hemophagocytic lymphohistiocytosis (HLH): CD8+ T cells and interferon gamma are essential for the disorder, Blood 104 (2004) 735–743.

45. D.J. Schaer, B. Schleiffenbaum, M. Kurrer, et al., Soluble hemoglobin-haptoglobin scavenger receptor CD163 as a lineage-specific marker in the reactive hemophagocytic syndrome, Eur. J. Haemotol. 74 (2005) 6–10.

46. M. Kristiansen, J.H. Graversen, C. Jacobsen, et al., Identification of the hemoglobin scavenger receptor, Nature 409 (2001) 198–201.

47. J. Bleesing, A. Prada, J. Villanueva, et al., The diagnostic significance of soluble CD163 and soluble IL2Rα chains in macrophage activation syndrome and untreated new onset systemic juvenile idiopathic arthritis,, Arthritis Rheum. 56 (2007) 965–971.

48. E.M. Behrens, T. Beukelman, M. Paessler, et al., Occult macrophage activation syndrome in patients with systemic juvenile idiopathic arthritis, J. Rheumatol. 34 (2007) 1133–1138.

49. N. Fall, M. Barnes, S. Thornton, et al., Gene expression profiling in peripheral blood in untreated new onset systemic juvenile idiopathic arthritis reveals molecular heterogeneity that may predict macrophage activation syndrome, Arthritis Rheum. 56 (2007) 3793–3804.

50. D.M. Komp, J. Mcnamara, P. Buckley, Elevated soluble interleukin-2 receptor in childhood hemophagocytic histiocytic syndromes, Blood 73 (1989) 2128–2132.

51. H.J. Moller, H. Aerts, H. Gronbaek, et al., Soluble CD163: a marker molecule for monocyte/macrophage activity in disease, Scand. J. Clin. Lab. Invest. 237 (2002) 29–33.

53. L. Fardet, P. Coppo, A. Kettaneh, et al., Low glycosylated ferritin, a good marker for the diagnosis of hemophagocytic syndrome, Arthritis Rheum. 58 (2008) 1521–1527.

54. K.J. Smith, H.G. Skeltom, J. Yeager, et al., Cutaneous, histopathologic, immunohistochemical, and clinical manifestations in patients with hemophagocytic syndrome, Arch. Dermatol. 128 (1992) 193–200.

55. A.P. Reiner, J.L. Spivak, Hematophagic Histiocytosis. A report of 23 new patients and a review of the literature, Medicine 67 (1998) 369–388.

59. A. Coca, K.W. Bundy, B. Marston, et al., Macrophage activation syndrome: serological markers and treatment with anti-thymocyte globulin, Clin. Immunol. 132 (2009) 10–18.

60. J.I. Henter, A. Horne, M. Arico, et al., HLH-2004:Diagnostic and therapeutic guidelines for hemopagocytic lymphohistiocytosis, Pediatr. Blood Cancer 48 (2007) 124–131.

61. A. Parodi, S. Davì, A.B. Pringe, et al., Macrophage Activation Syndrome in Juvenile Systemic Lupus Erythematosus. Multinational multicenter study of 38 patients, Arthritis Rheum. 60 (2009) 3388–3399.

63. R. Mouy, J.L. Stephan, P. Pillet, et al., Efficacy of cyclosporine A in the treatment of macrophage activation syndrome in juvenile arthritis: report of five cases, J. Pediatr. 129 (1996) 750–754.

64. A. Ravelli, F. De Benedetti, S. Viola, et al., Macrophage activation syndrome in systemic juvenile rheumatoid arthritis successfully treated with cyclosporine, J. Pediatr. 128 (1996) 275–278.

67. D. Fishman, M. Rooney, P. Woo, Successful management of reactive haemophagocytic syndrome in systemic-onset juvenile chronic arthritis, Br. J. Rheumatol. 34 (1995) 888.

77. C. Larroche, F. Bruneel, M.H. Andre, et al., Intravenously administered gamma-globulins in reactive hemophagocytic syndrome, Ann. Med. Interne. (Paris) 151 (2000) 533–539.

78. N.J. Balamuth, K.E. Nichols, M. Paessler, et al., Use of Rituximab in cinjunction with immunosuppressive chemotherapy for EBV-associated hemophagocytic lymphohistiocytosis, J. Pediatr. Hematol/Oncol. 29 (2007) 569–573.

79. S. Prahalad, K. Bove, D. Dickens, et al., Etanercept in the treatment of macrophage activation syndrome, J. Rheumatol. 28 (2001) 2120–2124.

Entire reference list is available online at www.expertconsult.com.

Chapter 46

SKELETAL MALIGNANCIES AND RELATED DISORDERS

James T. Cassidy and Ross E. Petty

Occasionally, a child in whom arthritis or a musculoskeletal pain syndrome has been erroneously diagnosed is discovered to have a bone tumor.[1] Although this unfortunate occurrence is rare, physicians must consider this possibility when examining any child with musculoskeletal pain. Musculoskeletal manifestations of malignancy in childhood may take one of four forms:

1. Primary benign or malignant tumors of bone, cartilage, fibrous or soft tissue, or miscellaneous origin
2. Metastatic bone tumors
3. Malignant infiltration of bone marrow: leukemia
4. Secondary effects of malignancy

Table 46–1 provides a classification of common bone tumors of childhood. This list is not comprehensive.[2-5] Overall, approximately one-half of bone tumors occurring in the first two decades of life are malignant.[6] This proportion contrasts sharply with the ratio in adulthood, when malignant tumors are much more frequent. Except for parosteal sarcoma, which is more frequent in girls, malignant bone tumors occur more frequently in boys, with a ratio of approximately 1.5:1; the male-to-female ratio is approximately 3:1 for osteoid osteomas and osteoblastomas.[2,3,7]

Bone tumors may be completely asymptomatic until a mass is detected by the patient or parent. They usually present with the insidious onset of tenderness, swelling, and localized pain accentuated at night or by weight-bearing. Local tenderness or bony swelling in the absence of trauma suggests the diagnosis. Systemic symptoms such as fever and weight loss are nonspecific but support the diagnosis of a malignant rather than a benign tumor.

A plain radiograph of the affected area is the best initial diagnostic evaluation.[8,9] It is important to notice if the lesion is osteolytic or osteogenic and whether there is a soft tissue reaction. Each tumor occurs in characteristic bones and locations (Table 46–2). Most benign or malignant tumors of a long bone arise in the metaphysis. Malignant tumors of the epiphysis are rare; Ewing sarcoma is the only malignant tumor commonly arising in the diaphysis.

The extent of the lesion can be estimated by computerized tomography (CT). Magnetic resonance imaging (MRI) delineates the soft tissue extent of early lesions, including involvement of the bone marrow.[10-12] Ultrasonography is valuable in assessing extraosseous extension.[13] Radionuclide scanning is useful in localizing a tumor or tumors, rather than in assisting with a specific diagnosis. Definitive diagnosis of a bone tumor rests on the histological evaluation of an open or fine-needle biopsy. The laboratory otherwise provides little assistance because anemia, leukocytosis, elevation of the erythrocyte sedimentation rate (ESR), and other indicators of inflammation are nonspecific and may be absent even in the presence of osseous malignancy. Serum alkaline phosphatase levels may be elevated beyond those associated with growth of the child.

PRIMARY TUMORS OF BONE, CARTILAGE, FIBROUS OR SOFT TISSUE, OR MISCELLANEOUS ORIGIN

Benign Tumors of Bone

Of the benign tumors, osteoid osteomas, osteochondromas, and chondromas are most common in the first two decades of life.[14,15] Approximately one-half of these lesions occur before the age of 20 years. Surgical treatment is often necessary.[16]

Osteoid Osteomas

Osteoid osteomas are benign tumors most common between the ages of 10 and 20 years, although they can also occur in younger children (Table 46–3).[17,18] The most common sites are the proximal femur, often in the neck and greater trochanter; the proximal tibia; and the pedicles, facets, and spinous processes of the vertebrae.[19]

Pain, the typical presentation, is described as a deep and penetrating ache usually worse at night, and may be dramatically responsive to low-dose aspirin or other nonsteroidal antiinflammatory drugs (NSAIDs). The site of the lesion is tender, and there may be marked muscle atrophy, weakness of that limb, or a limp. Lesions in the vertebrae may be associated with scoliosis with the concavity toward the site of the tumor. Occasionally, a synovial effusion is present if the tumor is adjacent to the hip or knee within the confines of the capsule. Signs of systemic illness are absent.

There are no abnormalities on laboratory evaluation; the diagnosis is based principally on radiological findings. On a plain radiograph, the typical lesion is a nidus of increased density within a ring of decreased density, which is surrounded by bone of increased density (Fig. 46–1). Histologically, the nidus is a mixture of osteoid,

Table 46–1

Classification of common bone tumors of childhood

Histological type	Benign	Malignant
Osteogenic	Osteoid osteoma	Osteosarcoma
	Osteoblastoma	Parosteal osteosarcoma
Chondrogenic	Osteochondroma	Chondrosarcoma
	Chondroma	—
	Chondroblastoma	—
	Chondromyxoid fibroma	—
Fibrogenic	Fibrous defect	Fibrosarcoma
Stromal	Giant cell tumor	—
Neuroectodermal	—	Ewing sarcoma
Hematopoietic	—	Reticulum cell sarcoma

Table 46–2

Most common types of tumors in specific bones*

Bone	Benign	Malignant
Femur	Osteochondroma	Osteosarcoma
Tibia	Osteoid osteoma	Osteosarcoma
	Osteochondroma	—
	Giant cell tumor	—
Innominate	Osteochondroma	Osteosarcoma
Humerus	Osteochondroma	Osteosarcoma
Vertebra	Osteoid osteoma	Reticulum cell sarcoma
Rib	Osteochondroma	Chondrosarcoma
Hand	Chondroma	Chondrosarcoma
Radius	Giant cell tumor	Osteosarcoma

*Listed in order of decreasing frequency.
Data from Dahlin DC, Unni KK: *Bone tumors: general aspects and data on 8,542 cases*, ed 4, Springfield, IL, 1986, Charles C Thomas.

Table 46–3

Osteoid osteoma

Characteristic	Description
Age at onset	Childhood to young adulthood
Sex ratio	Boys > girls
Symptoms	Localized aching or boring pain, mild at first, increasing in severity
	Worse at night, with rest, or with elevation
	Limpness, stiffness, or weakness
	Long history
Signs	Joint effusion occasionally
	Localized swelling or tenderness
Investigations	Solitary, lucent nucleus surrounded by sclerosis on radiographs
	Positive bone scan
Treatment	Pain is dramatically relieved by aspirin or nonsteroidal antiinflammatory drugs
	Excision

bone, and blood vessels surrounded by a fibrovascular layer that separates it from the surrounding sclerotic bone. This lesion is often difficult to identify by standard radiographic examination, especially in nondiaphyseal sites; other imaging techniques may be required for identification.[18] Technetium 99m bone scintigraphy is the diagnostic procedure of choice (Fig. 46–2). CT documents the precise extent of the lesion and its characteristic structure and is invaluable in planning a surgical approach. MRI may identify the nature of a soft tissue mass associated with an early lesion.[20-22]

The course of untreated osteoid osteoma varies. This tumor is not malignant, does not metastasize or cause death, and may spontaneously heal radiographically without surgical or other treatment.[17,23] However, the debility induced by the associated pain usually requires removal of the lesion. Excision is curative, and the recurrence rate is low. Aspirin or another NSAID can provide symptomatic relief and is occasionally justified on a long-term basis if the lesion is surgically inaccessible.

Osteoblastoma

The osteoblastoma is usually regarded as an osteoid osteoma larger than 1 to 2 cm in diameter.[23] It occurs much more often in boys than girls and is more frequent in adolescence than childhood. Pain is the presenting symptom. This tumor is most common in a vertebral arch and has an aggressive radiographical appearance with circumscribed erosion of the cortex. Malignant transformation has been reported. Surgical resection may be difficult because of the site or size of the lesion.

Benign Tumors of Cartilaginous Origin

Osteochondroma

Osteochondroma is the most common benign bone tumor occuring between the ages of 5 and 15 years.[2,3] It occurs with equal frequency in boys and girls. This tumor is often asymptomatic and presents as a painless exostotic mass that, by virtue of location and size, may induce local functional changes or result in pain because of pressure on neurovascular structures. An osteochondroma usually affects the metaphysis of a long bone and often arises at the site of a tendon insertion (most commonly around the knee in the distal femur or proximal tibia) or in the distal humerus. The osteochondroma extends away from the epiphysis as a bony outgrowth capped with cartilage up to 1 cm thick (Fig. 46–3). Some children with multiple lesions exhibit an autosomal dominant pattern of inheritance (i.e., multiple hereditary exostoses) (Fig. 46–4).[24] Treatment consists of surgical excision. Malignant change may occur in solitary or multiple osteochondromas.

Chondromas

Chondromas (i.e., enchondromas) make up about 10% of benign bone tumors. They occur with equal frequency in boys and girls and may affect young children and those in the second decade of life.[2,3] This cartilaginous tumor, which may represent overgrowth of normal epiphyseal hyaline cartilage, occurs most commonly in

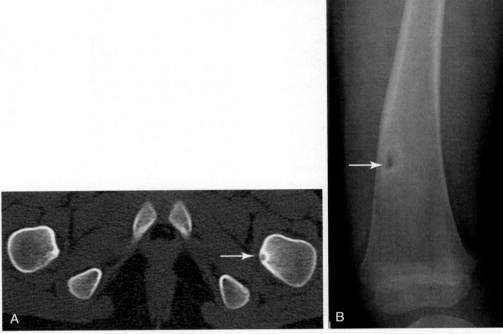

FIGURE 46–1   CT (transverse plane) showing osteoid osteoma *(arrow)* in a typical location in the left femoral neck **(A)** and radiograph demonstrating osteoid osteoma *(arrow)* in the distal femur **(B)**. (Courtesy Dr. L. Yewchuk).

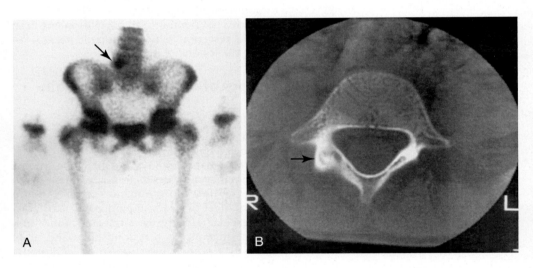

FIGURE 46–2   **A,** Increased uptake of technetium 99m in the region of an osteoid osteoma of the spine *(arrow).* **B,** Computerized tomography scan of the fourth lumbar vertebra delineates characteristics of the osteoid osteoma of the vertebral arch. Notice the sclerotic central nidus, surrounded by radiolucent granulation tissue *(arrow),* which is surrounded by sclerotic reactive bone.

the small tubular bones of the hand and foot, although other sites may be involved (Fig. 46–5). The radiographical appearance of a chondroma is that of a well-demarcated metaphyseal lesion of central destruction that may protrude from the surface of the bone or be confined within the medullary canal (i.e., enchondroma), usually with linear or speckled calcification. It often presents as a solitary, asymptomatic mass with a pathological fracture or is discovered as an incidental radiological finding. Prophylactic resection after biopsy confirmation is not usually considered necessary, but careful follow-up is warranted, because there is a low rate of malignant transformation to chondrosarcoma. Cytogenetic abnormalities are common and of value in tumor typing.[25]

Multiple enchondromatosis, or *Ollier disease,* commonly affects the hands and feet. Joint range of motion may be impaired, and the clinical presentation may be mistaken for arthritis. Growth deformities are common and require surgical management. Endochondromatosis in the presence of multiple cavernous hemangiomas is called *Maffucci syndrome* (Fig. 46–6). The frequency of malignant sarcomatous change is high (50%) in patients with Ollier or Maffucci syndrome.[3,26]

Periosteal Chondroma

Periosteal chondroma arises from the cortical surface and is most common in the proximal humerus and other long bones. Pain is often the presenting symptom. Wide excision is the treatment of choice.

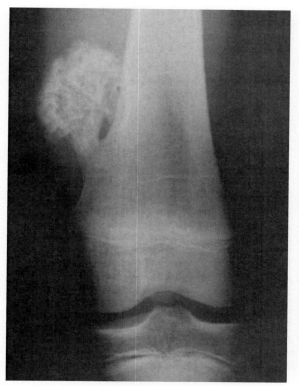

FIGURE 46–3 Osteochondroma of the distal femoral metaphysis. The tumor is directed away from the joint.

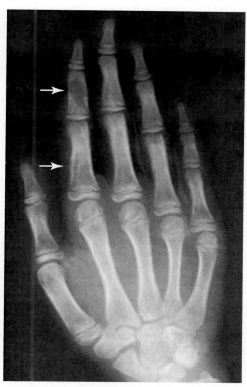

FIGURE 46–5 Radiograph of the hand of a child with enchondromas of the middle and proximal phalanges of the second finger *(arrows)*.

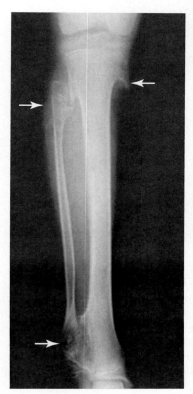

FIGURE 46–4 Radiograph of the tibia and fibula with multiple osteochondromas *(arrows)*.

Chondroblastoma

Chondroblastoma is an uncommon epiphyseal cartilaginous tumor of childhood; it is most common in the second and third decades of life and occurs in the hip, shoulder, or knee (Fig. 46–7).[27] The histopathology consists of polyhedral and giant cells with areas of fine calcifications. Foci of osteoid and bone may resemble a chondromyxoid fibroma. Most lesions are cured by excision and bone graft, but recurrences are a major concern. Growth disturbances and loss of function occur but are not common.

Chondromyxoid Fibroma

A chondromyxoid fibroma arises usually in the metaphyseal area with pain and tenderness as the most common presenting symptoms. It is an uncommon lesion and begins to occur in children at about the age of 10 years.[28] The radiographical appearance is one of an eccentric, sharply circumscribed zone of rarefaction, often with expansion of surrounding bone.

Benign Tumors of Fibrous Tissue

Fibrous Cortical Defect (Nonossifying Fibroma)

Nonossifying Fibromas are common between the ages of 4 and 8 years, occur more frequently in boys, and may affect up to 40% of children. They are significant

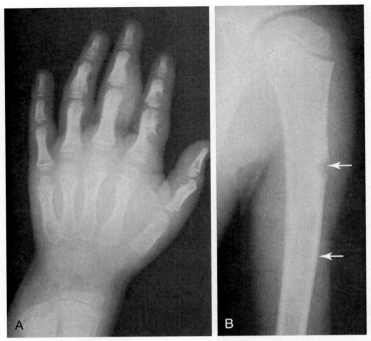

FIGURE 46–6   **A,** Characteristic changes of Maffucci syndrome. Notice the enchondromas of the proximal and middle phalanges of the second finger. The fusiform swelling of the third finger represents the soft tissue swelling of the hemangioma. The distal ulna is also involved. **B,** Radiograph of the humerus with the multiple enchondromas *(arrows)* of Maffucci syndrome.

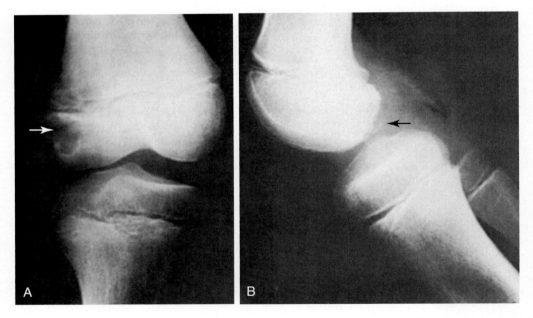

FIGURE   46–7 Chondroblastoma presenting as pain and effusion of the right knee of a 9 year-old boy. **A,** Anteroposterior view of a well-defined, oval, lytic lesion *(arrow)*. **B,** Lateral radiograph indicates that the lesion has eroded through the epiphysis *(arrow)* with small foci of calcification.

in that they may be mistaken for a more serious disease. There may be two or more fibromas, and they are usually an incidental finding (most often in the distal femur and proximal tibia) on radiographical evaluation.[8,9] The radiological appearance is virtually diagnostic, with a sharply marginated eccentric lucency in the metaphyseal cortex (Fig. 46–8). These lesions disappear with increasing age, leaving no significant residual defect. They rarely cause symptoms, and treatment is conservative; occasionally, pathological fractures occur.

Juvenile Fibromatosis

The disorders known as the *juvenile fibromatoses* are rare and include *juvenile aponeurotic fibroma, extraabdominal desmoid tumor,* and *diffuse infantile fibromatosis.* Lipomas and neurofibromas are occasionally associated with musculoskeletal symptoms, often resulting in the development of scoliosis. A variety of other forms of fibromatous soft tissue lesions have been described in children. *Infantile systemic hyalinosis* is a rare inherited disorder characterized by deposition of hyaline material in skin with

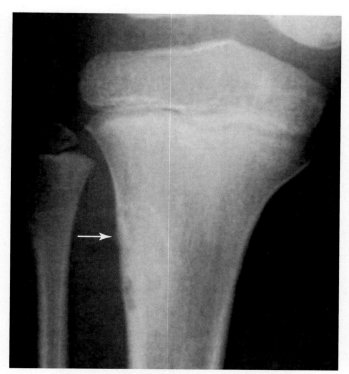

FIGURE 46–8 Benign fibrous cortical defect of the metaphysis of the tibia *(arrow)*. This lesion was detected as an incidental finding in a radiograph taken for evaluation of trauma.

the formation of nodules, in the musculoskeletal system with development of progressive joint contractures, and in viscera.[29] Death occurs by the age of 2 years. The basic defect is in mutations in the capillary morphogenesis protein 2.[30,31] Arabs, Japanese, and those living in the Indian subcontinent are particularly affected, thought by some to be a result of the frequency of consanguineous marriage among these ethnic groups.[32] Another subtype of the disorder is juvenile hyaline fibromatosis.[33] Both varieties are histologically similar and may represent a comparable or identical pathogenesis. Other names have included molluscum fibrosum and mesenchymal dysplasia.[34] The early onset of this disorder is in some ways similar to that of neonatal-onset multisystem inflammatory disorder.

Fibrous Dysplasia

Fibrous dysplasia is difficult to classify and probably represents a developmental abnormality or a benign neoplastic fibrous tissue lesion.[35] It is a relatively common disorder with a variable presentation mimicking that of almost any bone lesion. Monostotic disease, most commonly in a rib, occurs in approximately 85% of patients. Polyostotic fibrous dysplasia may be limited to two or three sites or result in extensive skeletal abnormalities. It is also part of the *McCune-Albright syndrome* in association with multiple endocrine abnormalities.[36]

The classic radiological appearance of fibrous dysplasia is an intramedullary diaphyseal lesion with a thinned, sometimes bulging cortex. An angular deformity of the bone is often present at the site of the lesion and may require surgical intervention, depending on its severity and the potential for pathological fracture. Most

monostotic lesions present no problem to the child, and resection is not indicated. Even with curettage, the recurrence rate is high. Bisphosphonates may be therapeutically indicated.[37-39] *Osteofibrous dysplasia* is a rare lesion of childhood that resembles monostotic disease.[40]

Ossifying Fibroma

Ossifying fibroma, or osteofibrous dysplasia, usually involves the mandible or tibia.[41] Although usually benign, it may be locally aggressive. Symptoms are often absent, and bony deformity prompts the consultation. Curettage is often unsuccessful, and observation alone is usually recommended after careful histopathological review.[42]

Benign Tumors of Soft Tissue

Pigmented Villonodular Synovitis

Pigmented villonodular synovitis (PVS) may represent a benign neoplasia, may be caused by an infectious process, or may be associated with repeated episodes of intraarticular hemorrhage. This condition is rare in childhood and is most common between the ages of 20 and 40 years. PVS affects males and females equally. It may present as recurrent swelling in a knee, ankle, or tendon sheath, and may be nodular or diffuse.[43-45] Nodular disease affects joints, bursae, or tendon sheaths; in diffuse PVS, a monarthritis of the knee, ankle, or less frequently, the hip is most common. Only rarely is the upper extremity affected.

The disorder is characterized by recurrent painless effusions and a slowly progressive destruction of cartilage and erosion of bone. A boggy fullness about the joint is present on clinical examination. The most striking feature is the presence of blood-stained, dark brown synovial fluid on joint aspiration. The synovium is dark and characterized by nodular areas of hypertrophy and hemosiderin-laden macrophages. There are proliferating synovial cells and fibroblasts, masses of stromal cells with frequent mitoses, and multinucleated giant cells.[46] MRI has aided in diagnostic evaluation. A characteristic finding is low signal density on T1- and T2-weighted MR studies.[47] Treatment often requires surgical excision, which is difficult with the nodular variety because of extension of the lesion into tendon sheaths. NSAIDs are useful in suppressing the inflammatory disease, and intraarticular glucocorticoids may have a role in management. Malignant PVS is rare, and its precise classification is controversial.[48]

Synovial Hemangioma

Synovial hemangioma is most common in the knee but is an infrequent lesion. It may present as intermittent hemarthrosis simulating monarticular arthritis. Synovial hemangioma may be associated with contiguous cutaneous hemangiomas, varicose veins, and bone and soft tissue hypertrophy (i.e., *Klippel-Trenaunay-Weber syndrome*)[49] or with capillary hemangiomas, thrombocytopenia, and depressed coagulation components (i.e., *Kasabach-Merritt syndrome*).[50] Bleeding from the hemangioma results in the sudden onset of painful joint swelling with effusion, often after minor local trauma. Recurrences are

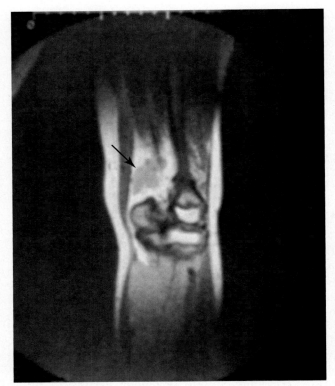

FIGURE 46–9   Magnetic resonance imaging study of the left knee of a 7 year-old boy with recurrent effusion and widespread cutaneous hemangiomata confirms the presence of a vascular mass just proximal to the knee joint *(arrow)*.

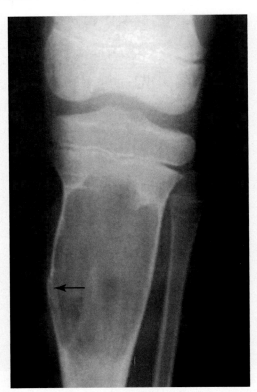

FIGURE 46–10   Radiograph of a pathological fracture *(arrow)* through the wall of a unicameral cyst of the tibia.

common and may result in chronic inflammatory synovitis and joint damage. Aspiration of synovial fluid at the onset of an effusion produces frank blood; later, the fluid may be xanthochromic and have a high bilirubin content. Radiographs demonstrate soft tissue swelling or a mass and, occasionally, phleboliths. The extent of the lesion is more accurately judged by MRI (Fig. 46–9).

Synovial Chondromatosis

In this unusual condition, synovial cartilaginous and osteocartilaginous bodies develop in the synovium and then are released free into the synovial fluid. Synovial chondromatosis is more common in boys and usually affects the knee. presenting symptoms are usually those of a loose body with intermittent pain, swelling, locking, and giving way. In early disease, radiographical studies are normal, but as the lesions calcify, they may be identified as discrete areas of stippled calcification. Treatment requires surgical excision. Malignant transformation is rare.[51,52]

Benign Tumors of Miscellaneous Origin

Unicameral (Solitary) Bone Cyst

Unicameral bone cyst is rare before the age of 3 years, occurs most commonly between the ages of 6 and 10 years, and is more frequently diagnosed in boys.[53] It usually arises in the metaphysis of a long bone and is often asymptomatic or causes only localized pain.[54] Because of

its size, it may result in localized swelling, a pathological fracture, or growth disturbance of the limb.[55] Radiography demonstrates a lucent lesion that adjoins but does not cross the physis or a fusiform widening of the bone (Fig. 46–10). These cysts usually require curettage and insertion of bone chips, although injection of the lesion with glucocorticoid has been effective.[53]

Aneurysmal Bone Cyst

Aneurysmal bone cyst is less common than the unicameral cyst, occurs more frequently in girls, and has its peak frequency in adolescence to early adulthood.[56] It presents most often as a reactive lesion with pain and swelling, commonly occurring in the metaphysis of a long bone or in a posterior element of the spine.[57] Onset may be insidious and prolonged over weeks to a few years. Radiographically, the lesion appears as a "bubble" with a circumscribed zone of rarefaction and surrounding destruction of the metaphyseal bone (Fig. 46–11). Differentiation from a unicameral cyst is aided by MRI.[58] Treatment requires surgical curettage, sometimes with resection or local irradiation or sclerotherapy.[53,59,60]

Giant Cell Tumor

Pain is usually the manifesting symptom of a giant cell tumor of bone. This tumor is most common in the second to third decades of life and occurs more frequently in girls. On radiographs, an expanding zone of eccentric radiolucency in the epiphysis of a long bone is characteristic.[2,3] Tumor size, location, and aggressiveness determine the outcome.[61]

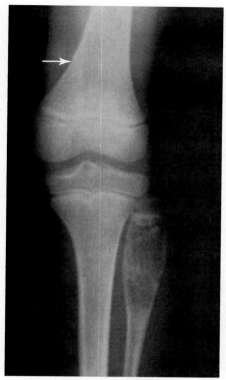

FIGURE 46–11 Radiograph of an aneurysmal bone cyst of the proximal fibula. Notice the benign cortical defect in the distal femur *(arrow)*. The two abnormalities are unrelated.

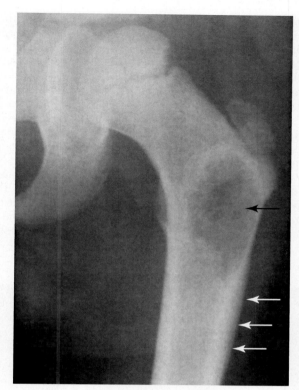

FIGURE 46–12 Radiograph of the femur with changes *(black arrow)* of Langerhans cell histiocytosis (i.e., eosinophilic granuloma). In addition to the lytic lesion, there is marked periosteal new-bone apposition *(white arrows)*.

Eosinophilic Granuloma

Eosinophilic granuloma, a lesion classified as a form of localized Langerhans cell histiocytosis (previously designated histiocytosis X) occurs predominantly in young children between the ages of 5 and 10 years and most commonly affects boys. Characteristic findings at onset are localized pain and swelling over a solitary mass.[62] The bones of the skull, spine, and pelvis and the diaphysis of the femur are most commonly affected. A radiograph demonstrates a discrete lytic lesion with cortical erosion and a periosteal reaction (Fig. 46–12). Percutaneous needle biopsy is indicated to establish the diagnosis.[63] Treatment requires surgical curettage, sometimes with low-dose radiation. It has been suggested that intralesional glucocorticoid may be a useful adjunct to therapy.[64] Other types of histiocytosis include *Hand-Schüller-Christian disease* and *Letterer-Siwe disease*.

MALIGNANT TUMORS

Malignant Tumors of Bone

Malignant musculoskeletal tumors of childhood account for 5% to 10% of malignant neoplasms; the most common of these lesions are osteogenic sarcoma, rhabdomyosarcoma, and Ewing sarcoma.[7,65] Osteogenic sarcoma is rare in the first decade of life but is the most common malignant bone tumor in the second

decade. The mean age of children with Ewing sarcoma is younger than that for any other primary tumor of bone. Survival rates (60% to 70%) have continued to improve modestly for these tumors.[66,67] There has also been progress in understanding their biology and genetic predisposition, especially in Ewing sarcoma and rhabdomyosarcoma.[68]

Osteosarcoma

Osteosarcoma (i.e., osteogenic sarcoma) accounts for 60% of all bone tumors in children.[69-73] It is most common at the time of maximal growth velocity in the second decade of life with 75% of cases occurring between the ages of 8 and 25 years of age, especially in taller children. The annual incidence of osteosarcoma is approximately 0.6 to 0.7 per 100,000 children.[74,75] It occasionally occurs in siblings.[76] Approximately 3% of these tumors develop in a field that has received previous irradiation. Osteosarcomas are also associated with certain acquired or genetic disorders such as retinoblastoma, enchondromatosis, hereditary multiple exostoses, and fibrous dysplasia. An increased risk of osteosarcoma is associated with the *Rothmund-Thomson syndrome*, a rare disorder characterized by short stature, telangiectases, small hands and feet, and hypoplastic thumbs.[77,78]

This tumor usually arises in the medullary canal of the bone, has a metaphyseal location, and occurs most often (60%) around the knee (e.g., distal femur, proximal tibia) and in the proximal humerus. Osteogenic sarcomas are highly malignant and metastasize early by hematogenous spread to many organs, especially the lungs, where they are a significant cause of secondary hypertrophic osteoarthropathy.[79]

Pain is the most common presenting symptom.[80] Swelling over the involved bone occurs a few weeks to months later. Secondary signs include local inflammation, involvement of regional lymph nodes, and loss of function of the limb. The presence of systemic signs such as weight loss, fever, or secondary hypertrophic osteoarthropathy suggests that skeletal and pulmonary metastases have already occurred.

Radiological investigations provide the most meaningful diagnostic information.[81] On plain radiographs, the lesion has a moth-eaten appearance with cortical destruction, periosteal elevation (i.e., Codman triangle), and a soft tissue mass (Fig. 46–13). The differential diagnosis may include osteomyelitis. Occasionally, two or more tumor sites are present, representing a multifocal origin or metastases to bone. Bone scintigraphy, CT, or MRI may be indicated to delineate the extent of the lesion. The diagnosis of osteogenic sarcoma is confirmed by the histological appearance on biopsy of marked cellular pleomorphism with spindle-shaped cells, chondrocytes, and osteoid. Osteosarcoma is commonly divided into five principal types: osteoblastic, chondroblastic, fibroblastic, telangiectatic, and a small-cell type that has features overlapping those of Ewing sarcoma.

The treatment of this tumor, with a five year survival rate of only 21%, has until recently included amputation of the limb.[66] Modification of the surgical approach, including segmental resection of the primary tumor[82] and the addition of adjuvant chemotherapy (including

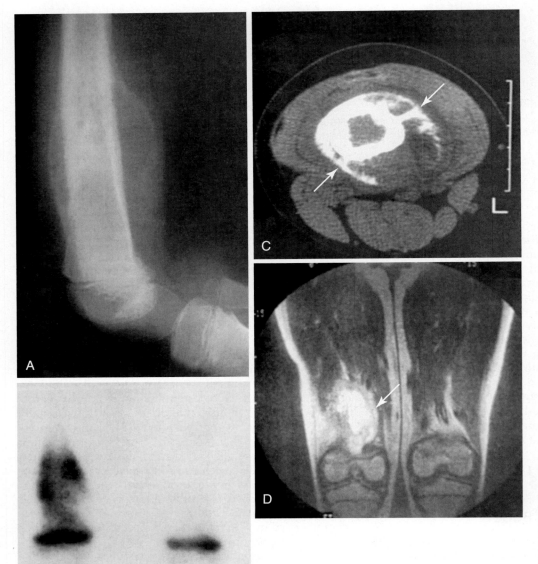

FIGURE 46–13 **A,** Radiograph of an osteosarcoma of the distal femoral metaphysis in a young boy. **B,** Technetium 99m bone scan of the femurs documents increased uptake of isotope by the osteosarcoma. **C,** Computerized tomography section through the thigh shows the extracortical bony densities *(arrows)* characteristic of osteosarcoma. **D,** Magnetic resonance imaging study demonstrates the tumor in the right thigh *(arrow).*

doxorubicin, cisplatin, and high-dose methotrexate with leucovorin rescue), has led to a disease-free survival rate of more than 50% at five years.[74,75,83,84] Prognostic features include the histological grade of the tumor, size of the initial lesion, and its response to preoperative treatment. Metastases at diagnosis are associated with a poor outcome (less than 20% survival). The rare *multifocal sclerosing osteosarcoma* has a poor prognosis.

Surface osteosarcomas do not involve the medullary cavity and often encircle the entire shaft of the bone.[85] They have been divided into two types: *parosteal* (or *juxtacortical*) and *periosteal*. These tumors behave differently from osteogenic sarcoma. The parosteal variety is more common in girls and occurs most often on the posterior surface of the distal femur. Malignant potential is low, it tends to metastasize late, and it has a much better prognosis. The periosteal type occurs more commonly in the tibia and is associated with an abundant proliferation of cartilage.

Malignant Tumors of Cartilage: Chondrosarcoma

Chondrosarcoma is a rare tumor (less than 5%) that develops in children from malignant transformation of a preexisting enchondroma or, later in life, in a patient with multiple heritable exostoses.[86] The initial symptoms are localized swelling or pain.[87] Radiographs are usually diagnostic with destruction of bone combined with mottled densities of calcification and ossification (i.e., "popcorn" appearance). Treatment consists of wide resection, adjuvant chemotherapy, and irradiation.[88]

Malignant Tumors of Fibrous Tissue: Fibrosarcoma

Fibrosarcoma is an uncommon tumor that occurs most often on a distal extremity as a soft, infiltrative mass with areas of hemorrhage or necrosis.[89,90] Histopathology confirms fibroblastic or myofibroblastic differentiation of all degrees.[91] There are two major patterns of presentation: *congenital fibrosarcoma* is most common in boys younger than 2 years; *postpubertal fibrosarcoma* is more aggressive.[89,92] Onset is characterized in most instances by painful swelling. No diagnostic radiographical features distinguish this tumor from osteosarcoma. In children younger than 2 to 5 years, congenital fibrosarcomas undergo rapid growth and extensive local invasion despite a relative lack of distant metastasis (7%). In children older than 10 years, the metastatic rate approaches 50%. Treatment involves surgical resection; approaches to treatment of the postpubertal type combine radical excision, postoperative irradiation, and adjuvant chemotherapy.[93] The overall combined survival rate is approximately 40% at five years and 30% at 10 years. Prognosis is obviously best for the more superficial and differentiated tumors. Fluorodeoxyglucose positron-emission tomography may have a role in identification and grading of these sarcomas of bone and soft tissue.[94]

Malignant Tumors of Soft Tissue

Rhabdomyosarcoma

Rhabdomyosarcomas are the most common soft tissue sarcomas in children and account for one-half of all soft tissue neoplasms in patients younger than 15 years.[87,95-98] They occur most often in children between the ages of 2 and 6 years or during adolescence, with an annual incidence of 0.4 to 0.9 per 100,000 children,[75] and are rare in older age groups. The tumor presents as a localized, painless, soft tissue mass. These tumors are most common in the head and neck but can arise in any striated muscle. Approximately 20% occur in the extremities, especially during adolescence. Rhabdomyosarcoma metastasizes early to the lung, bone, and bone marrow. It may erode into adjacent bone and produce a radiographical appearance of a soft tissue mass with an underlying periosteal reaction.[99] Treatment includes surgical excision, irradiation, and chemotherapy.[100-102] The five year survival rate is approximately 70%.[75,103,104]

Synovial Cell Sarcoma

Although rare in childhood, synovial cell sarcoma is the most common soft tissue sarcoma (6% to 10%) after the rhabdomyosarcomas.[105-108] This tumor rarely occurs within a joint; it usually develops in the periarticular soft tissue. Lower extremity involvement is most common, especially around the knee or foot or in the hand. The tumor may be associated with calcifications that suggest the diagnosis on radiographs. Tendon sheaths may also be involved.[109] Surgical excision, irradiation, and chemotherapy result in a seven-year survival rate of 60% to 70%. Prognosis is related to tumor size and ease of resection.[110-114] Most synovial sarcomas express a specific chromosomal abnormality: t(X;18) (p11.2;q11.2).[115]

Malignant Tumors of Miscellaneous Origin: Ewing Sarcoma

The Ewing sarcoma family of tumors probably arises from primitive multipotential mesenchymal or neural crest cell lineages in the medulla of bone or occasionally in soft tissue.[72,116,117] It is the most malignant of bone tumors and the second most common cancer of bone in children.[118] It accounts for 7% to 15% of all malignant bone tumors in childhood, with an annual incidence of 0.2 to 0.3 per 100,000 children.[75,119] This lesion is most common in white boys in the second decade of life (male to female ratio of 1.5:1), although the mean age at onset is somewhat younger than that for osteogenic sarcoma. It is uncommon in children of Asian or African descent. Ewing sarcoma often occurs in the diaphysis of the long bones (i.e., femur, humerus, or tibia) or in the innominate, but it can develop in any bone, including those of the axial skeleton, or even as an extra-skeletal lesion.[120] The tumor presents with pain, and local swelling systemic signs, including fever, are common, often occurring with abnormalities of laboratory indices of inflammation.[80]

The radiographic appearance is characteristically that of an aggressive, elongated, lytic lesion filling the medullary

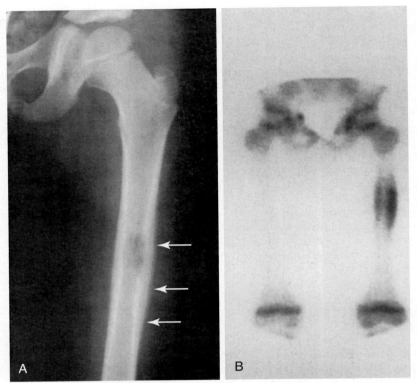

FIGURE 46–14 **A,** Radiograph of Ewing sarcoma in the diaphysis of the femur. The central lytic lesion is accompanied by periosteal reaction *(arrows).* **B,** Technetium 99m bone scan of the femurs of the same child, which shows localized increased uptake of the isotope in the tumor.

cavity, disrupting the cortex, and causing a roughening of the periosteum described as having an onion-skin or sunburst appearance (Fig. 46–14). This reaction may be easily confused with osteomyelitis. Ewing sarcoma eventually involves the entire shaft of the long bone and metastasizes to other bones and lungs. The histological appearance is that of sheets of small round cells that are positive on staining with periodic acid-Schiff reagent, sometimes with a perivascular pseudorosette appearance. Neural markers, chimeric fusion products, or a specific chromosomal translocation (t [11;22] [q24;q12]) in more than 95% of cases can be identified to differentiate this tumor from lymphoma, rhabdomyosarcoma, or neuroblastoma. Treatment combines surgical resection with irradiation and adjuvant chemotherapy.[93,121,122] The five year survival rate varies from 50% to 80%, depending on the site of the primary tumor.[123,124] Metastases to the lung or skeleton reduce the survival rate to 20% to 30%.[125,126] Allogenic or autologous stem cell transplantation has not improved survivorship.[127]

METASTATIC BONE TUMORS

In childhood, metastatic bone tumors are uncommon except for neuroblastoma. In a retrospective review of metastatic skeletal disease in childhood over a 38 year period, Leeson and coworkers[128] described 39 patients ranging in age from 18 months to 20 years. The tumors most commonly producing skeletal metastases were neuroblastoma (41%), rhabdomyosarcoma (18%), teratoma-carcinoma (10%), Wilms tumor (8%), and retinoblastoma (5%).

Neuroblastoma, a tumor of the sympathetic nervous system, has an incidence of 1.6 cases per 100,000 persons, primarily young children.[75] Bone metastases usually occur early and may be accompanied by fever but little else in the way of localizing abnormalities. The development of bone pain related to bony metastases or bone marrow infiltration soon follows. Neuroblastoma most commonly metastasizes to the spine (81%), skull (69%), femur (50%), ribs (44%), and pelvis (31%). Multiple bony metastases are the rule.

The radiographic appearance is that of a lytic lesion arising from the marrow cavity (Fig. 46–15). Scintigraphy is the most sensitive technique for determining the site and number of metastases and may document abnormal findings before radiographic changes on plain film are evident. Treatment includes surgical removal of the tumor together with irradiation and chemotherapy.[129] The survival rate at five years is approximately 55%.[75]

Wilms tumor is the most common retroperitoneal malignant tumor of childhood, with an incidence of two cases per 100,000 children.[75] It occurs most commonly in infants and young children (less than 4 years) in whom it usually presents as an abdominal mass. Tumors with a sarcomatous histology are particularly likely to metastasize to bone and may be associated with bone pain. Wilms tumor is frequently associated with several congenital anomalies, including sporadic aniridia, hemihypertrophy, genitourinary anomalies, and a deletion in chromosome 11.[130] Treatment includes nephrectomy, irradiation, and chemotherapy. The five year survival rate is approximately 80%.[75]

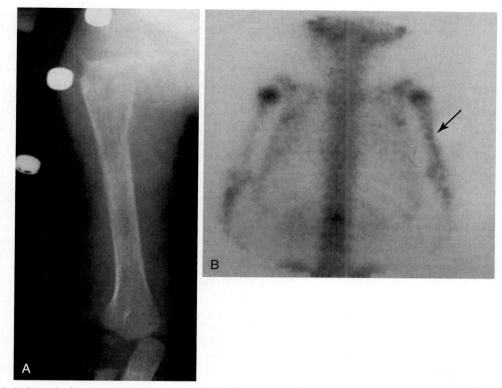

FIGURE 46–15   A, Radiograph of the humerus illustrates the moth-eaten appearance of extensive metastatic neuroblastoma in the proximal humerus. **B,** Technetium 99m bone scan shows increased uptake in the right humerus of the same child *(arrow).*

MALIGNANT INFILTRATION OF BONE MARROW: LEUKEMIA

Leukemia is the most common childhood malignancy that results in musculoskeletal pain and arthritis.[131-133] In most instances, the pain is diffusely localized to one area of the body, particularly over the metaphyses of the long bones (Table 46–4). Sometimes, a joint effusion occurs. Large joints, especially the knees, are most commonly affected, although small joints of the hands may be involved. The number of affected joints is usually relatively few. Associated periarticular disease is common.

The frequency of musculoskeletal signs or symptoms in childhood leukemia was evaluated in a two-year prospective study of 28 children.[131] Objective joint findings, often mild, were present in 50% of the children, most often at or near onset of the disease. In one half of the children, a single joint was involved, most often the knee; in the remainder, two or three joints, rarely more, were affected. Retrospective studies have usually indicated a lower prevalence of joint disease of 11% to 12%.[132,134]

A high index of suspicion is needed to confirm the diagnosis of leukemia in a child presenting with musculoskeletal pain.[135] The most distinctive diagnostic features of leukemia are the degree and location of the pain. In leukemia, pain is much more severe than in chronic arthritis and is characteristically metaphyseal in location rather than directly over a joint. Abnormally elevated levels of acute phase indices, such as the ESR, are out of proportion to the small number of affected joints.

Table 46–4	
Clinical characteristics of acute leukemia in children	
Characteristic	**Description**
Presentation	Low-grade fever, fatigue, pallor, weight loss
Pain	Often disproportionate to objective findings
	Diffuse musculoskeletal aching or pain and tenderness of metaphyses of long bones
	May be migratory joint pain or periarticular swelling or joint effusion
Hematological parameters	May be normal or with increased or decreased WBC count or platelet count, sometimes with blast cells in peripheral smear
	Increased ESR and lactate dehydrogenase and urate levels
Radiographs	Metaphyseal rarefaction, periosteal new-bone apposition

ESR, erythrocyte sedimentation rate; WBC, white blood cell.

Dissociation of the inflammatory indices (e.g., an elevated ESR with a normal or low platelet count), a low white blood cell count, or a striking increase in the serum level of lactic dehydrogenase or urate should also alert the physician to the possibility of leukemia. The hematological findings (i.e., complete blood count, white blood cell differential count, and platelet count) may be normal for weeks or months after the onset of symptoms, and repeated evaluations are essential. Blast cells in the peripheral blood may not be present at onset of the musculoskeletal symptoms, in which case bone marrow aspiration and biopsy are indicated. Antinuclear antibodies are occasionally detected in children with leukemia, and their presence should not be interpreted as an indication of inflammatory arthritis.[132]

Radiographical changes may be of assistance in the diagnosis. In addition to localized metaphyseal rarefaction (Fig. 46–16), there may be subperiosteal elevation or an elongated osteolytic reaction. Such changes, however, may be absent even in the presence of severe symptoms. Scintigraphy with technetium 99m documents an increased uptake in marrow, and in metaphyseal and periosteal areas. Differentiation from osteomyelitis or neoplasm (e.g., Ewing sarcoma) is paramount. Primary bone lymphoma, although rare, is best evaluated by MRI because plain radiograph films are often normal or near normal.[136]

SECONDARY EFFECTS OF MALIGNANCY

Secondary Hypertrophic Osteoarthropathy

The syndrome of secondary hypertrophic osteoarthropathy (SHO) consists of terminal clubbing, painful swelling of distal joints and soft tissues, profuse sweating, and radiographical evidence of periosteal new-bone formation affecting the hands, feet, and distal limbs. Although periosteal new-bone apposition can also be a radiological characteristic of early JIA or juvenile psoriatic arthritis, it is not associated in these children with the severe pain and tenderness of SHO.

Most cases of SHO in childhood are related to chronic pulmonary disease,[129] congenital heart disease, or, occasionally, the antiphospholipid antibody syndrome.[137] Associations with biliary atresia and regional enteritis have been reported. The pathogenesis of SHO is unknown, although hypoxic, endocrine, and neurogenic mechanisms have been suggested. SHO also occurs in the *POEMS syndrome* (i.e., polyneuropathy, organomegaly, endocrinopathy, M protein, and skin changes) in adults.[137] An important cause of SHO in childhood is pulmonary malignancy, most often caused by metastases from osteogenic sarcoma.[79,138] The typical clubbing and diffuse swelling of the joints and soft tissues of the hands, together with marked periosteal new-bone apposition along the proximal phalanges, metacarpals, and distal radius and ulna, are depicted in Figure 46–17. Scintigraphy with technetium 99m documents increased uptake in areas of involvement.

Children with symptomatic SHO are usually profoundly ill. The pain is severe, predominantly distal in location, and symmetrical in distribution. It is present during the daytime and may awaken the child at night. Medical treatment is usually unsatisfactory, although NSAIDs are sometimes temporarily effective. Resection of the pulmonary or pleural tumor may result in dramatic resolution of all signs and symptoms.

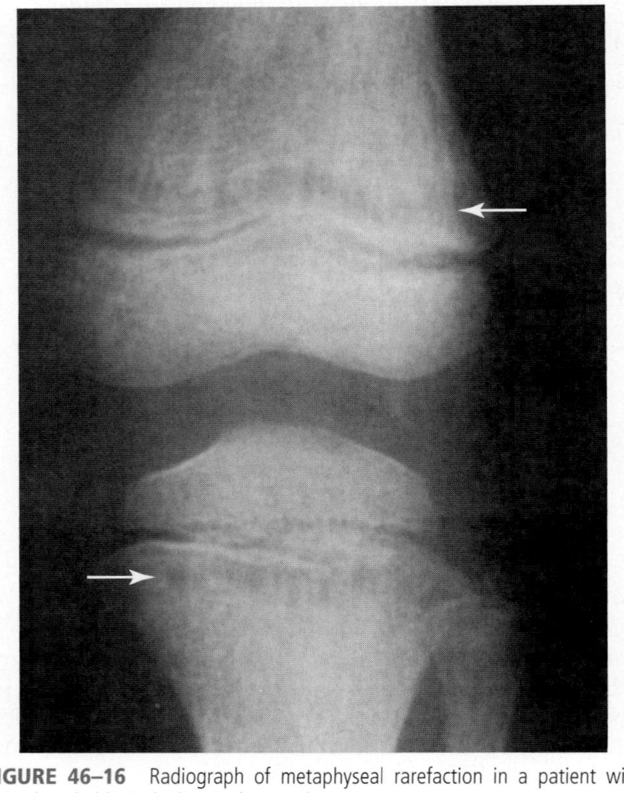

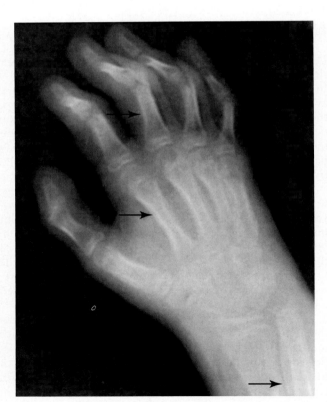

FIGURE 46–16   Radiograph of metaphyseal rarefaction in a patient with acute lymphoblastic leukemia *(arrows)*.

FIGURE 46–17   Secondary hypertrophic osteoarthropathy in a child with pulmonary metastases from osteosarcoma. Notice the marked periosteal new-bone apposition along the phalanges, metacarpals, and distal radius and ulna *(arrows)*.

Acanthosis Nigricans

Acanthosis nigricans is a rare disorder associated with a number of conditions, including malignancy, diabetes, obesity, various genetic syndromes, connective tissue diseases such as dermatomyositis, and glucocorticoid administration.[139,140] It may also occur in children with lipodystrophy or may be familial.[141] In juvenile dermatomyositis, it is associated with premature thelarche, lipodystrophy, and insulin resistance (see Chapter 24).

REFERENCES

1. R.C. Trueworthy, K.J. Templeton, Malignant bone tumors presenting as musculoskeletal pain, Pediatr. Ann. 31 (2002) 355–359.
2. J.M. Mirra, P. Picci, R.H. Gold, Bone tumors: clinical, radiologic, and pathologic correlations, Lea & Febiger, Philadelphia, 1989.
3. D.C. Dahlin, K.K. Unni, Dahlin's bone tumors: general aspects and data on 11,087 cases, ed 5, Lippincott-Raven, Philadelphia, 1996.
4. J.M. Herrera, A. Krebs, P. Harris, et al., Childhood tumors, Surg. Clin. North Am. 80 (2000) 747–760. xii.
6. C.A. Arndt, W.M. Crist, Common musculoskeletal tumors of childhood and adolescence, N. Engl. J. Med. 341 (1999) 342–352.
7. D.M. Parkin, C.A. Stiller, J. Nectoux, International variations in the incidence of childhood bone tumours, Int. J. Cancer 53 (1993) 371–376.
10. L.M. Fayad, D.A. Bluemke, K.L. Weber, et al., Characterization of pediatric skeletal tumors and tumor-like conditions: specific cross-sectional imaging signs, Skeletal Radiol. 35 (2006) 259–268.
11. S.L. Miller, F.A. Hoffer, Malignant and benign bone tumors, Radiol. Clin. North Am. 39 (2001) 673–699.
12. E.M. Azouz, Magnetic resonance imaging of benign bone lesions: cysts and tumors, Top Magn. Reson. Imaging 13 (2002) 219–229.
14. L. Copley, J.P. Dormans, Benign pediatric bone tumors. Evaluation and treatment, Pediatr. Clin. North Am. 43 (1996) 949–966.
15. J.S. Biermann, Common benign lesions of bone in children and adolescents, J. Pediatr. Orthop. 22 (2002) 268–273.
17. M.D. Cohen, T.M. Harrington, W.W. Ginsburg, Osteoid osteoma: 95 cases and a review of the literature, Semin. Arthritis Rheum. 12 (1983) 265–281.
19. G.N. Graham, H. Browne, Primary bony tumors of the pediatric spine, Yale. J. Biol. Med. 74 (2001) 1–8.
22. A. Drevelegas, D. Chourmouzi, G. Boulogianni, et al., Imaging of primary bone tumors of the spine, Eur. Radiol. 13 (2003) 1859–1871.
24. D.E. Porter, M.E. Emerton, F. Villanueva-Lopez, et al., Clinical and radiographic analysis of osteochondromas and growth disturbance in hereditary multiple exostoses, J. Pediatr. Orthop. 20 (2000) 246–250.
26. K.A. Pierz, R.B. Womer, J.P. Dormans, Pediatric bone tumors: osteosarcoma Ewing's sarcoma, and chondrosarcoma associated with multiple hereditary osteochondromatosis, J. Pediatr. Orthop. 21 (2001) 412–418.
30. S. Hanks, S. Adams, J. Douglas, et al., Mutations in the gene encoding capillary morphogenesis protein 2 cause juvenile hyaline fibromatosis and infantile systemic hyalinosis, Am. J. Hum. Genet. 73 (2003) 791–800.
33. B.H. Landing, R. Nadorra, Infantile systemic hyalinosis: report of four cases of a disease, fatal in infancy, apparently different from juvenile systemic hyalinosis, Pediatr. Pathol. 6 (1986) 55–79.
36. S. Lumbroso, F. Paris, C. Sultan, McCune-Albright syndrome: molecular genetics, J. Pediatr. Endocrinol. Metab. 15 (2002) 875–882.
37. J.P. Devogelaer, Treatment of bone diseases with bisphosphonates, excluding osteoporosis, Curr. Opin. Rheumatol. 12 (2000) 331–335.
38. R.D. Chapurlat, P.J. Meunier, Fibrous dysplasia of bone, Baillieres. Best Pract. Res. Clin. Rheumatol. 14 (2000) 385–398.
39. E. Schoenau, F. Rauch, Fibrous dysplasia, Horm. Res. 57 (2002) 79–82.
41. H.K. Williams, C. Mangham, P.M. Speight, Juvenile ossifying fibroma. An analysis of eight cases and a comparison with other fibro-osseous lesions, J. Oral Pathol. Med. 29 (2000) 13–18.
42. A.L. Folpe, S.W. Weiss, Ossifying fibromyxoid tumor of soft parts: a clinicopathologic study of 70 cases with emphasis on atypical and malignant variants, Am. J. Surg. Pathol. 27 (2003) 421–431.
44. E. de Visser, R.P. Veth, M. Pruszczynski, et al., Diffuse and localized pigmented villonodular synovitis: evaluation of treatment of 38 patients, Arch. Orthop. Trauma Surg. 119 (1999) 401–404.
45. N.S. Somerhausen, C.D. Fletcher, Diffuse-type giant cell tumor: clinicopathologic and immunohistochemical analysis of 50 cases with extraarticular disease, Am. J. Surg. Pathol. 24 (2000) 479–492.
47. F.J. Frassica, J.A. Khanna, E.F. McCarthy, The role of MR imaging in soft tissue tumor evaluation: perspective of the orthopedic oncologist and musculoskeletal pathologist, Magn. Reson. Imaging Clin. North Am. 8 (2000) 915–927.
48. F. Bertoni, K.K. Unni, J.W. Beabout, et al., Malignant giant cell tumor of the tendon sheaths and joints (malignant pigmented villonodular synovitis), Am. J. Surg. Pathol. 21 (1997) 153–163.
52. R. Sciot, P. Dal Cin, J. Bellemans, et al., Synovial chondromatosis: clonal chromosome changes provide further evidence for a neoplastic disorder, Virchows Arch. 433 (1998) 189–191.
54. F. Lokiec, S. Wientroub, Simple bone cyst: etiology, classification, pathology, and treatment modalities, J. Pediatr. Orthop. B 7 (1998) 262–273.
55. M. Clayer, C. Boatright, E. Conrad, Growth disturbances associated with untreated benign bone cysts, Aust. N. Z. J. Surg. 67 (1997) 872–873.
56. A. Leithner, R. Windhager, S. Lang, et al., Aneurysmal bone cyst. A population based epidemiologic study and literature review, Clin. Orthop. 363 (1999) 176–179.
61. S. Boutou-Bredaki, P. Agapios, G. Papachristou, Prognosis of giant cell tumor of bone. Histopathological analysis of 15 cases and review of the literature, Adv. Clin. Pathol. 5 (2001) 71–78.
65. F.A. Hoffer, Primary skeletal neoplasms: osteosarcoma and Ewing sarcoma, Top. Magn. Reson. Imaging 13 (2002) 231–239.
67. B.P. Himelstein, J.P. Dormans, Malignant bone tumors of childhood, Pediatr. Clin. North Am. 43 (1996) 967–984.
68. H. van den Berg, Biology and therapy of malignant solid tumors in childhood, Cancer Chemother. Biol. Response Modif. 20 (2002) 605–625.
69. N. Jaffe, Osteosarcoma, Pediatr. Rev. 12 (1991) 333–343.
73. M. Rytting, P. Pearson, A.K. Raymond, et al., Osteosarcoma in preadolescent patients, Clin. Orthop. 373 (2000) 39–50.
74. A.M. Goorin, H.T. Abelson, E. Frei III, Osteosarcoma: fifteen years later, N. Engl. J. Med. 313 (1985) 1637–1643.
75. W.M. Crist, L.E. Kun, Common solid tumors of childhood, N. Engl. J. Med. 324 (1991) 461–471.
77. A. Leonard, A.W. Craft, C. Moss, et al., Osteogenic sarcoma in the Rothmund-Thomson syndrome, Med. Pediatr. Oncol. 26 (1996) 249–253.
85. R.A. Vander Griend, Osteosarcoma and its variants, Orthop. Clin. North Am. 27 (1996) 575–581.
86. A. Kivioja, H. Ervasti, J. Kinnunen, et al., Chondrosarcoma in a family with multiple hereditary exostoses, J. Bone Joint Surg. Br. 82 (2000) 261–266.
88. F.Y. Lee, H.J. Mankin, G. Fondren, et al., Chondrosarcoma of bone: an assessment of outcome, J. Bone Joint Surg. Am. 81 (1999) 326–338.
90. H. Neville, C. Corpron, M.L. Blakely, et al., Pediatric neurofibrosarcoma, J. Pediatr. Surg. 38 (2003) 343–346.
91. W.G. Ward, P. Savage, C.A. Boles, et al., Fine-needle aspiration biopsy of sarcomas and related tumors, Cancer Control 8 (2001) 232–238.
92. R. Trobs, T. Meier, J. Bennek, et al., Fibrosarcoma in infants and children: a retrospective analysis—overdiagnosis in earlier years, Pediatr. Surg. Int. 15 (1999) 123–128.
93. J.G. Kennedy, P. Frelinghuysen, B.H. Hoang, Ewing sarcoma: current concepts in diagnosis and treatment, Curr. Opin. Pediatr. 15 (2003) 53–57.
94. E. Bastiaannet, H. Groen, P.L. Jager, et al., The value of FDG-PET in the detection, grading and response to therapy of soft tissue and bone sarcomas: a systematic review and meta-analysis, Cancer Treat. Rev. 30 (2004) 83–101.
95. G. Merlino, L.J. Helman, Rhabdomyosarcoma—working out the pathways, Oncogene 18 (1999) 5340–5348.

96. R. Dagher, L. Helman, Rhabdomyosarcoma: an overview, Oncologist 4 (1999) 34–44.
97. F.B. Ruymann, A.C. Grovas, Progress in the diagnosis and treatment of rhabdomyosarcoma and related soft tissue sarcomas, Cancer Invest. 18 (2000) 223–241.
98. R.B. Raney, Soft-tissue sarcoma in childhood and adolescence, Curr. Oncol. Rep. 4 (2002) 291–298.
99. M.B. McCarville, S.L. Spunt, A.S. Pappo, Rhabdomyosarcoma in pediatric patients: the good, the bad, and the unusual, Am. J. Roentgenol. 176 (2001) 1563–1569.
100. A.S. Pappo, D.N. Shapiro, W.M. Crist, Rhabdomyosarcoma. Biology and treatment, Pediatr. Clin. North Am. 44 (1997) 953–972.
101. R.J. Andrassy, Rhabdomyosarcoma, Semin. Pediatr. Surg. 6 (1997) 17–23.
104. H.P. McDowell, Update on childhood rhabdomyosarcoma, Arch. Dis. Child 88 (2003) 354–357.
105. D. Schmidt, P. Thum, D. Harms, et al., Synovial sarcoma in children and adolescents. A report from the Kiel Pediatric Tumor Registry, Cancer 67 (1991) 1667–1672.
106. A. Ferrari, M. Casanova, M. Massimino, et al., Synovial sarcoma: report of a series of 25 consecutive children from a single institution, Med. Pediatr. Oncol. 32 (1999) 32–37.
107. B. Skytting, Synovial sarcoma. A Scandinavian Sarcoma Group project, Acta. Orthop. Scand. (2000) 1–28.
108. R.J. Andrassy, M.F. Okcu, S. Despa, et al., Synovial sarcoma in children: surgical lessons from a single institution and review of the literature, J. Am. Coll. Surg. 192 (2001) 305–313.
111. B.T. Skytting, H.C. Bauer, R. Perfekt, et al., Clinical course in synovial sarcoma: a Scandinavian sarcoma group study of 104 patients, Acta. Orthop. Scand. 70 (1999) 536–542.
113. R.C. Thompson Jr., A. Garg, J. Goswitz, et al., Synovial sarcoma. Large size predicts poor outcome, Clin. Orthop. 373 (2000) 18–24.
114. J.J. Lewis, C.R. Antonescu, D.H. Leung, et al., Synovial sarcoma: a multivariate analysis of prognostic factors in 112 patients with primary localized tumors of the extremity, J. Clin. Oncol. 18 (2000) 2087–2094.
115. C. Fisher, Synovial sarcoma, Ann. Diagn. Pathol. 2 (1998) 401–421.
117. D.C. West, Ewing sarcoma family of tumors, Curr. Opin. Oncol. 12 (2000) 323–329.
118. R. Vlasak, F.H. Sim, Ewing's sarcoma, Orthop. Clin. North Am. 27 (1996) 591–603.
119. J.S. Miser, T.J. Triche, T.J. Kinsella, et al., Other soft tissue sarcomas of childhood, in: P.A. Pizzo, D.G. Poplack (Eds.), Principles and practice of pediatric oncology, ed 3, J. B. Lippincott-Raven, Philadelphia, 1997.
120. R. Ahmad, B.R. Mayol, M. Davis, et al., Extraskeletal Ewing's sarcoma, Cancer 85 (1999) 725–731.
121. A.G. Shankar, C.R. Pinkerton, A. Atra, et al., Local therapy and other factors influencing site of relapse in patients with localised Ewing's sarcoma. United Kingdom Children's Cancer Study Group (UKCCSG), Eur. J. Cancer 35 (1999) 1698–1704.
122. C.R. Pinkerton, A. Bataillard, S. Guillo, et al., Treatment strategies for metastatic Ewing's sarcoma, Eur. J. Cancer 37 (2001) 1338–1344.

123. P. Rosito, A.F. Mancini, R. Rondelli, et al., Italian Cooperative Study for the treatment of children and young adults with localized Ewing sarcoma of bone: a preliminary report of 6 years of experience, Cancer 86 (1999) 421–428.
124. T.W. McLean, C. Hertel, M.L. Young, et al., Late events in pediatric patients with Ewing sarcoma/primitive neuroectodermal tumor of bone: the Dana-Farber Cancer Institute/Children's Hospital experience, J. Pediatr. Hematol. Oncol. 21 (1999) 486–493.
126. R. Cardenas-Cardos, R. Rivera-Luna, N.A. Lopez-Facundo, et al., Ewing's sarcoma: prognosis and survival in Mexican children from a single institution, Pediatr. Hematol. Oncol. 16 (1999) 519–523.
127. S. Burdach, B. van Kaick, H.J. Laws, et al., Allogeneic and autologous stem-cell transplantation in advanced Ewing tumors: an update after long-term follow-up from two centers of the European Intergroup study EICESS. Stem-Cell Transplant Programs at Dusseldorf University Medical Center, Germany and St. Anna Kinderspital, Vienna, Austria, Ann. Oncol. 11 (2000) 1451–1462.
128. M.C. Leeson, J.T. Makley, J.R. Carter, Metastatic skeletal disease in the pediatric population, J. Pediatr. Orthop. 5 (1985) 261–267.
129. P. Losty, F. Quinn, F. Breatnach, et al., Neuroblastoma—a surgical perspective, Eur. J. Surg. Oncol. 19 (1993) 33–36.
130. N.E. Breslow, J.B. Beckwith, Epidemiological features of Wilms' tumor: results of the National Wilms' Tumor Study, J. Natl. Cancer Inst. 68 (1982) 429–436.
131. P.B. Costello, M.L. Brecher, J.I. Starr, et al., A prospective analysis of the frequency, course, and possible prognostic significance of the joint manifestations of childhood leukemia, J. Rheumatol. 10 (1983) 753–757.
132. F.T. Saulsbury, H. Sabio, Acute leukemia presenting as arthritis in children, Clin. Pediatr. (Phila.) 24 (1985) 625–628.
133. G. Jean-Baptiste, K. De Ceulaer, Osteoarticular disorders of haematological origin, Baillieres. Best Pract. Res. Clin. Rheumatol. 14 (2000) 307–323.
135. D.J. Gallagher, D.J. Phillips, S.D. Heinrich, Orthopedic manifestations of acute pediatric leukemia, Orthop. Clin. North Am. 27 (1996) 635–644.
136. A. Krishnan, A. Shirkhoda, J. Tehranzadeh, et al., Primary bone lymphoma: radiographic-MR imaging correlation, Radiographics 23 (2003) 1371–1383.
137. M. Martinez-Lavin, Hypertrophic osteoarthropathy, Curr. Opin. Rheumatol. 9 (1997) 83–86.
138. D.J. Roebuck, Skeletal complications in pediatric oncology patients, Radiographics 19 (1999) 873–885.
139. C.A. Stuart, M.S. Driscoll, K.F. Lundquist, et al., Acanthosis nigricans, J. Basic Clin. Physiol. Pharmacol. 9 (1998) 407–418.
140. J.S. Baird, J.L. Johnson, D. Elliott-Mills, et al., Systemic lupus erythematosus with acanthosis nigricans, hyperpigmentation, and insulin receptor antibody, Lupus 6 (1997) 275–278.

Entire reference list is available online at www.expertconsult.com.

Chapter 47

NONINFLAMMATORY MUSCULOSKELETAL PAIN CONDITIONS

Claire LeBlanc and Kristin Houghton

Musculoskeletal pain of noninflammatory origin is common in childhood and is a frequent cause of referral to pediatric rheumatologists, orthopedic surgeons, sports medicine specialists, and primary care physicians. Noninflammatory causes of pain are much more common than inflammatory ones, and early identification and differentiation from other causes of musculoskeletal pain, such as infection or malignancy, are essential to institute appropriate therapy and to avoid inappropriate investigations. Children and adolescents with inflammatory arthritis may develop mechanical pain secondary to muscle tendon imbalances exaggerated by anatomical alignment, neuromuscular or proprioceptive deficits, rapid growth, or change in activity level.

PAIN ASSOCIATED WITH HYPERMOBILITY

Generalized Hypermobility

The term benign joint hypermobility syndrome (BJHS) is applied to children with musculoskeletal pain associated with generalized hypermobility of the joints (or "double-jointedness") without any associated congenital syndrome or abnormality of connective tissue.[1-3] The criteria for hypermobility have evolved over the years, and currently most authors use either the nine-point Beighton scale or the modified criteria of Carter and Wilkinson (Table 47–1).[4,5] Beighton criteria for BJHS in particular have shown good reproducibility.[6] Estimates of the frequency of hypermobility range from 8% to 20% in white populations; Chinese, Arabic, Negroid, and Inuits have a much higher prevalence of hypermobility. Children ages 3- to 10-years-old are most strongly affected, because hypermobility decreases with age.[7-11] Girls are hypermobile about twice as often as boys are. Ballet dancers and musicians also appear to be affected.[12] A family history of hypermobility is common. Although many children fulfill the criteria for benign hypermobility, having widespread joint laxity, many more children are lax at only a few joints.[13] The cause of pain in hypermobile children with no evidence of structural joint damage is not clear. Altered proprioception or a disturbance in the autonomic nervous system may be factors leading to poor biomechanical loading and microtrauma in hypermobile knee joints.[14,15]

Hypermobility is frequently associated with intermittent pains following physical activities. Although there does not appear to be any correlation between hypermobility and low back pain in school children, it is correlated with adult back pain. It is not linked to progression of idiopathic scoliosis or spondylolisthesis.[15,16] Temporomandibular joint dysfunction may be a consequence of hypermobility.[17-19] Children with benign hypermobility are rarely disabled by the pain, although some evidence suggests it is associated with recurrent pain and fibromyalgia.[7,20-23] Mild joint effusions may be observed.[24] There does not appear to be a greater prevalence of joint dislocation among hypermobile youth, but more frequent ankle sprains have been reported.[25] Patients with patellofemoral pain (PFP) are more likely hypermobile than are control patients.[26]

Table 47–1

Criteria for hypermobility

Modified Criteria of Carter and Wilkinson

Three of five are required to establish a diagnosis of hypermobility:

  Touch thumb to volar forearm

  Hyperextend metacarpophalangeal joints so fingers parallel forearm

  >10° hyperextension of elbows

  >10° hyperextension of knees

Touch palms to floor with knees straight

Beighton Scale[†]

  ≥6 points defines hypermobility:

  Touch thumb to volar forearm (one point each for right and left)

  Extend fifth metacarpophalangeal joint to 90° (one point each for right and left)

  >10° hyperextension of elbow (one point each for right and left)

  >10° hyperextension of knee (one point each for right and left)

  Touch palms to floor with knees straight (one point)

Other noncriteria features of many children with hypermobility:

  Put heel behind head

  Excessive internal rotation to hip

  Excessive ankle dorsiflexion

  Excessive eversion of the foot

  Passively touch elbows behind the back

Carter C, Wilkinson J: Persistent joint laxity and congenital dislocation of the hip, *J Bone Joint Surg Br* 46:40-45, 1964.
[†]Beighton P, Solomon L, Soskolne C: Articular mobility in an African population, *Ann Rheum Dis* 32:413-418, 1973.

Although hypermobility is generally innocuous, several less benign associated syndromes are listed in Table 47–2; in most of these, it is immediately apparent that the child does not have straightforward BJHS, but conditions such as Marfan or Stickler syndrome can be overlooked if they are not specifically considered. Infants with hypermobility/floppiness often have delayed development of major motor skills, and this may lead to unnecessary anxiety and physiotherapy.[27,28] Joint pain, if not identified as related to hypermobility, may also lead to unnecessary laboratory investigations and treatments in a mistaken belief that the pains are rheumatic in origin.[29] Some studies suggest an association with skin extensibility and broad scar formation.[30,31] A benign bleeding tendency has been reported in children with hypermobile thumbs.[32] Both bladder and bowel problems due to "nonneurogenic sphincter dysfunction" may be more common in children with hypermobility.[33] Marfanoid habitus and eyelid laxity have not been consistently demonstrated in children with hypermobility.[12] Children with BJHS do not seem to be at an increased risk for aortic dilatation or mitral valve prolapse.[34-36] Premature osteoarthritis has been suggested due to hypermobility, but the evidence is not convincing.[37] Attempts to determine whether benign hypermobility is a risk factor for later joint disease may be confounded in cross-sectional studies by the fact that hypermobility in late adult life appears to be a marker of fitness,

with flexible older adults having less osteoarthritis and osteopenia.[38]

Treatment

Reassurance is the initial treatment of hypermobility. Supportive footwear is helpful for many. Some children benefit from a postactivity or evening dose of acetaminophen or a nonsteroidal antiinflammatory drug (NSAID). Older, more severely affected children may be helped by formal physical therapy that focuses on reestablishment of normal muscle power and overall reconditioning. Taping or bracing of troublesome joints and the use of orthotics may be beneficial.[39,40] Although hypermobility may enable a child to be a good gymnast or ballet dancer, injuries may be more frequent.[41-43] Currently, there is no scientific evidence to advise against specific vocational and sport selection.[12] Children who "crack their knuckles" are frequently hypermobile. Parents are often concerned that this activity might lead to joint damage, but it is probably not a cause of later osteoarthritis.[44]

Pes Planus

The flexible flat foot is normal in infants and the development of the arch is part of normal growth.[45] In children, particularly those with hypermobility, the arch may exist only when they are toe standing or lying but disappears on weight-bearing. The reported prevalence in young children (40% to 70%) is high but decreases with age. Boys and obese children are more commonly affected.[46] A patient with flat feet and hindfoot valgus is shown in Fig. 47–1.

Usually flexible flat feet are not a cause of significant discomfort. A study in adults found no relationship between pain scores and arch configuration.[47] Foot pain from weight-bearing on the talar head may occur in adolescents with a short Achilles tendon and hypermobile flat feet, but this is rare.[48,49] Pes planus (and pes cavus) in the athlete may be associated with discomfort and, more commonly, an overuse injury. A correlation between moderate-severe pes planus and low back pain or anterior knee pain has been reported.[50,51] However, neither pes planus nor pes cavus has been shown to be a significant predictor of injury in army recruits,[52] and one study reported fewer stress fractures in those with low arches.[53] Pes planus does not appear to impair athletic performance.[54]

Treatment is controversial. Wenger and associates[55] reported a prospective randomized trial of 98 children with flat feet who received no treatment or corrective orthopedic shoes, a Helfet heel-cup, or a custom-molded plastic insert. There was significant improvement in most children, irrespective of treatment group. Orthotic devices that involve only the hindfoot do not reduce the mediolateral ground forces in adults with pes planus.[56] Aggressive heel cord stretching and shoe modification may be initiated followed by a soft foot orthosis if needed.[49] Surgery to lengthen the heel cord is indicated only in the extreme cases in skeletally mature adolescents.[49,57]

In contrast to the mobile flat foot, a rigid flat foot is always pathological. This is defined by reduced range of motion of the tarsal and subtalar joints and a longitudinal arch that does not increase with toe raising. It may result from a tarsal coalition in which a fibrous bony connection

Table 47–2

Selected conditions associated with hypermobility

Marfan Syndrome
Tall and thin
Arm span greater than height
Lower ratio of upper-body segment to lower-body segment (long legs); normal ratio is 0.85 in whites and 0.92 in blacks
Arachnodactyly
Pectus excavatum or carinatum
Kyphoscoliosis
Dislocation of the lens of the eye
Aortic root dilatation
Heart murmurs, midsystolic click
Hernias
Autosomal dominant disorder due to mutations of fibrillin gene on chromosome 15

Homocystinuria
Marfanoid habitus
Major risk of thrombotic events
Autosomal recessive disorder usually associated with cystathionine β-synthase deficiency due to mutations of gene on long arm of chromosome 21

Stickler Syndrome
Marfanoid habitus
Typical facial appearance: malar hypoplasia, depressed nasal bridge, epicanthal folds, micrognathia
Cleft palate (Pierre Robin sequence)
Severe myopia (may lead to retinal detachment)
Sensorineural hearing loss
Mitral valve prolapse
Autosomal dominant disorder due to mutations of type II collagen gene on chromosome 12

Ehlers-Danlos Syndromes
Skin abnormalities: thin, hyperelastic, cigarette paper scars, easy bruising
Dislocation of joints
Rarely, artery aneurysms; hollow organ rupture
Heterogeneous conditions; at least nine types with different inheritance patterns

Osteogenesis Imperfecta
Blue sclerae
Fragile bones with multiple fractures and deformities
Short stature
Spinal deformity
Different types; usually autosomal dominant inheritance
Involves abnormalities of type I collagen

Williams Syndrome
Short stature
Characteristic elfin facial appearance
Hoarse voice
Friendly and loquacious
Developmental delay
Supravalvular stenosis
Occasionally hypercalcemia
Initially hypermobile but later become hypomobile without pain
Sporadic and inherited cases due to deletion of elastin allele on chromosome 7

Down Syndrome (Trisomy 21)
Hypotonia
Developmental delay
Characteristic facial appearance; epicanthal folds
Short stature
Endocardial cushion defects
Broad hands with simian creases
Brushfield (depigmented) spots of the iris
Usually inherited in a sporadic fashion

For further details about these conditions, the reader is referred to Jones KL: *Smith's recognizable patterns of human malformation,* ed 5, Philadelphia, 1997, Saunders. and Beighton P: *McKusick's heritable disorders of connective tissue,* ed 5, St. Louis, 1993, Mosby.

between two or more tarsal bones is present at birth (Fig. 47–2). It occurs in 1% of the population, affects boys twice as often as girls, and is often bilateral.[58,59] There is often a family history of this condition. Calcaneonavicular and talocalcaneal coalitions are most common. Pain and symptom onset usually occurs at the time of ossification: 8- to 12-years-old for calcaneonavicular and 12- to 16-years-old for talocalcaneal coalitions.[60] Children may report midfoot pain after repetitive running and jumping and frequent "ankle sprains." Clinically, there is restricted and possibly painful subtalar range of motion. Radiographs (oblique and axial views) may show calcaneonavicular coalitions but computerized tomography (CT) or magnetic resonance imaging (MRI) is needed for fibrous or cartilaginous coalition and other tarsal coalitions (see Fig. 47–2).[61] Children with symptomatic coalitions require orthopedic assessment for casting and/or orthoses, physiotherapy, and possible surgical excision of the bony bar.[59]

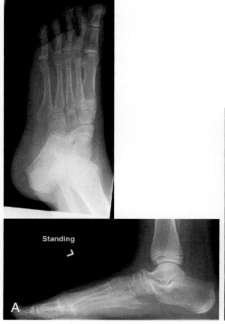

FIGURE 47–1   Pes Planus with hindfoot valgus.

Genu Recurvatum

Genu recurvatum, like pes planus, may be part of a generalized hypermobility syndrome or may occur as an isolated phenomenon. Symptoms are worse with standing or walking and are relieved by rest. Athletes may have particular difficulty.[62] Symptomatic genu recurvatum occurs most commonly in adolescent girls and is associated with popliteal pain and an increased incidence of anterior cruciate ligament injury.[62-64] Obese children are also more likely to be affected and suffer lower extremity pain.[65] Treatment includes orthotic correction of biomechanical faults, improving knee proprioception, muscle control (especially quadriceps strength) and gait, and maintaining good knee alignment during functional activities.[63,64]

PAIN ASSOCIATED WITH HYPOMOBILITY

Symptomatic generalized hypomobility is a relatively newly described entity consisting of decreased ranges of joint motion and pain in periarticular tissue probably caused by an increased stiffness in joint ligaments.[66] Exercise-induced lower extremity pain and habitual toe walking are typically associated with the hypomobility, and boys appear to be more frequently affected. Although familial hypomobility has been described, prevalence data are not yet available. This condition may be caused by changes in collagen metabolism, perhaps because of greater hydroxylation of lysine residues in collagen telopeptides due to an upregulation of telopeptice lysyl hydroxylase.[66] There are other relatively uncommon disorders, including hyalinosis and familial fibrosing serositis,[67,68] where pain may relate to very stiff joints (Table 47–3). Most children with marked stiffness/contractures due to conditions, such as arthrogryposis, Williams syndrome, and cerebral palsy,

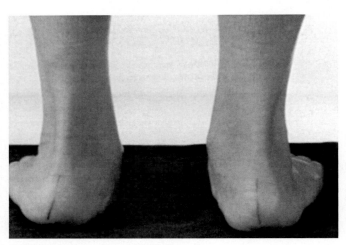

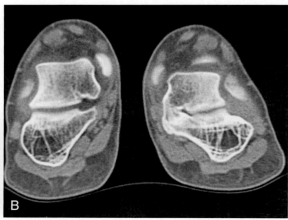

FIGURE 47–2   A, Standing lateral images of the left foot together with oblique images in this 10-year-old with left flat foot clinically. Alignment of mid and hind feet looks normal. There is, however, evidence of calcaneal-navicular coalition on the left associated with both talar and calcaneal beaking. (Courtesy of Dr. R. Cairns.) **B,** Computerized tomography illustrates the bony bridge between the calcaneus and talus on the right side. The left hindfoot is normal. This feature may not be detectable on plain radiographs. (Courtesy of Dr. R Cairns.)

Table 47–3

Selected conditions associated with hypomobility and joint contractures

Diabetes mellitus (diabetic cheiroarthropathy)
  Tightening of skin and soft tissues of fingers
  Short stature
Scleroderma and sclerodermalike conditions
Mucopolysaccharidoses and mucolipidoses with dysostosis multiplex
Autosomal recessive inheritance (except in Hunter syndrome, which is X-linked)
Hyalinosis
Familial fibrosing serositis
  Progressive contractures of fingers and toes
  Fibrosing pleuritis and constrictive pericarditis
  Probably autosomal recessive inheritance
Camptodactyly syndromes (several familial conditions including Blau syndrome)
Flexion contractures of fingers
Beals contractural arachnodactyly syndrome
  Marfanoid features
  Crumpled ears
  Cardiac abnormalities unusual
  Linked to fibrillinlike gene on chromosome 5 (autosomal dominant inheritance)
Winchester syndrome
  Multicentric osteolysis particularly of fingers, starting in infancy
  Autosomal recessive inheritance

For further details about the inherited conditions listed here, the reader is referred to Jones KL: *Smith's recognizable patterns of human malformation,* ed 5, Philadelphia, 1997, Saunders, and Beighton P: *McKusick's heritable disorders of connective tissue,* ed 5, St. Louis, 1993, Mosby.

do not seem to have arthralgias, so careful evaluation for other explanations for pain needs to be undertaken.

COMMON OVERUSE INJURIES

Soft Tissue Stress Injuries (Tenosynovitis, Tendinopathies, Muscle Strains)

Repetitive microtrauma can cause soft tissue and bone injuries. Muscle injuries include contusions, strains, tendinopathy, and complete rupture. Adolescents usually present with localized pain, which is aggravated by activity. Hamstring and quadriceps muscles are commonly affected in active young people, especially during the adolescent growth spurt when skeletal growth is greater than that of the muscle-tendon-unit. Avulsion injuries must always be considered in skeletally immature adolescents. On examination, there may be tenderness at the muscle attachment, musculotendinous junction, or in the muscle belly; swelling or ecchymoses; pain with passive stretch; and with resisted strength testing. Management includes rest, ice, compression, activity modification, and physiotherapy.

Although tenosynovitis commonly accompanies rheumatic disease, it can also occur because of unaccustomed repetitive movement, especially around the ankle (Achilles, tibialis anterior, and posterior tendons) or as stenosing tenosynovitis of the abductor pollicis longus or extensor pollicis brevis (de Quervain disease) at the wrists. There is often a history of increased activity or participation in a new sport.

The most common overuse tendinopathies involve the medial and lateral elbow epicondyles, patellar tendon, Achilles tendon, and rotator cuff. Adolescents with tendinopathy usually present with the insidious onset of localized pain coincident with increased activity. Pain initially occurs only at the initiation of activity but progresses to be present throughout activity and even at rest. The chronicity of symptoms suggests a degenerative, rather than inflammatory, process, and the term tendinopathy or tendinosis is preferred.[69] Management includes rest, ice, short term NSAIDs, eccentric strengthening and tendon sheath injection of corticosteroid in the acute phase. Extracorporeal shock wave therapy is of proven benefit for some chronic tendinopathies.[70]

Lower Extremity

Patellofemoral Pain Syndrome

PFP syndrome is a nonspecific descriptive term used to describe pain in and around the patella. Previous literature interchanged the term "chondromalacia patella" with anterior knee pain, but this term is now out of favor; chondromalacia patella is a surgical finding, not a diagnosis.

PFP affects active and nonactive children, is more common in girls, and is most common during the adolescent growth spurt (Table 47–4). Symptoms usually affect both knees with one side more suggestive than the other side. The etiology of PFP is unclear. There are currently two main theories: malalignment of the patella relative to the femoral trochlea with resultant articular cartilage abnormalities, and excessive mechanical loading.[71,72] Malalignment of the lower extremity influences patellar tracking and may include genu valgum, genu varum, genu recurvatum, leg length discrepancy, femoral anteversion, external tibial torsion, lateral displacement of the tibial tubercle, and excessive pronation of the subtalar joint.[72] Soft tissue tightness is common during the adolescent growth spurt with resultant inflexibilities (quadriceps, hamstrings, tensor fasciae latae, gastrosoleus complex) augmenting patellofemoral joint pain. Acute trauma, repetitive microtrauma/overuse, and malalignment may all lead to increased strain on the peripatellar soft tissues or increased patellofemoral joint stress.

The most common presenting complaint is dull, achy peripatellar or retropatellar pain and stiffness during and after activity, and after prolonged sitting with the knee in flexion ("theatre sign"). Aggravating factors include weight-bearing sport, stair use (descending worse than ascending), and squatting. Swelling is unusual. True instability does not occur, but patients often report "giving way" due to pain-related reflex inhibition of the quadriceps muscle or deconditioning. On examination, vastus medialis (VMO) wasting may be marked. There may be an increased Q-angle (angle formed between the line joining anterior superior iliac spine and center of the patella and the latter and tibial tuberosity), but its

Table 47–4	
Patellofemoral pain syndromes	
Age at onset	Adolescence to young adulthood
Sex ratio	Girls > boys
Symptoms	Insidious onset of activity related knee pain, difficulty descending stairs and squatting, need to sit with legs straight ("theatre sign")
Signs	VMO atrophy, patellar facet tenderness, positive quadriceps setting/grind and patellar compression tests, lateral tracking of patella. Weakness of the quadriceps, hip external rotators and abductors, and trunk muscles.

Table 47–5	
Mediopatellar plica syndrome	
Age at onset	Adolescence
Symptoms	Medial knee pain increased with activity, intermittent snapping, catching, giving way and locking.
Signs	Medial patellar retinaculum and anteromedial joint line tenderness, medial palpable band
MRI	Thickened synovial plica, occasional synovitis, changes in articular surface, and reactive changes in subchondral bone.

significance has been debated.[73] There may be superolateral or inferomedial retinacular or patellar facet tenderness. The lateral soft tissue patellar restraints are often tight with decreased passive medial patellar glide. A painful quadriceps setting/grind test (suprapatellar resistance while the patient performs isometrical quadriceps contraction with knee in full extension), and patellar compression test (direct compression of the patella into the trochlea) are diagnostic. There may be weakness of the quadriceps, hip external rotators and abductors, and trunk muscles.

Treatment

Reassurance and education are important components of therapy. Activity modification; cryotherapy; short-term NSAID therapy; flexibility exercises (hamstrings, quadriceps, iliotibial band (ITB), lateral retinaculum, gastrocnemius); and strengthening of the quadriceps (VMO), hip external rotators, abductors, and hamstrings are important. Patellar tracking exercises, patellofemoral orthoses or patellar taping, and shoe orthoses (subtalar pronation) are also proscribed. Gradual improvement and resolution of symptoms is the rule.

Patellofemoral Instability

Patellofemoral instability is due to lateral tracking of the patella in the femoral groove during knee flexion and extension. Children may complain of anterior knee pain, episodic giving way, and catching sensations associated with recurrent effusions. Dislocation results in an inability to straighten the leg with the knee held in a position of 20 to 30 degrees of flexion. Predisposing factors include hypermobility, patella alta, unifaceted or bipartite patella, shallow intercondylar groove, lateral attachment of the patellar ligament, and lower extremity malalignment.[74] On examination, findings are similar to PFP. The patellar apprehension test (contraction of the quadriceps muscle when the examiner attempts to displace the patella laterally) or frank lateral dislocation may be elicited. Treatment is the same as for PFP. Patellofemoral orthoses (stabilization braces) may prevent recurrent episodes of instability. Orthopedic referral and possible surgical management is recommended for acute and recurrent patellar dislocation.[74]

Synovial Plica

The knee has normal synovial folds that are residual embryonic remnants persisting from when the knee cavity was a septated structure. Occasionally, pathological conditions occur within the medial and lateral plica(e) due to local synovitis caused by acute, direct, or repetitive microtrauma. Rarely the membranes do not involute at all, leaving a complete septum. A nonperforated septum can result in unusual swelling that may mimic a soft tissue tumor.[75]

Synovial plica and its relationship to knee pain are controversial. This entity should be considered in those with PFP who do not respond to standard management. The mediopatellar plica syndrome is most common presenting with medial knee pain, patellar snapping, and catching during flexion (Table 47–5). Tenderness of the medial patellar retinaculum or anteromedial joint line may be found. The plica may be palpable as a tender thickened band when pressed against the edge of the condyle. MRI may show a thickened synovial plica occasionally accompanied by synovitis, changes in the patello-femoral articular surface, and reactive changes in the subchondral bone. Management includes patellar mobilization and massage; hamstrings, quadriceps, and gastrocnemius flexibility exercises; and NSAIDs with surgical removal of the plica reserved for recalcitrant symptoms.

Fat Pad Irritation/Impingement ("Hoffa Syndrome")

The infrapatellar fat pad is richly innervated, and injury may cause anterior knee pain. Impingement of the infrapatellar fat pad between the patella and the femoral condyle may be secondary to direct trauma or acute hyperextension injury. Chronic irritation may be associated with patellar tendinopathy, PFP, or recurrent synovitis. Pain is often present with knee extension, prolonged standing, and kneeling. On examination there is localized tenderness and swelling in the fat pad with posterior displacement of the inferior pole of the patella. Squatting, active extension of the knee or passive pressure into extension may reproduce pain. Associated predisposing biomechanical factors include genu recurvatum and anterior tilting of the pelvis. Treatment comprises local cryotherapy, taping the patella to reduce the amount of tilt and impingement, local muscle flexibility and strengthening exercises, and correcting lower limb biomechanics as in PFP. Surgery is usually not necessary.

Patellar Tendinopathy

"Jumper's knee" or patellar tendinopathy is a common cause of infrapatellar pain in skeletally mature individuals. Maximum discomfort is usually at the inferior patellar pole at the site of the proximal patellar tendon attachment, and is aggravated by jumping. On examination there is tenderness over the proximal patellar tendon; thickening or nodules may be palpable. There may be secondary PFP. Treatment requires load reduction (activity modification, biomechanical correction), cryotherapy, transfriction massage, and progressive eccentric strengthening.[76] Tenderness of quadriceps tendon attachment to the superior margin of the patella may also occur but is uncommon unless associated with underlying osteochondrosis. In skeletally immature children and adolescents the osteochondroses/traction apophysitis Osgood-Schlatter (OSD) and Sinding-Larsen-Johansson (SLJD) disease present similarly, but tenderness is at the tibial tuberosity and inferior patellar pole respectively. (See section on osteochondroses).

Iliotibial Band Syndrome

The ITB emanates from the tensor fasciae latae, gluteus medius and maximus muscles and extends laterally down the leg as a tight band of fascial tissue before attaching at Gerdy tubercle, which is just lateral to the tibial tubercle. The ITB slides anteriorly and posteriorly over the lateral femoral condyle as the knee moves from extension into flexion. Such repetitive movement may cause painless snapping, or pain and tenderness of an ITB bursa at the lateral knee. Occasionally adolescents localize pain proximally at the greater trochanter and may have an associated trochanteric bursitis. This condition is common in runners, especially those who have recently increased their distances, run downhill, or run on cambered roads. Risk factors include anatomical factors (genu varum, prominent lateral femoral condyle, subtalar pronation, internal tibial torsion), hip abductor weakness, and increased activity.[77-79] On examination, pain and snapping can often be reproduced by palpating over the lateral femoral condyle with passive movement of the knee through a 20 to 30 degree arc of flexion. ITB is often tight with a positive Ober test. Imaging is not usually necessary; ultrasound and MRI can confirm the diagnoses in difficult cases.[80] Management includes modified activity with relative rest, cryotherapy, ice, stretching of the ITB, physiotherapy emphasizing gluteal flexibility and strengthening, and, in refractory cases, surgical intervention may be required.

Apophysitis and Apophyseal Avulsion Injuries

Apophyseal injuries are common in young athletes, affect boys more often than girls, and are usually secondary to forceful or repetitive traction of the attached muscle. The apophyses of the pelvis appear and fuse later than physes in long bones. The physes are the weakest structures of the immature skeleton, placing adolescents at increased risk of apophyseal injury, especially during a "growth spurt". Adolescents have tight soft tissues during rapid growth, placing additional stress on the apophyses. Apophysitis

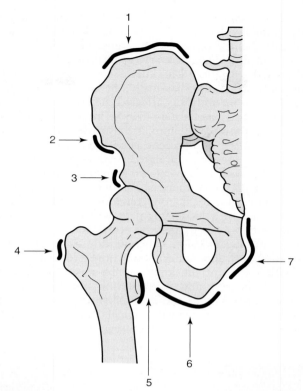

FIGURE 47–3 Hip and pelvis anatomy. 1 = Iliac crest (abdominal muscle attachment), 2 = Anterior superior iliac spine (sartorius attachment), 3 = Anterior inferior iliac spine (rectus femoris attachment), 4 = Greater trochanter (gluteal attachment), 5 = Lesser trochanter (psoas attachment), 6 = Ischial tuberosity (hamstring attachment), 7 = Pubic symphysis and inferior pubis ramus (gracilis and adductor attachments)

refers to an overuse stress injury at the insertion site of major abdominal and hip muscles around the pelvis. Adolescents usually present with dull, activity related pain. Radiographs are generally normal or show widening of the affected apophyses. Management includes rest, ice, modified activity, and physiotherapy. Most adolescents are able to return to sport within four to eight weeks.

Apophyseal avulsion fractures occur with sudden forceful muscle-tendon contraction. Common sites of avulsions are at the iliac crest (abdominal muscles), anterior superior iliac spine (sartorius), anterior inferior iliac spine (rectus femoris), ischial tuberosity (hamstrings), and lesser trochanter (iliopsoas) (Fig. 47–3). Adolescents usually present with localized pain, swelling, and reduced range of motion. Pain on resisted contractions of involved muscles, where hip joint motion is restricted, confirms pain is extrinsic to the hip joint. Radiographs demonstrate displacement of the apophyseal center, callus formation, and bony reaction. MRI is useful in suspected avulsion injuries with normal radiographs.[81] Management is usually nonoperative and includes rest, ice, modified activity, and physiotherapy. Most adolescents are able to return to sport within four to eight weeks.

Osteochondritis Dissecans

Osteochondritis dissecans (OCD) is an idiopathic lesion of bone and cartilage, resulting in bone necrosis and loss of continuity with subchondral bone. There may be partial or complete separation of articular cartilage with or without involvement of subchondral bone. Proposed etiologies include acute trauma, repetitive microtrauma, vascular insufficiency, primary ossification defect, or normal growth variant.[82] The knee (75% of cases) is most commonly affected.[83] Classically, the lateral aspect of the medial femoral condyle is affected, but the lateral femoral condyle and patella may also be involved. The ankle (talus) and elbow (capitellum) are also affected. OCD may be asymptomatic and present as an incidental finding on radiographs done for unrelated reasons, or adolescents may present with activity related pain and swelling. Locking may be present if there is instability of the fragment. On examination, focal bony tenderness, joint effusion, and evidence of a loose fragment with extension block or palpable loose body may be noted. Radiographs may show a radiolucent lesion, subchondral fracture, potential separation with subchondral bone, and a loose body.[82]

OCD lesions of the knee can be missed on routine nonweight-bearing anterior/posterior and lateral radiographs; tunnel (notch) and axial (skyline patellar profile) views are required to view the articular surfaces of the distal femoral condyles and patella (Fig. 47–4).[84] MRI may

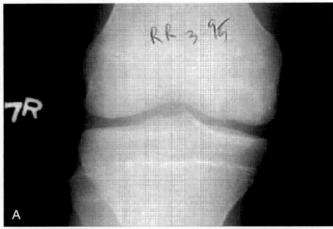

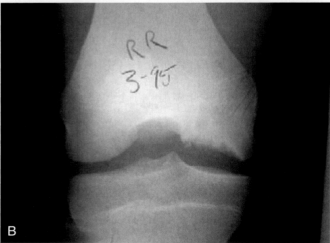

FIGURE 47–4 A, Anterior posterior radiograph shows minimal cystic changes affecting the lateral condyle. **B,** Tunnel or notch views show the cystic changes more clearly. (Redrawn from Wall E, Von Stein D: Juvenile osteochondritis dissecans, *Orthop Clin North Am* 34:341-353, 2003.

show cartilage changes earlier with contrast enhancement of intact cartilage lesions.[85] Staging of lesions has been done based on radiographic,[86] MRI,[87] and arthroscopic[88] appearance. The Berndt and Harty classification characterizes OCD lesions based on radiographical appearance.[86] Stage I reflects small areas of compression, Stage II lesions are separate fragments, Stage III includes detached hinged fragments, and Stage IV lesions are loose bodies.[86] Treatment depends on the site and stage of the lesion and the skeletal maturity of the patient with early lesions in skeletally immature patients having the best prognosis.[85] Conservative treatment is generally reserved for stable, nondetached, smaller lesions in children with open physes. This includes protective weight-bearing, immobilization, cryotherapy, NSAIDs, and up to six to 18 months of rehabilitation.[89] Surgical treatment is reserved for those who fail conservative measures and for those with symptomatic stable lesions, closed physes or approaching skeletal maturity, large lesions, detached unstable lesions, or loose bodies. Surgical options include "microfracture" (subchondral drilling), debridement and fragment excision, fragment fixation with screws, biodegradable pins, autologous bone sticks and osteochondral plugs, osteochondral autologous transplantation, and autologous chondrocyte implantation.[89]

Shin Splints (Posteromedial Tibial Stress Syndrome)

Activity related pain and tenderness along the posteromedial border of the tibia is often referred to as "shin splints" or periostitis. Posteromedial tibial stress syndrome is an apt anatomical description of the periostitis and fascitis caused by repetitive traction at the origins of the muscle fascial attachments along the middle and distal posterior medial tibia. Adolescents usually complain of shin pain at onset and towards the end of weight-bearing activity that resolves with rest. Alignment (hindfoot pronation), relative inflexibility (tight gastrosoleus complex), recent increase in activity levels, and change in footwear may be contributing factors.[90] Physical examination demonstrates generalized tibial boney tenderness. Radiographs are normal and radionuclide bone scans show diffuse increased uptake classically at the junction of the middle and distal one third of the posteromedial tibia. The differential diagnoses include stress fracture and posterior compartment syndrome. Management includes rest, ice, modified activity, improving gastrosoleus and posterior tibialis strength and flexibility, change in footwear or orthotic, and correction of any training errors.

Stress Fractures

Stress fracture occurs when normal stress is applied to abnormal bone or abnormal stress is applied to normal bone and represents a disturbance between bone resorption and bone regeneration. In the case of normal bones, it is believed to be a fatigue fracture or overuse injury. They are more common in youth who report a recent increase in activity, poor nutrition, and females with amenorrhea.[91] The distal to middle third of the tibia is the most common site. The second and third metatarsals are commonly injured in older adolescents and adults (runners, dancers) and represent the classic "March

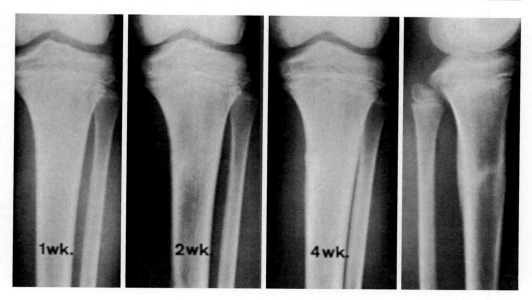

FIGURE 47-5 Serial radiographs document the evolution of a stress fracture in a 10-year-old girl. Two weeks after the onset of leg pain, the fracture line is evident. After four weeks, the fracture callus is seen. (Courtesy of Dr. RN Hensinger.)

fracture" seen in the military.[92] Several site specific stress fractures are high risk for nonunion, complete fracture, or avascular necrosis (AVN), including the proximal fifth metatarsal, tarsal navicular, scaphoid, and femoral neck. Pediatric stress fractures usually present with progressively worsening pain, aggravated by weight-bearing activity and relieved with rest. Some patients report pain at rest or even at night. There may be associated swelling. On examination, the fracture site is tender to palpation. Early radiographs may be normal, and late radiographs detect callus formation (Fig. 47-5), physeal widening, or apophyseal fragmentation. Early lesions are best detected by MRI and radionucleotide bone scan.[93] CT is useful for evaluation of high risk stress fractures. Management depends on symptoms and the site of injury. Treatment includes activity modification and if required a short period of nonweight-bearing and immobilization. High risk stress fractures often require nonweight-bearing immobilization for six to eight weeks, or surgical intervention.[58,94]

Upper Extremity

Little League Shoulder

Overuse injuries of the shoulder are common in young athletes involved in throwing sports, tennis, and swimming. Little league shoulder is described as a stress fracture of the proximal humeral physis, which likely occurs because of poor throwing techniques and a greater susceptibility of the immature skeleton to injury. Significant rotational stresses and distraction forces on the physis may be etiological factors. Of these, excessive external rotation forces likely play a greater role in the deformation the proximal humeral cartilage.[95] The children usually present with pain in the lateral proximal humerus. Tenderness and swelling are noted over the anterior and lateral shoulder. Many have reduced internal rotation of the dominant shoulder, which may be due to contracture of the posterior inferior capsule, as seen in adult

throwers.[96] Radiographs demonstrate widening of the proximal humeral physis. Treatment is typically nonsurgical, consisting of relative rest from shoulder activity and rehabilitation focused on progressive stretching and strengthening of the rotator cuff. Prior to return to play, modification in throwing technique, intensity, and frequency needs to be addressed. Prevention is the key, and, for young baseball pitchers, Little League Baseball Inc., recommends an age-appropriate restriction in number of pitches per day and mandatory rest periods between pitching appearances.[97]

Tennis Elbow

Overuse of the arm related to excessive wrist extension can cause lateral elbow pain, which is commonly called "tennis elbow" or lateral epicondylitis. One percent to 3% of the general population are affected with peak prevalence at the ages of 40- to 60-years-old.[98] The pathological process consists of tendinosis of the extensor carpi radialis brevis tendon. Patients present with lateral elbow pain with maximal tenderness 1 to 2 cm distal to the lateral epicondyle. The discomfort is reproduced by resisted wrist extension, especially with the wrist pronated and radially deviated. Resisted extension of the middle finger is also painful. Although generally not required to confirm diagnosis, MRI demonstrates a thickened common extensor tendon with increased signal intensity.[99] Most cases are asymptomatic at one year, regardless of treatment. Relative rest, ice, massage, and short course NSAIDS followed by rehabilitative physical therapy may provide benefit. Resilient cases may improve with steroid injection,[100] nitric oxide patch,[101] acupuncture,[102] autologous blood injection,[103] and possibly botulinum toxin injection.[104] Surgery is rarely required. Prior to returning to sport, correction of inappropriate sport technique and equipment and the use of a counterforce brace are recommended.[105] Children are more likely to suffer a valgus compressive injury to the bony aspect of the lateral elbow. Recurrent injury can lead to Panner osteochondrosis, which usually affects children between the ages

5- and 11-years-old. The ossific nucleus becomes flattened and fragmented, but the condition resolves with no long-term sequelae.[106] OCDs of the capitellum is another possible sequelae; it may present with lateral elbow pain, swelling, and inadequate extension in older youth. Rest and immobilization can allow adequate healing, but surgery may be necessary. The key to the reduction of elbow pain in young throwing athletes is prevention. In baseball, limiting the number of pitches per day and avoiding more stressful throws (curveball or slider) until close to skeletal maturity is recommended.[107]

Golfer Elbow

Overuse of the arm may also result in medial elbow pain or "golfer elbow." This condition is less common than "tennis elbow" with a prevalence of 0.2% to 0.5% in the adult population.[98] This condition is due to a flexor/pronator tendinopathy in the skeletally mature. These individuals have localized tenderness at or below the medial epicondyle with pain on resisted wrist flexion and forearm pronation, especially when a passive stretch is placed on the tendon.[99] MRI may be useful to demonstrate a thickened or abnormally thin common flexor tendon with increased signal intensity.[99] Treatment is similar to tennis elbow, although careful application of ice or corticosteroid injection is important to avoid injury to the ulnar nerve.

Medial elbow pain is more common than lateral in skeletally immature throwing athletes. Repeated valgus stress to the medial epicondyle typically presents with local swelling and tenderness. Radiographs may be normal or show fragmentation and sometimes avulsion of the medial epicondyle. MRI may detect stress injury of the medial epicondyle apophysis before radiographical changes occur.[99] Treatment consists of rest until asymptomatic followed by gradual stretching and strengthening to regain full range of motion and power. Surgery is rarely necessary but is indicated for avulsions displaced greater than 5 mm. Prevention of this injury is key.[107]

Disorders of the Trunk

Chest Pain

Chest pain is a frequent complaint in the pediatric population. Rowe and coworkers reported that six of 1000 children's emergency department visits were for chest pain,[108] and these visits occurred with equal frequency in boys and girls. Of 366 patients, 28% were diagnosed with chest wall pain; only 1% had cardiac causes (Table 47–6). Precordial catch syndrome, previously known as Texidor twinge, is a very underrecognized condition in which there is a history of recurrent, well-localized, sharp chest wall pain of sudden onset lasting a few seconds to minutes, with negative findings on examination or laboratory testing.[109]

Costochondritis

Costochondritis is a poorly understood condition characterized by anterior chest wall pain. It is usually acute and stabbing, is often related to position or deep breathing, and is common in adolescents, constituting the reason for

Table 47–6

Causes of chest pain in children presenting to an emergency department

Category	%	Conditions Included
Chest wall	28	Costochondritis, Tietze syndrome, musculoskeletal pain, breast tenderness
Lung/pleura	19	Asthma, infection, embolism, pleurisy, pneumothorax
Trauma	15	Contusion, abrasion
Psychogenic	5	Depression, anxiety, conversion disorder, hyperventilation
Other	21	Esophagitis, gastritis, upper respiratory tract infection, constipation, cardiac causes
Unknown	12	Chest pain of undetermined cause

Adapted and reprinted from Rowe BH, Dulberg CS, Peterson RG et al: Characteristics of children presenting with chest pain to a pediatric emergency department, *Can Med Assoc J* 143:388, 1990, by permission of the publisher. Adapted from Brower AC: The osteochondroses, *Orthop Clin North Am* 14:99, 1983; Resnick D: The osteochondroses. In Resnick D, Niwayama G, editors: *Diagnosis of bone and joint disorders*, Philadelphia, 1981, Saunders; and other sources.

4% of outpatient visits.[110] It may be caused by repetitive trauma or idiopathic inflammation.[111] On examination, tenderness of one or more of the 2nd to 5th costal cartilages is noted without associated swelling, heat, or erythema. Restriction of the corresponding costovertebral and costotransverse joints may be found.[112] Results of investigations (inflammatory markers or imaging) have been inconsistent to date. The syndrome can be self-limited or chronic and intermittent, but most resolve by one year. Local anesthetic injections, NSAIDS, acupuncture, mobilization/manipulation, and taping may provide symptomatic relief.[113,114]

Tietze Syndrome

This is also another benign condition of the anterior chest wall, but unlike costochondritis it is associated with swelling (not erythema or warmth) of the 2nd and 3rd costochondral junctions.[114] Etiology is unknown, but microtrauma and inflammation may play a role. Injury, septic arthritis, spondyloarthritis, and malignancies may present similarly and should be excluded.[113] Plain films are usually normal, but bone scan may demonstrate focal increased uptake, and CT may show sclerosis of the sternal manubrium. MRI reveals a spectrum of changes including enlarged and edematous cartilage and rapid contrast enhancement of subchondral bone.[115] Treatment consists of reassurance, analgesia, and for recalcitrant cases local corticosteroid injections.[116]

Slipping Rib Syndrome

This syndrome is believed to be due to hypermobility of the 8th to 12th (false) ribs and may be caused by direct trauma or repetitive trunk motion during certain sports.[113,117] These rib cartilages attach to each other by fibrous tissue, rather than directly to the sternum, such that interruption of this tissue permits a rib to impinge on the adjacent superior one. This causes a click and severe sharp chest or abdominal pain, which may be from intercostal nerve irritation, sprain of the costal cartilage, or strain of the intercostal muscle. Pain may fade over a few hours or persist as a lesser dull ache. Exacerbations occur with periodic resubluxations precipitated by vigorous physical activity, trauma, or coughing. Physical findings include tenderness of the affected ribs, worsening pain on direct pressure over these ribs, and asymmetry of rib position. The physician can reproduce symptoms by hooking fingers under the inferior margins of the affected ribs and pulling anteriorly "positive hooking maneuver" usually with an intercostal nerve block.[118,119] Radiological imaging does not confirm the diagnosis but helps to exclude other conditions.[114] Treatment consists of reassurance, avoidance of exacerbating movements, taping, manipulation, and injection of local anesthetic. In severe cases, excision of the anterior rib end and costal cartilage may be required.[120]

Back Pain

Back pain in the general pediatric population is common in developed countries. Studies from Denmark, Switzerland, and Iceland report 44% to 74% of teenagers had one episode of back pain, whereas 21% had weekly symptoms.[121,122,123] The incidence of low back pain in this age group ranges from 16% to 22%. It is more common in girls and rates rise with increasing age. One large cohort study suggested persistent low back pain in early adolescence is a strong predictor of similar symptoms in later life.[124] Most children have mild and self-limiting symptoms and, although they frequently report difficulty with some functional tasks, few miss school or sports participation.[125] The etiology of back pain in children is believed to be multifactorial. Although several papers reviewed by Trevelyan reported greater odds of low back pain in children with a positive parental history,[126] a large Finnish twin study suggested genetic factors play a minor role. They reported symptoms seemed to be related more to shared and unshared environmental factors.[127] Height of the child, trunk muscle weakness, body mass index, excess sedentary activity, and heavy backpacks do not appear to be associated with later onset of low back pain. Competitive sports activities are associated with greater risk of low back pain.[126] Evidence suggests children with back pain are more likely to report negative psychosocial experiences, and those with anxiety and depression are at greater risk of future onset back pain.[128,129]

Relatively little is known about the most effective way to treat idiopathic back pain in children. In one study, 47% attributed onset to a traumatic, sport-related event.[130] In a longitudinal study, more than 50% of children who reported back pain initially denied ever having had back pain when reinterviewed two years later, indicating that for many children back pain resolves spontaneously.[131] Regular physical activity may also be beneficial. In a recent Danish accelerometry study, 364 nine year olds were followed prospectively, and those with back pain at baseline that participated in high levels of physical activity were less likely to have back pain at the age of 12-years-old. Those with highest levels of physical activity were least likely to develop low back pain in follow-up.[132]

In contrast, back pain is a relatively infrequent reason for referral to a pediatric orthopedic surgeon,[133] accounting for 2% of consultations. Among those children seen because of low back pain, no specific cause could be found in almost half; Scheuermann disease was present in 15%, spondylolysis in 13%, infection in 8%, tumor, and disk prolapse in 6%.[133]

Lumbar Disk Herniation

Disk protrusion (primarily L4-5 or L5-S1) in adolescents only accounts for 1% to 4% of all herniations. Indeed of 1920 patients who underwent disk surgery, only 0.5% were children, and none was under the age of 12-years-old.[134] Family history of lumbar disk herniation is common. Boys may be more frequently affected than girls may be.[135-137] Low back pain with or without sciatica occurs after trauma or exertion in 50%, which may reflect a preexisting disk lesion.[138,139] Coughing, sneezing, and bending may aggravate the pain. Examination reveals limitation of forward bending, straight-leg raising, and, in 25%, weakness of the plantar flexors.[139] Diagnosis is confirmed by MRI or CT myelography, and careful inspection for apophyseal fracture is recommended in this age group, especially those with large or central herniations.[140] Conservative treatment with rest, analgesics, and physical therapy is successful in up to 80% of cases.[141] Operative therapy is indicated with persistent or progressive neurological deficit.[139,140,142] The success of surgery in adolescents is quite good.[136,137] However, in one study of 129 children younger than the age of 18-years-old, at a mean follow-up of 12.4-years-old, the outcome was excellent in only 40%, good in 47%, and poor in 13%, with reintervention required in 10%.[143]

Diskitis

Diskitis is a well-recognized entity in children under 10-years–old, usually affecting the disk space between the 3rd and 4th lumbar vertebrae. Pediatric referral centers report an incidence of about one to two cases per year. The pathological mechanism of diskitis is unclear with trauma, increased vascularity of the vertebrae, and infection all implicated.[144,145] Children may present with back pain, limp, neck stiffness, fever, irritability, and gastrointestinal upset. Toddlers often refuse to stand or sit. Tenderness on palpation of the spinous processes is infrequently found, and the complete blood count and inflammatory markers are normal or mildly elevated, hence diagnosis is often delayed four to six weeks.[146] Plain radiographs demonstrate disk space narrowing and irregular endplates of adjacent vertebrae by two to four weeks; bone scan shows increased focal uptake within one week of symptoms, but MRI is the investigation of choice as it detects early diskitis and can exclude spinal tumors.[142] Since many authors attribute the etiology to staphylococcal infection, antibiotic treatment is recommended, and only those who do not improve should undergo CT guided needle biopsy. The natural course of the disease is benign with the majority asymptomatic by three weeks. Chronic low back pain and spinal fusion may occur, hence ongoing follow-up is suggested.[147]

Calcific diskitis is a relatively uncommon childhood condition that presents with acute onset of neck pain, torticollis, and calcification of the cervical or thoracic intervertebral disks. The etiology is unclear, but interruption of a tenuous blood supply is suggested. Plain radiographs and MRI are usually diagnostic.[148]

Spondylolysis and Spondylolithesis

Spondylolysis is a defect in the pars interarticularis and most commonly affects the fifth (85% to 95%) and fourth (5% to 15%) lumbar vertebrae. The majority of cases of pediatric spondylolysis are isthmic and represent stress fracture.[149] Congenital dysplastic spondylolysis (defect in the orientation of the facets L5/S1) is usually a painless incidental radiographical finding. Spondylolysis is rare before the age of 5-years-old and usually affects athletic teenage boys. The cited incidence is 6% in adults and 8% to 15% in athletes.[149] There is a genetic predisposition to spondyloysis among certain ethnic groups with the prevalence among the Inuit in Northern Canada as high as 20% to 50%.[150] Spondylolysis is more commonly associated with participation in sports involving repetitive extension, flexion, and rotation, such as gymnastics, dance, and soccer. Both acute and overuse injuries occur, although overuse injuries are more common. Factors that increase lumbar lordosis (weak abdominal muscles, tight hip flexors, tight thoracolumbar fascia) may increase stress on the posterior elements of the spine. There is also an association between spina bifida occulta, and spondylolysis.[151]

Spondylolithesis occurs with bilateral pars defects and is defined by forward translation of one vertebra on the next caudal segment.[149] Spondylolithesis is graded based on the percentage of slip of one vertebral body on the vertebra below (grade 1 slip [0% to 25% slip], grade 2 [25% to 50%], grade 3 [50% to 75%] and grade 4 [>75%]).[152] Spondylolithesis is less common than spondylolysis, is more common in females, and typically occurs during the adolescent growth spurt. Progression of slip is rare after skeletal maturity.[152]

The usual presentation of spondylolysis and spondylolithesis is the insidious onset of extension related low back pain. Symptoms generally increase over months, and there may be radiation of pain to the buttocks and posterior thigh. If there are radicular symptoms of numbness and weakness, spondylolithesis and disk herniation need to be considered. On examination, there may be lumbar hyperlordosis, ipsilateral paraspinal muscle spasm, and tight hamstrings with posterior thigh pain on forward flexion. Discomfort is worsened by hyperextension of the spine and may localize to the affected side on single-leg extension. There is usually focal tenderness to palpation over the site of the pars lesion and may be a step-off at the lumboscaral junction with slip. Strength, sensation, and lower extremity reflexes are normal in most cases. Abnormal findings may be found with associated nerve root irritation. Radiographs (standing lateral, coned lateral of the lumbosacral junction, AP) are the first line of investigation (Fig. 47–6). The value of oblique views is debated.[153] A single-photon emission computerized tomography (SPECT) bone scan is more sensitive and identifies lesions with active bone turnover. CT scans are often used to confirm lesions and acuity.[154] The role of MRI is not yet clear with some studies citing a high rate

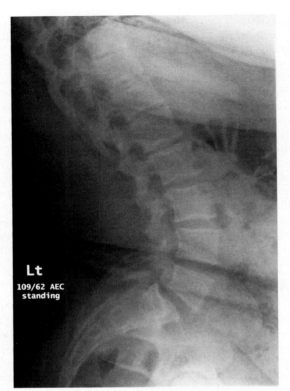

FIGURE 47–6 Spondylolysis of L5 is visible on this lateral radiograph. There is also Grade 1 spondylolisthesis with anterior slip of L5 on S1. Endplate changes are seen throughout the lumbar spine. (Courtesy of Dr. R. Cairns.)

of false positives and others showing good correlation with SPECT and CT.[154,155]

The goals of management are to achieve bony or fibrous union, relieve pain, optimize and restore function, and prevent or minimize the degree of spondylolisthesis. Initial management includes avoidance of activities that cause pain. Physiotherapy includes antilordotic exercises and strategies to improve abdominal and hip flexor strength and hamstring flexibility. The use of thoracolumbar orthoses (to limit extension and rotation) is variable and largely physician- and center-specific. There are no randomized controlled trials, but cohort studies show significant improvement with bracing.[156] Adolescents can return to sport (with or without a brace) when they are pain-free, usually within a few months. Standing lateral radiographs should be done at four to six month intervals until skeletal maturity to assess for progression of spondylolisthesis. Adolescents with greater than 50% slip (Grade 3 or 4) warrant orthopedic referral.

Scheuermann Disease

Scheuermann disease is the most common cause of (relatively) fixed kyphotic deformity in adolescence with an incidence of 0.4% to 10%. It is most frequently diagnosed between the ages of 12- and 15-years-old and has no gender preference.[157] The pathogenesis is unclear, but disorders in vertebral ossification or collagen aggregation, genetic factors, and biomechanical abnormalities may play a role. Most patients are asymptomatic and concerned about cosmetic appearance, but pain may be noted, especially in athletes with high demands on their back. The

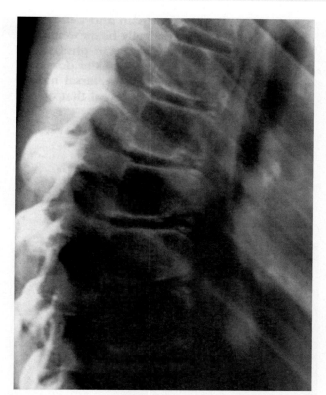

FIGURE 47–7 Lateral radiograph of the spine illustrating the abnormalities of the anterior margins of the vertebral bodies that are characteristic of Scheuermann disease and result in anterior wedging. (Courtesy of Dr R. Cairns.)

thoracic pattern with nonstructural hyperlordosis of the lumbar and cervical spine is the most common variant and is often associated with moderate scoliosis. The thoracolumbar form occurs infrequently, but patients experience more pain and restriction in exercise, which are more likely to progress into adulthood. Tightness of the pectoral and hamstring muscles has been noted.[106] Neurological deficits are rare, and cardiopulmonary insufficiency occurs only with severe curves measuring >100 degrees.[158] Classic standing lateral radiological features include anterior wedging of at least three adjacent vertebral bodies each by 5 or more degrees, end plate irregularities, loss of disk space height, and Schmorl nodes (Fig. 47–7).[159] Some investigators recommend radiographical criteria should include any thoracic kyphosis of at least 45 degrees associated with ≥1 vertebra wedged 5 degrees or more, while others suggest diagnosis depends on the rigidity of the kyphotic curve on lateral hyperextension spine films.[160]

Treatment should be selected on a case by case basis. For skeletally immature patients with a reducible curve of <65 degrees, treatment usually consists of simple analgesia, exercise, and, occasionally, the use of a back brace to prevent flexion. A review of three retrospective studies demonstrated brace treatment could improve the degree of kyphosis, but compliance is essential, since progressive worsening is noted out of the brace.[161] Overall, nonsurgical outcome is very good. Surgical intervention is rarely indicated (70 to 75 degrees kyphosis) but appears to be the best method to significantly correct this deformity. A 30 to 40 degree correction of the degree of kyphosis

is usually achieved postoperatively but tends to worsen by a few degrees over time.[161-163] There is no correlation between functional and radiographical outcome.[163] A cohort study of all 63 patients treated in a single institution by exercise and observation only, Milwaukee bracing, or surgical fusion using Harrington rods failed to find any statistical difference in quality of life, pain, function, or degree of curve after a mean of 14 years.[164] Patients with curves exceeding 70 degrees at follow-up had inferior function.

OSTEOCHONDROSES

Osteochondroses are unique to the growing skeleton and are believed to be due to AVN caused by repetitive stress and disruption of the vascular supply to bone. Articular sites are most common, but nonarticular and physeal osteochondroses also occur.[165,166] There are over 70 osteochondroses, and they have been named after individuals who first described them (Table 47–7).[167] The etiology is unclear and probably includes normal variants of development, stress injury, and vascular insufficiency.[168] The typical presentation is localized pain aggravated by exercise and/or swelling. With the exception of Freiberg disease (2nd and 3rd metatarsal), they are more common in boys than in girls. Onset of symptoms is related to skeletal maturity with girls usually presenting earlier than boys do. Kienbock disease is the only osteochondroses to occur after skeletal maturity. The natural history is usually resolution of symptoms over several months to two years. Some sites are associated with long-term problems secondary to bony incongruity and subsequent positional deformity or early degenerative osteoarthritis. Some of the more common osteochondroses are discussed.

Osgood-Schlatter and Sinding-Larsen-Johansson

OSD and SLJD disease are microavulsion fractures due to the patellar tendon traction forces on the apophyses. OSD involves the growth plate of the tibial tuberosity at the inferior attachment of the patellar ligament and is more common than SLJD, which occurs at the inferior pole of the patella at the superior attachment of the patellar ligament. Both conditions present in adolescence during growth spurt and are characterized by localized pain aggravated by exercise, particularly running and jumping (Table 47–8). They are more common in athletes with one study reporting a 21% incidence of OSD in a group of athletes vs 4.5% in age-matched nonathletes.[169] On examination, there is localized tenderness and soft tissue swelling. Tightness of surrounding muscles (quadriceps, hamstrings, gastrocnemius) is common. Radiographs are not usually required, but if pain is severe or there is marked swelling, radiographs can exclude bony tumor, fracture, or infection. Typical radiographs of OSD show enlargement and fragmentation of the tubercle (Fig. 47–8). Radiographs of SLJD may show ossification and calcification of the inferior patellar pole (Fig. 47–9). Clinical and laboratory evaluation show no evidence of

Table 47–7

The osteochondroses

Type	Condition/Eponym	Site
Articular Upper extremity	Kienbock	Lunate
	Thiemann	Basal phalanges
	Mauclaire	Second metacarpal head
	Prieser	Carpal navicular
	Burns	Distal ulna
	Brailsford	Radial head
	Panner	Capitellum
	Osteochondritis dissecans (OCD)	Capitellum
	Hass	Head of humerus
	Friedrich	Sternal end clavicle:
Articular lower extremity	Legg-Calvé-Perthes	Femoral head
	Meyer dysplasia	Femoral epiphysis
	Diaz	Talus
	Kohler	Tarsal navicular
	Frieberg	Metatarsal head (2nd, 3rd)
	Köhler	Primary patellar center
	Buscke	Medial cuneiform
	Osteochondritis dissecans (OCD)	Femoral condyles, talar dome
Nonarticular upper extremity	Adams	Medial epicondylosis
Nonarticular lower extremity	Osgood-Schlatter Disease (OSD)	Tibial tuberosity
	Sinding-Larsen Johansson (SLJD)	Inferior pole of patella
	Sever	Calcareous
	Iselin	Fifth MT tuberosity
	Milch	Ischial apophysis
	Buchman	Iliac crest
	Oldberg	Ischiopubic region
	Van Neck	Pubic symphysis
	Mandl	Greater trochanter
	Liffert-Arkin	Distal tibia
Spine	Schmorl	Disk
	Calve	Vertebral body
Physeal	Scheuermann	Thoracic spine epiphysis
	Blount	Proximal tibia
Normal variation		

Adapted from Brower AC: The osteochondroses, *Orthop Clin North Am* 14:99, 1983; Siffert RS: Classification of the osteochondroses, *Clin Orthop Rel Res* 158, 1981; and other resources.

Table 47–8

Osgood-schlatter disease

Age at onset	Adolescence
Sex ratio	Boys > girls
Symptoms	Pain localized to tibial tuberosity worsened by running and jumping, pain with kneeling
Signs	Tenderness and swelling over tibial tuberosity at site of inferior patellar tendon attachment, tightness of surrounding muscles
Radiographs	Soft tissue swelling, enlarged and sometimes fragmented tubercle

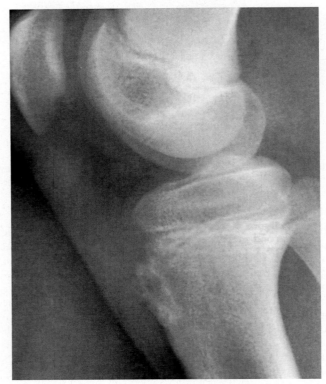

FIGURE 47–8 Radiograph of the knee of a boy with Osgood-Schlatter disease. In addition to fragmentation of the apophysis, the soft tissues overlying the tibial tubercle are thickened. (Courtesy of Dr R. Cairns.)

chronic inflammation, and there is no association with human leukocyte antigen-B27, so it is not a form fruste of enthesitis related juvenile idiopathic arthritis (JIA).[170]

Management is conservative; these are self-limited conditions that resolve with skeletal maturity, but symptoms may persist for up to 24 months. Treatment includes activity modification, local cryotherapy, local muscle stretching and strengthening (quadriceps, hamstrings, gastrocnemius), and correction of any predisposing biomechanical factors (e.g., subtalar pronation) with physical therapy, bracing, and/or orthotics. Occasionally in OSD, symptoms may persist after skeletal maturity due to non-\union of the tibial tuberosity. Excision of a symptomatic ossicle often relieves the symptoms.[171]

Sever Disease

Sever disease (calcaneal apophysitis) is a traction apophysitis of the os calcis at the insertion of the Achilles tendon. It affects children aged 7- to 14-years-old[172] who present with pain that increases with running and jumping. On examination, there may be swelling and

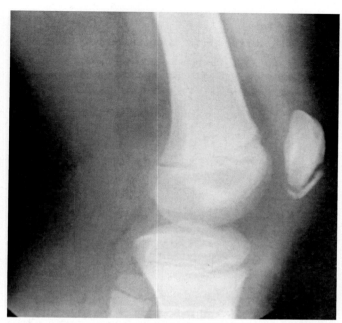

FIGURE 47–9 Radiograph of the knee of a boy with Sindling-Larsen-Johansson disease. The lower pole of the patella has been separated from the patella. (Courtesy of Dr. R. Cairns.)

tenderness over the posterior heel, pain with medial and lateral squeeze of the calcaneal apophysis, weakness of ankle dorsiflexion, and contracture of the Achilles tendon.[173] Radiographs demonstrate a normally irregular apophysis, but lucencies and fragmentation are more commonly associated with pain.[174] Management includes Rest, Ice, Compression, Elevation (RICE), NSAIDS, activity modification, Achilles stretching, strengthening of the ankle dorsiflexors, physiotherapy and short-term use of a heel lift or heel cup in footwear. Children who do not respond to usual therapies require further imaging with MRI. Ogden and colleagues showed children with persistent pain had metaphyseal trabecular stress fracture not traction apophysitis[175] and required immobilization.

Iselin Disease

Iselin disease refers to traction apophysitis of the tuberosity of the fifth metatarsal. The apophysis is within the peroneus brevis tendon insertion site. The secondary ossification center usually fuses by age 11-years-old in girls and 14-years-old in boys. Pain with weight-bearing activity, tenderness over the base of the fifth metatarsal, and pain with resisted eversion are common. Radiographs differentiate Iselin disease from avulsion fracture: the apophysis is parallel to the long axis of the fifth metatarsal, and fractures are usually transverse.[176] Technetium bone scan may help confirm apophysitis. Management includes RICE, modified activity, immobilization, and physiotherapy. Fractures at the metaphyseal-diaphyseal junction (Jones fracture) are significant injuries and require nonweight-bearing immobilization and orthopedic referral for open reduction and internal fixation.

Köhler Disease

Köhler disease is an osteochondroses of the tarsal navicular that affects children between 5- and 9-years-old and may be bilateral in up to 25% of cases.[177] Children usually complain of midfoot pain that worsens with weight-bearing activity. On examination, there is localized swelling, erythema, and tenderness over the navicular. Children characteristically weight bear on the lateral aspect of the foot.[178] Radiographs show increased sclerosis of the navicular, but irregular ossification is also common in normal growth, so clinical correlation is required for diagnosis. Management includes RICE, NSAIDs, activity modification, and immobilization in a walking boot for severe cases. Complete resolution of symptoms is the rule and persistent or late-onset foot complaints are usually caused by other, unrelated pathology.[179]

Freiberg Disease

Freiberg disease is an osteonecrosis of the second or third metatarsal head, occurring most frequently in athletic adolescent females, especially dancers.[177,180] Gradual onset forefoot pain that worsens with weight bearing activity is typical. On examination, there is focal pain and tenderness and occasional swelling over the affected metatarsal head. Radiographs show initial widening of the MTP joint space, followed by collapse and sclerosis of the articular surface of the metatarsal head, which eventually reossifies. The process takes two to three years. Freiberg infarction has been ascribed to trauma,[181] but a review of 31 patients (33 feet) found only 15% of cases were precipitated by trauma. Pedbarographical studies failed to show high pressure at the affected metatarsal head. However, the affected metatarsal was the longest in the foot in 85% of cases, leading the authors to hypothesize this may predispose to vascular insufficiency and infarction of the metatarsal head.[182] Management includes RICE, activity modification, footwear modification, and immobilization. Surgical management is reserved for those failing conservative strategies.[183]

Thiemann Disease

Thiemann disease is a rare osteochondrosis of the phalangeal epiphyses, which has an unknown etiology but may be familial. Onset is typically during adolescence affecting the PIP joint of the middle finger but later may involve adjacent digits symmetrically. Distal interphalangeal joints of the hands and the interphalangeal joints of the first toes may also be affected. Flexion contractures of the large joints also occur.[184,185] Fusiform swelling and tenderness of the affected joint characterize it, and pain, if present, may worsen with exposure to cold. The affected epiphyses demonstrate sclerosis, flattening, cup-shaped widening, and eventually fragmentation in radiographs. Acute phase reactants are normal. Histological study demonstrates aseptic necrosis with normal vessels and no inflammation. Thiemann disease often follows a benign course with normalization of the phalangeal dimensions after growth plate closure. Trauma may worsen the prognosis.[184,186-191]

DEVELOPMENTAL CONDITIONS

Legg-Calvé-Perthes disease

Legg-Calvé-Perthes (LCP) disease was independently and simultaneously described by Legg,[192] Calvé,[192] and Perthes[193] in 1909. It is an idiopathic AVN/osteonecrosis of the femoral epiphysis that usually affects 4- to 10-year-olds, peaking between 5- and 7-years-old. It affects about four boys for each girl affected and is bilateral in 10% to 15%.[194] There is an increased incidence among family members; it is more common in Caucasians and occurs more frequently in urban than in rural dwellers.[195,196] LCP has been associated with delayed skeletal maturation and growth hormone anomalies.[197,198] The pathogenesis of LCP has been described as arterial infarction or abnormal venous drainage.[199,200] The cause is not known, but a disturbance of the fibrinolytic system is believed to play a role. This includes hemoglobinopathies such as sickle cell disease and thalassemia,[201-203] thrombophilias mediated by protein C or S deficiencies,[204] hypofibrinolysis or high level of lipoprotein a.[204,205] Passive smoking is also a risk factor.[206]

Children usually present with a limp or pain in the hip, thigh, or knee. Examination reveals limited and painful internal rotation and abduction of the affected hip. Trendelenburg may be positive. Four radiographical stages are described (1) the earliest signs include decreased size or increased density of the proximal femoral epiphyses on an AP view, widening of the joint space and crescent sign (a subchondral fracture that correlates with the extent of necrosis) on the lateral view; (2) a fragmentation stage, at which the bony epiphysis begins to soften and deform with patchy areas of increased radiolucency and radiodensity; (3) a reossification and healing stage, at which new bone grows into the femoral heard, normal bone density returns, and radiodensities develop in previously radiolucent areas, and abnormalities of the shape of the femoral head, and neck appear; and (4) the residual stage, at which the femoral head is healed and bone density is normal, but the head is deformed (Fig. 47–10). These changes may take several years to complete. MRI has greater sensitivity to detect early changes. Bilateral Perthes' disease is usually asynchronous; apparently synchronous bilateral Perthes' should raise the suspicion of an alternative diagnosis, such as epiphyseal dysplasia.

Treatment consists of rest from aggravating activities and exercises to preserve hip range of motion; orthoses or surgery may be required. The aim of all forms of treatment is to maintain the femoral head well covered within the acetabulum and to minimize the deformity of the head. Generally, with early intervention the condition resolves, and children return to their activities. The main long-term concern is early osteoarthritis. A recent study of 610 children with LCP disease found that only 24% of untreated patients had a spherical femoral head at follow-up.[207] Timing of treatment is also important since of 97 children who underwent femoral osteotomy, those who had surgery during AVN (stage 1) or in the early part of fragmentation (stage 2) had better outcomes than in those operated on later.[208] A Norwegian prospective study with

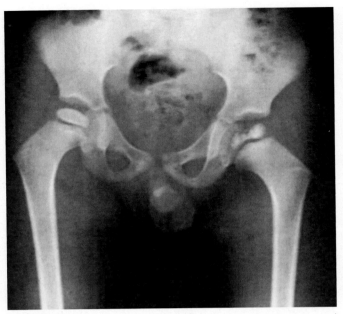

FIGURE 47–10 Legg-Calvé-Perthes disease. On the right side, the capital femoral epiphysis is flattened and sclerotic; on the left, it is fragmented. The femoral metaphyses are widened, especially on the left side.

five year follow-up on 358 children reported more than 50% of femoral head involvement was the strongest predictor of poor outcome. Age greater than 6-years-old also conferred worse prognosis than younger children.[209] The Herring or lateral pillar classification also strongly correlates with outcome. In Lateral Pillar Group A, there is no loss of height in the lateral one third of the head and little density change; in Lateral Pillar Group B, there is lucency and loss of less than 50% of the lateral height; in the B/C border group, there is loss of 50% of the original height of the lateral pillar, and in Lateral Pillar Group C, there is more than 50% loss of lateral height.[210] A prospective multicenter study with follow-up at skeletal maturity on 345 patients with 337 affected hips found that children aged 8-years-old (6-years-old skeletal age) or older at onset and lateral pillar B group or B/C border group had better outcome with surgical treatment than with nonoperative treatment. Children with Group B hips under age 8-years-old at onset had a good outcome regardless of treatment, whereas those with Group C hips had poor outcome.[211] Osteonecrosis of the proximal femoral epiphyses may be associated with systemic disease (leukemia, lymphoma, systemic lupus erythematosus), hemoglobinopathies, coagulopathies, and as a complication of corticosteroid treatment or trauma.

Slipped Capital Femoral Epiphyses

Slipped Capital Femoral Epiphyses (SCFE), displacement of the proximal femoral epiphysis on the femoral neck, is more common in obese children, boys, African Americans, Hispanics, and Asian of Pacific islanders.[212,213] It is more frequently associated with skeletal immaturity and is bilateral in 20% to 40%.[214] A U.S. study found the combined age of onset for 1997 and 2000 databases was 12.7-years-old (boys) and 11.2-years-old (girls),[212] which

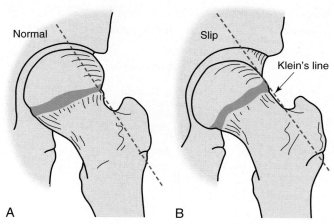

FIGURE 47–11 Klein line in normal situation versus in slipped capital femoral epiphysis. Klein line is drawn along the radiographical border of the neck of the femur. This line should intersect the epiphysis. **A,** Klein line in normal situation. **B,** Alignment of Klein's line with slip: the epiphysis is out of alignment. (Redrawn from Reynolds RA: Diagnosis and treatment of slipped capital femoral epiphysis, *Curr Opin Pediatr* 11:76-79, 1999

is lower than previously reported.[215] A similar study in Scotland showed a trend of increased rates of SCFE and younger age at onset which reflects the secular trend in increased obesity rates.[216] Children and adolescents usually present with a limp and may have hip, groin, or knee pain. An acute slip may develop after a moderate injury, resulting in more severe pain and inability to weight bear. The affected hip is often preferentially held in abduction and external rotation with decreased active and passive internal rotation and adduction. Trendelenburg may be positive reflecting gluteus medius weakness. Patients are classified as having a stable or unstable slip based on their ability to weight bear on the affected leg.[217] Radiographs (AP and frog leg lateral) of the hip may show widening and irregularity of the physis with posterior inferior displacement of femoral head. On the AP view, a line drawn from the superior femoral neck (Klein line) should intersect some portion of the femoral head (Fig. 47–11). Standard radiographs may underestimate the severity of SCFE and MRI can be helpful in diagnosing a "pre-slip" and may show physeal widening, synovitis, periphyseal edema, and joint effusion. Technetium bone scan and MRI are also useful in the early detection of osteonecrosis and chondrolysis, known complications of SCFE.

SCFE may compromise the vascular supply to the femoral head and lead to AVN; all cases warrant urgent orthopedic referral. Unstable SCFE have a much greater risk of AVN. A Canadian study of 87 patients demonstrated one AVN (1.4%) in 73 stable slips and three AVN (21.4%) in 14 unstable slips.[218] Pretreatment bone scan and MRI appear to be a sensitive predictor for the development of AVN.[219] Treatment includes nonweight-bearing, traction and surgery with epiphyseal fixation and osteotomy. Most patients do well after surgical fixation. Complications include AVN and chondrolysis and may occur in both treated and untreated cases.[220] Patients require long-term follow-up as SCFE may develop within 12 to 18 months in the contralateral hip, if prophylactic pinning is not performed.[221] Children under age 10-years-old or

over age 16-years-old and thin children who do not fit the typical profile for SCFE should undergo evaluation for endocrinopathies (thyroid disease, growth hormone abnormalities) associated with SCFE.[222]

Bipartite Patella

The patella ossifies between the ages of 3- and 5-years-oldwith gradual coalescence of multiple ossification centers. Accessory ossification centers often occur, especially in the superolateral patella. A bipartite patella is usually an asymptomatic, incidental radiographical finding. Radiographs show regular smooth fragment margins with no evidence of soft tissue swelling, differentiating the lesion from acute fracture. Occasionally bipartite patella may cause anterior knee pain. Clinically there is soft tissue tenderness at the superolateral patellar pole. Initial treatment is conservative with modified activity and local flexibility and strengthening exercises. Surgical options include excision or fixation of the bipartite patella or release of the vastus lateralis insertion.[223]

Sesamoid Pathology

The medial and lateral sesamoid bones act as pulleys for the flexor hallucis brevis tendons and help stabilize the first MTP joint. Sesamoid disease includes inflammation, fracture or sprain of bipartite sesamoid. Bipartite or multipartite sesamoids are present in 10% to 33% of feet.[177] Injury is usually seen in young athletes who repetitively push off the ball of their feet during jumping or ballet.[177] Children and adolescents usually complain of pain with forefoot weight bearing and may walk on the lateral foot border. On exam there may be localized tenderness and swelling. Treatment includes RICE, NSAIDS, modified activity, modified footwear (wide toe box, stiff sole, low heel), orthoses (cut-out), and physiotherapy. Surgical excision of a sesamoid bone should be avoided unless significant osteonecrosis occurs.

Accessory Bones of the Foot

Accessory navicular is the most common accessory bone in the foot, occurring in 4% to 14% of the general population.[60] A bony prominence may be visible in the proximal medial arch. It is usually asymptomatic but may become painful with ossification. Adolescents may present with medial foot pain, synchondrosis disruption or posterior tibialis tendinopathy, and dysfunction. On examination, tenderness is localized over the navicular and resisted strength testing of posterior tibialis (inversion, plantarflexion) reproduces pain. Anteroposterior or 45 degrees eversion oblique radiographs confirm an accessory navicular and technetium bone scan may show localized increased uptake. Conservative treatment with physiotherapy and/or boot and rigid orthotics is usually successful. Surgical excision is considered for recalcitrant cases.

The secondary ossification center at the posterior aspect of the talus appears at age 8-years-old to 10-years-old in girls and 11- to 13-years-old in boys. Failure to fuse creates an os trigonum. It is usually unilateral and occurs in 10% of the population.[60] It can be congenital (persistent separation of secondary ossification center) or acquired (fracture nonunion). Most are asymptomatic; but children participating in sport involving repetitive ankle plantarflexion or inversion may complain of pain in the posterolateral ankle. On examination, there may be tenderness over the posterior ankle and calcaneus and pain with forced plantarflexion. Radiographs of the ankle, including lateral view in plantar flexion show os trigonum. Posterior impingement of the talus may involve synovium, hypertrophied capsule, and flexor hallucis longus tendon. Management of posterior impingement syndrome includes rest, NSAIDS, physiotherapy, taping, and orthopedic referral for possible resection.

Miscellaneous

Traumatic Arthritis

Joint swelling associated with trauma occurs in older school-aged children and adolescents. Overuse syndromes or structurally abnormal joints are the usual causes of such transient joint swelling. Acute injury may result in hemorrhage from an intraarticular fracture, joint dislocation, or tear of a large intraarticular ligament. JIA is far more common than traumatic arthritis in the very young.

Chondrolysis

Idiopathic chondrolysis of the hip is characterized by pain and limp in adolescence, with progressive loss of articular cartilage space by an undefined but presumed inflammatory process. It can occur as an apparently idiopathic event or secondary to other hip pathology, particularly SCFE or LCP disease and has also been described in association with prolonged immobilization, severe trauma, and septic arthritis, rheumatoid arthritis, and Stickler syndrome. An association with spondyloarthropathy has been postulated but not confirmed; other authors consider this condition an independent subform of juvenile arthritis.[224] Girls are affected more than boys are, and African Americans may be more severely affected than other racial groups. Symptoms of pain and stiffness are commonly unilateral. There are no systemic features and investigations (hematological, microbiological, immunological, and acute phase reactants) are normal. Early radiographs may be normal, and late radiographs commonly show regional osteoporosis, premature closure of the femoral capital physis, narrowing of the joint space, and lateral overgrowth of the femoral head. Early MRI findings include a geometrical region of abnormal signal intensity centered in the proximal femoral epiphysis, accompanied by ipsilateral ill-defined acetabular bone marrow edema, mild synovial hypertrophy, and minimal if any joint fluid.[225] Some patients recover, but many go on to develop painful and disabling osteoarthritis of the hip. In one study, all 11 patients, a mean of 13 years after presentation, had constant pain and stiffness with severe radiological damage.[226] Management includes protective weight-bearing, NSAIDs, physiotherapy, and orthopedic intervention as necessary.[227] The role of intraarticular steroid injections

is unclear, and there is no current treatment regimen with proven benefit.

Growing Pains

The term growing pains is a misnomer, because the peak incidence of pain does not coincide with the peak growth period.[228-230] The authors prefer the term benign nocturnal pains of childhood; however, no generally accepted alternative term exists.[231-233] Growing pains should be restricted to identification of a fairly narrow spectrum of complaints (Table 47–9). Children who have unusual symptoms or abnormal findings on examination such as tenderness, local swelling, or erythema should not be diagnosed with this condition.

Surveys of school-aged children have indicated that as many as 10% to 20% had growing pains.[231,232,234] It is most likely to occur in preschool- to school-aged children. The pain is generally nonarticular, affecting both lower extremities, and is often located deep in the thigh, shin, and calf or behind the knee. Benign pain in the groin, back, or upper extremity is far less frequent. It may be precipitated by exercise and is usually relieved by massage. Evenings or nighttime is when the pain occurs, lasting minutes to hours and often interrupting sleep but disappearing by morning. The frequency of attacks varies from daily to once every few months often following a day of high physical activity.[235] Growing pains are never associated with fever, weight loss, night sweats, easy bruising, or a limp. Children with such pain have completely normal patterns of activity and normal physical examinations during and after the episode. Results of laboratory studies and radiography are normal.

The etiology and pathophysiology of the pain is unknown. Theories include lower pain threshold, overuse, decreased bone strength, biomechanical abnormalities and maternal anxiety.[236] Long clinical experience with such pains in many children, however, has proved they do not portend serious illness. Successful management includes education of the child and family about the benign nature of the problem. Gentle massage with or without analgesics is usually effective. In children with frequent attacks, administration of an evening dose of either acetaminophen or an NSAID may be preventive. Passive stretching can also be of benefit.[237] Those with underlying mechanical abnormalities, such as hypermobility or pes planus, may benefit from shoe inserts.[238]

Table 47–9

Growing pains (benign nocturnal pains of childhood)

Age at onset	4 to 12 years
Sex ratio	Probably equal, slightly more girls in some series
Symptoms	Deep aching, cramping pain in thigh or calf, usually in the evening or during the night; never present in the morning; bilateral; responds to massage; and analgesia
Signs	Physical examination results are normal
Investigations	Laboratory and radiographical studies (if done) have normal results

Restless Legs Syndrome

Restless legs syndrome (RLS) is a sensorimotor disorder characterized by a strong irresistible urge to move the lower extremities. Adult prevalence is 5% to 10% (U.S. and Western Europe), and pediatric prevalence is 2%. Boys and girls are equally affected.[239,240] Young children may not meet diagnostic criteria because they have difficulty expressing typical symptoms. Criteria in children include meeting all four adult criteria (urge to move legs, worse during rest and at night, relief with movement) and a description of characteristic leg discomfort in their own words. The cause of this condition is unknown, but genetic factors; dopamine dysfunction, and low-iron stores have been proposed.[241] Adult literature reports 40% to 92% of RLS onset before 35- to 40-years old is familial, but the exact mode of inheritance is controversial. A positive parental history of RLS has been noted in 53% to 77% of pediatric cases.[239] Large genome-wide association studies detected an association of variants in 4 genes: MEIS1, BTBD9, MAP2K5, LBXCOR1.[242,243] Some children with "growing pains" may really have the RLS, but this is unlikely for the majority.[244] Hyperactivity/attention deficit disorder appears more common in children with RLS.[245] Management requires the identification and discontinuation of medication or other triggering factors. These include selective serotonin reuptake inhibitors, metoclopramide, diphenhydramine, nicotine, caffeine, and alcohol and sleep deprivation. Drug therapy might include iron supplementation, if iron stores are low, and dopaminergic medication, especially if ADHD coexists. Slow progression of the disease with periods of stability has been reported.[246]

Carpal Tunnel Syndrome

Carpal tunnel syndrome is a rare condition in children. A review of 64 cases found that about 50% were secondary to various lysosomal storage diseases, and 25% were idiopathic.[247] The children often had long-standing, rather nonspecific symptoms, such as poor manual dexterity. By the time of diagnosis, clinical findings of weakness and thenar wasting are often marked, thus it is important to have a low threshold of suspicion, particularly in children with skeletal abnormalities. Physical exam should include provocative median nerve testing. A controlled study in adults with electrophysiologically proven carpal tunnel syndrome found that the wrist-flexion test (Phalen maneuver) was the most sensitive, whereas the nerve-percussion or compression test (Tinel sign) was least sensitive but most specific.[248] In children, these clinical tests are often normal, hence electrophysiological testing is essential.[247] Importantly electrophysiological tests often show bilateral abnormalities in children, even if only one hand is affected clinically. Some authors suggest clinical or electrophysiological screening be performed in children with mucopolysaccaridoses and mucolipidoses, even before symptoms develop.[249] Operative release is often the only effective treatment in children, and some suggest that early surgery should be performed to minimize damage.[250]

Cervical Neuropraxia ("Stinger")

A "stinger" may be the most common symptomatic upper extremity nerve injury seen in competitive contact (especially American football) sports. It is typically described as a transient shooting pain or paresthesia radiating down one arm with or without weakness after contact with the head and/or shoulder. Typically there is a C5/C6 dermatomal distribution. Neck pain and bilateral upper extremity involvement should prompt a search for cervical spinal cord damage rather than "stinger". The mechanisms of injury include traction on the brachial plexus or cervical nerve root (especially in younger athletes) or direct compression on these structures.[251,252] Imaging is not required unless symptoms persist, there are neurological deficits, or the athlete has two or more episodes. MRI is helpful to identify foraminal narrowing or disk herniation and can distinguish areas of compression on the brachial plexus or enlargement of the "stretched" neural structures with increased T2 signal intensity.[253] CT myelography may provide more detail about the extent of central canal stenosis. Electrodiagnostic studies may be useful in differentiating cervical radiculopathy from brachial plexopathy for those with persistent weakness. Most athletes are able to continue contact sport after a single "stinger" that resolves quickly. For those with more complex episodes or persistence of symptoms, the extent and recovery of any associated neurological deficit, recurrence pattern, and anatomical factors determine return to play.[253]

Neuralgic Amyotrophy

Neuralgic amyotrophy (NA) (brachial plexus neuropathy) is rare with an annual incidence rate of one to two per 100,000 individuals.[254] It is more common in adults but occasionally affects older children. NA almost always manifests as an acute onset of severe shoulder pain, followed by weakness and localized muscle wasting, without restricted passive range of motion and little or no additional sensory complaints.[255-259] Up to 30% of cases may be bilateral.[260] Preceding infection is reported in up to 50% of patients with exercise, surgery, vaccination, orthopedic conditions and underlying arthritis, vasculitis, or connective tissue disease possible precipitating factors.[261] A rare autosomal dominant form associated with SEPT9 mutation presents similarly to idiopathic NA, but onset occurs at an earlier age; dysmorphic features and a relapsing-remitting course are seen.[262] Idiopathic neuralgic amyotrophy may be recurrent in over 25% of patients within two years of disease onset.[260] The pathogenesis is unclear, but inflammatory, vascular insufficiency and traumatic theories are postulated.[261] Acute pain responds best to long-acting NSAIDS and narcotics. Corticosteroids may reduce time to recovery. The overall prognosis is good, but patients may take many months or years to recover, and physiotherapy is needed to minimize the risk of permanent joint contracture.

Brachial neuritis follows a similar pattern as NA but is accompanied by paralysis. Similarly lumbosacral plexus neuropathy can occur, leading to leg pain and paralysis.[196] Characteristic electromyographic findings of damage to both the nerve roots, and the peripheral nerves usually confirm the diagnosis. Treatment consists of supportive care, analgesics, and immobilization for pain control followed by rehabilitation. This is a self-limiting disorder, which does not tend to recur, but patients may take a few years to recover.[263]

REFERENCES

1. J.A. Kirk, B.M. Ansell, E.G. Bywaters, The hypermobility syndrome. Musculoskeletal complaints associated with generalized joint hypermobility, Ann. Rheum. Dis. 26 (1967) 419–425.

4. P. Beighton, L. Solomon, C.L. Soskolne, Articular mobility in an African population, Ann. Rheum. Dis. 32 (1973) 413–418.

7. M. Mikkelsson, J.J. Salminen, H. Kautiainen, Joint hypermobility is not a contributing factor to musculoskeletal pain in pre-adolescents, J. Rheumatol. 23 (1996) 1963–1967.

34. M.B. Mishra, P. Ryan, P. Atkinson, et al., Extra-articular features of benign joint hypermobility syndrome, Br. J. Rheumatol. 35 (1996) 861–866.

39. N. Adib, K. Davies, R. Grahame, et al., Joint hypermobility syndrome in childhood. A not so benign multisystem disorder? Rheumatology 44 (2005) 744–750.

45. L.T. Staheli, D.E. Chew, M. Corbett, The longitudinal arch, A survey of eight hundred and eighty-two feet in normal children and adults, J. Bone Joint Surg. Am. 69 (1987) 426–428.

58. T.L. Pommering, L. Kluchurosky, S.L. Hall, Ankle and foot injuries in pediatric and adult athletes, Prim. Care 32 (2005) 133–161.

59. K.A. Vincent, Tarsal coalition and painful flatfoot, J. Am. Acad. Orthop. Surg. 6 (1998) 274–281.

60. M.L. Omey, L.J. Micheli, Foot and ankle problems in the young athlete, Med. Sci. Sports Exerc. 31, 1999.

63. J.K. Loudon, H.L. Goist, K.L. Loudon, Genu recurvatum syndrome, J. Orthop. Sports Phys. Ther. 27 (1998) 361–367.

66. R.H. Engelbert, C.S.P.M. Uiterwaal, E. van de Putte, et al., Pediatric generalized joint hypomobility and musculoskeletal complaints: a new entity? Clinical, biochemical, and osseal characteristics, Pediatrics 113 (2004) 714–719.

69. J.J. Wilson, T.M. Best, Common overuse tendon problems: A review and recommendations for treatment, Am. Fam. Physician 72 (2005) 811–818.

72. C. LaBella, Patellofemoral pain syndrome: evaluation and treatment, Prim. Care 31 (2004) 977–1003.

74. R.Y. Hinton, K.M. Sharma, Acute and recurrent patellar instability in the young athlete, Orthop. Clin. North Am. 34 (2003) 385–396.

81. T.G. Sanders, M.B. Zlatkin, Avulsion injuries of the pelvis, Semin. Musculoskelet. Radiol. 12 (2008) 42–53.

82. R.C. Schenck Jr., J.M. Goodnight, Osteochondritis dissecans.[see comment], J. Bone Joint Surg. Am. 78 (1996) 439–456.

85. E. Wall, D. Von Stein, Juvenile osteochondritis dissecans, Orthop. Clin. North Am. 34 (2003) 341–353.

89. M.S. Kocher, R. Tucker, T.J. Ganley, et al., Management of osteochondritis dissecans of the knee: current concepts review, Am. J. Sports Med. 34 (2006) 1181–1191.

90. P.M. Kortebein, K.R. Kaufman, J.R. Basford, et al., Medial tibial stress syndrome, Med. Sci. Sports Exerc. 32 (2000) 27S–33S.

94. K.G. Harmon, Lower extremity stress fractures, Clin. J. Sport. Med. 13 (2003) 358–364.

98. R. Shiri, E. Viikari-Juntura, H. Varonen, et al., Prevalence and determinants of lateral and medial epicondylitis: a population study, Am. J. Epidemiol. 164 (2006) 1065–1074.

100. N. Smidt, D.A. van der Windt, W.J. Assendelft, et al., Corticosteroid injections, physiotherapy, or a wait-and-see policy for lateral epicondylitis: a randomised controlled trial [see comment] [summary for patients in Aust J Physiother 48:239, 2002; PMID: 12369566], Lancet 359 (2002) 657–662.

106. R. Jawish, P. Rigault, J.P. Padovani, et al., Osteochondritis dissecans of the humeral capitellum in children, Eur. J. Pediatr. Surg. 3 (1993) 97–100.

108. B.H. Rowe, C.S. Dulberg, R.G. Peterson, et al., Characteristics of children presenting with chest pain to a pediatric emergency department, CMAJ. 143 (1990) 388–394.

110. R.T. Brown, Costochondritis in adolescents, J. Adolesc. Health Care 1 (1981) 198–201.

113. E.C. Sik, M.E. Batt, L.M. Heslop, Atypical Chest Pain in Athletes, Curr. Sports Med. Rep. 8 (2009) 0–6.

119. D.A. Saltzman, M.L. Schmitz, S.D. Smith, et al., The slipping rib syndrome in children, Paediatr. Anaesth. 11 (2001) 740–743.

121. C. Leboeuf-Yde, K.O. Kyvik, At what age does low back pain become a common problem? A study of 29,424 individuals aged 12-41 years, Spine 23 (1998) 228–234.

129. G.T. Jones, A.J. Silman, G.J. Macfarlane, Predicting the onset of widespread body pain among children, Arthritis Rheum. 48 (2003) 2615–2621.

133. P.G. Turner, J.H. Green, C.S. Galasko, Back pain in childhood, Spine 14 (1989) 812–814.

137. P.J. Papagelopoulos, W.J. Shaughnessy, M.J. Ebersold, et al., Long-term outcome of lumbar discectomy in children and adolescents sixteen years of age or younger, J. Bone Joint Surg. Am. 80 (1998) 689–698.

145. S.D. Early, R.M. Kay, V.T. Tolo, Childhood diskitis [Review], J. Am. Acad. Orthop. Surg. 11 (2003) 413–420.

149. M.J. Herman, P.D. Pizzutillo, R. Cavalier, Spondylolysis and spondylolisthesis in the child and adolescent athlete, Orthop. Clin. North Am. 34 (2003) 461–467.

152. J.E. Lonstein, Spondylolisthesis in children. Cause, natural history, and management, Spine 24 (1999) 2640–2648.

154. R.S. Campbell, A.J. Grainger, I.G. Hide, et al., Juvenile spondylolysis: a comparative analysis of CT, SPECT and MRI, Skeletal Radiol. 34 (2005) 63–73.

157. P.M. Murray, S.L. Weinstein, K.F. Spratt, The natural history and long-term follow-up of Scheuermann kyphosis, J. Bone Joint Surg. Am. 75 (1993) 236–248.

161. T.G. Lowe, B.G. Line, Evidence based medicine: analysis of Scheuermann kyphosis [Review], Spine 32 (2007) S115–S119.

165. G.E. Omer Jr., Primary articular osteochondroses, Clin. Orthop. Relat. Res. 158 (1981) 33–40.

166. J.F. Katz, Nonarticular osteochondroses, Clin. Orthop. Relat. Res. 158 (1981) 70–76.

170. D.D. Sherry, R.E. Petty, S. Tredwell, et al., Histocompatibility antigens in Osgood-Schlatter disease, J. Pediatr. Orthop. 5 (1985) 302–305.

173. D.M. Peck, Apophyseal injuries in the young athlete, Am. Fam. Physician 51 (1996) 1891–1895.

177. E.G. Manusov, W.A. Lillegard, R.F. Raspa, et al., Evaluation of pediatric foot problems: Part I. The forefoot and the midfoot, Am. Fam. Physician 54 (1996) 592–606.

184. A.C. Allison, B.S. Blumberg, Familial osteoarthropathy of the fingers, J. Bone Joint Surg. Br. 40 (1958) 538.

193. L.F. Peltier, The classic: concerning arthritis deformans juvenilis. Professor Georg C. Perthes, Clin. Orthop. Relat. Res. 158 (1981) 5–9.

194. A. Catterall, The natural history of Perthes' disease, J. Bone Joint Surg. Br. 53 (1971) 37–53.

207. B. Joseph, G. Varghese, K. Mulpuri, et al., Natural evolution of Perthes disease: a study of 610 children under 12 years of age at disease onset, J. Pediatr. Orthop. 23 (2003) 590–600.

209. O. Wiig, T. Terjesen, S. Svenningsen, Prognostic factors and outcome of treatment in Perthes' disease: a prospective study of 368 patients with five-year follow-up, J. Bone Joint Surg. Br. 90 (2008) 1364–1371.

210. J.A. Herring, H.T. Kim, R. Browne, Legg-Calve-Perthes disease. Part I: Classification of radiographs with use of the modified lateral pillar and Stulberg classifications, J. Bone Joint Surg. Am. 86 (2004) 2103–2120.

211. J.A. Herring, H.T. Kim, R. Browne, Legg-Calve-Perthes disease. Part II: Prospective multicenter study of the effect of treatment on outcome [see comment], J. Bone Joint Surg. Am. 86 (2004) 2121–2134.

212. C.L. Lehmann, R.R. Arons, R.T. Loder, et al., The epidemiology of slipped capital femoral epiphysis: an update, J. Pediatr. Orthop. 26 (2006) 286–290.

214. R.A. Reynolds, Diagnosis and treatment of slipped capital femoral epiphysis, Curr. Opin. Ped. 11 (1999) 76–79.

217. R.T. Loder, B.S. Richards, P.S. Shapiro, et al., Acute slipped capital femoral epiphysis: the importance of physeal stability, J. Bone Joint Surg. Am. 75 (1993) 1134–1140.

224. N. Adib, K.L. Owers, J.D. Witt, et al., Isolated inflammatory coxitis associated with protrusio acetabuli: a new form of juvenile idiopathic arthritis? Rheumatology 44 (2005) 219–226.

228. J.M. Naish, J. Apley, "Growing pains": a clinical study of non-arthritic limb pains in children, Arch. Dis. Child 26 (1951) 134–140.

239. D.L. Picchietti, H.E. Stevens, Early manifestations of restless legs syndrome in childhood and adolescence, Sleep Med. 9 (2008) 770–781.

243. J. Winkelmann, B. Schormair, P. Lichtner, et al., Genome-wide association study of restless legs syndrome identifies common variants in three genomic regions, Nat. Genet. 39 (2007) 1000–1006.

247. P.M. Lamberti, T.R. Light, Carpal tunnel syndrome in children [Review], Hand Clin. 18 (2002) 331–337.

254. D.I. Rubin, Neuralgic amyotrophy: clinical features and diagnostic evaluation, Neurologist 7 (2001) 350–356.

Entire reference list is available online at www.expertconsult.com.

Chapter 48

PAIN AMPLIFICATION SYNDROMES

David D. Sherry

Pediatric rheumatologists encounter children with a wide variety of musculoskeletal pains, including those with acute and chronic pain for which an overt primary cause for the pain cannot be found or surmised. In these disorders, frequently the pain seems excessive or amplified to the examining physician. In this chapter the approach and evaluation of pain in children will be addressed first, followed by a review of the presentation and treatment of children with amplified musculoskeletal pain syndromes.

EVALUATION OF MUSCULOSKELETAL PAIN

Pain is the subjective expression of an unpleasant sensation or emotional experience associated with actual or perceived tissue damage.[1] It is difficult, if not impossible, for an observer to know with any certainty to what extent another person is in pain. Even experienced observers, such as nurses or parents, may differ in their assessments of the degree of pain a child is experiencing. Although parents and children tend to make a similar assessment of the degree of pain, parents may over- or underestimate their child's pain in relation to the child's own self-report. An important premise in the evaluation and management of a child in pain is that the child's report of pain and its severity must be accepted at face value. "Pain is what the patient says it is, and exists when he says it does."[2] Prolonged malingering in childhood is exceedingly rare. Effective management requires that the child knows that he or she is believed. Many interacting issues determine whether a child's pain disturbs the child's and the family's functioning, and when, if ever, medical help is sought (Fig. 48–1).

Assessment of Musculoskeletal Pain

History and Physical Examination

In obtaining a history, answers to the following questions should be sought:
- What is the character of the pain?
- Are there any other symptoms?
- Is there a family history of musculoskeletal or other significant conditions or chronic pain?
- What are the family, social, emotional, and educational circumstances?

More detailed questions addressing these four general areas are listed in Table 48–1. In addition to a history of pain-related symptoms, a complete past history and review of systems are essential to document the child's overall health status. This may be quite time-consuming but is especially important in children with amplified pains; it is the initial step in establishing a trusting relationship with the child and family, who often feel that their concerns have not been considered seriously and that no one is looking at the child as a whole. The answers elicited by the questions will allow a directed clinical examination, enabling the physician to develop a focused differential diagnosis. The physician can then reasonably determine whether further investigations are indicated. A few key observations to be made during the physical examination are listed in Table 48–2.

Laboratory Examination

It is important to have a clear rationale for undertaking any investigation. In many situations, no testing is required. A large number of investigations increases the likelihood of false-positive results that may obfuscate. Usually an evaluation of indices of inflammation (complete blood count, erythrocyte sedimentation rate, and C-reactive protein) is appropriate. It is suspect to make a diagnosis of a noninflammatory condition in a child with an abnormal blood count or increased acute-phase reactants unless the abnormalities can be clearly ascribed to an intercurrent illness. Tests for antinuclear antibodies and rheumatoid factors are of little value in the absence

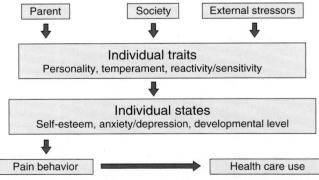

FIGURE 48–1 Factor influencing pain expression and the seeking of health care

Table 48–1

History of musculoskeletal pain

What is the character of the pain?
  Which body parts are painful?
  How long has the pain been present?
  Is the pain getting better, worse, or staying the same?
  What makes the pain better?
  What makes the pain worse?
  Is there diurnal variation in the severity of the pain?
  Is the pain present at night and, if so, does it wake the
    child?
  Does the pain interfere with function, and, if so, what
    specifically?
  Is the pain sharp, aching, deep, boring, etc?
  Does the pain radiate, migrate, or spread?
  Is the painful area tender to touch or clothing?
  Is the painful area either cold or hot to the touch?
  Does the painful part look abnormal or swollen?
  What is the child's or parent's assessment of the pain
    severity?
Are there other symptoms?
  Fever?
  Rash?
  Change in gastrointestinal function?
  Weight loss?
  Upper or lower respiratory tract symptoms?
  Muscle weakness?
  Sleep disturbance?
  Depression?
  Anxiety?
Family and social history
  Ankylosing spondylitis, reactive arthritis, or inflammatory
    bowel disease?
  Back pain, heel pain, or acute iritis?
  Psoriasis?
  Fibromyalgia or other chronic pain condition?
  Is there an identifiable stressor in the family, school, or peer
    group?
  Are there significant or recent life changes?
  Where is the child sleeping?
  What activities does the child participate in?
  How do the parents describe the child's personality?

Table 48–2

The clinical examination: several key observations

Does the child look well or ill?
Is the child's affect commensurate with the level of reported
  pain?
Does the child have an air of *la belle indifference* about him
  or her?
Is there any joint swelling?
Is there any muscle weakness or atrophy?
Is there any tenderness to palpation and, if so, is it over joints,
  entheses, or muscles?
Is there any body area of allodynia, and, if so, is the area
  constant or does it vary over time?
Is there any color, temperature, or perspiration change?
Are there any inconsistencies in the examination?
Is there any neurological dysfunction?
Are there abnormal child-parent interactions, such as
  enmeshment, hostility, or berating?
Is there evidence of concurrent conversion symptoms?
In children with back pain, are signs of nonorganic back pain
  present?

of clinical evidence of inflammatory disease, and false-positive antinuclear antibody seropositivity in particular may lead to unnecessary investigations.[3-5] Imaging studies should be directed specifically to rule in or out a specific diagnosis (e.g., plain radiographs or bone scintigraphy for trauma or tumor and magnetic resonance imaging for spinal cord lesions).

Pain Assessment

A number of methods are available to assess pain in children. Because pain is a complex state, influenced by many factors, no single instrument can provide a complete evaluation. Nonetheless, application of one or more of the available instruments will aid in understanding pain in the individual child and in groups of children with similar diseases.

Physiological Measures

A number of physiological measures may be useful to assess pain in very young children or in older children who have limited communication skills. These include heart rate, blood pressure, palmar sweating, transcutaneous oxygen tension, and cutaneous blood flow. Most of these tests have little or no data, however, to support their reliability, validity, sensitivity, specificity, or practicality.[6] Therefore, it is only with great suspect that one should rely on these measures as a gauge of the degree of pain a child is experiencing.

Behavioral Measures

Physicians routinely interpret the child's behavior as an indicator of the severity of pain. However, perhaps because behavioral measurements are integrated into the assessment almost subconsciously, and because of inherent biases about what constitutes appropriate responses to pain, such behavioral assessments may be misleading. Nevertheless, it is important to be able to quantify pain behaviors because they represent important indicators of how a child is dealing with or responding to noxious or perceived noxious stimuli. Furthermore, pain behaviors may themselves positively or negatively affect a child's and a family's pain-coping mechanisms, so an ability to measure these behaviors may help to understand and better manage the child's pain.[7]

A number of different scales of pain behavior have been developed. These include various assessments of crying or other verbal responses, facial expressions, and limb movements.[7] The Children's Hospital of Eastern Ontario Pain Scale (CHEOPS)[8] is validated and widely used. However, this instrument is not sensitive to change in children who have been in pain for several hours, presumably because pain behaviors habituate if the pain persists. In this situation, CHEOPS scores are generally low and correlate poorly with self-report measures.[9] Using a standardized observational method with videotapes, Jaworski and colleagues[10] measured pain behaviors in 30 children with juvenile rheumatoid arthritis and concluded that this method was a reliable and valid measure of pain. They stated that measures of pain behavior might be particularly useful in outcome studies because these behaviors were, notably, relatively independent of depression.

Self-Report Measures

A number of both unidimensional and multidimensional self-report instruments for children were developed during the 1990s.[11]

UNIDIMENSIONAL PAIN MEASURES

The most frequently used simple unidimensional pain scale is the visual analog scale (VAS). For older children and adults, this is usually a 10-cm horizontal or vertical line anchored by phrases such as "no pain" at one end and "the worst imaginable pain" at the other. The patient puts a mark along the line to represent the level of pain. This mark is measured in millimeters from the "no pain" end to give a value that can be compared over time. For younger children, the VAS is usually anchored by a cartoon happy face at one end and a crying face at the other. Variants of the VAS for children include pain thermometers[12] or pain ladders.[13] Other unidimensional scales include Likert scales, in which the pain is rated on a 4-, 5-, or 6-point verbal scale, such as no pain, mild pain, moderate pain, or severe pain,[14] or as a number from 1 to 10. A Faces Rating Scale[15] is a nonverbal nonnumerical Likert scale for younger children.

MULTIDIMENSIONAL PAIN MEASURES

Multidimensional instruments are questionnaires that collect information about a number of domains relevant to pain, including pain severity; psychological well-being, such as levels of anxiety and depression; coping strategies; and self-efficacy. The best known of these is the Varni/Thompson Pediatric Pain Questionnaire.[16] Other questionnaires are designed to assess pain-coping strategies[17] and competency.[18] Often these self-report measures are filled in by health care providers or parents, rather than by the children themselves, but the evidence that such observer, or proxy, evaluations are accurate is equivocal at best.[19,20]

Amplified Musculoskeletal Pain

Many children with severe musculoskeletal pain do not have an identified inflammatory disease or mechanical derangement to cause their degree of pain and debility. These children have usually been seen by multiple physicians and have undergone multiple investigations before the correct diagnosis is made. Unfortunately, attempts to identify an increasingly rare and unlikely cause for the pain help perpetuate it. An experienced physician can often recognize the condition promptly and, by halting further medical investigations and initiating appropriate therapy, provide great service to the child and family.

HISTORICAL REVIEW

Chronic musculoskeletal pain in children received virtually no attention until the latter half of the 20th century. In 1951, Naish and Apley[21] published a study on pediatric limb pains due to nonarthritic causes. Since then, doctors have increasingly recognized that a significant number of children suffer from both chronic and amplified musculoskeletal pain.[22,23] Reflex neurovascular dystrophy (complex regional pain syndrome, type I) was first described in a child in 1971[24] and fibromyalgia in 1985.[25] These two disorders are the subject of most studies whereas other, less clearly classified amplified musculoskeletal pain conditions are less frequently reported.[26-28]

Definition and Classification

Current terms used to describe these conditions are inadequate and confusing because many children have features shared among different subsets.[26,28] Authors have separated these children depending on physical features (such as the presence of overt autonomic signs,[1] or number of painful points with a variety of systemic symptoms)[25,29] or location (localized or diffuse).[26] The terminology used is, in one sense, moot because evaluation and treatment are similar between subsets.[27,30]

In this chapter, the term *amplified musculoskeletal pain* is used because it is descriptive, does not presume an etiology, and differentiates these children from adults with chronic pain. The word amplified refers to the idea that the body amplifies the pain in much the same way feedback is a viscous cycle between microphone and speaker. It does not imply that the child is willfully hyperbolizing. When reading a particular study, it is important to know what criteria were used to classify children with various forms of amplified musculoskeletal pain (Table 48–3). Discrete subsets exist in each of the groups. Specifically, children who fulfill the criteria for fibromyalgia are included with those with diffuse idiopathic musculoskeletal pain, and those with complex regional pain syndrome are included with those with localized idiopathic musculoskeletal pain. There is a subset of children with intermittent amplified musculoskeletal pain in whom the criterion for duration is not satisfied; they are nevertheless included in some reports due to the severity of their pain and marked dysfunction that may reoccur over years.[31]

EPIDEMIOLOGY

Incidence and Prevalence

Population surveys of school children confirm that musculoskeletal pain is common; back pain is as frequent as 20%,[32] and limb pain has been reported in 16%.[22,33] Fibromyalgia has been reported to have a frequency in children and adolescents of 2% to 6%.[34,35] There are no specific data regarding the other amplified musculoskeletal pain syndromes, but 5% to 8% of new patients presenting to North American pediatric rheumatology centers most likely have a form of amplified musculoskeletal pain.[5,36] Although it may be selection and referral bias, many pediatric rheumatologists believe they have been seeing increasing numbers of children with amplified musculoskeletal pain in the past two decades.

Age at Onset

Amplified musculoskeletal pain has been described in patients as young as 2-years-old, but the majority of reports involve children in late childhood and

Table 48–3

Criteria for different subsets of amplified musculoskeletal pain

Complex Regional Pain Syndrome, Type I[1]
Criteria 2-4 must be satisfied.
1. The presence of an initiating noxious event, or a cause of immobilization
2. Continuing pain, allodynia, or hyperalgesia with which the pain is disproportionate to any inciting event
3. Evidence at some time of edema, changes in skin blood flow, or abnormal sudomotor activity in the region of the pain
4. This diagnosis is excluded by the existence of conditions that would otherwise account for the degrees of pain and dysfunction

Complex Regional Pain Syndrome, Type II[1]
All three criteria must be satisfied.
1. The presence of continuing pain, allodynia, or hyperalgesia after a nerve injury, not necessarily limited to the distribution of the injured nerve
2. Evidence at some time of edema, changes in skin blood flow, or abnormal sudomotor activity in the region of the pain
3. This diagnosis is excluded by the existence of conditions that would otherwise account for the degrees of pain and dysfunction

1990 American College of Rheumatology Criteria for Fibromyalgia[29]
Both criteria must be satisfied.
1. Widespread pain (bilateral, and above and below the waist and axial pain) present for at least 3 months
2. Pain (not tenderness) on digital palpation with 4 kg of pressure on 11 of the following 18 sites:
    a. Occiput: at insertion of suboccipital muscle
    b. Low cervical: at anterior aspect of the intertransverse spaces of C5-C7
    c. Trapezius: at the midpoint of the upper border
    d. Second rib: just lateral to the second costochondral junction at the upper rib border
    e. Scapula: the medial border just above the spine of the scapula
    f. Lateral epicondyle: 2 cm distal to the epicondyle
    g. Gluteal: in the upper outer quadrant of the buttocks
    h. Greater trochanter: 1 cm posterior to the trochanteric prominence
    i. Knees: at the medial fat pad 1 cm proximal to the joint mortise

Yunus and Masi Criteria for Childhood Fibromyalgia[25]
All 4 major and 3 minor, OR the first 3 major, 4 painful sites, and 5 minor need to be satisfied.
Major:
1. Generalized musculoskeletal aching at 3 or more sites for 3 or more months
2. Absence of underlying condition or cause
3. Normal laboratory tests
4. Five or more typical tender points (see sites under 1990 ACR criteria above)
Minor:
1. Chronic anxiety or tension
2. Fatigue
3. Poor sleep
4. Chronic headaches
5. Irritable bowel syndrome
6. Subjective soft tissue swelling
7. Numbness
8. Pain modulation by physical activities
9. Pain modulation by weather factors
10. Pain modulation by anxiety or stress

Diffuse Idiopathic Pain[26]
Both criteria must be satisfied.
1. Generalized musculoskeletal aching at 3 or more sites for 3 or more months
2. Exclusion of disease that could reasonably explain the symptoms.

Localized Idiopathic Pain[26]
All 3 criteria must be satisfied.
1. Pain localized to one limb persisting
    a. 1 week with medically directed treatment OR
    b. 1 month without medically directed treatment
2. Absence of prior trauma that could reasonably explain the symptoms
3. Exclusion of diseases that could reasonably explain the symptoms

adolescence.[25,26,28,37-41] The mean age at onset is generally 12- or 13-years-old. Older adolescents may be underrepresented, presumably because they are referred to adult specialists.

Female to Male Ratio

All large series agree that girls predominate over boys in a ratio of approximately 4:1.[25,26,28,37,39-41] Since women seek medical advice more often than men, there may be a selection bias; however, given the disability involved, this is most likely not a major factor in children. It is the author's experience that the sex ratio has changed over the years, with relatively more boys presenting of late. It used to be 80% of children with amplified musculoskeletal pain syndrome were female, but more recently it has dropped to 65% female.

Geographical and Racial Distribution

There have been no formal investigations regarding the relationship of amplified pain syndromes to ethnicity; however, a series from Philadelphia reported a disproportionate number of white patients (15 of 15).[42] All reports are from developed countries, and comparisons with developing nations are impossible.[43]

ETIOLOGY AND PATHOGENESIS

The cause, or causes, of the different amplified musculoskeletal pain syndromes is unknown. Childhood pain syndromes differ significantly from those occurring in adults; there is a distinct difference between technetium bone scintigraphy in children and adults with complex regional pain syndrome type I, and children do not have the classic three phases (edema and erythema, cyanosis and coolness, and atrophy and dystrophic changes) of complex regional pain syndrome observed in adults.[44] Children respond more readily to physical and occupational therapy.[28,31,37,39,42,45] Nevertheless, in many children, these syndromes seem to be causally related to injury, illness, or psychological distress, either singly or in combination.

Injury, including surgery, frequently precedes complex regional pain syndrome in adults, and minor injury is commonly reported in children. Rarely, more overt trauma may be the inciting event.[46-49] Six children in British Columbia developed complex regional pain syndrome type 1 following hepatitis B vaccine; this was thought to be either due to the injection trauma or to constituents of the vaccine.[50] Minor trauma may play a role in localizing the site of amplified musculoskeletal pain. Children who are hypermobile may be at increased risk of developing the fibromyalgia form of amplified musculoskeletal pain, perhaps due to chronic microtrauma; however, there is uncertainty about this.[51-54]

Illness, such as myocardial infarction, has been associated in adults with the complex regional pain syndrome, and arthritis may coexist with amplified pain in children.[27,55] Amplified musculoskeletal pain has been observed in children with a variety of illnesses, including cerebral palsy, muscular dystrophy, new-onset diabetes, and leukemia. These associations may or may not be coincidental.

Psychological distress is a recurring theme in most reports of children with amplified musculoskeletal pain, although controlled studies are lacking.[21,28,37,40,54,56-64] Clearly, there are children and families who are overtly psychologically dysfunctional or distressed, but whether this is the cause of, the effect of, or unrelated to the development of an amplified musculoskeletal pain syndrome is not known. However, not all families with a painful, dysfunctional child are inappropriately distressed.

The role of hormonal or environmental factors is uncertain. The observation that girls are more frequently affected may reflect the fact that girls have lower pain thresholds, increased levels of hypermobility, increased frequency of sleep disorders than boys, and differences in coping and cultural expectations (especially in Western countries).[65-67] The social history may document multiple recent major life events, such as moving, changes in the nuclear family, family illness and deaths, or school stress.[28,40] There is commonly a role model (usually a parent) for either chronic pain or disability. Interdependency, or enmeshment, between the patient and the parent (usually the mother) is striking in many families; even when the physician directly addresses a question to the child, the parent will answer.[28,40]

The pathophysiology of amplified musculoskeletal pain is unknown, but in some children, especially those with localized or regional pain, it may be related to either increased sympathetic nervous system activity or increased α-adrenoceptor responsiveness.[68-73] Diffuse amplified pain, particularly fibromyalgia, has been extensively studied in adults, and a wide variety of hypotheses have been suggested, including abnormal muscle anatomy and physiology, altered sleep pattern, abnormal serotonin metabolism, hypothalamic-pituitary-adrenal axis hypofunction, decreased cerebral blood flow, trauma, and psychological distress. Two recent studies of a small number of adults with fibromyalgia suggest that they have a deranged sympathetic response to orthostatic stress.[74,75] There is no convincing evidence that any of these factors is of primary importance.[76]

Additionally, there are suggestive data regarding the role of central mechanisms for complex regional pain syndrome. Recently, functional magnetic resonance imaging in children with complex regional pain syndrome suggest pain-induced activation of endogenous pain modulatory systems manifested by activation in the basal ganglia and parental lobe may be at play.[77] These changes persist once the complex regional pain syndrome is resolved. Rommel and colleagues found hemisensory impairment beyond the painful area and more allodynia and movement disorders in patients with sensory deficits, suggesting a central mechanism for complex regional pain syndrome.[78] In the rat model of complex regional pain syndrome, only animals older than 33-days-old (analogous to 8-years-old in humans) can be induced to develop the symptom complex, indicating that the nervous system has to obtain as certain level of maturity before complex regional pain syndrome can develop.[79]

GENETIC BACKGROUND

Amplified musculoskeletal pain syndromes occurs in siblings,[80,81] parent/child pairs,[57,82,83] spouses, and multiple family members.[84,85] Buskila and colleagues[86] reported that 28% of 58 offspring from 20 mothers had fibromyalgia,[86] and Pellegrino and colleagues identified that 52% of 50 subjects from 17 families had fibromyalgia, and another 22% had clinical evidence of abnormal muscle consistency, with a set of identical twins developing fibromyalgia within six months of each other.[83] Other researchers have noted that not only fibromyalgia but also other chronic pain conditions are more common in family members of children with fibromyalgia.[87] In the Netherlands, 31 families were identified with multiple members (up to five family members) affected with complex regional pain syndrome,[88] but a clear mode of inheritance was not observed. No particular gene has been implicated, although one small study of complex regional pain syndrome type 1, suggested that women with human leukocyte antigen-DR2 (HLA-DR2)[15] may be more resistant to treatment.[89] If genetic factors are important in amplified pain conditions, it is probable multiple genetic polymorphisms are involved that predispose the individual to develop amplified pain when inciting environmental and cultural factors are present.

CLINICAL MANIFESTATIONS

Although there are differences between localized and diffuse amplified musculoskeletal pain syndromes, the medical history and physical examination are surprisingly consistent. In children with localized amplified musculoskeletal pain, minor trauma that might not be clearly recalled is common ("someone must have stepped on my foot"). The pain and consequent disability increase over time regardless of medication. A cast or splint may increase the pain or, at best, minimize the pain while it is worn, but immobilization is an important factor in perpetuating the pain. Autonomic signs (edema, cyanosis, coolness, increased perspiration) may be persistent or transient or may not occur. In one study of 70 children with complex regional pain syndrome, all had pain, 86% had allodynia, 77% edema, 77% coolness to the limb, 73% cyanosis, and only 31% hyperhidrosis.[41] Allodynia (pain generated by normally nonpainful stimuli) can be marked ("the breeze of someone walking by hurts") and can lead to significant impairment. This phenomenon, too, can be transient. Any body part can be involved, and the child may have several areas of pain. The lower extremity is more commonly involved than the upper, and peripheral body parts are more commonly involved than central areas. Occasionally, only one small area is involved, such as a finger, the nose, or a tooth.[90] Localized pain is usually continuous.

In diffuse amplified musculoskeletal pain, the onset is usually more gradual and can be vague in location and character. There is an absence of autonomic signs, but affected children complain of poor sleep and depression more often than do those with localized pain.[76] However, there is a significant number of children with diffuse amplified musculoskeletal pain who start out with very localized pain or even clear cut complex regional pain syndrome that then spreads and may involve the entire body. Children with diffuse amplified musculoskeletal pain frequently report a multiplicity of symptoms. The pain is often centrally located, involving the back, chest, abdomen, head, and extremities.

In all children with amplified musculoskeletal pain, conversion symptoms are not uncommon.[27,28,91] Numbness is frequently reported, but these children can manifest paralysis, nonepileptic episodes (pseudoseizures), muscle shaking or rigidity, blindness, or a bizarre (histrionic) gait. Eating disorders can be present,[92,93] and a high index of suspicion for these need to be maintained. Even when reporting severe pain or other somatic symptoms, the child often has a markedly incongruent affect, smiling even when reporting severe pain (up to 10 out of 10), and can have a *la belle indifference* about the pain and dysfunction it causes. A few children, usually but not exclusively those with localized amplified musculoskeletal pain, will demonstrate marked pain behaviors such as crying or screaming. Affected children often seem to be mature for their age, are accomplished in school and extracurricular activities, and are described by their parents as perfectionistic, empathetic, and pleasers.

Notable points on physical examination include the absence of findings suggesting an underlying disease, a normal neurological examination, and the presence of allodynia. Careful sensory testing, with special attention to dermatomal and peripheral nerve innervation, is required. Allodynia is present if pain is reported when lightly touching the skin or gently pinching a fold of skin. The border of the allodynia can vary dramatically. Signs of autonomic dysfunction, especially coolness and cyanosis, may only be present after exercising the limb or may become apparent if the limb is held in a dependent position for a few minutes.

The distribution of painful points is outlined in Table 48–3 and illustrated in Figure 48–2. Control points, such as the forehead, shin, and thumbnail, will define how widespread the pain is.[94] It is not uncommon for children with diffuse amplified musculoskeletal pain to report that their entire body is painful, even to the point of having pain from gently touching their hair. A number of children with diffuse amplified pain do not have the painful points of fibromyalgia, although they are otherwise indistinguishable from those fulfilling criteria.

Prolonged back pain in childhood is often due to a serious illness and should be carefully investigated.[95] However, there is a subset of children with nonorganic back pain, usually in conjunction with diffuse amplified musculoskeletal pain. Distinguishing signs include the axial loading test, distracted straight leg raising, passive rotation test, overreaction, and allodynia (Table 48–4).[96]

PATHOLOGY

There is virtually no information concerning the histopathology of connective or nerve tissues from children with amplified musculoskeletal pain syndromes. Three children with complex regional pain syndrome type I had findings on biopsies of skin, muscle, and nerve consistent with ischemic injury.[97] Endothelial swelling, basement

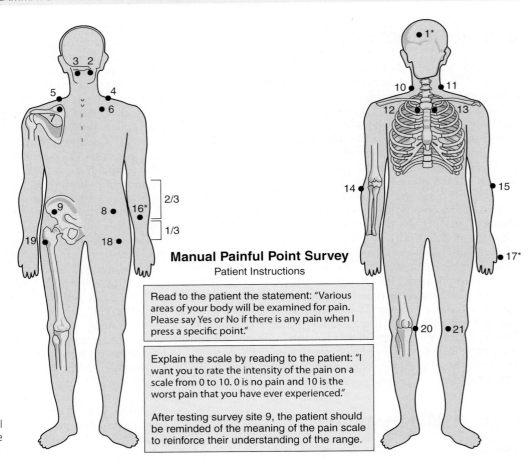

Manual Painful Point Survey
Patient Instructions

Read to the patient the statement: "Various areas of your body will be examined for pain. Please say Yes or No if there is any pain when I press a specific point."

Explain the scale by reading to the patient: "I want you to rate the intensity of the pain on a scale from 0 to 10. 0 is no pain and 10 is the worst pain that you have ever experienced."

After testing survey site 9, the patient should be reminded of the meaning of the pain scale to reinforce their understanding of the range.

FIGURE 48–2 Diagram of painful points in fibromyalgia as defined by the American College of Rheumatology.[29]

Table 48–4	
Signs of nonorganic back pain	
Test	**Description**
Axial loading test	A positive test occurs when back pain is reported while the examiner exerts downward pressure on the top of a standing patient's head. Neck pain may be elicited and is not a positive test.
Distracted straight leg raising	In a positive test, flexion of the hip causes back pain when the patient is supine but not when sitting.
Passive rotation test	A positive test occurs when the patient reports back pain with passive rotation at the ankles and knees, keeping the pelvis, back, and shoulders in the same plane.
Overreaction	Overreaction is defined as excessive wincing, muscle tremors, screaming, or collapsing with pain. "Excessive" is quite subjective and may vary based on age, mental status, cultural influences, or fear.
Allodynia	Report of pain to light touch or a gentle pinch of the skin, usually with a border that varies on repeat testing.

Data from Waddell G, McCulloch JA, Kummel E, et al: Nonorganic physical signs in low-back pain, *Spine* 5:117-125, 1980.

membrane thickening and reduplication, and patchy fiber atrophy of muscle were observed. The author had one patient with complex regional pain syndrome with ischemic changes present in the synovium of her knee.

DIFFERENTIAL DIAGNOSIS

A number of other painful conditions need to be considered in the evaluation of a child who may have an amplified musculoskeletal pain syndrome. Table 48–5 lists disorders confused with amplified pain syndromes, many of which are discussed in other chapters. One condition commonly misdiagnosed as an amplified pain syndrome is the seronegative enthesopathy arthropathy syndrome, especially in children with back pain. The most common misdiagnoses for children who actually have an amplified pain syndrome are trauma, mechanical pain, or arthritis.

GENERAL ASSESSMENT OF PAIN IN CHILDREN WITH AMPLIFIED MUSCULOSKELETAL PAIN

There are two major independent variables to consider when assessing pain: (1) the quality and quantity of the pain complaint itself, and (2) the amount of dysfunction as a consequence of the pain. The report of pain is always valid because, by definition, pain is subjective.[1] Therefore, the most useful measurement of pain is the self-report on a verbal or visual analog scale. The quality of pain can be assessed using various instruments such as the McGill Pain Questionnaire or Pediatric Pain Questionnaire.[16,98]

Table 48–5

Differential diagnosis in children presenting with marked pain

Diagnosis	Typical Age	Distinguishing Characteristics
Fabry disease	Adolescents	Episodic, excruciating burning pain in the distal extremities; blue maculopapular, hyperkeratotic lesions clustered on the lower trunk and perineum; erythrocyte sedimentation rate is usually elevated
Neoplasia	Any	Episodic or migratory pain or arthritis, generalized malaise, anorexia, and bone pain
Spinal cord tumors	Any	Abnormal neurological examination, altered gait, or spinal curvature
Erythromelalgia	Adolescents	Pain with erythematous, warm, swollen hands or feet that is eased by cold to the point that patients refuse to remove ice or cold water from their affected limbs
Pernio (chilblains)	Any	Burning pain with associated red to purple, swollen papules on exposed fingers or toes after cold injury
Raynaud disease	Adolescents	Tricolor change (white, blue, red), associated with tingling; usually not very painful
Hypermobility	Children	Intermittent nocturnal pains that may occur after certain activities
Restless legs syndrome	Adolescents	Nocturnal discomfort in, and an inability to keep from moving, the legs; paresthesias, not pain per se, are common and rarely cause awakening
Myofascial pain	Adolescents	Sustained contraction of part of a muscle, especially those about the head, jaw, and upper back; pain well localized and reproduced when that part of the muscle is palpated
Chronic recurrent multifocal osteomyelitis	Any	Specific point tenderness
Chronic compartment syndrome	Adolescents	Severe muscle pain (usually calf) after exercising
Progressive diaphyseal dysplasia	Adolescents	Severe leg pain, fatigue, headaches, weight loss, weakness, and an abnormal, waddling gait; radiographs show cortical thickening and sclerosis of the diaphysis of the long bones
Peripheral mononeuropathy	Adults	Posttraumatic mononeuropathy
Transient migratory osteoporosis	Adolescents	Rapidly developing, painful osteoporosis
Vitamin D deficiency	Adults	Hyperesthetic pain in debilitated patients with multiple reasons to be deficient in vitamin D
Thyroid disease	Any	Widespread musculoskeletal pain with either hypothyroidism or hyperthyroidism with associated symptoms of thyroid dysfunction

The amount of reported pain does not directly correlate with the degree of incapacity, which can vary from almost none to being bedridden. An important observation is that, with treatment, function usually returns before the pain diminishes. Functional measurements vary depending on the location of the pain and the presence of coexisting conditions, such as arthritis or, more commonly, conversion symptoms. Children with both amplified musculoskeletal pain and conversion paralysis can be extremely dysfunctional.

Children with amplified musculoskeletal pain suffer more than children with other musculoskeletal conditions do, which may indicate the degree to which the disorder is a manifestation of psychological distress. In one comparison of the degree of well-being, children with complex regional pain syndrome type 1 ranked themselves as significantly more disabled as measured by a visual analog scale than those with juvenile rheumatoid arthritis.[40]

Psychological dysfunction is almost universally present by the time these children are identified.[28,37,40,54,99,100] Even though these syndromes are not psychological in cause, the psychological toll on the child and family is often severe. The degree of psychosocial pathology is highly variable and may range from anxiety or poor coping to borderline personality disturbance, or may involve siblings and other family members.

LABORATORY EXAMINATION

Often, after taking a history and performing an examination, the diagnosis of an amplified pain syndrome is certain, and no further investigations are required. If done, tests of blood and urine are normal. The most common "abnormal" test is a low-titer positive antinuclear antibody (1:40 to 1:160), which should be discounted.[3] There may be normal or slightly slowed nerve conduction velocity in patients with complex regional pain syndrome type 1.[101,102] Any laboratory testing should be done with caution; the more tests performed, the more likely the occurrence of false positive results is, leading to unjustified doubt about the diagnosis, anxiety concerning more serious illnesses, and delay in initiating treatment.

RADIOGRAPHICAL EXAMINATION

Radiographical findings are normal or demonstrate disuse osteoporosis, depending on the duration and degree of disability; rarely will children have the spotty osteoporosis that occurs in adults with complex regional pain syndromes.[37] Technetium radionuclide bone scans are probably the most useful study if the diagnosis is in doubt.[42,45] The most frequent abnormality is decreased radionuclide uptake in the affected limb. A normal study is evidence against an underlying bone disease, such as osteomyelitis, osteoid osteoma, or a stress fracture, but abnormal scans are subject to differing interpretations, especially if the findings are subtle.[103] Magnetic resonance images (MRI) in children with localized amplified pain document regional bone marrow edema with T1-weighted MR images of low signal intensity and T2-weighted MR images with high signal intensity; it has been reported that MRI is more sensitive than scintigraphy[104,105] but early on has a difficulty distinguishing between the edema of amplified musculoskeletal pain and the edema of subtle fractures.

TREATMENT

The plethora of widely disparate treatments attests that there are no proven therapies demonstrated by well-controlled therapeutic trials in children with amplified musculoskeletal pain.[27,64] Many reports describe a single child or a very small group of children. Therefore, treatment is based largely on clinical experience.

Treatment should have two goals: restoration of function and relief of pain. Anything less is not ideal, although, because pain is subjective and not directly amenable to specific treatment, there are patients in whom restoration to full function without total pain relief has to be accepted. Helping the child develop skills to cope with the pain is often effective in relieving distress and dysfunction, even if the pain persists.

Most publications deal with localized amplified musculoskeletal pain, specifically complex regional pain syndrome type I. Of these, most report benefit, in order of success, with physical and occupational therapy, transcutaneous electrical nerve stimulation, lidocaine patches, and sympathetic blocks.[28,37,39-41,48,81,101,102,106-114] Most authors advocate aggressive physical and occupational therapy aimed at reversing immobility and increasing function. Treatments used less commonly and with variable results include glucocorticoids,[41,47] tricyclic antidepressants, anticonvulsants, opioids, sympathectomy, biofeedback, behavioral modification, and psychotherapy.[41,47,115,116] Steroids were not helpful in six children[117] and have been associated with marked morbidity; therefore, they should not be used in children. Wilder and colleagues advocated a combination of multiple physical and medical approaches, including sympathetic blocks and sympathectomy, with pain resolution in less than one half of their patients.[41] A recent Cochrane systematic analysis could not make a conclusion regarding the effectiveness of sympathetic blocks in complex regional pain syndrome,[118] and a randomized double-blind placebo study of guanethidine regional blocks was stopped early due to side effects; however, the data showed no difference in outcome between drug and placebo.[119] Bernstein and colleagues successfully treated 23 children with physical and occupational therapy alone and reported long-term follow-up on 20; 12 were without any pain, five had occasional discomfort without any physical signs, two had moderate discomfort with swelling, and one had a recurrence of neurovascular dystrophy.[37] Sherry and colleagues treated 103 patients with an intense physical and occupational therapy program without medications, and 95 (92%) resolved all pain and all regained function.[39] At follow-up five years later, 88% remained symptom-free.

There are few reports of treatment of diffuse amplified musculoskeletal pain in children. Studies in adults with fibromyalgia have found combination therapy with education, mild aerobic exercise, a low-dose tricyclic antidepressant, and a nonsteroidal antiinflammatory drug (NSAID) helpful but not curative.[25,51,120-123] Eleven of 15 children (73%) with fibromyalgia judged cyclobenzaprine to be helpful, but the durability of benefit was not reported.[121] Another study reported that only three of 33 children with fibromyalgia indicated that they would recommend cyclobenzaprine to other individuals with similar pain.[123] An intense physical and occupational therapy program in children with fibromyalgia resolved all symptoms in one study and was very successful in the author's experience.

All drug treatment of amplified musculoskeletal pain in children is off-label and possesses more than minimal risk, and that the vast majority of children respond to physical and occupational therapy, invasive therapies including epidural infusions, lidocaine infusions, nerve and ganglion blocks, spinal cord stimulators, pain pumps, and ketamine coma have a vanishingly small role. The author has had children subjected to all these therapies without durable benefit, and a few with marked side effects. There are reports of amputation for pain and the author has seen it done to one child.[124] The philosophy of such therapies is that the physician is going to actively stop the pain rather than have the child work through the pain and resolve it, more or less, on their own.

Psychological support has been advocated.[62,100,120,125] Using progressive muscle relaxation and guided imagery, Walco and Ilowite treated five girls with fibromyalgia in four to nine sessions, and four reported no pain in an average of 10 months later.[125] Gedalia and colleagues reported that only two of five children with fibromyalgia found cognitive behavioral therapy helpful.[52] However, Long and coworkers stated that more of a focus should be on the parents whose protective responses to the child's pain may inadvertently promote greater disability and symptoms.[126] Formal psychotherapy based on an initial psychological evaluation has been advocated by some.[30,87,127] It is the author's experience that children benefit to a degree from cognitive behavioral therapy, but it does not often lead to complete resolution of symptoms. A recent Cochrane analysis concluded that psychological treatments are effective for long-term pain control in children with a headache, and psychological treatments may improve pain control in children with musculoskeletal and recurrent abdominal pain, but there is little evidence available to estimate effects on disability or mood.[128] More traditional psychotherapy may be beneficial; children with fibromyalgia are less prone to depression than adults but have a high incidence of anxiety that may interfere with function[129] and may warrant psychiatric evaluation for medication.

Sleep disturbance is frequently mentioned as an important aspect childhood fibromyalgia; however, no data exist about whether treating sleep is of benefit. Good sleep hygiene (Table 48–6) is always advocated, but the

Table 48–6

Elements of good sleep hygiene

- No caffeine
- No television or radio in the bedroom
- Have a set bedtime and awake same time 7 days a week
- Have the bedroom completely dark
- Do not exercise within 2 hours before bedtime
- If not asleep in 30 minutes, get up and do a quiet, boring activity without disturbing the parents (only use the bed for sleeping)

degree of effectiveness is not known. Low-dose tricyclic antidepressant medication has been recommended to facilitate sleep initiation,[120,123] but it is not needed in most children with fibromyalgia or other amplified musculoskeletal pain syndromes. It is paramount for the physician to not take on the sleep issues, since usually the children have a sleep complaint, not a sleep disorder per se. The vast majority of children with very poor sleep do not fall asleep during the day, so the sleep complaint does not need to be specifically treated. The goal is not to have the child feel like he or she has slept well, but rather to be functional and, eventually, resolve the pain, not the sleeping symptoms.

The author has been successful with a team approach with psychological evaluation and therapy (if indicated) for children with both localized and diffuse amplified musculoskeletal pain, which involves intense physical and occupational therapy directed to the restoration of full function.[28,30,31,39,130,131] This therapy is generally for five to six hours on weekdays for a mean of three to four weeks. The children are treated one-on-one with the therapist who is encouraging both speed and quality of movement. Exercises are focused on normal function and aerobic training, such as walking times, rope jumping, climbing stairs, dressing, and other activities of daily living.[27,30,39,130] Allodynia is treated with desensitization using towel and lotion rubs, vibration, and wearing normal clothing and footwear. Most children are day patients and are expected to engage in normal family activities at night and weekends while doing a home exercise program. Children who are very dysfunctional, or have severe postexercise pain behaviors, require inpatient treatment. Others have used a more prolonged inpatient treatment program (three months) with graded physical exercises, graded activities, and counseling with good outcomes.[132]

Children with persistently poor sleep habits may benefit from a sleep study, especially if sleep apnea is suspected. Analgesics, physical therapy modalities such as transcutaneous nerve stimulation and acupuncture, sympathetic blocks, and glucosteroids are, in the author's experience, not required and have been associated with untoward reactions. Children with clinical depression need an evaluation by a psychiatrist. Psychological testing is helpful not only in ascertaining whether there are significant family or other environmental stress factors (such as learning disabilities) and whether the child is depressed, but also as a foundation for cognitive behavioral therapy to teach pain coping strategies.

Children with amplified musculoskeletal pain frequently use alternative treatments, but there are no data regarding benefit. Children have tried herbal therapy, massage, magnet therapy, homeopathy, reflexology, aromatherapy, elimination diets, hyperbaric oxygen, to name a few, and, in the author's experience, these have been uniformly ineffective; none can be recommended.

COURSE AND PROGNOSIS

No studies of the natural history are available. Some children have amplified pain that persists for years, and yet there are children with self-limited involvement who are never evaluated in a tertiary center. Many children have spontaneous remission of illness; 11 of 15 children incidentally diagnosed with fibromyalgia were asymptomatic after 30 months.[133] However, 92% of children diagnosed with fibromyalgia in a pediatric rheumatology center still had significant pain 15 to 60 months (mean, 33 months) later.[134] Siegel and colleagues reported that 33 or 35 patients (94%) treated with low dose tricyclic antidepressant medication, mild exercise, and NSAIDs still had diffuse pain and poor sleep after one year, although their overall well-being improved 1.8 points on a 1 to 10 point scale.[123]

The author has experienced much better short- and long-term outcomes.[30,39] In general, children fulfilling criteria for complex regional pain syndrome type 1 do better than those children with regional pain without signs of autonomic dysfunction, who, in turn, do better than those with diffuse amplified musculoskeletal pain. After a mean of five years, 88% of children with complex regional pain syndrome type 1 were free of pain and fully functional.[39] Most (90%) of those without autonomic signs were functional, but only 78% were without pain.[28] Initially, 90% of the group with fibromyalgia were pain free, but this success declined to 50% over five years. However, 90% still remained fully active in school or employment. A difference in outcome between girls and boys or in younger children compared with older adolescents was not observed.

The frequency of relapses is rarely reported but occurs in all forms of amplified musculoskeletal pain. The clinical manifestation of the second episode may be different from the first, even changing between localized and diffuse disease.[26,28] In the author's experience, children with relapses are more likely to have significant underlying psychopathology, specifically, a prior suicide attempt. The age, sex, and duration of symptoms did not predict relapses. In adult women who sustain a wrist fracture, the prevalence of complex regional pain syndrome can be reduced from 10% to 2% by giving vitamin C for 50 days postinjury.[135] Although it is a bit of an extrapolation, the author recommends 1000 mg of vitamin C in children who have had an amplified musculoskeletal pain syndrome if they suffer an injury or undergo surgery.

In addition to recurrent episodes of amplified musculoskeletal pain, children may develop chronic pain involving other organ systems, especially headaches or abdominal pains, and other psychological problems, including conversion disorders (blindness, paralysis), suicide attempts, panic attacks, incapacitating dizziness or fatigue, or eating disorders. Controlled studies have not been done, so it is unclear whether these problems occur at a greater frequency than in the general population.

CONCLUSION

Musculoskeletal pain is common in childhood, and an accurate diagnosis of the cause and a logical and consistent approach to its management are important. A careful history and examination combined with judicious laboratory or radiographical investigations can usually allow an accurate diagnosis to be made. The use of a few simple measures of pain intensity, particularly self-report scales, can help the physician assess how the child and the parent perceive the pain and thereby enable institution of the most appropriate management. Once the diagnosis of amplified musculoskeletal pain is made, reassurance about the nature of condition and treatment with appropriate physiotherapy should be promptly introduced. However, many children with amplified musculoskeletal pain need complex medical and psychological management involving a multidisciplinary team approach. It is challenging to care for these children, but the outcome is generally very rewarding. The treating team can help these children with their immediate problem by helping them resolve the pain and dysfunction but also help many with long-term and, perchance, more important issues by improving the psychological functioning of the child and family.

REFERENCES

1. H. Merskey, N. Bogduk, Classification of chronic pain: descriptions of chronic pain syndromes and definitions of pain terms, second ed. IASP Press, Seattle, 1994.
14. M.C. Savedra, M.D. Tesler, Assessing children's and adolescents' pain, Pediatrician 16 (1989) 24–29.
16. J.W. Varni, K.L. Thompson, V. Hanson, The Varni/Thompson Pediatric Pain Questionnaire. I. Chronic musculoskeletal pain in juvenile rheumatoid arthritis, Pain 28 (1987) 27–38.
19. A.M. Kelly, C.V. Powell, A. Williams, et al., Parent visual analogue scale ratings of children's pain do not reliably reflect pain reported by child, Pediatr. Emerg. Care 18 (2002) 159–162.
21. J. Nash, J. Apley, "Growing pains": a clinical study of non-arthritic limb pains in children, Arch. Dis. Child 26 (1951) 134–140.
25. M.B. Yunus, A.T. Masi, Juvenile primary fibromyalgia syndrome. A clinical study of thirty-three patients and matched normal controls, Arthritis Rheum. 28 (1985) 138–145.
26. P.N. Malleson, M. al-Matar, R.E. Petty, Idiopathic musculoskeletal pain syndromes in children, J. Rheumatol. 19 (1992) 1786–1789.
28. D.D. Sherry, T. McGuire, E. Mellins, et al., Psychosomatic musculoskeletal pain in childhood: clinical and psychological analyses of 100 children, Pediatrics 88 (1991) 1093–1099.
29. F. Wolfe, H.A. Smythe, M.B. Yunus, et al., The American College of Rheumatology 1990 Criteria for the Classification of Fibromyalgia. Report of the Multicenter Criteria Committee, Arthritis Rheum. 33 (1990) 160–172.
30. D.D. Sherry, Pain syndromes, in: J.I. Miller (Ed.), Adolescent rheumatology, Martin Duntz, London, 1998.
34. D. Buskila, J. Press, A. Gedalia, et al., Assessment of nonarticular tenderness and prevalence of fibromyalgia in children, J. Rheumatol. 20 (1993) 368–370.
37. B.H. Bernstein, B.H. Singsen, J.T. Kent, et al., Reflex neurovascular dystrophy in childhood, J. Pediatr. 93 (1978) 211–215.
39. D.D. Sherry, C.A. Wallace, C. Kelley, et al., Short- and long-term outcomes of children with complex regional pain syndrome type I treated with exercise therapy, Clin. J. Pain 15 (1999) 218–223.
40. D.D. Sherry, R. Weisman, Psychologic aspects of childhood reflex neurovascular dystrophy, Pediatrics 81 (1988) 572–578.
41. R.T. Wilder, C.B. Berde, M. Wolohan, et al., Reflex sympathetic dystrophy in children. Clinical characteristics and follow-up of seventy patients, J. Bone Joint Surg. Am. 74 (1992) 910–919.
42. D.P. Goldsmith, F.B. Vivino, A.H. Eichenfield, et al., Nuclear imaging and clinical features of childhood reflex neurovascular dystrophy: comparison with adults, Arthritis Rheum. 32 (1989) 480–485.
44. E.C. Tan, B. Zijlstra, M.L. Essink, et al., Complex regional pain syndrome type I in children, Acta Paediatr. 97 (2008) 875–879.
45. R.M. Laxer, R.C. Allen, P.N. Malleson, et al., Technetium 99m-methylene diphosphonate bone scans in children with reflex neurovascular dystrophy, J. Pediatr. 106 (1985) 437–440.
52. A. Gedalia, J. Press, M. Klein, et al., Joint hypermobility and fibromyalgia in schoolchildren, Ann. Rheum. Dis. 52 (1993) 494–496.
53. M. Mikkelsson, J.J. Salminen, H. Kautiainen, Joint hypermobility is not a contributing factor to musculoskeletal pain in preadolescents, J. Rheumatol. 23 (1996) 1963–1967.
54. G.J. Reid, B.A. Lang, P.J. McGrath, Primary juvenile fibromyalgia: psychological adjustment, family functioning, coping, and functional disability, Arthritis Rheum. 40 (1997) 752–760.
55. P.H. Veldman, H.M. Reynen, I.E. Arntz, et al., Signs and symptoms of reflex sympathetic dystrophy: prospective study of 829 patients, Lancet 342 (1993) 1012–1016.
56. A. Aasland, B. Flato, I.H. Vandvik, Psychosocial factors in children with idiopathic musculoskeletal pain: a prospective, longitudinal study, Acta Paediatr. 86 (1997) 740–746.
57. F. Balague, M.L. Skovron, M. Nordin, et al., Low back pain in schoolchildren. A study of familial and psychological factors, Spine 20 (1995) 1265–1270.
58. S. Bruehl, C.R. Carlson, Predisposing psychological factors in the development of reflex sympathetic dystrophy. A review of the empirical evidence, Clin. J. Pain 8 (1992) 287–299.
59. B. Flato, A. Aasland, I.H. Vandvik, et al., Outcome and predictive factors in children with chronic idiopathic musculoskeletal pain, Clin. Exp. Rheumatol. 15 (1997) 569–577.
60. G.T. Jones, A.J. Silman, G.J. Macfarlane, et al., Predicting the onset of widespread body pain among children, Arthritis Rheum. 48 (2003) 2615–2621.
62. M. Mikkelsson, J.J. Salminen, H. Kautiainen, Non-specific musculoskeletal pain in preadolescents, Prevalence and 1-year persistence, Pain 73 (1997) 29–35.
64. K.P. White, M. Harth, An analytical review of 24 controlled clinical trials for fibromyalgia syndrome (FMS), Pain 64 (1996) 211–219.
65. D.K. Brazier, H.E. Venning, Conversion disorders in adolescents: a practical approach to rehabilitation, Br. J. Rheumatol. 36 (1997) 594–598.
66. F. Cicuttini, G.O. Littlejohn, Female adolescent rheumatological presentations: the importance of chronic pain syndromes, Aust. Paediatr. J. 25 (1989) 21–24.
68. J.M. Arnold, R.W. Teasell, A.P. MacLeod, et al., Increased venous alpha-adrenoceptor responsiveness in patients with reflex sympathetic dystrophy, Ann. Intern. Med. 118 (1993) 619–621.
73. P. Procacci, F. Francini, M. Maresca, et al., Skin potential and EMG changes induced by cutaneous electrical stimulation II, Subjects with reflex sympathetic dystrophies, Appl. Neurophysiol. 42 (1979) 125–134.
77. A. Lebel, L. Becerra, D. Wallin, et al., fMRI reveals distinct CNS processing during symptomatic and recovered complex regional pain syndrome in children, Brain 131 (2008) 1854–1879.
78. O. Rommel, M. Gehling, R. Dertwinkel, et al., Hemisensory impairment in patients with complex regional pain syndrome, Pain 80 (1999) 95–101.
82. D. Buskila, Fibromyalgia in children—lessons from assessing nonarticular tenderness, J. Rheumatol. 23 (1996) 2017–2019.
85. A. Mailis, W. Furlong, A. Taylor, Chronic pain in a family of 6 in the context of litigation, J. Rheumatol. 27 (2000) 1315–1317.
86. D. Buskila, L. Neumann, I. Hazanov, et al., Familial aggregation in the fibromyalgia syndrome, Semin. Arthritis Rheum. 26 (1996) 605–611.
87. L.E. Schanberg, F.J. Keefe, J.C. Lefebvre, et al., Social context of pain in children with Juvenile Primary Fibromyalgia Syndrome: parental pain history and family environment, Clin. J. Pain 14 (1998) 107–115.

88. A.M. de Rooij, M. de Mos, M.C. Sturkenboom, et al., Familial occurrence of complex regional pain syndrome, Eur. J. Pain 13 (2009) 171–177.

93. T.J. Silber, Eating disorders and reflex sympathetic dystrophy syndrome: is there a common pathway? Med. Hypotheses 48 (1997) 197–200.

94. A. Okifuji, D.C. Turk, J.D. Sinclair, et al., A standardized manual tender point survey I. Development and determination of a threshold point for the identification of positive tender points in fibromyalgia syndrome, J. Rheumatol. 24 (1997) 377–383.

96. G. Waddell, J.A. McCulloch, E. Kummel, et al., Nonorganic physical signs in low-back pain, Spine 5 (1980) 117–125.

99. J. Apley, One child, in: J. Apley, C. Ounsted (Eds.), One child, JB Lippincott, Philadelphia, 1982.

100. L.E. Schanberg, F.J. Keefe, J.C. Lefebvre, et al., Pain coping strategies in children with juvenile primary fibromyalgia syndrome: correlation with pain, physical function, and psychological distress, Arthritis Care Res. 9 (1996) 89–96.

103. M. Schurmann, J. Zaspel, P. Lohr, et al., Imaging in early posttraumatic complex regional pain syndrome: a comparison of diagnostic methods, Clin. J. Pain 23 (2007) 449–457.

109. B.H. Lee, L. Scharff, N.F. Sethna, et al., Physical therapy and cognitive-behavioral treatment for complex regional pain syndromes, J. Pediatr. 141 (2002) 135–140.

111. T.J. Silber, M. Majd, Reflex sympathetic dystrophy syndrome in children and adolescents. Report of 18 cases and review of the literature, Am. J. Dis. Child 142 (1988) 1325–1330.

112. R.P. Stanton, J.R. Malcolm, K.A. Wesdock, et al., Reflex sympathetic dystrophy in children: an orthopedic perspective, Orthopedics 16 (1993) 773–779, discussion 9-80.

117. S.B. Ruggeri, B.H. Athreya, R. Doughty, et al., Reflex sympathetic dystrophy in children, Clin. Orthop. Relat. Res. (1982) 225–230.

120. K.K. Anthony, L.E. Schanberg, Juvenile primary fibromyalgia syndrome, Curr. Rheumatol. Rep. 3 (2001) 165–171.

123. D.M. Siegel, D. Janeway, J. Baum, Fibromyalgia syndrome in children and adolescents: clinical features at presentation and status at follow-up, Pediatrics 101 (1998) 377–382.

125. G.A. Walco, N.T. Ilowite, Cognitive-behavioral intervention for juvenile primary fibromyalgia syndrome, J. Rheumatol. 19 (1992) 1617–1619.

127. I.H. Vandvik, K.O. Forseth, A bio-psychosocial evaluation of ten adolescents with fibromyalgia, Acta Paediatr. 83 (1994) 766–771.

128. C. Eccleston, T.M. Palermo, A.C. Williams, et al., Psychological therapies for the management of chronic and recurrent pain in children and adolescents, Cochrane Database Syst. Rev. (2009) CD003968.

129. S. Kashikar-Zuck, I.S. Parkins, T.B. Graham, et al., Anxiety, mood, and behavioral disorders among pediatric patients with juvenile fibromyalgia syndrome, Clin. J. Pain 24 (2008) 620–626.

130. D.D. Sherry, Amplified musculoskeletal pain in children. Diagnosis and treatment. A guide for physical and occupational therapists, 2002. Retrieved from www.childhoodrnd.org.

132. A.C. de Blecourt, H.R. Schiphorst Preuper, C.P. Van Der Schans, et al., Preliminary evaluation of a multidisciplinary pain management program for children and adolescents with chronic musculoskeletal pain, Disabil. Rehabil. 30 (2008) 13–20.

133. D. Buskila, L. Neumann, E. Hershman, et al., Fibromyalgia syndrome in children—an outcome study, J. Rheumatol. 22 (1995) 525–528.

135. P.E. Zollinger, W.E. Tuinebreijer, R.S. Breederveld, et al., Can vitamin C prevent complex regional pain syndrome in patients with wrist fractures? A randomized, controlled, multicenter dose-response study, J. Bone Joint Surg. Am. 89 (2007) 1424–1431.

Entire reference list is available online at www.expertconsult.com.

Chapter 49

SKELETAL MATURATION AND BONE MINERALIZATION IN THE PEDIATRIC RHEUMATIC DISEASES

Rolando Cimaz and Fernanda Falcini

NORMAL SKELETAL MATURATION

An understanding of bone biology is essential to an appreciation of skeletal growth and adaptation to mechanical stresses throughout life.[1-4] Bone can be divided into two primary types: *cortical* bone, which consists of compact bone in the long bones of the appendicular skeleton; and *trabecular* bone, which is the primary component of vertebral bodies and the flat bones of the skull and pelvis.[5] Trabecular bone has a much greater surface than cortical bone and is metabolically more active. Bones change remarkably in size, shape, and microstructure throughout the period of growth.[6,7] Bones of the appendicular and axial skeletons develop initially by ossification of preexisting cartilage from mesenchymal condensations in the embryo *(enchondral ossification)*. In contrast, bones of the face, skull, and initially the mandible and clavicle develop by ossification of fibrocellular tissue *(membranous ossification)*. All axial and appendicular bones also undergo secondary membranous ossification; the diaphyseal cortex is continuously modified by periosteal new bone apposition.

Anatomy of Bone

Long bones consist of four parts. The *diaphysis* is the long tubular midportion of bone that ends in the *metaphysis*, the flared portion of bone that is separated from the *epiphysis* by the growth plate or *physis*. At birth, the diaphysis is relatively short. It grows in length by enchondral ossification. Cartilage cells proliferate toward the ends of bones; those closest to the middle of the bone ossify. Periosteal deposition of new bone increases the diameter of the diaphysis. The newborn diaphysis consists of laminar bone that lacks the *Haversian canal system* characteristic of mature bone; as the child ages, the intercellular matrix increases, porosity decreases, and the hardness of the bone increases.[8] All epiphyses, except that of the distal femur, are completely cartilaginous at birth. The cartilage is gradually replaced by bone until only

the articular cartilage remains unossified in the mature skeleton.

The physis is a cellular zone in which mitoses are frequent and new cells are being formed. Factors influencing growth at the physis include thyroxine, growth hormone, and testosterone. Growth hormone and insulin-like growth factor I (IGF-I) act together to facilitate the achievement of peak bone mass during puberty. Testosterone stimulates the physis to undergo rapid cell division, with resultant physeal widening during the growth spurt (the anabolic effect), but it eventually slows growth (androgenic effect). Estrogens suppress the growth rate by increasing calcification of the matrix, a prerequisite to epiphyseal closure.

The relative contributions of individual physes to limb length are summarized in Table 49–1. Growth of the appendicular skeleton ceases with completion of ossification of the iliac apophyses, although height of the vertebral bodies may continue to increase and contribute to overall height of the body until the third decade of life.[9] Skeletal bone age can be determined by radiographical identification of the onset of secondary ossification in the long bones and by physeal closure. In general, ossification centers appear earlier, and physes fuse earlier, in girls than in boys.

Bone Mineral Metabolism

The complex structure and composition of bone is directly related to the two primary functions of the skeleton: *to support the tissues of the body in order to permit locomotion and to provide a reservoir of ions critical to metabolic functions.*[10-13] Bone is composed of 70% mineral and 30% organic constituents. *Hydroxyapatite*, constituted primarily of calcium and phosphorus, accounts for 95% of the mineral content. Magnesium, present in smaller amounts, is also important in homeostasis. The organic component consists of 98% matrix, which is predominantly type I collagen. Noncollagenous proteins, such as osteocalcin, fibronectin, osteonectin, and osteopontin, make up 5% of the matrix. Cells occupy the remaining 2% of the organic component of bone and are responsible for formation, resorption, and maintenance of the remodeling cycle. *Osteoclasts* are derived from mononuclear cells and resorb bone. *Osteoblasts* form osteoid and osteoid matrix. *Osteocytes* differentiate from osteoblasts and maintain the integrity of bone through a network of canaliculi.

Biochemical Markers of Bone Formation and Resorption

Bone turnover in a growing skeleton is a linked phenomenon of facilitating bone formation and limiting bone resorption in order for skeletal growth to occur. Studies

of bone mineral metabolism generally assay a specific set of markers of bone formation and resorption in blood or urine.[14-16] Table 49–2 summarizes the principal characteristics of commonly used biochemical markers of bone remodeling. However, there are many confounding factors in using these measures (e.g. urinary acidity, medications, magnesium concentration, and renal function). Moreover, additional difficulties are intrinsic in the interpretation of pediatric measurements, mainly because these markers reflect growth and remodeling. Therefore, geographical reference data for age, sex, and ethnicity are essential. Although these markers cannot be used for the *diagnosis* of osteoporosis, they are important in the study of bone turnover in pathological conditions, and they can be useful in the follow-up of patients during antiosteoporotic treatment, for evaluation of compliance, and possibly for prognosis.

Measures of bone formation include the activity of *bone-specific alkaline phosphatase* which is released during osteoblastic activity. Osteocalcin (also called bone-gla protein) is a vitamin K-dependent, γ-carboxylated protein derived from osteoblasts. Its serum concentration reflects the portion of newly synthesized protein that does not bind to the mineral phase of bone and is released into the circulation. Serum *carboxylterminal propeptide of type I procollagen (PICP)* is also a marker of bone formation.[17] PICP is a globular protein cleaved by a specific peptidase at the C-terminal end of the procollagen triple helix. Its concentration in blood directly reflects the number of collagen fibrils formed.

Plasma *tartrate-resistant acid phosphatase* is a marker of bone resorption.[18,19] This labile enzyme is released during osteoclastic activity. The urinary concentration of the *deoxypyridinoline crosslinked telopeptide of type I collagen* represents hydroxylysyl and lysyl post-translational components of the crosslinkage of type I collagen that

Table 49–1		
Relative contributions of individual physes to length of bone and limb		
Contribution to Total Growth (%)		
Growth Area	**Of Bone**	**Of Limb**
Humerus		
Proximal	80	40
Distal	20	10
Radius/ulna		
Proximal	20	10
Distal	80	40
Femur		
Proximal	30	15
Distal	70	40
Tibia/fibula		
Proximal	55	27
Distal	45	18

Table 49–2	
Biochemical markers of bone remodeling	
Markers of Bone Formation	
Alkaline phosphatase (ALP)	Enzyme secreted by osteoblasts, but also by other cells (e.g. liver, gut, kidneys). In children, about 80% of ALP is derived from bone. Bone-specific ALP is a constituent of osteoblast membrane and can be assayed in serum (no circadian variations)
Osteocalcin	Small noncollagenous protein synthesized by osteoblasts and chondrocytes and deposited in the extracellular bone matrix. A small amount enters the circulation and can be measured in serum. It is a sensitive and specific marker of bone formation
Procollagen type I propeptides	N-terminal and C-terminal extension peptides are cleaved during the extracellular processing of type I collagen, prior to fibril formation, and can be measured in serum
Markers of Bone Resorption	
Tartrate-resistant acid phosphatase (TRAP)	Enzyme present in the osteoclast and released during osteoclastic activity. Serum TRAP is not bone-specific
Hydroxyproline	Amino acid found in collagenous proteins of bones and other soft connective tissue. A product of post-translational hydroxylation of proline in the procollagen chain. Can be measured in urine, but not specific (can be released by noncollagenous proteins and dietary proteins)
Collagen crosslinks (pyridinoline, deoxypyridinoline)	Pyridinoline and deoxypyridinoline are generated from lysine and hydroxylysine during post-translational modification of collagen. They are released during matrix resorption and excreted in urine, but new assays are available for serum determination. Of the two, deoxypyridinoline is more specific for bone
Collagen type I N-terminal (Ntx) and C-terminal (ICTP or Ctx) telopeptides	Derived from degradation of type I collagen. Ntx is more sensitive. Both can be measured in serum and Ntx also in urine

stabilize the molecule. It is measured in the urine in relation to the concentration of creatinine. These crosslinks are reflective of mature collagen breakdown and are also a marker of bone resorption.[20] Deoxypyridinoline is found in large amounts in only type I collagen; therefore, its urinary excretion reflects the metabolic breakdown of that molecule. Urinary hydroxyproline has been used similarly. The *urinary calcium/creatinine ratio* is also a marker of bone resorption.

Calcium-Regulating Hormones

Assessment of bone mineral metabolism includes assays for calcium-regulating hormones such as *parathyroid hormone (PTH), 25-hydroxyvitamin D_3 [25-(OH)D_3], and 1,25-dihydroxyvitamin D_3 [1,25-(OH)$_2D_3$].*[21] The primary function of PTH is to maintain the ionized calcium concentration of the blood within a narrow physiological range. Hypocalcemia results in stimulation of PTH secretion, whereas hypercalcemia suppresses its secretion. PTH regulates calcium homeostasis by acting on the major calcium reservoir of the body, the skeleton. It stimulates osteoclastic activity and thereby bone resorption. It also stimulates the conversion of 25-(OH)D_3 to 1,25-(OH)$_2D_3$. The principal source of 25-(OH)D_3 is dietary vitamin D_2. Ultraviolet light also endogenously stimulates the production of vitamin D_3 from 7-dehydrocholesterol in the skin. 25-(OH)D_3 is biologically inactive and is hydroxylated in the kidneys to the 1,25-(OH)$_2D_3$ hormone. This hormone, *calcitriol*, stimulates intestinal absorption of calcium, thereby elevating the serum calcium concentration. Receptors for 1,25-(OH)$_2D_3$ are present on intestinal cells. Care must be taken in interpreting the results of measurement of the vitamin D hormones, because diet, malnutrition, the presence of diseases leading to malabsorption or a catabolic state, and geographical location and season of the year (sun exposure) influence the results.

The RANK, RANK-L, Osteoprotegerin System

The osteoclast, a cell derived from the monocyte/macrophage hematopoietic lineage, is one of the pivotal effectors in bone resorption. Discovery of the RANK signaling pathway in the osteoclast provided insight into the mechanisms of osteoclastogenesis and activation of bone resorption.[22-29] Osteoprotegerin (OPG), receptor activator of nuclear factor-κB (RANK), and the RANK ligand (RANKL) are parts of a family of biologically related tumor necrosis factor receptor (TNFR)/TNF-like proteins that regulate osteoclast function. RANK, a transmembrane signaling receptor, is mainly expressed by monocytes and macrophages; it is essential for osteoclast differentiation and activation and therefore for bone resorption. Its activation depends on binding with RANKL. OPG is a soluble protein that acts as a decoy receptor of RANKL, inhibiting osteoclast differentiation and activation, and thereby reduces bone resorption. To maintain bone homeostasis, balance in the RANKL, RANK, OPG system is required. The mature osteoclast, in response to activation of RANK by RANKL, undergoes internal structural changes that enables it to resorb bone.

Skeletal Maturation and Peak Bone Mass

Bone mineralization during childhood and adolescence is highly correlated with anthropometric parameters, such as age, weight, height, and Tanner stage.[30-33] Rapid skeletal accretion occurs during intrauterine growth of the fetus and the early months of infancy. Thereafter, skeletal growth is linear throughout childhood. Before puberty, there is no substantial difference between boys and girls in bone mass of the axial or appendicular skeleton. Early puberty and adolescence are characterized by accelerated skeletal maturation and account for at least 40% of the total adult skeletal mass. During this period, sex differences in bone mass become expressed;[34-36] skeletal growth correlates closely with sexual maturation, because epiphyseal closure is under hormonal control.

In North America, girls reach puberty at the approximate age of 11.15 ± 1.10-years-old. Menarche occurs soon after at 13.5 ± 1.02-years-old, and epiphyseal closure is complete at approximately 16-years-old. Puberty in boys begins a half year later, at 11.64 ± 1.07-years-old, and lasts approximately one year longer than in girls. Lumbar bone mineral density (BMD) increases 35% to 70% during adolescence in both boys and girls, but a more prolonged bone maturation period in males results in a larger increase in bone size and cortical thickness.[37-41] Several studies have documented the critical importance of puberty in achievement of peak bone mass, and evidence suggests that bone mass accrual in females essentially ceases within a few years after menarche.[42-46] Also, it has been reported that the age at onset of menstruation might predict BMD in the lumbar spine.[47]

Peak bone mass is defined as the level of bone mass achieved at the end of skeletal maturation. The precise age in normal individuals at which peak bone mass is reached is still uncertain and may depend on the site studied and the method used.[48] Studies by dual x-ray absorptiometry (DXA) indicate that peak bone mass is reached for the most part in late adolescence within the second decade of life. At the lumbar spine, areal BMD progressively increases during childhood and adolescence, reaching a plateau at approximately 15- and 17-years-old in girls and boys, respectively. At the femoral neck, areal BMD reaches a peak at approximately 14.5-years-old in girls and 16.5-years-old in boys; thereafter, it remains stable or declines slightly. At the distal one third of the radius, BMD, assessed by single-photon absorptiometry, progressively increases up to 18- to 19-years-old in boys and 15- to 16-years-old in girls, but a slight additional increase may be evident until the third decade of life.[35,49] The skull mass never peaks, increasing throughout life, as a result of continuous periosteal expansion. Total body BMD continues to increase modestly after epiphyseal closure in boys and plateaus in girls.[39]

A recent study[50] indicated that the age of attaining peak bone mass at the hip is younger than at the spine, and bone mineral content (BMC) and bone surface area at the spine might continue to increase throughout the early 30s in females. BMD was assessed by DXA in 300 healthy females aged 6- to 32-years-old. At the spine, femoral neck, greater trochanter, and Ward triangle, the highest BMD level was observed at 23.0 ± 1.4, 18.5 ± 1.6, 14.2 ± 2.0, and 15.8 ± 2.1-years-old, respectively.

Determinants of Bone Mass

Determinants of peak bone mass include *intrinsic factors,* such as heredity, sex, and hormones,[51] *extrinsic factors,* such as nutrition (calcium, vitamins, calories, protein), and *mechanical influences* related to body weight and physical activity.[52-54] Although weight-bearing exercise appears to enhance bone mineral accrual in children, particularly during early puberty, it remains unclear as to what constitutes the optimal exercise program. Moreover, the specific exercise intervention that will provide the optimal stimulus for peak bone mineral accretion is unclear. A school-based exercise intervention program during the first school years in prepubertal girls showed increased accrual of BMC and areal BMD and gain in bone width. These data support that physical activity could be recommended as a strategy to increase peak bone mass and increase the bone resistance to fractures.[55] Moreover, a recent longitudinal study assessing the effects of jumping on skeletal development over four-years in peripubertal children showed that short-term high impact exercise in the prepubertal period has a persistent effect over and above those of normal growth and development. If the benefits are sustained until BMC plateaus in early adulthood, this could have substantial effects on fracture risk.[56]

It is estimated that heredity determines up to 75% to 85% of the skeletal mass.[57-61] Environmental variables, including those related to endocrine and nutritional influences, mechanical forces, and risk factors, account for the remainder. The genetic basis at the molecular level by which bone mass and strength are determined have yet to be fully elucidated. Many genes may be involved, and several polymorphisms have been implicated, including those for interleukin-6 (IL-6), vitamin D receptors, calcitonin receptor, transforming growth factor-β, estrogen receptor-α, osteocalcin, apolipoprotein E, OPG, androgen receptor, osteopontin, osteonectin, and type I collagen.[61,62] Data suggest that genetic variations at multiple genetic loci are important in bone accrual, and that the combination of genotypes at several loci may have a major role in determining BMD and BMC.[62] Among extrinsic factors, an adequate intake of calcium and vitamin D is a relatively important factor in achievement of peak bone mass.[63-66] Calcium is, however, a threshold nutrient.[67]

Addition of calcium citrate malate (approximately 1000 mg/day) to the diet over a three-year period produced measurable increases in both appendicular and axial bone density in the supplemented twin of 70 pairs of monozygotic twins.[68] In the treatment group, significant incremental bone formation at several measured sites of cortical and trabecular bone was documented in 22 prepubertal children but did not occur in 23 postpubertal or pubertal children.

Vitamin D intake in peripubertal girls is also important in achievement of optimal peak bone mass,[69] and polymorphisms in vitamin D receptor genes are important in the achievement of optimal BMD.[70-72] Finally, skeletal loading associated with body weight is an additional crucial variable that is an independent determinant of peak BMD.[73-75]

DIAGNOSTIC METHODS

Definition of Osteoporosis and Osteopenia and Measurement of Bone Density

Osteoporosis is a disorder characterized by parallel loss of matrix and BMC and microarchitectural deterioration of bone tissue. *Osteopenia* is a low bone mass for age or, more specifically, for skeletal age and stage of sexual maturation. Osteoporosis and osteopenia in adults are defined at levels relative to a "normal" young adult population. The World Health Organization (WHO) developed criteria for the diagnosis of osteoporosis in 1994. These criteria assess the risk of osteoporosis by determining the number of standard deviations between normal peak bone mass and BMD measured with DXA at any skeletal site. This "T score" defines normal bone density (T score between 0 and –1), osteopenia (between –1 and –2.5), and osteoporosis (less than –2.5).[76]

There are currently no accepted definitions for osteoporosis and osteopenia in childhood, because the WHO definition is based on the T score (obtained by comparison with young adults) and not on a Z score (obtained by comparison with age- and sex-matched geographical controls). In children and adolescents who have not yet achieved peak bone mass, BMD should be referred to as a Z score, which is calculated by the following formula: *(BMD of the patient – mean BMD of the control group) ÷ standard deviation of the control group.* In contrast to adults, there are no studies that identify a fracture threshold in children for any specific Z score.

No evidence-based definition of osteoporosis in children is available, partly because no data on the estimation of fracture risk based on standard deviations of bone mass exist. In addition, for a pathogenesis-oriented approach to musculoskeletal alterations in children, a detailed description of skeletal alterations and muscle mass and force might be superior to a definition of osteoporosis based on Z-scores of bone mass alone. In a child with a reduction of bone mass (with or without a fracture), the following variables should be assessed:

- Bone mass in relation to body height
- If possible trabecular density, cortical density, and geometrical variables of bone
- Muscle mass in relation to body height
- Bone mass in relation to muscle mass

The International Society for Clinical Densitometry has recently produced a position statement on bone densitometry in children, which states that the diagnosis of osteoporosis in children and adolescents should not be made based on densitometric criteria alone. According to this definition, the diagnosis of osteoporosis requires the presence of a clinically significant fracture history and a low BMC or BMD. A clinically significant fracture is defined as one or more of the following: long bone fracture of the lower extremities, vertebral compression fracture, or two or more long bone fractures of the upper extremities. Low BMC or BMD is defined as a BMC or areal BMD Z-score less than or equal to –2, adjusted for age, gender, and body size, as appropriate. A Z-score between –1 and –2 is defined as the low range of normality.[77]

Bone mass depends on both the size and density of skeletal bone; and osteoporosis is usually determined relative to bone density. However, with current diagnostic techniques, such as DXA, it is not possible to measure true bone density, because this method measures only a cross-sectional area of the scan, not a true volume. To measure the true density, the depth (volume) of the bone would need to be known and taken into account.

Dual-Energy X-Ray Absorptiometry

Absorptiometry is a means of assessing BMC or density of various areas of the skeleton. *Single-photon absorptiometry* uses an iodine 125 source and is restricted to measuring BMC at the one-third and one-tenth distal radial sites of the forearm. This technique is used primarily for assessment of the appendicular skeleton. Although bone width can be calculated by single-photon absorptiometry, estimations of BMD are not accurate.

Dual-photon absorptiometry uses a gadolinium source with photons of 44 and 100 KeV measured simultaneously in order to calculate BMC or BMD of any area of the skeleton by a computerized subtraction of tissue density from that of bone. Although this method is applicable to children and is accurate, measurement time is prolonged, at least 35 to 45 minutes for a complete skeletal survey, and therefore this technique is no longer in use.

The technique most appropriate for children because of low radiation (= 3 mrem), speed, and accuracy is DXA. DXA employs two beams of 70 and 140 KeV to distinguish soft tissue from bone (Fig. 49–1). The introduction of DXA has increased knowledge of skeletal maturation and the pediatric diseases that affect bone metabolism. The ratio of cortical to trabecular bone differs in various parts of the skeleton; therefore, DXA measures a composite of trabecular and cortical bone mass. Sites often measured clinically by absorptiometry include the one-third distal radius (95% cortical and 5% trabecular), the one-tenth distal radius (25% cortical and 75% trabecular), the lumbar vertebral bodies (5% cortical and 95% trabecular), the femoral neck (75% cortical and 25% trabecular), and the greater trochanteric area of the femur (50% cortical and 50% trabecular).

DXA has been widely accepted as a noninvasive method for measurement of BMD. However, this diagnostic procedure has some limitations in childhood, especially because it measures only a two-dimensional computation of BMC (i.e., divided by surface area): the *areal BMD*. A three-dimensional estimate of skeletal density can be obtained when both anteroposterior and lateral measurements are correlated for skeletal size (cubic centimeters), *the volumetric BMD*. The latter value is seldom available in published data. Areal BMD results as obtained from DXA are influenced by bone size. *The growth of an individual can increase the areal BMD without any actual increase in true bone density; failure to adjust for bone size can therefore lead to erroneous interpretations of DXA values.*

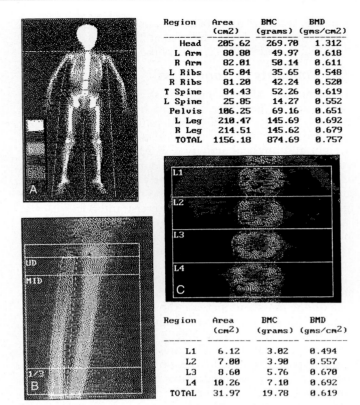

Region	Area (cm2)	BMC (grams)	BMD (gms/cm2)
Head	205.62	269.70	1.312
L Arm	80.88	49.97	0.618
R Arm	82.01	50.14	0.611
L Ribs	65.04	35.65	0.548
R Ribs	81.20	42.24	0.520
T Spine	84.43	52.26	0.619
L Spine	25.85	14.27	0.552
Pelvis	106.25	69.16	0.651
L Leg	210.47	145.69	0.692
R Leg	214.51	145.62	0.679
TOTAL	1156.18	874.69	0.757

Region	Area (cm2)	BMC (grams)	BMD (gms/cm2)
L1	6.12	3.02	0.494
L2	7.00	3.90	0.557
L3	8.60	5.76	0.670
L4	10.26	7.10	0.692
TOTAL	31.97	19.78	0.619

FIGURE 49–1 Dual energy x-ray absorptiometry (DXA) of an 8-year old girl with juvenile rheumatoid arthritis. **A,** Whole body. **B,** Radius. **C,** L1-L4 vertebral bodies. BMC, bone mineral content; BMD, bone mineral density, UD = ultradistal.

Moreover, with BMD measurements in children, there are general problems not specific to the diagnostic technique. When interpreting clinical results, one must consider that in growing children, even a stable BMD value (i.e., a lack of an increase during a period of skeletal growth) represents an abnormality of bone metabolism. Also, areal BMD should be interpreted not only in relation to age-matched controls, but also with corrections for height, weight, and geographical matching. Unfortunately, published pediatric standards for BMD are limited, and the lack of normal control values often makes the interpretation of data difficult. Finally, pubertal status (Tanner stage), frequently delayed in children with chronic rheumatic diseases, is fundamental in the process of bone acquisition and should always be taken into account when comparing patients and controls.

Other Diagnostic Methods

Evaluation of mineralized bone mass using simple radiography is insensitive. Bone mass may have already diminished by 30% to 40% by the time osteoporosis is detectable on conventional x-ray films. Several additional noninvasive methods for measuring bone mass and mineral content have been developed. Table 49–3 includes the characteristics of the most commonly used methods of measuring bone density.

Quantitative computerized tomography (QCT) is applicable to measurement with the axial skeleton with a radiation exposure comparable to that of plain radiography.

Table 49–3

Comparison of different methods for bone density measurement

Method	Site	Dose (mRem)	Average Time for Scanning (Min)	Comments
SPA	Radius	5-18	15	Rarely used
DPA	Lumbar spine, femur	1-15	20-45	Rarely used
DXA	Lumbar spine, hip, radius, total body	1-3 (0.1 if peripheral, i.e., distal radius)	<5 for lumbar spine	Gold standard (best method available today)
QCT	Lumbar spine	100-1000	10-20	True volumetric density can be measured
PQCT	Radius, tibia	6	10	Allows for selective measurements of cortical and trabecular density, bone area, cortical area, cortical thickness, periosteal and endosteal circumferences, muscle cross-sectional area, and biomechanical strain strength indices. Not available yet for clinical routine use.
US	Phalanxes, heel, tibia	0	1-2	Ease of scan, fast, no radiation, inexpensive, portable. Downsides: operator-dependent, needs standardization and more reference data

DPA, Dual-photon absorptiometry; DXA, dual-energy X-ray absorptiometry; PQCT, peripheral quantitative computed tomography; QCT, quantitative computerized tomography; SPA, single-photon absorptiometry; US, ultrasound.

Peripheral QCT has lower radiation exposure and permits analysis of volumetric bone density of appendicular cortical and trabecular sites.

Peripheral QCT (pQCT) has become very important in recent years. Measurements can be done at the radius or the tibia. Radiation exposure is very low, less than 0.3 µSv. It is currently the only technique in clinical use that differentiates between trabecular and cortical bone and determines bone density, bone geometry, and muscle cross-sectional area. Variables of bone geometry like cortical thickness, marrow area, and bone area are particularly suitable as indicators of bone strength, which is the most important outcome variable in the assessment of pediatric bone.

In younger children, the precision of pQCT measurements might be compromised by the partial volume effect. This term reflects the fact that partially filled voxels will not be included in the data analysis. As the voxel size is fixed, the cortical bone mass may be underestimated in a young child with a relatively thinner cortical thickness. Another point of concern is whether pQCT measurements at the appendicular skeleton adequately reflect the situation of the whole skeleton, including axial sites.[78] However, this technique is promising, and clinical studies for juvenile idiopathic arthritis (JIA) have already been performed.[79,80]

Quantitative high-frequency sonography (ultrasonography) is a new and noninvasive method of estimating bone quality. This radiation-free procedure measures the transmission of ultrasound waves through bones and has been proposed for the assessment of bone density. Two parameters can be simultaneously determined from the measured signal: *speed of sound and broadband ultrasound attenuation (BUA)*. BUA measures the loss of sound caused by bone as a function of frequency; in normal adults and children, it may be the parameter that demonstrates the highest correlation with BMD determined by DXA. In addition, sonographic measurements of bone may provide additional information about bone quality, such as stiffness and

elasticity. Normative values for healthy children have been published.[81,82] Also, pilot studies in children with rheumatic diseases have provided relatively good correlations between ultrasonographic bone density measured in the calcaneum[83] or at the midtibia[84] and BMD determined by DXA, supporting the clinical use of ultrasound densitometry. This technique is a promising tool to assess bone mass and quality in children in view of the absence of radiation exposure, low cost, and portability of the equipment.[85-89]

BONE MINERALIZATION IN THE RHEUMATIC DISEASES

Low Bone Mass in Children with Chronic Arthritis

Failure to develop adequate bone mineralization is common in children with chronic arthritis. Juxtaarticular osteopenia can be evident in plain radiographs even in early disease, whereas diffuse osteopenia or osteoporosis can develop later and lead to the risk of vertebral collapse and long-bone fractures after minimal trauma.

Multiple risk factors are known to be associated with decreased bone mass (Table 49–4), and many studies have been published on this subject.[90-110] Active arthritis has an osteopenic effect, both around affected joints and systemically, by means of a complex and still partly unknown network of proinflammatory cytokines. In particular, IL-6 is known to have a profound effect on bone metabolism.[111,112]

Pepmueller and colleagues[104] measured BMC and BMD in 41 children with juvenile rheumatoid arthritis (JRA) and 62 healthy geographical controls and analyzed serum markers of bone metabolism. Decreased BMD was found at all sites in the patient group with a negative correlation between measures of disease severity and bone mass.

Table 49–4
Risk factors for osteoporosis in children with chronic arthritis
Active inflammatory disease
Glucocorticoid treatment
Decreased mobility
Protein/caloric malnutrition
Inadequate calcium/vitamin D intake
Decreased sun exposure
Decreased height and weight
Pubertal delay

These researchers hypothesized that decreased mineralization rather than increased resorption was the primary pathophysiological mechanism. However, the balance between bone formation and resorption is controlled by a variety of factors, and further studies on this subject have yielded conflicting results.[102,113] Although BMD may be decreased at all sites in children with arthritis, the appendicular skeleton is predominantly affected.[114]

Henderson and coworkers[108] evaluated predictors of BMD in prepubertal patients with JRA who had not been treated with glucocorticoids. Almost 30% of mild to moderately ill patients had low total body BMD. Parameters of disease severity (number of swollen joints, articular severity score, erythrocyte sedimentation rate) exerted a negative effect on bone mineralization. In another study of postpubertal females who had never received systemic glucocorticoids, approximately 30% of the subjects with mild to moderate disease demonstrated low bone mass.[109] A stepwise logistic regression model was used to identify contributing factors, and the only variable that significantly contributed to BMC was lean body mass, which accounted for the majority of the variance in total body BMC. This decreased lean body mass could be the result of altered body composition, which often occurs in chronic inflammatory arthritis.

Lien and colleagues evaluated with a two-year controlled study of bone mass and bone turnover 108 children with early JRA matched with 108 healthy children for age, sex, race, and county of residence. Bone mass and changes in total body, spine, femur, and forearm BMD and BMC, body composition, growth, and biochemical parameters of bone turnover were examined at baseline and at follow-up a mean of 24 months later. Low or very low total body BMC was observed in 24% of the patients and 12% of the healthy children. Bone formation, bone resorption, and weight-bearing activities were reduced in patients when compared to controls. Total body BMC was lower in patients with polyarticular onset than in those with oligoarticular disease onset. Patients with JIA have moderate reductions in bone mass gains, bone turnover, and total body lean mass early in the disease course.[115]

A recent study using pQCT of the tibia was performed in 101 patients with JIA and 830 healthy control subjects, all aged 5 to 22-years-old, with the aim of identifying determinants of musculoskeletal deficits, muscle cross-sectional area [mCSA], trabecular volumetric bone mineral density [vBMD], and cortical bone strength, and to determine if cortical bone strength is appropriately adapted to muscle forces. Outcomes of pQCT were expressed as sex- and race-specific Z scores. Multivariable linear regression models assessed mCSA and bone status in patients compared with controls and identified factors associated with musculoskeletal deficits in JIA. Marked deficits in vBMD and bone strength occurred in JIA in association with severe and longstanding disease.[79]

Roth and colleagues assessed 25 JIA patients by pQCT longitudinally with a median of 48 months between measurements. Patients showed some improvement in mCSA and muscle force, and an increase in cortical thickness. The marrow area remained enlarged, but by increasing the cortical thickness bone strength increased. In addition to efficient disease control, training modalities to improve muscle strength and subsequent bone development have to be included in therapeutic approaches.[80]

Effects of Childhood Arthritis on Bone Mass in Adulthood

Diseases occurring during childhood and adolescence associated with a loss of bone mass may predispose patients to premature osteoporosis and fractures during adulthood, if the predetermined peak bone mass is not established during skeletal maturation by late adolescence. Chronic inflammatory diseases can potentially have a detrimental effect on future BMD and fracture risk.

Zak and colleagues[116] assessed BMD of the hip and spine in 65 young adults (mean age, 32.2-years-old) with a history of juvenile chronic arthritis. They found that BMD was significantly lower in these patients than in age-, sex-, height-, and weight-matched healthy controls. Moreover, significantly more patients than expected had osteopenia and osteoporosis. Factors associated with a lower BMD included active disease at the time of the study, baseline erosions, higher Steinbrocker functional class, polyarticular course, and chronic steroid treatment. The presence of juvenile chronic arthritis by itself explained about 20% of BMD variation.

French and coworkers[117] also determined the extent of osteopenia in a population-based cohort of adults with a history of JRA. Forty-one percent of the patients had a T score of 1 or lower at either the lumbar spine or the femoral neck. In another study,[118] the impact of disease activity on peak bone mass was assessed in 229 young adults in their mid-20s with juvenile arthritis at a mean of 15 years after disease onset. Patients with persistent disease had a significantly lower BMD than did healthy subjects, whereas patients whose disease was in remission had overall a normal bone mass. However, even in women with only a history of arthritis in childhood, total body BMD was significantly lower, although this was not true for the lumbar spine or radius. In a later report,[119] a large proportion (41%) of adolescents with early-onset disease were found to have a low bone mass more than 10 years after onset, and their low BMC was related to the duration of active disease, disease severity, measures of bone resorption, and anthropometric parameters such as height and weight.

Other Connective Tissue Diseases

Children and adolescents with systemic lupus erythematosus (SLE), juvenile dermatomyositis (JDM), and the vasculitides are also at risk for the development of osteopenia and osteoporosis, both from the disease itself and from its medical treatment. Glucocorticoid therapy, often in high doses and for prolonged periods, is the basis of treatment for most of these disorders. Avoidance of sun exposure and limited mobility in these patients can also contribute to decreased mineralization. A report from 15 patients with JDM showed low BMD values in the majority and persistent or worsening osteopenia in patients with ongoing active disease.[120]

Another recent study on 10 girls aged 7- to 16-years-old with JDM reported that lumbar BMD was significantly lower than age-matched healthy controls. A correlation was observed between BMD and weight, suggesting that reduced bone mass in JDM may be related to other intrinsic mechanisms in addition to steroid treatment and that some aspects of the disease itself may contribute to this condition.[121]

In SLE, despite evidence that in adults osteopenia is common,[122] scant pediatric data exist.[123] Recent reports in childhood-onset SLE provide evidence of a high frequency of osteopenia, a lower peak bone mass, and a higher risk of osteoporosis later in life because the disease develops before achieving peak bone mass. The lumbar spine was the most seriously affected skeletal site, followed by the femoral neck. Higher cumulative steroid doses were associated with lower bone mass.[124,125] In another study, Compeyrot and colleagues studied 64 consecutive patients with juvenile SLE (JSLE) in whom routine DXA scanning was performed to determine the prevalence of low BMD and to identify associated risk factors. Lumbar spine osteopenia was defined as a BMD Z score comprised between –1 and –2.5, and osteoporosis as a BMD Z score of <2.5. Their results indicated that osteopenia and osteoporosis are common in JSLE and are associated more closely with increased disease duration than with cumulative steroid dose.[126]

Lately, lean mass has been identified as a major determinant of bone density, suggesting that muscle rehabilitation may be an additional target for bone therapeutic intervention in reducing the risk of fractures in JSLE.[127] In addition to the same risk factors that exist for chronic arthritis, renal impairment, reduced sun exposure, and endocrine dysfunction in SLE can all contribute to a low bone mass.

Effect of Drug Treatment on Bone Mineral Density

The relationship between glucocorticoid therapy and vertebral fractures in the rheumatic diseases of childhood is well known.[128] Figure 49–2 shows a vertebral collapse in a young patient with SLE who had been treated with oral prednisone. Steroids have profound effects on the skeleton and on bone formation, mainly through a depletion of bone-forming cells and a decrease in their function.[129] Impaired osteoblastic cell differentiation, associated with an increase in apoptosis, causes a decrease in bone-forming

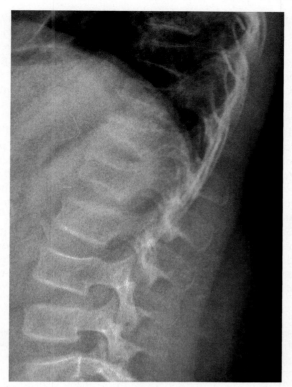

FIGURE 49–2 Vertebral crush fractures in a girl with systemic lupus erythematosus treated with oral prednisone for three years.

cells. Moreover, glucocorticoids shift the differentiation of stromal cells away from the osteoblastic and toward the adipocytic lineage;[130] in addition to causing depletion of mature osteoblasts, they inhibit the function of differentiated cells. Histomorphometric analysis of bone biopsies from patients receiving glucocorticoids demonstrate increased bone resorption as well.[131]

Significant bone loss occurs after the initial exposure to steroids, and even modest doses of these agents increase the risk of fractures.[132] However, it is important to note that patients taking glucocorticoids often have an underlying inflammatory disease that leads to bone resorption.

A recent study from children with JIA showed reductions in BMD and a 10% prevalence of vertebral compression fractures in steroid-treated children. Despite the satisfactory average BMD and height Z scores, the high prevalence of vertebral fractures indicates that osteoporosis remains a concern in children with JIA. This prompts preventive measures, such as optimizing vitamin D and Ca intake, and encourages weight-bearing physical activity.[133] Reyes and coworkers assessed the factors that contribute to a decreased Z-score of volumetric spine BMD and the development of vertebral fractures in children receiving chronic steroid therapy. Children who were not ambulatory, on methotrexate (MTX), or growth retarded had higher rates of vertebral fractures.[134]

Among other effects, glucocorticoids decrease gastrointestinal calcium absorption and increase its urinary excretion, leading to the development of secondary hyperparathyroidism. They also affect IGFs, mainly decreasing synthesis of IGF-I, and inhibit the synthesis of type I collagen, with a consequent decrease in bone matrix available for mineralization.[135] Recent research has provided new insights into the mechanisms of these glucocorticoid actions at the cellular and molecular levels.[136-139] Another important effect on bone is mediated by RANKL and OPG. Glucocorticoids increase the expression by human osteoblastic and stromal cells in culture of RANKL and decrease that of OPG.[140]

The osteopenic effect of MTX has been described in children with malignancies treated with high-dose protocols and confirmed by in vitro studies.[141-144] However, lower-dose MTX is not associated with this osteopenic effect.[108,109,145] Most likely, the significant beneficial effect on arthritis counterbalances in vivo the demonstrated inhibitory effect on osteoblasts.

Biological drugs have shown to significantly reduce inflammation in JIA patients. A recent study provided evidence that one year of etanercept therapy induced a sustained benefit on bone loss in children with JIA by controlling the underlying disease activity.[146]

PRIMARY AND SECONDARY BONE MINERALIZATION DISORDERS

Osteoporosis in an otherwise healthy child or adolescent is rare, although idiopathic osteoporosis is a well-known entity. Rather, pediatric osteoporosis is increasingly recognized in the setting of acute or, more often, chronic illness. Table 49–5 summarizes the primary and secondary pediatric disorders associated with low bone mass.

PREVENTION

Prevention of osteopenia and osteoporosis during the critical developmental stages of skeletal maturation is fundamental in order to decrease osteoporosis and fracture risk later in life. Optimal dietary calcium intake is important, because it accounts for 5% to 10% of the variance in peak bone mass. An adequate calcium intake is

---

Table 49–5

Pediatric disorders associated with low bone mass

Primary

Idiopathic juvenile osteoporosis	A demineralization disorder of unknown etiology. Usually manifests in early puberty. Clinical findings include pathological fractures, bone pain, and difficulty walking. Diagnosis of exclusion. Spontaneous recovery within 3 to 4 years (coinciding with sexual maturation)
Osteogenesis imperfecta	Heritable (autosomal dominant or recessive) disorders of connective tissue. Different types with varying degree of severity (from mild to lethal). Fragile bones, blue sclerae, deafness, short stature, abnormalities of skin and teeth, and spinal deformity are all parts of the spectrum. Treatment with pamidronate leads to substantial improvement

Secondary

Disease	Pathophysiology of Bone Mass Impairment
Connective tissue (chronic arthritis, SLE, JDM, vasculitis, etc.)	Mainly proinflammatory cytokines, glucocorticoid use. Also nutritional defects, reduced mobility and sun exposure.
Gastrointestinal (inflammatory bowel disease, celiac disease, liver disorders)	As above, in addition to malabsorption (hence calcium and vitamin D deficiencies)
Endocrine (Turner syndrome, diabetes mellitus, growth hormone deficiency, delayed puberty, Cushing disease, hypothyroidism, hypopituitarism, hyperparathyroidism, hypogonadism)	Excess or deficiency of hormones in bone metabolism (e.g., T3, T4, PTH, GH, IGF-I, glucocorticoids, sex steroids). Also exercise-induced amenorrhea in osteopenic female athletes
Hematological (thalassemia, thrombophilia)	In thalassemia, hypogonadism is present (from transfusion-induced iron overload). Anticoagulants, such as heparin, have a detrimental effect on bone mass
Oncological	Neoplastic infiltration of endocrine organs, tumor cell production of humoral factors, toxicity of chemotherapy (e.g. methotrexate) and radiotherapy
Metabolical (glycogen-storage disease, lysosomal-storage disorders such as Gaucher disease, homocystinuria)	Interference with type I collagen fibrils, decreased mechanical load, organ infiltration
Renal (chronic renal failure)	Nutritional deficiencies, vitamin D, PTH, and calcium/phosphate metabolical abnormalities, growth failure
Neurological (cerebral palsy, paraplegia, epilepsy, myopathies)	Immobilization, decreased mechanical load, nutritional defects, anticonvulsive medications
Cystic fibrosis	Pancreatic insufficiency (malabsorption), respiratory involvement (glucocorticoid use), hypogonadism
Psychiatric (bulimia, anorexia nervosa)	Low body mass index, malnutrition, low estrogen
Asthma	Secondary to steroid treatment. Even inhaled steroids reduce acquisition of bone mineral in prepubertal children

SLE, systemic lupus erythematosus and JDM, juvenile dermatomyositis.

recommended for all children, according to the published guidelines (800 mg/day from the ages of 1- to 5-years-old, 1200 mg/day from 6- to 10-years-old, and 1500 mg/day from 11- to 24-years-old); during steroid treatment, supplemental daily doses might be required. It has been demonstrated that calcium supplementation enhances bone mineral acquisition in postmenarcheal girls with low calcium intake.[147] Likewise, vitamin D intake should be maximized to at least 400 units a day, and, if not contraindicated by the underlying disease, sun exposure should be recommended to facilitate vitamin D synthesis. Control of chronic illness, adequate general protein-calorie nutrition, and appropriate weight-bearing activity are other determinants of bone accretion. Finally, smoking and excessive alcohol consumption in adolescents should be avoided, because they are likely to be risk factors for a decreased peak bone mass.

The American College of Rheumatology has published revised guidelines for the prevention and treatment of glucocorticoid-induced osteoporosis in adult patients that may also be relevant to children and adolescents.[148] Recommendations include modification of lifestyle factors, weight-bearing physical exercise, calcium and vitamin D supplementation, avoidance or reduction of alcohol and tobacco consumption, and periodic measurement of BMD. A baseline measurement of BMD at the lumbar spine is recommended at the initiation of long-term (longer than six months) glucocorticoid therapy, and longitudinal measurements may be repeated periodically during treatment to monitor bone status.

TREATMENT

Studies of the medical treatment of osteoporosis in childhood are relatively new. It is difficult to perform controlled trials in uncommon diseases, and additional caution should be used when interpreting the results of published studies. Bone loss tends to taper or plateau after six to 12 months of steroid treatment, and during this period any given therapy might show benefit. Moreover, there are methodological problems, some of which are specific to childhood (see earlier discussion of the limitations of diagnostic tools and interpretation of results).

Calcium and vitamin D supplementation might have some benefit in mild disease, but severely affected patients need more potent interventions. There is a paucity of interventional studies on calcium/vitamin D supplementation in pediatric rheumatic diseases, and pharmacological interventions with vitamin D in children with chronic arthritis have yielded conflicting results.[103,149,150]

A recent prospective, randomized, placebo-controlled study in children with JRA showed that 1000 mg of calcium carbonate and 400 international unit of vitamin D per day for 24 months produced a small but significant increase in BMD compared with placebo and 400 international unit of vitamin D per day. Dietary supplementation with calcium in this study population of JRA patients with mild-to-moderate disease provided a small but measurable increase in BMD. However, this increase was seen in patients whose baseline BMD was normal. The effect of this small increase in BMD over a two-year study may

or may not be related to a change in the frequency of bone fractures. Given the high frequency of normal BMD at baseline, normal progression of BMD seen in patients receiving placebo, and a significant but small increase in BMD seen in those receiving calcium supplementation, routine calcium supplementation for children with JRA who are not being treated with steroids is not recommended.[150] Among other candidates for treatment, growth hormone[151,152] and calcitonin[153,154] have both been tried with satisfactory results. Of the newer agents in clinical use, bisphosphonates seem to be the most promising. Bisphosphonates, which are analogues of pyrophosphate characterized by P-C-P bonds, were first studied in humans about 30 years ago. Several chemical features contribute to their biological action: the P-C-P moiety facilitates the ability of these compounds to adsorb to hydroxyapatite, and therefore target the bone, while variations in their side chains determine the potency and spectrum of action of each individual compound (Fig. 49–3). Bisphosphonates are selectively concentrated in bone and inhibit bone resorption by interfering with the action of osteoclasts. Some of the biochemical mechanisms that account for these effects have been elucidated.[155-160]

Until recently, the use of bisphosphonates in pediatrics has been limited because of fear of adverse effects on a growing skeleton, because of potential risks to a fetus if administered to a girl approaching child-bearing age, and because the drug is not appreciably eliminated in the short- to medium-term. More recently, bisphosphonates have been judged to be safe, at least in the short-term, even in pediatric practice, and their use expanded.[156,161-164]

Lately, Thornton and colleagues reviewed a total of 59 papers, where treatment durations were up to three years. The most common side effect was a flulike reaction with intravenous treatment. This occurred during the first infusion and was transient; the symptoms were managed with paracetamol and did not occur during subsequent cycles. They concluded that bisphosphonates are a promising treatment for low BMD and fragility fractures in children with JIA, although the quality of the current evidence is variable, and better studies are needed to more clearly assess their role.[165]

Table 49–6 lists the observed and the possible adverse effects of pediatric use of bisphosphonates. Untoward effects in children have not been reported in greater frequency than in adults. With the newer, nitrogen-containing bisphosphonates, secondary osteomalacia is not a problem. Hypocalcemia and fever are infrequent and transient, and mild abdominal discomfort or dyspepsia are only occasional complaints. Radiological abnormalities described in prepubertal patients include

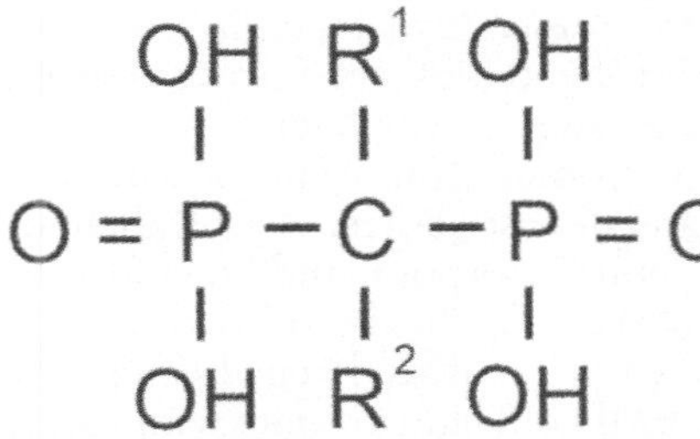

FIGURE 49–3 Chemical structure of bisphosphonates. R^1 and R^2, side chains.

Table 49–6

Adverse effects of bisphosphonates

Observed

Increase in body temperature following intravenous infusion, flulike symptoms

Nausea, dyspepsia, esophagitis, abdominal pain, diarrhea, constipation

Hypocalcemia, hypophosphatemia, hypomagnesemia

Transient lymphopenia

Iritis, uveitis, scleritis, conjunctivitis

Mineralization defects (with etidronate), transient skeletal pain, epiphyseal and metaphyseal radiological sclerosis in growing bones

Feared but not Observed

Irreversible and permanent effect on bone remodeling

Impaired healing and nonunion of fractures

Damage to growth plates and impairment in linear growth

Fetal abnormalities

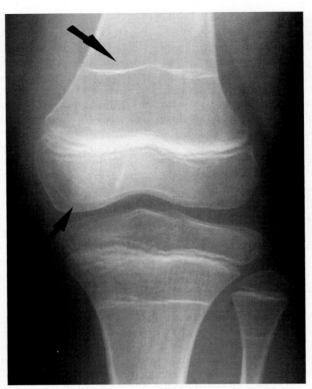

FIGURE 49–4   Radiological alterations (metaphyseal dense lines) following treatment with oral alendronate in a prepubertal child. This patient had previously received intravenous pamidronate (the previous dense lines have migrated; see *arrows*).

bandlike metaphyseal sclerosis (Fig. 49–4) and concentric epiphyseal and apophyseal sclerosis.[166] After drug discontinuation, these abnormalities tend to disappear. No adverse effects on growth have been noted, even after long follow-up. Bone biopsies have demonstrated no signs of mineralization defects and a normal bone structure.[167]

An open, multicenter, prospective study of safety and efficacy of alendronate in children with rheumatic diseases has been published.[168] To be included, patients had to be receiving chronic steroid treatment or had to have a low BMD determined by DXA. Forty-three patients (30 females and 13 males) with JIA (17 patients), SLE (12), JDM (7), or other connective tissue diseases (7) were studied. The mean age was 12.9 ± 3.7-years-old; 14 patients were postpubertal. Alendronate was administered orally at a daily dosage of 5 or 10 mg (for children with body weight less than or greater than 20 kg, respectively). Baseline Z scores ranged from –1.3 to –5.3. Each patient also underwent serial clinical and laboratory evaluations. Lumbar spine BMD was measured at baseline and after six and 12 months by a standardized protocol and with cross-calibration of all instruments. Z scores were calculated by comparing results with age- and sex-matched controls. A substantial increase of bone mass was observed in all children with an average BMD increase of 14.2 ± 10% after one year. One third of the patients attained a normal BMD. Height increased by an average of 4.3 ± 3.7 cm. In comparison, BMD had increased by only 1% in 16 patients who were monitored during the year immediately preceding alendronate therapy. Knee radiographs in the prepubertal children demonstrated an absence of rickets and the presence of metaphyseal lines. Alendronate was well tolerated except for occasional abdominal pain and one episode of esophagitis.

In a follow-up study, variations in parameters of bone metabolism and disease activity were evaluated.[169] Parameters of both bone resorption and bone formation significantly decreased during the first 12 months, whereas none of the disease activity indices changed significantly. Z-score variations in BMD did not correlate with variations of the inflammatory parameters (erythrocyte sedimentation rate,

matrix metalloproteinase-3, IL-6, C-reactive protein). It was concluded that the observed increase in BMD was not secondary to a change in disease activity but was most likely an effect of treatment with alendronate.

Many questions still remain unanswered, and, in particular, the long-term adverse effects in a growing skeleton are unknown at this time. Also, potential risks for young women in their childbearing years with respect to fetal toxicity cannot be disregarded. Therefore, bisphosphonate therapy in pediatric patients remains controversial because of inadequate long-term efficacy and safety data. Current data are inadequate to support their use in children to treat reductions in bone mass/density alone. For osteoporosis associated with chronic illness, bisphosphonate treatment is recommended only in the setting of clinical trials or as compassionate therapy for children with reductions in bone mass/density associated with low-trauma extremity fractures and symptomatic vertebral compression.[170]

REFERENCES

16. S.P. Robins, S.A. New, Markers of bone turnover in relation to bone health, Proc. Nutr. Soc. 56 (1997) 903–914.
23. L.C. Hofbauer, A.E. Heufelder, Role of receptor activator of nuclear factor-kB and osteoprotegerin in bone cell biology, J. Mol. Med. 79 (2001) 243–253.
27. B. Bolon, V. Shalhoub, P.J. Kostenuik, et al., Osteoprotegerin: an endogenous antiosteoclast factor for protecting bone in rheumatoid arthritis. Arthritis Rheum. 46 (2002) 3121–3135.
29. W.J. Boyle, W. Scott Simonet, D.L. Lacey, Osteoclast differentiation and activation, Nature 423 (2003) 337–342.

47. E. Lazcano-Ponce, J. Tamayo, A. Cruz-Valdez, et al., Peak bone mineral area density and determinants among females aged 9 to 24 years in Mexico, Osteoporosis Int. 14 (2003) 539–547.

50. Y.C. Lin, R.M. Lyle, C.M. Weaver, et al., Peak spine and femoral neck bone mass in young women, Bone 32 (2003) 546–553.

54. T. Kuroda, Y. Onoe, Y. Miyabara, et al., Influence of maternal genetic and lifestyle factors on bone mineral density in adolescent daughters: a cohort study in 387 Japanese daughter-mother pairs, J. Bone Miner. Metab. 27 (2009) 379–385.

56. Gunter, A.D.K. Baxter-Jones, R.L. Mirwald, et al., Jump starting skeletal health: A 4-year longitudinal study assessing the effects of jumping on skeletal development in pre and circumpubertal children, Bone 42 (2008) 710–718.

62. M.C. Willing, J.C. Torner, T.L. Burns, Gene polymorphisms, bone mineral density and bone mineral content in young children: the Iowa bone development study, Osteoporosis Int. 14 (2003) 650–658.

76. J.A. Kanis, L.J. Melton, C. Christiansen, et al., The diagnosis of osteoporosis, J. Bone Miner. Res. 9 (1994) 1137–1140.

77. F. Rauch, H. Ploktin, L. Di Meglio, et al., Fracture prediction and definition of Osteoporosis in children and adolescents: The ISCD 2007 Pediatric Official Position, J. Clin. Densitom. 11 (2007) 22–28.

78. B. Zemel, S. Bass, T. Binkley, et al., Peripheral quantitative computed tomography in children and adolescents: the 2007 ISCD Pediatric official position, J. Clin. Densitometry 11 (2008) 59–74.

79. J.M. Burnham, J. Shults, S.E. Dubner, et al., Bone density, structure, and strength in juvenile idiopathic arthritis. Importance of disease severity and muscle deficits, Arthritis Rheum. 58 (2008) 2518–2527.

80. J. Roth, M. Linge, N. Tzaribachev, et al., Musculoskeletal abnormalities in juvenile idiopathic arthritis—a four year longitudinal Study, Rheumatology (Oxford) 46 (2007) 1180–1184.

84. C.F. Njeh, N. Shaw, J.M. Gardner-Medwin, et al., Use of quantitative ultrasound to assess bone status in children with juvenile idiopathic arthritis: a pilot study, J. Clin. Densitom. 3 (2000) 251–260.

85. F. Falcini, G. Bindi, G. Simonini, et al., Bone status evaluation with calcaneal ultrasound in children with chronic rheumatic diseases. A one year followup study, J. Rheumatol. 30 (2003) 179–184.

90. R. Cimaz, M. Biggioggero, Osteoporosis, Curr. Rheum. Reports 3 (2001) 365–370.

91. J.T. Cassidy, C.B. Langman, S.H. Allen, et al., Bone mineral metabolism in children with juvenile rheumatoid arthritis, Ped. Clin. North Am. 42 (1995) 1017–1033.

96. L. Hillman, J.T. Cassidy, L. Johnson, et al., Vitamin D metabolism and bone mineralization in children with juvenile rheumatoid arthritis, J. Pediatr. 121 (1994) 910–916.

97. R. Hopp, J. Degan, J.C. Gallagher, et al., Estimation of bone mineral density in children with juvenile rheumatoid arthritis, J. Rheumatol. 18 (1991) 1235–1239.

102. E.C. Rabinovich, Bone mineral status in juvenile rheumatoid arthritis, J. Rheumatol. 27 (2000) 34–37.

104. P.H. Pepmueller, J.T. Cassidy, S.H. Allen, et al., Bone mineralization and bone mineral metabolism in children with juvenile rheumatoid arthritis, Arthritis Rheum. 39 (1996) 746–757.

108. C.J. Henderson, G.D. Cawkwell, B.L. Specker, et al., Predictors of total body bone mineral density in non-corticosteroid-treated prepubertal children with juvenile rheumatoid arthritis, Arthritis Rheum. 40 (1997) 1967–1975.

109. C.J. Henderson, B.L. Specker, R.I. Sierra, et al., Total-body bone mineral content in non-corticosteroid-treated postpubertal females with juvenile rheumatoid arthritis. Frequency of osteopenia and contributing factors, Arthritis Rheum. 43 (2000) 531–540.

114. J.T. Cassidy, L.S. Hillman, Abnormalities in skeletal growth in children with juvenile rheumatoid arthritis, Rheum. Dis. Clin. North Am. 23 (1997) 499–522.

115. G. Lien, A.M. Selvaag, B. Flatø, et al., A two-year prospective controlled study of bone mass and bone turnover in children with early juvenile idiopathic arthritis, Arthritis Rheum. 52 (2005) 833–840.

116. M. Zak, C. Hassager, D.J. Lovell, et al., Assessment of bone mineral density in adults with a history of juvenile chronic arthritis: a cross-sectional long-term follow-up study, Arthritis Rheum. 42 (1999) 790–798.

117. A.R. French, T. Mason, A.M. Nelson, et al., Osteopenia in adults with a history of juvenile rheumatoid arthritis. A population based study, J. Rheumatol. 29 (2002) 1065–1070.

118. M. Haugen, G. Lien, B. Flatø, et al., Young adults with juvenile arthritis in remission attain normal peak bone mass at the lumbar spine and forearm, Arthritis Rheum. 43 (2000) 1504–1510.

119. G. Lien, B. Flatø, M. Haugen, et al., Frequency of osteopenia in adolescents with early-onset juvenile idiopathic arthritis. A long-term study of one hundred five patients, Arthritis Rheum. 48 (2003) 2214–2223.

120. W.A. Stewart, P.D. Acott, S.R. Salisbury, et al., Bone mineral density in juvenile dermatomyositis: assessment using dual x-ray absorptiometry, Arthritis Rheum. 48 (2003) 2294–2298.

124. V. Lilleby, G. Lien, K. Frey Frøslie, et al., Frequency of osteopenia in children and young adults with childhood-onset systemic lupus erythematosus, Arthritis Rheum. 52 (2005) 2051–2059.

125. V. Lilleby, Bone status in juvenile systemic lupus erythematosus, Lupus 16 (2007) 580–586.

126. S. Compeyrot-Lacassagne, P.N. Tyrrell, E. Atenafu, et al., Prevalence and etiology of low bone mineral density in juvenile systemic lupus erythematosus, Arthritis Rheum. 56 (2007) 1966–1973.

127. P. Regio, E. Bonfá, L. Takayama, et al., The influence of lean mass in trabecular and cortical bone in juvenile onset systemic lupus erythematosus, Lupus 17 (2008) 787–792.

132. T.P. Van Staa, H.G.M. Leufkens, L. Abenhaim, et al., Use of oral corticosteroids and risk of fractures, J. Bone Miner. Res. 15 (2000) 993–1000.

133. H. Valta, P. Lahdenne, H. Jalanko, et al., Bone health and growth in glucocorticoid-treated patients with juvenile idiopathic arthritis, J. Rheumatol. 34 (2007) 831–836.

136. F.S. Weinstein, J.R. Chen, C.C. Powers, et al., Promotion of osteoclast survival and antagonism of bisphosphonate-induced osteoclast apoptosis by glucocorticoids, J. Clin. Invest. 109 (2002) 1041–1048.

145. M.L. Bianchi, R. Cimaz, E. Galbiati, et al., Bone mass change during methotrexate treatment in patients with juvenile rheumatoid arthritis, Osteoporosis Int. 10 (1999) 20–25.

146. G. Simonini, T. Giani, S. Stagi, et al., Bone status over 1 yr of etanercept treatment in juvenile idiopathic arthritis, Rheumatology (Oxford) 44 (2005) 777–780.

148. American College of Rheumatology ad hoc Committee on glucocorticoid-induced osteoporosis, Recommendations for the prevention and treatment of glucocorticoid-induced osteoporosis—2001 update, Arthritis Rheum. 44 (2001) 1496–1503.

150. R. Carrasco, D.J. Lovell, E.D. Giannini, et al., Biochemical markers of bone turnover associated with calcium supplementation in children with juvenile rheumatoid arthritis. Results of a double-blind, placebo-controlled intervention trial, Arthritis Rheum. 58 (2008) 3932–3940.

152. D. Simon, N. Lucidarme, A.M. Prieur, et al., Effects on growth and body composition of growth hormone treatment in children with juvenile idiopathic arthritis requiring steroid therapy, J. Rheumatol. 30 (2003) 2492–2499.

156. F.H. Glorieux, N.J. Bishop, H. Plotkin, et al., Cyclic administration of pamidronate in children with severe osteogenesis imperfecta, N. Engl. J. Med. 339 (1998) 947–952.

165. J. Thornton, D.M. Ashcroft, M.Z. Mughal, et al., Systematic review of effectiveness of bisphosphonates in treatment of low bone mineral density and fragility fractures in juvenile idiopathic arthritis, Arch. Dis. Child 91 (2006) 753–761.

166. E.L. Van Persijn van Meerten, H.M. Kroon, S.E. Papapoulos: Epi- and metaphyseal changes in children caused by administration of bisphosphonates, Radiology 184 (1992) 249–254.

167. C. Brumsen, N.A. Hamdy, S.E. Papopoulos, Long-term effects of bisphosphonates on the growing skeleton: studies of young patients with severe osteoporosis, Medicine (Baltimore) 76 (1997) 266–283.

168. M.L. Bianchi, R. Cimaz, M. Bardare, et al., Efficacy and safety of alendronate for the treatment of osteoporosis in diffuse connective tissue diseases in children, Arthritis Rheum. 43 (2000) 1960–1966.

169. R. Cimaz, M. Gattorno, M.P. Sormani, et al., Changes in markers of bone turnover and inflammatory parameters during alendronate therapy in pediatric patients with rheumatic diseases, J. Rheumatol. 29 (2002) 1786–1792.

170. L.K. Bachrach, L.M. Ward, Clinical Review: Bisphosphonate use in childhood osteoporosis, J. Clin. Endocrinol. Metab. 94 (2009) 400–409.

Entire reference list is available online at www.expertconsult.com.

Chapter 50

PRIMARY DISORDERS OF BONE AND CONNECTIVE TISSUES

Deborah Wenkert

A pediatric rheumatologist must be able to differentiate primary disorders of bones and joints from those of a predominantly inflammatory etiology.[1,4,9-17] There are hundreds of pediatric bone disorders, and this chapter is not intended to be comprehensive but will provide an approach to the recognition and characterization of non-inflammatory skeletal conditions to provide a framework for establishing a differential diagnosis. Detailed clinical, biochemical, pathophysiological, and genetic information is available for genetic diseases in the Online Mendelian Inheritance in Man (OMIM). Therefore, in this chapter, each disease is followed by an OMIM designation to direct the reader to this continually updated, referenced website (www.ncbi.nih.gov/omim) with links to pubmed. The website www.genetests.org directs the clinician to current reviews of genetic disorders and laboratories for specific genetic analyses. An international working group frequently updates a classification of osteochondrodysplasias.[17] The website http://ghr.nlm.nih.gov/ provides current information for families.

BONES AND THEIR DEVELOPMENT

Bones of the skeleton have diverse origins. The craniofacial skeleton derives from neural crest ectodermal cells.[18] The ribs and vertebrae develop from the sclerotome division of somites.[19] The appendicular skeleton stems from the lateral plate mesoderm.[20,21] These origins are sometimes reflected in the distribution of involved bones in disorders of somatic mosaicism (see later discussion).

Types of Bone Formation

The skull, clavicles, pelvis and much of the spine develop by *intramembranous or mesenchymal ossification* from the direct transformation of a vascular membrane.[20] Intramembranous ossification occurs in several steps: First, primary (disorganized, weak, woven) bone is formed by an early primary Haversian system that is subsequently replaced by a more slowly formed, well organized, lamellar, and compact bone.

In contrast, elongation of long bones and the ossification of the epiphyses of long bones, carpal, and tarsal bones, of the center of the vertebrae, and of the sternum occur by *endochondral ossification* from vascular invasion and resorption of a virtually avascular hyaline cartilage.[20] However, long bone formation starts with a periosteal bone collar formed by intramembranous ossification of the mesenchyme on the diaphyseal surface of embryonic long bones. The formation is then penetrated by a vascular channel to permit the development of bone marrow and to allow the introduction of osteogenic precursors. The core of the diaphysis then undergoes endochondral ossification, with the creation of a bone island within the calcified cartilage of the anlagen. This initial bone created by endosteal growth is also eventually replaced by the thick trabeculae of the cancellous bone. The elongation at the growth plate of long bones occurs through endochondral ossification in a well-organized series of steps, culminating in the hypertrophy of chondrocytes in the zone of cartilage transformation. That step is followed by vascular invasion, the death of many of the chondrocytes, and the transformation of others to osteoblasts. In the zone of ossification, a layer of bone is formed over the mineralized cartilage. Sex hormones are important in bone development[22,23] and estrogen is necessary for epiphyseal closure in both sexes.[24] Androgens seem to stimulate bone formation, either directly or indirectly through their impact on muscle tissue.[25]

Three Dimensional Bone Structure

Within each long bone, two types of bone structure are found: cortical (or compact) and trabecular, (cancellous or spongy) bone (Fig. 50–1).[26] Cortical bone comprises most of the pediatric skeleton and an even larger percentage of the adult skeleton. The cortical bone forms a shell around the cancellous bone at the metaphysis, but the majority is found in the diaphysis, where it increases its diameter via periosteal apposition and creates the marrow cavity by endosteal resorption. Cortical bone differs from trabecular bone in its rate of turnover (3% a year versus 25% a year in adults), its porosity, and its responsiveness

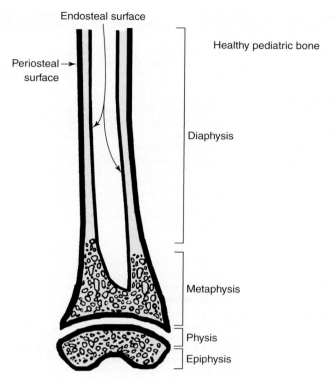

Endosteal surface

Periosteal → surface

Healthy pediatric bone

Diaphysis

Metaphysis

Physis

Epiphysis

Figure 50–1   Healthy pediatric bone.

to hormonal influences. The rate of turnover of bone and the percentage of cortical versus trabecular bone varies during childhood.[27] Trabecular bone is more responsive to acute deficiency states as a source of needed minerals. It is found in the metaphyses of long bones and other locations including the body of the vertebrae, the inner portions of the pelvis, and the jaw. Ninety percent of the lateral lumbar spine bone density as measured by dual x-ray absorptiometry (DXA) represents trabecular bone, whereas 95% of the distal radius DXA measurement represents cortical bone.[28]

Cellular Components of Bone

Cells of the skeleton include osteoblasts, osteocytes, and osteoclasts (5%, 95%, and 1% of the cells of the adult skeleton respectively).[28] These cells communicate with each other by direct cell contact and/or through signaling molecules. Disruption of the function of one cell can impact the others.[29]

Osteoblasts and chondrocytes both derive from the same mesenchymal stem cell, the osteochondrogenic precursor (Table 50–1).[30,31] Axial patterning, recruitment, and differentiation to osteoblasts requires β catenin[32] and is regulated by a number of factors, including bone morphogenetic proteins (BMPs) and other members of the transforming growth factor-beta (TGF-β) superfamily, fibroblast growth factor, Core-binding Factor Runt domain alpha subunit 1 (CBFA1), additional transcription factors, and Indian hedgehog (Ihh). Osteoblasts have many receptors allowing a response to multiple factors including calcitriol, sex hormones, thyroid hormone, interleukin-1 (IL-1), tumor necrosis factor-alpha (TNF-α)[33] and prostaglandins.[34] Growth hormone and parathyroid hormone (PTH) have

significant anabolic effects. Other factors such as serotonin, whose synthesis in the enterochromaffin cells in the duodenum is inhibited by low density lipoprotein (LDL) receptor related protein 5, can inhibit the proliferation of osteoblasts.[35] The nervous system also impacts osteoblasts. Neurons can stimulate the release of receptor activator of nuclear factor κ B ligand (RANKL) (see later discussion) by osteoblasts, thus upregulating osteoclasts. Hereditary sensory and autonomic neuropathy, type V (HSAN5; OMIM #608654), a congenital insensitivity to pain syndrome caused by mutation in the nerve growth factor beta gene, features painless fractures and delayed healing. Head trauma, through unknown mechanisms, is an inciting factor for heterotopic bone formation at the hip.[36]

Osteoblasts produce multiple factors including prostaglandins, IL-6, Insulin-like Growth Factor (IGF), vascular endothelial growth factor (VEGF),[37] and BMPs.[34] Most osteoblasts are found lining the surfaces of bone; some eventually undergo apoptosis, and others are destined to become osteocytes.

Osteocytes are embedded in lacunae in bone. They interconnect through dendritic processes in the canaliculi. Mechanical forces transmitted onto the fluid in the canaliculae are detected by osteocytes,[38] which then signal osteoblasts and osteoclasts to respond to mechanical loading. Additionally, osteocytes play an important role in phosphate homeostasis and matrix mineralization,[39,40] and may play a role in glucocorticoid-induced bone fragility.

Osteoclasts (Table 50–2) are bone resorbing cells seen on the bone surface and derived from bone marrow macrophages.[41] Osteoclasts use the cytoskeleton to move along the surface of bone and create a resorptive pit by tight association with the bone matrix (using primarily the $\alpha_v\beta_3$ integrin associating with actin) creating a sealing zone. Osteoclasts release acid (formed with carbonic anhydrase II) using a proton pump and chloride channel into the resorptive pit to demineralize the bone. They then discharge the lysosomal matrix metalloproteinase (MMP) cathepsin K to degrade the organic matrix. A layer of glycoprotein-rich material is laid down on the resorbed surface, the so-called "cement line," to which the new osteoblasts can adhere. Osteopontin is a key protein in this process and in migration. Two related cytokines, macrophage colony stimulating factor, secreted by osteoblast precursors, and RANKL, secreted by osteoblasts, are responsible for osteoclastogenesis.[41] RANKL, also called osteoclast differentiating factor, is identical to a factor involved in the interaction of T cells and dendritic cells called tumor necrosis factor-related activation-induced cytokine (TRANCE). Other cytokines such as TNF-α, IL-1, IL-6, and IL-17 can upregulate the activation of osteoclast activity.[41] TGF-β and estrogen can inhibit osteoclastogenesis.[41] Estrogen deprivation and glucocorticoid excess lead to an excess of osteoclasts. Estrogen exposure increases TGF-β, which stimulates osteoclast apoptosis.[42]

Osteoclasts are responsible for repair of microfractures, release of minerals from bone in response to PTH, clearing cartilage from the growth plate of long bones, modeling the bones properly as they grow (Fig. 50–2), and creating sufficient intramedullary space for the bone marrow. Hematopoietic production moves from the liver and the spleen in fetal life to the bone marrow.[41,43]

Table 50–1

Clinical examples of dysregulation of osteoblasts

Name of Disease	OMIM #	Gene	Significance and Characteristics
Demonstrating Impact on Endochondral vs. Intramembranous Bone Formation			
Aromatase enzyme deficiency	+107910	Aromatase enzyme deficiency (that converts androgen to estrogen)	Even boys need estrogen to close growth plates – Even males have delayed bone age, delay in epiphyseal closure, excessive tall stature, osteoporosis
Cleidocranial dysplasia	#119600	Runx2 or CBFA1 inactivating mutation (AD)	CBFA1 has a greater impact on intramembranous ossification than endochondral ossification – Endochondral: short stature and osteopenia; membranous: absent or partially absent clavicles, hypoplastic iliac wings, dental abnormalities, and delayed closure of the fontanelle—remaining patent into adulthood
Activation of Osteoblast			
Progressive diaphyseal dysplasia	#131300	*TGFβ1* activating mutation (AD)	TGFβ1 impact on osteoblasts – Thick cortices and progressive diaphyseal widening along with an elevated ESR, leg pain, muscle weakness and hearing loss
Fibrodysplasia ossificans progressiva	#135100	*ACVR1* (activin receptor IA, a BMP type I receptor) activating mutations (AD)	BMP impact on osteoblasts – Extensive, extraskeletal ossification (true bone) progressing caudal to ventral, especially in areas of trauma (elevated ESR, during flares). Short hallux valgus and progressive cervical vertebral fusion begin at birth (ifop.org).
Progressive osseous heteroplasia or pseudopseudohypoparathyroidism	#166350	*GNAS1* (guanine nucleotide binding protein alpha subunit) important for hormone signaling (including PTH) paternally inherited, inactivating mutations (AD)	PTH impact on osteoblasts – Dermal ossification in infancy, progressive bone formation in muscle and fascia, +/– features of maternally inherited mutations (Albright hereditary osteodystrophy [OMIM #103580]: short stature, mental deficiency, hypothyroidism, hypogonadism, acquired short 4th and 5th metacarpals from premature fusion in phalangeal epiphyses).
Autosomal dominant endosteal hyperostosis	#144750	*LRP5* activating mutations (AD)	LRP5 impact on osteoblasts: Dense, good quality bone resistant to fracture, large mandible, torus palatinus, headaches from Chiari malformations
Type I van Buchem disease and sclerosteosis	#269500; #239100	*SOST* (an inhibitor of BMPs, sclerostin) inactivating mutations (AR)	An antibody to sclerostin is in clinical trials for the treatment of osteoporosis: Mild to moderate gigantism, broad dense clavicles, ribs and scapulae, prominent mandible and cranial hyperostosis +/– cranial nerve palsies
myositis ossificans (trauma induced ectopic ossification)	-	-	Sometimes trauma leads to extraskeletal ossification rather than calcification: trauma induced bone formation (from burns, joint replacement, repetitive injury)
Inactivation of Osteoblast			
Cleidocranial dysplasia			See endochondral vs. intramembranous previously
Osteoporosis pseudoglioma syndrome (OPPG)	#259770	*LRP5* inactivating mutations (AR)	LRP5 impacts not only on osteoblasts: Congenital blindness, hypermobility and progressive childhood osteoporosis +/– other organ involvement

Extracellular Matrix: Proteins

The majority of bone is comprised of extracellular matrix (minerals, proteins, and lipids).[28] Type I collagen serves as the scaffolding in the extracellular matrix (Tables 50–3 and 50–4). Bundles of type I collagen are arranged as a triple-helical structure made of two identical α 1 (I) chains and one α 2 (I) chain. It is the most predominant protein in bone and binds and orients other proteins and minerals. Collagen is deposited in a lamellar fashion and strengthened by multiple crosslinks, both within and between the triple-helical collagen molecules. These pyridinoline crosslinks, which are resistant to degradation, are

Table 50–2

Clinical examples of dysregulation of osteoclasts

Activation of Osteoclast			
Name of Disease	**OMIM #**	**Gene**	**Significance and Characteristics**
Juvenile Paget's Disease	#239000	OPG (the decoy receptor for RANKL) deactivating mutation (AR)	Impact of the RANK/RANKL/OPG pathway – Bone pain, fragility and deformation of entire skeleton with expanded osteoporotic bones, elevated ESR and deafness.
Expansile Skeletal Hyperphosphatasia, Familial Expansile Osteolysis and Paget Disease of Bone 2	#174810, #602080	RANK activating mutation (AD)	Expansile osteolytic bone disease with bone fragility and deformation of a few bones and deafness.
Hyperparathyroidism	Multiple	Multiple	Impact of PTH on osteoclasts – Osteoporosis, lytic areas in bone, fractures.

Inactivation of Osteoclast			
Name of Disease	**OMIM #**	**Gene**	**Significance and Characteristics**
Osteopetrosis	#259700	The vacuolar proton pump inactivating mutations (AR)	Impact of acidification of the lacunae – Babies develop a dense, fracture prone skeleton with widened metaphyses, cranial nerve impingement with blindness and deafness, hepatosplenomegally with failure of hematopoesis. In these forms of osteopetrosis, the defect lies in the osteoclast. Excessive numbers of osteoclasts are seen on bone biopsy ('osteoclast rich osteopetrosis') and patients respond to bone marrow transplant (BMT) since osteoclasts are bone marrow derived.
	#259730	Carbonic anhydrase II inactivating mutations (AR)	
	#259710	RANK inactivating mutations (AR)	
	#612301	RANKL inactivating mutations (AR)	Impact of inactivation of RANK/RANKL/OPG pathway – In this 'osteoclast poor' form, the defect is in cells of mesechymal lineage, and BMT should be more problematic.
Alber Schoenberg Disease, 'Mild' Osteopetrosis	#166600	*CLCN7* (Chloride Channel 7)	Impact of mild dysfunction of osteoclasts – Dense, fracture prone skeleton with widened metaphyses +/- cranial nerve impingement
Bisphosphonate induced osteopetrosis			Impact of medicinal oversuppression of osteoclasts – Dense, fracture prone skeleton with widened metaphyses

Other diseases of insufficient osteoclast activity with osteopetrotic features also exist (eg. Pyknodyostosis from deactivating cathepsin-K activity, #265800).
An antibody to RANKL is in clinical trials for treatment of osteoporosis as is a cathepsin-K inhibitor.

released during bone resorption, and (along with collagen I C- and N-terminal telopeptides) may reflect bone turnover[44] when measured in serum and urine. Collagen undergoes multiple steps of post-translational modification,[45] including crosslinking initiated by lysyl oxidase[46] and requiring prolyl hydroxylase.[47] Degradative enzymes of collagen include matrix MMPs, cathepsins, and serine proteinases. Fibrils contain type V collagen and ColA1 and ColA2. Non-collagenous proteins comprise 10% to 15% of bone protein.[28] They include serum derived proteins (one fourth of non-collagenous proteins), such as albumin, which bind to bone matrix by their acidic affinity for hydroxyapatite; and bone derived proteins, which regulate mineralization, act as growth factors, and influence cell-cell or cell-matrix interactions, collagen organization, or cellular function.

Mineralization

Bone mineralization is regulated by serum concentrations of calcium (detected by Calcium Sensing Receptor (CaSR)) and phosphorus, which influence and are influenced by PTH.[48] Other hormonal regulators including estrogen, androgens, cortisol, thyroid hormone, growth hormone, 1,25 dihydroxyvitamin D, calcitonin, PTH related peptide (PTHrP1), and the phosphatonins, including fibroblast growth factor 23 (FGF-23), dentin

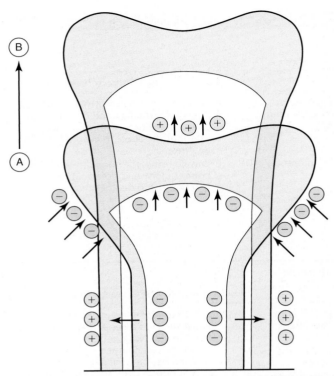

Figure 50–2 Pediatric bone has the additional task of shaping (modeling) long bones as they grow. Failure of osteoclast from hereditary disorders (osteopetrosis) or from medicinal oversuppression can lead to inhibition of physiological inwaisting.

matrix acidic phosphoprotein (DMP1), phosphate regulating endopeptidase homolog x-linked (PHEX), polypeptide N-acetyl galactosamonyl transfer (GALNT3), fibroblastic growth factor receptor 1 (FGFR1), Klotho, and the sodium/phosphate co-transporter in the kidney (Table 50–5).[49,50] These hormones impact mineral homeostasis in the gut, bone, and kidney. Severe calcium deprivation, vitamin D deficiency, and multiple hereditary disorders cause rickets[43] with expanded ankles, knees, and wrists, rachitic rosary, and progressive genu valgum or varum from soft, undermineralized bone (Table 50–5 and Fig. 50–4). Excess FGF-23 production leading to rickets, as occurs in these disorders and tumor induced osteomalacia, is also sometimes seen in McCune-Albright syndrome (Fig. 50–5), fibrous dysplasia, epidermal nevus syndrome, and neurofibromatosis.[43] Mineralization is also impacted by an inhibitor of mineralization, inorganic pyrophosphate (PPi), the concentration of which is regulated by alkaline phosphatase on the surface of osteoblasts; homolog of ank, named for the progressive ankylosis mouse (ANKH), which facilitates the transport of PPi across the plasma membrane into the extracellular compartment; and ectonucleotide pyrophosphatase/phosphodiesterase 1, which generates extracellular PPi through the cleavage of adenosine triphosphate also regulates PPi concentrations.[51] Serum calcium levels are also influenced by dietary factors including acid load, excessive oxalates, sodium, protein, and phytate (elevated in soy, nuts and seeds), and calcium binders.[52]

Generalized ectopic mineralization (metastatic calcification) occurs in conditions in which the calcium x phosphorus product is elevated[36] (e.g., hypercalcemia from hypervitaminosis D, sarcoidosis, hyperparathyroidism, renal failure or hyperphosphatemia from hypoparathyroidism, cell lysis following chemotherapy for leukemia, renal failure, when there is a decreased concentration of the inhibitor of mineralization, PPi) (see Table 50–5). Localized, dystrophic calcification occurs in areas of repetitive injury, neoplasm, infection (including intracranial calcification with prenatal infection with TORCH (Toxoplasmosis, other (Syphilis), Rubella, Cytomegalovirus, Herpes simplex virus) infections, some autoimmune diseases (juvenile dermatomyositis, scleroderma variants), and calcinosis cutis.[53]

Other minerals such as magnesium, copper, cadmium, and zinc also play an important role in bone metabolism as enzymatic cofactors. Two multi-organ system disorders, Menkes disease (OMIM #309400) and X-linked cutis laxa (OMIM # 304150), which result from mutation of a copper transporter gene, feature osteoporosis, either metaphyseal flaring or exostoses, and bony shaping abnormalities, thus demonstrating the importance of copper in bone metabolism.[43]

APPROACH TO THE DIAGNOSIS OF PRIMARY SKELETAL DISORDERS

The child with a primary skeletal disorder may present to the pediatric rheumatologist for a variety of reasons, including musculoskeletal pain, hypermobility of joints, congenital or acquired restriction of range of joint motion, gait abnormalities, muscle weakness, or because of the suspicion of the presence of an inflammatory arthropathy. Determination of the cause of the complaint requires careful clinical assessments and focused radiological and laboratory evaluations.

Clinical Evaluation

The clinical presentations of primary disorders of the skeleton and connective tissues can be quite complex. An approach to the history and physical examination of the child with a suspected skeletal disorder is shown in Table 50–6. Abnormalities of maternal health and the prenatal history may suggest a specific diagnosis. A detailed dietary history and history of prescribed or alternative medication is particularly important in children with bone pain or myalgia. The presence of co-morbidities often suggests specific diagnostic possibilities. Developmental delay is seen in disorders such as many of the storage diseases. A history of intrauterine or frequent fractures points to a variety of diagnostic possibilities, including metabolic disease and child abuse. A family history of consanguinity supports the possibility of an autosomal recessive disease; family members with short stature or manifestations similar to those of the patient support the presence of a genetically determined disease.

In addition to a general physical examination and standard measurements, the child with a suspected skeletal

Table 50-3

Dysregulation of bone matrix: Decreased or malformed structural protein

COL1A1 and COL1A2 Related Diseases

Significance	Name of Disease	OMIM #	Gene and inheritance	Characteristics
Osteogenesis imperfecta (OI) is the most common cause of primary osteoporosis in children (incidence of 1 in 10,000-20,000). Each type of OI can be associated with fragility fractures, easy bruising, hypermobility, increased sweating, dental carries, scoliosis and deafness, wormian bones, and gracile long bones. Intrafamily variability may be due to other genetic influences, episodes of prolonged immobility, or differences in lifestyle (fracture prone behavior, inadequate nutrition, smoking, excessive weight). Bisphosphonates have been efficacious for troublesome OI. Fig. 50-3	Type I OI	#166200	COL1A1 or COL1A2 (severity seems related to the particular mutation)	Mildest of the first four forms of OI; normal stature, blue sclerae, normal teeth, low-normal to very low bone mineral density, few too many fragility fractures,
	Type IV OI	#166220		Normal to gray sclerae, short stature, dentinogenesis imperfecta (DI), low bone mineral density, tibial bowing, and typically more fractures than seen in type I.
	Type III OI	#259420	(AD)	Macrocephaly, micrognathia, dwarfism, +/− blue sclerae, barrel chest, short bowed extremities, and characteristic high pitched voice. Radiographs reveal very low BMD, unrecognized fractures, widened metaphyses, "popcorn calcifications," protrusio acetabulae, and basilar impression. Diagnosed in utero with short-limbed dwarfism or fractures
	Type II OI	#166210		Perinatal lethal, long bone bowing with fractures are apparent in utero or at birth.
See Table 50-4 for further information on Ehlers Danlos Syndromes (EDS).	EDS arthrochalasia type (VIIA and VIIB)	#130060	COL1A1 or COL1A2 mutation preventing conversion of type I procollagen to collagen (AD)	Short stature, fractures, hypermobility, congenital bilateral hip dislocation, poor wound healing, and atrophic scars
	Caffey Disease	#114000	R836C substitution in COL1A1 (AD)	Fever, elevated ESR and cortical hyperostosis appearing ≤5-months of age, resolving by age of 2 years of age; hypermobility, and skin with atrophic scars
The importance of posttranslational modification: Prolyl 3-hydroxylase 1 (LEPRE1 gene product) complexes with cartilage-associated protein (CRTAP) and cyclophilin B to hydroxylate a single proline of COL1A1; Procollagen-lysine, 2-oxoglutarate 5-dioxygenase 2 (PLOD2) catalyzes lysyl residues in collagen.	Type VII and Type IIB OI	#610682, #610854	CRTAP (AR)	Lethal/severe OI; microcephaly, proptosis, white or light blue sclerae, undertubulation of long bones
	Type VIII OI	#610339	LEPRE1 (AR)	Lethal/severe OI; white sclerae, round face, severe growth deficiency and osteoporosis, bulbous metaphyses
	Bruck syndrome 2	#609220	PLOD2 (AR)	Osteopenia, fractures, wormian bones, congenital contractures of knees and elbows

Continued

Table 50–3—cont'd

Dysregulation of bone matrix: Decreased or malformed structural protein

Significance	Name of Disease	OMIM #	Gene and inheritance	Characteristics
COL2A1 Related Diseases				
Type II collagen is found primarily in hyaline cartilage, the nucleus pulposus, and the vitreous of the eyes. Thus, COL2 mutations often affect the eyes, joints, height, and the spine. There are ≥40 different genes encoding ≥27 different collagens; six are present in the eyes and cartilage and are absent in the majority of other adult tissues.	Stickler syndrome	#108300 #604841 #184840	*COL2A1*, AD *COL11A1*, AD *COL11A2*, AD	Variably associated with marfanoid habitus, hyperextensibility, myopia, cataracts, congenital glaucoma, retinal detachment, scoliosis, kyphosis, hearing loss, spondyloepiphyseal dysplasia, early-onset osteoarthritis, midface hypoplasia including cleft palate and micrognathia. Knee, ankle and wrist enlargement (often congenital) can be misdiagnosed as JIA or CINCA/NOMID.
	Kniest syndrome	#156550	*COL2A1*, AD	Kniest, or Swiss-cheese cartilage, syndrome is more severe.
	Spondyloepiphyseal dysplasia congenita	#183900	*COL2A1*, AD	Diminished joint mobility, short stature, characteristic abnormalities of the pelvis and vertebral bodies, platyspondyly, and equinovarus deformities of the feet are common. Radiographs show dysplastic and late-developing femoral heads. An associated immunodeficiency has been reported in some patients.
Fibrillin Related and Mimics for Marfan Syndrome				
Fibrillin 1 is ubiquitously expressed in the connective tissue of skin, heart, muscle, cornea, tendon, vasculature, lungs, kidneys, and bone. Fibrillin 2 plays a larger role in prenatal life.	Marfan Syndrome	#154700	*Fibrillin 1, (FBN1)* AD	Tall stature, long legs, arm span exceeds height, arachnodactyly, and variably associated with osteoporosis, hypotonia, joint pain and effusion, upward dislocation of the lens and iridodonesis, striae distensae and elastosis perforans serpiginosa and in 30% of patients aortic root dilation, aneurysm formation, mitral valve prolapse, and/or conduction defects.
	Congenital Contractural Arachnodactyly	#121050	*Type 2 fibrillin (FBN2)*, AD	Long hands and feet, accelerated linear growth ear helix abnormality, an early progressive kyphoscoliosis, an elongated head, and congenital contractures of the knees, elbows, and proximal interphalangeal joints, which tend to improve during childhood.
Early identification is crucial because the thrombosis and mental retardation that accompany the disorder can be ameliorated in some individuals through targeted dietary restriction and medicinal intervention.	Homocystinuria	#236200	cystathionine β-synthase (CBS), inactivating AR	Mimics Marfan syndrome in body habitus, osteoporosis, and lens ectopia (but downward dislocation occurring in homocystinuria by age 8-years-old). Hypotonia is present, but the joints are usually stiff rather than hyperextensible.

Types V and VI OI (OMIM %610967, %610968) are similar to Type IV OI but without dentinogenesis or known etiology and with unique bone histologies. Type V is distinguished by congenital dislocation of the radial head, hypertrophic callus formation and calcification of the intraosseous membranes during late childhood, restricting supination. Type VI OI is distinctive for a lack of wormian bones, and an elevated alkaline phosphatase. A chromosomal location for Type V OI has recently been identified. Osteoporosis Pseudoglioma Syndrome (OPPG), Hypophosphatasia (HPP) (see table), and a number of other disorders resemble OI.

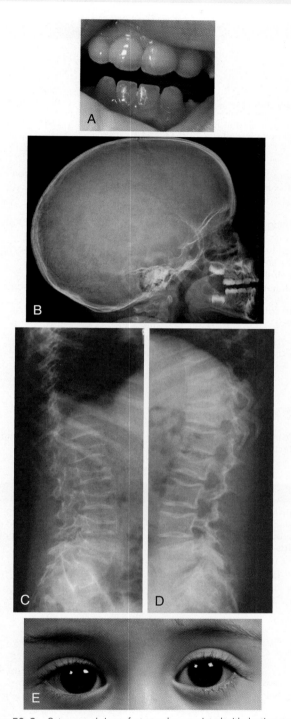

Figure 50–3 Osteogenesis Imperfecta can be associated with dentinogenesis imperfecta **A,** Wormian bones **B,** on lateral skull radiograph, vertebral compression fractures **C,** which can sometimes improve spontaneously **D,** or with the use of medicinal intervention, and **E,** sometimes blue sclera.

as seen in some types of Ehlers Danlos syndromes, or pseudo-sclerodermatous changes, as in melorheostosis.

The skeleton serves multiple simultaneous functions: It acts as a reservoir for minerals and carbonate, a scaffold for muscle (including respiratory muscles), an endocrine organ,[49] an environment for bone marrow, and a protector of internal organs. When evaluating a patient with a skeletal disease, it is important to determine several characteristics of the affected bones: Which bones are affected? Do the affected bones share a common embryogenesis? Are the affected bones formed by endochondral or membranous ossification? Which part of the bone is affected: the diaphysis (periosteal vs. endosteal surface), metaphysis, physis, or epiphysis? Is cortical or trabecular bone affected? Are the abnormalities congenital or acquired? Is the major abnormality one of osteoblasts or osteoclasts, structural protein or mineral? Are the observed abnormalities most likely the result of genetic, mechanical, nutritional, environmental, or endocrine aberrations? In answering these questions, clinical evaluation is accompanied by a radiological assessment.

Radiological Assessment

Evaluation of a child with a suspected primary skeletal abnormality should begin with plain radiographs. Radiographs should be evaluated for shaping abnormalities of bone, fractures, density, cortical thickness, location of involvement (axial vs. appendicular, proximal vs. distal and diaphyseal, metaphyseal, physeal, or epiphyseal), the presence of periosteal elevation or osteolytic lesions, and the presence of calcinosis vs. exostoses vs. ectopic bone. A lateral radiograph of the skull and antero-posterior (AP) and lateral radiographs of an entire infant may identify a bone disease, but are not sufficient to evaluate possible child abuse. For older children, lateral radiographs of the skull to include proximal cervical spine, lateral views of the thoracic and lumbar spine; postero-anterior (PA) view of hands and wrists; and AP views of the pelvis, lower extremities and feet are recommended in addition to any area of clinical concern.[54] Some radiographical abnormalities are present at birth;[55] others evolve[56] or improve with time.[57] Bilateral views help differentiate symmetrical from asymmetrical disorders but do not imply a lack of pathology when findings are symmetrical. Comparable radiographs of the parents can reveal the presence of a dominantly inherited disorder. It is important to recognize that a high bone mineral density score implies pathology, that DXA provides no information about bone quality, and that in evaluating children with skeletal dysplasias, DXA scan values need to be adjusted for body size.[53]

Laboratory Assessment

The laboratory assessment of a child with a suspected primary disorder of the skeleton can help to exclude inflammatory diseases, investigate causes of osteoporosis and rickets, and guide the clinician to tailoring dietary intake to the child's skeletal uptake of minerals. Although inflammatory indices are usually normal or only slightly

disorder requires a more detailed evaluation of body proportions, determination of abnormalities of the hair or skin, and determination of the presence of hyper- or hypo-mobility. Examination of the joints should exclude swollen or deformed joints, and examination of the skin may show hyper-elasticity, and characteristic scarring

Table 50–4A

Ehlers Danlos Syndromes

EDS Subtype	Previous EDS Designation	OMIM	Biochemical Defect	Gene Defect and Inheritance	Skeletal Phenotype
Classic type	Type I (gravis)	#130000	50% from Type V collagen; 50% unknown	46% *COL5A1*; 4% *COL5A2*; rarely *COL1A1* (AD)	Osteopenia
	Type II (mitis)	#130010			NA
Hypermobility type	Type III (benign)	#130020; #606408	Most unknown; few with tenascin X insufficiency	Most unknown (AD); few with *TNXB* (AR, AD)	Osteopenia
Vascular type	Type IV (arterial)	#130050	Type III collagen	98-99% *COL3A1* (AD, AR)	Acroosteolysis
Kyphoscoliotic	Type VI (ocular)	#225400	Procollagen-lysine, 2-oxoglutarate 5-dioxygenase 1	*PLOD1* (lysyl hydroxylase 1) (AR)	Osteoporosis
Arthrocalasia (cardiac valvular)	Type VIIa	#130060	Type I collagen (conversions of type I procollagen to collagen is inhibited)	*Col1A1* (AD)	Osteopenia
	Type VIIb			*Col1A2* (AR)	
Dermatosparaxis (tearing of skin)	Type VIIc	#225410		Procollagen protease *ADAMTS2* (AR)	
Other forms without known mutations at the time of the classification (1997)	Type V	%305200	Previously thought to be due to lysyl oxidase deficiency	XL	NA
	Type VIII (periodontitis)	%130080		AD	NA
	Type X	225310	Fibronectin		NA
	Type XI	%147900'		AD	NA
	Progeroid EDS	#130070	Xylosylprotein 4-β-galactosyltransferase	*XGPT1* AR	Osteopenia

Table 50–4B

EDS Subtype	Minor Criteria					
Classic type	Soft, velvety skin	Molluscoid pseudotumors	Subcutaneous spheroids	Pes planus, dislocations, sprains, and other complications of joint hypermobility	Muscle hypotonia, delayed gross motor development	Easy bruising
Hypermobility type	Narrow high arched palate	Recurrent dislocations	Chronic joint limb, back pain	Postural hypotension or tachycardia	Functional bowel disorder	Easy bruising
Vascular type	Chronic dislocation	Congenital hip dislocation	Talipes equinovarus (clubfoot)	AV carotid-cavernous sinus fistula	Pneumothorax/ pneumohemothorax	Easy bruising
Kyphoscoliotic	Wide atrophic scars	Marfanoid habitus	Rupture of medium-sized arteries	Mild to moderate delay of gross motor skills		
Arthrocalasia (cardiac valvular)	Hyperextensible skin	Tissue fragility including atrophic scars, easy bruising	Muscle hypotonia	Kyphoscoliosis		
Dermatosparaxis (tearing of skin)	Soft doughy skin texture	Premature rupture of fetal membranes, large hernias	Easy bruising			

Table 50–4A—cont'd

Diagnostic Criteria	Major Criteria				
	1	2	3	4	5
High specificity when first 3 major criteria are met	Skin hyperextensibility	Wide atrophic scars	Joint hypermobility	Positive family history	NA
All 3 major criteria met	Soft skin with normal or only slightly increased extensibility	No fragility or significant skin or soft tissue abnormalities	Joint hypermobility	NA	NA
Any 2 major criteria	Arterial rupture	Intestinal rupture	Uterine rupture in pregnancy	FH of Vascular EDS	NA
3 major criteria	Hyperextensible, friable easily bruised skin	Severe muscle hypotonia at birth	Generalized joint laxity	Progressive scoliosis present within 1st year of life	Scleral fragility and globe rupture
	Severe generalized joint hypermobility with recurrent subluxations	Congenital bilateral hip dislocation			
	Severe skin fragility	Sagging redundant skin			

Table 50–4B—cont'd

Minor Criteria					
Manifestations of tissue extensibility: hiatal hernia, anal prolapse in childhood, cervical insufficiency	Surgical complications (postoperative hernia)				
Positive family history without more severe EDS phenotype	Dental crowding				
Characteristic facial appearance (thin lips and philtrum, small chin, thin nose, large eyes)	Gingival recession	Thin translucent skin (especially chest and abdomen)	Acrogeria (aged appearing extremities)	Small joint hypermobility	Tendon/muscle rupture	Early onset varicose veins

elevated, they can be significantly increased in a few disorders (e.g., Camurati-Engelmann [OMIM #131300], Caffey [OMIM#114000], and Juvenile Paget disease [OMIM #239000]). Serum levels of calcium, phosphate, and alkaline phosphatase are usually unremarkable in congenital skeletal dysplasias but can provide useful clues to diagnosis and treatment in disorders of bone mineral metabolism. Laboratory abnormalities to aid in identifying primary disorders of the skeleton are listed in Table 50–7.

Genetic Basis of Primary Disorders of Bone and Connective Tissues

The patterns of inheritance of bone disorders include classic autosomal dominant, or recessive or X-linked inheritance with activating versus inactivating mutations. Many mutations demonstrate variable penetrance, in which disease is present in only some of the individuals carrying a mutation within a family,[58,59] and the appearance of dominant or recessive inheritance depends on the severity of the mutation.[60] Imprinting may be observed, in which the disease phenotype depends on whether the abnormal gene is inherited from mother or father.[61] In a contiguous gene syndrome, haplo-insufficiency of more than one gene leads to a phenotype of more than one disease.[62] Pseudoautosomal dominant inheritance occurs when there is haplo-insufficiency of a gene on the X chromosome, which escapes X inactivation and has a functional Y chromosome homolog.[63] In addition, new mutations can occur in a single egg or sperm, thereby creating the first individual in a family with a genetic disease who could then pass on the mutation to offspring. In gonadal mosaicism, mutation of the germline cells of the mother or father represents a recurrence risk to siblings of the first affected individual.[64] In somatic mosaicism, mutation occurs in only some of the cells of the embryo during embryogenesis.[65] Thus, genetic counseling is important, even in cases of a "new" mutation.

SELECTED SYNDROMES

Examples of Syndromes Characterized by Joint Hypermobility

Joint mobility is affected in many primary skeletal disorders. Hypermobility (see Table 50–6) is more common in children with musculoskeletal pain and is characteristic of many bone diseases[66] and disorders of poor muscle tone. Children have greater joint mobility than adults, and adult normal ranges should not be used in assessing a child for hypermobility. The subject of so-called benign hypermobility is discussed in detail in Chapter 47. A search for an underlying disease is appropriate in children who have excessive hypermobility. (e.g., have the ability to put their feet behind their head, approximate the thumb to the forearm) or who also have (or have a family history of) short stature, nephrolithiasis, hearing loss, frequent fractures, fish-mouthed scars, poor wound healing, or frequent dislocations

(e.g., Ehlers-Danlos syndrome), or dental abnormalities, osteoporosis, dysmorphic appearance, or other organ system involvement (especially the kidneys, heart, eyes, central nervous system, and skin).

Stickler Syndrome

Autosomal dominant and recessive Stickler syndrome (STL) is variably associated with marfanoid habitus and mitral valve prolapse (type I STL), sensorineural hearing loss and skeletal problems (scoliosis, joint hyperextensibility, spondyloepiphyseal dysplasia (SED), and premature osteoarthritis), ophthalmologic (myopia, cataracts, congenital glaucoma, and retinal detachment), and facial abnormalities (midface hypoplasia, cleft palate, and micrognathia). Intelligence is normal. Four genes account for most cases of STL. For autosomal dominant STL, Type I STL (OMIM #108300) occurs from mutations of type II collagen (*COL2A1*); type II STL (OMIM #60841) and type III STL (OMIM #184840) occur from disruption of the genes encoding Collagen XI (*COL11A1*, and *COL11A2* respectively). Autosomal recessive STL occurs from COL9A1 mutation (see later discussion for allelic disorders).

Ehlers Danlos Syndromes

The Ehlers Danlos syndromes are caused by defects in genes encoding collagen or collagen modifiers and characterized in most types by joint hypermobility and/or skin laxity. Details of the genetic defects and clinical presentations are presented in Table 50–4A and B.

Examples of Syndromes Associated with Joint Hypomobility

Hypomobility may reflect the effects of inflammatory joint or muscle disease, or result from misshapen ends of long bones (e.g., from skeletal dysplasias, rickets, or previous fracture), which can lead to an often symmetrical restricted range of motion. Bowing deformities can mimic flexion contractures (e.g., anterior femoral bowing, appearing to be a flexion contracture of the knee).

Kniest Syndrome and Spondyloepiphyseal Dysplasia Congenita

Kniest Syndrome and SED congenita are autosomal dominant disorder resulting from mutations of *COL2A1*, the same gene associated with type I STL. Kniest, or Swiss-cheese cartilage, syndrome (OMIM #156550) is characterized by congenitally short limbs and trunk, macrocephaly with a round face and a depressed nasal bridge,[67] progressive stiffness of the fingers, dislocation of the hips, and kyphoscoliosis. Like type I STL there is cleft palate, myopia, retinal detachment, deafness, and enlargement of the joints, but it is more severe. Significant contractures interfere with mobility and are associated with pain. In SED congenita (OMIM #183900), diminished joint mobility, short stature, platyspondyly, and equinovarus deformities of the feet are common. Radiographs show dysplastic and late-developing femoral heads. An associated immunodeficiency has been reported in some patients.

Table 50–5

Clinical examples of dysregulation of mineralization

Name of Disease	OMIM #	Gene and inheritance	Significance	Characteristics
Undermineralization				
X-linked hypophosphatemic rickets	#307800	PHEX inactivating (XD)	A few of the hereditary hypophosphatemic rickets. Each features Genu valgum or varum, bone pain, short stature, tooth abscesses +/− craniosynostosis	Also features the most common form of rickets
Autosomal dominant hypophosphatemic rickets	#193100	FGF-23 activating, (AD)		Also features weakness (childhood or adult onset).
Autosomal recessive hypophosphatemic rickets	#241520	DMP1 inactivating, (AR)		Also features deafness and osteosclerosis
Vitamin D dependent rickets, type 1A	#264700	25-hydroxyvitamin D3-1-alpha-hydroxylase (CYP27B1) inactivating (AR)		Also features weakness and enamel hypoplasia
Vitamin D dependent rickets, type 2A	#277440	Vitamin D receptor, inactivating (AR)		Also features weakness and enamel hypoplasia
Hypophosphatasia (HPP)		Tissue nonspecific ALP, inactivating	Rickets or osteomalacia with low alkaline phosphatase (ALP) levels but without low levels of calcium or phosphorus	Each subtype features hypermobility and early tooth exfoliation (before age 5, with the root still attached) +/- craniosynostosis
Odonto HPP	#146300	AD or AR	Excess of PPi, an inhibitor of mineralization, and a substrate of ALP, leads to hypophosphatasia (HPP). Severity depends on the number and severity of mutation(s). Unlike hypophosphatemic rickets, it is not amenable to treatment with phosphate and 1,25 OH vitamin D.	The mildest form no rickets
Childhood HPP	#241510	AD or AR		Also features rickets and weakness
Infantile HPP	#241500	AR		Also features failure to thrive with 50% mortality rate
Perinatal lethal HPP		AR		Death in utero or shortly after birth
Overmineralization				
Familial hyperphosphatemic tumoral calcinosis	#211900	FGF-23 or Klotho (or GALNT3), inactivating (AR)		Calcium phosphate crystal deposition in skin and subcutaneous tissue (with hyperphosphatemia)
Generalized arterial calcification of infancy	#208000	ENPP1, Inactivating (AR)	By deposition with PPi in conditions with increased PPi (in adulthood).	

Neutralizing antibodies to FGF-23 are in clinical trials for treatment of hypophosphatemic rickets; bone targeted alkaline phosphatase is in clinical trials for enzyme replacement therapy in HPP.

Disorders Characterized by Tall Stature

Marfan Syndrome

Dominant mutation of fibrillin 1 leads to Marfan syndrome (OMIM #154700), which is highly variable in severity, is characterized by tall stature, with the arm span exceeding height, and arachnodactyly. It is variably associated with high arched palate, kyphoscoliosis, joint hypermobility, pectus carinatum or excavatum, hypotonia, joint pain and effusion.[68] Fibrillin 1 is ubiquitously expressed in the connective tissue of the skin, heart, muscle, cornea, tendon, vasculature, lungs, kidney, and bone. Clinical difficulties involve the skeleton, the eyes (upward dislocation of the lens and iridodonesis), the skin (striae distensae and elastosis perforans serpiginosa), and, in 30% of patients, the cardiovascular system (aortic root dilation and aneurysm formation, mitral valve prolapse, and conduction defects). Affected patients can die unexpectedly from cardiac complications. Overviews of the management of Marfan syndrome are provided by Keane and Pyeritz[69] and Dean.[70]

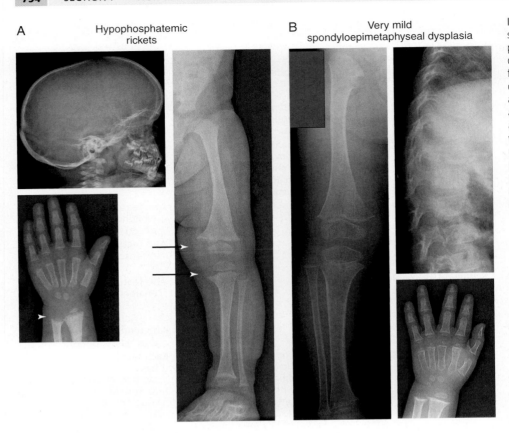

A   Hypophosphatemic rickets

B   Very mild spondyloepimetaphyseal dysplasia

Figure 50–4   **A,** Premature fusion of the saggital suture frequently occurs in hypophosphatemic rickets, leading to a high forehead and dochiocephaly, as seen this patient. Metaphyseal flaring, growth plate widening, and irregularity of the provisional zone of calcification (arrows) are also seen. Untreated patients typically have an elevated alkaline phosphatase and will have a subnormal fasting phosphorus for age, even when receiving calcitriol and phosphate supplementation. **B,** Metaphyseal flaring without growth plate widening, dochiocephaly, or biochemical disturbances, but with spinal shaping abnormalities differentiate spondyloepimetaphyseal dysplasia from rickets.

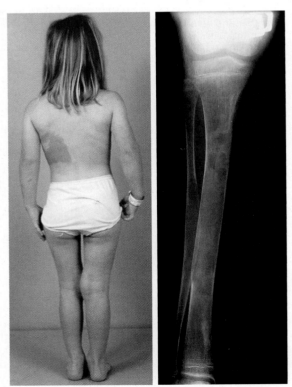

Figure 50–5   McCune Albright Syndrome from somatic mosaicism of GNAS1 inactivating mutations, leading to hormone resistance and large "Coast of Maine" appearing café au lait spots and sometimes, as seen in this girl, fibrous dysplasia.

Congenital Contractural Arachnodactyly

Type 2 fibrillin (*FBN2*) plays a large role in prenatal life. Autosomal dominant mutation of *FBN2* leads to congenital contractural arachnodactyly (OMIM #121050), a condition confused with Marfan syndrome.[71] Congenital contractures of the knees, elbows, and proximal interphalangeal joints tend to improve during childhood. Long hands and feet and accelerated linear growth occur in both syndromes. There is an associated ear helix abnormality, an early progressive kyphoscoliosis, and an elongated head.

Homocystinuria

Recessively inherited homocystinuria caused by cystathionine β-synthase (CBS) deficiency (OMIM #236200) mimics Marfan syndrome in body habitus, and the presence of osteoporosis. Downward dislocation of the lens occurs in homosystinuria by the age of 8 years. Hypotonia is present, but the joints are usually stiff rather than hyperextensible. Early identification is crucial in CBS deficient patients since the thrombosis and mental retardation that accompanies the disorder can be ameliorated in some individuals through targeted dietary restriction (methionine) and/or medicinal intervention (pyridoxine).[72]

Melorheostosis

Tight, bound-down skin occurs in sporadic melorheostosis (OMIM #155950), a rare, idiopathic, sclerosing bone disease, (Fig. 50–8b) typically affecting one or

Table 50–6

History and physical examination

	Question	Example of Relevance
Birth History	Prenatal ultrasound abnormalities	In utero bowing, fractures +/– poor mineralization (e.g., HPP and OI) or small for gestational age (dwarfism).
	Gestational age	Significant mineralization of the skeleton occurs during the third trimester. Premature infants can be misdiagnosed as having an intrinsic bone disease.
	Alcohol, drug use, or infections in mom	Fetal alcohol syndrome, in utero drug exposure, and infections can present with bony abnormalities.
	Previous pregnancies and miscarriages	Some recessive disorders can lead to death in utero and a milder phenotype in similarly affected siblings or in siblings with only one mutation.
	Any congenital anomalies	Multiple bone disorders are associated with congenital anomalies (club foot, cleft palate, cardiac malformations, and contractures).
Dietary History	Nursed vs. formula during first year of life	Vitamin D insufficiency can occur in nursing babies.
	General nutrition	Poor nutrition can exacerbate or lead to bone disease.
	Calcium intake (Note: 8 oz. of milk = 2 slices of cheese =~300 mg calcium).	Laboratory results impacted by calcium intake should be interpreted in context of % RDA consumed (RDA is 500mg/d (1-4 yrs), 800 mg/d (4-9 yrs), and 1300mg/d (9-19 yrs).
	Soda (soft drink) intake	Soda, particularly dark high phosphate containing soda, appears to demineralize the skeleton.
	Excess vitamin or fluoride intake (e.g., from excess tea or toothpaste) or alternative therapies	Vitamin D insufficiency is common and can account for bone pain and fibromyalgia-like symptoms in some patients. Excess vitamins, fluoride, heavy metals can cause radiographical and symptomatic bone disease.
Medications	Current or previous medications	Prednisone and other medications (anticonvulsants, heparin, MTX, radiotherapy) are associated with lowered bone mass.
Other Medical Disorders	Inflammatory disorder	Vasculitis, JIA, type I diabetes, inflammatory bowel disease, and celiac disease have all been associated with osteoporosis; CINCA/NOMID has a characteristic patellar overgrowth and can be associated with metaphyseal dysplasia.
	Endocrine disorder	Osteoporosis occurs with hyperthyroidism, diabetes, or deficiencies of growth hormone, estrogen, or testosterone. Unique bone phenotypes occur in polyglandular autoimmune disease (candidiasis, adrenal insufficiency, hypoparathyroidism, diabetes mellitus) and Albright hereditary osteodystrophy (see text).
	Ocular or cardiac abnormalities	Eye +/– cardiac abnormalities occur in Osteoporosis Pseudoglioma, Stickler and Marfan syndromes, and Homocystinuria (see tables).
	Pancreatic	Shwachman-Diamond syndrome (OMIM #260400): metaphyseal dysplasia, pancreatic insufficiency, neutropenia, and infections.
	Frequent infections	Adenosine deaminase deficiency (OMIM #102700): metaphyseal dysplasia, deficient immunoglobulins, and B and T cell function.
	Respiratory	Hypertrophic osteoarthropathy occurs with pulmonary or liver disease; in osteomalacia or type III OI, poor rib formation can jeopardize pulmonary function.
	Dental history (including age of primary tooth exfoliation)	Dentinogenesis imperfecta in OI types III and IV; enlarged pulp chambers, and abscessed teeth in XLH; early tooth loss (<age 5-years-old) in HPP; pulp chamber stones in hereditary tumoral calcinosis.
	Liver disease	Vitamin A toxicity (see natural or alternative therapies previously)
	Skin	Hernias, nevi, striae and bruising are each associated with bone disorders.
	Renal disease	Elevated P and PTH in renal failure; proteinuria in one type of IMO (confused with JIA); nephrocalcinosis, or nephrolithiasis from elevated urine Ca × P.
	Deafness	From involvement of middle ear bones (OI), cochlear destruction (Juvenile Paget Disease), or cranial nerve encroachment (osteopetrosis).
	GI	Malabsorption leading to nutritional deficiencies; inflammatory GI diseases.
	Weakness	Most forms of rickets (excluding XLH) are associated with weakness. Coxa valga and overtubulation are associated with weakness.

Continued

Table 50–6—cont'd

History and physical examination

	Question	Example of Relevance
Developmental Milestones	Gross motor skills	Delay may indicate weakness (as a primary or secondary problem), bone pain, or be part of global developmental delay (as seen in mucopolysaccharidoses, NOMID/CINCA, and Albright Hereditary Osteodystrophy).
	Verbal skills	Speech therapy frequently needed in craniosyostosis patients; also see above
Fracture History	Fracture history	27% of girls, 42% of boys fracture by age 16-years-old (most commonly in the forearm). Recurrent fractures affect 12%-20%. Minimal trauma, unusual location, or excessive fracture rate should prompt investigation.
	Length of interval between fractures	Casting or immobilization demineralizes bone, temporarily predisposing the immobilized bone(s) to recurrent fracture.
	Bones that have been involved in fracture	In the absence of significant trauma, vertebral compression fractures (VCF) are pathological. VCFs occur in cancer, lymphangiomatosis, mucopolysaccharidoses, and all causes of osteoporosis.
	Fracture healing rate	Delayed healing is characteristic of rickets and diseases with slow remodeling (osteopetrosis).
Family History	Ethnic background	Disease prevalence differs among ethnic groups for many hereditary disorders.
	Consanguinity	Recessive disorders are more common with consanguinity.
	Blood relatives with: short stature (<5 ft for women;<5″4″ for men) or any of difficulties listed above	Some bone diseases skip generations (x-linked recessive or variable penetrance). Therefore, the history in distant relatives may be important.
	Type of difficulty and to what extent other affected family members have had difficulty	Although sometimes of variable penetrance, heritable disorders often run true in a family (same mutation and epigenetic influences). Family history can help with anticipatory guidance. If a child has increased morbidity compared with his affected family members, a search for secondary causes may be indicated.
Social History	Who lives at home, stress at home?	Nonaccidental trauma must always be considered in a patient with frequent fractures, even if there is a known underlying bone disease.
	Where do you live?	Toxin exposure, particularly heavy metals
Physical Exam	Standard PE	Attention to organ systems listed previously
	Height	Excessive tall or short stature occurs in many hereditary bone diseases.
	Sitting height	Exclude rhizomelic shortening
	Arm span	Arm span > height from long extremities (Marfan syndrome) or short torso (VCF)
	Head shape and circumference	Craniosynostosis may alter head shape and size.
	Bone deformity (including genu valgum or varum) or tenderness	Silent fractures, compromised chest shape or circumference
	Equal hip heights, shoulder heights	Exclude leg length discrepancy, scoliosis
	Finger and toenail clubbing	From any cause of acroosteolysis (pachydermoperiostosis [OMIM #259100] with arthritis, osteoporosis, ptosis, and marfanoid habitus)
	Digital lengths	Hallux valgus in FOP, short 4th and 5th digits in AHO or POH, arachnodactyly in Marfan Syndrome
	Hair	Alopecia: vitamin D dependent rickets II (OMIM #277440); Slow growing: trichorhinophalangeal syndrome (OMIM #190350), AD, with cone shaped epiphyses, joint swelling; coarse: Hajdu-Cheney (OMIM %102500) with acroosteolysis, deafness, osteoporosis
	Skin	Café au lait spots: McCune Albright (OMIM #174800), striae (Cushing syndrome), laxity: EDS
	Hypermobility Beighton Criteria: a total score of ≥ 5	Diagnosis of EDS and other genetic disorders rely on Beighton Criteria
	1 point if unilateral, 2 if bilateral	Passive dorsiflexion of the 5th finger >90 degrees
	1 point if unilateral, 2 if bilateral	Passive flexion of the thumb to the forearm
	1 point if unilateral, 2 if bilateral	Hyperextension of the elbow past 10 degrees
	1 point if unilateral, 2 if bilateral	Hyperextension of the knee past 10 degrees
	1 point	Trunk forward flexion with knees fully extended and palms resting on the floor

Table 50–7

Laboratory and radiographical evaluation

Standard laboratory evaluation

Fasting Blood

Calcium (Ca)	High and low Ca should be adjusted for albumin concentration and interpreted in light of PTH and urinary Ca levels.
Ionized Ca	Handling and processing can invalidate result; however, if collected and run properly, a better indicator of available blood Ca
Phosphorus (P)	Normal range varies across childhood. Low values for age are associated with hypophosphatemic rickets. High values are seen in a number of bone and mineral diseases.
Magnesium	Important cofactor of many enzymes. Hypomagnesaemia increases PTH secretion but, when severe, can lead to PTH resistance and hypocalcemia.
Alkaline Phosphatase	And/or bone alkaline phosphatase. Derived from osteoblast (bone formation marker); normal range varies across childhood. Both high (rickets, fracture, or disease with high remodeling rate) and low values (hypophosphatasia, celiac disease, and glucocorticoid excess) are significant.
Parathyroid hormone (PTH)	A suppressed fasting PTH with a normal to elevated fasting serum Ca and elevated 24 hour urine Ca is consistent with excessive Ca (or vitamin D) intake for that patient (i.e., the patient's bones are unable to use the excess Ca, thus suppressing PTH, which may be disadvantageous to the growing skeleton).
25-OH Vitamin D	Both low and high values are significant. A normal range has not been established for children. Impact of low 25-OH Vit D on bone mineralization first occurs at 25-OH vitamin D levels below 10-20 ng/mL.
CMP	To assess extraskeletal manifestations of disease and/or secondary cause of bone disease
CBC with Diff and PLT	

Urine

Urinalysis: 24-hour urine for	To assess extraskeletal manifestations of disease and/or secondary cause of bone disease
Ca **P**	Elevated Ca × P product may predispose the child to nephrocalcinosis or nephrolithiasis. Hypercalcuria (especially with suppressed PTH) may indicate a skeletal inability to absorb mineral (vitamin D insufficiency, small skeletal mass, excessive calcium, or vitamin D intake). Hyperphosphatemia is better assessed with TMP/GFR or TRP (see later discussion).
Creatinine	To assess renal function and to assess mineral excretion in comparison with creatinine excretion (perhaps less useful in very young patients or those with low muscle mass)
Sodium	Excessive salt intake leads to excessive salt excretion with an obligatory calcium loss

Additional laboratory evaluation when warranted

Fasting Blood

Osteocalcin		Bone formation marker
PINP	Type I collagen N-terminal propeptide	Bone formation marker
TRAP	Tartrate resistant acid phosphatase	Bone resorption marker but elevated with osteoclast dysfunction (osteopetrosis)
BB-CK	Brain isoform of creatine kinase also present in osteoclasts (marker of osteoclast dysfunction as in osteopetrosis)	
1, 25-OH Vitamin D	Activated form of Vitamin D. Dependent on 25-OH vitamin D. Useful for assessment of hypercalcemia	
ESR	Elevated ESR can occur in primary and secondary bone disease.	Primary osteoporosis is uncommon in children; secondary causes should be sought.
Anti-tissue transglutaminase (IgA)	Celiac disease can be associated with osteoporosis. IgA anti-TTG has a high specificity but only if the child is not IgA deficient.	
Total IgA		
TSH, free T4	Hypothyroidism is associated with osteoporosis.	
Cortisol	Progressive osteoporosis occurs in Cushing syndrome	
FSH, LH, Testosterone	Evaluate disturbances as extraskeletal manifestation of or as cause of bone disease.	
Homocysteine	To screen for homocysteinuria and carrier state for methyltetrahydrofolate reductase (MTHFR) polymorphism (C677T): both associated with osteoporosis.	

Continued

Table 50–7—cont'd

Review Available Family Laboratory Test Results	Similar laboratory abnormalities in even an asymptomatic parent can support the diagnosis of an autosomal dominant disorder (e.g., familial hypocalciuric hypercalcemia Type I [OMIM #145980], benign familial hyperphosphatasemia [OMIM %171720], or hypophosphatasia [#146300])	
24 hour urine for:		
Deoxypyridinoline	Crosslink degradation product of collagen	Bone resorption marker higher in children; must use age appropriate norms; elevated in disorders of high bone turnover.
NTX & CTX	N- and C-terminal telopeptides of type I procollagen	
Homocysteine	To screen for homocysteinuria	

2 hour urine for P handling: Adult normal ranges do not apply in childhood (low age adjusted values occur in hypophosphatemic rickets; high age adjusted values occur in tumoral calcinosis and other disorders with high serum P)

TMP/GFR	Tubular maximum for phosphate corrected for GFR	TmP/GFR (mg/dL) = Plasma phosphate – ([urine phosphate × plasma creatinine]/urine creatinine)
TRP	Tubular reabsorption of phosphate	TRP (%) = 100 – fractional excretion of phosphate

Standard Radiographs

Radiograph	Extra Comments when Ordering	Clinical Relevance
Lateral skull	Include proximal cervical spine (C1, C2)	Wormian bones are seen with early onset osteoporosis; basilar impression can occur with osteoporosis; underdevelopment of the odontoid and C1, C2 instability occur in some bone dysplasias; premature craniosynostosis, a feature of a number of dysplasias, can be detected for the coronal suture or inferred by dochiocephalic shape for the sagittal suture on this view; beaten copper appearance of the anterior skull is worrisome for increased intracranial pressure as can occur in craniosynostosis.
Lateral thoracic and lumbar spine	Two separate x-rays unless in an infant	Shaping abnormalities (dysplasia), vertebral compression fractures (osteoporosis), spondylolysis, and spondylolithesis.
PA hand	Outstretched hand to include the wrist and distal radius.	Diaphysis, metaphysis, physis and epiphysis of the radius, ulna, and all of the long bones of the hand can be assessed for a generalized involvement typical to a dysplasia or metabolic disturbance, such as rickets.
AP knee	Assess shaping, thickness, and mineralization.	Evaluation of diaphysis, metaphysis, physis, and epiphysis in a weight bearing bone.
AP pelvis	Assess for evidence of bone dysplasia.	Shaping abnormalities (dysplasia), sclerosis.
Review Previous Radiographs	Radiographical appearance of bone at time of fracture.	Was the child osteoporotic at the time of fracture? After immobilization for the treatment of a fracture, osteopenia or osteoporosis can develop. Did the child fracture through a normally shaped bone?
	What type of fracture?	Chalk stick (straight across) vs. spiral fracture, single vs. multiple. Does the fracture match the trauma? Was the child casted for a certain fracture or possible fracture (e.g., Salter I) vs. sprain?

Additional Radiographical Evaluation When Warranted

Area of pain	Rule out focal abnormality	
DXA	Adjustments should be made for body size. Image should be viewed to see if the appropriate area was circumscribed. Attention should be given to low Z-scores, high Z-scores, or changing Z-scores. Total BMD and BMC should always be increasing during childhood. T scores do not apply to children.	
Review available family radiographs and BMD	To assess for hereditary abnormality	NOTE: 60%-80% of BMD is accounted for by genetics.

Table 50–8

Heritable disorders with skeletal disturbances that may manifest as arthritis

Disorder	OMIM #	Joint and Bone Abnormalities seen in Childhood	Other Features (Sometimes)	Gene(s)
CACP (camptodactyly, arthropathy, coxa vara, pericarditis) syndrome	#208250	Polyarthritis with contractures, camptodactyly at birth	Pericarditis, coxa vara	Proteoglycan-4 gene AR
Carpal-tarsal osteolyses	Including #259600 and #166300	"Arthritis" in wrists, ankles, and elbows; knees with pain; swelling; AM stiffness; limitation of motion; rapid destruction of carpals; tarsals; "sucked candy" appearance of metacarpals; and metatarsals	With or without hirsuitism, short stature, osteoporosis, nephropathy, dysmorphic appearance	MMP2 or other genes AR & AD
Nail-patella syndrome	#161200	Symmetrical polyarthritis, hypoplastic patellae, thumbnails, scoliosis, restricted elbow range, radial head dislocations, iliac horns, and club feet	Short stature, glomerulonephritis, flat facies, cleft palate, epicanthal folds, ptosis, myopia, cleft palate, hearing loss	LIM-homeodomain protein AD
Mucopolysaccharidoses, mucolipidoses, mannosidosis, fucosidosis, gangliosidosis, sialidosis, sialic storage disease, galactosialidosis, and mucosulfatidosis	Multiple	Dysostosis multiplex (odonto hypoplasia, j shaped sella, broad oar shaped ribs, oval vertebrae with gibbus, pelvic and femoral head abnormalities); joint effusions, stiffness, and/or hypermobility	With or without: progressive face coarsening, corneal clouding, mental retardation, hernias, and hepatosplenomegaly	
Stickler syndrome	#108300 #604841 #184840	Spondyloepiphyseal dysplasia, scoliosis, osteoarthritis, "Legg-Perthes disease"	Marfanoid habitus, hearing loss, visual loss, mitral valve prolapse, flat face, small mandible, cleft palate	COL2A1; COL11A1; COL11A2; COL9A1(AD and AR)
Progressive pseudorheumatoid arthritis of childhood	#208230	Arthritis, periarticular osteoporosis, coxa vara, platyspondyly, flattened enlarged epiphyses, wide metaphyses	Disease onset: age 3- to 8-years old, progressive disorder; muscle weakness with waddling gait	WNT-1-inducible signaling pathways protein 3 (AR)
Metaphyseal and epiphyseal dysplasias	Multiple	Osteoarthritis	Variable with and without spine involvement	Multiple
Trichorhinophalangeal syndrome	#190350, #150230 and #190351	Enlarged proximal interphalangeal joints, coned epiphyses, short fourth and fifth metacarpals, progressive hip arthritis, scoliosis	Bulbous nose, thin hair, large ears, micrognathia, short stature, "Legg-Calve-Perthes" and in type II: exostoses +/− mental retardation	Putative transcription factor (TRPS1) (type 1 and 3) or TRPS1 and EXT1 (type 2) (AD)
Glycogen storage diseases	Including +232200, #232220, and #232500	With osteoporosis and gouty arthritis (glycogen storage disease I) or arthrogryposis multiplex (in glycogen storage disease IV)	Decreased muscle mass, short stature, xanthoma, multiple organ system difficulties	Multiple
Pachydermoperiostosis	#259100	Teenage onset, joint effusions and pain, enlarged hands feet and digits, periostitis, acroosteolysis (with digital clubbing)	Progressively coarse face, thick facial skin with gyri, hyperhidrosis, redundant skin on the scalp, cheeks, forehead, eyelids, palms and soles oily skin, striae, and acne.	15-alpha hydroxy-prostaglandin dehydrogenase type I (AD)

only a few neighboring long bones. Although sometimes asymptomatic, melorheostosis can be associated with intermittent swelling and pain around joints, asymmetrical growth, unilateral Raynaud-like symptoms, soft tissue fibrosis, vascular anomalies, and contractures.[73] Buschke-Ollendorff Syndrome (osteopoikilosis with dermatofibrosis lenticularis disseminata—orange papular skin lesions of increased elastin fibers) (OMIM #166700) results from an autosomal dominant mutation in *LEMD3*, and can be associated with areas of dermal fibrosis and foreshortened limbs and contractures, and rarely with melorheostotic lesions.[73,74]

Examples of Mimics of Arthritis

Primary disorders of connective tissue (including some of those discussed previously) may present with arthritis or what can be mistaken for arthritis[74,75] (see Table 50–8); often with pain worsening with activity. Some mimics of arthritis, however, have elevated erythrocyte sedimentation rates[43,75] and/or morning stiffness, gelling phenomena (personal observation), and may appear to respond to nonsteroidal anti-inflammatory drugs.[74,75] A congenital or hereditary arthropathy is suggested if there are multiple affected family members, parental consanguinity, and absence of autoantibodies (rheumatoid factor or antinuclear antibody),[66] symmetry of abnormalities, or multiple organ involvement. Osteoarthritis can occur in children who have abnormal cartilage.[76] Irregular joint surfaces, ligamentous laxity, or poor alignment can lead to osteoarthritis in early adulthood, especially in the weight-bearing joints. Orthopaedic intervention with growth plate stapling (epiphysiodesis) can allow a patient to "outgrow" a lower extremity malalignment (genu valgum or varus) or length discrepancy if intervention is taken long enough before growth plate fusion.

Dysostosis Multiplex

Although classified as osteochondrodysplasias, the dysostosis multiplex group of disorders differs from other osteochondrodysplasias in that they are storage disorders.[77,78] They include mucopolysaccharidoses, mucolipidoses, mannosidosis, fucosidosis, gangliosidosis, sialidosis, sialic storage disease, galactosialidosis, and mucosulfatidosis. These progressive diseases, resulting from an accumulation of substrate within the lysosomes of the cells that normally express the missing enzyme. They variably include the development of corneal clouding, dwarfism, mental retardation, joint effusions, face coarsening, stiffness or hypermobility, skeletal dysplasia of skull, thorax, vertebrae, pelvis, hands, and feet; and, in the case of Morquio disease, odontoid hypoplasia. Early intervention with bone marrow transplantation and enzyme replacement, available for some of these disorders, may interrupt some aspects of the otherwise unrelenting, devastating progressive mental and multisystem degeneration.[79]

Mucopolysaccharidoses

The mucopolysaccharidoses are genetically determined deficiencies of enzymes involved in the metabolism of glycosaminoglycans (Table 50–9).[80] Progressive skeletal dysplasia particularly affects the vertebrae, hips, and hands.[80,81] In the more severe types, such as Hurler

---

Table 50–9

Mucopolysaccharidoses

Type	Name	Inheritance	MPS	Enzyme Defect	Clinical Features
IH	Hurler	AR	DS, HS	α-L-iduronidase	Corneal clouding, dysostosis multiplex, heart Disease, severe mental retardation, death in childhood
IS	Scheie*	AR	DS, HS	α-L-iduronidase	Milder skeletal disease, normal intelligence, normal life span (?)
II	Hunter	XR	DS, HS	Iduronate sulfatase	Milder than type I; no corneal clouding
IIIA	Sanfilippo	AR	HS	Heparan-N-sulfatase	Mild skeletal, severe CNS abnormalities
IIIB				N-acetyl-α-D-glucosaminidase	
IIIC				Acetyl-CoA-glucosaminidase acetyltransferase	
IIID				N-acetyl-glucosamine-6-sulfatase	
IVA	Morquio	AR	KS	N-acetylgalactosoamine-6-sulfatase	Severe skeletal changes; corneal clouding; normal intelligence
IVB				β-Galactosidase	
VI	Maroteaux-Lamy	AR	DS	N-acetylgalactosoamine-4-sulfatase	Severe skeletal changes, corneal clouding, heart disease, normal intelligence
VII	Sly	AR	DS, HS	β-Glucuronidase	Dysostosis multiplex, variable intelligence, hepatosplenomegaly, white blood cell inclusions

*Formerly classified as Type V.
DS, Dermatan sulfate; HS, heparan sulfate; KS, keratan sulfate; MPS, mucopolysaccharide found in urine.
Modified from Beighton P: *McKusick"s heritable disorders of connective tissue*, ed 5, St. Louis, 1993, Mosby-Year Book.

syndrome (i.e., mucopolysaccharidosis [MPS] type IH), dwarfism, and marked coarsening of the facial features develops. Deposition of mucopolysaccharide leads to mental retardation and corneal clouding. A claw-hand deformity is often the first clue to the diagnosis.

Two of these storage diseases (Morquio and Scheie Syndromes) mimic inflammatory arthritis. The comparatively mild dysostosis but severe dwarfing of the autosomal recessive, Morquio Syndrome (MPS Type IVA OMIM #253000; MPS Type IVB OMIM #253010; Morquio Syndrome Type C OMIM #252300) may suggest juvenile idiopathic arthritis (JIA). Children with this syndrome, who have normal intelligence, may present with an effusion of a large joint (particularly the knee) or with progressive musculoskeletal stiffness, usually by the age of 3- or 4-years. The small joints of the hands become enlarged and stiff, a valgus deformity of the knees develops, and the gait becomes stiff and waddling. The joints are not always hypomobile, however, and some joints (such as the wrists), although enlarged, may be hypermobile. A pectus deformity and barrel chest are usual features. Characteristic radiographical findings include platyspondyly and odontoid hypoplasia and should help differentiate this disorder from the various forms of SED.[82]

In an autosomal recessive, mild form of Hurler disease, Scheie syndrome (MPS type IS) (OMIM #607016), intelligence is normal, the face is without coarsening, and stature is preserved. However, without intervention, there is a progressive restriction of range of motion the joints of the hands, elbows, and knees without swelling or pain. Corneal clouding and cardiac valvular disease develop generally in adulthood. Enzyme replacement or hematopoietic stem cell transplantation may mitigate the skeletal and cardiovascular abnormalities. All acute phase reactants are normal and urinary excretion of dermatan sulfate is increased, but a demonstration of decreased enzymatic activity of alpha-L-iduronidase activity is a more reliable screening test, and genetic testing is available.

Mucolipidoses

The term mucolipidosis (ML) is applied to a group of four disorders characterized by the intracellular accumulation of glycosaminoglycans and sphingolipids but without excess urinary glycosaminoglycan excretion. Progressive neurological and ocular abnormalities occur in all of these autosomal recessive disorders (Table 50–10).[83]

ML type I (OMIM #256550), an isolated neuraminidase (sialidase) deficiency, causes a Hurler-like syndrome with joint contractures, short trunk and stature, and dysostosis multiplex (see previously). Urinary excretion of sialated urinary oligosaccharides (bound sialic acid) is markedly elevated.

I-cell disease (ML type II α/β) (OMIM #252500) also causes a Hurler-like syndrome with progressive limitation of joint range of motion. The name is derived from the presence of prominent intra-cytoplasmic inclusions in cultured fibroblasts. I-cell disease[84] and pseudo-Hurler polydystrophy (ML type III α/β) (OMIM #252600)[85] are caused by mutations in the GNPTAB (the α/β subunit of the UDP-N-acetylglucosamine lysosomal-enzyme

Table 50–10

Mucolipidoses

Type	Name	Enzyme Defect	Musculoskeletal Features
I	Sialidase deficiency	Sialidase deficiency	Contractures, short stature, dysostosis multiplex
II	I-cell disease	Phosphotransferase deficiency	Progressive limitation of range of motion
III	Pseudo-Hurler polydystrophy	Phosphotransferase deficiency	Progressive limitation of range of motion; dysostosis multiplex
IV	Sialolipidosis	Uncertain	No characteristic skeletal changes

N-acetylglucosamine-1-phosphotransferase) gene. In pseudo-Hurler polydystrophy, restriction of joint mobility becomes apparent by the age of 2 years, but there is no inflammatory arthritis. Radiological findings are those of dysostosis multiplex. By the age of 6 years, features of Hurler syndrome dominate the clinical picture. A number of other primary disorders of the skeleton are characterized by the presence of stiff or enlarged joints and may be confused with inflammatory arthritis.

Diastrophic Dysplasias

Diastrophic dysplasia (OMIM #222600, #600972) and its variants, achondrogenesis type IB (#600972), multiple epiphyseal dysplasia 4 (OMIM #226900), and atelosteogenesis type II (OMIM #256050) are caused by autosomal recessive mutation in the sulfate transporter gene.[86-89] These are characterized by short limbs, small chest, radial dislocation, enlarged joints (particularly the knees), hitchhiker thumb, gap between first and second toes, clubfoot, and limitation of finger movement. Features include progressive fragmentation and calcification of the cartilage with swelling and eventual fusion of the joints, particularly the small joints of the phalanges. Calcification of the cartilage occurs in the ears, trachea, and costochondral junctions.

Dyggve-Melchior-Clausen dysplasia (OMIM #223800) and Smith-McCort dysplasia (OMIM #607326) are rare autosomal recessive disorders caused by deactivating mutation of the ubiquitously expressed dymeclin gene. Affected newborns present with some limitation of movement. Patients are often short, have an exaggerated lumbar lordosis and sternal prominence, and have progressive mental retardation. They develop claw-hand deformities. Radiographs show platyspondyly, epiphyseal dysplasia, irregular metaphyses, and a lacy appearance of the iliac crests. Biopsy shows widened cisternae of rough endoplasmic reticulum in chondrocytes.[90]

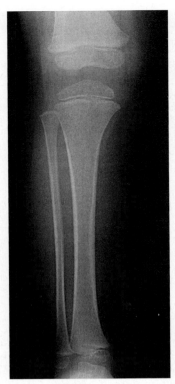

Figure 50–6 Widening of the metaphyses in a child with platyspondyly and progressive pseudorheumatoid arthropathy.

Progressive Pseudorheumatoid Arthropathy

This autosomal recessive disorder (OMIM #208230) presents between the ages of 3 and 8-years in healthy appearing children and is caused by mutation in *WISP3* (WNT1 inducible signaling pathway protein 3, felt to play a role in BMP and WNT signaling). It is a progressive disorder manifesting with stiffness, swelling, weakness with waddling gait, joint-space narrowing, and periarticular osteopenia, and progresses to metaphyseal enlargement, contractures, and kyphoscoliosis with platyspondyly (Fig. 50–6). This disorder is sometimes labeled "rheumatoid arthritis with Scheuermann disease" but has none of the laboratory abnormalities of JIA.

Trichorhinophalangeal Syndrome

Trichorhinophalangeal syndrome type 1 and the more severe type 3 are autosomal dominant disorders (OMIM #190350 and #190351), arising from mutation of a putative transcription factor (TRPS1). Both disorders are characterized by craniofacial and skeletal abnormalities, including a bulbous nose, short stature, sparse hair, enlarged interphalangeal joints, cone-shaped epiphyses, short metacarpals and metatarsals, and small, flat, fragmented capital femoral epiphyses suggestive of Legg-Calvé-Perthes disease.[91,92] Trichorhinophalangeal syndrome type II, the Langer-Giedion syndrome (OMIM #150230), is a contiguous gene syndrome deriving from the deletion of TRPS1 as well as its neighboring gene, EXT1. It is additionally associated with multiple exostoses, causing pain when occurring around joints and variably associated with mental retardation.

Disorders Characterized by Abnormal Bone Density

Osteoporosis is increasingly becoming a concern of rheumatologists, and new pharmaceuticals are being developed to treat this condition that are likely to have unique unrecognized side effects in children. Knowing the complications of hereditary skeletal disorders in which the same pathways are disrupted allows the clinician to anticipate additional potential problems. The pediatric rheumatologist should gain an understanding of these rare disorders before prescribing these drugs.

Generalized Deficiencies of Bone Mineralization

Abnormalities of bone mineralization are frequent features of primary skeletal disorders. Decreased bone density from overactive osteoclasts, underactive osteoblasts, or defects in structural proteins or mineralization requires different therapeutic approaches.[1] Since 60% to 80% of BMD is inherited,[7] finding a similar BMD in a parent may help differentiate secondary osteoporosis from primary causes. Osteoporosis is discussed in grater detail in Chapter 49.

Localized Abnormalities of Bone Density

DENSE BONE

Increased bone density can occur from disruption of the balance between osteoblasts, osteoclasts, and mineralization, and from fluorosis.[93,94] Bone pain, fractures, spinal stenosis, deafness, and other sequelae of nerve entrapment are among the difficulties that can complicate diseases associated with a radiodense skeleton (see Tables 50–1 and 50–2; Fig. 50–8).

LYTIC BONE LESIONS

True lytic bone diseases appear radiographically as hypodense areas within the skeleton and occur in metastatic cancer and a number of inherited syndromes, often with a distinctive distribution and sometimes with other organ system involvement.

The *idiopathic osteolyses* are grouped according to the area predominantly affected. Cherubism (OMIM #118400) manifests at the ages of 3 or 4 years with jaw osteolysis; other osteolyses involve phalangeal[95] or carpal/tarsal bones,[96,97] or are multicentric.[98] Acro-osteolysis (progressive loss of tips of distal phalanges) occurs as a feature of a number of different disorders.[99] Carpal-tarsal osteolysis syndromes, (Fig. 50–9) begin before the age of 1 year with restricted joint mobility, swelling and pain of the proximal interphalangeal joints, and enlargement of the wrists.[100-102] They result from mutation in type IV collagenase (MMP2) in Torg-Winchester and Nodulosis-Arthropathy-Osteolysis syndromes (OMIM #259600). These disorders are also complicated by the development of corneal clouding, coarsening of the face, joint contractures, osteoporosis, bone erosion, and atlantoaxial subluxation. Carpal/tarsal osteolysis associated with nephropathy has also been described.[37,96,103,104] Early radiographs of the wrists in carpal/tarsal osteolyses are often misinterpreted as showing a delayed bone age.[37]

Figure 50–7 Failure of tubulation with persistence of sclerosis and neo-osseous osteopenia is seen six years after the cessation of bisphosphonates in this 17-year-old with bisphosphonate-induced osteopetrosis.

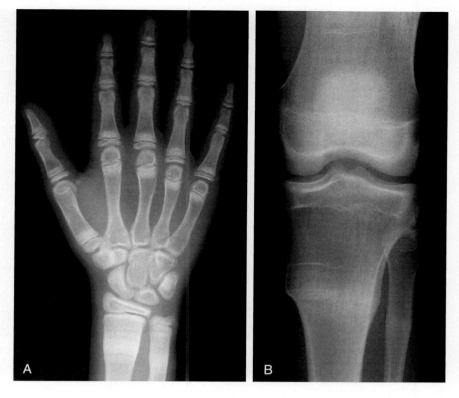

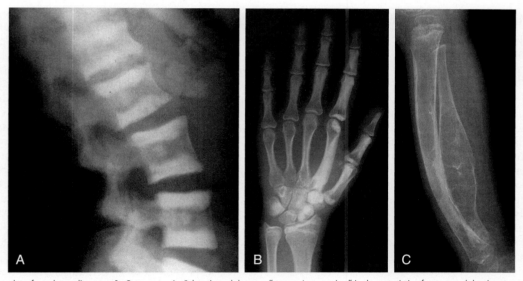

Figure 50–8 Examples of rare bone diseases. **A,** Osteopetrosis. Sclerotic endplates or "rugger Jersey spine" is characteristic of autosomal dominant osteopetrosis. **B,** Melor-rheostosis. Endosteal hyperostosis occurring in one or a few neighboring bones in a sclerotomal distribution is characteristic for melorrheostosis in childhood. This patient had shortened first and second digits, smaller thenar eminence, overlying bound down skin, and Raynaud-like phenomena affecting one hand. Later radiographs typically show a "melted candle wax" appearance when the hyperostosis becomes periosteal. **C,** Juvenile Paget Disease (Osteoprotegrin (OPG) deficiency), with a wide, expanded "pagetic" appearance, affecting the entire skeleton, as demonstrated in this 4-year-old boy's tibia and fibula. An elevated ESR and pain typically accompany the disorder.

Phantom bone disease (i.e., Gorham disease) occurs between the ages of 5 and 10 years and is not hereditary.[105] A carpal/tarsal osteolysis is usual. Osteolysis can also occur from overactivation of osteoclasts (see Table 50–2). Other disorders, such as neurofibromatosis Type I (OMIM #162200), can be misinterpreted as showing osteolysis. Metaphyseal enchondromas (at risk for malignant transformation) occurs in multiple enchondromatosis (OMIM #166000), including Ollier and Maffucci syndromes, cystic angiomatosis of bone (OMIM 123880), and disorders of metaphyseal undermineralization (see Table 50–6).

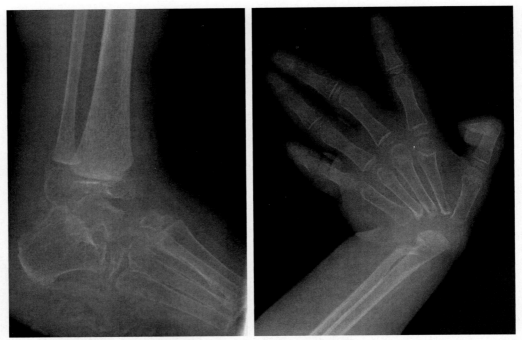

Figure 50–9 Idiopathic multicentric osteolysis (IMO), the progressive loss of carpal and tarsal bones, occurs during childhood with eventual destruction of the metacarpals, metatarsals, distal tibia, radius, and ulna, as can be seen in this 4-year-old with IMO and nephropathy. Early in the course of the disease, hand films can be misread as showing "delayed bone age."

ENVIRONMENTAL FACTORS AFFECTING BONE

Mechanical Factors

Unloading the skeleton (from bed rest, or immobilization or space travel) is associated with a significant reversible adverse effect on bone.[106] This must be considered when interpreting radiographs. Obesity can exacerbate bowing deformity in soft, undermineralized bone, but even normal bone can bow when exposed to excessive weight.[107] Blount disease is a disorder of lower extremity bowing which can mimic a localized metaphyseal dysplasia or rickets.[107] Although individuals with increased body mass index develop an increase in body mineral density, this does not compensate for the increase in body weight.[108]

Nutritional and Environmental Factors

A number of nutritional and environmental factors influence bone and mineral metabolism (see Chapter 49). Insufficiency of calcium, vitamin D, vitamin C, or copper can lead to physeal abnormalities.[109] Anorexia and cessation of menses are risk factors for osteopenia.[110] Toxicities can occur from excessive intake of aluminum containing antacids (causing hypophosphatemic rickets),[111] vitamin A (causing premature growth plate fusion),[109,112] fluoride (present in tea, causing dense, painful bones),[113] vitamin D (hypercalcemia),[114] and calcium (predisposing to nephrolithiasis).[115] Maternal disease and nutrition and toxic exposure can impact the skeletal health of the fetus.

Genetic disorders,[116] maternal vitamin K deficiency,[117] warfarin-induced embryopathy,[118] maternal lupus embryopathy,[119,120] and congenital rubella syndrome[121] lead to a radiographical appearance of chondrodysplasia punctata (stippling of the vertebrae and epiphyses and asymmetrical growth). Hypoparathyroidism and vitamin D deficiency in the mother can lead to a self-limited secondary hyperparathyroidism (with associated radiographical features) in the fetus and newborn.[122,123] Children with fetal alcohol syndrome[124] have mental, cardiac, and growth disturbances and a characteristic facial appearance (midface flattening, short palpebral fissures, and smooth, elongated upper lip) and may have flexion contractures of the elbows, restricted motion of the metacarpophalangeal joints, camptodactyly, and clinodactyly.

REFERENCES

1. C.R. Scriver, A.L. Beaudet, W.S. Sly (Eds.), The metabolic basis of inherited disease, ed 6., McGraw-Hill, New York, 1989.
2. U.S. National Institute of Health: Clinical Trials: www.clinicaltrials.gov.
3. M. Cheung, Drugs used in paediatric bone and calcium disorders, Endocr. Dev. 16 (2009) 218–232.
4. N.C. Walsh, T.N. Crotti, S.R. Goldring, et al., Rheumatic diseases: the effects of inflammation on bone, Immunol. Rev. 208 (2005) 228–251.
9. M.M. Reeder, Reeder and Felson's gamuts in bone, joint, and spine radiology: comprehensive lists of roentgen differential diagnosis, Springer-Verlag, New York, 1993.
10. R.S. Lachman, Radiology of syndromes, metabolic disorders and skeletal dysplasia, fifth ed., Mosby Year Book, St. Louis, 2006.
11. R. Wynne-Davies, C.M. Hall, A.G. Apley, Atlas of skeletal dysplasias, Churchill Livingstone, Edinburgh, 1985.
12. L.J. Deftos, Clinical essentials of calcium and skeletal disorders, Professional Communications, Caddo, 1998.
13. K.L. Jones, Smith's recognizable patterns of human malformation, ed 6., Saunders, Philadelphia, 2005.

15. R. Smith, P. Wordsworth, Clinical and biochemical disorders of the skeleton, Oxford University Press, New York, 2005.
16. P.M. Royce, B. Steinmann (Eds.), Connective tissue and its heritable disorders molecular, genetic, and medical aspects, Wiley-Liss, New York, 2002.
17. A. Superti-Furga, S. Unger, and the Nosology Group of the International Skeletal Dysplasia Society, Nosology and classification of genetic skeletal disorders: 2006 revision, Am. J. Med. Genet. 143A (2007) 1–18.
20. A. Erlebacher, E.H. Filvaroff, S.E. Gitelman, et al., Toward a molecular understanding of skeletal development, Cell 80 (1995) 371–378.
21. B.R. Olsen, A.M. Reginato, W. Wang, Bone development, Annu. Rev. Cell Dev. Biol. 16 (2000) 191–220.
23. O. Nilsson, R. Marino, F. De Luca, et al., Endocrine regulation of the growth plate, Horm. Res. 64 (2005) 157–165.
27. A.M. Parfitt, R. Travers, F. Rauch, et al., Structural and cellular changes during bone growth in healthy children, Bone 27 (2000) 487–494.
28. C.F. Rosen (Ed) Primer on the Metabolic Bone Diseases and Disorders of Mineral Metabolism, ed 7., Washington DC, American Society for Bone And Mineral Research (2009).
29. K. Henriksen, A.V. Neutzsky-Wulff, L.F. Bonewald, et al., Local communication on and within bone controls bone remodeling, Bone 44 (2009) 1026–1033.
30. E. Zelzer, B.R. Olsen, The genetic basis for skeletal diseases, Nature 423 (2003) 343–348.
31. G. Karsenty, E.F. Wagner, Reaching a genetic and molecular understanding of skeletal development, Dev. Cell 2 (2002) 389–406.
33. Y. Tanaka, S. Nakayamada, Y. Okada, Osteoblasts and osteoclasts in bone remodeling and inflammation, Curr. Drug Targets Inflamm. Allergy 4 (2005) 325–328.
34. D.J. Hadjidakis, Androulakis II, Bone remodeling, Ann. N. Y. Acad. Sci. 1092 (2006) 385–396.
35. V.K. Yadav, J.H. Ryu, N. Suda, et al., Lrp5 controls bone formation by inhibiting serotonin synthesis in the duodenum, Cell 135 (2008) 825–837.
36. D. Wenkert, M.P. Whyte, Heterotopic ossification and calcinosis in bone disease in rheumatology, in: M. Maricic, O. Gluck (Eds.), Lippincott, Williams & Wilkins, Philadelphia, 2005.
38. S. Weinbaum, S.C. Cowin, Y. Zeng, A model for the excitation of osteocytes by mechanical loading-induced bone fluid shear stresses, J. Biomech. 27 (1994) 339–360.
43. McKusick-Nathans Institute of Genetic Medicine, Johns Hopkins University (Baltimore, MD) and National Center for Biotechnology Information, National Library of Medicine (Bethesda, MD): Online Mendelian Inheritance in Man, OMIM (TM) www.ncbi.nlm.nih.gov/omim.
44. F. Pagani, C.M. Francucci, L. Moro, Markers of bone turnover: Biochemical and clinical perspectives, J. Endocrinol. Invest. 28 (2005) 8–13.
47. J.C. Marini, W.A. Cabral, A.M. Barnes, et al., Components of the collagen prolyl 3-hydroxylation complex are crucial for normal bone development, Cell Cycle 6 (2007) 1675–1681.
48. J.T. Potts, Parathyroid hormone: past and present, J. Endocrinol. 187 (2005) 311–325.
49. S. Fukumoto, T.J. Martin, Bone as an endocrine organ, Trends. Endocrinol. Metab. 20 (2009) 230–236.
50. T.M. Strom, H. Jüppner, PHEX, FGF23, DMP1 and beyond, Curr. Opin. Nephrol. Hypertens. 17 (2008) 357–362.
51. M. Murshed, D. Harmey, J.L. Millán, et al., Unique coexpression in osteoblasts of broadly expressed genes accounts for the spatial restriction of ECM mineralization to bone, Genes Dev. 19 (2005) 1093–1104.
52. D.S. Goldfarb, Prospects for dietary therapy of recurrent nephrolithiasis, Adv. Chronic Kidney Dis. 16 (2009) 21–29.
54. N.D. Kellogg, American Academy of Pediatrics Committee on Child Abuse and Neglect: Evaluation of suspected child physical abuse, Pediatrics 119 (2007) 1232–1241.
60. C.A. Moore, J.C. Ward, M.L. Rivas, et al., Infantile hypophosphatasia: autosomal recessive transmission to two related sibships, Am. J. Med. Genet. 36 (1990) 15–22.
61. E.M. Shore, J. Ahn, S. Jan de Beur, et al., Paternally inherited inactivating mutations of the GNAS1 gene in progressive osseous heteroplasia, N. Engl. J. Med. 346 (2002) 99–106.
62. J. Hou, J. Parrish, H. Ludecke, et al., A 4-megabase YAC contig that spans the Langer-Giedion syndrome region on human chromosome 8q24.1: use in refining the location of the trichorhinophalangeal syndrome and multiple exostoses genes (TRPS1 and EXT1), Genomics 29 (1995) 87–97.
66. E.C. Chalom, J. Ross, B.H. Athreya, Syndromes and arthritis, Rheum. Dis. Clin. North Am. 23 (1997) 709–727.
78. J.E. Wraith, The mucopolysaccharidoses: a clinical review and guide to management, Arch. Dis. Child 72 (1995) 263–267.
79. J. Muenzer, J.E. Wraith, L.A. Clarke, International Consensus Panel on Management and Treatment of Mucopolysaccharidosis I: Mucopolysaccharidosis I: management and treatment guidelines, Pediatrics 123 (2009) 19–29.
96. D. Wenkert, S. Mumm, S.M. Wiegand, et al., Absence of MMP2 mutation in idiopathic multicentric osteolysis with nephropathy, Clin. Orthop. Relat. Res. 462 (2007) 80–86.
109. J. Lawson, Drug-induced metabolic bone disorders, Semin. Musculoskelet. Radiol. 6 (2002) 285–297.
111. E.K. Pivnick, N.C. Kerr, R.A. Kaufman, et al., Rickets secondary to phosphate depletion. A sequela of antacid use in infancy, Clin. Pediatr. (Phila) 34 (1995) 73–78.
114. P. Koutkia, T.C. Chen, M.F. Holick, Vitamin D intoxication associated with an over-the-counter supplement, N. Engl. J. Med. 345 (2001) 66–67.
115. D. Feldman, F.H. Glorieux, J.W. Pike (Eds.), Vitamin D, Academic Press, San Diego, 1997.
120. T.E. Kelly, B.A. Alford, K.M. Greer, Chondrodysplasia punctata stemming from maternal lupus erythematosus, Am. J. Med. Genet. 83 (1999) 397–401.

Entire reference list is available online at www.expertconsult.com.

INDEX

Page numbers followed by f, t or b indicate figures, tables, or boxes, respectively.

Cutaneous Assessment Tool, 165
Cutaneous leukocytoclastic angiitis, 480t
Cutaneous polyarteritis nodosa, 502–503, 502f
Cutaneous sclerosis
  diffuse. *See* Diffuse cutaneous systemic sclerosis
  limited, 435–436
Cutaneous vasculitis, 224
Cyclic hematopoiesis, 655–656, 656t
Cyclooxygenase(s)
  COX-1, 50, 72
  COX-2. *See* COX-2
  function of, 50
  isoforms of, 50, 72
Cyclophosphamide
  administration of, 105t, 106
  adverse effects of, 106
  antiinflammatory effects of, 106
  bladder toxicity caused by, 106
  central nervous system vasculitis treated with, 540
  chemical structure of, 131f
  fertility effects, 106–107
  guidelines for, 106t
  interstitial lung disease treated with, 431–432
  intravenous, 105t
  luteinizing hormone–releasing hormone and, 107
  malignancy risks, 107
  mechanism of action, 105–106
  polyarteritis nodosa treated with, 501–502
  in pregnancy, 107
  rapidly progressive glomerulonephritis treated with, 489
  renal function-impaired patients treated with, 106t
  syndrome of inappropriate antidiuretic hormone associated with, 106
  systemic lupus erythematosus treated with, 320t, 338
  Wegener granulomatosis treated with, 526–529
Cyclosporine, 107–108
  Behçet disease-related ocular disease treated with, 556
  chemical structure of, 131f
  description of, 107
  guidelines for, 108t
  juvenile dermatomyositis treated with, 408
  juvenile rheumatoid arthritis treated with, 108
  in pregnancy, 108
  systemic lupus erythematosus treated with, 320t, 338
  uveitis treated with, 312
Cyclosporine-A
  macrophage activation syndrome treated with, 679
  systemic juvenile idiopathic arthritis treated with, 246
Cystathionine ß-synthase deficiency, 756
Cysteine proteinases, 11, 11t
Cystic fibrosis, 624, 625t
Cystinosis, 615, 617f
Cystoid macular edema, 308–309, 310f
Cytokine(s)
  activation induced by, 49f
  adaptive immunity, 47t–48t
  biological therapies that affect, 113–120
  characteristics of, 54
  classification of, 45–46
  counterregulatory, 34
  definition of, 45–46

Cytokine(s) *(Continued)*
  in diffuse cutaneous systemic sclerosis, 417
  fibroblast behavior regulated by, 416t
  in inflammation, 45–50, 54–55
  innate immunity, 47t
  in juvenile idiopathic arthritis, 54–55, 216–217
  in juvenile psoriatic arthritis, 291
  proinflammatory, 42
  rheumatoid arthritis and, 54
  in polyarticular juvenile idiopathic arthritis, 55
  in rheumatoid factor–negative polyarthritis, 250
  in systemic juvenile idiopathic arthritis, 55, 237–238
  types of, 47t–48t
Cytokine receptors, 45–50
Cytolytic T lymphocyte-associated antigen, 383
Cytolytic T lymphocyte-associated antigen-4, 30–31, 111–112, 634
Cytotoxic drugs, 103–109
  azathioprine, 103–104, 104t, 131f, 320t, 338, 556
  mycophenolate mofetil. *See* Mycophenolate mofetil
Cytotoxic T cells, 24, 28–29, 33–34, 676

D

Dactylitis, 290f, 293
Damage-associated molecular patterns, 628
  calcium-binding proteins, 54
  description of, 17–18, 41, 53–54
Data collation, 141
Decision analysis, 134
Decision errors, 148, 148t
"Deep sequencing," 66–67
Deep venous thrombosis
  in acute osteomyelitis, 568
  in antiphospholipid syndrome, 351
Defensins, 24
Deficiency of interleukin-1 receptor antagonist, 49, 657, 658f, 669t, 670–671, 670f
Deflazacort, 100
Degrees of freedom, 150
Dehydroepiandrosterone, 217
Delayed gadolinium-enhanced magnetic resonance imaging, 179
Delayed-type hypersensitivity, 45
Demyelinating diseases and syndromes, 117, 541
Dendritic cells
  adaptive inflammatory response and, 55
  description of, 20–21
  functions of, 20
  immature, 38
  medullary thymic epithelial cells as, 36
  plasmacytoid, 20–21
    in autoimmunity, 40f
    functions of, 40
  in systemic lupus erythematosus, 39–40
Dependent variables, 147
Dermatan sulfate, 9
Dermatitis
  in juvenile dermatomyositis, 384–386
  in neonatal lupus erythematosus, 369
Dermatomyositis. *See* Juvenile dermatomyositis
Dermatomyositis-like syndrome, 640
Dermatosparaxis, 753t–754t
Descriptive epidemiology, 129
Descriptive statistics, 144–145
Detection bias, 144
Developmental hip dysplasia, 178f

Dexamethasone
  chemical structure of, 129f
  description of, 101
Diabetes mellitus, 622t–624t, 621f, 622–624
Diabetic cheiroarthropathy, 427, 621f, 623–624
Diabetic osteopathy, 624
Diagnosis of disease, 131
Diapedesis, 42
Diaphysis, 732
Diarthrodial joints, 7–8
Diastrophic dysplasia, 763
Diclofenac
  dosing of, 73t
  mechanism of action, 72
Differential misclassification bias, 144
Diffuse cutaneous systemic sclerosis, 414–435
  anemia associated with, 427
  anti–Scl-70 antibodies, 427
  assessment of, 429
  bibasilar pulmonary fibrosis associated with, 428–429
  cardiac function in, 427–428
  classification of, 414–415, 415t
  clinical manifestations of, 418–422
    acrosclerosis, 419, 419f
    calcinosis, 419–420, 421f
    cardiac disease, 421
    central nervous system disease, 422
    digital pitting, 419, 421f
    digital ulcers, 431
    edema, 419
    gastrointestinal disease, 420–421, 428, 429f, 433
    hypertension, 422, 432
    interstitial lung disease, 431–432
    musculoskeletal disease, 420, 433
    pulmonary arterial hypertension, 432
    pulmonary disease, 421–422, 424f, 431–432
    Raynaud phenomenon, 420, 430–431, 468
    renal disease, 422, 424, 432–433
    Sjogren syndrome, 422
    skin disease, 419–420, 432
    telangiectasias, 419, 420f
  collagen abnormalities, 418
  course of, 433–435
  cytokines in, 417
  deaths caused by, 434–435, 435t
  definition of, 414
  differential diagnosis of, 424–427
    chemically induced sclerodermalike disease, 425–426
    chronic graft-versus-host disease, 424–425
    diabetic cheiroarthropathy, 427
    local idiopathic fibroses, 426–427
    nephrogenic systemic fibrosis, 425
    phenylketonuria, 426
    porphyria cutanea tarda, 427
    pseudosclerodermas, 426–427
    scleredema, 427
  endothelial cells, 417
  epidemiology of, 415
  etiology of, 415–418
  experimental therapies for, 433
  gender ratios, 415
  genetic background of, 418
  histopathology of, 423–424, 423f–424f
  historical review of, 414
  immunological factors, 416–417, 416t
  incidence of, 415
  laboratory examination of, 427–428

Oligoarticular disease, 102
Oligoarticular juvenile idiopathic arthritis
　clinical manifestations of, 266
　cytokines in, 55
　diagnosis of, 266
　enthesitis-related arthritis vs., 279
　hip joint arthritis associated with, 266
　oligoarthritis caused by, 266
　onset of, 211
Oligonucleotide microarrays, 66–68
Ollier disease, 685
Omeprazole, 78
One-sample statistical tests, 150
One-sample *t* test, 150
One-tailed hypothesis, 129
One-way analysis of variance, 151
Open randomized, actively controlled trial, 139
Open studies, 137–138
Opsoclonus-myoclonus syndrome, 541
Ordinal variables, 143
Organizations, 175
Orthopedic surgery, 230
Osgood-Schlatter disease, 279, 705,
　711–712, 712f, 712t, 759t–760t
Ossifying fibroma, 687
Osteitis, 670
Osteoblastoma, 683, 683t
Osteoblasts, 732–733, 745, 746t
Osteocalcin, 733, 733t, 759t–760t
Osteochondritis dissecans, 705–706, 706f
Osteochondrodysplasia, 624–625, 746t
Osteochondroma, 683–684, 685f, 759t–760t
Osteochondroses, 711–713, 712t
　definition of, 711
　Freiberg disease, 713
　Iselin disease, 713
　Köhler disease, 713
　Osgood-Schlatter disease, 759t–760t, 279,
　　705, 711–712, 712f, 712t
　Sever disease, 712–713
　Sinding-Larsen-Johansson disease, 279,
　　705, 711–712, 713f
　Thiemann disease, 713
Osteoclasts, 732–733, 745, 749t–750t,
　765f–766f
Osteocytes, 732–733, 745
Osteofibrous dysplasia, 687
Osteogenesis imperfecta, 701t, 738t, 749t–
　750t, 751f
Osteogenic sarcoma, 689–690
Osteoid osteoma, 682–683, 683t, 684f
Osteomalacia, 755t
Osteomyelitis, 567–572
　acute, 567–568, 571f
　Brodie abscess associated with, 568, 568t,
　　569f
　chronic, 567–569
　chronic recurrent multifocal. *See* Chronic
　　recurrent multifocal osteomyelitis
　classification of, 567
　clinical manifestations of, 567–568, 568t
　course of, 569
　definition of, 567
　diagnosis of, 569, 570f
　epidemiology of, 567
　etiology of, 567
　laboratory examination of, 569
　magnetic resonance imaging of, 569, 570f
　metaphysis predilection of, 567–568
　neonatal, 568
　pathogenesis of, 567
　prognosis for, 569
　radiographic evaluation of, 569, 570f
　septic arthritis vs., 563
　sites affected by, 568t

Osteomyelitis *(Continued)*
　Streptococcus pneumoniae as cause of, 567
　subacute, 568
　treatment of, 569
　vertebral, 570
Osteonecrosis, 622
Osteopathy, 89, 740
Osteopenia, 180, 224
　definition of, 735
　glucocorticoid-induced, 406–407, 741
　in juvenile dermatomyositis, 404f, 405
　low bone mass associated with, 738t
　methotrexate and, 740
　prevention of, 740–741
Osteopetrosis, 765f
Osteoporosis
　in articular disease, 299, 737t
　bisphosphonates for, 741, 741f, 742t
　definition of, 735–736
　glucocorticoid-induced, 97–98, 98f,
　　100–101, 406–407, 741
　idiopathic juvenile, 757t–758t
　juvenile dermatomyositis, 403–404, 404f
　in juvenile dermatomyositis, 389
　prevention of, 740–741
　risk factors for, 737t
　in systemic lupus erythematosus, 339,
　　739
　treatment of, 741–742, 741f, 742t
　vitamin D for prevention of, 100
　World Health Organization criteria for,
　　735
Osteoporosis pseudoglioma syndrome, 746t
Osteoprotegerin, 389, 734, 765f
Osteosarcoma, 683t, 690, 691f
Outcomes
　core set measures, 159, 160t
　hierarchy of, 159
　measurement tools for, 207
　terminology associated with, 158t
Outcomes research, 130, 134
Overall quality of life, 159, 165
Overreaction test, 726t
Oxaprozin, 73t, 76t
Oxicams, 73t

P

P values, 148
Pachydermoperiostosis, 624–625, 761t
Paget disease, 765f
Pain
　amitriptyline for, 122
　amplified. *See* Amplified musculoskeletal
　　pain
　antidepressants for, 122
　assessment of, 198, 221
　behaviors associated with, 193, 195–196,
　　198
　biobehavioral model of, 192–194
　chronic, 198, 204f
　chronic arthritis and, 221–222
　cognitive factors, 193
　cognitive-behavioral treatments for, 194
　complex regional pain syndrome, 472,
　　723t, 724
　COX-2 and, 72–74
　definition of, 720
　emotions and, 193
　expression of, 221
　factors that affect, 221, 720f
　gate control theory of, 192
　interferential therapy for, 201–202
　leukemia-related, 683t, 693–694
　measures of, 194–196, 195f–196f

Pain *(Continued)*
　musculoskeletal. *See* Musculoskeletal pain
　neuroleptics for, 123
　nonpharmacological techniques for,
　　199–200
　prevalence of, 192
　psychological interventions for, 194
　quality of life affected by, 198, 204f
　transcutaneous electrical nerve stimulation
　　for, 201–202
Pain pathways, 192, 193f
Pain-amplification syndrome, 221. *See also*
　Amplified musculoskeletal pain
Paired groups, 147–148
Pancreatitis, 337, 624
Pancytopenia, 88
PANDAS. *See* Pediatric autoimmune neu-
　ropsychiatric disorders associated with
　streptococcal infections
Panniculitis, 388–389, 547
Pannus, 179
Pansclerotic morphea, 438–439
Papillary necrosis, 79
Parallel group design, 139
Parametric test, 149
Paramyxovirus, 574–575
Parathyroid hormone, 734
Parotid biopsy, 462
Parotitis, 458–459, 459t
Paroxysmal nocturnal hemoglobinuria, 24
Parry Romberg syndrome, 438
Pars planitis, 305, 311
Parsonage-Turner syndrome, 472
Parvovirus B19, 217–218, 316, 573–574
Passive cell death, 35–36
Passive range of motion, 205
Passive rotation test, 726t
Patellar tendinopathy, 705
Patellofemoral instability, 704–707
Patellofemoral pain syndrome, 703–704,
　704t
Pathergy, 553–554
Pathogen-associated molecular patterns, 17,
　17t, 628
Patient education, 170
Patient preference, 158t
Patient-oriented research, 134–142
　clinical trials. *See* Clinical trials
　population, 137
　regulatory affairs, 134
Pattern recognition receptors, 17–20, 17t,
　18f, 24, 53–54
Pauciarticular juvenile rheumatoid arthritis
　description of, 262, 264
　follow-up, 269
　joint space narrowing associated with, 267
　outcomes of, 269
Peak bone mass, 734–735
Peak concentration, 136
Pearson product-moment correlation, 152
Pediatric autoimmune neuropsychiatric
　disorders associated with streptococcal
　infections, 606
Pediatric Gait, Arms, Leg, Spine screen, 222
Pediatric investigation plan, 137
Pediatric Pain Questionnaire, 194–195,
　195f–196f
Pediatric Quality of Life Inventory, 160t, 164
Pediatric Research Equity Act, 137
Pediatric rheumatologist, 170t
Pediatric rheumatology
　advances in, 3–4
　ambulatory clinics, 3t
　challenges in, 3–4
　history of, 1